*Principles of*

# ATHLETIC TRAINING

## A Guide to Evidence-Based Clinical Practice

### SIXTEENTH EDITION

## William E. Prentice, PhD, ATC, PT, FNATA

Professor, Coordinator Sports Medicine Program
Department of Exercise and Sport Science
The University of North Carolina at Chapel Hill
Chapel Hill, North Carolina

Mc
Graw
Hill
Education

PRINCIPLES OF ATHLETIC TRAINING: A GUIDE TO EVIDENCE-BASED CLINICAL PRACTICE, SIXTEENTH EDITION

4 5 6 7 8 9 LWI 21 20 19 18

ISBN 978-1-259-82400-5
MHID 1-259-82400-4

Chief Product Officer, SVP Products & Markets: *G. Scott Virkler*
Vice President, General Manager, Products & Markets: *Marty Lange*
Managing Director: *David Patterson*
Brand Manager: *Penina Braffman, Jamie Laferrera*
Product Developer: *Anthony McHugh*
Marketing Manager: *Meredith Leo*
Director, Content Design & Delivery: *Terri Scheisl*
Program Manager: *Jennifer Shekleton*
Content Project Managers: *Melissa M. Leick, George Theofanopoulos, Sandra Schnee*
Buyer: *Laura Fuller*
Design: *Studio Montage, Inc.*
Content Licensing Specialists: *Lori Slattery*
Cover Image: © *Science Photo Library / Alamy Stock Photo*
Design Elements: Clipboard: © *Mcgraw-Hill Education*
Magnifying glass: © *juliardi/Getty Images RF*
Compositor: *MPS Limited*
Printer: *LSC Communications*

**Library of Congress Cataloging-in-Publication Data**

Prentice, William E.
   Principles of athletic training : a guide to evidence-based clinical
   practice / William E. Prentice, PhD, ATC, PT, FNATA, professor,
   coordinator of Sports Medicine Program, Department of Exercise and Sport
   Science, The University of North Carolina at Chapel Hill, Chapel Hill,
   North Carolina.
   Sixteenth edition. | New York, NY : McGraw-Hill Education,
   [2017] | Subtitle changed from previous edition. | Includes
   bibliographical references and index.
   LCCN 2016040018 | ISBN 9781259824005 (alk. paper)
   LCSH: Athletic trainers. | Physical education and training.
   LCC RC1210 .A75 2017 | DDC 613.7—dc23
   LC record available at https://lccn.loc.gov/2016040018

mheducation.com/highered

# Brief Contents

# Contents

# Appendixes

# Preface

## PHILOSOPHY

Since the first edition of *Principles of Athletic Training* was published in 1963, the profession of athletic training has experienced amazing growth, not only in numbers but also in the associated body of knowledge. During all those years and in fifteen previous editions, the authors of this text, Daniel Arnheim, John Klafs, and now Bill Prentice, have taken it as a personal responsibility to provide the reader with the most current clinical information in athletic training and sports medicine. It has always been based on the most current research evidence and, consequently, it has endured as one of the preeminent textbooks for athletic training students and professionals for more than 50 years.

The text is designed to lead the student from general foundations to specific concepts relative to injury prevention, evaluation, management, and rehabilitation. As with other health care professions, the gold standard for athletic trainers is to make decisions about the clinical care of individual patients based on the current best available evidence in the professional literature to achieve the most optimal patient outcomes. It has always been important for this text to address all of the competencies and clinical proficiencies that the profession has identified as critical relative to both the education of our students and to the practice of athletic training. The changes, updates, and additions to this sixteenth edition are a reflection of my commitment and passion toward continuing Dan Arnheim's and John Klafs's tradition.

## THE ATHLETIC TRAINER AS A HEALTH CARE PROVIDER

Over the years since the origins of the athletic training profession in the 1930s, the majority of athletic trainers have been employed at colleges and universities, and in secondary schools, providing services almost exclusively to an athletic population. Historically, this work environment has been referred to as the "traditional setting" for employment for athletic trainers.

During the past decade, the role of the athletic trainer has gradually evolved into one that is unquestionably more aligned with that of a health care provider. Today, more than 40 percent of certified athletic trainers are employed in clinics and hospitals or in industrial and occupational settings, working under the direction of a physician as physician extenders. Although many athletic trainers continue to work in colleges, universities, and secondary schools, others can be found working as health care providers in all kinds of professional sports, including rodeo and NASCAR; in performing arts and the entertainment industry; in medical

equipment sales and support; in the military; with law enforcement departments; and with government agencies, including NASA, the U.S. Senate, and the Pentagon.

This expansion of potential employment settings has forced the profession not only to change the methods by which health care is delivered to a variety of patient populations but also to change athletic training education programs to teach and/or establish professional competencies and proficiencies that are universal to all settings.

Depending on the employment settings in which they work, athletic trainers no longer provide health care only to athletes, nor do they only provide health care to individuals who are injured as a result of physical activity. Thus, the athletic trainer is more closely aligned with other allied health professionals, and athletic training has gained recognition as a clinical health care profession.

## WHO IS IT WRITTEN FOR?

*Principles of Athletic Training: A Guide to Evidence-Based Clinical Practice* should be used by athletic trainers in courses concerned with the scientific, evidence-based, and clinical foundations of athletic training and sports medicine. Practicing athletic trainers, physical therapists, and other health care professionals involved with physically active individuals will also find this text valuable.

## CONTENT ORGANIZATION

The 29 chapters in the sixteenth edition are organized into six sections: Professional Development and Responsibilities, Risk Management, Pathology of Sports Injury, Management Skills, Musculoskeletal Conditions, and General Medical Conditions.

As in previous editions, developing the sixteenth edition included serious consideration and incorporation of suggestions made by students, as well as detailed feedback from reviewers and other respected authorities in the field. Consequently, this sixteenth edition reflects the major dynamic trends in the field of athletic training and sports medicine. Furthermore, it is my hope that this newest edition will help prepare students to become competent health care professionals who will continue to enhance the ongoing advancement of the athletic training profession.

In addition to the inclusion of material that focuses on evidence-based practice, this newest edition continues to undergo changes in content. The changes and additions are reflective of the ever-increasing body of knowledge that is expanding the scope of practice for the athletic trainer.

Throughout the text, information relevant to athletic trainers working in a variety of employment settings is included. As is the case for those working in secondary schools and colleges or universities, athletic trainers working in clinical, hospital, corporate, or industrial settings must be competent in preventing and recognizing injuries, and supervising injury rehabilitation programs. However, staff athletic trainers working in these settings treat and rehabilitate a wider range of patients both in terms of age and physical condition. The athletic trainer may provide care to pediatric, adolescent, young adult, adult, and geriatric patients. Patients may have physical ailments that may or may not be related to physical activity.

## WHAT IS NEW IN THIS EDITION?

This latest edition of *Principles of Athletic Training: A Guide to Evidence-Based Clinical Practice* continues to evolve in concert with the profession. Historically, the authors have tried diligently to stay on the cutting edge of the athletic training profession with regard not only to presenting a comprehensive and ever expanding body of knowledge but also with the latest techniques of delivering educational content to students. Most evident in this edition is the replacement of many of the older photos, and the addition of new photos to better illustrate the injuries, conditions, or clinical techniques described in the text. In addition to the hard copy of this text, the author has created an online library of approximately 1,400 instructional videos that clearly demonstrate specific clinical techniques, injury evaluation skills, rehabilitative exercises, and manual therapy skills that are used by experienced athletic trainers. There is also an online eBook version of this text that will facilitate direct access to the instructional videos from within the body of the text.

## CHAPTER-BY-CHAPTER ADDITIONS

One of the objectives throughout this text has been to incorporate the best available evidence to support the recommendations being made relative to patient care. The strength of those recommendations (SoR) based on the NATA Position, Official, and Consensus statements is identified within the text and can easily be found next to the reference where appropriate.

For the special tests presented in Chapters 18 to 25, the specificity, sensitivity, and positive and negative likelihood ratios are included wherever possible to show the usefulness and diagnostic accuracy of each of those tests based on the best available evidence in the literature.

### Chapter 1

- Added information on the Youth Sport Safety Alliance and their Secondary School Student Athletes Bill of Rights
- Added new information on the athletic trainer's role in managing athletes with disabilities
- Updated the information on rating the levels of evidence and the strength of recommendations
- Expanded the section on patient-related outcome measures

- Added new table listing the outcome measures most often used by sports medicine professionals
- Added information on the CAATE decision to establish the entry-level degree for professional practice for athletic trainers at the masters level
- Update Board of Certification requirements for certification and continuing education

### Chapter 2

- Added new information on establishing a crisis management plan
- Updated information on electronic medical records
- Reorganized, expanded, and updated the information on pre-participation exams
- Replaced old versions with new updated medical history and physical examination forms

### Chapter 3

- Clarified information on negligence
- Added new information and a focus box explaining the Affordable Care Act
- Replaced outdated form with a new Student-Athlete Insurance Information form

### Chapter 4

- Updated information on newest guidelines and recommendations for continuous training relative to intensity of the activity
- Updated information on high-intensity interval training
- Updated information on fartlek training
- Updated information on weight-bearing exercises

### Chapter 5

- Updated new 2016 Food label
- Updated information on vegetarian diets
- Updated the calorie table for fast foods
- Added new section on Dual Energy X-ray Absorptiometry (DXA)
- Added new information on binge eating disorder

### Chapter 6

- Updated NCAA-mandated guidelines for acclimatization in preseason football practices
- Updated revised information from the NATA 2015 position statement on exertional heat illness
- Changed classification of hyponatremia, which is no longer classified as an exertional heat illness
- Updated information on lightning safety

### Chapter 7

- Updated table on equipment regulatory agencies
- Updated information on the selection and fitting of the newest available football helmets
- Included updated information on the effectiveness of soccer headgear

## Chapter 8
- Updated the information on the effectiveness of using ankle braces versus ankle taping

## Chapter 9
- Updated information on the cause of muscle cramps
- Revised information on tendinopathies to clarify the differences between tendinitis and tendinosis

## Chapter 10
- Revised and clarified information on the gate control theory of pain management

## Chapter 11
- Updated information on mental disorders
- Updated the keys for referring patients with mental disorders for further care

## Chapter 12
- Added new information on medical "time-outs"
- Reorganized and updated new 2015 guidelines for CPR
- Added new acronym POLICE and updated discussion of acute care for musculoskeletal injuries
- Added new inter-association recommendations for removal of facemask, helmet, and shoulder pads
- Added new recommendation for treating patients with suspected cervical spine injuries, including immobilization and placing the patient on a spineboard, scoop stretcher, or vacuum mattress

## Chapter 13
- Reorganized the order of topic presentation throughout to create a more logical flow of information
- Added a new discussion and photos of various functional screening tests
- Added a new discussion on applying the best available evidence in clinical decision making, including sensitivity, specificity, likelihood ratios, and more.
- Updated information and replaced all of the photos for various imaging techniques
- Added new information on refractometers

## Chapter 14
- Updated the most current information regarding the immune system
- Updated the most recent worldwide and U.S. statistics in HIV and AIDS

## Chapter 15
- Updated the section on shortwave diathermy
- Added new discussion of dry needling technique
- Replaced most of the pictures with updated photos of the latest therapeutic modality devices

## Chapter 16
- Added new information on the mental aspects of dealing with the stress of rehabilitating an injury
- Updated information on the Graston technique
- Added new information on structural integration
- Added new information on postural restoration

## Chapter 17
- Updated the table of the list of drug classifications and definitions
- Updated the athletic trainers guide to frequently used drugs

## Chapter 18
- Introduced the concept of the "core" in the foot
- Clarified the functions of absorption and propulsion in the foot as they apply to pronation and supination
- Added new special tests: Mulder's test and the Dorsiflexion-Eversion test
- Updated information on using orthotics to enhance foot control

## Chapter 19
- Added new special test for the ankle: the Cotton test.
- Added clinical prediction rules for the ankle joint
- Updated information on the most recent management and rehabilitation techniques for ankle sprains
- Emphasized the importance of balance training in patients with chronic ankle instability

## Chapter 20
- Added clinical prediction rules for the knee
- Updated information on shoe types and the relationship to knee injuries
- Updated most recent information on the mechanisms that cause injuries to the ACL
- Updated information on the most current strategies for preventing knee injuries

## Chapter 21
- Updated information about the mechanism and treatment of hamstring injuries
- Added additional special test for the hip including: flexion-internal rotation test, scour test, patellar-pubic percussion test, resisted hip abduction test, and Craig's test
- Added new clinical prediction rules for the hip

## Chapter 22
- Added new special test: the Rent test
- Added new clinical prediction rules for the shoulder

## Chapter 23

- Added new special tests: the elbow-extension test and moving valgus stress test
- Updated etiology for ulnar collateral ligament injury
- Updated information on medial and lateral epicondylitis

## Chapter 24

- Added clinical prediction rule for carpal tunnel syndrome
- Updated and replaced the majority of the photos

## Chapter 25

- Added new tests: Stork test, Gillet test, Gaenslen's test, thigh thrust rest, sacral thrust test, and prone instability test
- Added clinical prediction rules for the spine

## Chapter 26

- Updated the ever-changing information on prevention, assessment, and management of concussion
- Added the latest version of the Sport Concussion Assessment Tool 3 (SCAT3)
- Updated information where appropriate on facial, dental, eye, ear, and nasal injuries

## Chapter 28

- Replaced almost all of the photos depicting the various types of skin diseases and disorders

## Chapters 27 and 29

- Updated both chapters with the latest medical information on organs and body systems, general medical conditions to help the athletic trainer with recognition, management, and referral decisions

# INSTRUCTOR RESOURCES

These resources include invaluable information to accompany the sixteenth edition of *Principles of Athletic Training*, including key terminology, lecture outlines, and worksheets with the accompanying answer keys. It also integrates the text with image clips. These components can be accessed via the Instructor Resources tab within Connect®.

## Test Bank

The test bank includes approximately 2,000 examination questions. Each chapter contains true-false, multiple choice, and completion test questions. The worksheets in each chapter also include a separate test bank of matching, short-answer, listing, essay, and personal or injury assessment questions that can be used as self-testing tools for students or as additional sources for examination questions.

## Computerized Test Bank

McGraw-Hill's EZ Test is a flexible and easy-to-use electronic testing program. The program allows instructors to create tests from book specific items. It accommodates a wide range of question types and instructors may add their own questions. Multiple versions of the test can be created, and any test can be exported for use with course management systems such as WebCT, BlackBoard, or PageOut. The program is available for Windows and Macintosh environments.

## PowerPoint Presentation

A comprehensive and extensively illustrated PowerPoint presentation accompanies this text for use in classroom discussion. The PowerPoint presentation may also be converted to outlines and given to students as a handout. You can easily download the PowerPoint presentation from the Instructor Resources tab in Connect®.

## Instructional Videos

Instructional videos are available on Connect® *for Principles of Athletic Training*. These visual aids are designed to illustrate key concepts, promote critical thinking, and engage students on the most relevant topics in athletic training.

## Connect® for *Principles of Athletic Training*.

**Connect** is an online learning system composed of interactive exercises and assessments, like those that appear on the new Board of Certification exam. Videos, animations, and other multimedia features enable students to visualize complicated concepts and practice skills. All of the activities are automatically graded and can be submitted to the instructor's grade book. For more information, visit connect.mheducation.com

Connect® for Principles of Athletic Training was developed by Amanda Benson, PhD, ATC, from Louisiana State University, and Linda Bobo, PhD, ATC, from Stephen F. Austin Slate University, and has been updated for the new edition. Connect® is a Web-based assignment and assessment platform that gives students the means to better connect with their coursework, their instructors, and the important concepts that they need to know for success now and in the future. Students can practice important skills at their own pace and on their own schedule, receive instant feedback on their work, and track performance on key activities. With Connect®, students get 24/7 online access to an eBook—an online edition of the text—to aid them in successfully completing their work, wherever and whenever they choose. With Connect®, instructors can deliver assignments, graphing questions, quizzes, and tests easily online.

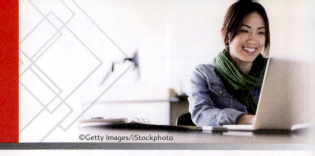

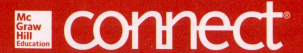

**Required=Results**

©Getty Images/iStockphoto

## McGraw-Hill Connect® Learn Without Limits

Connect is a teaching and learning platform that is proven to deliver better results for students and instructors.

Connect empowers students by continually adapting to deliver precisely what they need, when they need it, and how they need it, so your class time is more engaging and effective.

> 73% of instructors who use **Connect** require it; instructor satisfaction **increases** by 28% when **Connect** is required.

# Analytics

## Connect Insight®

Connect Insight is Connect's new one-of-a-kind visual analytics dashboard—now available for both instructors and students—that provides at-a-glance information regarding student performance, which is immediately actionable. By presenting assignment, assessment, and topical performance results together with a time metric that is easily visible for aggregate or individual results, Connect Insight gives the user the ability to take a just-in-time approach to teaching and learning, which was never before available. Connect Insight presents data that empowers students and helps instructors improve class performance in a way that is efficient and effective.

# Mobile

Connect's new, intuitive mobile interface gives students and instructors flexible and convenient, anytime–anywhere access to all components of the Connect platform.

### Connect's Impact on Retention Rates, Pass Rates, and Average Exam Scores

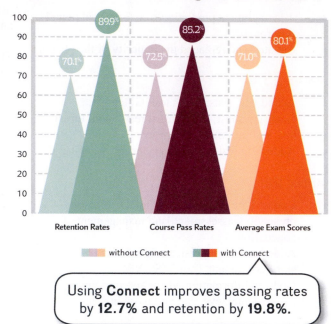

| | Retention Rates | Course Pass Rates | Average Exam Scores |
|---|---|---|---|
| without Connect | 70.1% | 72.5% | 71.0% |
| with Connect | 89.9% | 85.2% | 80.1% |

> Using **Connect** improves passing rates by **12.7%** and retention by **19.8%**.

### Impact on Final Course Grade Distribution

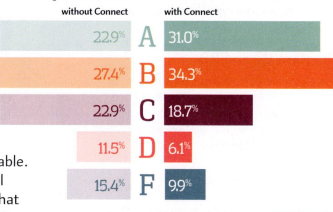

| | without Connect | | with Connect |
|---|---|---|---|
| A | 22.9% | | 31.0% |
| B | 27.4% | | 34.3% |
| C | 22.9% | | 18.7% |
| D | 11.5% | | 6.1% |
| F | 15.4% | | 9.9% |

> Students can view their results for any **Connect** course.

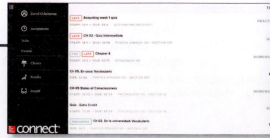

# Adaptive

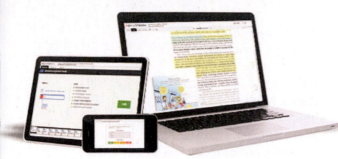

©Getty Images/iStockphoto

## THE **ADAPTIVE READING EXPERIENCE** DESIGNED TO TRANSFORM THE WAY STUDENTS READ

More students earn **A's** and **B's** when they use McGraw-Hill Education **Adaptive** products.

## SmartBook®

Proven to help students improve grades and study more efficiently, SmartBook contains the same content within the print book, but actively tailors that content to the needs of the individual. SmartBook's adaptive technology provides precise, personalized instruction on what the student should do next, guiding the student to master and remember key concepts, targeting gaps in knowledge and offering customized feedback, and driving the student toward comprehension and retention of the subject matter. Available on smartphones and tablets, SmartBook puts learning at the student's fingertips—anywhere, anytime.

Over **5.7 billion questions** have been answered, making McGraw-Hill Education products more intelligent, reliable, and precise.

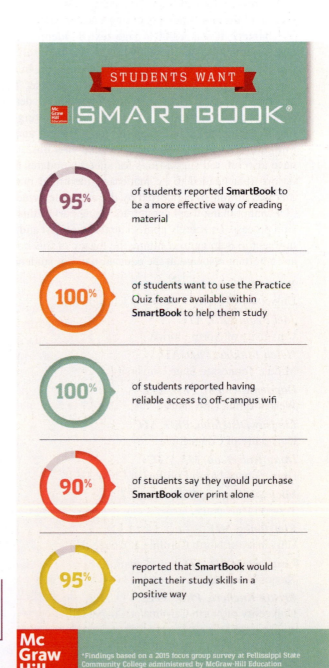

STUDENTS WANT

**SMARTBOOK®**

**95%** of students reported **SmartBook** to be a more effective way of reading material

**100%** of students want to use the Practice Quiz feature available within **SmartBook** to help them study

**100%** of students reported having reliable access to off-campus wifi

**90%** of students say they would purchase **SmartBook** over print alone

**95%** reported that **SmartBook** would impact their study skills in a positive way

Mc Graw Hill Education

*Findings based on a 2015 focus group survey at Pellissippi State Community College administered by McGraw-Hill Education

www.mheducation.com

# Acknowledgments

I would like to express my sincere appreciation to my Developmental Editor, Gary O'Brien who, as always, has provided invaluable guidance throughout the development of this edition. In truth, Gary should share authorship with me on this project. Through his efforts he has demonstrated ownership and a personal investment in making this text the best it can be. His input, patience with me, and dedication to this project has been indispensable and I truly respect his opinions and direction on all of our projects. I would be hard pressed to complete any of our projects without his help.

For this revision, instead of having a reviewer take on the daunting and time-consuming task of reviewing all 29 chapters of this 1,000+ page text, I identified specific individuals who have distinguished themselves as content experts to review a specific chapter or, in some cases, chapters related to their area of expertise. These reviewers have provided critical, constructive, detailed comments and suggestions relative to the existing content in each chapter based on the most current and best available evidence in the professional literature. They have also offered suggestions for specific updates or additions that needed to be made and identified material that was no longer supported by the available evidence.

I cannot thank them enough for being part of this revision process. I sincerely appreciate their interest and commitment in helping to continue the legacy of this book as an important resource in the education of our students.

**Bruce Baldwin, OD, PhD**
University of North Carolina at Chapel Hill

**Joel Beam EdD, ATC**
University of North Florida

**Helen Binkley, PhD, ATC**
Middle Tennessee State University

**Damien Clement, PhD, ATC**
West Virginia University

**Lindsay Distefano, PhD, ATC**
University of Connecticut

**Doug Halverson, MA, ATC**
University of North Carolina at Chapel Hill

**Michael Higgins, PhD, ATC, PT**
Towson University

**Kim Jones, MD**
University of North Carolina at Chapel Hill

**Lisa Jutte, PhD, ATC**
Xavier University

**Kristin Kuchera, PhD, ATC**
University of North Carolina at Chapel Hill

**James "Mick" Lynch, MD**
Florida Southern University

**Jill Manners, EdD, ATC**
Western Carolina University

**Janis Matson, MA**
University of North Carolina at Chapel Hill

**Patrick McKeon, PhD, ATC**
Ithaca College

**Johna Mihalik, PhD, ATC**
University of North Carolina at Chapel Hill

**Jennifer O'Donoghue, PhD, ATC**
North Carolina State University

**Barbara Osborne, JD**
University of North Carolina at Chapel Hill

**Sakiko Oyama, PhD, ATC**
University of Texas San Antonio

**Jody Padua, OT**
Occupational Therapy Consultant-Chapel Hill

**Kathryn Pietrosimone, PhD**
University of North Carolina at Chapel Hill

**Eric Rivera, DDS**
University of North Carolina at Chapel Hill

**Christine Rosenbloom, PhD, RD**
Nutrition Consultant- Atlanta Georgia

**Amy Sauls, PharmD**
University of North Carolina at Chapel Hill

**Jason Scibek, PhD, ATC**
Duquesne University

**Jay Scifers, DsPT, ATC, PT**
Moravian College

**Carrie Shearer, MS, PT, ATC**
University of North Carolina at Chapel Hill

**Abbie Smith-Ryan, PhD**
University of North Carolina at Chapel Hill

**Erik Swartz, PhD, ATC**
University of New Hampshire

**Tim Uhl, PhD, ATC, PT**
University of Kentucky

**Erik Wikstrom, PhD, ATC**
University of North Carolina at Chapel Hill

**Gary Wilkerson, PhD, ATC**
University of Tennessee at Chattanooga

**Steve Zinder, PhD, ATC**
University of South Florida

Finally, I want to thank my wife, Tena, and our sons, Brian and Zach, for their enduring support and encouragement. They constantly help me to keep my perspective on both my professional and personal life.

*William E. Prentice*

# Applications at a Glance

# PART I

# Professional Development and Responsibilities

# 1

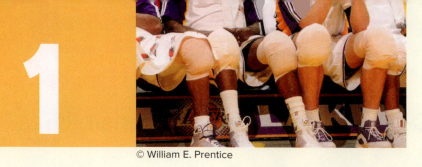

© William E. Prentice

# The Athletic Trainer as a Health Care Provider

## ■ Objectives

*When you finish this chapter you should be able to*

- Recognize the historical foundations of athletic training.
- Identify the various professional organizations dedicated to athletic training and sports medicine.
- Identify various employment settings for the athletic trainer.
- Differentiate the roles and responsibilities of the athletic trainer, the team physician, and the coach.

- Define evidence-based practice as it relates to the clinical practice of athletic training.
- Explain the function of support personnel in sports medicine.
- Discuss certification and licensure for the athletic trainer.

## ■ Outline

## ■ Key Terms

patient
athletic training clinic
evidence-based practice

PICO
ATC

## ■ Connect Highlights   connect

*Visit connect.mcgraw-hill.com for further exercises to apply your knowledge:*

- Clinical application scenarios covering professional role responsibilities
- Click-and-drag question format covering professional organizations, BOC domains, and support personnel
- Multiple-choice questions covering history of athletic training, employment settings, and certification and licensure for the athletic trainer

Athletic trainers are health care professionals who specialize in preventing, recognizing, managing, and rehabilitating injuries. In cooperation with physicians, other allied health personnel, administrators, coaches, and parents, the athletic trainer functions as an integral member of the health care team in clinics, secondary schools, colleges and universities, professional sports programs, and other athletic health care settings. As you will see throughout the course of this text, athletic trainers provide a critical link between the medical community and individuals who participate in all types of physical activity (Figure 1–1).

> The certified athletic trainer is a highly educated and skilled professional specializing in health care for the physically active.

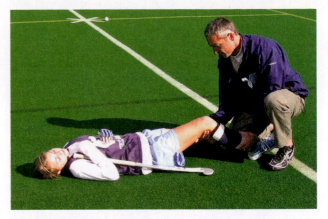

FIGURE 1–1    The field of athletic training provides a critical link between the medical community and the physically active individual.
© William E. Prentice

## HISTORICAL PERSPECTIVES

### Early History

The drive to compete was important in many early societies. Sports developed over a period of time as a means of competing in a relatively peaceful and nonharmful way. Early civilizations show little evidence of highly organized sports. Evidence indicates that in Greek and Roman civilizations there were coaches, trainers (people who helped the athlete reach top physical condition), and physicians (such as Hippocrates and Galen) who assisted the athlete in reaching optimum performance. Many of the roles that emerged during this early period are the same in modern sports.

> The history of athletic training draws on the disciplines of exercise, medicine, physical therapy, physical education, and sports.

For many centuries after the fall of the Roman Empire, there was a complete lack of interest in sports activities. Not until the beginning of the Renaissance did these activities slowly gain popularity. Athletic training as we know it came into existence during the late nineteenth century with the firm establishment of intercollegiate and interscholastic athletes in the United States. Because the first athletic trainers of this era possessed no technical knowledge, their athletic training techniques usually consisted of a rub, the application of some type of counterirritant, and occasionally the prescription of various home remedies and poultices. It has taken many years for the athletic trainer to attain the status of a well-qualified allied health care professional.[69]

### Evolution of the Contemporary Athletic Trainer

The terms *training* and *athletic training, trainer,* and *athletic trainer* are often used interchangeably and are frequently confused with one another. Historically, *training* implies the act of coaching or teaching. In comparison, athletic training has traditionally been known as the field that is concerned with the athlete's health and safety. A trainer is someone who trains dogs or horses or functions in coaching or teaching areas. The *certified athletic trainer* is one who is a specialist in athletic training. Athletic training has evolved over the years to play a major role in the health care of a variety of patient populations in general and the athlete in particular. This evolution occurred rapidly after World War I with the appearance of the athletic trainer in intercollegiate athletics. During this period, the major influence in developing the athletic trainer as a specialist in preventing and managing athletic injuries came from the work of S. E. Bilik, a physician who wrote the first major text on athletic training and the care of athletic injuries, called *The Trainer's Bible,* in 1917.[8]

> A certified athletic trainer provides health care to physically active individuals.

In the early 1920s, the Cramer family in Gardner, Kansas, started a chemical company and began producing a liniment to treat ankle sprains. Over the years, the Cramers realized that there was a market for products to treat injured athletes. In an effort to enhance communication and facilitate an exchange of ideas among coaches, athletic trainers, and athletes, Cramer began publication of *First Aider* in 1932. The members of this family were instrumental in the early development of the athletic training profession and have always played a prominent role in the education of athletic training students.[70]

During the late 1930s, an effort was made, primarily by several college and university athletic trainers, to establish a national organization named the National Athletic Trainers' Association (NATA). After struggling for existence from 1938 to 1944, the association essentially disappeared during the difficult years of World War II.

Between 1947 and 1950, university athletic trainers once again began to organize themselves into separate regional conferences, which would later become district organizations within NATA. In 1950, some 101 athletic trainers from the various conferences met in Kansas City, Missouri, and officially formed the National Athletic Trainers' Association. The primary purpose for its formation was to establish professional standards for the athletic trainer.[70] Since NATA was formed in 1950, many individuals have made contributions to the development of the profession.

After 1950, the growth of the athletic training profession has been remarkable. In 1974, when NATA membership numbers were first tracked, there were 4,500 members. Today those numbers have grown to more than 42,000 members. Certified athletic trainers can be found internationally with more than 500 working in 25 countries outside the United States. The majority of these are in Japan and Canada.[22] As the athletic training profession has grown and evolved over the last 50 years, many positive milestones have occurred that have collectively shaped the future direction of the profession, including the establishment of a certification exam; recognition of athletic trainers as health care providers; increased diversity of practice settings; the passage of practice acts that regulate athletic trainers in most states; third-party reimbursement for athletic training services; and ongoing reevaluation, revision, and reform of athletic training educational programs.

## The Changing Face of the Athletic Training Profession

Over the years since the origins of the athletic training profession in the 1930s, the majority of athletic trainers have been employed at colleges and universities and in secondary schools, providing services almost exclusively to an athletic population. Historically, this work environment has been referred to as the "traditional setting" for employment for athletic trainers.

Today the role of the athletic trainer has gradually evolved into one that is unquestionably more aligned with that of a health care provider. More than 40 percent of certified athletic trainers are employed in clinics and hospitals, or in industrial and occupational settings working under the direction of a physician as athletic trainers in physician practice. Although many athletic trainers continue to work in colleges, universities, and secondary schools, others can be found working as health care providers in hospitals; all kinds of professional sports, including rodeo and NASCAR; in industrial settings; in performing arts and the entertainment industry; in medical equipment sales and support; in the military; with law enforcement departments; and with government agencies, including NASA, the U.S. Senate, and the Pentagon.

This expansion of potential employment settings has forced the profession not only to change the methods by which health care is delivered to a variety of patient populations but also to change athletic training education programs to teach and/or establish professional competencies and proficiencies that are universal to all settings.

Depending on the employment settings in which they work, athletic trainers no longer provide health care only to athletes, nor do they provide health care only to individuals who are injured as a result of physical activity. Additionally, the desire to align the athletic trainer more closely with other allied health professionals and to establish athletic training as a clinical health care profession has necessitated changes in terminology that has been "traditionally" accepted as appropriate.

Certainly, athletic trainers continue to work with athletes. It has been suggested that a more appropriate term to use when treating an athlete who sustains an injury is **patient** or *client*. Thus, throughout this text the term *athlete* is used to refer to a physically active individual who participates in recreational or organized sport activities who is not currently injured. Any individual who is ill or injured who is being treated by an athletic trainer is referred to as a *patient*.

It has also been recommended that instead of referring to treating athletes in the athletic training room, it is more appropriate to refer to treating patients in the athletic training clinic or facility. Thus, the term **athletic training clinic** is used to refer to a health care facility for treating individuals who have an illness or injury.

# SPORTS MEDICINE AND ATHLETIC TRAINING
## The Field of Sports Medicine

The term *sports medicine* refers generically to a broad field of health care related to physical activity and sport. The field of sports medicine encompasses a number of more specialized aspects of dealing with the physically active or athletic populations that may be classified as relating either to performance enhancement or to injury care and management (Figure 1–2). Those areas of specialization that are primarily concerned with performance enhancement include exercise

> Athletic training must be considered a specialization under the broad field of sports medicine.

physiology, biomechanics, sport psychology, sports nutrition, strength and conditioning coaches, and personal fitness training. Areas of specialization that focus more on injury care and management specific to the athlete are the practice of medicine, athletic training, sports physical therapy, sports massage therapy, sports dentistry, osteopathic medicine, orthotics/prosthetics, chiropractic, podiatry, and

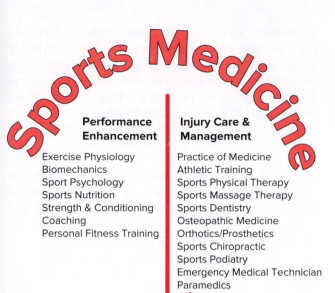

## Sports Medicine

| Performance Enhancement | Injury Care & Management |
|---|---|
| Exercise Physiology | Practice of Medicine |
| Biomechanics | Athletic Training |
| Sport Psychology | Sports Physical Therapy |
| Sports Nutrition | Sports Massage Therapy |
| Strength & Conditioning | Sports Dentistry |
| Coaching | Osteopathic Medicine |
| Personal Fitness Training | Orthotics/Prosthetics |
| | Sports Chiropractic |
| | Sports Podiatry |
| | Emergency Medical Technician |
| | Paramedics |

FIGURE 1–2 Areas of specialization under the sports medicine "umbrella."

emergency medical technology. The American College of Sports Medicine (ACSM) has defined sports medicine as multidisciplinary, including the physiological, biomechanical, psychological, and pathological phenomena associated with exercise and sports.[3] The clinical application of the work of these disciplines is performed to improve and maintain an individual's functional capacities for physical labor, exercise, and sports. Sports medicine also includes the prevention and treatment of diseases and injuries related to exercise and sports.

## Growth of Professional Sports Medicine Organizations

The twentieth century brought with it the development of a number of professional organizations dedicated to athletic training and sports medicine. Professional organizations have many goals: (1) to upgrade the field by devising and maintaining a set of professional standards, including a code of ethics; (2) to bring together professionally competent individuals to exchange ideas, stimulate research, and promote critical thinking; and (3) to give individuals an opportunity to work as a group with a singleness of purpose, thereby making it possible for them to achieve objectives that, separately, they could not accomplish. The organizations identified below are presented in chronological order according to their year of establishment. Addresses, phone numbers, and/or Web sites for these and other related sports medicine organizations can be found in Appendix A in the back of this text.

> Many professional organizations that are dedicated to achieving health and safety in sports developed in the twentieth century.

Several of these professional organizations also disseminate information to the general public about safe participation in sport activities in the form of guidelines or position statements. See *Focus Box 1–1:* "Key National Athletic Trainers Association Position, Official, Consensus, and Support Statements" for a list of statements addressing the practice of athletic training.

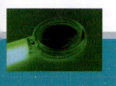

# FOCUS 1–1 Focus on Healthcare Administration and Professional Responsibilities

## Key National Athletic Trainers Association Position, Official, Consensus, and Support Statements

**Consensus Statements** (www.nata.org /news-publications/pressroom /statements/consensus)

*Inter-Association Consensus Statement on Best Practices for Sports Medicine Management for Secondary Schools and Colleges* (January 2014)

*Appropriate Medical Care for Secondary School-Age Athletes* (2003)

**Official Statements** (www.nata.org/news -publications/pressroom/statements /official)

*Proper Supervision of Secondary School Student Aides* (2014)

*Full-Time On-Site Athletic Trainer Coverage for Secondary School Athletic Programs* (2004)

*Providing Quality Health Care and Safeguards to Athletes of All Ages and Levels of Participation* (December 2011)

*Use of Qualified Athletic Trainers in Secondary Schools* (2004)

**Support Statements** (www.nata.org/news -publications/pressroom/statements /support)

*American Academy of Family Physicians' Support of Athletic Trainers for High School Athletes* (2007)

*NCAA Support of Recommendations and Guidelines for Appropriate Medical Coverage of Intercollegiate Athletics* (August 2003)

*American Medical Association's Support of Athletic Trainers in Secondary Schools* (1998)

Appendix B provides a complete listing of all position, consensus, official, and support statements developed by or with support from the National Athletic Trainers Association. Also listed in this appendix are specific Web sites where these statements may be found.

**International Federation of Sports Medicine** Among the first major organizations was the Fédération Internationale de Médecine du Sport (FIMS). In English it is called the International Federation of Sports Medicine. It was created in 1928 at the Olympic Winter Games in St. Moritz, Switzerland, by Olympic medical doctors with the principal purpose of promoting the study and development of sports medicine throughout the world. FIMS is made up of the national sports medicine associations of more than 100 countries. This organization includes many disciplines that are concerned with the physically active individual. To some degree, the ACSM has patterned itself after this organization.

**American Academy of Family Physicians** The American Academy of Family Physicians (AAFP) was founded in 1947 to promote and maintain high-quality standards for family doctors who are providing continuing comprehensive health care to the public. AAFP is a medical association of more than 100,000 members. Many team physicians are members of this organization. It publishes *American Family Physician.*

**National Athletic Trainers' Association** Before the formation of the National Athletic Trainers' Association in 1950, athletic trainers occupied a somewhat insecure place in the athletic program. Since that time, as a result of the raising of professional standards and the establishment of a code of ethics, there has been considerable professional advancement. The stated mission of NATA is

> To enhance the quality of health care provided by certified athletic trainers and to advance the athletic training profession.

The association accepts as members only those athletic trainers who are properly qualified and who are prepared to subscribe to a code of ethics and to uphold the standards of the association. NATA currently has more than 42,000 members. It publishes a quarterly journal, *The Journal of Athletic Training,* and *Athletic Training Education Journal* online, and holds an annual convention at which members have an opportunity to keep abreast of new developments and to exchange ideas through clinical programs. The organization is constantly working to improve both the quality and the status of athletic training.

**American College of Sports Medicine** As discussed previously, the ACSM is interested in the study of all aspects of sports. Established in 1954, ACSM has a membership of more than 45,000, composed of medical doctors, doctors of philosophy, physical educators, athletic trainers, coaches, exercise physiologists, biomechanists, and others interested in sports. The organization holds national and regional conferences and meetings devoted to exploring the many aspects of sports medicine, and it publishes a quarterly magazine, *Medicine and Science in Sports and Exercise.* This journal includes articles in French, Italian, German, and English, and provides complete translations in English of all articles. It reports recent developments in the field of sports medicine on a worldwide basis.

**American Orthopaedic Society for Sports Medicine** The American Orthopaedic Society for Sports Medicine (AOSSM) was created in 1972 to encourage and support scientific research in orthopedic sports medicine; the organization works to develop methods for safer, more productive, and more enjoyable fitness programs and sports participation. Through programs developed by the AOSSM, members receive specialized training in sports medicine, surgical procedures, injury prevention, and rehabilitation. AOSSM's 3,000 members are orthopedic surgeons and allied health professionals committed to excellence in sports medicine. Its official bimonthly publication is the *American Journal of Sports Medicine.*

**National Strength and Conditioning Association** The National Strength and Conditioning Association (NSCA) was formed in 1978 to facilitate a professional exchange of ideas in strength development as it relates to the improvement of athletic performance and fitness and to enhance, enlighten, and advance the field of strength and conditioning.

NSCA has a membership of more than 30,000 professionals in 52 countries, including strength and conditioning coaches, personal trainers, exercise physiologists, athletic trainers, researchers, educators, sport coaches, physical therapists, business owners, exercise instructors, fitness directors, and students training to enter the field. In addition, the NSCA Certification Commission offers two of the finest and the only nationally accredited certification programs: the Certified Strength and Conditioning Specialist (CSCS) and the NSCA Certified Personal Trainer (NSCA-CPT). NSCA publishes both the *Journal of Strength and Conditioning Research* and *Strength and Conditioning.*

**American Academy of Pediatrics, Council on Sports Medicine and Fitness** The American Academy of Pediatrics, Sports Committee was organized in 1979. Its primary goal is to educate all physicians, especially pediatricians, about the special needs of children who participate in sports. Between 1979 and 1983, this committee developed guidelines that were incorporated into a report, *Sports Medicine: Health Care for Young Athletes,* edited by Nathan J. Smith, M.D.

**American Physical Therapy Association, Sports Physical Therapy Section** In 1981, the Sports Physical Therapy Section of the American Physical Therapy Association (APTA) was officially established. The mission of the Sports Physical Therapy Section is "to provide a forum to establish collegial relations between physical therapists, physical therapist assistants, and physical therapy students interested in sports physical therapy." The Section and its 6,000 members promote the prevention, recognition, treatment, and rehabilitation of injuries in an athletic and physically active population through special interest groups (SIGs); provide educational opportunities through sponsorship of continuing education programs and publications; promote the role of the sports physical therapist to other health professionals; and support research to further establish the scientific basis for sports physical therapy. The Section's official journal is the *Journal of Orthopaedic and Sports Physical Therapy.*

**NCAA Committee on Competitive Safeguards and Medical Aspects of Sports** The National Collegiate Athletic Association (NCAA) Committee on Competitive Safeguards and Medical Aspects of Sports collects and develops pertinent information about desirable training methods, prevention and treatment of sports injuries, utilization of sound safety measures at the college level, drug education, and drug testing; disseminates information and adopts recommended policies and guidelines designed to further the objectives just listed; and supervises drug-education and drug-testing programs. Each year, this committee publishes the *Sports Medicine Handbook* that contains a wealth of continuously updated information related to sports medicine, which can be very useful to the athletic trainer.

**National Academy of Sports Medicine** The National Academy of Sports Medicine (NASM) was founded in 1987 by physicians, physical therapists, and fitness professionals; it focuses on the development, refinement, and implementation of educational programs for fitness, performance, and sports medicine professionals. According to its mission statement, "NASM is dedicated to transforming lives and revolutionizing the health and fitness industry through its unwavering commitment to deliver innovative education, solutions and tools that produce remarkable results." In addition to offering a fitness certification (Certified Personal Trainer) and performance certification (Performance Enhancement Specialist), NASM offers advanced credentials and more than 20 continuing education courses in a variety of disciplines. NASM serves more than 100,000 members and partners in 80 countries.

**Other Health-Related Organizations** Many other health-related professions, such as dentistry, podiatristry, and chiropractic, have, over the years, become interested in the health and safety aspects of sports. Besides national organizations that are interested in athletic health and safety, there are state and local associations that are extensions of the larger bodies. National, state, and local sports organizations have all provided extensive support to the reduction of illness and injury risk to the athlete.

**Other Sports Medicine Journals** Other journals that provide an excellent service to the field of athletic training and sports medicine are *The International Journal of Sports Medicine,* which is published in English by Thieme-Stratton, Inc., New York; *The Journal of Sports Medicine and Physical Fitness,* published by Edizioni Minerva Medica SPA, ADIS Press Ltd., Auckland 10, New Zealand; the *Journal of Sport Rehabilitation* and *Athletic Therapy and Training,* both published by Human Kinetics Publishers, Inc., Champaign, Illinois; the *Physician and Sportsmedicine,* published by McGraw-Hill, Inc., New York; *Physical Therapy* and *Clinical Management,* both published by the American Physical Therapy Association, Fairfax, Virginia; *Physical Medicine and Rehabilitation Clinics* and *Clinics in Sports Medicine,* both published by W. B. Saunders, Philadelphia; *Training and Conditioning,* published by MAG, Inc., Ithaca, New York; *Sports Health*: *A Multidisciplinary Approach,* published by Sage in Thousand Oaks, California; and *Athletic Training and Sports Health Care*: *The Journal for the Practicing Clinician,* published by Slack Inc., in Thorofare, New Jersey.

There is a significant number of other journals that relate in some way to sports medicine. They are listed in Appendix C located at the end of this text.

# EMPLOYMENT SETTINGS FOR THE ATHLETIC TRAINER

Opportunities for employment as an athletic trainer have changed dramatically in recent years. Athletic trainers no longer work only in athletic training clinics at the college, university, or secondary-school level. The employment opportunities for athletic trainers are more diverse than ever.[46] A discussion of the various employment settings follows (Table 1–1).

## Clinics and Hospitals

Today, more than 40 percent of certified athletic trainers are employed in clinics and hospitals—more than in any other employment setting. The role of the athletic trainer varies from one clinic to the next. Athletic trainers may be employed in an outpatient ambulatory rehabilitation clinic working in general patient care; in hospital emergency rooms: as health, wellness, or performance enhancement specialists; or as clinic administrators. Their job may also involve ergonomic assessment, work hardening, CPR training, or occasionally overseeing drug-testing programs. They may also be employed by a hospital but work in a clinic. Other clinical athletic trainers are employed by a hospital, but work only in local secondary schools or small colleges for practice, game, or single event coverage. For the most part, private clinics have well-equipped facilities in which

> The largest percentage of certified athletic trainers are employed in clinics and hospitals.

**TABLE 1–1** **Employment Settings for Athletic Trainers***

**Clinic**

- Hospital-based (employed by hospital; work in a clinic)
  - General patient care
  - Health/wellness/performance enhancement
  - Occupational/industrial (100%/split)
  - Administration
- Outpatient/ambulatory/rehabilitation clinic
  - General patient care
  - Health/wellness/performance enhancement
  - Occupational/industrial (100%/split)
  - Administration
- Physician-owned clinic (patient care or administration)
  - Orthopedic
  - Primary care
  - Family practice
  - Pediatric
  - Physiatry
  - Other
- Secondary school/clinic (employed by clinic; work in school)
  - Secondary school (100%)
  - Secondary school (split)
- Clinic, other

**Hospital (work in a hospital but not in a hospital-based clinic)**

- Administration
- Emergency department
- Orthopedics
- Other

**Industrial/occupational (work on-site at an industrial or occupational facility)**

- Clinic
- Ergonomics
- Health/wellness/fitness
- Other

**Corporate (work for company that sells to the profession or in patient care for that company)**

- Business/sales/marketing
- Ergonomics
- Health/wellness/fitness
- Patient care

**College/university**

- Professional staff/athletics/clinic
- Faculty/academic/research
- Split appointment
  - Division 1
  - Division 1AA
  - Division 2
  - Division 3
- Administration

**Two-year institution**

- Professional staff/athletics/clinic
- Faculty/academic/research
- Split appointment
- Administration

**Secondary school (employed by school or district)**

- High school (teacher/clinical/split)
  - Public
  - Private
- Middle school (teacher/clinical/split)
  - Public
  - Private

**Professional sports**

- Baseball, M
- Basketball, M/W
- Football, M
- Hockey, M
- Soccer, M/W
- Lacrosse, M
- Softball, W
- Golf, M/W
- Tennis, M/W
- Wrestling
- Boxing
- Rodeo
- Auto racing (NASCAR, Indy Car)

**Amateur/recreational/youth sports**

- Amateur (work for NGB, USOC, or amateur athletics)
- Recreational (work for municipal or recreational league or facility)
- Youth sports (AAU)

**Performing arts**

- Dance
- Theater
- Entertainment industry (Disney, casinos, tour bands)

**Military/law enforcement/government**

- Military (Air Force, Army, Navy, Marines, Coast Guard, Merchant Marines, National Guard)
  - Active duty/civilian
- Academy
- Administration
- Law enforcement
  - Local department or agency (police/fire/rescue)
  - State department or agency (police/investigation)
  - Federal department or agency (FBI, CIA, ATF)
- Government
  - Local
  - State
  - Federal (Senate, House, judicial)
  - Agencies (NASA, FDA)
- Hospital/clinic
- Other

**Health/fitness/sports/performance enhancement clinics/clubs (work for franchise, chain, or independent club)**

**Independent contractor (work for themselves and are not employees)**

*Modified from National Athletic Trainers' Association.

to work. In many sports medicine clinics, the athletic trainer may be responsible for formulating a plan to market or promote athletic training services offered by that clinic throughout the local community[30] (Figure 1–3A).

**Athletic Trainers in Physician Practice** Some athletic trainers work in clinics that are owned by physicians. Although virtually all athletic trainers work under the direction of a physician, those employed as an athletic trainer in physician practice actually work in the physician's office, where patients of all ages and backgrounds are being treated.[66] The educational preparation for athletic trainers allows them to function in a variety of domains, including injury prevention, evaluation, diagnosis, management and rehabilitation, health education, nutrition, training and conditioning, preparticipation physicals, and maintenance of essential documentation.[104] Although the contact with only the physically active population may not be as great as in other employment settings, the athletic trainer in physician practice can expect regular hours, few weekend or evening responsibilities, opportunity for growth, and, in general, better pay.[26,31] All these factors collectively make athletic trainer in physician practice positions attractive for the athletic trainer. Potentially, many new jobs can be created as physicians become more and more aware of the value that an athletic trainer, functioning as an athletic trainer in physician practice, can provide to their medical practice[24] (Figure 1–3B).

## Industrial/Occupational Settings

It is becoming relatively common for industries to employ athletic trainers to oversee fitness and injury rehabilitation programs for their employees.[1] The athletic trainer working in an industrial or occupational setting must have a sound understanding of the principles and concepts of workplace ergonomics, including inspecting, measuring, and observing dimensions of the work space, as well as specific tasks that are performed at the workstation.[23] Once a problem has been identified, the athletic trainer must be able to implement proper adjustments to workplace ergonomics to reduce or minimize possible risks for injury. In addition to these responsibilities, athletic trainers may be assigned to conduct wellness programs and provide education and individual counseling. It is likely that many job opportunities will exist for the athletic trainer in industrial/occupational settings in the next few years (Figure 1–3C&D).

## Corporate Settings

Opportunities are expanding for athletic trainers to use their educational background as preparation for working in business, sales, or marketing of products that other athletic trainers may use. Athletic trainers might also be employed by a company to administer health, wellness, and fitness programs or to provide some patient care to their employees.

## Colleges or Universities

At the college or university level, clinical positions for athletic trainers vary considerably from institution to institution. In smaller institutions, the athletic trainer may be a half-time teacher in physical education and half-time athletic trainer. In some cases, if the athletic trainer is a physical therapist rather than a teacher, he or she may spend part of the time in the school health center and part of the time in athletic training. Increasingly at the college level, athletic training services are being offered to members of the general student body who participate in intramural and club sports. In most colleges and universities, the athletic trainer is full-time, does not teach, works in the department of athletics, and is paid by the institution. However, it has been suggested that athletic trainers at colleges and universities should be employed by the campus or student health services rather than by the athletic department.[15]

In February 1998, the NATA created the Task Force to Establish Appropriate Medical Coverage for Intercollegiate Athletics (AMCIA) to establish recommendations for the extent of appropriate medical coverage to provide the best possible health care for all intercollegiate student-athletes. Essentially, the AMCIA task force made recommendations for the number of athletic trainers who should be employed at a college or university based on a mathematical model created by a number of variables existing at each institution. These guidelines were revised and updated in 2003. (For directions to determine the recommended number of athletic trainers, consult "Recommendations and Guidelines for Appropriate Medical Coverage of Intercollegiate Athletics,"[68] see *Focus Box 1–1*.) In August 2003, the NCAA Committee on Competitive Safeguards and Medical Aspects of Sports (CSMAS) recommended that NCAA institutions "examine the adequacy of their sports medicine coverage"[54]—in particular, whether the increased time demands placed on certified athletic trainers reduces their ability to provide high-quality care to all student-athletes. After reviewing the *Recommendations and Guidelines*, the CSMAS "encouraged NCAA institutions to reference the NATA AMCIA in their assessment of the adequacy of their sports medicine coverage . . . and share the responsibility to protect student athlete health and safety through appropriate medical coverage of its sports and supporting activities."

A number of athletic trainers working at colleges and universities are employed as faculty members.[40] These individuals may or may not be assigned clinical responsibilities. Instead, in addition to teaching responsibilities, these faculty members may serve as program directors and/or as researchers.

## Secondary Schools

There are more than 42,000 public and private secondary schools in the United States. It would be ideal to have

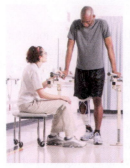
**A:** Clinics and Hospitals

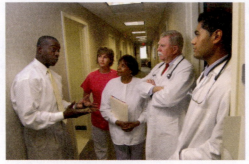
**B:** Athletic Trainer in Physician Practice

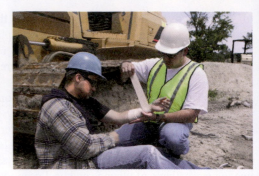
**C:** Industrial-Rehabilitation

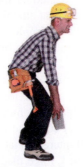
**D:** Work Hardening/Occupational

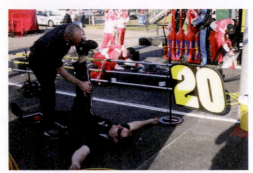
**E:** Professional Sports—NASCAR

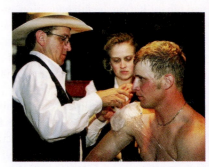
**F:** Professional/Sports—Rodeo

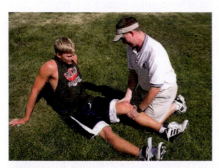
**G:** Youth Sports

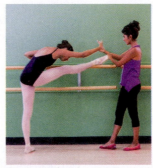
**H:** Performing Arts

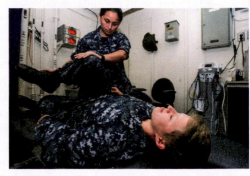
**I:** Military

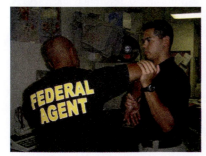
**J:** Law Enforcement

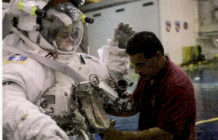
**K:** NASA

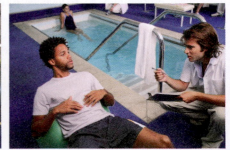
**L:** Health Clubs

**FIGURE 1−3** Athletic trainers work in a variety of employment settings.

(a) © Ingram Publishing/AGE Fotostock; (b) © Thinkstock/Getty Images; (c) © aabejon/Getty Images; (d) © YAY Media AS/Alamy; (e) Courtesy Logan Stewart; (f) Courtesy Dwayne Durham; (g) © William E. Prentice; (h) © Marc Romanelli/Blend Images LLC; (i) US Navy; (j) Courtesy The National Athletic Trainers' Association; (k) NASA-JSC; (l) © Fuse/Getty Images

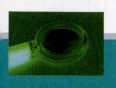

# FOCUS 1–2  Focus on Healthcare Administration and Professional Responsibilities

## Full-time, on-site athletic trainer coverage for secondary-school athletic programs

"The National Athletic Trainers' Association, as a leader in health care for the physically active, believes that the prevention and treatment of injuries to student-athletes are a priority. The recognition and treatment of injuries to student-athletes must be immediate. The medical delivery system for injured student-athletes needs a coordinator within the local school community who will facilitate the prevention, recognition, treatment and reconditioning of sports related injuries. Therefore, it is the position of the National Athletic Trainers' Association that all secondary schools should provide the services of a full-time, on-site, certified athletic trainer (ATC) to student-athletes."

From NATA official statement *Full time, on-site athletic trainer coverage for secondary-school athletic programs* (2004) (http://www.nata.org/sites/default/files/SecondarySchool.pdf). Reprinted with permission from the National Athletic Trainers' Association.

certified athletic trainers serve every secondary school and middle school in the United States.[49] Many of the physical problems that occur later from improperly managed sports injuries could be avoided initially if proper care from an athletic trainer had been provided.[7] If a secondary school or middle school hires an athletic trainer, it is very often in a faculty–athletic trainer capacity.[73] This individual is usually employed as a teacher who carries a reduced teaching load and performs athletic training duties. In this instance, compensation usually is on the basis of both teaching, a stipend as an athletic trainer, or both.[41] Salaries for the secondary-school athletic trainer are continuing to improve.[5]

Some school districts have found it effective to employ a centrally-placed certified athletic trainer. In this case, the athletic trainer, who may be full- or part-time, is a nonteacher who serves a number of schools. The advantage is savings; the disadvantage is that one individual cannot provide the level of service usually required by a typical school. A less desirable means of obtaining secondary-school athletic training coverage is using a certified graduate student from a nearby college or university. However, this practice may prevent a school from employing a certified athletic trainer on a full-time basis.

In 1995, the NATA adopted an official statement on hiring athletic trainers in secondary schools that appears in *Focus Box 1–2:* "Full-time, on-site athletic trainer coverage for secondary-school athletic programs." Based on a proposal from the American Academy of Pediatrics, in 1998 the American Medical Association adopted a policy calling for certified athletic trainers to be employed in all secondary-school athletic programs (see Appendix B). Although this policy was simply a recommendation and not a requirement, it was a very positive statement supporting the efficacy of athletic trainers in the secondary schools (*Focus Box 1–1*). To date Hawaii is the only state that requires an athletic trainer to be employed at each school.

Following the adoption of this policy, the NATA provided a second official statement on certified athletic trainers in secondary schools, which appears in *Focus Box 1–3:* "The use of qualified athletic trainers in secondary schools."

In 2008, the NATA published a consensus statement "Appropriate medical care for the secondary-school-age athlete" in which recommendations were provided for handling specific medical situations that can arise in the secondary-school setting (see *Focus Box 1–1*).[2]

In 2013, a group called the Youth Sports Safety Alliance, composed of more than 100 professional organizations, released a list of proposed rules and recommendations called the Secondary School Student Athletes' Bill of Rights. This "Bill" focuses on protecting students who participate in secondary-school sports. It calls for health providers such as athletic trainers and/or doctors to be available at every secondary school participating in interscholastic athletics. *Focus Box 1–4* shows the recommendations included in the "Secondary school student athletes' bill of rights."

Most recently in 2014, an inter-association consensus statement on the best practices for sports medicine management of secondary schools and colleges was released that defined the roles and responsibilities of the athletic trainer working in the secondary schools (http://natajournals.org/doi/pdf/10.4085/1062-6050-49.1.06).

## Professional Sports

Although the availability of positions for athletic trainers working at the professional level is limited, opportunities to work in this setting continue to expand. Virtually every professional team, regardless of the sport, employs at least one and occasionally as many as four certified athletic trainers. Athletic trainers work with both male and female professional teams, including football, basketball, baseball, hockey, soccer, lacrosse, softball, golf, and tennis. They are also employed in professional rodeo, auto racing (NASCAR), and wrestling. The athletic trainer for professional sports teams usually performs specific team athletic training duties for 6 to 8 months out of the year; the other 4 to 6 months

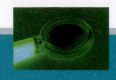

## FOCUS 1–3 Focus on Healthcare Administration and Professional Responsibilities

### The use of qualified athletic trainers in secondary schools

"The National Athletic Trainers' Association (NATA) is confident the best way to protect the public is to allow only Board of Certification–certified athletic trainers and state licensed athletic trainers to practice as athletic trainers. NATA is not alone in these beliefs. The American Medical Association has stated that certified athletic trainers should be used as part of a high school's medical team. The American Academy of Family Physicians agrees and states on its Web site, 'The AAFP encourages high schools to have, whenever possible, a BOC-certified or registered/licensed athletic trainer as an integral part of the high-school athletic program.

"In states with athletic training regulation, allowing other individuals to continue practicing as athletic trainers without a valid state license or BOC certification places the public at risk. Athletic trainers have unique education and skills that allow them to properly assess and treat acute and traumatic injuries in high-school athletics. In coordination with the team physician, they routinely make decisions regarding the return-to-play status of student-athletes. Other allied health professionals are not qualified to perform these tasks. Finally, most situations encountered by athletic trainers should not be left to a coach or layperson who does not have the necessary education and medical and emergency care training."

From NATA Official statement Use of qualified athletic trainers in secondary schools (2004) (http://www.nata.org/sites/default/files/ATsInHSs.pdf) Reprinted with permission from the National Athletic Trainers' Association.

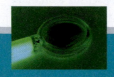

## FOCUS 1–4 Focus on Healthcare Administration and Professional Responsibilities

### Secondary-school student athletes' bill of rights

I. Student Athletes have the right to be coached by individuals who are well trained in sport-specific safety and to be monitored by athletic health care team members.

II. Student Athletes have the right to quality, regular preparticipation examinations and each athlete has the right to participate under a comprehensive concussion management plan.

III. Student Athletes have the right to participate in sporting activities on safe, clean playing surfaces, in both indoor and outdoor facilities.

IV. Student Athletes have the right to utilize equipment and uniforms that are safe, fitted appropriately and routinely maintained, and to appropriate personnel trained in proper removal of equipment in case of injury.

V. Student Athletes have the right to participate safely in all environmental conditions where play follows approved guidelines and medical policies and procedures, with a hydration plan in place.

VI. Student Athletes have the right to a safe playing environment with venue-specific emergency action plans that are coordinated by the athletic health care team and regularly rehearsed with local emergency personnel.

VII. Student Athletes have the right to privacy of health information and proper referral for medical, psychosocial and nutritional counseling.

VIII. Student Athletes have the right to participate in a culture that finds "playing through pain" unacceptable unless there has been a medical assessment.

IX. Student Athletes have the right to immediate, on-site injury assessments with decisions made by qualified sports medicine professionals.

X. Student Athletes have the right, along with their parents, to the latest information about the benefits and potential risks of participation in competitive sports, including access to statistics on fatalities and catastrophic injuries to youth athletes. Reprinted with permission from the National Athletic Trainers' Association.

are spent in off-season conditioning and individual rehabilitation. The athletic trainer working with a professional team is involved with only one sport and is paid according to contract, much as a player is. Playoff and championship money may be added to the yearly income (Figure 1–3E&F).

### Amateur/Recreational/Youth Sport

Athletic trainers are working at all levels of amateur sport. The United States Olympic Committee employs athletic trainers and interns at three training centers. Every national governing body (NGB) for each of the

Olympic sports employs either a single athletic trainer or a group of athletic trainers to work with the national teams and developmental programs for younger athletes. Some municipal or community-based recreational programs employ athletic trainers either full-time or as independent contractors to cover their programs. The Amateur Athletic Union (AAU) also employs athletic trainers to cover its tournaments (Figure 1–3G).

## Performing Arts

A relatively new and expanding employment opportunity exists in the performing arts and entertainment industry. Athletic trainers can be found working with dance companies and theater performance groups. They are employed by Disney television shows, movie sets, and the large casinos. Some touring bands even employ athletic trainers to work with their performers and road crew who sustain injuries while traveling (Figure 1–3H).

## The Military/Law Enforcement/Government

The United States military, particularly the Navy, the Marines, and the Army, have demonstrated increased emphasis on injury prevention and health care for the troops.[64] Treatment centers are being developed that closely resemble and, to a great extent, function as athletic training clinics. The centers are staffed by sports medicine physicians, orthopedists, athletic trainers, physical therapists, and support staff. Injured personnel are seen as soon as possible by an athletic trainer, who evaluates an injury, makes decisions on appropriate referral, and begins an immediate rehabilitation program. Currently, over 100 athletic trainers are in the military as either active duty or reserve personnel.[64] Occasionally, some contract positions are available. It is likely that the role of the athletic trainer in the military will increase substantially over the next several years (Figure 1–3I).

Opportunities are increasing for athletic trainers to become involved with local, state, and federal law enforcement groups and agencies. Athletic trainers are working with police and firefighters as well as with agencies such as the FBI and the American Federation of Teachers (AFT) (Figure 1–3J). Other athletic trainers are employed by government agencies such as the United States Senate, NASA, and the Pentagon (Figure 1–3K).[45]

## Health and Fitness Clubs

It is likely that a significant number of job opportunities for athletic trainers exist in health and fitness clubs. Some clubs may offer patient care, but it is more likely that the athletic trainer is a performance-enhancement specialist or an instructor. These clubs may be a chain, a franchise, or an independent club (Figure 1–3L).

## Treating Physically Active Populations

In the various employment settings, athletic trainers no longer treat only athletes, but instead a physically active population. *Physically active* individuals engage in athletic, recreational, or occupational activities that require physical skills and utilize strength, power, endurance, speed, flexibility, range of motion, and agility. *Physical activity* consists of athletic, recreational, or occupational activities that require physical skills and utilize strength, power, endurance, speed, flexibility, range of motion, and agility.

**The Adolescent Athlete** Children have always been physically active. But in today's society, playtime or physical activity for many adolescents is focused on organized competition. Certainly, many relevant sociological issues arise in answer to questions such as how old children should be when they begin to compete and when a child should begin training and conditioning. Skeletally immature adolescents present a particular challenge to the athletic trainer involved in some aspect of their health care. Adolescents cannot be approached either physically or emotionally in the same manner as adults. Thus, the athletic trainer must be aware of patterns of growth and development and all the special considerations that this process brings with it.

**The Aging Athlete** Aging involves a lifelong series of changes in physiological and performance capabilities. These capabilities increase as a function of the growth process throughout adolescence, peak sometime between the ages of 18 and 40 years, then steadily decline with increasing age. However, this decline may be due as much to the sociological constraints of aging as to biological effects. In most cases, after age 35, qualities such as muscular endurance, coordination, and strength tend to decrease. Recovery from vigorous exercise requires a longer amount of time. Regular physical activity, however, tends to delay and in some cases prevent the appearance of certain degenerative processes.

It is possible for individuals to maintain a relatively high level of physiological functioning if they maintain an active lifestyle. Consistent participation in vigorous physical activity can result in improvement of many physiological parameters regardless of age. The effects of exercise on the aging process and the long-term health benefits of exercise have been convincingly documented.

Generally, exercise is considered a safe activity for most individuals. ACSM has recommended that individuals under age 40 who are apparently healthy with no significant risks can generally begin an exercise program without further medical evaluation, as long as the exercise program progresses gradually and moderately, and no unusual signs or symptoms develop.[3] Individuals who are over age 40 or who are at high risk should have a complete medical examination and undergo an exercise test before beginning an exercise program.

**The Occupational Athlete** The occupational, industrial, or worker "athlete" often engages in strenuous, demanding, or repetitive physical activities while performing his or her job. Like other athletes, these activities can lead to accidents and injuries. Although an objective of any athletic trainer remains the immediate, accurate, and appropriate medical care of those injured in physical activity, the significant reduction of workers' compensation costs and improved employee productivity becomes critically important in the corporate or industrial world. Training a worker to use appropriate ergonomic techniques while engaging in the physical demands of the job is essential for preventing or at least minimizing the incidence of injury. Should injury occur, intervention strategies that correct faulty body mechanics, strength deficits, or lack of flexibility can help the worker return to performing his or her normal job.

**Athletes with Disabilities** Over the past several decades there has been increased emphasis on the role of physical activity and sport in enhancing health and quality of life of individuals with disabilities and chronic illnesses. Most recently, sport for athletes with disabilities has transitioned away from a medical rehabilitation model and moved toward a recreational, competitive, and even an elite-level sports model. Athletes with amputations, with spinal cord injuries who are confined to wheelchairs, with cerebral palsy, with visual or hearing impairments, with mental or other impairments have special needs when engaging in sport activities. Athletic trainers working with these individuals need advanced knowledge and understanding of these conditions and illnesses to be able to provide for the needs of athletes with special challenges. Opportunities to work with athletes who have disabilities are certainly increasing.

# ROLES AND RESPONSIBILITIES OF THE ATHLETIC TRAINER

Of all the professionals charged with injury prevention and health care provision for an injured patient, perhaps none is more intimately involved than the athletic trainer. The athletic trainer is the one individual who deals with the patient throughout the period of rehabilitation, from the time of the initial injury until the patient's complete, unrestricted return to activity. Certainly, providing effective health care for an injured athlete requires input from a cadre of individuals who compose the sports medicine team, including the physicians, coaches, and many other support personnel.[11] The athletic trainer is most directly responsible for all phases of health care, including preventing injuries from occurring, providing initial first aid and injury management, evaluating injuries, and designing and supervising a timely and effective program of rehabilitation that can facilitate the safe and expeditious return to activity.

The athletic trainer must be knowledgeable and competent in a variety of specialties encompassed under the umbrella of "sports medicine" if he or she is to be effective in preventing and treating injuries. The specific roles and responsibilities of the athletic trainer differ and to a certain extent are defined by the situation in which he or she works.[10]

## Board of Certification Domains of Athletic Training

In 2015 the Board of Certification (BOC)* completed the latest Practice Analysis (7th Edition),** which defines the profession of athletic training.[10] The latest Practice Analysis replaced the Role Delineation Study (6th edition) and went into effect in 2017. This Practice Analysis was designed to examine the primary tasks performed by the entry-level athletic trainer and the knowledge and skills required to perform each task.

> **Five Domains of Athletic Training**
> - Injury/illness prevention and wellness promotion
> - Examination, assessment, and diagnosis
> - Immediate and emergency care
> - Therapeutic intervention
> - Healthcare administration and professional responsibilities

The panel determined that the roles of the practicing athletic trainer could be divided into five major domains: (1) injury/illness prevention and wellness promotion; (2) examination, assessment, and diagnosis; (3) immediate and emergency care; (4) therapeutic intervention; and (5) healthcare administration and professional responsibilities.

**Injury/Illness Prevention and Wellness Promotion** A primary responsibility of the athletic trainer is to make the competitive environment as safe as possible to minimize the risk of injury. If injury can be prevented initially, there will be no need for first aid and subsequent rehabilitation. The athletic trainer should educate all of those individuals who are in some way either directly or indirectly responsible for the health care of the athlete.

The athletic trainer can minimize the risk of injury by (1) conducting

> An athletic trainer has taken a job at a sports medicine clinic that has four physical therapists and two physical therapy assistants. This clinic has never employed an athletic trainer before, and there is some uncertainty among the physical therapists as to exactly what role the athletic trainer will play in the function of the clinic.
>
> **?** How does the role of the athletic trainer working in the clinic differ from the responsibilities of the athletic trainer working in a university setting?

---

*The Board of Certification (BOC) has been responsible for the certification of athletic trainers since 1969. Upon its inception, the BOC was The Certification Committee for NATA, the profession's membership association. However, in 1989, the BOC became an independent nonprofit corporation. Formerly known as the NATABOC, the BOC officially changed its name in 2004.

**The 2015 Practice Analysis went into effect in 2017 and continues through 2022.

preparticipation exams; (2) ensuring appropriate training and conditioning of the athlete; (3) monitoring environmental conditions to ensure safe participation; (4) selecting, properly fitting, and maintaining protective equipment; (5) making certain that the athlete is eating properly; and (6) making sure the athlete is using medications appropriately, while discouraging substance abuse.

***Conducting Preparticipation Physical Examinations*** The athletic trainer, in cooperation with the team physician, should obtain a medical history and conduct physical examinations of the athletes before participation as a means of screening for existing or potential problems (see Chapter 2). The medical history should be reviewed closely, and clarification should be sought for any point of concern.

The preparticipation examination should include the measurement of height, weight, blood pressure, and body composition. The physician examination should concentrate on cardiovascular, respiratory, abdominal, genital, dermatological, and ear, nose, and throat systems, and may include blood work and urinalysis. A brief orthopedic evaluation would include range of motion, muscle strength, and functional tests to assess joint stability. When the athletic trainer knows at the beginning of a season that an athlete has a physical problem that may predispose that athlete to an injury during the course of the season, he or she may immediately implement corrective measures that may significantly reduce the possibility of additional injury.

***Developing Training and Conditioning Programs*** Perhaps the most important aspect of injury prevention is making certain that the athlete is fit and thus able to handle the physiological and psychological demands of competition. The athletic trainer works with the coaches to develop and implement an effective training and conditioning program for the athlete (see Chapter 4). It is essential that the athlete maintain a consistently high level of fitness during the preseason, the competitive season, and the off-season. This consistent level of fitness is critical not only for enhancing performance parameters but also for preventing injury and reinjury. An athletic trainer must be knowledgeable in the area of applied physiology of exercise, particularly with regard to strength training, flexibility, improvement of cardiorespiratory fitness, maintenance of body composition, weight control, and nutrition. Many colleges and most

All-American High School is considering hiring an athletic trainer instead of using an emergency medical technician. However, the administrators do not completely understand why an athletic trainer may be more beneficial for their athletes. A group of area athletic trainers will be holding a meeting to discuss the potential change.

**?** What reasons should the athletic trainers use to persuade the administrators to hire an athletic trainer?

professional teams employ full-time strength coaches to oversee this aspect of the total program. The athletic trainer, however, must be acutely aware of any aspect of the program that may have a negative impact on an athlete or a group of athletes and must offer constructive suggestions for alternatives when appropriate. At the secondary-school level, the athletic trainer may be totally responsible for designing, implementing, and overseeing the fitness and conditioning program for the athletes.

***Ensuring a Safe Playing Environment by Minimizing Safety Hazards*** To the best of his or her ability, the athletic trainer must ensure a safe environment for competition. This task may include duties not typically thought to belong to the athletic trainer, such as collecting trash, picking up rocks, or removing objects (e.g., hurdles, gymnastics equipment) from the perimeter of the practice area, all of which might pose potential danger to the athlete. Athletic trainers must also identify safety hazards involving issues such as workplace ergonomics, equipment considerations, maintenance, and sanitation. The athletic trainer should call these potential safety hazards to the attention of an administrator. The interaction between the athletic trainer and a concerned and cooperative administrator can greatly enhance the effectiveness of the sports medicine team.

The athletic trainer should also be familiar with the potential dangers associated with practicing or competing under inclement weather conditions, such as high heat and humidity, extreme cold, or electrical storms. Practice should be restricted, altered, or canceled if weather conditions threaten the health and safety of the athlete. If the team physician is not present, the athletic trainer must have the authority to curtail practice if the environmental conditions become severe (see Chapter 6).

***Selecting, Fitting, and Maintaining Protective Equipment*** The athletic trainer works with coaches and equipment personnel to select protective equipment and is responsible for maintaining its condition and safety (see Chapter 7). Because liability lawsuits have become the rule rather than the exception, the athletic trainer must make certain that high-quality equipment is purchased and that it is constantly being worn, maintained, and reconditioned according to specific guidelines recommended by the manufacturers.

Protective equipment and devices can consume a significant portion of the athletic budget. The person responsible for purchasing protective equipment is usually inundated with marketing literature on a variety of braces, supports, pads, and other types of protective equipment. Decisions on purchasing specific pieces or brands should be based on research data that clearly document effectiveness in reducing or preventing injury (Figure 1–4).

Equipment is expensive, and schools are certainly subject to budgeting restrictions. However, purchasing decisions about protective equipment should always be made in the best interest of the athlete. Most colleges and

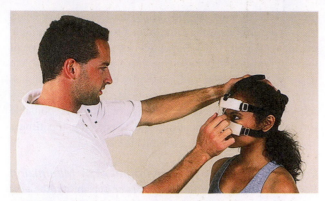

FIGURE 1–4  The athletic trainer should be responsible for taping and for the fitting of protective devices.
© William E. Prentice

professional teams hire full-time equipment managers to oversee this area of responsibility, but the athletic trainer must be knowledgeable about and aware of the equipment being worn by each athlete.

The design, building, and fitting of specific protective orthopedic devices are also responsibilities of the athletic trainer. Once the physician has indicated the problem and how it may be corrected, the athletic trainer should be able to construct an orthopedic device to correct it.

### Explaining the Importance of Diet and Lifestyle Choices
Good nutrition can have a substantial impact on health and well-being. Poor nutritional habits can certainly have a negative effect on ability to perform at the highest level possible. However, for all the attention that athletes, coaches, and athletic trainers direct at practicing sound nutritional habits, good nutritional decisions are still subject to a tremendous amount of misunderstanding, misinformation, and occasionally quackery. An athletic trainer is often asked for advice about matters related to diet, weight loss, and weight gain and is occasionally asked about disordered eating. The athletic trainer does not need to be an expert on nutrition but must possess some understanding of the basic principles of nutrition[101] (see Chapter 5). The athletic trainer should also be able to discuss nonhealth lifestyle habits, such as alcohol, tobacco, and drug use. They must educate and encourage patients to make healthy lifestyle choices.

### Using Medications Appropriately
The athlete, like anyone else, may benefit greatly from using medications prescribed for various medical conditions by qualified physicians. Under normal circumstances, an athlete would be expected to respond to medication just as anyone else would. However, because of the nature of physical activity, the athlete's situation is unique; intense physical activity requires that special consideration be given to the effects of certain types of medication.

For the athletic trainer who is overseeing the health care of the athlete, some knowledge of the potential effects of certain types of drugs on performance is essential. Occasionally, the athletic trainer must make decisions regarding the appropriate use of medications based on knowledge of the indications for use and of the possible side effects in athletes who are involved in training and conditioning as well as in injury rehabilitation programs. The athletic trainer must be cognizant of the potential effects and side effects of over-the-counter and prescription medications on the athlete during rehabilitation as well as during competition (see Chapter 17).

In addition, the athletic trainer should also be aware of the problems of substance abuse, both in ergogenic aids that may be used in an effort to enhance performance and in the abuse of so-called recreational or street drugs. The athletic trainer may be involved in drug testing of the athlete and should thus be responsible for educating the athlete in drug use and substance abuse.

### Examination, Assessment, and Diagnosis
Frequently, the athletic trainer is the first person to see a patient who has sustained an injury. The athletic trainer must be skilled in recognizing the nature and extent of an injury through competency in injury evaluation. Once the injury has been diagnosed, the athletic trainer must be able to provide the appropriate first aid and then refer the patient to appropriate medical personnel.

The athletic trainer must be able to efficiently and accurately diagnose an injury and illnesses. Information obtained in an initial evaluation may be critical later on when swelling, pain, and guarding mask some of the functional signs of the injury.

It is essential that the athletic trainer be alert and observe, as much as possible, everything that goes on in practice. Invaluable information regarding the nature of an injury can be obtained by seeing the mechanism of the injury.

The subsequent off-the-field examination should include (1) a brief medical history of exactly what happened, according to the athlete; (2) observation; (3) palpation; and (4) special tests, which might include tests for range of motion, muscle strength, or joint stability or a brief neurological examination. Information obtained in this initial examination should be documented by the athletic trainer and given to the physician once the athlete is referred. The team physician is ultimately responsible for providing medical diagnosis of an injury. The initial clinical diagnosis often provides the basis for this medical diagnosis (see Chapter 13).

### Understanding the Pathology of Injury and Illness
The athletic trainer must be able to recognize both general medical conditions and the various types of musculoskeletal and nervous system injuries that can occur in the physically active population. Based on this knowledge of different injuries, the athletic trainer must possess some understanding of both the sequence and time frames for the various phases of healing, realizing that certain physiological events must occur during each of the phases (see Chapter 10). Anything done during training and conditioning or during a rehabilitation program that interferes with this healing process will likely delay a return to full

activity. The healing process must have an opportunity to accomplish what it is supposed to. At best, the athletic trainer can only try to create an environment that is conducive to the healing process. Little can be done to speed up the process physiologically, but many things may be done to impede healing both during training and conditioning and during rehabilitation.

**Referring to Medical Care** After the initial management of an injury, the athletic trainer should routinely refer the patient to a physician for further evaluation and to confirm the diagnosis. If an athlete requires treatment from medical personnel other than the team physician, such as a dentist or an ophthalmologist, the athletic trainer should arrange appointments as necessary. Referrals should be made after consultation with the team physician.

**Referring to Support Services** If needed, the athletic trainer must be familiar with and should have access to a variety of personal, school, and community health service agencies, including community-based psychological and social support services available to the patient. With assistance and direction from these agencies, the athletic trainer, together with the athlete, should be able to formulate a plan for appropriate intervention following injury.

**Immediate and Emergency Care** The athletic trainer is often responsible for the initial on-the-field injury assessment and diagnosis following acute injury. Once this initial diagnosis is done, the athletic trainer then must assume responsibility for administering appropriate first aid and for making correct decisions in the management of acute injury (see Chapter 12). Although the team physician is frequently present at games or competitions, in most cases he or she cannot be at every practice session, where injuries are more likely to occur. Thus, the athletic trainer must possess sound skills not only in the initial recognition and evaluation of potentially serious or life-threatening injuries and/or illnesses but also in emergency care.

The athletic trainer must be certified in cardiopulmonary resuscitation and the use of automated external defibrillators (AEDs) by the American Red Cross, the American Heart Association, or the National Safety Council. Athletic trainers must also consider seeking certification in first aid by the American Red Cross or the National Safety Council. Many athletic trainers have gone beyond these essential basic certifications and have completed emergency medical technician (EMT) requirements.

The athletic trainer should establish well-defined emergency action plans in cooperation with local rescue squads and the community hospitals that can provide emergency treatment.[75] Emergency care is expedited, and the injured athlete's frustration and concern are lessened if arrangements regarding transportation, logistics, billing procedures, and appropriate contacts are made before an injury occurs.

**Therapeutic Intervention** An athletic trainer must work closely with and under the direction of the team physician with respect to designing rehabilitation and reconditioning protocols that make use of appropriate therapeutic exercise, rehabilitative equipment, manual therapy techniques, or therapeutic modalities. The athletic trainer should then assume the responsibility of overseeing the rehabilitative process, ultimately returning the patient to full activity (see Chapter 16).

*Designing Rehabilitation Programs* Once an injury or illness has been evaluated and diagnosed, the rehabilitation process begins immediately. In most cases, the athletic trainer designs and supervises an injury rehabilitation program, modifying that program based on the healing process. It is critical for an athletic trainer to have a sound background in anatomy. Without this background, an athletic trainer cannot evaluate an injury. And if the athletic trainer cannot evaluate an injury, there is no point in the athletic trainer knowing anything about rehabilitation because he or she will not know at what phase the injury is in the healing process. The athletic trainer must also understand how to incorporate therapeutic modalities and appropriate therapeutic exercise techniques into the rehabilitation program if it is to be successful.

*Supervising Rehabilitation Programs* The athletic trainer is responsible for designing, implementing, and supervising the rehabilitation program from the time of initial injury until return to full activity. It is essential that the athletic trainer has a solid foundation in the various techniques of therapeutic exercise and an understanding of how those techniques can be incorporated most effectively into the rehabilitation program. The athletic trainer must also be familiar with the skills and normal biomechanics necessary for optimal performance on particular sport activity. The athletic trainer must establish both short-term and long-terms goals for the rehabilitation process and then be able to modify the program to meet those goals. The athletic trainer should constantly reassess the status of an existing injury so that correct decisions can be made

A high-school basketball player suffers a grade 2 ankle sprain during midseason of the competitive schedule. After a 3-week course of rehabilitation, most of the pain and swelling have been eliminated. The athlete is anxious to get back into practice and competitive games as soon as possible, and subsequent injuries to other players have put pressure on the coach to force the athlete's return. Unfortunately, the athlete is still unable to perform the functional tasks (cutting and jumping) essential in basketball.

**?** Who is responsible for making the decision regarding when the athlete can fully return to practice and game situations?

about altering and/or progressing the rehabilitation program. All those individuals who are in some way involved with the rehabilitative process, such as coaches, parents, administrators, and other health care professionals, should be consistently informed of the patient's progress toward full return to activity, while maintaining the necessary confidentiality regarding the patient's injury.

***Incorporating Therapeutic Modalities*** Athletic trainers use a wide variety of therapeutic modalities in the treatment and rehabilitation of injuries. Modality use may involve a relatively simple technique, such as using an ice pack as a first-aid treatment for an acute injury, or may involve more complex techniques, such as the stimulation of nerve and muscle tissue by electrical currents. Certainly, therapeutic modalities are useful tools in injury rehabilitation, and when used appropriately these modalities can greatly enhance the patient's chances for a safe and rapid return to athletic competition. It is essential for the athletic trainer to possess knowledge about the scientific basis and the physiological effects of the various modalities on a specific injury (see Chapter 15). Modalities, though important, are by no means the single most critical factor in injury treatment. Therapeutic exercise that forces the injured anatomical structure to perform its normal function is the key to successful rehabilitation. However, therapeutic modalities play an important role in reducing pain and are extremely useful as an adjunct to therapeutic exercise.

***Offering Psychosocial Intervention*** The psychological aspect of dealing with an injury is a critical yet often neglected aspect of the rehabilitation process. Injury and illness produce a wide range of emotional reactions. Therefore, the athletic trainer needs to develop an understanding of the psyche of each patient (see Chapter 11). Patients vary in terms of pain threshold, cooperation and compliance, competitiveness, denial of disability, depression, intrinsic and extrinsic motivation, anger, fear, guilt, and ability to adjust to injury. Principles of sport psychology may be used to improve total performance through visualization, self-hypnosis, and relaxation techniques. The athletic trainer plays a critical role in social support for the injured patient.[6] Athletic trainers should recognize that patients may exhibit abnormal social, emotional, and mental behaviors. Athletic trainers should also be able to recognize the role of mental health in injury and recovery, and use intervention strategies to maximize the connection between mental health and restoration of participation. If the athletic trainer recognizes that a problem exists, he or she should refer the patient to the appropriate medical personnel for intervention.

**Healthcare Administration and Professional Responsibilities** The athletic trainer is responsible for the organization and administration of the training clinic, including the maintenance of health and injury records for each patient, the requisition and inventory of necessary supplies and equipment, maintenance and safety of equipment, the supervision of assistants or athletic training students, and the establishment of policies and procedures for day-to-day operation of the athletic training program (see Chapter 2).[5]

***Record Keeping*** Accurate and detailed record keeping—including medical histories, preparticipation examinations, injury reports, treatment records, and rehabilitation programs—are critical for the athletic trainer, particularly in light of the number of lawsuits directed toward malpractice and negligence in health care. Maintaining accurate records may also be a requirement of many state licensing boards. Many athletic trainers are responsible for filing insurance claims for reimbursement. Although record keeping may be difficult and time consuming for the athletic trainer who treats and deals with a large number of patients each day, it is an area that simply cannot be neglected.

***Ordering Equipment and Supplies*** Although tremendous variations in operating budgets exist, depending on the level and the institution, decisions regarding how the available money may best be spent are always critical. The athletic trainer must keep on hand a wide range of supplies to enable him or her to handle whatever situation may arise. At institutions with severe budgetary restrictions, prioritization based on experience and past needs must become the mode of operation. A creative athletic trainer can make do with very little equipment, which should include at least a taping and treatment table, an ice machine, and a few free weights. As in other health care professions, the more tools available for use, the more effective the practitioner can be, as long as he or she understands how to use those tools most effectively.

***Supervising Personnel*** In an athletic training environment, the quality and efficiency of the certified assistant athletic trainers and graduate assistants and athletic training students in carrying out their specific responsibilities are absolutely essential.[14] The person who supervises these individuals has a responsibility to design a reasonable work schedule that is consistent with their other commitments and responsibilities outside the clinic. It is the responsibility of the head athletic trainer to provide an environment in which assistants and athletic training students can continually learn and develop professionally.[18] The supervision of athletic training students necessitates constant visual and auditory interaction and the ability to intervene physically on behalf of the patient or student.

***Establishing Policies for the Operation of an Athletic Training Program*** Although the athletic trainer must be able to easily adjust and adapt to a given situation, it is essential that specific policies, procedures, rules, and regulations be established to ensure the smooth and consistent day-to-day operation of the athletic training program. A plan should be established for emergency management of injury. Appropriate channels for referral after injury and emergency treatment should be used consistently.

Policies and procedures must be established and implemented that reduce the likelihood of exposure to infectious agents by following universal precautions, which can prevent the transmission of infectious diseases (see Chapter 2).

# PROFESSIONAL RESPONSIBILITIES OF THE ATHLETIC TRAINER

## The Athletic Trainer and Continuing Education

As the clinical competencies for a practicing athletic trainer continue to expand, the certified athletic trainer should assume personal responsibility for continuously expanding his or her own knowledge base and expertise within the field. This professional development may be accomplished by attending continuing education programs offered at state, district, and national meetings. Athletic trainers must also routinely review professional journals and consult current textbooks to stay abreast of the most up-to-date techniques. The athletic trainer should also make an effort to be involved professionally with national, regional, or state organizations that are committed to enhancing the continued growth and development of the profession.

> A young athletic trainer has taken his first job at All-American High School. The school administrators are extremely concerned about the number of athletes who get hurt playing various sports. They have charged the athletic trainer with the task of developing an athletic training program that can effectively help prevent the occurrence of injury to athletes in all sports at that school.
>
> **?** What actions can the athletic trainer take to reduce the number of injuries and to minimize the risk of injury in the competitive athletes at that high school?

## The Athletic Trainer as an Educator

The athletic trainer must take time to help educate athletic training students. The continued success of any profession lies in its ability to educate its students. Education should not simply be a responsibility; it should be a priority.

To be an effective educator, the athletic trainer needs an understanding of the basic principles of learning and pedagogy (the methods and practice of teaching). The athletic trainer should seek and develop competence in presenting information to students through the use of a variety of instructional techniques.[48] The athletic training educator should also make an effort to stay informed about the availability of relevant audiovisual aids, multimedia, newsletters, journals, workshops, and seminars that can enhance the breadth of the students' educational experience.[103] The athletic trainer must also be able to evaluate student knowledge and competencies through the development and construction of appropriate tests.[18] The athletic training educator should also assume some responsibility for helping the students secure a professional position following graduation. Guiding the athletic training student in constructing an appropriate resume will help in this effort (see Appendix D at the end of this text).

Students of athletic training must be given a sound academic background in a curriculum that stresses the competencies that are outlined in this chapter and presented in detail throughout this text. As a health care provider, the athletic trainer must understand the importance of teaching students how to incorporate the best available research-based evidence with clinical experience and individual patient values to achieve optimal patient outcomes.

Athletic trainers should provide students with the rationale for practicing patient-centered care with regard to the psychosocial barriers that patients and clinicians face with injury/disease, the importance of effective patient education, and strategies for open collaboration/communication between the patient and his or her health care network.

They should help students develop the knowledge needed to continuously improve the quality of care they are providing to the patient by learning how to consistently identify a treatment objective, incorporate an appropriate clinical intervention, and determine the extent to which that intervention enhanced the quality of care resulting in an improved patient outcome.

Athletic trainers should expose students to the knowledge base and skill sets specific to various exercise scientists and health care providers, including physical therapists, nutritionists, physicians, dentists, podiatrists, nurse practitioners, radiologists, chiropractors, and pharmacologists, so that they may gain an understanding of and an appreciation for the value that appropriate interprofessional referral can have in delivering optimal care to their patients.

Athletic trainers should help students learn how to use online databases to access the most recent evidence pertaining to optimal patient care, to use electronic medical records and software programs to manage clinical data, and to use e-mail, texting, and social media to more efficiently communicate with patients and other clinicians.

Finally, they should expose students to, and gain an appreciation for the behavioral characteristics and the leadership qualities that an individual needs to possess to portray a positive professional impression of themselves, the health care team, and the profession of athletic training to their patients and colleagues. They must be able to translate the theoretical base presented in the classroom into practical application in a clinical setting if they are to be effective in treating patients.[14] The athletic training educator accomplishes this application by organizing appropriate laboratory and/or clinical experiences to evaluate the students' clinical competencies.[80] Certainly, the preceptors can have a significant impact on the development of the athletic training student.[48]

The athletic trainer must also educate the general public, in addition to a large segment of the various allied medical health care professions, as to exactly what athletic trainers are and the scope of their roles and responsibilities. This education is perhaps best accomplished by organizing workshops and clinics in the community and with corporate and industrial groups, holding professional seminars, meeting with local and community organizations, publishing research in both scholarly and popular journals, and, most important, doing a professional job of providing quality health care to an injured patient.

## The Athletic Trainer as a Counselor

The athletic trainer should take responsibility for informing parents and coaches about the nature of a specific injury and how it may affect the ability of the patient to compete. The athletic trainer should be concerned primarily with counseling and advising the patient not only with regard to the prevention, rehabilitation, and treatment of specific injuries but also on any matter that might be of help to the patient.[61,62] Perhaps one of the most rewarding aspects of working as an athletic trainer can be found in the relationships that the athletic trainer develops with individual patients.

During the period of time that athletes are competing, the athletic trainer has the opportunity to get to know them very well on a personal basis because he or she spends a considerable amount of time with them. Athletes often develop a degree of respect for and trust in the athletic trainer's judgment, which carry over from their athletic life into their personal life. It is not uncommon for an athletic trainer to be asked questions about a number of personal matters, at which point he or she crosses a bridge from athletic trainer to friend and confidant. This considerable responsibility is perhaps best handled by first listening to the problems, presenting several options, and then letting the athlete make his or her own decision. Certainly, the role of counselor and advisor cannot be taken lightly.[81,84]

## The Athletic Trainer as a Researcher

As the athletic training profession continues to gain credibility as an allied health care profession, it is essential that athletic trainers work to enhance their visibility and credibility by engaging in research and scholarly publication.[96] Certainly, not everyone who works as an athletic trainer, in every employment setting, would be expected to engage in publishing research as part of his or her job responsibilities. Although it is true that many clinical athletic trainers publish case studies, assist in large research studies, and even conduct their own research, most often the research that is published in professional journals is conducted by individuals who are program directors, faculty members, or doctoral students employed in colleges and universities.[89] These individuals, along with graduate students seeking masters degrees at most

CAATE-accredited Post-Professional Athletic Training Education Programs are required to conduct research either as part of their job description or as a requirement for attaining their degree. It is likely that, as the numbers of educators, academicians, and graduate students continue to increase, more and more scholarly papers will be submitted for publication in professional journals.[95] Regardless of whether an individual possesses the inclination or the ability to conduct research, each certified athletic trainer must at the very least take responsibility for developing some comprehension of basic research design and statistical analysis and thus be able to interpret and evaluate new research. The athletic training profession cannot continue to move forward unless its members generate their own specific body of knowledge.[72]

Although the transition to evidence-based practice will be difficult for some, it is absolutely essential that the entire athletic training profession must become familiar and comfortable with that process as it is now the gold standard in our clinical practice.[50]

## The Importance of Engaging in Evidence-Based Practice for the Athletic Trainer

Athletic trainers, like other health care professionals, must routinely integrate evidence-based practice into patient care. Most simply, **evidence-based practice** is making decisions about the clinical care of individual patients based on the current best available evidence in the professional literature.[90] Practicing evidence-based medicine means integrating external clinical evidence from systematic research with clinical expertise while focusing on patient values and preferences (Figure 1–5). Individual clinical expertise is the proficiency and judgment that individual clinicians acquire through clinical experience and clinical practice.[77] External clinical evidence is clinically relevant research either from the basic sciences or medicine, or from patient-centered clinical research into the accuracy and precision of preventive, therapeutic, and rehabilitative techniques.[56] For athletic trainers, the evidence-based approach raises questions about

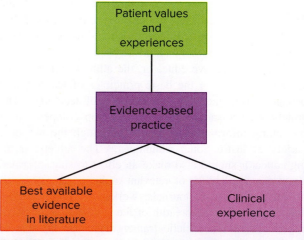

FIGURE 1–5   The evidence-based practice model.

clinical techniques such as specific evaluative tests, certain rehabilitation techniques, or the effectiveness of using therapeutic modalities.[13] External clinical evidence often invalidates previously accepted clinical techniques and treatments and replaces them with new ones that are more appropriate and efficient.[100] Without making use of the current best available evidence, clinical practice is in danger of becoming rapidly out of date, and this will undoubtedly have a negative impact on patient outcomes.[3]

In evidence-based practice, there are five steps that athletic training clinicians should take when attempting to determine the efficacy of using a specific clinical technique: (1) develop a clinical question; (2) search the literature to find the best evidence; (3) evaluate the strength of that evidence; (4) apply the best-available evidence in the literature to clinical experience and specific patient needs; and (5) assess the outcome or effectiveness of the treatment.[90]

**Developing a Clinical Question** When developing a clinical question, a **PICO** format which is based on three or four specific components should be used. PICO is an acronym for (1) **P**atient problems or condition; (2) **I**nterventions that are possible treatment options; (3) a **C**omparison of the alternatives that might be used in the intervention (a clinical question does not always need a specific comparison, in which case the acronym would simply be **PIO**); and (4) the **O**utcome that you want the patient to achieve.[90]

**Searching the Literature** When conducting a literature search, several different bibliographic databases will likely be used most often by athletic trainers, including Articles Plus, Google Scholar, PubMed/MEDLINE, CINAL, SPORTDiscus, and EBSCO host. These databases are called "pre-appraised," or EBP, databases.

Enter key words from the clinical question you are interested in answering into a search within the database. For example, if your clinical question is *"Is ultrasound effective in treating ankle sprains?"* enter the key term "ultrasound," which would be what is referred to as a *medical subject heading term* (MeSH). If you enter "ultrasound AND/OR ankle sprains" you would be using a *Boolean Operator* that searches for articles that include both terms.[82]

**Evaluating the Strength of the Evidence** When evaluating the strength of the evidence found in the literature, it is important to understand that many different types of research studies exist that have different purposes and individual strengths and weaknesses.[47] Among the different types of research, study designs are randomized controlled trials, including meta-analyses and systematic reviews; cohort studies that include outcomes research; case-control studies; case studies; and anecdotal evidence often based on expert opinion. Case studies provide the least scientific rigor while a meta-analysis is more rigorous and allows for less bias or systematic error.[56] The type of study can certainly have an effect on the quality of the information that study provides relative to the original clinical question.

***Critical assessment of results*** When critically assessing the results of a study, the evidence-based medicine approach requires you to answer three primary questions:

1. Are the results valid, and did the study measure what it was supposed to measure?
2. If the study is valid, what is the clinical significance of the study?
3. If the results are valid and clinically important, are the results applicable to the patient?

Critical appraisal papers (CAPs) or critical appraisal topics (CATs) are scholarly papers that analyze the level or quality of the evidence of a specific research study or topic, which is developed and written based on these three questions.[55] Scholarly journals are beginning to include the publication of CAPs and CATs as stand-alone papers.

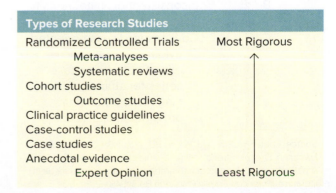

**Rating levels of evidence and levels of recommendation** There are three commonly used scales that assess the level or quality of the evidence in a specific research study.[54] The three scales are the *Strength of Recommendation Taxonomy (SORT)*, the *Level of Evidence* from the *Oxford Centre for Evidence-Based Medicine (CEBM)*, and the *Grading of Recommendations Assessment Development and Evaluation (GRADE)*. These scales look at the level of evidence that is based on the validity of the study. All of these scales are used to indicate the degree of confidence in the evidence to be recommended for use in clinical practice.

The SORT scale was developed by the American Academy of Family Physicians[20] and has been adopted for use by the National Athletic Trainers Association. The SORT scale uses letters A, B, and C to rate the strength of the evidence (A is highest) (Table 1–2).

The CEBM scale assigns a number from 1 to 5 (1 is highest) to rate its quality based on the type of research study (Table 1–3). Levels 1, 2, and 3 of evidence are further subdivided into subcategories a, b, and c, again based on the type of study. The GRADE uses four grades, from A to D, to rate the quality of the evidence from High to Very Low[58] (Table 1–4).

> **Strength of recommendations (SoR) based on the NATA Position, Official, and Consensus statements published since 2008 are identified throughout the text and can be easily found next to the reference in bold text where appropriate.**

**Using Systematic Reviews** Several additional databases publish systematic reviews and meta-analyses of the existing research. These systematic reviews provide clinicians with pre-filtered evidence, save time, and minimize the need for appraisal expertise. They provide the "state-of-the-art" information relative to a given research question.[82] The *Cochrane Database of Systematic Reviews* currently contains the largest database, and it is recommended that athletic trainers begin their search of systematic reviews here. *Scientific American Medicine* and the *ACP Journal Club* are databases that provide systematic overviews of the literature relative to a specific clinical question. These databases identify, review, synthesize, and appraise all of the high-level research evidence, to provide the clinician with recommendations as to which techniques should be incorporated into clinical practice. But simply locating these systematic reviews is only part of the process. The clinician must be able to further distinguish those systemic reviews that are high quality and those that are not. The type of research study design, the analysis of data, and the way the data are reported determine the overall quality of the study.

> **The Cochrane Database is the most comprehensive collection of systematic reviews.**

There are a number of scales and systems that rate the quality of these systematic reviews and meta-analyses.[97] Among the more commonly used scales to rate study quality are the Physiotherapy Evidence Database (PEDro), the Jadad Scale, and the New Castle—Ottawa Scale (NOS). These scales cannot be universally applied to all types of research designs. For example, the

| TABLE 1–3 | Levels of Evidence* |
|---|---|
| **Level** | **Type of Study** |
| 1. | Randomized controlled trials |
| | a. Meta-analysis/systematic reviews of randomized controlled trials |
| | b. Randomized controlled studies with small standard deviation |
| | c. All or none randomized controlled studies |
| 2. | Cohort studies |
| | a. Systematic reviews of cohort studies |
| | b. Individual cohort studies with low-quality randomized controls |
| | c. Outcomes research |
| 3. | Case-control studies |
| | a. Systematic reviews of case-control studies |
| | b. Individual case-control studies |
| 4. | Case reports/studies |
| 5. | Anecdotal evidence, expert opinions without critical appraisal |

*From the Centre for Evidence-Based Medicine, Oxford.

| TABLE 1–2 | Strength of Recommendation Taxonomy (SORT) |
|---|---|
| **Strength of Recommendation** | **Definition** |
| A | Consistent, good-quality, patient-oriented evidence |
| B | Inconsistent or limited-quality, patient-oriented evidence |
| C | Consensus, disease-oriented evidence, usual practice, expert opinion, or case series for studies of diagnosis, treatment, prevention, or screening |

Source: Ebell, MH, Siwek, J, Weiss, BD, Woolf, SH, Susman, J, Ewigman, B, et al.: Strength of recommendation taxonomy (SORT): A patient-centered approach to grading evidence in the medical literature, *American Family Physician* 69(3):548–556, 2004.

| TABLE 1-4 | Grading of Recommendations Assessment, Development and Evaluation (GRADE) | |
|---|---|---|
| Code | Quality of Evidence | Definition |
| A | High | Further research is very unlikely to change our confidence in the estimate of effect.<br>• Several high-quality studies with consistent results<br>• In special cases: one large, high-quality multi-center trial |
| B | Moderate | Further research is likely to have an important impact on our confidence in the estimate of effect and may change the estimate.<br>• One high-quality study<br>• Several studies with some limitations |
| C | Low | Further research is very likely to have an important impact on our confidence in the estimate of effect and is likely to change the estimate.<br>• One or more studies with severe limitations |
| D | Very low | Any estimate of effect is very uncertain.<br>• Expert opinion<br>• No direct research evidence<br>• One or more studies with very severe limitations |

Source: New Evidence Plus, 2016. Courtesy of John Wiley & Sons.

PEDro scale is designed to be used with systematic reviews and randomized controlled trials, whereas the NOS is designed to review nonrandomized studies with meta-analyses. The scales have totally different scoring systems, and scores from one scale cannot be compared to scores from a different scale.[97]

Standardized reporting guidelines assist authors with organizing critical pieces of information to include in doing a systematic review, and include Quality of Reports of Meta-Analyses of Randomized Controlled Trials (QUORUM), Standards for the Reporting of Diagnostic Accuracy Studies (STARD), Quality Assessment of Studies of Diagnostic Accuracy included in Systematic Reviews (QUADAS), Consolidated Standards of Reporting Trials (CONSORT), and Strengthening the Reporting of Observational Studies in Epidemiology (STROBE).

**Applying the Best Available Evidence in Making Clinical Decisions** Once the research that appears in the literature has been evaluated to determine the level of evidence and a level of recommendation for incorporating a specific technique into clinical practice, it becomes the responsibility of the clinician to understand those recommendations if they are to be correctly applied.[85] Additionally, the clinician must then define the circumstances unique to each patient, and ask the patient whether he or she has any other existing problems that might influence the effectiveness or the safety of the treatment. The patient's preferences, values, and rights should also be taken into consideration. The best available research evidence should be integrated with the patient's specific clinical circumstances and wishes to come up with a correct and meaningful decision about management.[57]

It is critical to bridge the barriers between research evidence and clinical decision making to ensure that patients receive optimal treatment. It is recommended that the current best available evidence be expeditiously incorporated into clinical decision making to minimize the delay between the generation of evidence and its clinical application.[32] This should serve to increase the number of patients who can potentially benefit from the current best clinical treatments available.

**Assessing the Outcomes of a Treatment** After the clinician has implemented a treatment technique that is supported by the best available evidence in the research literature, there needs to be some assessment of the effectiveness of that intervention on the ability of a patient to function normally. Outcomes research is done in an attempt to understand the end results of specific health care practices and interventions. In athletic training, examples of interventions could involve the use of a particular special test in evaluating an injury, a specific treatment technique, or the effectiveness of using a therapeutic modality.

Outcomes assessment measures change in a patient's functional status. These assessments may be based on either disease or condition-oriented evidence or patient-oriented evidence. Traditionally, disease or condition-oriented evidence has focused on mechanisms of the condition or injury, pathophysiology (ligament injury), impairments (strength, ROM, swelling), prevalence, functional limitations, and prognosis, and are based primarily on *clinician-centered outcome measures (CCO)*. The most recent trend in outcomes research has become to focus more on patient-oriented evidence that looks at the effects of the disease on the patient's overall health status (physical and mental health) and quality of life (social, emotional and physical well-being). Patient-oriented evidence takes into consideration the patient's perceptions and experiences from *patient-centered/rated outcome measures (PROMs)* on variables that are important to the patient. If clinicians can systematically identify clearly defined patient-centered goals, they will be more likely to provide treatment and care that is patient-centered. As a result, the approach may be more effective in determining whether a treatment or intervention meets the established goals.[98]

**The Disablement Model** Clinical outcomes are the end result of health care services. Clinical outcomes assessment is based on the conceptual framework of the *disablement model* that looks at functional loss due to a specific impairment and the associated impact on quality of life instead of focusing solely on a medical diagnosis. This model also serves as the measurement method for the collection of patient-oriented evidence, a concept central to evidence-based practice.[98] A number of disablement models have been proposed, including the Nagi Model, the National Center for Medical Rehabilitation Research Disablement Model (NCMRR), and, the World Health Organization International Classification of Functioning Model (IFC). Although differences exist among their terminology, all models consistently stress the whole individual beginning with the *origin* of the existing pathology (what type of tissue is injured); the *organ* level, which describes specific impairments associated with that body system; the *person* level, which looks at specific functional limitations; and the *social* implications created by the patient's disability and its effect on quality of life (Figure 1–6). Disablement models should help the athletic training clinician to a more comprehensive view of overall health-related quality of life (HRQOL), rather than a concentration on specific functional impairments.[88]

**Patient–Reported Outcome Scales (PROs)** Although the disablement model serves as the foundation for outcomes research, clinician-centered outcomes (CCOs) are measures that provide insight into the physiology of illness or injury. Clinician-centered outcomes are generally more important to the clinician than the patient.[60] Patient-centered/rated outcome measures (PROMs) gather information directly from the patient using structured questionnaires that have been demonstrated to provide meaningful, quantitative assessments of how the patient feels and how they are able to function with their disorders as a result of a treatment or intervention.[97] They serve to influence patient care, provide meaningful information regarding the effectiveness of interventions, contribute to the process of clinical reasoning, enhance communication, and motivate patients.[97]

Patient-derived scores that reflect changes in a clinical intervention that are meaningful for the patient are referred to as the *minimal clinically important difference (MCID)*. The MCID is a published value of change in an instrument that indicates the *clinical bottom line*, which is the minimum amount of change required for your patient to feel a difference in the variable being measured.[37] Several different types of PROMs are available to look at health status and quality of life:

- *Generic* instruments look at a broad range of aspects of health status and the consequences of illness or conditions that may be found in a wide range of primarily healthy populations (e.g., SF-36—Medical Outcomes Study 36-Item Short-Form Health Survey, Musculoskeletal Function Assessment). These should be used in initial examinations and then follow-ups and reevaluations.
- *Dimension-specific instruments* focus on one specific aspect of health status concentrating primarily on psychological well-being (e.g., McGill Pain Questionnaire).
- *Disease-specific* instruments are specific to a particular patient group that share a common disease (e.g., The Asthma Quality of Life Scale).
- *Site or region specific* instruments assess health problems in a specific part of the body (e.g., The Oxford Hip Score).
- *Summary-item* instruments include single items and may be specific to either a region or disease.[98]

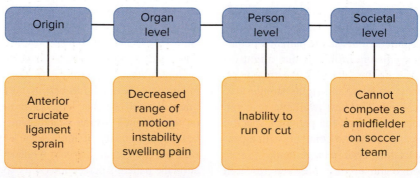

FIGURE 1–6    Disablement model.

Table 1–5 lists the existing outcome measures that are currently being used by athletic trainers and other sports medicine professionals.

***Global Rating of Change Scales*** Athletic trainers commonly ask their patients whether their injury has gotten better or worse with treatment, and then they use this information to determine the efficacy of a particular treatment or to guide future injury management decisions. *Global rating of change (GRC)* scales are commonly used in clinical research particularly with musculoskeletal injuries.[39] With GRC scales the patient must assess a particular aspect of their current health status (e.g., pain), then also be able to recall that status at a previous point in time, and finally to calculate the difference between the two. The magnitude of this difference is then scored on a balanced 7–11 point numerical or visual scale with written descriptors on the ends and at the midpoint. The *minimum detectable change* of a measure gives an indication of the degree to which scores change. However, what the clinician is really interested in is the *minimally clinically important change*, which is the change that is likely to be clinically relevant to a patient. The simplicity, ease of administration, and ease of interpretation of GRC scales makes them an attractive alternative to the more complex and time-consuming PROs (e.g., SF-36) for use in clinical practice.[43]

Patient-centered clinical outcomes assessments are a critical component in evidence-based practice. Athletic training clinicians and researchers must make concerted efforts to focus on patient-based outcomes that ultimately guide and direct the practice of athletic training.[83,88,97,100]

## Professional Behaviors of the Athletic Trainer

**Personal Qualities** There is probably no field of endeavor that can provide more work excitement, variety of tasks, and personal satisfaction than athletic training.[42] A person contemplating going into this field should love sports and should enjoy the world of competition, in which there is a level of intensity seldom matched in any other area.

An athletic trainer's personal qualities, not the facilities and equipment, determine his or her success.[4] Personal qualities are the many characteristics that identify individuals in regard to their actions and reactions as members of society. Personality is a complex mix of the many characteristics that together give an image of the individual to those with whom he or she associates.[76] The personal qualities of athletic trainers are important, because they in turn work with many complicated and diverse personalities. Although no attempt

| Personal qualities of the athletic trainer: |
| --- |
| • Stamina and ability to adapt |
| • Empathy |
| • Sense of humor |
| • Ability to communicate |
| • Intellectual curiosity |
| • Ethics |

**TABLE 1–5** **List of Available Patient-Related Outcome Measures Used in Sports Medicine\***

**Generic Instruments**
- Disablement in the Physically Active Scale (DPA)
- Patient Specific Functional Scale (PSFS)

**Generic Lower Extremity Instruments**
- Lower Extremity Functional Scale (LEFS)

**Generic Upper Extremity Instruments**
- Disabilities of the Arm, Shoulder, and Hand (DASH)
- Quick Disabilities of the Arm, Shoulder, and Hand Questionnaire (QuickDASH)
- Upper Extremity Functional Index (UEFI)
- Global Rating of Change Scale (GROC)

**Pain Instruments**
- Numeric Pain Rating Scale (NPRS)
- Short-form McGill Pain Questionnaire (SF-MPQ-2)

**Anatomy Specific Instruments**
*Neck*
- Neck Disability Index (NDI)
- Neck Bournemouth Questionnaire (NBQ)

*Shoulder*
- Shoulder Pain and Disability Index (SPADI)
- Disabilities of the Arm, Shoulder, and Hand (DASH)
- Quick Disabilities of the Arm, Shoulder, and Hand Questionnaire (QuickDASH)

*Elbow*
- Patient-Rated Tennis Elbow Evaluation (PRTEE)

*Hip*
- Western Ontario and McMaster Universities Arthritis Index (WOMAC)
- Oxford Hip Scale (OHS)
- International Hip Outcome Tool (iHOT)

*Knee*
- Cincinnati Knee Rating System
- Knee Injury and Osteoarthritis Outcomes Score (KOOS)
- Anterior Knee Pain Rating Scale (AKPS)

*Ankle*
- Foot and Ankle Disability Index (FADI), also used with FADI sport
- FADI sport
- Foot and Ankle Ability Measure (FAAM)

*Lumbar Spine*
- Oswestry Disability Index
- Quebec Back Pain Disability Scale
- Roland-Morris Disability Questionnaire

*\*Courtesy of Jennifer O'Donoghue PhD, LAT, ATC, CSCS, Department of Sports Medicine, North Carolina State University; and Rich Patterson MS, ATC, Department of Athletic Training, University of Charleston.*

has been made to establish a rank order, the qualities discussed in the following paragraphs are essential for a good athletic trainer.

***Stamina and Ability to Adapt*** Athletic training is not the field for a person who likes an 9-to-5 job. Long, arduous hours of often strenuous work will sap the strength of anyone not in the best of physical and emotional health. Athletic training requires abundant energy, vitality, and physical and emotional stability.[86] Every day brings new challenges and problems that must be solved. The athletic trainer must be able to adapt to new situations with ease.[17]

> As a member of a helping profession, the athletic trainer is subject to burnout.

A problem that can happen in any helping profession and does on occasion occur among athletic trainers and athletic training students is burnout.[102] This problem can be avoided if addressed early. The term *burnout* is commonly used to describe feelings of exhaustion and disinterest toward work.[44] Clinically, burnout is most often associated with the helping professions; however, it is seen in athletes and other types of individuals engaged in physically or emotionally demanding endeavors.[44] Most persons who have been associated with sports have known athletes, coaches, or athletic trainers who just drop out.[16] Such workers have become dissatisfied with and disinterested in the profession to which they have dedicated a major part of their lives.[94] Signs of burnout include excessive anger, blaming others, guilt, being tired and exhausted all day, sleep problems, high absenteeism, family problems, and self-preoccupation.[44] Athletic trainers who have high levels of perceived stress tend to experience higher emotional exhaustion and depersonalization and lower levels of personal accomplishment.[33] Persons experiencing burnout may cope by consuming drugs or alcohol.

The very nature of athletic training is one of caring about and serving the patient. When the emotional demands of work overcome the professional's resources to cope, burnout may occur.[25] Too many athletes to care for, coaches' expectations to return an injured athlete to action, difficulties in caring for chronic conditions, and personality conflicts involving athletes, coaches, physicians, or administrators can leave the athletic trainer physically and emotionally drained at the end of the day. Sources of emotional drain include little reward for one's efforts, role conflicts, lack of autonomy, and a feeling of powerlessness to deal with the problems at hand. Commonly, the professional athletic trainer is in a constant state of high emotional arousal and anxiety during the working day.

Individuals entering the field of athletic training must realize that it is extremely demanding. Even though the field is often difficult, they must learn that they cannot be "all things to all people." They must learn to say no when their health is at stake, and they must make leisure time for themselves beyond their work.[42] Perhaps most important, athletic trainers must make time to spend with their family, friends, and loved ones.[53]

***Empathy*** Empathy is the capacity to enter into the feeling or spirit of another person. Athletic training is a field that requires both the ability to sense when an athlete is in distress and the desire to alleviate that stress.

***Sense of Humor*** Many patients rate having a sense of humor as the most important attribute that an athletic trainer can have. Humor and wit help release tension and provide a relaxed atmosphere. The athletic trainer who is too serious or too clinical will have problems adapting to the often lighthearted setting of the sports world.[87]

***Ability to Communicate*** Athletic training requires a constant flow of both oral and written communication. As an educator, a psychologist, a counselor, a therapist, and an administrator, the athletic trainer must be a good communicator. The athletic trainer must communicate on a daily basis with athletes, coaches, physicians, administrators, school boards, and members of the patient's family.

***Intellectual Curiosity and Critical Thinking Ability*** The athletic trainer must always be a student. The field of athletic training is so diverse and ever changing that it requires constant study. The athletic trainer must have an active intellectual curiosity. Through reading professional journals and books, communicating with the team physician, and attending professional meetings, the athletic trainer stays abreast of the field. The athletic trainer is constantly challenged to think critically and problem solve when making clinical decisions relative to patient care. This is essential in achieving optimal patient outcomes.

***Ethics*** The athletic trainer must act at all times with the highest standards of conduct and integrity.[19,28,38,79,92,99] To ensure this behavior, the NATA has developed a code of ethics, which was approved in 1993 and was most recently revised in 2013.[65] The complete code of ethics appears in Appendix E. The four basic ethics principles are as follows:

1. Members shall respect the rights, welfare, and dignity of all.
2. Members shall comply with the laws and regulations governing the practice of athletic training.
3. Members shall maintain and promote high standards in their provision of services.
4. Members shall not engage in conduct that could be construed as a conflict of interest or that reflects negatively on the profession.

Members who act in a manner that is unethical or unbecoming to the profession can ultimately lose their certification.

***Professional Memberships*** It is essential that an athletic trainer become a member of and be active in professional organizations. Such organizations are continuously upgrading and refining the profession. They provide an ongoing source of information about changes occurring in the profession and include the NATA, district associations within the NATA, various state athletic training organizations, and ACSM. Some athletic trainers are also physical therapists. Increasingly, physical therapists are becoming interested in working with physically active individuals. Physical therapists and athletic trainers often have a good working relationship. Other athletic trainers may also be occupational therapists (OTs), physician assistants (PAs), certified strength and conditioning specialists (CSCS), nurses, or performance enhancement specialists (PESs).

## The Athletic Trainer and the Athlete

The major concern of the athletic trainer should always be the injured patient. It is essential to realize that decisions made by the physician, coach, and athletic trainer ultimately affect the athlete. Athletes are often caught in the middle between coaches telling them to do one thing and medical staff telling them to do something else. Thus, the injured athlete must always be informed and made aware of the why, how, and when that collectively dictate the course of an injury rehabilitation program.

The athletic trainer should make it a priority to educate the athlete about injury prevention and management. Athletes should learn about techniques of training and conditioning that may reduce the likelihood of injury. They should be well informed about their injuries and taught how to listen to what their bodies are telling them to prevent reinjury.

**The Athletic Trainer and the Athlete's Parents** In the secondary-school setting, the athletic trainer must take the time to explain to and inform the parents about injury management and prevention.[27] With a patient of secondary-school age, the parents' decisions regarding health must be a primary consideration.

In certain situations, particularly at the secondary school and middle-school levels, many parents will insist that their child be seen by their family physician rather than by the individual designated as the team physician. It is also likely that the choice of a physician that the athlete can see will be dictated by the parents' insurance plan (that is, their HMO or PPO). This creates a situation in which the athletic trainer must work and communicate with many different "team physicians." The opinion of the family physician must be respected even if the individual has little or no experience with injuries related to sports.

The coach, athletic trainer, and team physician should make certain that the athlete and his or her family are familiar with the Health Insurance Portability and Accountability Act (HIPAA), which regulates how individuals who have health information about an athlete can share that information with others and not be in violation of the privacy rule.[39] HIPAA was created to protect a patient's privacy and limit the number of people who can gain access to medical records. HIPAA regulations are discussed in more detail in Chapter 2.

## The Athletic Trainer and the Team Physician

In most situations, the athletic trainer works primarily under the direction of the team physician, who is ultimately responsible for directing the total health care of the athlete (Figure 1–7). In cooperation with the team physician, the athletic trainer must make decisions that ultimately have a direct effect on the patient.

From the viewpoint of the athletic trainer, the team physician should assume a number of roles and responsibilities with regard to injury prevention and the health care of the athlete.[51] (See *Focus Box 1–5:* "Duties of the team physician.")

The physician should be an advisor to the athletic trainer.[35] However, the athletic trainer must be given the flexibility to function independently in the decision-making process and must often act without the advice or direction of the physician. Therefore, it is critical that the team physician and the athletic trainer share philosophical opinions regarding injury management and rehabilitation programs; this cohesion will help minimize any discrepancies or inconsistencies that may exist.[59] Most athletic trainers would prefer to work with, rather than for, a team physician.

**Compiling Medical Histories** The team physician should be responsible for compiling medical histories and conducting physical examinations for each athlete, both of which can provide critical information that may reduce the possibility of injury. Preparticipation screening done by both the athletic trainer and the physician are important in establishing baseline information to be used for comparison, should injury occur during the season.

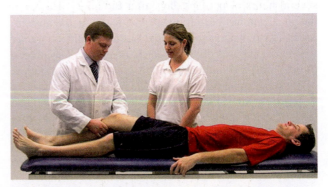

FIGURE 1–7　The athletic trainer carries out the directions of the physician.
© William E. Prentice

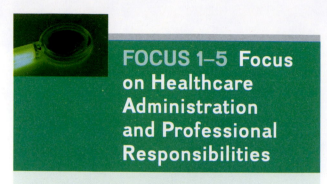

## FOCUS 1–5 Focus on Healthcare Administration and Professional Responsibilities

### Duties of the team physician

- Seeing that a complete medical history of each athlete is compiled and is readily available and determining the athlete's health status through a physical examination
- Diagnosing and treating injuries and illnesses
- Directing and advising the athletic trainer about health matters
- If possible, attending all games, athletic contests, scrimmages, and practices
- Deciding when, on medical grounds, athletes should be disqualified from participation and when they may be permitted to reenter competition
- Serving as an advisor to the athletic trainer and the coach and, when necessary, as a counselor to the athlete
- Working closely with the school administrator, school dentist, athletic trainer, coach, and health services personnel to promote and maintain consistently high standards of care for the athlete
- Acting, when necessary, as an instructor to the athletic trainer, assistant athletic trainer, and student athletic trainers about special therapeutic methods, therapeutic problems, and related procedures

**Diagnosing Injury** The team physician should assume responsibility for making a medical diagnosis of an injury and should be keenly aware of the program of rehabilitation as designed by the athletic trainer after the diagnosis. Athletic trainers should be capable of doing an accurate initial evaluation after acute injury and determining a clinical diagnosis. Input from that evaluation may be essential to the physician, who may not see the patient for several hours or perhaps days after the injury. However, the physician has been trained specifically to diagnose injuries and to make recommendations to the athletic trainer for treatment based on that medical diagnosis. The athletic trainer, with a sound background in injury rehabilitation, designs and supervises an effective rehabilitation scheme. The closely related yet distinct roles of the physician and the athletic trainer require both cooperation and close communication if they are to be optimized.

**Recommendations for Disqualification and Return to Play** The physician determines when a recommendation should be made that an athlete be disqualified from competition on medical grounds and must have the final say as to when an injured athlete may return to activity.[34]

Any decision to allow an athlete to resume activity should be based on recommendations from the athletic trainer.[52] An athletic trainer often has an advantage in that he or she knows the injured athlete well, including how the athlete responds to injury, how the athlete moves, and how hard to push to return the athlete safely to activity. The physician's judgment must be based not only on medical knowledge but also on knowledge of the psychophysiological demands of a particular sport.[93]

> Team physicians must have absolute authority in determining the health status of an athlete who wishes to participate in the sports program.

**Attending Practices and Games** A team physician should make an effort to attend as many practices, scrimmages, and competitions as possible. This attendance obviously is difficult at an institution that has twenty or more athletic teams. Thus, the physician must be readily available, should the athletic trainer (who generally is at most practices and games) require consultation or advice.

If the team physician cannot attend all practice sessions and competitive events or games, it is sometimes possible to establish a plan of rotation involving a number of physicians. In this plan, any one physician needs to be present at only one or two activities a year. The rotation plan has proved practical in situations in which the school district is unable to afford a full-time physician or has so limited a budget that it must ask for volunteer medical coverage. In some instances, the attending physician is paid a per-game stipend.

**Commitment to Sports and the Athlete** Most important, the team physician must have a strong love of sports and must be generally interested in and concerned about the young people who compete. Colleges and universities typically employ someone to act as a full-time team physician. Secondary schools most often rely on a local physician who volunteers his or her time. To serve as a team physician for the purpose of enhancing social standing in the community can be a frustrating and potentially dangerous situation for everyone involved in the athletic program.

When a physician is asked to serve as a team physician, arrangements must be made with the employing educational institution about specific required responsibilities. Policies must be established regarding emergency care, legal liability, facilities, personnel relationships, and duties.[21] It is essential that the team physician at all times promotes and maintains consistently high-quality care for the athlete in all phases of the sports medicine program.

**Academic Program Medical Director** Accredited athletic training education programs must have a physician medical director who is responsible for the coordination and guidance of the medical aspects of the program. The medical director—who may or may not be the team physician—should provide input to the program's educational content and provide classroom, laboratory, and/or clinical instruction.

## The Athletic Trainer and the Coach

It is critical for the coach to understand the specific roles and responsibilities of each individual who could be involved in treating an injured patient. This is even more critical if there is no athletic trainer to oversee the health care and the coach is forced to assume this responsibility. Individual states differ significantly in the laws that govern what nonmedical personnel can and cannot do when providing health care. **It is the responsibility of coaches to clearly understand the limits of their ability to function as a health care provider in the state where they are employed.**

The coach is directly responsible for preventing injuries by seeing that athletes have undergone a preventive injury conditioning program. The coach must ensure that sports equipment, especially protective equipment, is of the highest quality and is properly fitted. The coach must also make sure that protective equipment is properly maintained. A coach must be keenly aware of what produces injuries in his or her sport and what measures must be taken to avoid them (Figure 1–8). When necessary, a coach should be able to apply proper first aid. This knowledge is especially important in serious head and spinal injuries. **All coaches (both head and assistant) should be certified in cardiopulmonary resuscitation (CPR) and AED** by the American Red Cross, the American Heart Association, or the National Safety Council. **Coaches should also be certified in first aid** by the American Red Cross or the National Safety Council.[78] For the coach, obtaining these certifications is important so that he or she is able to provide correct and appropriate health care for the injured athlete. But it is also true that not having these certifications can have some negative legal implications for the coach and his or her employer.

> All head and assistant coaches should be certified in CPR, AED, and first aid.

It is essential that a coach have a thorough understanding of the skill techniques and environmental factors that may adversely affect the athlete. Poor biomechanics in skill areas such as throwing and running can lead to overuse injuries of the arms and legs, whereas overexposure to heat and humidity may cause death. Just because a coach is experienced in coaching does not mean that he or she knows proper skill techniques. Coaches must engage in a continual process of education to further their knowledge in their sport. When a sports program or specific sport is without an athletic trainer, the coach very often takes over this role.

Coaches work closely with athletic trainers; therefore, both must develop an insight into each other's problems, so that they can function effectively. The athletic trainer must develop patience and must earn the respect of the coaches, so that his or her judgment in all medical matters is fully accepted. In turn, the athletic trainer must avoid questioning the abilities of the coaches in their fields and must restrict opinions to athletic training matters. To avoid frustration and hard feelings, the coach must coach, and the athletic trainer must conduct athletic training matters. In terms of the health and well-being of the athlete, the physician and the athletic trainer must have the last word. This position must be backed at all times by the athletic administrator.

This is not to say, however, that the coach should not be involved with the decision-making process. For example, during the time the athlete is rehabilitating an injury, there may be drills or technical instruction sessions that the athlete can participate in that will not exacerbate the existing problem. Thus, the coach, the athletic trainer, and the team physician should be able to negotiate what the athlete can and cannot do safely in the course of a practice.

Any personal relationship takes some time to grow and develop. The relationship between the coach and the athletic trainer is no different. The athletic trainer must demonstrate to the coach his or her capability to correctly manage an injury and guide the course of a rehabilitation program. It will take some time for the coach to develop trust and confidence in the athletic trainer. The coach must understand that what the athletic trainer wants for the athlete is exactly the same as what the coach wants— to get an athlete healthy and back to practice as quickly and safely as possible.

## REFERRING THE PATIENT TO OTHER MEDICAL AND NONMEDICAL SUPPORT SERVICES AND PERSONNEL

In certain situations, an individual may require treatment from or consultation with a variety of both medical and nonmedical services or personnel other than the athletic trainer or team physician. After the athletic trainer consults with the team physician about a particular matter,

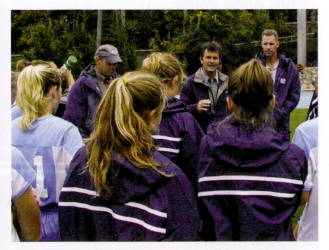

FIGURE 1–8  The coach, in conjunction with other members of the sports medicine team, is responsible for preventing injuries in his or her sport.
© William E. Prentice

either the athletic trainer or the team physician can arrange for appointments as necessary. When referring an athlete for evaluation or consultation, the athletic trainer must be aware of the community-based services available and the insurance or managed care plan coverage available for that athlete.

A number of support health services and personnel may be used. These services and personnel include school health services; nurses; physicians, including orthopedists, neurologists, internists, family medicine specialists, ophthalmologists, pediatricians, psychiatrists, dermatologists, gynecologists, and osteopaths; dentists; podiatrists; physician's assistants; physical therapists; strength and conditioning specialists; biomechanists; exercise physiologists; nutritionists; sport psychologists; massage therapists; occupational therapists; social workers; emergency medical technicians; sports chiropractors; orthotists/prosthetists; equipment personnel; and referees.

## School Health Services

Colleges and universities maintain school health services that range from a department operating with one or two nurses and a physician available on a part-time basis to an elaborate setup comprised of a full complement of nursing services with a staff of full-time medical specialists and complete laboratory and hospital facilities. At the secondary-school level, health services are usually organized so that one or two nurses conduct the program under the direction of the school physician, who may serve a number of schools in a given area or district. This organization poses a problem, because it is often difficult to have qualified medical help at hand when it is needed. Local policy determines the procedure for referral for medical care. If such policies are lacking, the athletic trainer should see to it that an effective method is established for handling all athletes requiring medical care or opinion. The ultimate source of health care is the physician. The effectiveness of athletic health care service can

> **Support personnel concerned with the athlete's health and safety:**
>
> - School health services
> - Nurse
> - Physician
> - Dentist
> - Podiatrist
> - Physician's assistant
> - Physical therapist
> - Strength and conditioning specialist
> - Biomechanist
> - Exercise physiologist
> - Nutritionist
> - Sport psychologist
> - Massage therapist
> - Occupational therapist
> - Emergency medical technician and paramedic
> - Sports chiropractors
> - Orthotist/prosthetist
> - Equipment personnel
> - Referee
> - Social worker

be evaluated only to the extent to which it meets the following criteria:

1. Availability at every scheduled practice or contest of a person qualified and delegated to render emergency care to an injured or ill participant
2. Planned access to a physician by phone or nearby presence for prompt medical evaluation of the health care problems that warrant this attention
3. Planned access to a medical facility, including plans for communication and transportation

## Nurse (RN, LPN, NP)

As a rule, the nurse is not usually responsible for the recognition and management of sports injuries. However, in certain institutions that lack an athletic trainer, the nurse may assume the majority of the responsibility in providing health care for the athlete. The nurse works under the direction of the physician. It is essential that the nurse works in liaison with the athletic trainer and the school health services. A nurse practitioner (NP) is a registered nurse with advanced education and clinical training. NPs diagnose and treat common acute and chronic problems, and prescribe and manage medications.

## Physician (MD)

A number of physicians with a variety of specializations can aid in treating the patient (see *Focus Box 1–6:* "Specializations for physicians").

## Osteopath (DO)

An osteopath is a trained physician who emphasizes the role of the musculoskeletal system in health and disease using a holistic approach to the patient. An osteopath incorporates a variety of manual and physical treatment interventions in the prevention and treatment of disease.

## Dentist (DDS, DMD)

The role of team dentist is somewhat analogous to that of team physician. He or she serves as a dental consultant for the team and should be available for first aid and emergency care. Good communication between the dentist and the athletic trainer should ensure a good dental program. There are three areas of responsibility for the team dentist:

1. Organizing and performing the preseason dental examination
2. Being available to provide emergency care when needed
3. Conducting the fitting of mouth protectors

## Podiatrist (DPM)

Podiatry, the specialized field dealing with the study and care of the foot, has become an integral part of sports health care. Many podiatrists are trained in surgical

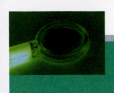

## Specializations for physicians

**Dermatologist** A dermatologist should be consulted for problems and lesions occurring on the skin.

**Family medicine physician** A physician who specializes in family medicine supervises or provides medical care to all members of a family. Many team physicians in colleges and universities, and particularly at the secondary-school level, are engaged in family practice.

**Gynecologist** A gynecologist is consulted when health issues in the female reproductive system are of primary concern.

**Internist** An internist is a physician who specializes in the practice of internal medicine. An internist treats diseases of the internal organs by using methods other than surgery.

**Neurologist** A neurologist specializes in treating disorders of and injuries to the nervous system. There are common situations in athletics in which consultation with a neurologist is warranted, such as for head injury or peripheral nerve injury.

**Ophthalmologist** Physicians who manage and treat injuries to the eye are ophthalmologists. An optometrist evaluates and fits patients with glasses or contact lenses.

**Orthopedist** The orthopedist is responsible for treating injuries and disorders of the musculoskeletal system. Many colleges and universities have a team orthopedist on their staff.

**Osteopath (DO)** An osteopath emphasizes the role of the musculoskeletal system in health and disease, using a holistic approach to the patient. An osteopath incorporates a variety of manual and physical treatment interventions in the prevention and treatment of disease.

**Pediatrician** A pediatrician cares for and treats injuries and illnesses that occur in young children and adolescents.

**Physiatrist** Physical Medicine and Rehabilitation (PM&R) is a branch of medicine that provides integrated care in the prevention, diagnosis, and treatment of disorders related to the brain, muscles, and bones, spanning from traumatic brain injury to lower back pain.

**Psychiatrist** Psychiatry is a medical practice that deals with the diagnosis, treatment, and prevention of mental illness.

---

procedures, foot biomechanics, and the fitting and construction of orthotic devices for the shoe. Like the team dentist, a podiatrist should be available on a consulting basis.

## Physician Assistant (PA)

Physician assistants (PAs) are trained to assume many of the responsibilities for patient care traditionally done by a physician. A physician assistant is licensed to triage, conduct patient evaluations, diagnose and treat patients, arrange for various hospital-based diagnostic tests, and prescibe appropriate medications without conferring with or being seen by a physician. PAs have a physician supervisor but there are several levels of supervision to include the physician being available by phone. A number of athletic trainers have also become PAs in recent years.

## Physical Therapist (PT)

Some athletic trainers use physical therapists to supervise the rehabilitation programs for injured athletes, whereas the athletic trainer concentrates primarily on getting a player ready to practice or compete. In many sports medicine clinics, athletic trainers and physical therapists work in teams, jointly contributing to the supervision of a rehabilitation program. A number of athletic trainers are also physical therapists. A physical therapist can be certified as a sports certified specialist (SCS). The physical therapist is prepared to treat a variety of patient populations with different types of injuries, whereas the athletic trainer is focused primarily on treating and working with the physically active population.

## Strength and Conditioning Specialist (CSCS)

Many colleges and universities and some secondary schools employ full-time strength coaches to advise athletes on training and conditioning programs. Athletic trainers should routinely consult with these individuals and advise them about injuries to a particular athlete and exercises that should be avoided or modified relative to a specific injury. A strength coach can be certified by the National Strength and Conditioning Association as a CSCS.

## Biomechanist

An individual who possesses some expertise in the analysis of human motion can also be a great aid to the athletic trainer. The biomechanist uses sophisticated video and computer-enhanced digital analysis equipment to study movement. By advising the athlete, coach, and athletic trainer on matters such as faulty gait patterns or improper throwing mechanics, the biomechanist can reduce the likelihood of injury to the athlete.

## Exercise Physiologist

The exercise physiologist can significantly influence the athletic training program by giving input to the athletic trainer regarding training and conditioning techniques, body composition analysis, and nutritional considerations. Exercise physiologists monitor and assess cardiovascular and metabolic effects and mechanisms of exercise, replenishment of fluids during exercise, and exercise for cardiac and musculoskeletal rehabilitation.

## Nutritionist (RD)

Increasingly, individuals in the field of nutrition are becoming interested in athletics. Many college athletic training programs have sports dietitians who are engaged as consultants, either part-time or full-time. These dietitians are registered dietitians (RDs) that are also certified as specialists in sports dietetics (CSSD) programs that are geared to the needs of a particular sport. He or she also assists individual athletes who need special nutritional counseling.

## Sport Psychologist

The sport psychologist can advise the athletic trainer on matters related to the psychological aspects of the rehabilitation process. The way the athlete feels about the injury and how it affects his or her social, emotional, intellectual, and physical dimensions can have a substantial effect on the course of a treatment program and how quickly the athlete may return to competition. The sport psychologist uses different intervention strategies to help the athlete cope with injury. Sport psychologists can seek certification through the Association for the Advancement of Sport Psychology.

## Massage Therapist (NCBTMB)

The mission of the American Massage Therapy Association (AMTA) is "to serve its members while advancing the art, science, and practice of massage therapy." Many massage therapists choose to become nationally certified in massage therapy, whereas others are required by their states to pass a national certification exam administered by the National Certification Board for Therapeutic Massage and Bodywork (NCBTMB). National certification indicates that these massage therapists possess core skills, abilities, knowledge, and attributes to practice safely and competently, as determined by the NCBTMB. The massage therapy profession is regulated in most states in the form of either a license, registration, or certification making it illegal for anyone to work as a massage therapist unless he or she has a license.

## Occupational Therapist (OT)

Occupational therapists work with patients who have conditions that are mentally, physically, developmentally, or emotionally disabling to improve their ability to perform tasks in their daily living and working environments. Some occupational therapists treat individuals whose ability to function in a work environment has been impaired. These practitioners arrange employment, evaluate the work environment, plan work activities, and assess the client's progress.

## Emergency Medical Technician (EMT) and Paramedic

There are four levels of emergency medical service (EMS) providers: Emergency Medical Responder (EMR), Emergency Medical Technician (EMT), Advanced EMT (AEMT), and Paramedic. Emergency Medical Responders are the first to arrive at the scene of an incident and are trained to provide basic emergency medical care. The EMT is trained to care for patients at the scene of an accident and while transporting patients by ambulance to the hospital under medical direction. An Advanced EMT (AEMT) has more advanced training that allows the administration of intravenous fluids, the use of manual defibrillators, and the application of advanced airway techniques. Paramedics provide the most extensive prehospital care by administering drugs orally and intravenously, interpreting electrocardiograms (ECGs), performing endotracheal intubations, and using monitors and other complex equipment.

## Sports Chiropractor (DC)

Chiropractors emphasize diagnosis and treatment of mechanical disorders of the musculoskeletal system, believing that these disorders affect general health by way of the nervous system. Chiropractors make use of spinal and extremity manipulations in their treatments.

## Orthotist/Prosthetist (ROT)

These individuals custom fit, design, and construct braces, orthotics, and support devices based on physician prescriptions.

## Equipment Personnel

Sports equipment personnel are becoming specialists in the purchase and proper fitting of protective equipment. They work closely with the coach and the athletic trainer.

## Referee

Referees must be highly knowledgeable regarding rules and regulations, especially those that relate to the health and welfare of the athlete. They work cooperatively with the coach and the athletic trainer. They must be capable of checking the playing facility for dangerous situations and equipment that may predispose the athlete to injury. They must routinely check athletes to ensure that they are wearing adequate protective pads.

## Social Worker

Occasionally, athletes or their families need a referral for social support services within the community. Social workers can offer counseling and support for a variety of personal or family difficulties, such as substance abuse or family planning.

# RECOGNITION AND ACCREDITATION OF THE ATHLETIC TRAINER AS AN ALLIED HEALTH CARE PROFESSIONAL

In June 1990, the American Medical Association (AMA) officially recognized athletic training as an allied health care profession. The primary purpose of this recognition was to have the profession of athletic training recognized in the same context as other allied health care professions and to be held to similar professional and educational expectations, as well as to allow for the accreditation of educational programs.[29] Overseen by NATA's Professional Education Committee (PEC), since 1969 athletic training education programs became the responsibility of the AMA. The AMA's Committee on Allied Health Education and Accreditation (CAHEA) was charged with developing the requirements (*Essentials and Guidelines*) for the structure and function of academic programs to prepare entry-level athletic trainers. The Joint Review Committee on Athletic Training (JRC-AT) was originally charged with evaluating athletic training education programs seeking accreditation and making recommendations to CAHEA as to whether those educational programs met the necessary criteria to become an accredited program in athletic training education. The JRC-AT was made up of representatives from the NATA, the American Academy of Pediatrics, the American Orthopedic Society for Sports Medicine, and the American Academy of Family Physicians. As of 1993, all entry-level athletic training education programs became subject to the CAHEA accreditation process.

In June 1994, CAHEA was dissolved and was replaced immediately by the Commission on Accreditation of Allied Health Education Programs (CAAHEP). The CAAHEP is recognized as an accreditation agency for allied health education programs by the Council for Higher Education Accreditation (CHEA). CHEA is a private, nonprofit national organization that coordinates accreditation activity in the United States. Formed in 1996, its mission is to promote academic quality through formal recognition of higher education accreditation bodies and to work to advance self-regulation through accreditation. Recognition by CHEA affirms that standards and processes of accrediting organizations are consistent with the quality, improvement, and accountability expectations that CHEA has established. Entry-level bachelors and masters

> **Evolution of athletic training education accreditation bodies:**
> - PEC, 1969
> - Recognition of ATC as an allied health professional, 1990
> - CAHEA, 1993
> - CAAHEP, 1994
> - JRC-AT, 2003
> - CAATE, 2006

athletic training education programs that were at one time approved by NATA, and subsequently accredited by CAHEA, were accredited by CAAHEP through 2005.

In 2003, the JRC-AT leadership decided that the profession of athletic training had matured and outgrown the structure and constraints of CAAHEP and that the profession would be better served if the JRC-AT became an independent accrediting agency like those in the other allied health professions. This change meant that, instead of the JRC-AT making accreditation recommendations to CAAHEP, the JRC-AT would accredit athletic training education programs. In 2006, the JRC-AT had officially become the Committee for Accreditation of Athletic Training Education (CAATE). As of 2014, CAATE was officially recognized by the Council for Higher Education Accreditation (CHEA). Through recognition by CHEA, CAATE is in the same context/level as CAAHEP and other national accreditors.

The effects of CAATE accreditation are not limited to just educational aspects. In the future, this recognition may affect regulatory legislation, the practice of athletic training in nontraditional settings, and insurance considerations. This recognition will continue to be a positive step in the development of the athletic training profession.

## Other Health Care Organization Accrediting Agencies

Although CAATE is the accrediting organization for athletic training, other organizations accredit various health care agencies and organizations.

**Joint Commission on Accreditation of Healthcare Organizations** The Joint Commission on Accreditation of Healthcare Organizations (JCAHO) is the nation's largest standards-setting and accrediting body in health care. JCAHO accredits more than 18,000 health care organizations and programs in the United States. Its mission is to improve the quality of care provided to the public through the provision of health care accreditation and related services that support performance improvement in health care organizations.

**Commission on Accreditation of Rehabilitation Facilities** The Commission on Accreditation of Rehabilitation Facilities (CARF) is an accrediting organization that promotes quality rehabilitation services by establishing standards of quality for organizations to use as guidelines in developing and offering their programs or services to consumers. CARF uses the standards to determine how well an organization is serving its consumers and how it can improve. CARF standards are developed with input from consumers, rehabilitation professionals, state and national organizations, and funders. Every year the standards are reviewed and new ones are developed to keep pace with changing conditions and current consumer needs.

## CAATE Accredited Entry-Level Athletic Training Education Programs

Since 2006, the CAATE has been responsible for accrediting entry-level athletic training education programs at both the graduate and undergraduate levels. Subsequently, the CAATE assumed responsibility for accrediting post-professional masters degree and residency programs as well, both of which are designed to provide certified athletic trainers an advanced clinical, research, and scholarly experience beyond the entry-level professional degree. In 2015, the CAATE with the support of the NATA Board of Directors, the Board of Certification, and the NATA Research and Education Foundation made the decision to establish the entry-level degree for professional practice at the masters level. Using a medical-based model, athletic training students are educated to serve in the role of allied health care professionals, with an emphasis on clinical reasoning skills.

**Professional Education Committee (PEC) Competencies and Clinical Proficiencies** In 1996, the leadership of the NATA established the Executive Committee for Education to dictate the course of educational preparation for the athletic training student.

In the *Role Delineation Study,* the Board of Certification (BOC) defined the minimum competencies required to practice as an athletic trainer and thus reflects the contemporary standards of practice. The Professional Education Committee (a subcommittee of the Executive Committee for Education) determines the competencies that should be taught in CAATE-accredited education programs. Entry-level athletic training education programs use a evidence-based approach both in the classroom and in clinical settings.

Educational content is based on knowledge and skills and clinical integrated proficiencies. In the document "Athletic Training Education Competencies" (5th edition), the Professional Education Council has assigned the competencies to eight areas.[63] These competencies are required for both curriculum development and the education of students enrolled in entry-level athletic training education programs. They define the educational content that students enrolled in these programs must master. The eight areas currently established by the Professional Education Committee are (1) evidence-based practice, (2) prevention and health promotion, (3) clinical examination and diagnosis, (4) acute care of injury and illness, (5) therapeutic interventions, (6) psychosocial strategies and referral, (7) health care administration, and (8) professional development and responsibility.

***Foundational Behaviors of Professional Practice***
These affective competencies can be found in every aspect of the educational program, including lecture, laboratory, and clinical instruction. They represent the "people" components of professional practice.[63] Some are easily defined; others must be modeled by instructors. Foundational behaviors include the following:

1. Recognizing that the primary focus of practice should be the patient
2. Understanding that competent health care requires a team approach
3. Being aware of the legal components of patient care
4. Practicing in an ethical manner[71]
5. Advancing the knowledge base in athletic training
6. Appreciating the cultural diversity of individual patients
7. Being an advocate and model for the athletic training profession

## Post-Professional Athletic Training Education Programs

Post-Professional Athletic Training Education Programs are currently accredited by CAATE. The CAATE-accredited Post-Professional Athletic Training Education Programs are designed to enhance the academic and clinical preparation of individuals who are already certified athletic trainers and those who have completed the requirements for certification.

## Specialty Certifications

The NATA is in the process of developing specialty certifications to further enhance the professional development of certified athletic trainers by expanding their scope of practice. Entry-level athletic training education programs provide a general educational foundation, whereas specialty certifications build on this foundation. Specialty certifications in athletic training will be voluntary areas of postgraduate study, and certification in areas more advanced than entry level. According to the NATA Postprofessional Athletic Training Education Committee, the purpose is to "provide the athletic trainer with an advanced clinical practice credential that demonstrates the attainment of knowledge and skills that will enhance the quality of patient care, optimize clinical outcomes, and improve patients' health-related quality of life, in specialized areas of athletic training practice." Specialization in any field of health care requires significant clinical experience in a specific content area and a continuous training effort, which ultimately results in a credential that signifies clinical expertise.

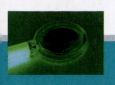

## FOCUS 1–7  Focus on Healthcare Administration and Professional Responsibilities

### Board of Certification requirements for certification as an athletic trainer

*Purpose of certification*

The Board of Certification (BOC) was incorporated in 1989 to provide a certification program for entry-level athletic trainers and recertification standards for certified athletic trainers. The purpose of this entry-level certification program is to establish standards for entry into the profession of athletic training. Additionally, the BOC has established the continuing education requirements that a certified athletic trainer must satisfy to maintain current status as a BOC-certified athletic trainer.

*The process*

Annually, the Board of Certification reviews the requirements for certification eligibility and standards for continuing education. Additionally, the board reviews and revises the certification examination in accordance with the test specifications of the BOC role delineation study, which is reviewed and revised every 5 years.

*Requirements for candidacy for the BOC certification examination*

Candidates who are enrolled and/or registered in their final semester/

quarter prior to graduation are eligible to sit for the BOC exam. Qualified candidates for the BOC exam must have received confirmation on their exam application by the Program Director recognized by the CAATE that they have earned or will earn their Bachelor's or Master's degree. Candidates who graduated with a Bachelor's or Master's degree from a CAATE (previously JRC-AT) accredited program in 2003 or later meet the education requirements for the BOC exam.

## REQUIREMENTS FOR CERTIFICATION AS AN ATHLETIC TRAINER

An athletic trainer who is certified by the BOC is a highly qualified health care professional educated and experienced in dealing with the injuries that occur with physical activity. Candidates for certification are required to have an extensive background of both formal academic preparation and supervised practical experience in a clinical setting, according to CAATE guidelines.[29] The guidelines listed in *Focus Box 1–7:* "Board of Certification requirements for certification as an athletic trainer" have been established by the BOC.[10] Since 2004, the only way that a candidate can become certified is by completing an entry-level athletic training education program that has been accredited by CAATE.

### The Certification Examination

Once the requirements have been fulfilled, applicants are eligible to sit for the certification examination. The certification examination was developed by the BOC in conjunction with an independent examination development and administration company and is currently administered at various locations throughout the United States.[67] In 2007, the certification examination became a computer-based exam (CBE). The CBE tests for knowledge and skill in five major domains: (1) injury/illness prevention and wellness protection; (2) clinical evaluation and diagnosis; (3) immediate and emergency care; (4) treatment and rehabilitation; and (5) organizational and professional health and well-being. Successful

performance on the certification examination leads to BOC certification as an athletic trainer with the credential of **ATC**. (For the latest information on certification requirements, visit the BOC Web site at www.bocatc.org) BOC certification is a prerequisite for licensure in most states.

### Continuing Education Requirements

To ensure the ongoing professional growth and involvement by the certified athletic trainer, BOC has established requirements for continuing education.[9,72] The purposes of the requirements are to encourage certified athletic trainers to continue to obtain current professional development information, to explore new knowledge in specific content areas, to master new athletic training–related skills and techniques, to expand approaches to effective athletic training, to further develop professional judgment, and to conduct professional practice in an ethical and appropriate manner.

To maintain certification, all certified athletic trainers must document a minimum of 50 continuing education units (CEUs), 10 of which must be approved evidence-based practice programs or courses, attained during each 2-year recertification term. CEUs may be awarded for attending symposiums, seminars, workshops, or conferences; completing webinars or home study courses; serving as a speaker, panelist, or certification exam writer; authoring a research article in a professional journal; authoring or editing a textbook; and completing postgraduate course work. All certified athletic trainers must also demonstrate proof of current CPR/AED certification.

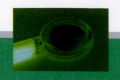

## FOCUS 1–8 Focus on Healthcare Administration and Professional Responsibilities

### State regulation of the athletic trainer*

| | | |
|---|---|---|
| Alabama (L) | Massachusetts (L) | South Carolina (C) |
| Alaska (L) | Michigan (L) | South Dakota (L) |
| Arizona (L) | Minnesota (R) | Tennessee (L) |
| Arkansas (L) | Mississippi (L) | Texas (L) |
| Colorado (E) | Missouri (L) | Utah (L) |
| Connecticut (L) | Montana (L) | Vermont (L) |
| Delaware (L) | Nebraska (L) | Virginia (L) |
| Florida (L) | Nevada (L) | Washington (L) |
| Georgia (L) | New Hampshire (L) | West Virginia (R) |
| Hawaii (E) | New Jersey (L) | Wisconsin (L) |
| Idaho (L) | New Mexico (L) | Wyoming (E) |
| Illinois (L) | New York (C) | |
| Indiana (L) | North Carolina (L) | States with no regulation: California |
| Iowa (L) | North Dakota (L) | |
| Kansas (L) | Ohio (L) | *As of 2016. |
| Kentucky (C) | Oklahoma (L) | E = exempt from existing licensure standards; C = certification; R = registration; L = licensure. For additional information about individual state regulating boards, visit www.nata.org. |
| Louisiana (C) | Oregon (R) | |
| Maine (L) | Pennsylvania (C) | |
| Maryland (L) | Rhode Island (L) | |

## STATE REGULATION OF THE ATHLETIC TRAINER

During the early 1970s, the leadership of the NATA realized the necessity of obtaining some type of official recognition by other medical allied health organizations of the athletic trainer as a health care professional. Laws and statutes specifically governing the practice of athletic training were nonexistent in most states.

> **Forms of state regulation:**
> - Licensure
> - Certification
> - Registration
> - Exemption

Based on this perceived need, the athletic trainers in many states organized their efforts to secure recognition by seeking some type of regulation by state licensing agencies. To date, this ongoing effort has resulted in 49 of the 50 states enacting some type of regulatory statutes governing the practice of athletic training.[69]

Rules and regulations governing the practice of athletic training vary tremendously from state to state. Regulation may be in the form of licensure, certification, registration, or exemption (see *Focus Box 1–8:* "State regulation of the athletic trainer").

For the most part, legislation regulating the practice of athletic training has been positive and to some extent protects the athletic trainer from litigation. In 2016 the U.S. House of Representatives passed H.R. Bill 921 which clarifies medical liability rules for licensed athletic trainers and other medical professionals allowing them to legally treat their athletes while traveling in other states. This bill ensures that they will be deemed to have satisfied any licensure requirements of the secondary state thus protecting them from litigation.

### Licensure

Licensure limits the practice of athletic training to those who have met minimal requirements established by a state licensing board. Through this licensing board, the state limits the number of individuals who can perform functions related to athletic training as dictated by the practice act. Requirements for licensure vary from state to state, but most require a specific educational and training background, evidence of good moral character, letters of recommendation from current practitioners, and minimal acceptable performance on a licensing examination. Licensure is the most restrictive of all the forms of regulation. Individuals who are providing health care services to an athlete cannot call themselves athletic trainers in a particular state unless they have met its requirements for licensure.[12]

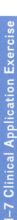

**1–7 Clinical Application Exercise**

A certified athletic trainer moves to a different state to take a new job. She discovers that in that state the ATC must be licensed to practice athletic training.

**?** Because she was registered as an athletic trainer in the other state, must she go through the process of licensure in her new state?

## Certification

State certification as an athletic trainer differs from certification as an athletic trainer by the BOC. An individual who has passed the BOC exam does not automatically obtain a state certification. Although certification does not restrict the use of the title of athletic trainer to those certified by the state, it can restrict the performance of athletic training functions to only those individuals who are state certified. State certification indicates that a person possesses the basic knowledge and skills required in the profession and has passed a certification examination. Many states that offer certification use the BOC exam as a criterion for granting state certifi.[12]

## Registration

Registration means that, before an individual can practice athletic training, he or she must register in that state. The individual has paid a fee for being placed on an existing list of practitioners. The state may or may not have a mechanism for assessing competency. However, registration does prevent individuals who are not registered with the state from calling themselves athletic trainers.[12]

## Exemption

Exemption means that a state recognizes that athletic trainers perform functions similar to those of other licensed professions (e.g., physical therapy) yet allows them to practice athletic training despite the fact that they do not comply with the practice acts of other regulated professions. Exemption is most often used in those states in which there are not enough practitioners to warrant the formation of a state regulatory board.[12]

# FUTURE DIRECTIONS FOR THE ATHLETIC TRAINER

Certified athletic trainers possess a strong, highly structured academic background in addition to a substantial amount of closely supervised clinical experience in their chosen area of expertise. The athletic trainer continues to gain credibility and recognition as a health care professional. Certainly, recognition as an allied health profession by the American Medical Association in 1990 was a major milestone for the profession. In the future, this recognition may affect regulatory legislation, the practice of athletic training in nontraditional settings, and third-party reimbursement. Without question, this recognition will continue to be a positive factor in the development of the athletic training profession.

Future directions for athletic training will be determined by the efforts of the NATA and its membership and will likely include the following:

- Athletic trainers, like other health care professionals, routinely integrate evidence-based practice into patient care.
- Ongoing reevaluation, revision, and reform of athletic training education programs will continue to be a priority.
- Recognition of CAATE by the Council for Higher Education Accreditation will further enhance the credibility of athletic training as an allied health profession.
- Athletic trainers must continue to actively seek third-party reimbursement for athletic training services provided.
- Eventually, every state will regulate the practice of athletic training, and there will be a move to standardize the state practice acts to make them more consistent from state to state.
- Athletic trainers will seek and achieve specialty certifications to better assist in expanding their scope of practice.
- It is very likely that the greatest number of job opportunities during the next decade will be in public and private secondary and middle schools.
- Although the largest percentage of athletic trainers currently work in clinical settings, the number of clinics owned and staffed by athletic trainers will increase.
- Recognition of the athletic trainer in physician practice, who can be incorporated into the daily operations of a physician's office will increase.
- The potential for expansion of athletic trainers in the military is great.
- The potential exists for increasing job opportunities for certified athletic trainers in industrial and corporate settings.
- There will be opportunities for athletic trainers to work with children and teenagers as sport performance specialists.
- Opportunities for athletic trainers working in fitness and wellness settings will increase.
- As the general population continues to age, opportunities for athletic trainers to work with the elderly physically active population will increase.
- Athletic trainers must continue to enhance their visibility through research efforts and scholarly publication. Certified athletic trainers must strive to develop some comprehension of basic research design and statistical analysis to be able to interpret new research.
- Athletic trainers should continue to make themselves available for local and community meetings to discuss the health care of the athlete.
- The certified athletic trainer will become recognized internationally as a health care provider and will be found in Canada, South America, Europe, Asia, and Australia.
- Most important, athletic trainers must continue to focus on injury prevention and to provide appropriate, high-quality health care to physically active individuals regardless of the setting in which injury occurs.

## SUMMARY

- Athletic trainers are health care professionals who specialize in preventing, recognizing, managing, and rehabilitating injuries.
- A number of organizations dedicated to athletic training and sports medicine have developed over the years. They devise and maintain professional standards of practice, exchange ideas, stimulate research, and collectively work toward a common goal. Among these organizations are the National Athletic Trainers' Association and the American College of Sports Medicine.
- Athletic trainers are employed in a variety of settings, including clinics, hospitals, industries, corporations, colleges and universities, secondary schools, professional sports, amateur and youth sports, the performing arts, the military, law enforcement, the government, and health or fitness clubs.
- The primary roles of an athletic trainer include injury/illness prevention and wellness promotion, examination, assessment, and diagnosis, immediate and emergency care, therapeutic intervention, and health-care administration and professional responsibilities.
- Practicing evidence-based health care means integrating external clinical evidence from systematic research with clinical expertise while focusing on patient values and preferences.
- Athletic trainers should exhibit professional behavior characteristics that will allow them to communicate and work in cooperation with patients, clients, athletes, administrators, physicians, parents, and coaches.
- They may refer to or consult with variety of both medical and nonmedical services and/or personnel to obtain help and advice in overseeing the health care needs of the physically active population.
- Educational programs for athletic trainers are accredited by the Committee for Accreditation of Athletic Training Education (CAATE). Once an individual completes an accredited program, she or he is eligible to become certified as an athletic trainer (ATC). In most states, a state licensing board regulates certified athletic trainers' practices.

## WEB SITES

National Athletic Trainers' Association: www.nata.org
*This site describes the athletic training profession, how to become involved in athletic training, and the role of an athletic trainer.*

American Sports Medicine Institute: www.asmi.org
*The American Sports Medicine Institute's mission is to improve through research and education the understanding, prevention, and treatment of sports-related injuries. In addition to stating this mission, the site provides access to current research and journal articles.*

American Academy of Orthopaedic Surgeons: www.aaos.org
*This site provides some information for the general public as well as information to its members. The public information is in the form of patient education brochures; the site also includes a description of the organization and a definition of orthopedics.*

American Orthopaedic Society for Sports Medicine: www.sportsmed.org
*This site is dedicated to educating health care professionals and the general public about sports medicine. The site provides access to the American Journal of Sports Medicine and a wide variety of links to related sites.*

Athletic Trainer.com: www.athletictrainer.com
*This Web site is specifically designed to give information to athletic trainers, including students, and those interested in athletic training. It provides access to interesting journal articles and links to several informative Web sites.*

National Collegiate Athletic Association: www.ncaa.org
*This site gives general information about the NCAA and the publications that the NCAA circulates. This site may be useful for those working in the collegiate setting.*

Commission on Accreditation of Athletic Training Education: www.caate.net
*This site contains information on accreditation for athletic training education programs.*

Board of Certification: www.bocatc.org
*This site provides up-to-date information on requirements for certification as well as a listing of certification test dates and sites.*

## SOLUTIONS TO CLINICAL APPLICATION EXERCISES

1–1  To some extent, the role of the clinical athletic trainer is dictated by that state's regulation of the practice of athletic training. Certainly, the clinical and academic preparation of athletic trainers should enable them to effectively evaluate an injured patient and guide that patient through a rehabilitative program. The athletic trainer should treat only those individuals who have sustained injury related to physical activity and not patients with neurological or orthopedic conditions. The athletic trainer may work part-time in the clinic and then cover one or several secondary schools around the area. The athletic trainer and physical therapist should work as a team to maximize the effectiveness of patient care.

1–2  Although emergency medical technicians are qualified to handle emergency situations, an athletic trainer is able to provide comprehensive health care to the All-American High School athletes. An athletic trainer is responsible for the prevention of athletic injuries; the recognition, evaluation, and assessment of injuries; and the treatment and rehabilitation of athletic injuries.

1–3 Ultimately, the team physician is responsible for making that decision. However, that decision must be made based on collective input from the athletic trainer, the coach, and the athlete. Remember that everyone on the sports medicine team has the same ultimate goal—to return the athlete to full competitive levels as quickly and safely as possible.

1–4 To help prevent injury, the athletic trainer should (1) arrange for physical examinations and preparticipation screenings to identify conditions that predispose an athlete to injury; (2) ensure appropriate training and conditioning of the athletes; (3) monitor environmental conditions to ensure safe participation; (4) select and maintain properly fitting protective equipment; and (5) educate parents, coaches, and athletes about the risks inherent in sport participation.

1–5 The athletic trainer should make use of an evidence-based practice approach to find an answer to her clinical question "Can incorporating a jump-landing training program reduce the number of ACL injuries in female athletes?" The next step is to search the literature to find the best evidence and then evaluate the strength of that evidence. She needs to apply the evidence that she finds in the literature and use her clinical experience to address the specific goal of reducing the incidence of ACL tears. Finally she needs to assess the outcome or effectiveness of having integrated this jump-landing training program in reducing ACL injuries in her female athletes.

1–6 As of 2004, everyone must graduate from a CAATE-accredited program to take the BOC exam and become a certified athletic trainer. Therefore, she must transfer to an institution that offers an entry-level CAATE-approved program, in which she must complete course work and directly supervised clinical experience.

1–7 The laws regarding regulation of the certified athletic trainer vary from state to state. It is likely that she will have to apply for a license through the athletic training licensing board in her new state to get a license to practice in that state. It is not likely that there is reciprocity between the two states.

## REVIEW QUESTIONS AND CLASS ACTIVITIES

1. How do modern athletic training and sports medicine compare with early Greek and Roman approaches to the care of the athlete?

2. What professional organizations are important to the field of athletic training?

3. Why is athletic training considered a team endeavor? Contrast the coach's, athletic trainer's, and team physician's roles in athletic training.

4. Define evidence-based practice as it relates to athletic training clinical practice.

5. What qualifications should the athletic trainer have in terms of education, certification, and personality?

6. What are the various employment opportunities available to the athletic trainer?

7. Explain the criteria for becoming certified as an athletic trainer.

8. Discuss the methods by which different states regulate the practice of athletic training.

## REFERENCES

1. Albensi R: The impact of health problems affecting worker productivity in a manufacturing setting. *Athletic Therapy Today* 8(3):13, 2003.

2. Almquist J: Summary statement: Appropriate medical care for the secondary school–aged athlete, *J Athl Train* 43(4):417, 2008.

3. American College of Sports Medicine: ACSM's resource manual: For guidelines for exercise testing and prescription, Baltimore, 2009, Lippincott, Williams & Wilkins.

4. Arnold B: Importance of selected athletic trainer employment characteristics in collegiate, sports medicine clinic, and high school settings, *J Athl Train* 33(3):254, 1998.

5. Arnold B: 1994 athletic trainer employment and salary characteristics, *J Athl Train* 31(3): 215, 1996.

6. Barefield S: Social supports in the athletic training room: Athletes' expectations of staff and student athletic trainers, *J Athl Train* 32(4): 333, 1997.

7. Berry J: High school athletic therapy, Part 2, *Athletic Therapy Today* 3(1):47, 1998.

8. Bilik S: *The trainer's bible,* New York, 1956, Reed (originally published 1917).

9. Board of Certification (BOC), Continuing Education Office: *Continuing education file 2012–2015,* Dallas, 2007, BOC.

10. Board of Certification, Inc.: *Practice Analysis, 7th Edition,* Omaha, Nebraska, 2015, Board of Certification.

11. Brukner P: Sports medicine: The team approach. In Brukner P: *Clinical sports medicine,* ed 3, Sydney, 2010, McGraw-Hill.

12. Campbell D: Regulation of athletic training. In Konin J: *Clinical athletic training,* Thorofare, NJ, 1997, Slack.

13. Casa D: Question everything: The value of integrating research into an athletic training education (editorial), *J Athl Train* 40(3):138, 2005.

14. Coker C: Consistency of learning styles of undergraduate athletic training students in the traditional classroom versus the clinical setting, *J Athl Train* 35(4):441, 2000.

15. Courson R, et al.: Inter-association consensus statement on best practices for sports medicine management for secondary schools and colleges, *J Athl Train* 49(1):128–137, 2014.

16. Craig, D: Educating students on athletic training political involvement, *Athletic Therapy and Training* 14(2):3, 2009.

17. Cuppett M: A survey of physical activity levels of certified athletic trainers, *J Athl Train* 37(3):281, 2002.

18. Curtis N: Student athletic trainer perceptions of clinical supervisor behaviors: A critical incident study, *J Athl Train* 33(3):249, 1998.

19. Dunn, W: Ethics in sports medicine, *The American Journal of Sports Medicine* 35(5):840–844, 2007.

20. Ebell M: Strength of Recommendation Taxonomy (SORT): A patient-centered approach to grading evidence in the medical literature, *Am Fam Physician* 69(3):548–556, 2004.

21. Editorial: The ethics of selecting a team physician. "Show me the money" shouldn't be part of the process, *Sports Med Digest* 23(4):37, 2001.

22. Ferrara M: Globalization of the athletic training profession, *J Athl Train* 41(2):135, 2006.

23. Fícca M: Injury prevention in the occupational setting, *Athletic Therapy Today* 8(3):6, 2003.

24. Finkam S: The athletic trainer or athletic therapist as physician extender, *Athletic Therapy Today* 7(3):50, 2002.

25. Giacobbi P: Low burnout and high engagement levels in athletic trainers: Results of a nationwide random sample, *J Athl Train* 44(4): 370–77, 2009.

26. Green J: Athletic trainers in an orthopedic practice, *Athletic Therapy Today* 9(5):62, 2004.

27. Gould T: Secondary-school administrators' knowledge and perceptions of athletic training, *Athletic Therapy Today* 8(1):57, 2003.

28. Graber G: Ethics 101, *Athletic Therapy Today* 8(2):6, 2003.

29. Grace P: Milestones in athletic trainer certification, *J Athl Train* 34(3):285, 1999.

30. Gray R: The role of the clinical athletic trainer. In Konin J: *Clinical athletic training,* Thorofare, NJ, 1997, Slack.

31. Hajart A: The financial impact of an athletic trainer working as a physician extender in orthopedic practice, *The Journal of Medical Management Practice,* 29(4):250–54, 2013.

32. Haynes B: Barriers and bridges to evidence based clinical practices, *British Medical Journal* 317(7135):273–76, 1998.

33. Hendrix A: An examination of stress and burnout in certified athletic trainers at division 1-A universities, *J Athl Train* 35(2):139, 2000.

34. Herring S, et al.: Sideline preparedness for the team physician: A consensus statement, *Med Sci Sports Exerc* 33(5):846, 2001.

35. Herring, S: Team physician consensus statement: 2013 Update, *Medicine and Science in Sports and Exercise,* 45(8):1618–22, 2013.

36. Hertel J: Research training for clinicians: The crucial link between evidence-based practice and third-party reimbursement (editorial), *J Athl Train* 40(2):69, 2005.

37. Jaeschke R: Ascertaining the minimal clinically important difference. *Controlled Clinical Trials* 10(4):407–15,1989.

38. Jonas J: Ethics in injury management, *Athletic Therapy Today* 11(1):28, 2006.

39. Jones D: HIPAA: Friend or foe to athletic trainers? *Athletic Therapy Today* 8(2):17, 2003.

40. Judd M: Athletic training education program directors' perceptions on job selection, satisfaction, and attrition, *J Athl Train* 39(2):185, 2004.

41. Kahanov L, Andrews L: A survey of athletic training employers' hiring criteria, *J Athl Train* 36(4):408, 2001.

42. Kaiser D: Finding satisfaction as an athletic trainer, *Athletic Therapy Today* 10(6):18, 2005.

43. Kamper S: Global rating of change scales: A review of strengths and weaknesses and considerations for design, *Journal of Manual and Manipulative Therapy* 17(3):163–70, 2009.

44. Kania M: Personal and environmental characteristics predicting burnout among certified athletic trainers at National Collegiate Athletic Association institutions, *J Athl Train* 44(1): 58–66, 2009.

45. Kirkland M: A case study of athletic training at the Kennedy Space Center, *Athletic Therapy Today* 8(3):9, 2003.

46. Kirkland M: Increasing diversity of practice settings for athletic trainers, *Athletic Therapy Today* 10(5):1, 2005.

47. Knight K: Study/experimental/research design: Much more than statistics, *J Athl Train* 45(1): 98–100, 2010.

48. Laurent T: Clinical instructors and student athletic trainers' perceptions of helpful clinical instructor characteristics, *J Athl Train* 36(1):58, 2001.

49. Lyznicki J: Certified athletic trainers in secondary school: Report of the Council on Scientific Affairs, American Medical Association, *J Athl Train* 34(3):272, 1999.

50. Manspeaker S: Overcoming barriers to implementation of evidence-based practice concepts in athletic training education: Perceptions of select educators, *J Athl Train* 46(5):514–22, 2011.

51. Matheson G: Advocating injury prevention: The team physician's role, *Physician Sportsmed* 33(8):1, 2005.

52. Matheson G: Return-to-play decisions: Are they the team physician's responsibility? *Clinical Journal of Sport Medicine* 21(1):25, 2011.

53. Mazerolle S: Assessing strategies to manage work and life balance of athletic trainers working in the National Collegiate Athletic Association Division I setting, *J Athl Train* 46(2):194–205, 2011.

54. Mitten M: Support for certified athletic trainers in intercollegiate athletics, Memorandum from National Collegiate Athletic Association, August 14, 2003.

55. McKeon P: Assessment of the quality of clinically relevant research, *Athletic Therapy and Training* 14(3):4–9, 2009.

56. McKeon P: Hierarchy of research design in evidence-based sports medicine, *Athletic Therapy Today* 11(4):42, 2006.

57. McKeon P: Finding context: A new model for interpreting clinical evidence, *Athletic Therapy and Training* 16(5):10–13, 2011.

58. Medina J: Rating the levels of evidence in sports medicine research, *Athletic Therapy Today*, 11(1):38–41, 2006.

59. Mellion M: The team physician. In Mellion M: *Sports medicine secrets*, Philadelphia, 2002, Hanley-Balfus.

60. Michener L: Patient-and clinician-rated outcome measures for clinical decision making in rehabilitation, *Journal of Sport Rehabilitation*, 20(1):37, 2011.

61. Misasi S: Academic preparation of athletic trainers as counselors, *J Athl Train* 31(1):39, 1996.

62. Moulton M: The role of counseling collegiate athletes, *J Athl Train* 32(2):148, 1997.

63. National Athletic Trainers' Association: Athletic training competencies , ed 5, Dallas, 2010, National Athletic Trainers' Association.

64. National Athletic Trainers' Association: A closer look at the military setting, *NATA News* 12:30, 2003.

65. National Athletic Trainers' Association: *NATA code of ethics*, NATA, Dallas, 2013.

66. National Athletic Trainers' Association: What is the physician extender? *NATA News* 1:12, 2004.

67. National Athletic Trainers' Association Board of Certification: *Study guide for the NATA BOC entry-level athletic trainer certification examination*, Philadelphia, 1995, Davis.

68. National Athletic Trainers' Association Education Council: *NCAA Recommendations and Guidelines for Appropriate Medical Coverage for Intercollegiate Athletics*, 2003, National Athletic Trainers' Association.

69. National Athletic Trainers' Association Government Affairs & Advocacy: http://www.nata.org /government-affairs-advocacy.

70. O'Shea M: *A history of the National Athletic Trainers' Association*, Greenville, NC, 1980, National Athletic Trainers' Association.

71. Peer K: Ethics education: The cornerstone of foundational behaviors of professional practice, *Athletic Therapy Today* 12(1):2, 2007.

72. Pittney W: Continuing education in athletic training: An alternative approach based on adult learning theory. *J Athl Train* 33(1):72, 1998.

73. Pittney W: A qualitative examination of professional role commitment among athletic trainers working in the secondary school setting, *J Athl Train* 45(2):198–204, 2010.

74. Pitney W: Qualitative inquiry in athletic training: Principles, possibilities, and promises. *J Athl Train* 36(2):185–89, 2001.

75. Potter B: Developing professional relationships with emergency medical services providers, *Athletic Therapy Today* 11(3):18, 2006.

76. Raab S: Characterizations of a quality certified athletic trainer, *J Athl Train* 46(5):672–79, 2011.

77. Raina P: Athletic therapy and injury prevention: Evidence-based practice, *Athletic Therapy Today* 9(6):10, 2004.

78. Ransone J: Assessment of first-aid knowledge and decision making of high school athletic coaches, *J Athl Train* 34(3):267, 1999.

79. Ray R: Ethical practice in athletic training: A thing of the past? *Athletic Therapy Today* 8(2):1, 2003.

80. Rich V: Clinical instructors' and athletic training students' perceptions of teachable moments in an athletic training clinical education setting, *J Athl Train* 44(3):294–303, 2009.

81. Rock J: A preliminary investigation into the use of counseling skills in support of rehabilitation from sport injury, *J Sport Rehabil* 11(4):284, 2002.

82. Rosenberg W: Evidence-based medicine: An approach to clinical problem-solving, *BMJ* 310:1122, 1995.

83. Sauers E: A team approach: Demonstrating sport rehabilitation's effectiveness and enhancing patient care through clinical outcomes assessment. *Journal of Sport Rehabilitation* 20(1):3, 2011.

84. Scriber K: The challenge of balancing our professional and personal lives, *Athletic Therapy Today* 10(6):14, 2005.

85. Sexton, P: Clinical decision making: Assumptions made in the absence of evidence, *Athletic Therapy and Training* 16(2):1–3, 2011.

86. Shelley G: Practical counseling skills for athletic therapists, *Athletic Therapy Today* 8(2):57, 2003.

87. Shibinski K: The role of humor in enhancing the classroom climate, *Athletic Therapy and Training* 15(5): 27–29, 2010.

88. Snyder A: Using disablement models and clinical outcomes assessment to enable evidence-based athletic training practice, Part I: Disablement models, *J Athl Train* 43(4):428–36, 2008.

89. Starkey C: Scholarly productivity of athletic training faculty members, *J Athl Train* 36(2):156, 2001.

90. Steves R: Evidence-based medicine: What is it and how does it apply to athletic training? *J Athl Train* 39(1):83, 2002.

91. Stiller-Ostrowski J: Recently certified athletic trainers' undergraduate educational preparation in psychosocial intervention and referral, *J Athl Train* 44(1):67–75, 2009.

92. Swisher J: Professionalism & ethics—ethical issues in athletic training: A foundational descriptive investigation, *Athletic Therapy and Training* 14(2), 2009.

93. Team physician consensus statement, *Med- Sci Sports Exerc* 32(4):877, 2002.

94. Terranova A: National Collegiate Athletic Association division and primary job title of athletic trainers and their job satisfaction or intention to leave athletic training, *J Athl Train* 46(3):312–18, 2011.

95. Turocy P: Overview of athletic training education research publications, *J Athl Train* 37(4S):s162, 2002.

96. Turocy P: Survey research in athletic training: The scientific method of development and implementation, *J Athl Train* 37(4S):s174, 2002.

97. Valier A: Beyond the basics of clinical outcomes assessment: Selection appropriate patient-rated outcome instruments for patient care, *Athletic Training Education Journal* 10(1), 91–100, 2015.

98. Valovich McLeod, T: Using disablement models and clinical outcomes assessment to enable evidence-based athletic training practice, Part II: Clinical outcomes assessment, *Journal of Athletic Training* 43(4):437–45, 2008.

99. Velasquez BJ: Sexual harassment in the athletic training room: Implications for athletic trainers, *Athletic Therapy Today* 8(2):20, 2003.

100. Vesci B: Current evidence guiding clinical practice in athletic training, *Athletic Training & Sports Health Care: The Journal for the Practicing Clinician* 2(2):57, 2010.

101. Vinci DM: Nutrition communication and counseling skills, *Athletic Therapy Today* 6(4):34, 2001.

102. Walter J: An assessment of burnout in undergraduate athletic training education program directors, *J Athl Train* 44(2):190–96, 2009.

103. Wiksten D: Effective use of multimedia technology in athletic training education, *J Athl Train* 37(4S):213, 2002.

104. Xerogeanes J: The athletic trainer as orthopedic physician extender, *Athletic Therapy Today* 12(1):1, 2007.

# ANNOTATED BIBLIOGRAPHY

Amato H, Cole S, Hawking C: *Clinical skills documentation guide for athletic training*, Thorofare, NJ, 2006, Slack.

*Reflects the standards and specific outcomes of the NATA Clinical Proficiencies by presenting clinical skills set following a checklist design format.*

Bilik SE: *The trainer's bible,* ed 9, New York, 1956, Reed.

*A classic book, first published in 1917, by a major pioneer in athletic training and sports medicine.*

Board of Certification: *Role delineation study,* ed 5, Philadelphia, 2010, F.A. Davis.

*Contains a complete discussion of the 2004 role delineation study that redefined the responsibilities of the athletic trainer.*

Cartwright L, Pittney W: *Athletic training for student assistants,* Champaign, IL, 2001, Human Kinetics.

*A practical guide for student athletic training assistants, including their roles and responsibilities within the sports medicine team.*

Hannum S: *Professional behaviors in athletic training,* Thorofare, NJ, 2000, Slack.

*Focuses on essentials of effective career development. Addresses many of the skills students will require to build their image as health care professionals, such as communication, critical thinking, networking, interpersonal skills, and recognition of cultural differences.*

Laurent T: *Athletic training clinical education guide 2009,* Delmar Learning.

*Provides a structured format for goal setting, reflection, skills verification, and journaling.*

Long B, Hale C: *Athletic Training Exam review*. Baltimore, 2009, Lippincott, Williams & Wilkins.

*Provides a framework for athletic students to begin their certification examination preparation.*

Mueller F, Ryan A: *Prevention of athletic injuries: the role of the sports medicine team,* Philadelphia, 1991, F.A. Davis.

*Provides an in-depth discussion of the various members of the sports medicine team.*

National Athletic Trainers' Association: *Far beyond a shoe box: fifty years of the National Athletic Trainers' Association,* Dallas, 1999, National Athletic Trainers' Association.

*An interesting text about the history of NATA that should be read by any student interested in athletic training as a career.*

VanLunen, B, Hankemeier, D, Welch, C: *Evidence guided practice: a framework for clinical decision making in athletic training,* Thorofare, NJ, 2015, Slack.

*This text will help students and practicing clinicians to incorporate evidence-based concepts into clinical practice.*

Van Ost L, Manfre K: *Athletic training exam review: a student guide to success,* Thorofare, NJ, 2009, Slack.

*Emphasizes the roles and responsibilities of student athletic trainers necessary to make them successful as health care professionals.*

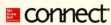

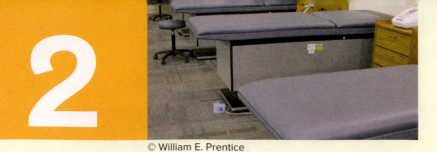
© William E. Prentice

# Health Care Organization and Administration in Athletic Training

## ■ Objectives

*When you finish this chapter you should be able to*

- Establish a strategic plan for conducting an athletic training program in secondary-school, collegiate, professional, clinic, corporate, and industrial settings.
- Plan a functional, well-designed athletic training clinic for a secondary-school, collegiate, or professional setting.
- Discuss issues relative to operating an athletic training program in secondary-school, collegiate, professional settings, clinic, hospital, corporate, and industrial settings.

- Identify policies and procedures that should be enforced in the athletic training clinic.
- Explain the importance of the preparticipation physical examination.
- Construct the necessary records that must be maintained by the athletic trainer.
- Describe current systems for gathering injury surveillance data.

## ■ Outline

## ■ Key Terms

accident                injury                epidemiology

## ■ Connect Highlights    connect

*Visit connect.mcgraw-hill.com for further exercises to apply your knowledge:*

- Clinical application scenarios covering athletic training clinic design, risk management, policies, and procedures
- Click-and-drag questions covering budgeting, athletic training clinic design, and preparticipation physical examination
- Multiple-choice questions covering preparticipation physical examination, maintaining records, and developing a strategic plan for an athletic training clinic
- Selection questions covering preparticipation physical examination and classification of sport

O perating an effective athletic health care program requires careful organization and administration regardless of whether the setting is a secondary school, college, university, or professional team or a clinical, hospital, or industrial facility. Besides being a clinical practitioner, the athletic trainer must be an administrator who performs both managerial and supervisory duties.[12] This chapter looks at the administrative tasks required of the athletic trainer for successful operation of the program, including facility design, policies and procedures, budget considerations, personnel management, administration of physical examinations, record keeping, and injury data collection.

# ESTABLISHING A SYSTEM FOR ATHLETIC TRAINING HEALTH CARE

## Developing a Strategic Plan

Perhaps the first step in establishing a health care program in athletic training is to determine why such a program is needed and what the goals of this program should be.[19] The basic questions in the strategic planning process must be answered by clinic, hospital, or school administrators; medical directors; athletic directors; or school boards who, in most cases, will ultimately be responsible for funding and supporting the health care program in athletic training.[21,44] The depth of the commitment from these decision makers toward providing quality health care will, to a large extent, determine the size of the staff, the size of the facility, and the scope of operation of the health care program. Clearly written Mission and Vision statements will help focus the direction of the program and should be an outcome of the strategic planning process.[32]

Strategic planning should involve many individuals, including administrators, other allied health care providers, student-athletes, coaches, physicians, staff athletic trainers, patients, parents, and community-based health leaders. Including many individuals in the planning process will help secure allies who are committed to seeing the program succeed.[44]

Strategic planning should be an ongoing process that takes a critical look at the strengths and weaknesses of the program and then takes immediate action to correct deficiencies. The *SWOT* analysis—which looks at Strengths, Weaknesses, Opportunities, and Threats underlying planning[42]—is a useful and effective technique in strategic planning for existing athletic health care programs. Administrators should take a close

look at a cost-effectiveness analysis of operating an athletic health care program to determine the value of the return on their investment.

## Developing a Policies and Procedures Manual

Once the strategic planning process is complete and some consensus has been reached by those involved in the process, the next step is to create a detailed policies and procedures manual based on the mission and vision

> Every athletic training program must develop policies and procedures that carefully delineate the daily routine of the program.

statements. This manual will be used by everyone who is involved with providing some aspect of health care, including the athletic training staff, physicians, other allied health personnel, and administrators.[4] *Policies* are clear and accurate written statements that identify the basic rules and principles (the what and why) used to control and expedite decision making. Policies are essential for operating the athletic training clinic. *Procedures* describe the process by which something is done (the how). *Focus Box 2–1:* "Items to include in a policies and procedures manual" includes recommendations for topics to be included.

# ISSUES SPECIFIC TO ATHLETIC TRAINING PROGRAM OPERATION IN THE SECONDARY-SCHOOL, COLLEGE, OR UNIVERSITY SETTING

It is imperative that every athletic program develop policies and procedures that carefully delineate the daily routine of the program.[20]

## The Scope of the Athletic Training Program

An important consideration in any athletic training program is to determine who is to be served by the athletic training staff.[55] The individual athlete/patient, the institution, and the community are considered.

**The Athlete** The athletic trainer must decide the extent to which the athlete/patient will be served. For example, will prevention and care activities be extended to athletes for the entire year, including summer and other vacations, or only during the competitive season? Also, the athletic trainer must decide what care will be rendered. Will it extend to all systemic illnesses or just to musculoskeletal problems?

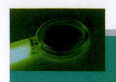

## FOCUS 2–1 Focus on Healthcare Administration and Professional Responsibilities

### Items to include in a policies and procedures manual

*Program Operation*

- Goals and objectives
- Mission statement
- Vision statement
- Organizational structure
- Scope of operation
- Hours of operation
- Patient scheduling
- Patient billing
- Patient referral
- Facility cleaning, sanitation, and hygiene
- Equipment use, maintenance, and repair
- Documentation and maintenance of medical records
- Release of medical records
- Budget and purchasing
  - Supplies
  - Equipment
- Emergency procedures
  - Fire
  - Code (cardiac arrest)

- Emergency action plan
- Disaster plan (tornado)
- Active shooter plan
- Safety and security considerations
  - Access to facility
  - OSHA guidelines
- Inclement weather
- Incident reports

*Human Resources Issues*

- Job descriptions
- Hiring practices
- Quarterly and yearly employee evaluations
- Licensure and certification
- Dress code
- Vacation policy
- Benefits
- Sexual harassment
- Termination policy
- Staff attendance

**The Institution** A policy must be established as to who will be served by the athletic training program. Often, legal concerns and the school liability insurance dictate who, beyond the athlete, is to be served. A policy should make it clear whether students other than athletes/patients, athletes from other schools, faculty, and staff are to receive care. If so, how are they to be referred and medically directed? Also, it must be decided whether the athletic training program will act as a clinical setting for athletic training students.

**The Community** A decision must be made as to which, if any, outside group(s) or people in the community will be served by the athletic training staff. Again, legality and the institution's insurance program must be taken into consideration when making this decision. If a policy is not delineated in this matter, outside people may abuse the services of the athletic training clinic and staff.

## Providing Health Care Services

**Health Care Services for Facility Personnel** A concern of any athletic department is whether proper health care services are provided for the athletic training clinic and specific sports. If a school has a full-time athletic training staff, an athletic training clinic could, for example, operate from 6 A.M. to 11 P.M. Mornings are commonly reserved for treatments and exercise rehabilitation; early afternoons are for treatment, exercise rehabilitation and preparation

for practice or a contest; and late afternoons and early evenings are spent in injury management. Secondary schools with limited available supervision may be able to provide athletic training clinic coverage only in the afternoons.

**Health Care Services for Sports** Ideally, all sports should have a certified and licensed athletic trainer in attendance at all practices and contests, both at home and away. Many colleges and universities have sufficient personnel to provide coverage to a variety of sports simultaneously. At the secondary-school level, however, only one or occasionally two athletic trainers may be available to cover every sport that the secondary school offers. Thus, it is impossible for the athletic trainer to be in several places at one time. The athletic trainer in this difficult situation must make some decisions about where the greatest need for coverage is, based on the potential risk of a particular sport and the number of athletes involved.[40]

## Hygiene and Sanitation

The practice of good hygiene and sanitation is of the utmost importance in an athletic training program. The prevention of infectious diseases is a direct responsibility of the athletic trainer, whose duty it is to see that all athletes/patients are surrounded by the

> Good hygiene and sanitation are essential for an athletic training program.

most hygienic environment possible and that each individual is practicing sound health habits. Chapter 14 discusses the management of bloodborne pathogens. The athletic trainer must be aware of and adhere to guidelines for the operation of an athletic care facility as dictated by the Occupational Safety and Health Administration (OSHA).

**The Athletic Training Clinic** The athletic training clinic should be used only for the prevention and care of sports injuries.[27] Too often, the athletic training clinic becomes a meeting or club room for the coaches and athletes. Unless definite rules are established and practiced, cleanliness and sanitation become an impossible chore. Unsanitary practices or conditions must not be tolerated. The following are some important athletic training clinic policies:

1. No cleated shoes are allowed. Dirt and debris tend to cling to cleated shoes; therefore, athletes should remove cleated shoes before entering the athletic training clinic.
2. Game equipment is kept outside. Because game equipment, such as balls and bats, add to the sanitation problem, they should be kept out of the athletic training clinic. Coaches and athletes must be continually reminded that the athletic training clinic is not a storage room for sports equipment.
3. Shoes must be kept off treatment tables. Because of the tendency of shoes to contaminate treatment tables, they must be removed before any care is given to the patient.
4. Athletes should shower with antimicrobial soap, after every practice before receiving treatment.[59] **SoR:B** The athlete should make it a habit to shower before being treated if the treatment is not an emergency. This procedure helps keep tables and therapeutic modalities sanitary.
5. Roughhousing and profanity should not be allowed. Athletes must be continually reminded that the athletic training clinic is for injury care and prevention. Horseplay and foul language lower the basic purpose of the athletic training clinic.
6. No food or smokeless tobacco should be allowed.
7. Cell phones must not be used for photos or other social media posts due to issues with HIPAA and patient privacy.

General cleanliness of the athletic training clinic, the locker rooms, and the athletic venues must be constantly maintained. Through the athletic trainer's example, the athlete may develop an appreciation for cleanliness and in turn develop wholesome personal health habits. Cleaning responsibilities in most schools are divided among the athletic training staff, equipment managers, and the custodial staff. The custodial staff, equipment managers, and the athletic training staff should work closely together to make certain that all duties relative to cleanliness are covered. Ultimately, the athletic trainer is responsible for making sure that a lack of cleanliness of the facilities and equipment is not a threat to the health and well-being of the athletes. Care of permanent building structures and trash disposal are usually the responsibilities of custodians, whereas the upkeep of specialized equipment falls within the responsibilities of both the athletic trainers and the equipment managers. Used, dirty clothing, including practice gear, undergarments, outerwear, and uniforms, must be laundered on a daily basis.[59] **SoR:B** Equipment, including knee sleeves and braces, ankle braces, etc., should be disinfected in the manufacturer's recommended manner on a daily basis.[58]

The division of routine cleaning responsibilities may be generally organized as follows:

1. Custodial staff
   a. Sweeps floors daily
   b. Cleans and disinfects sinks and built-in tubs daily
   c. Mops and disinfects hydrotherapy area twice a week
   d. Refills paper towel and drinking cup dispensers as needed
   e. Empties wastebaskets and disposes of trash daily
2. Athletic training staff
   a. Cleans and disinfects treatment tables daily
   b. Cleans and disinfects hydrotherapy modalities daily
   c. Cleans and polishes other therapeutic modalities weekly
   d. Disinfects equipment, including knee sleeves and braces, and the like, according to the manufacturer's recommendations, on a daily basis.[59] **SoR:C**
3. Equipment managers
   a. Clean and disinfect frequently touched surfaces such as wrestling mats, locker room benches, and floors.[59] **SoR:A**
   b. Have all practice and game gear, including soiled clothing, practice gear, undergarments, outerwear, and uniforms, laundered daily.[59] **SoR:B**

**The Gymnasium** Maintaining a clean environment is a continual battle in the secondary-school, college, and university settings.[48] Practices such as passing a common towel to wipe off perspiration, using common water bottles, disposable razors, and hair clippers, and failing to change dirty clothing for clean are prevalent violations of sanitation in sports.[59] **SoR:A** The following is a suggested cleanliness checklist that may be used by the athletic trainer:

1. Facilities cleanliness
   a. Are the gymnasium floors swept daily?
   b. Are drinking fountains, showers, sinks, urinals, and toilets cleaned and disinfected daily?
   c. Are lockers aired and sanitized frequently?
   d. Are mats cleaned routinely (wrestling mats and wall mats cleaned daily)?

2. Equipment and clothing issuance
   a. Are equipment and clothing fitted to the athlete and properly maintained to avoid skin irritations?
   b. Is swapping of equipment and clothes prevented?
   c. Is clothing laundered and changed frequently?
   d. Is wet clothing allowed to dry thoroughly before the athlete wears it again?
   e. Is individual attention given to proper shoe fit and upkeep?
   f. Is protective clothing provided during inclement weather or when the athlete is waiting on the sidelines?
   g. Are clean, dry towels provided each day for each athlete?

**The Athlete** To promote good health among the athletes, the athletic trainer should encourage sound health habits. The following checklist may be a useful guide for coaches, athletic trainers, and athletes:

1. Promptly report injuries, illnesses, open wounds, and skin disorders to the athletic trainer.
2. Practice good daily living habits of resting, sleeping, and proper nutrition.
3. Shower after practice.
4. Dry thoroughly and cool off before departing from the gymnasium.
5. Avoid drinking from a common water dispenser.
6. Avoid using a common towel.
7. Avoid exchanging workout clothes with teammates.
8. Practice good foot hygiene.
9. Avoid contact with teammates who have a contagious disease or infection.
10. Understand the role exercise can play in maintaining a healthy lifestyle and preventing chronic disease.

## Emergency Telephones

Every individual responsible for overseeing an athletic health care program as well as athletic personnel who are conducting practices or competitions should all have access to wireless phones for the purpose of contacting or communicating with emergency services or medical health care providers should a need arise. Also note that in certain calling areas outside of the wireless area code, 911 calls are routed back to the originating service area code, which does no good in an emergency situation. Cell phone reception and connectivity should be routinely assessed. Walkie-talkies are also useful when practices or games occur at several different facilities simultaneously. These devices can greatly enhance communication capabilities. It may be necessary to at least have access to a land line just in case wireless service is disrupted.

## Budgetary Concerns

A seemingly ongoing problem that athletic trainers face is to obtain a budget of sufficient size to permit them to perform an adequate job of providing athletic health care.[39] Most secondary schools provide only limited budgetary provisions for athletic training, except for the purchase of tape, ankle wraps, and an athletic training kit that contains a minimum amount of supplies.[7] Many fail to provide a room and any of the special facilities that are needed to establish an effective athletic training program. Some school boards and administrators fail to recognize that the functions performed in the athletic training clinic are an essential component of the athletic program.[7] Colleges and universities face similar problems, but not to the extent of secondary schools. By and large, athletic training at the college level is recognized as an important aspect of the athletic program.

A major problem facing many athletic trainers is a budget of insufficient size.

Budgetary needs vary considerably within programs; some require only a few thousand dollars, whereas others spend hundreds of thousands of dollars. The amount spent on building and equipping an athletic training clinic, of course, is entirely a matter of local option. In purchasing equipment, immediate needs and the availability of personnel to operate specialized equipment should be kept in mind.

Budgeting should be a continuous process involving prioritizing, planning, documenting, and evaluating the goals of the athletic training program and formulating a plan for how available resources can be utilized and expended during the next budget period.[42]

Budget records should be kept on file, so that they are available for use in projecting the following year's budgetary needs. The records present a picture of the distribution of current funds and substantiate future budgetary requests.

**Supplies** The supplies that the athletic trainer uses to carry out daily tasks may be classified as either expendable or nonexpendable. Some athletic trainers spend much of their budget on expendable supplies, which cannot be reused. Supplies that are expendable are used for injury prevention, first aid, and management. Examples of expendable supplies are adhesive tape, adhesive bandages, and hydrogen peroxide. Nonexpendable supplies are those that can be reused. Examples are compression wraps, scissors, and neoprene sleeves. An annual inventory must be conducted at the end of the year or before supplies are ordered. Accurate records must be kept to justify future requests.

Supplies may be expendable or nonexpendable.

**Equipment** The term *equipment* refers to items that may be used in the athletic training clinic for a number of years. Equipment may be further divided into nonconsumable capital and capital equipment. Nonconsumable capital equipment is not usually removed from the athletic training clinic. Examples of nonconsumable capital equipment are ice machines, treatment tables, isokinetic machines, and electrical therapeutic modalities. Capital equipment includes crutches, coolers, and athletic training kits.

> Equipment may be nonconsumable capital or capital.

**Purchasing Systems** The purchase of supplies and equipment must be done through either direct buy or competitive bid. For expensive purchases, an institutional purchasing agent is sent out to competing vendors, who quote a price on specified supplies or equipment. Orders are generally placed with the lowest bidder. Smaller purchases and emergency purchases may be made directly from a single vendor.[7]

> Purchasing may be done through direct buy or competitive bid.

An alternative to purchasing expensive equipment is to lease it. Many manufacturers and distributors are willing to lease equipment on a monthly or yearly basis. Over the long run, purchasing equipment is less costly. In the short term, however, if a large capital expenditure is not possible, a leasing agreement should be considered.[42]

**Additional Budget Considerations** In addition to supplies and equipment, the athletic trainer must also consider other costs included in the operation of an athletic training program; these include telephone and postage, program. These include utilities, contracts with physicians or clinics for services, professional liability insurance, memberships in professional organizations, professional journals or textbooks, travel and expenses for attending professional meetings, and clothing to be worn in the athletic training clinic.[42,44]

> The principal at All-American High School has received a mandate from the school board to develop a risk management plan for the athletic program. The principal asks the athletic trainer to chair a committee to develop this plan.
>
> **?** What considerations are important for inclusion in this risk management plan?

## Developing a Risk Management Plan

The athletic trainer, working in conjunction with the appropriate administrative personnel, must be responsible for developing a risk management plan that covers security issues, fire safety, electrical and equipment safety, and emergency action plans.[3,4,14,17,51,52]

**Security Issues** The athletic trainer must decide who will have access to the athletic training clinic. In addition to the staff athletic trainers, the team physician must have keys to access the athletic training clinic. Graduate assistant athletic training students may also be given keys as necessary at the collegiate level; at the secondary-school level, however, athletic training students should be in the athletic training clinic only when directly supervised. At the collegiate level, coaches do not need to have access to the athletic training clinic; however, at the secondary-school level, coaches might need to have a key to get into the clinic at times when the athletic trainer is not available. Access to areas of the building other than the athletic training clinic should be strictly limited.

**Fire Safety** The athletic trainer should establish and clearly post a plan for evacuating the athletic training clinic, should a fire occur. Smoke detectors and fire alarm systems must be tested periodically and inspected to make certain that they are functioning normally.

**Electrical Equipment Safety** Electrical safety in the athletic training setting should be of primary concern to the athletic trainer. Accidents can be avoided by taking some basic precautions and acquiring some understanding of the power distribution system and electrical grounds. *Focus Box 2–2:* "Safety when using electrical equipment" lists considerations for electrical safety.

**Emergency Action Plan** In cooperation with existing community-based emergency health care delivery systems, the athletic trainer should develop a systematic plan for accessing the emergency medical system and subsequent transportation of injured athletes to an emergency care facility.[5] Meetings should be scheduled periodically with EMTs or paramedics who work in the community to make certain that they understand the role of the athletic trainer as a provider of emergency health care.[23] It is important to communicate the special considerations for dealing with athletic equipment issues before an emergency arises. Chapter 12 discusses the emergency action plan in detail.

**Crisis Management Plan** Crisis management must be a central component of an institution's risk management program. It is unfortunate that a climate currently exists in the United States in which educational institutions can be affected either directly or indirectly at any moment by some type of crisis situation. A crisis could be caused by weather, public health, or act of terror emergencies. Crisis management involves knowing how to respond to a crisis situation quickly and efficiently to protect and ensure the health, safety, and well-being of all those who might inadvertently become victims of the crisis. Everyone at that institution must know exactly what needs to be done immediately to mitigate the threat of injury to specific individuals and the general population. Administrators, health care providers, and community-based emergency management and public safety personnel

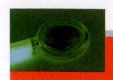

### Safety when using electrical equipment

- The entire electrical system of the building or athletic training clinic should be designed or evaluated by a qualified electrician.
- Problems with the electrical system may exist in older buildings or in situations in which rooms have been modified to accommodate therapeutic devices (e.g., putting a whirlpool in a locker room in which the concrete floor is always wet or damp).
- It should not be assumed that all three-pronged wall outlets are grounded. The ground must be checked. Ground fault interrupters (GFIs) should be installed, particularly in those areas in which water and electricity are used together (e.g., whirlpools, hydrocollator, electric stimulation).
- The athletic trainer should become very familiar with the equipment being used and with any problems that exist or may develop.

- Any defective equipment should be labeled and removed immediately from the clinic.
- The plug should not be jerked out of the wall by pulling on the cable.
- Extension cords or multiple adapters should never be used.
- Equipment should be reevaluated on a yearly basis and should conform to *National Electrical Code* guidelines. A clinic that is not in compliance with this code has no legal protection in a lawsuit.
- Common sense should always be exercised when using electrotherapeutic devices. A situation that appears to be potentially dangerous may, in fact, result in injury or death.

must collectively be involved in the planning and documentation of specifically how all parties should act and react in a crisis situation.

### Accessing Community-Based Health Services

In addition to the community-based emergency medical services personnel, the athletic trainer should become familiar with existing local and regional community health services and agencies that may be accessed, should a need arise to refer an athlete for psychological or sociological services. Referrals should be made with input and assistance from the team physician. The family of an athlete requiring referral for psychological or sociological counseling must be informed of the existing problems, particularly when the athlete is a minor.

**2-2 Clinical Application Exercise**

State University has an opening for an assistant athletic trainer in its Department of Athletics. The athletic director has asked the head athletic trainer to be in charge of the recruitment and hiring process for the new position.

**?** What factors must be considered in hiring a new employee?

### Human Resources and Personnel Issues

Putting together the appropriate personnel to accomplish program goals and objectives is critical to success. Any program is only as good as the group of individuals who make up the team. Recruiting, hiring, and retaining the

most qualified personnel is essential if the athletic training program is to be effective.[22]

- Specific policies dealing with recruitment, hiring and firing, performance evaluations, and promotions are mandated by federal law (Equal Employment Opportunity Commission). The policies for recruitment and hiring clearly mandate that all qualified applicants should receive equal consideration regardless of their race, gender, sexual preference, religion, or nationality. Athletic trainers who are in a position to hire new staff must strictly adhere to these mandates.[24]
- Once an individual has been hired, it is important for everyone to understand what his or her roles and responsibilities are. Individual job descriptions and job specifications that describe qualifications, accountability, a code of conduct, and the scope of that position should be written. A well-defined organizational chart should be created to show the chain of command.[44]
- The head athletic trainer must serve as a supervisor for the staff assistants, graduate students, and undergraduate athletic training students.[30] The supervisor should strive to improve the job performance and enhance the professional development of those being supervised. *Focus Box 2-3:* "Models of supervision for the head athletic trainer" defines supervisory models.[44]
- Performance evaluations should be done at regularly scheduled intervals to analyze the quality of the work being performed. Evaluations should focus first on the positive aspects of job performance and then on any weaknesses.[30]

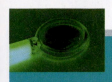

Each of these policies relative to personnel issues should be included in the policies and procedures manual.

## Designing an Athletic Training Clinic

Maximizing the use of facilities and effectively using equipment and supplies are essential to the function of any athletic program.[43] The athletic training clinic must be designed to meet the many requirements of the athletic training program (Figure 2–1).[11,37,46] The size and layout of the athletic training clinic will depend on the scope of the athletic training program, including the size and number of teams and athletes and what sports are offered.[40] The hospital/clinical setting has a much broader patient population than a secondary-school or university athletic training clinic, and thus the requirements for equipment and supplies are somewhat different.[37] To accommodate the various functions of an athletic training program, the athletic training clinic must serve as a health care center for patients.[11]

> The athletic training clinic is a multipurpose area used for first aid, therapy and rehabilitation, injury prevention, medical procedures (such as preparticipation physical examinations), and athletic training administration.

**Size** The size of the athletic training clinic can range anywhere from a large storage closet in some secondary schools to 15,000 + square-foot (1,394 sq.m) sports medicine complexes in some universities. Certainly, the size of the clinic can have a major impact on how the athletic training program is managed. But the most important consideration is to organize the athletic training program in a manner that most efficiently takes advantage of the space available. When designing a new athletic training clinic, the athletic trainer should work closely with design architects to communicate the specific needs of the institution and the number of athletes who will be served.[45]

**Location** The athletic training clinic should have an outside entrance from the athletic field or court. It should also have direct access to courts and fields to provide practice and game setup as well. This arrangement makes it unnecessary to take injured athletes in through the building and possibly through several doors; it also permits access when the rest of the building is not in use. All entrances must be ADA handicapped accessible. A double door at each entrance is preferable to allow easy passage of a wheelchair or a stretcher. A ramp at the outside entrance is safer and far more functional than are stairs.

The athletic training clinic should be near the locker rooms if possible, so that showers are readily available to athletes/patients going in for treatment following practice. Toilet facilities should be located adjacent to the athletic training clinic and should be readily accessible through a door in the athletic training clinic.

Because the athletic training clinic is where emergency treatment is given, its light, heat, and water sources should be independent from those for the rest of the building.

> **2–3 Clinical Application Exercise**
>
> The members of the school board at All-American High School voted to allocate $25,000 to renovate a 25' × 40' storage space and to purchase new equipment for an athletic training clinic. The athletic trainer has been asked to provide the school principal with a wish list of what should be included in this facility. The physical renovation will cost approximately $17,000.
>
> ? How can this space be best used, and what type of equipment should be purchased to maximize the effectiveness of the new facility?

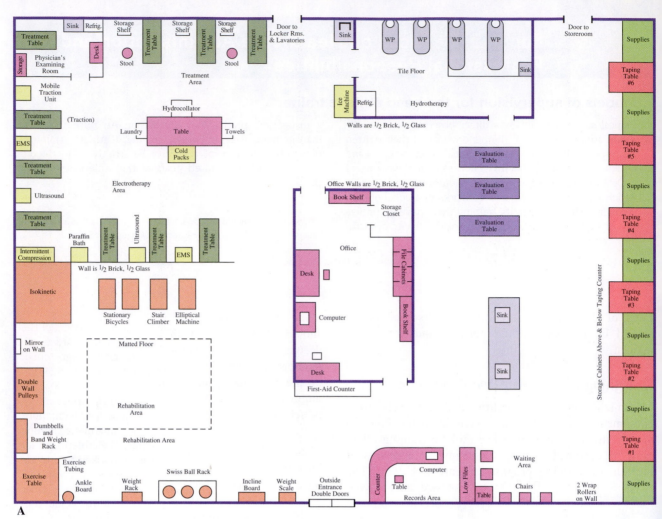

**FIGURE 2–1** The ideal athletic training clinic should be well designed to maximize its use. A, Larger athletic training clinic at a college or university.

© William E. Prentice

*Continued*

**Illumination** The athletic training clinic should be well lighted throughout. Lighting should be planned with the advice of a technical lighting engineer. Obviously, certain areas need to be better lit than others. For example, the wound care, taping, evacuation, and treatment areas need better lighting than is necessary in the rehabilitation area. Ceilings and walls act as reflective surfaces to help provide an equitable distribution and balance of light. Natural lighting through windows or skylights can be helpful.

**Special Service Areas** Apart from the storage and office space, a portion of the athletic training clinic should be divided into special sections, preferably by half walls or partial glass walls. Space, however, may not permit a separate area for each service section, and an overlapping of functions may be required.

**Treatment Area** The treatment area should include a number of treatment tables, preferably of adjustable height, that can be used during the application of therapeutic modalities. Adjustable stools on rollers should also be readily

available. The hydrocollator unit and ice bags should be easily accessible to this area.

**Electrotherapy Area** The electrotherapy area is used for treatment by ultrasound, diathermy, or electrical stimulating units. Equipment should include treatment tables, wooden chairs, dispensing tables for holding supplies, shelves, and a storage cabinet for supplies and equipment. The area should contain a sufficient number of grounded outlets, preferably in the walls and several feet above the floor. It is advisable to place rubber mats or runners on each side of the treatment tables as a precautionary measure. This area must be under supervision at all times, and cabinets used for storage of equipment and supplies should be kept locked when not in use.

**Hydrotherapy Area** In the hydrotherapy area, the floor should slope toward a centrally located drain to prevent standing water. Equipment may include whirlpool baths (one permitting complete immersion of the body), several lavatories, and storage shelves. Because some of this equipment is electrically operated, many precautions

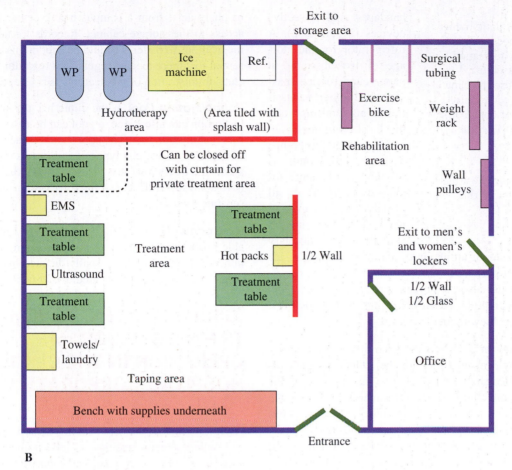

FIGURE 2–1 **continued,** B. Small athletic training clinic at a secondary-school.
© William E. Prentice

must be taken. All electrical outlets should be placed 4 to 5 feet (1.2 to 1.5 m) above the floor and should have spring-locked covers and water spray deflectors. All cords and wires must be kept clear of the floor to eliminate any possibility of electrical shock. To prevent water from entering the other areas, glass should be used to separate the hydrotherapy area from the rest of the clinic due to noise, heat, humidity while still allowing visibility. When an athletic training clinic is planned, ample outlets must be provided; under no circumstances should two or more devices be operated from the same outlet. All outlets must be properly grounded using ground fault interrupters (GFIs).[36]

### Rehabilitation and Reconditioning Area

Ideally, an athletic training clinic should accommodate injury reconditioning under the strict supervision of the athletic trainer. Selected pieces of resistance equipment should be made available. Depending on the existing space, dumbbells and free weights; exercise machines for knee, ankle, shoulder, hip, and so forth; isokinetic equipment; devices for balance and proprioception; and space for using resistance bands may all be available for use.

### Taping, Bandaging, and Orthotics Area

Each athletic training clinic should provide a place in which taping, bandaging, and applying orthotic devices can be executed. This area should have taping tables, a sink, and a storage cabinet.

### Physician's Examination Room

In most clinics, colleges and universities, the team physician/medical director has a room in which examinations and treatments may be given. This room contains an examining table, a sink, locking storage cabinets for medications and supplies, and a small desk with a desktop computer. At all times, this clinic must be kept locked to outsiders.

### Storage Facilities

Many athletic training clinics lack ample storage space. Often, storage facilities are located a considerable distance away, which is extremely inconvenient. In addition to the storage cabinets and shelves provided in each of the three special service areas, a small storage closet should be placed in the athletic trainer's office. All these cabinets should be used for the storage of general supplies as well as for the small, specialized equipment used in the respective areas. A large storage area is a necessity for the storage of bulky equipment, medical supplies, adhesive tape,

> It is essential to have adequate storage space available for supplies and equipment.

A clinical athletic trainer is approached by the community recreation department with a request to use the clinic to treat its community-based recreational football and basketball league participants who are injured.

❓ How should the athletic trainer deal with this request?

bandages, and protective devices (Figure 2–2). A refrigerator for the storage of frozen water in paper cups for ice massage and other necessities is also an important piece of equipment. In small sports programs, a large refrigerator is probably sufficient for all ice needs. If at all possible, an ice-making machine should be installed in an auxiliary area to provide an ample and continuous supply of ice for treatment purposes.

There should also be storage spaces provided for patients in which to place their belongings (e.g., book bags, clothes) while they are being treated.

**Athletic Trainer's Office** A space at least 10 feet by 10 feet (3 by 3 m) is ample for the athletic trainer's office. The office should be located so that all areas of the athletic training clinic can be well supervised without the athletic trainer having to leave the office. Glass partitions on two sides permit the athletic trainer to observe all activities even while seated at the desk. A desk, desktop computers, a tackboard for clippings and other information, telephones, and a record file are the basic equipment. The office should have an independent lock-and-key system so that it is accessible only to authorized personnel.

**Additional Areas** If space is available, several other areas could be included as part of an athletic training clinic.

*Pharmacy Area* A separate room that can be secured for storing and administering medications is helpful. All medications, including over-the-counter drugs, should be kept under lock and key. If prescription medications are kept in the athletic training clinic, only the team physician

or pharmacist from a campus health center should have access to the storage cabinet. Records for administering medications to patients should be kept in this area. It is essential to adhere to state regulations regarding the storage and administration of medications (see Chapter 17).

*Rehabilitation Pool* If the clinic has the space and the institution can afford one, a pool can be an extremely useful rehabilitation tool. The pool should be accessible to individuals with various types of injuries. It should have a graduated depth to at least 7 feet (2.1 m), the deck should have a nonslip surface, and the filter system should be in a separate room.[42]

*Restrooms* There should be at least one restroom available in the athletic training clinic. Requirements for the number of restrooms are usually dictated by the building code occupancy limits assigned to that facility.

# ISSUES SPECIFIC TO ATHLETIC TRAINING PROGRAM OPERATION IN THE CLINIC, HOSPITAL, CORPORATE, OR INDUSTRIAL SETTING

As is the case for those working in secondary schools and colleges or universities, athletic trainers working in clinical, hospital, corporate, and industrial settings must be competent in preventing and recognizing injuries and supervising injury rehabilitation programs. However, staff athletic trainers working in these settings treat and rehabilitate a wider range of patients in terms of age and physical condition. The athletic trainer may provide care to pediatric, adolescent, young adult, adult, and geriatric patients. The patients have physical ailments that may or may not be related to physical activity. In addition, athletic trainers who work in clinical, corporate, or industrial facilities may find themselves in the role of an entrepreneur who owns a clinic facility or practice; an administrator who oversees the day-to-day operations; a marketing director; or a community outreach coordinator. They must also be knowledgeable regarding administrative and management skills, marketing, fiscal responsibilities, reimbursement, documentation, and outcomes assessment.[30]

## Scope of Practice

Athletic trainers who work in a clinic, hospital, or ambulatory care center will likely see a patient population that is diverse not only in age but also in the variety of injuries, illnesses, and conditions. Athletic trainers in hospitals may be involved in inpatient, outpatient, or ambulatory care.

For the most part, the owner of an outpatient clinic or its chief administrator will dictate the patient population that the clinic will treat (i.e., orthopedic, sports, occupational, cardiac, etc.). Athletic trainers working

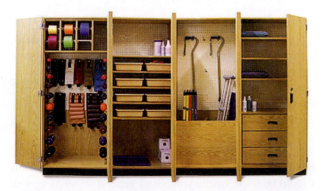

FIGURE 2–2 An effective athletic training program must have appropriate storage facilities that are highly organized.
Courtesy Hausmann Industries

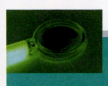

## FOCUS 2–4 Focus on Healthcare Administration and Professional Responsibilities

### Additional certifications for athletic trainers working in a clinic or hospital

| Certification | Association/Organization |
|---|---|
| Orthopedic technologist (OT) | National Association of Orthopedic Technologists |
| Orthotics and prosthetics (ABC) | American Board for Certification in Orthotics and Prosthetics |
| Certified surgical technologist (CST) | Association of Surgical Technologists |
| Certified professional ergonomist (CPE) | Board of Certification for Professional Ergonomists |
| Certified strength and conditioning specialist (CSCS) | National Strength and Conditioning Association |
| Performance enhancement specialist (PES) | National Academy of Sports Medicine |
| Corrective exercise specialist (CES) | National Academy of Sports Medicine |
| Certified clinical research associate (CRA) | Association of Clinical Research Professionals |

in either a privately owned clinic or a corporate/industrial setting may be involved in individual patient care, working in on-site employee fitness centers, working in ergonomic and occupational work hardening safety programs, supervising employee drug-testing programs, overseeing wellness programs, or overseeing and engaging in outreach programs and athletic event coverage, which essentially helps market the clinic to the community.

Regardless of the setting, limitations and restrictions on what an athletic trainer can do and who can be treated are in large part determined by the regulatory statutes governing professional practice in individual states. It is the responsibility of both the administrator and the athletic trainer to know the limits of practice.

**Location of the Clinic** Because most privately owned clinics are in business to make a profit, it is essential to build a patient base. Certainly, the location of the facility is a key to attracting patients and making it a successful business.[37] Several other factors may determine whether the chosen location is good:

- What are the zoning laws in the area?
- Is there any type of traffic problem that would create an accessibility issue for potential patients?
- Are there doctors in the area who will refer patients to this clinic?
- Will these doctors use an athletic trainer to treat their patients?
- Are there businesses in the area for which this clinic could provide industrial rehabilitation or on-site workplace assessment?
- Are there schools in the area that could use sports medicine coverage by an athletic trainer?
- Are there any other clinics or hospitals that provide similar services that may directly or indirectly compete with the new business?

**Hours of Operation** To most effectively meet the scheduling needs of potential patients, the clinic must be open at times that do not conflict with normal school or work hours. This means that the clinic must be open early in the morning and remain open at least into the early evening, so patients can get to the facility either before or immediately after school or work. Also, it is important to maintain hours of operation at least one day over the weekend.[37]

## Clinic Personnel and Human Resources Issues

The athletic trainer must work with a number of different health care providers in the clinical or corporate setting, including physicians, physician's assistants, physical therapists, physical therapy assistants, occupational therapists, occupational therapy assistants, nutritionists, and nurses. Additionally, if the clinic is in a hospital, respiratory therapists, speech therapists, recreational therapists, and pharmacists may also be involved in patient care. Each of these individuals should have a formal, specific job description developed by human resources personnel. The most effective treatment models seem to involve a team approach and require communication and cooperation on the part of all involved in providing some aspect of health care.

Athletic trainers who work in a clinical or hospital setting may seek additional certifications that can expand the scope of their roles and responsibilities. *Focus Box 2–4: "Additional certifications for athletic trainers working in a clinic or hospital"* lists those certifications.

## Potential Athletic Training Duties

**Ergonomic Assessment** Ergonomics is the science of designing products, machines, and systems to maximize the comfort, efficiency, and safety of the people who use them.[56] Ergonomics is based on the principles of anthropometry (the science of human measurement) and biomechanics (the study of muscular activity) applied to industrial engineering to adapt or alter the design of products and workplaces to an individual's physical strengths, limitations, size, and shape.

One of the primary goals of ergonomics is the prevention of accidents and injuries in the workplace by attempting to minimize risk factors, such as repetition, vibration, force, and awkward/static postures as they relate to musculoskeletal disorders.[56] Ergonomists work to eliminate these problems by designing workplaces, such as assembly lines, computer workstations and to prevent injuries. They position machinery and tools to be accessible without twisting, reaching, or bending. They design adjustable desks, chairs, and workbenches to comfortably accommodate workers of many different sizes, preventing the need to continuously lean or overextend the arms.

An athletic trainer may work with an occupational therapist or an ergonomist to provide an ergonomic assessment, an evaluation of a workstation and the physical environment and its interaction with the employee.[50] This assessment involves not only adjusting and making recommendations regarding the employee's workstation but also providing instruction on injury prevention techniques, including suitable stretches, strengthening exercises, and suggested rest breaks. An ergonomic assessment report outlines the results of the assessment and is forwarded to the injured employee, workplace manager or administrator, medical practitioner, and other involved parties.[56] A follow-up review may be conducted to ensure that the recommendations have been implemented (Figure 2–3).

**Work Hardening/Conditioning Programs** Athletic trainers may supervise or participate in work hardening or conditioning programs that involve intensive outpatient

therapy for individuals injured on the job. The goal is to regain functionality and return to work in a full-duty capacity. The starting point for these patients is a musculoskeletal evaluation of their strength, posture, flexibility, gait, sensation, and reflexes.[50] This is followed by a functional capacity evaluation to determine skill deficits as measured against physical job requirements. The following skills may be evaluated in a functional capacity evaluation:[50]

- Tolerance for prolonged sitting and standing
- Hand grip strength and coordination
- Repetitive lifting capacity at various levels
- Repetitive push, pull, and carrying capacities
- Lifting biomechanics and proper postures/mechanics in the workplace
- Repetitive squat
- Prolonged trunk flexion or rotation in sitting and standing
- Prolonged crawling, kneeling, and crouch positions
- Maximum walking, stairs, and stepladder capacity
- Balance

The athletic trainer then discusses the results and recommendations of these evaluations with the patient. This collective information is used to develop a rehabilitation plan to allow the patient to return to work at the appropriate level of performance.

*Work conditioning* refers to intensive rehabilitation offered 3 hours a day for 3 days a week, whereas *work hardening* refers to intensive therapy offered 8 hours a day for 5 days a week. Treatments may involve simulated work, education about avoiding reinjury, and job site analysis to assist the employer in making appropriate equipment modifications for an employee returning to work after an injury (Figure 2–4).

**Wellness Center** Athletic trainers may supervise a wellness center and assume responsibility for organizing wellness screenings, workshops, and employee health

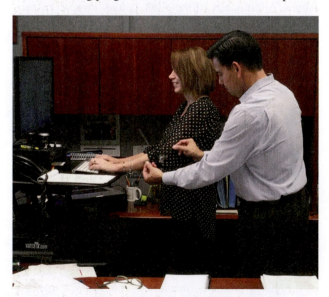

FIGURE 2–3   Ergonomic assessment.
© William E. Prentice

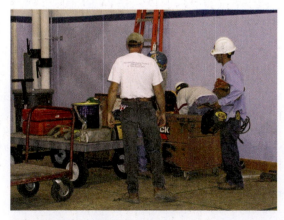

FIGURE 2–4   Work hardening.
© William E. Prentice

fairs. Worksite health screenings may be offered for asthma, hypertension, diabetes, cholesterol, osteoporosis, prostate cancer, skin cancer, glaucoma, weight loss, smoking cessation, and stroke. Early detection can save both the employees and a company the emotional and financial costs of medical conditions that have advanced because they went undetected. Results may be given directly to employees or sent to their homes with a detailed explanation.

Wellness workshops raise employees' awareness about their health, help them understand their susceptibility to disease, and motivate them to seek medical consultation or make important changes that will reduce their risks and enhance the quality of their lives. Workshop topics might include nutrition, men's health, women's health, skin care, fitness and exercise, family and personal development, and workplace health and safety.

Health fairs are an effective and enjoyable means of educating employees about various health issues. In addition to offering multiple screening services at various booths, employees can obtain health education materials at information tables while learning from and interacting with health professionals.

**Community Outreach and Marketing** When employed by some clinics or a hospital, athletic trainers may see patients or have other in-house responsibilities during part of the day. But in the afternoons or evenings they may be assigned to provide athletic training coverage for an athletic program at a local secondary school or college. They may also cover single athletic events in the community. These outreach programs not only provide a valuable service to athletes in the community but also serve as an effective marketing tool to promote and advertise the clinic. This marketing strategy helps provide visibility for the clinic to physicians, other health care providers, parents, and other schools at all levels, as well as other potential patients from throughout the community.

**Corporate Fitness Programs** Athletic trainers working in corporate settings are commonly charged with the responsibility of overseeing in-house employee fitness programs.[32] Physical fitness offers a variety of proven health benefits, including a decreased risk of heart disease and heart attack. Physically fit employees can also handle physical work tasks better and deal with stressful situations more easily, and they tend to be less susceptible to illness and injuries. Corporations offer fitness programs to their employees to reduce health costs, increase productivity, reduce absenteeism, decrease turnover, improve morale, lower health care expenditures, and reduce sick leave (Figure 2–5).

After an initial consultation, the athletic trainer administers fitness evaluations for all participating employees to determine their baseline fitness levels for

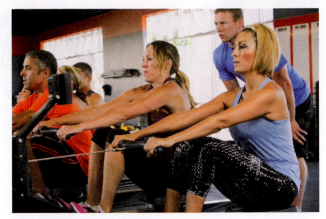

FIGURE 2–5    A corporate fitness program.
© Erik Isakson/Blend Images LLC

cardiorespiratory endurance, body composition, flexibility, muscle strength, and endurance. Based on information from the initial consultation and fitness evaluation, an individual exercise prescription may be developed for each participating employee. Typical exercise sessions may include warm-up activities, aerobic conditioning, strength training, flexibility exercises, and cool-down. Training sessions should teach safe, effective exercise techniques and educate employees on training intensity, frequency, and progression to maximize results and reduce injuries. By following these guidelines, employees can meet their fitness goals, while the corporation benefits from a healthier workforce.[34]

**Drug-Testing Programs** An athletic trainer working in a corporate or a clinic setting may be asked to oversee a drug-testing program for employees. A drug-testing program can deter employees from coming to work unfit for duty. It also discourages drug abusers from applying to a company in the first place. A corporation may require a full-service testing program to comply with federal requirements or a simple preemployment screening program. Legal defensibility is the most important aspect of any drug-testing program. The corporation should use federally certified laboratories and confirm and verify all positive results through a medical review department.

## Fiscal Management

When an athletic trainer is employed by a for-profit business, such as a clinic or a hospital, he or she must have some understanding of basic business practices and fiscal management.[44] Certainly, if the athletic trainer is an administrator or an owner of a clinic, it is even more critical to understand how to run a profitable business.

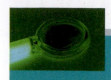
**Information contained in medical records**

*Medical History*

Family history
Social history
Habits
Immunization history
Growth chart and developmental history
Substance abuse inquiry
   Surgical history
   Obstetric history

*Medical Encounters*

Chief complaint
History of the present illness
   Complete physical examination
   Assessment and plan

*Orders and Prescriptions*

*Progress Notes*

*Results of Previous Diagnostic Tests*

For the most part in the health care industry, businesses rely on billing a patient's insurance company and being reimbursed for services provided to that patient. Third-party reimbursement and issues with managed care are discussed in detail in Chapter 3. Maintaining a positive accounts payable to accounts receivable (AP/AR) ratio, in which more money is being collected than must be paid out in expenses, is the goal of every successful business. Other responsibilities include financial planning, which assesses the goals and objectives of the company; establishing contractual obligations with payors and providers; developing an efficient billing and collection system; formulating a budget, which requires the coordination of resources and expenditures; and deciding on expenditures for necessary equipment and supplies.

## RECORD KEEPING

For athletic trainers, as for all health care providers, keeping accurate, updated medical records is essential.

> Keeping adequate records is critical for any athletic trainer.

Some athletic trainers object to keeping records and filling out forms, stating that they have neither the time nor the inclination to be bookkeepers. Nevertheless, because lawsuits are the rule rather than the exception, accurate and up-to-date records are an absolute necessity. Medical records are also critical for accurate and timely assessment and evaluation of practices and for documentation of practices and activities to ensure that responsibilities and expectations are being met. *Focus Box 2–5* lists the type of information usually found in standard medical records. Medical records, injury reports, treatment logs, personal information cards, injury evaluations and progress notes, supply and equipment inventories, and annual reports are essential records that should be maintained by the athletic trainer.

### Electronic Versus Paper Medical Records

An electronic health record (EHR) or electronic medical record (EMR) is a digital version of the paper records used in the past, which contains all of a patient's medical history; medications and allergies; immunizations; lab test results; images; vital signs; demographics, such as age, height, weight, and other relevant data; and insurance and billing information. EMRs can be easily shared among different health care providers. An EHR provides a long-term collection of an individual's health care information, whereas an EMR is a patient record that is created and used for specific visits in a clinic, hospital, or physician's office in an institution that can be accessed by health care providers within the institution. Electronic medical records can certainly simplify the process for any health care provider who may need to review a complete medical record for an individual patient between facilities. It seems fairly clear that using electronic medical records improves overall efficiency, reduces errors, and reduces costs. The downside to using electronic medical records is that the improved portability and accessibility creates security issues that threaten patient privacy.

### Patient File Management Systems

Effective management of patient records and supporting documents is a critical factor in the efficiency of operation an athletic training program. Optimally, athletic trainers should use some type of comprehensive patient-file management system for appropriate chart documentation, risk management, outcomes, and billing.

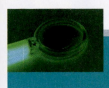

### HIPAA authorization

Following is a list of core elements that must be present for a disclosure authorization to be valid:

- A description of the information to be used or disclosed
- Identification of the persons or class of persons authorized to make use of or disclosure of the protected health information
- Identification of the persons or class of persons to whom the covered entity is authorized to provide or disclose information
- A description of each purpose of the use or disclosure
- An expiration date or event
- The individual's signature and date
- If signed by a personal representative, a description of his or her authority to act for the individual

## Maintaining Confidentiality in Record Keeping

**Release of Medical Records** The athletic trainer may not release a patient's medical records to anyone without written consent. If the patient/athlete wishes to have medical records released to professional sports organizations, insurance companies, the news media, or any other group or individual, the athlete must sign a waiver that specifies which information is to be released. The only exception to this is the appropriate disclosure of information among those professionals who are involved in providing health care to the injured individual.

**Health Insurance Portability and Accountability Act (HIPAA)** The Health Insurance Portability and Accountability Act (HIPAA) regulates how athletic trainers, physicians, administrators, and other allied health personnel with private health information (PHI) about patients can share that information with others.[26] The regulation guarantees that patients have access to their medical records, gives them more control over how their protected health information is used and disclosed, and provides a clear avenue of recourse if their medical privacy is compromised.[31] Authorization by a patient to release medical information is not necessary on a per-injury basis.[25] A written blanket authorization signed by the patient at the beginning of the year will suffice for all injuries and treatments during the course of participation for that year. These one-time, blanket authorizations must indicate what information may be released, to whom, and for what length of time.[25] *Focus Box 2–6:* "HIPAA authorization" is a list of core elements that must be present for the authorization to be valid.

**Family Educational Rights and Privacy Act (FERPA)** The Family Educational Rights and Privacy Act (FERPA) protects the privacy of student educational records. It has been suggested that in some instances medical records should be kept along with a student's educational records; thus, the right to privacy of medical records would be protected under FERPA instead of HIPAA.[26] FERPA gives parents certain rights with respect to their children's educational records. These rights transfer to the student when he or she reaches the age of 18 or attends a school beyond the secondary-school level. Students to whom the rights have been transferred are "eligible students." Parents and eligible students have the right to inspect and review the student's educational records maintained by the school. Parents and eligible students have the right to request that a school correct records that they believe to be inaccurate or misleading. Schools must have written permission from the parent or eligible student to release any information from a student's educational records.

## Preparticipation Examinations (PPE)

The first piece of information that the athletic trainer should collect on each athlete is obtained from an initial preparticipation examination before the start of practice.[29] The primary purpose of the preparticipation exam is to identify an athlete who may be at risk before he or she participates in a specific sport.[1] It also allows comparisons from one year to the next with regard to growth and development, weight gain/loss, and the like. The preparticipation examination should consist of a medical history, and a physical examination, which includes a cardiovascular screening, orthopedic screening, general medical screening, neurologic screening (only if warranted), and, a wellness screening.[41] In addition, if the athlete indicates a history of concussion on the medical history form, a thorough neurologic assessment should be done to rule out other neurologic conditions such

> **Preparticipation health examination:**
>
> - Medical history
> - Physical examination
> - Cardiovascular screening
> - Maturity assessment
> - Orthopedic screening
> - Wellness screening

A sports medicine clinic has agreed to organize and conduct preparticipation exams for All-American High School, which offers 18 sports–6 in the fall, 6 in the winter, and 6 in the spring. There are a total of approximately 500 athletes, and approximately 200 of them are involved in the fall sports. The athletic trainer who works in the clinic is charged with arranging and administering preparticipation examinations so that each athlete can be cleared for competition.

**?** How can the athletic trainer most efficiently set up the preparticipation exams to clear 200 athletes for competition in the fall sports?

as seizure disorder, cervical spine stenosis, or spinal cord injury.[13] **SoR:C** Information obtained during this examination establishes a baseline to which comparisons may be made after injury. It may also reveal conditions that could warrant disqualification from certain sports.[29] The examination also satisfies insurance and liability issues.

The NATA has published a position statement "Preparticipation Physical Examinations and Disqualifying Conditions" (www.nata.org /sites/default/files/Conley .pdf) that provides guidelines for conducting preparticipation exams.

In 2010, the NCAA instituted mandatory testing for sickle cell trait for all athletes in Division I. Students are given a blood test to screen for the sickle cell trait prior to the first season that they are eligible to compete. Under the current rules, athletes can avoid testing by proving they have previously been tested or by signing a waiver releasing the NCAA and their university from liability. The NATA has published a consensus statement, "Sickle Cell Trait and the Athlete" (www.nata.org/sites/default /files/SickleCellTraitAndTheAthlete.pdf) that provides guidelines and precautions for modifying workouts in athletes with sickle cell trait.

***Cardiovascular Screening*** In 1996, the American Heart Association (AHA) published recommendations concerning the cardiovascular component of the preparticipation exam in competitive athletes.[49] The critical task of the preparticipation cardiac examination is identifying life-threatening conditions from

> **Potentially lethal cardiovascular conditions:**
> - Hypertrophic cardiomyopathy
> - Aortic stenosis
> - Marfan's syndrome

specific questions regarding risk factors and symptoms of cardiovascular disease asked when obtaining the medical history.[13] **SoR:C** Although the cardiac examination need not involve complex tests, it must permit the recognition of abnormal heart sounds, heart murmurs, and other signs of pathology through auscultation.[13] **SoR:C** It has been suggested that an electrocardiogram (ECG) should be mandatory in the preparticipation screening of athletes.[10] However, while there is a general consensus that an ECG would certainly increase the diagnostic accuracy of the screening exam, it is not currently considered to be cost-effective in screening athletes.

The vast majority of exams are negative, but the physician should be alert to such potentially lethal conditions as hypertrophic cardiomyopathy, aortic stenosis, and Marfan's syndrome. A history of symptoms during exertion, certain features of physical appearance, and clinical findings require referral to a cardiologist.[49] Cardiac testing using ECG or exercise stress testing is not a routine aspect of the PPE unless warranted by findings from the personal and family history.[13] **SoR:B** Some physicians have advocated for the addition of an echocardiogram to the screening process even though an ECG is easier to administer and has a lower cost.

***Orthopedic Screening*** Orthopedic screening may be done as part of the physical examination or separately by the athletic trainer. A quick orthopedic screening exam is accurate in detecting existing musculoskeletal injuries usually takes about 90 seconds[13] **SoR:A** (Figure 2–8).[1] A more detailed, site-specific orthopedic examination may

**Medical History** A comprehensive medical and family history form is perhaps the most important part of the preparticipation exam and should be completed before the physical examination and orthopedic screening. Its purpose is to identify any past or existing medical problems.[1] And to identify any underlying condition that might predispose an athlete to injury.[13] **SoR:B** For younger athletes it may be necessary to have input from parents to ensure the accuracy of the history. This form should be updated for each individual every year. Medical histories should be closely reviewed by both the physician and the athletic trainer with the athlete, so that personnel can be prepared, should a medical emergency arise.[13] **SoR:C** Necessary participation release forms and insurance information should be collected along with the medical history (Figure 2–6).[33]

**Physical Examination** The physical examination should include an assessment of height, weight, body composition, blood pressure, and pulse rate. The general medical screening portion of the physical exam should include vision, musculoskeletal, skin, dental, ear, nose, throat, heart and lung function, abdomen, lymphatics, genitalia (males only), and maturation index. The use of routine laboratory tests such as urinalysis, complete blood count (CBC), lipid profile, ferritin level, and others may be included as part of the physical exam but is not necessary unless specific concerns arise from the medical history.[13] **SoR:B** (Figure 2–7).[33]

# MEDICAL HISTORY FORM

NAME: _____ ID#: _____
BIRTHDATE: _____ SPORT: _____TODAY'S DATE: _____
STATUS: NEW_____ RETURNING _____ SIGNATURE_____

Please answer all questions and explain the yes answers.
1. Have you ever had or been told you have any of the following? Circle your response, date beside yes answers, and explain below.

| | | | |
|---|---|---|---|
| YES/NO Heat Exhaustion | YES/NO Lung Disease | YES/NO Ulcers | YES/NO Frequent Diarrhea |
| YES/NO Heat Stroke | YES/NO Kidney Disease/Stones | YES/NO Bleeding from Rectum | YES/NO Migraine Headaches |
| YES/NO Heart Murmur | YES/NO Rheumatic Fever | YES/NO Blood in Urine | YES/NO Hayfever |
| YES/NO Heart Palpitations | YES/NO Eating Disorder | YES/NO Unusual Bruising | YES/NO Mononucleosis |
| YES/NO Diabetes | YES/NO Skin Problems/Rash | YES/NO Unusual Bleeding | YES/NO Weight Loss |
| YES/NO High Blood Pressure | YES/NO Muscle Cramps (greater than 10 lbs) | YES/NO Hernia | YES/NO High Cholesterol |
| YES/NO Epilepsy or Seizures | YES/NO Recurring Infections (skin, sinus, etc.) | YES/NO Depression | |
| YES/NO Anemia | YES/NO Asthma | YES/NO Recurring Anxiety | |

Explain: _____
_____

YES/NO  2. Have you had any other major illnesses? Date and Explain: _____
_____

YES/NO  3. Have you ever had surgery? Date and Explain: _____
_____

YES/NO  4. Have you ever been hospitalized for a reason other than surgery? Date and Explain: _____

YES/NO  5. Are you missing any of the following: kidney, eye, testicle (or undescended testicle), or any other organ?
Explain: _____

YES/NO  6. Have you ever experienced significant or recurrent cough, shortness of breath, wheezing, chest pain, chest tightness, or near fainting with exercise? Explain: _____

YES/NO  7. Do you ever feel your heart beating irregular, too fast, or skipping beats? Explain: _____

YES/NO  8a. Are you allergic to any medicines? Explain: _____

YES/NO  8b. Do you have any other allergies (i.e., insect bites, foods, etc.)? Explain: _____

YES/NO  9. Have you been tested for sickle cell trait? Result: _____

YES/NO  10. Do you wear glasses or contact lenses while participating in sports? _____

YES/NO  11. Do you have a broken, chipped, loose, or missing tooth or dental plate? Explain: _____

YES/NO  12. Have you ever fainted? When? _____ Explain: _____

YES/NO  13. Have you ever had a concussion (head injury with or without loss of consciousness)? How many? _____
Date(s): _____

YES/NO  14. Have you ever suffered a neck injury, stinger, or burner? Date(s): _____
Did you have numbness, tingling, weakness, or paralysis? _____

YES/NO  15. Have you ever broken/dislocated a bone/joint (include stress fractures)? Date: _____ Which bone/joint: _____
Date: _____ Which bone/joint: _____

YES/NO  16. Have you had any musculoskeletal injury in the past 3 years? Explain: _____
Is it completely healed? _____

YES/NO  17. Does any joint feel as if it is slipping? _____

YES/NO  18. Do you have a pin, plate, screw or anything metal in your body? _____

YES/NO  19. Do you wear any protective or assistive devices? (e.g., Knee brace) _____

20. Is there a family history of: Family members (e.g., Father, Sister)
YES/NO Heart Disease or Marfan's Syndrome _____       YES/NO High Cholesterol _____
YES/NO Cancer _____                                   YES/NO Diabetes ___
YES/NO High Blood Pressure _____                      YES/NO Other Significant Illnesses or Conditions____
YES/NO Heart Attack or Cardiac Death before Age 50 _____

YES/NO  21. Have you ever been medically disqualified or restricted from participation in a sport or exercise program?
Explain: _____

YES/NO  22. Are you taking any medications currently or routinely (including birth control)? _____
Drug Dose Times/Day_____

YES/NO  23. Are you currently taking supplements to improve performance or for weight control?_____

YES/NO  24. Do you use any tobacco products (cigarettes, chewing tobacco, cigars)? Explain: _____

YES/NO  25. Do you use alcohol? If yes, how much and how often? _____

YES/NO  26. Has anyone ever suggested you need to cut down on your drinking or have you ever had any negative consequences from drinking (injury, ER visit, citation, DUI, etc.)? _____

YES/NO  27. Do you use recreational drugs? If yes, what do you use? _____

YES/NO  28. Do you feel stressed or under pressure? _____

YES/NO  29. Do you experience periods of depression, sadness, or hopelessness? Explain: _____

YES/NO  30. Do you have concerns about your weight? _____

YES/NO  31. Have you ever had issues with disordered eating ?_____

## FOR WOMEN ONLY

32. Date of last menstrual period _____

YES/NO  33. Have you ever had a PAP smear? If so, when?_____

34. My periods are now (circle one):
Regular (every 28–35 days)        Irregular (every 36 days or more/or less than 21 days)        Absent (no periods for 3 months)

YES/NO  35. Do you take birth control pills for any reason? Explain: _____

YES/NO  36. Do you have any gynecological problems (i.e., cramps, PMS, discharge, etc.) Explain: _____

YES/NO  37. Have you ever missed your period for 6 months or more? Explain: _____

YES/NO  38. Have you ever had a sexually transmitted disease? Explain: _____

## DO NOT WRITE BELOW THIS LINE

REQUIRED IMMUNIZATIONS VERIFIED? YES/NO
CLEARED /NOT CLEARED/ PENDING
CLINICIAN'S COMMENTS: _____
_____
CLINICIAN'S SIGNATURE: _____ DATE: _____

FIGURE 2–6   Sample medical history form.

# PHYSICAL EXAMINATION FORM

NAME: _____ ID#: _____

BIRTHDATE: _____ SPORT: _____ TODAY'S DATE: _____

STATUS: NEW_____ RETURNING _____ SIGNATURE: _____

HEIGHT: _____

WEIGHT: _____ BODY MASS INDEX (BMI): _____ % Body Fat: _____

RESTING PULSE: _____

BLOOD PRESSURE (Seated): _____ (Supine): _____ (Standing): _____

VISION: Right Eye 20/_____ Corrected? Yes/No

Glasses_____ Contacts_____

Left Eye 20/_____ Corrected? Yes/No

Glasses_____ Contacts_____

PUPILS: Equal_____ Reactive to Light_____

## MUSCULOSKELETAL REGIONS

|  | Normal | Problems |
|---|---|---|
| Neck |  |  |
| Back |  |  |
| Shoulder |  |  |
| Elbow |  |  |
| Wrist |  |  |
| Hand/Finger |  |  |
| Hip |  |  |
| Knee |  |  |
| Ankle/Lower Leg |  |  |
| Foot/Toes |  |  |

## GENERAL MEDICAL

|  | Normal | Problems |
|---|---|---|
| Heart |  |  |
| Respiratory/Lungs |  |  |
| Lymph Nodes |  |  |
| Neurological |  |  |
| Skin |  |  |
| Breast |  |  |
| Genital |  |  |
| Eyes |  |  |
| Ears, Nose, Throat |  |  |
| Urinary |  |  |
| Psych |  |  |

COMMENTS: _____
_____
_____

Physician/ Athletic Trainer Signature _____ Date: _____

FIGURE 2−7   Sample physical examination form.

| Orthopedic Screening Examination | |
|---|---|
| **Activity and Instruction** | **To Determine** |
| Stand facing examiner | Acromioclavicular joints; general habitus |
| Look at ceiling, floor, over both shoulders; touch ears to shoulders | Cervical spine motion |
| Shrug shoulders (examiner resists) | Trapezius strength |
| Abduct shoulders 90° (examiner resists at 90°) | Deltoid strength |
| Full external rotation of arms | Shoulder motion |
| Flex and extend elbows | Elbow motion |
| Arms at sides, elbows 90° flexed; pronate and supinate wrists | Elbow and wrist motion |
| Spread fingers; make fist | Hand or finger motion and deformities |
| Tighten (contract) quadriceps; relax quadriceps | Symmetry and knee effusion; ankle effusion |
| "Duck walk" four steps (away from examiner with buttocks on heels) | Hip, knee, and ankle motion |
| Stand with back to examiner | Shoulder symmetry; scoliosis |
| Knees straight, touch toes | Scoliosis, hip motion, hamstring tightness |
| Raise up on toes; raise heels | Calf symmetry, leg strength |

FIGURE 2–8   Orthopedic screening. Equipment that may be needed includes reflex hammer, tape measure, pin, and examining table.

be conducted to assess strength, range of motion, and stability at various joints (Figure 2–9).

**General Medical Screening** In addition to a physical screening of the eyes, mouth, ear, nose, throat, thorax, abdomen, lymph nodes, urinary system, and skin, several additional assessments may be necessary.

A maturity assessment should be part of the physical examination as a means of protecting the young, physically developing athlete.[35] The most commonly used methods are circumpubertal (sexual maturity), skeletal, and dental assessments. Of the three, Tanner's five stages of maturity assessment, indicating the maturity of secondary sexual characteristics, is the most expedient for use in the station method of examination.[53] The Tanner approach evaluates pubic hair and genitalia development in boys and pubic hair and breast development in girls (Figure 2–10). Other indicators are facial and axillary hair. Stage 1 indicates that puberty is not evident, and stage 5 indicates full development. The crucial stage in terms of collision and high-intensity noncontact sports is stage 3, in which the fastest bone growth occurs. In this stage, the growth plates are two to five times weaker than the joint capsule and tendon attachments.[34] Young athletes in grades 7 through 12 must be matched by maturity, not age.[53]

An assessment of all medications and dietary supplements currently being used by the athlete should be closely reviewed by the physician and athletic trainer. The athletic trainer should be able to provide the athlete with up-to-date information regard the use of dietary supplements (see Chapter 5).[13] **SoR:B**

Athletes who report feelings of depression, sadness, hopelessness, or stress on the medical history form should be referred to mental health practitioners for more in-depth assessment when appropriate.[13] **SoR:C**

For those athletes who report a history of anemia, abnormal menstrual cycles, diabetes, asthma, elevated cholesterol or lipid levels, or other such symptoms will require additional laboratory tests and referral to a physician who specializes in that condition.[13] **SoR:C**

**Wellness Screening** Some preparticipation exams include a screening for wellness. The purpose is to determine whether the athlete is engaging in healthy lifestyle behaviors and should include questions about diet, rest, exercise, and weight control, as well as questions about lifestyle habits that pose a threat to wellness such as alcohol, drug, and tobacco use, and stress. A number of wellness screening tools are available. Figure 2–11 provides an example of a wellness screening questionnaire.

**Health Maintenance and Personal Hygiene Screening** A screening tool for assessing the general principles of health maintenance and personal hygiene, should include questions about skin care, dental hygiene and dental care, sanitation, immunizations, avoiding infectious and contagious diseases, and sleep habits.

**Administering the Preparticipation Exam** Currently a standardized and universally accepted process for administering a preparticipation exam (PPE) does not exist. It is recommended that a complete PPE be administered to all new athletes initially. Once an initial PPE has been administered, for subsequent seasons, at minimum, an update and review of the medical history should be conducted.[13] **SoR:C** Ideally, the PPE should be administered 4 to 6 weeks before the preseason to allow time for proper

# ORTHOPEDIC SCREENING FORM

Name_____ ID#_____

| Posture | Normal | Asymmetrical /Abnormal | Comments |
|---|---|---|---|
| Head Tilt | | | |
| Shoulders Level | | | |
| Spinal Curves-Cervical Thoracic, Lumbar | | | |
| Scapular winging | | | |
| Pelvis, hips, knees, ankles level | | | |
| Leg length | | | |

| Joint/Movement | ROM | | | Strength | | |
|---|---|---|---|---|---|---|
| **Shoulder:** | Normal | Asymmetrical | Comments | Normal | Asymmetrical | Comments |
| Abduction | | | | | | |
| Adduction | | | | | | |
| Extension | | | | | | |
| Flexion | | | | | | |
| Internal rotation | | | | | | |
| External rotation | | | | | | |
| **Elbow:** | | | | | | |
| Flexion | | | | | | |
| Extension | | | | | | |
| **Wrist:** | | | | | | |
| Flexion | | | | | | |
| Extension | | | | | | |
| Flexion | | | | | | |
| **Hip:** | | | | | | |
| Flexion | | | | | | |
| Extension | | | | | | |
| Internal Rotation | | | | | | |
| External Rotation | | | | | | |
| Adduction | | | | | | |
| Abduction | | | | | | |
| **Knee:** | | | | | | |
| Flexion | | | | | | |
| Extension | | | | | | |
| **Ankle:** | | | | | | |
| Dorsiflexion | | | | | | |
| Plantar flexion | | | | | | |
| Inversion | | | | | | |
| Eversion | | | | | | |
| **Trunk:** | | | | | | |
| Flexion | | | | | | |
| Extension | | | | | | |
| Rotation | | | | | | |
| Lateral flexion | | | | | | |

| Joint Instability | Comments |
|---|---|
| Shoulder | |
| Elbow | |
| Hip | |
| Knee | |
| Ankle | |

**Evaluator's Signature**　　　　　　　　**Date**

FIGURE 2–9   Sample of a detailed orthopedic screening form.

## Males

*Stage 1.* No evidence of pubic hair.

*Stage 2.* Slightly pigmented hair laterally at the base of the penis. Usually straight.

*Stage 3.* Hair becomes darker and coarser, begins to curl, and spreads over the pubic region.

*Stage 4.* Hair is adult in type but does not extend onto thighs.

*Stage 5.* Hair extends onto the thighs and frequently up the linea alba.

## Females

*Stage 1.* No evidence of pubic hair.

*Stage 2.* Long, slightly pigmented, downy hair along the edges of the labia.

*Stage 3.* Darker, coarser, slightly curled hair spread sparsely over the mons pubis.

*Stage 4.* Adult type of hair but it does not extend onto thighs.

*Stage 5.* Adult distribution, including spread along the medial aspects of the thighs.

FIGURE 2–10    Tanner's five stages of maturity.[53]

---

1. Circle the appropriate response for each question.
2. Add the total number of points for each section.

| BEHAVIOR | Almost Always | Sometimes | Almost Never | | Almost Always | Sometimes | Almost Never |
|---|---|---|---|---|---|---|---|
| **TOBACCO USE** | | | | **STRESS CONTROL** | | | |
| If you never smoke or use tobacco products, enter a score of 10 for this section and go to the next section on Alcohol and Drugs. | | | | 1. I have a job or do other work that I enjoy. | 2 | 1 | 0 |
| 1. I avoid smoking cigarettes and chewing tobacco. | 2 | 1 | 0 | 2. I find it easy to relax and to express my feelings freely. | 2 | 1 | 0 |
| 2. I smoke only low-tar and low-nicotine cigarettes, or I smoke a pipe or cigars. | 2 | 1 | 0 | 3. I anticipate and prepare for events or situations likely to be stressful for me. | 2 | 1 | 0 |
| **Tobacco Use Score: \_\_\_\_** | | | | 4. I have close friends, relatives, or others with whom I can discuss personal matters and call on for help when needed. | 2 | 1 | 0 |
| **ALCOHOL AND DRUGS** | | | | 5. I participate in group activities (such as church and community organizations) or hobbies that I enjoy. | 2 | 1 | 0 |
| 1. I avoid drinking alcoholic beverages or I drink no more than one or two a day. | 4 | 1 | 0 | **Stress Control Score: \_\_\_\_** | | | |
| 2. I avoid using alcohol or other drugs (especially illegal drugs) as a way of handling stressful situations or problems in my life. | 2 | 1 | 0 | **SAFETY** | | | |
| 3. I am careful not to drink alcohol when taking certain medicines (e.g., medicine for sleeping, pain, colds, and allergies) or when pregnant. | 2 | 1 | 0 | 1. I wear a seat belt when riding in a car. | 2 | 1 | 0 |
| 4. I read and follow the label directions when using prescribed and over-the-counter drugs. | 2 | 1 | 0 | 2. I avoid driving while under the influence of alcohol and other drugs. | 2 | 1 | 0 |
| **Alcohol and Drug Score: \_\_\_\_** | | | | 3. I obey traffic rules and the speed limit when driving. | 2 | 1 | 0 |
| **EATING HABITS** | | | | 4. I am careful when using potentially harmful products or substances (such as household cleaners, poisons, and electrical devices). | 2 | 1 | 0 |
| 1. I eat a variety of foods each day, such as fruits and vegetables, whole-grain breads and cereals, lean meats, dairy products, dry peas and beans, and nuts and seeds. | 4 | 1 | 0 | 5. I avoid smoking in bed. | 2 | 1 | 0 |
| 2. I limit my intake of fat, saturated fat, and cholesterol (including fat in meats, eggs, butter and other dairy products, shortenings, and organ meats, such as liver). | 2 | 1 | 0 | 6. I am not sexually active or I have sex with only one mutually faithful, uninfected partner, or I always engage in safe sex (using condoms), and I do not share needles to inject drugs. | 2 | 1 | 0 |
| 3. I limit the amount of salt I eat by cooking with only small amounts, not adding salt at the table, and avoiding salty snacks. | 2 | 1 | 0 | **Safety Score: \_\_\_\_** | | | |
| 4. I avoid eating too much sugar (especially frequent snacks of sticky candy or soft drinks). | 2 | 1 | 0 | **WHAT YOUR SCORES MEAN** | | | |
| **Eating Habits Score: \_\_\_\_** | | | | Scores of 9 and 10: Excellent. Your answers show that you are aware of the importance of this area to your health. | | | |
| **EXERCISE/FITNESS HABITS** | | | | Scores of 6 to 8: Good. Your health practices in this area are good, but there is room for improvement. | | | |
| 1. I maintain a desired weight, avoiding overweight and underweight. | 3 | 1 | 0 | Scores of 3 to 5: Fair. Your health risks are showing. | | | |
| 2. I do vigorous exercises for 15–30 minutes at least three times a week (examples include running, swimming, and brisk walking). | 3 | 1 | 0 | Scores of 0 to 2: Poor. Your answers show that you may be taking serious and unnecessary risks with your health. Perhaps you are not aware of the risks and what to do about them. You can easily get the information and help you need to improve, if you wish. | | | |
| 3. I do exercises that enhance my muscle tone for 15–30 minutes at least three times a week (examples include yoga and calisthenics). | 2 | 1 | 0 | If you have questions or concerns, you should consult your athletic trainers for advice. | | | |
| 4. I use part of my leisure time participating in individual, family, or team activities that increase my level of fitness (such as gardening, bowling, golf, and baseball). | 2 | 1 | 0 | | | | |
| **Exercise/Fitness Score: \_\_\_\_** | | | | | | | |

FIGURE 2–11    Wellness screening questionnaire.

Source: Modified from Health Style: A Self-Test, U.S. Department of Health and Human Services, Public Health Service, National Clearing House, Washington, DC.

follow-up on any findings that cause concern. In some instances, the PPE may be administered on the same day or the day before preseason begins. However, this makes it difficult to make certain that all of the athletes are cleared to participate on the first day of practice.[13] **SoR:C**

The preparticipation exam may be effectively administered either on an individual basis by a personal physician, or it may be done using a station examination system with a team of examiners.[13,54] **SoR:C** Examination by a personal physician has the advantage of yielding an in-depth history and an ideal physician–patient relationship. A disadvantage of this type of examination is that it may not be directed to the detection of the factors that predispose the athlete to a sports injury. The most thorough and sport-specific type of preparticipation examination is the station examination (Table 2–1). This method can provide the athlete with a detailed examination in a short period of time. A team may include physicians, osteopaths, nurses, athletic trainers, physical therapists, or physician's assistants, exercise physiologists, nutritionist, and athletic training students.

Privacy must be respected at all times when the findings of the PPE are communicated. HIPAA regulations require written authorization from the athlete, or the legal guardian if the athlete is a minor, before any private health information may be released.[13] **SoR:C**

**Clearance to Participate** The purpose of the preparticipation exam is to identify the athlete who may be at risk for injury before he or she participates in a specific sport. It is the responsibility of the physician and the athletic trainer to make decisions regarding the appropriate interventions to remediate and ultimately alleviate those medical issues that are of concern before clearing an athlete to fully engage in or return to sport activity. Decisions to clear an athlete for participation must be based on the best available evidence and should always be in the best interest of the athletes' health and well-being.

## Sport Disqualification

As discussed previously, sports participation involves risks. Certain injuries and conditions warrant concern on the part of both the athlete and sports medicine personnel about continued participation in sport activities. Table 2–2 lists those conditions.[2] A team physician and institution have the legal right to restrict an individual from participating in athletics as long as the decision is individualized, reasonably made, and based on competent medical evidence.[13] Most conditions that potentially warrant disqualification should be identified by a preparticipation examination and noted in the medical history.[1] The NATA has published a position

| TABLE 2–1 | Suggested Components of a Preparticipation Physical Examination |
|---|---|
| **Station** | **Points Noted** |
| 1. Individual history (reviewed); height, weight, body composition, body mass index (BMI) | "Yes" answers are probed in depth; height and weight relationships |
| 2. Snellen test, vision | Upper limits of visual acuity—20/40 |
| 3. Oral (mouth), ears, nose, throat | Dental prosthesis or caries; abnormalities of the ears, nose, throat |
| 4. Chest, heart, lungs | Heart abnormalities, blood pressure, pulse, murmurs, clarity of lungs |
| 5. Abdomen | Masses, tenderness, organomegaly |
| 6. Genitalia (male only) | Abnormalities of genitalia, hernia |
| 7. Skin | Suspicious rashes or lesions |
| 8. Musculoskeletal | Postural asymmetry, decreased range of motion or strength, abnormal joint laxity |
| 9. Urinalysis | Lab test for sugar and protein |
| 10. Blood work | Lab test to determine hematocrit and sickle cell trait (mandated by NCAA |
| Review | History and physical examination reports are evaluated and the following decisions are made: <br>(a) No sports participation <br>(b) Limited participation (no participation in specific activities or sports) <br>(c) Clearance withheld until certain conditions are met (e.g., additional tests taken, rehabilitation completed) <br>(d) Full, unlimited participation allowed |

Source: Adapted from Myers, GC and Garrick, JG: The preseason examination of school and college athletes. In Strauss, RH (ed.): Sports medicine, Philadelphia: WB Saunders, 1984.

## TABLE 2–2  Recommendations for Activity Restriction and Disqualification

| | Noncontact | | | Contact | |
| --- | --- | --- | --- | --- | --- |
| | Strenuous | Moderately Strenuous | Nonstrenuous | Contact/Collision | Limited Contact/Collision |
| Atlantoaxial instability | Yes* | Yes | Yes | No | No |
| Acute illnesses | * | * | * | * | * |

*Needs individual assessment (e.g., contagiousness to others, risk of worsening illness)

| | Strenuous | Moderately Strenuous | Nonstrenuous | Contact/Collision | Limited Contact/Collision |
| --- | --- | --- | --- | --- | --- |
| Cardiovascular | | | | | |
| Carditis | No | No | No | No | No |
| Hypertension | | | | | |
| Mild | Yes | Yes | Yes | Yes | Yes |
| Moderate | * | * | * | * | * |
| Severe | * | * | * | * | * |
| Congenital heart disease | † | † | † | † | † |

*Needs individual assessment

†Patients with mild forms can be allowed a full range of physical activities; patients with moderate or severe forms or who are postoperative should be evaluated by a cardiologist before athletic participation.

| | Strenuous | Moderately Strenuous | Nonstrenuous | Contact/Collision | Limited Contact/Collision |
| --- | --- | --- | --- | --- | --- |
| Eyes | | | | | |
| Absence or loss of function of eye | * | * | * | * | * |
| Detached retina | † | † | † | † | † |

*Availability of American Society for Testing and Materials (ASTM)–approved eye guards may allow competitor to participate in most sports, but this must be judged on an individual basis.

†Consult ophthalmologist.

| | Strenuous | Moderately Strenuous | Nonstrenuous | Contact/Collision | Limited Contact/Collision |
| --- | --- | --- | --- | --- | --- |
| Inguinal hernia | Yes | Yes | Yes | Yes | Yes |
| Kidney: absence of one | Yes | Yes | Yes | No | Yes |
| Liver: enlarged | Yes | Yes | Yes | No | No |
| Musculoskeletal disorders | * | * | * | * | * |

*Needs individual assessment

| | Strenuous | Moderately Strenuous | Nonstrenuous | Contact/Collision | Limited Contact/Collision |
| --- | --- | --- | --- | --- | --- |
| Neurological status | | | | | |
| History of serious head or spine trauma, repeated concussions, or craniotomy | Yes | Yes | Yes | * | * |
| Convulsive disorder | | | | | |
| Well controlled | Yes | Yes | Yes | Yes | Yes |
| Poorly controlled | Yes† | Yes | Yes†† | No | No |

*Needs individual assessment

†No swimming or weight lifting

††No archery or riflery

| | Strenuous | Moderately Strenuous | Nonstrenuous | Contact/Collision | Limited Contact/Collision |
| --- | --- | --- | --- | --- | --- |
| Ovary: absence of one | Yes | Yes | Yes | Yes | Yes |
| Respiratory status | | | | | |
| Pulmonary insufficiency | * | * | Yes | * | * |
| Asthma | Yes | Yes | Yes | Yes | Yes |

*May be allowed to compete if oxygenation remains satisfactory during a graded stress test

| | Strenuous | Moderately Strenuous | Nonstrenuous | Contact/Collision | Limited Contact/Collision |
| --- | --- | --- | --- | --- | --- |
| Sickle-cell trait | Yes | Yes | Yes | Yes | Yes |
| Skin: Boils, herpes, impetigo, scabies | Yes | Yes | Yes | * | * |

*No gymnastics with mats, martial arts, wrestling, or contact sports until not contagious

| | Strenuous | Moderately Strenuous | Nonstrenuous | Contact/Collision | Limited Contact/Collision |
| --- | --- | --- | --- | --- | --- |
| Spleen: enlarged | No | Yes | Yes | No | No |
| Testicle: absent or undescended | Yes | Yes | Yes | Yes* | Yes* |

*Certain sports may require protective cup.

Source: Data from Committee on Sports Medicine: Pediatrics 81:738, 1988.

statement "Preparticipation Physical Examinations and Disqualifying Conditions" (www.nata.org/sites /default/files/Conley.pdf) that provides guidelines for recommending disqualification of injured athletes.

## Personal Information Card

Always on file on the desktop or tablet in the athletic trainer's office or on the more portable smartphone is the athlete's personal information file. This file is created by the athlete at the time of the health examination and serves as a means of contacting the athlete's family, personal physician, and insurance company in case of emergency.

## Injury Reports and Injury Disposition

An injury report serves as a record for future reference (Figure 2–12). If the emergency procedures followed are

---

# ATHLETE/PATIENT INJURY RECORD FORM

Name _____ Sport _____ Date:___ /___ /___ Time: _____ Injury record number: _____

Player I.D. _____ Age: _____ Location: _____ Intercollegiate—nonintercollegiate

Initial injury     Recheck     Reinjury          Preseason—Practice—Game          Incurred while participating in sport: yes____ no____

Description: How did it happen? _____

_____

Initial impression: _____

_____

_____

| SITE OF INJURY | BODY PART | | STRUCTURE | Treatment Plan _____ |
|---|---|---|---|---|
| 1  Right | 1  Head | 25  MP joint | 1  Skin | _____ |
| 2  Left | 2  Face | 26  PIP joint | 2  Muscle | _____ |
| 3  Proximal | 3  Eye | 27  Abdomen | 3  Fascia | _____ |
| 4  Distal | 4  Nose | 28  Hip | 4  Bone | _____ |
| 5  Anterior | 5  Ear | 29  Thigh | 5  Nerve | _____ |
| 6  Posterior | 6  Mouth | 30  Knee | 6  Fat pad | _____ |
| 7  Medial | 7  Neck | 31  Patella | 7  Tendon | _____ |
| 8  Lateral | 8  Thorax | 32  Lower leg | 8  Ligament | _____ |
| 9  Other | 9  Ribs | 33  Ankle | 9  Cartilage | _____ |
| _____ | 10  Sternum | 34  Achilles tendon | 10  Capsule | _____ |
| | 11  Upper back | 35  Foot | 11  Compartment | |
| **SITE OF EVALUATION** | 12  Lower back | 36  Toes | 12  Dental | |
| 1  Health Service | 13  Shoulder | 37  Other | 13  _____ | |
| 2  Athletic Trn Clinic | 14  Rotator cuff | _____ | | **Medication** _____ |
| 3  Site-Competition | 15  AC joint | _____ | _____ | _____ |
| 4  _____ | 16  Glenohumeral | _____ | _____ | _____ |
| | 17  Sternoclavicular | **NONTRAUMATIC** | **NATURE OF INJURY** | _____ |
| **PROCEDURES** | 18  Upper arm | 1  Dermatological | 1  Contusion | _____ |
| 1  Physical exam | 19  Elbow | 2  Allergy | 2  Strain | _____ |
| 2  X-ray | 20  Forearm | 3  Influenza | 3  Sprain | _____ |
| 3  Splint | 21  Wrist | 4  Urinary | 4  Fracture | _____ |
| 4  Wrap | 22  Hand | 5  Genitourinary | 5  Rupture | _____ |
| 5  Cast | 23  Thumb | 6  Systemic Infection | 6  Tendonitis | _____ |
| 6  Aspiration | 24  Finger | 7  Local Infection | 7  Bursitis | |
| 7  Other | | 8  Other | 8  Myositis | **Prescription Administered** |
| _____ | | | 9  Laceration | 1  Antibiotics      5  Muscle relaxant |
| _____ | | | 10  Concussion | 2  Antiinflammatory  6  Enzyme |
| | | | 11  Avulsion | 3  Decongestant    7 |
| | _____ | _____ | 12  Abrasion | 4  Analgesic    _____ |
| | _____ | _____ | 13  _____ | |
| **DISPOSITION** | **REFERRAL** | **DISPOSITION OF INJURY** | | **INJECTIONS** |
| 1  Health Service | 1  Orthopedic | 1  No part. | | 1  Corticosteroids |
| 2  Athletic Trainer | 2  Neurological | 2  Part part. | Degree | 2  Antibiotics |
| 3  Hospital | 3  Int. Med. | 3  Full part. | 1    2    3 | 3  Analgesics |
| 4  Physician | 4  Mental Health | | | 4  _____ |
| 5  Other | 5  ENT | | | |
| _____ | 6  Dentist | | | |
| | 7  Other | Previous injury _____ | | |
| | _____ | | | |

Physician/Athletic Trainer Signature

FIGURE 2–12   Athletic injury record form.

questioned at a later date, an athletic trainer's memory of the details may be somewhat hazy, but a report completed at the time of injury provides specific information. In a litigation situation, an athletic trainer may be asked questions about an injury that occurred three years in the past. All injury reports should be filed in the athletic trainer's office and in the patient's medical records.

## Patient Treatment Log

Each athletic training clinic should maintain individual daily treatment logs for each patient who receives any service. Emphasis is placed on recording the treatments for the patient who is receiving daily therapy for an injury. Like accident records and injury dispositions, these records often have the status of legal documents and are used to establish certain facts in a civil litigation, an insurance action, or a criminal action after injury.

**Injury Evaluation and Progress Notes** Injuries should be evaluated by the athletic trainer, who must record information obtained in some consistent format. The SOAP format (*S*ubjective, *O*bjective, *A*ssessment, *P*lan for treatment) is a concise method of recording the initial evaluation and progress notes for the injured athlete and is discussed in detail in Chapter 13. The subjective portion of the SOAP note refers to what the patient tells the athletic trainer about the injury relative to the history or what he or she felt. The objective portion documents information that the athletic trainer gathers during the evaluation, such as range of motion, strength levels, patterns of pain, and so forth. The assessment records the athletic trainer's professional opinion about the injury based on the information obtained during the subjective and objective portions. The plan for treatment indicates how the injury will be managed and includes short- and long-term goals for rehabilitation.

## Supply and Equipment Inventory

The athletic trainer is responsible for managing a budget, most of which is spent on equipment and supplies. Every year an inventory must be conducted and recorded on such items as new equipment needed, equipment that needs to be replaced or repaired, and the expendable supplies that need replenishing.

> The athletic trainer has requested that the school purchase a new computer to be housed in the athletic training room. The administrator indicates that funds are tight; however, the athletic trainer is asked to develop a written proposal to justify the purchase.
>
> **?** What information can the athletic trainer include in the request that could justify purchasing a new computer for the athletic training room?

## Annual or Seasonal Reports

Both clinic administrators and athletic administrators require an annual or seasonal report on the functions of the athletic training program. This report serves as a means for making program changes and improvements. It commonly includes the number of patients served, a survey of the number and types of injuries, an analysis of the program, and recommendations for future improvements.

# COMPUTERS, TABLETS, AND SMARTPHONES AS TOOLS FOR THE ATHLETIC TRAINER

As is the case in all of our society, computers, tablets, and smartphones have become indispensable tools for the athletic trainer and have completely revolutionized the way information is managed. A great deal of information can be efficiently located and stored for immediate and future use because of constant improvement in storage and retrieval capacities. Software packages are available to help store and retrieve any type of relevant records or information.[18]

The first step in integrating computers, tablets, and smartphones into an athletic training program is to decide exactly how and for what purposes they will be used. It is essential to seek advice from expert professionals or consultants prior to purchasing a system to ensure that the hardware and corresponding operating system are capable of supporting the software that will make them useful information management and communication tools.

> **Computers facilitate the record-keeping process.**

Thousands of software programs are available that will allow the user to store, manipulate, and retrieve information; create written documents through word processing; analyze data statistically; and communicate with many individuals in a variety of forms.

Record keeping is a time-consuming but essential chore for all athletic trainers regardless of whether they work at a college or university, at a secondary school, in the clinical setting, or in industry. Several software packages are available specifically for managing injury records in the athletic training setting. A problem that athletic trainers must address is ensuring security and protecting the confidentiality of medical records stored on a computer, tablet, or smartphone. Databases that contain such information must be accessible only to the athletic trainer or team physician/medical director and must be protected by a password.

Besides record keeping, software can also be used for budgeting and inventory; managing a personal schedule or calendar; and creating a database or a spreadsheet from which injury data can be organized, retrieved, or related to specific injury situations or other injury records for statistical analysis. Other software can analyze and provide information about nutrition, body composition, and injury risk profiles based on other anthropometric measures and can be used to record isokinetic evaluation and exercise.[36]

The use of educational software to assist in teaching and the academic preparation of athletic training students has become an integral component in the majority of athletic training educational programs. New instructional and educational software with interactive capabilities of eBooks has made the multimedia presentation of instructional material, and thus learning, more interesting and effective for the athletic training student.

The Internet and the World Wide Web have impacted and changed all of our lives. We live in a world where any kind of information is immediately accessible to anyone who knows how to use the system. The sports medicine community in general and the athletic trainer specifically can access thousands of Web sites and apps that have direct application to clinical practice, to the education of athletic training students, and to the general base of knowledge that is relevant to the field.

# COLLECTING INJURY DATA

Because of the vast number of physically active individuals involved with organized and recreational sports, some knowledge relative to the number and types of injuries sustained during participation in these activities is essential.[47] Although methods are much improved over the past, many weaknesses exist in systematic data collection and analysis of sports injuries.[28]

## The Incidence of Injuries

An **accident** is an unplanned event capable of resulting in loss of time, property damage, injury, disablement, or even death.[57] An **injury** may be defined as damage to the body that restricts activity or causes disability to such an extent that the patient is not able to practice or compete the next day.[57]

Injury data may be analyzed by looking at several factors. The *incidence* of injury analyzes the risk of sustaining an injury during some specified time period (i.e., practice, games). Injury *prevalence* analyzes the total number of injuries in a specific population. *Incidence rate* is the number of new injuries that occur in a particular population during a specified time period. Injury *exposure rates* look at the incidence of injuries per the number of individual athlete exposures during a specific time period. Risk factors that might potentially contribute to the incidence of injury can be analyzed using outcome studies to determine the strength of their relevance and whether modifying these risk factors is effective in reducing injury rates.[6,58]

> The epidemiological approach toward injury data collection provides the most information.

> Risk of injury is determined by the type of sport—contact or collision, limited contact, or noncontact.

There is little doubt that a *case study* approach, which looks at one incidence of an injury, can yield some critical information about the cause and subsequent efficacy of treatment for that injury. However, an approach that analyzes a large number of similar injuries can provide the greatest amount of information. In general, the incidence of sports injuries can be studied epidemiologically from many points of view—in terms of age at occurrence, gender, body regions that sustain injuries, or the occurrence in different sports.[58] Sports are usually classified according to the risk, or chances, of injuries occurring under similar circumstances and are broadly divided into contact or collision, limited contact, or noncontact[2] (Table 2–3).

Athletes in all sports, recreational and organized, who participate in sports in the span of one year face a 50 percent chance of sustaining some injury. Of the 50 million estimated sports injuries per year, 50 percent require only minor care and no restriction of activity.[28] Approximately 90 percent of injuries are muscle contusions, ligament sprains, and muscle strains; however, 10 percent of these injuries lead to microtrauma complications and eventually to a severe, chronic condition in later life.

Of the sports injuries that must be medically treated, sprains or strains, fractures, dislocations, and contusions are the most common.[28] In terms of the body regions most often injured, the knee has the highest incidence, with the ankle second and the upper limb third. For both males and females the most commonly injured body part is the knee, followed by the ankle; however, males have a much higher incidence of shoulder and upper-arm injuries than do females.

## Catastrophic Injuries

Although millions of individuals participate in organized and recreational sports, there is a relatively low incidence of fatalities or catastrophic injuries. Ninety-eight percent of individuals with injuries requiring

| TABLE 2–3 | Classification of Sports* | |
|---|---|---|
| **Noncontact** | **Limited Contact** | **Contact or Collision** |
| Weight lifting | Windsurfing or surfing | Wrestling |
| Track | Volleyball | Water polo |
| Tennis | Ultimate Frisbee | Team handball |
| Table tennis | Squash | Soccer |
| Swimming | Softball | Ski jumping |
| Shot put | Snowboarding | Rugby |
| Scuba diving | Skiing (cross-country, downhill, water) | Rodeo |
| Sailing | Skating (ice, in-line, roller) | Martial arts |
| Running | Skateboarding | Lacrosse |
| Rope jumping | Racquetball | Ice hockey |
| Riflery | Pole vault | Football (tackle) |
| Race walking | Horseback riding | Field hockey |
| Power lifting | High jump | Diving |
| Orienteering | Handball | Boxing |
| Javelin | Gymnastics | Baseball |
| Golf | Football (flag) | |
| Field events | Floor hockey | |
| Discus | Field events | |
| Dancing (ballet, modern, Jazz) | Fencing | |
| Curling | Cheerleading | |
| Crew or rowing | Canoeing or kayaking (white water) | |
| Canoeing or kayaking (flat water) | Bicycling | |
| Bowling | Baseball | |
| Bodybuilding | | |
| Badminton | | |
| Archery | | |

Source: Data from the American Academy of Pediatrics Committee on Sports Medicine and Fitness: Medical conditions affecting sports participation, Pediatrics 107(5):1205, 2001.

hospital emergency room medical attention are treated and released.[9] Deaths have been attributed to chest or trunk impact with projectiles, other players, or nonyielding objects (e.g., goalposts). Deaths have occurred when players were struck in the head by sports implements (bats, golf clubs, hockey sticks) or by missiles (baseballs, soccer balls, golf balls, hockey pucks). Death has also resulted when an individual received a direct blow to the head from another player or the ground. On record are a number of sports deaths in which a playing structure, such as a goalpost or backstop, fell on a participant.

The highest incidence of indirect sports death stems from heatstroke. Less common indirect causes include cardiovascular and respiratory problems or congenital conditions not previously known. Catastrophic injuries leading to cervical injury and quadriplegia are seen mainly in American football. Although the incidence is low for the number of players involved, it could be lowered even further if more precautions were taken.[38]

In most popular organized and recreational sports activities, the legs and arms have the highest risk factor for injury, with the head and face next. Muscle strains, joint sprains, contusions, and abrasions are the most frequent injuries sustained by the active sports participant. The major goal of this text is to provide the reader with the fundamental principles necessary for preventing and managing illnesses and injuries common to the athlete.

## Current National Injury Data-Gathering Systems

The state of the art of sports injury surveillance is unsatisfactory.[57] Currently, most local, state, and federal systems are concerned with the accident or injury only after it has happened, and they focus on injuries requiring medical assistance or those that cause time loss or restricted activity.

The ideal system takes an epidemiological approach.[57] **Epidemiology** is the scientific study of factors affecting the health and illness of individuals and populations.[58] Epidemiology takes an evidence-based approach for identifying risk factors for injury and determining optimal treatment methods in clinical practice. It serves as the foundation for interventions made in the interest of public health and preventive medicine. When considering the risks inherent in a particular sport, both extrinsic and intrinsic factors must be studied. [42] Thus, information is gleaned from both epidemiological data and the individual measurements of the athlete. The term *extrinsic factor* refers to the type of activity that is performed, the amount of exposure to injury, factors in the environment, and the equipment. The term *intrinsic factor* refers directly to the athlete and includes age, gender, neuromuscular aspects, structural aspects, performance aspects, and mental and psychological aspects.

Over the years, a number of athletic injury surveillance systems have been implemented; most have collected data for a few years and then ceased to exist. The currently active systems that are most often mentioned are the National Safety Council, the Annual Survey of Football Injury Research, the National Center for Catastrophic Sports Injury Research, the NCAA Injury Surveillance System, the National Electronic Injury Surveillance System (NEISS), and the National High School Sports-Related Injury Surveillance Study.

**National Safety Council** The National Safety Council* is a nongovernmental, nonprofit public service organization. It draws sports injury data from a variety of sources, including educational institutions.

**Annual Survey of Football Injury Research** In 1931, the American Football Coaches Association (AFCA) conducted its first Annual Survey of Football Fatalities. Since 1965, this research has been conducted at the University of North Carolina. In 1980, the survey's title was changed to the Annual Survey of Football Injury Research. Every year, with the exception of 1942, data have been collected about public school, college, professional, and sandlot football. Information is gathered through personal contact interviews and questionnaires. The sponsoring organizations of this survey are the AFCA, the NCAA, and the National Federation of State High School Associations (NFHS).

This survey classifies football fatalities as direct or indirect. Direct fatalities are those resulting directly from participation in football. Indirect fatalities are produced by systemic failure caused by the exertion of playing football or by a complication that arose from a nonfatal football injury.

**National Center for Catastrophic Sports Injury Research** In 1977, the NCAA initiated the National Survey of Catastrophic Football Injuries. As a result of the injury data collected from this organization, several

significant rule changes have been incorporated into collegiate football. Because of the success of this football project, the research was expanded to all sports for both men and women, and a National Center for Catastrophic Sports Injury Research was established at the University of North Carolina. With support from the NCAA, the NFHS, the AFCA, and the Section on Sports Medicine of the American Association of Neurological Sciences, this center compiles data on catastrophic injuries at all levels of sport.[9]

**NCAA Injury Surveillance System** The NCAA Injury Surveillance System (ISS) was established in 1982 primarily for the purpose of studying the incidence of football injuries, so that rule change recommendations could be made to reduce the injury rate.[16] Since that time, this system has been greatly expanded and now collects data on most major sports. For the most part, athletic trainers are primarily involved in the collection and transmission of injury data.

The ISS had previously relied on the willingness of athletic trainers to submit paper forms reporting injuries in various NCAA-sponsored sports. In Fall 2004, the ISS fully converted to a Web-based data-collection system that can compile far more data than ever before, providing member institutions with a low-cost means of tracking medical information and analyzing injury trends.

> A collegiate athletic trainer is approached by the school administration to determine the potential risk of injury to their football team.
>
> **?** What approach is best suited to gather this information?

**National Electronic Injury Surveillance System** In 1972, the federal government established the Consumer Product Safety Act (CPSA), which created and granted broad authority to the Consumer Product Safety Commission to enforce the safety standards for more than 10,000 products that may be risky to the consumer.[57] To perform this mission, the National Electronic Injury Surveillance System (NEISS)† was established. Data on injuries related to consumer products are monitored 24 hours a day from a selected sample of 5,000 hospital emergency rooms nationwide. Sports injuries represent 25 percent of all injuries reported by NEISS. It should be noted that a product may be related to an injury, but not be the direct cause of that injury.[57]

---

*National Safety Council, Itasca, IL.

†National Electronic Injury Surveillance System, U.S. Consumer Product Safety Commission, Directorate for Epidemiology, National Injury Information Clearinghouse, Washington, DC.

Once a product is considered hazardous, the commission can seize the product or create standards to decrease the risk. Also, manufacturers and distributors of sports recreational equipment must report to the commission any product that is potentially hazardous or defective. The commission can also research the reasons that a sports or recreational product is hazardous.

## National High School Sports-Related Injury Surveillance Study

The National High School Sports-Related Injury Surveillance Study, administered through the Center for Injury Research and Policy, was first implemented in 2005 and has collected data annually since then. It was first established as the high-school version of the NCAA Injury Surveillance System. Known as High School RIO™, it is an Internet-based data collection tool that looks at time-loss injuries in a national sample of U.S. high-school athletes. This system collects data weekly on athlete exposure, injury type, and the injury event, using certified, licensed athletic trainers to provide data.[57] The data collected meets the needs of the high-school sports community that includes student-athletes, parents, pediatric sports medicine clinicians, high-school athletic directors, local/state high-school athletic associations/administrators, and the NFHS (National Federation of State High School Associations).[15]

## Using Injury Data

Valid, reliable sports injury data can materially help decrease injuries. If properly interpreted, the data can be used to modify rules, assist parents, coaches, and players in understanding risks, and help manufacturers evaluate their products against the overall market. The public, especially parents, should understand the risks inherent in a particular sport, and insurance companies that insure athletes must know risks in order to set reasonable costs.

## SUMMARY

- The administration of a program of health care demands a significant portion of the athletic trainer's time and effort. The efficiency and success of the athletic training program depend in large part on the administrative abilities of the athletic trainer in addition to the clinical skills required to treat the injured patient.
- The athletic training health care program may best serve the athlete; the hospital, clinic, or corporation; and the community by establishing specific policies, procedures, and regulations governing the use of available services.
- An athletic training program in secondary schools, colleges, and universities should decide whom the program will serve and how coverage will be provided, establish rules for hygiene and sanitation of the facility, develop a budget, develop a risk management plan, and address human resources and personnel issues.
- The athletic training program can be enhanced by designing or renovating a facility to maximize the potential use of the space available. Space designed for injury treatment, rehabilitation, modality use, office space, physician examination, record keeping, and storage of supplies should be designated within each facility.
- An athletic training program in the hospital, clinical, corporate, or industrial setting must decide what type of patients will be treated in that facility; how that facility can best serve that patient population; how to resolve clinic personnel and human resources issues; exactly what an athletic trainer might be responsible for in the day-to-day operation of that facility; and the fiscal management issues in a for-profit clinic.
- Preparticipation exams must be given to athletes and should include a medical history, a general physical examination, and orthopedic screenings.
- The athletic trainer must maintain accurate and up-to-date medical records in addition to the other administrative tasks that are necessary for the operation of the athletic training program in all settings in which an athletic trainer may work.
- Computers, tablets, and smartphones are extremely useful tools that enable athletic trainers to retrieve and store a variety of records.
- A number of data-collection systems tabulate the incidence of sports injuries. The systems mentioned most often are the National Safety Council, the Annual Survey of Football Injury Research, the National Electronic Injury Surveillance System, the NCAA Injury Surveillance System, the National Center for Catastrophic Sports Injury Research, and the National High School Sports-Related Injury Surveillance Study.

## WEB SITES

National Athletic Trainers Association Position, Official, Consensus, and Support Statements

*Preparticipation Physical Examinations and Disqualifying Conditions:* www.nata.org/sites/default/files/Conley.pdf

*Skin Diseases:* www.nata.org/sites/default/files/position-statement-skin-disease.pdf

*Sickle Cell Trait and the Athlete:* www.nata.org/sites/default/files/SickleCellTraitAndTheAthlete.pdf

*Appropriate Medical Care for Secondary School-Age Athletes:* www.nata.org/sites/default/files/appropriatemedicalcare4secondaryschoolageathletes.pdf

*Emergency Planning in Athletics:* www.nata.org/sites/default/files/EmergencyPlanningInAthletics.pdf

## SOLUTIONS TO CLINICAL APPLICATION EXERCISES

2–1 The athletic trainer should work in conjunction with the appropriate administrative personnel to develop a risk management plan that includes security issues, fire safety, electrical and equipment safety, and emergency injury management.

2–2 Federal law mandates specific policies for recruitment, hiring, and firing. All qualified applicants should receive equal consideration regardless of their race, gender, religion, or nationality. The head athletic trainer must strictly adhere to these mandates.

2–3 The athletic training clinic should have specific areas designated for taping and preparation, treatment and rehabilitation, and hydrotherapy. It should have an office for the athletic trainer and adequate storage facilities positioned within the space to allow for an efficient traffic flow. Equipment purchases might include four or five treatment tables and two or three taping tables (these could be made in-house, if possible), a large-capacity ice machine, a combination ultrasound/electrical stimulating unit, a whirlpool, and various free weights and exercise tubing.

2–4 The athletic trainer should take this request to the clinic administrator to have it approved. They must decide on a fee for treating these patients and hours for treatment. A decision should also be made about personnel for game and event coverage. A budget should also be developed for supplies and equipment.

2–5 The preparticipation examination should consist of a medical history, a physical examination, and a brief orthopedic screening. The preparticipation physical may be effectively administered using a station examination system with a team of examiners. A station examination can provide the athlete with a detailed examination in a short period of time. A team of people is needed to examine this many individuals. The team should include several physicians, medically trained nonphysicians (nurses, athletic trainers, physical therapists, or physician's assistants), and managers, athletic training students, or assistant coaches.

2–6 The athletic trainer should explain that the computer can be used for maintaining medical records, word processing, planning a budget, managing a personal schedule or calendar, and creating a database containing injury data that can be organized, retrieved, or related to specific injury situations or to other injury records for analysis. Additional software can provide the athletic trainer with analysis and information about nutrition, body composition, and injury risk profiles.

2–7 The athletic trainer should do a simple study in which one-half of the players are randomly placed in the ankle braces while the other half continue to play in their high-top shoes. By comparing the number of ankle injuries in the group wearing the braces with those in the group without the braces, the athletic trainer can make a decision as to the effectiveness of the braces in preventing ankle injuries. Collecting and analyzing injury data is helpful in determining the efficacy of many of the techniques used by the athletic trainer.

2–8 The NCAA Injury Surveillance System would best suit this purpose. This system of information can also be used to prevent injuries by presenting information to coaches, referees, and administrators to enforce necessary changes to the football program.

## REVIEW QUESTIONS AND CLASS ACTIVITIES

1. What are the major administrative functions that an athletic trainer must perform?
2. Design two athletic training clinics—one for a secondary school and one for a large university.
3. Observe the activities in the athletic training clinic. Pick both a slow time and a busy time to observe.
4. Why do hygiene and sanitation play an important role in athletic training? How should the athletic training clinic be maintained?
5. Fully equip a new medium-size secondary-school, college, or clinical athletic training clinic. Pick equipment from current catalogs.
6. Establish a reasonable budget for a small secondary school, a large high school, and a large college or university.
7. Identify the groups or individuals to be served in a collegiate athletic training clinic.
8. What job duties and responsibilities might an athletic trainer be assigned when working in a clinic, hospital, corporate, or industrial setting?
9. Help organize a preparticipation health examination for ninety football players.
10. Record keeping is a major function in athletic training. What records are necessary to keep? How can a computer help?
11. Debate what conditions constitute good grounds for medical disqualification from a sport.
12. Discuss the epidemiological approach to recording sports injury data.

## REFERENCES

1. American Academy of Pediatrics: *Preparticipation physical evaluation,* ed 4, Elk Grove Village, IL, 2010, American Academy of Pediatrics.
2. American Academy of Pediatrics Committee on Sports Medicine and Fitness: Medical conditions affecting sports participation, *Pediatrics* 107(5):1205, 2001.
3. Ammon R: *Sport facility management: Organizing events and mitigating risks,* Morgantown, WV, 2010. Fitness Information Technology.
4. Anderson B: Policies and philosophies related to risk management in the athletic setting, *Athletic Therapy Today,* 11(1):10, 2006.
5. Anderson J, et al.: National Athletic Trainers' Association Position Statement: Emergency planning in athletics, *J Athl Train* 37(1):99, 2002.
6. Armsey T: Medical aspects of sports: Epidemiology of injuries, preparticipation physical examination, and drugs in sports, *Clin Sports Med* 23(2):255–79, 2004.
7. Bagnall D: Budget planning key in secondary schools, *NATA News,* January 15, 2001.

8. Barker A: Developing a crisis management plan. *Athletics Administration* 40(2):41, 2005.

9. Boden, B: Catastrophic injuries in pole-vaulters, *Am J Sports Med* 29(1):50, 2001.

10. Borjesson M: Is there evidence for mandating electrocardiogram as part of the pre-participation examination?, *Clinical Journal of Sports Medicine* 21(1):13–17,2011.

11. Brown J: Athletic training facilities. In Sawyer T, editor: *Facilities planning for health, fitness, physical activity, recreation & sports* , Champaign, IL, 2013, Sagamore Publishing.

12. Claiborne T: Certified athletic trainers provide effective care in the high school setting, *Athletic Therapy Today* 12(2):34, 2007.

13. Conley K, et al. National Athletic Trainers' Association position statement: Preparticipation physical examinations and disqualifying conditions, *Journal of Athletic Training*, 49(1):102–20, 2014.

14. Curtis N: Risk management, *Athletic Therapy Today* 11(1):34, 2006.

15. Darrow, C: Epidemiology of severe injuries among United States high school athletes 2005–2007, *American Journal of Sports Medicine* 37(9):1798–1805, 2009.

16. Dick R: NCAA injury surveillance system: A tool for health and safety risk management, *Athletic Therapy Today* 11(1):42, 2006.

17. Eickhoff-Shemek J: *Risk management for health/fitness professionals: Legal issues and strategies*, Baltimore, MD: 2008, Lippincott, Williams & Wilkins.

18. Eng J: Computerizing clinical documentation, *Phys Ther* 14(6):36, 2006.

19. Fried G: *Managing sport facilities*. Champaign, IL, 2015, Human Kinetics.

20. Goforth M: Understanding organization structures of the college, university, high school, clinical, and professional settings. *Clinics in Sports Medicine* 26(2):201, 2007.

21. Gratto J: *Management principles for health professionals*, Burlington, MA, 2011, Jones and Bartlett Learning.

22. Harrelson G: *Administrative topics in athletic training: Concepts to practice*, Thorofare, NJ, 2009, Slack.

23. Herbert D: Emergency preparedness recommendations for high school and college athletic programs. *Sports, Parks & Recreation Law Reporter* 21(1):71, 2007.

24. Jonas J: Ethics in injury management, *Athletic Therapy Today* 11(1):28, 2006.

25. Jones D: HIPAA: Friend or foe to athletic trainers? *Athletic Therapy Today* 8(2):17, 2003.

26. Keil J: HIPAA and FERPA: Competing or collaborating? *Journal of Allied Health* 39(4):161–65, 2010.

27. Knight K: Athletic training clinic operations. In Knight K, editor: *Developing clinical proficiency in athletic training,* ed 3, Champaign, IL, Human Kinetics, pp. 14–19, 2009.

28. Knowles S: Issues in estimating risks and rates in sports injury research, *J Athl Train* 41(2):207, 2006.

29. Koester M: Preparticipation screening of high school athletes: Are recommendations enough? *Physician Sportsmed* 31(8):330, 2003.

30. Konin J: The athletic trainer as a personnel manager. In Konin J, editor: *The clinical athletic trainer,* Gaithersburg, MD, 1997, Slack.

31. Krager C: HIPAA for health care professionals, Independence, KY, 2008, Cengage Learning.

32. Kurtz M: Leadership in athletic training: Implications for practice and education in allied health care, *Journal of Allied Health* , 39(4):265–79, 2010.

33. Landry G: Preparticipation physical examination. In Landry G, editor: *Essentials of primary care sports medicine,* Champaign, IL, 2003, Human Kinetics.

34. Marshall A: Challenges and opportunities for promoting physical activity in the workplace, *Journal of Science and Medicine in Sport* 7(1 Supplement):60, 2004.

35. Mirwald R: An assessment of maturity from anthropometric measurements. *Med Sci Sports Exerc* 34(4):689, 2002.

36. Moss R: Facilities and foibles, *Athletic Therapy Today* 7(1):22, 2002.

37. Moyer-Knowles J: Planning a new athletic facility. In Konin J, editor: *The clinical athletic trainer,* Gaithersburg, MD, 1997, Slack.

38. Mueller F: Fatal and catastrophic injuries in athletics: Epidemiological data and challenging circumstances. In Casa D, editor: *Preventing sudden death in sport and physical activity*, Sudbury, MA, 2012, Jones and Bartlett.

39. Oliver, C: Athletic training room essentials. Interscholastic, *Athletic Administration* 28(4):21, 2002.

40. Peterson E: Insult to injury: Feeling understaffed, underequipped and undervalued, athletic trainers say minimum of space and equipment will yield extensive benefits, *Athletic Business* 23(1):57, 1999.

41. *Physician and sportsmedicine: Preparticipation physical evaluation monograph*, ed 3, New York, 2004, McGraw-Hill.

42. Rankin J: *Athletic training management: Concepts and applications,* St. Louis, 2006, McGraw-Hill.

43. Ray R: Where athletic trainers work: Facility design and planning. In Ray R, Konin J, editors: *Management strategies in athletic training*, ed 4, Champaign, IL, 2011, Human Kinetics.

44. Ray R, Konin J, editors: *Management strategies in athletic training,* ed 4, Champaign, IL, 2011, Human Kinetics.

45. Sabo J: *Athletic training room design and layout.* In Proceedings, National Athletic Trainers' Association 50th Annual Meeting and Clinical Symposium, June 16–19, 1999, Kansas City, MO, 1999, Human Kinetics.

46. Sabo J: Design and construction of an athletic training facility, *NATA News,* May 10, 2001.

47. Schiff M: Soccer injuries in female youth players: Comparison of injury surveillance by certified athletic trainers and Internet, *J Athl Train*, 45(3):238–42, 2010.

48. Schwartz E: *Sport facility operations management*. St. Louis, 2010, Elsevier.

49. Shappy J: Preparticipation exam to identify risk for sudden cardiac death, *Athletic Training and Therapy* , 14(6):13–16, 2009.

50. Shephard R: Supervision of occupational fitness assessments, *Canadian Journal of Applied Physiology* 28(2):225, 2003.

51. Streator S: Risk management in athletic training, *Athletic Therapy Today* 6(2):55, 2001.

52. Swann E: Managing risk in an athletic training education program, *Athletic Therapy Today* 11(1):17, 2006.

53. Tanner M: *Growth of adolescence,* ed 2, Oxford, England, 1962, Blackwell Scientific.

54. Von Fange T: The preparticipation physical exam. In Hoffman R, editor: *Common musculoskeletal problems*, New York, 2010, Springer.

55. Wham G: Key factors for providing appropriate medical care in secondary school athletics: Athletic training services and budget, *J Athl Train* 45(1):75–86, 2010.

56. Wilson A: *Effective management of musculoskeletal injury: A clinical ergonomics approach to prevention, treatment, and rehabilitation,* Philadelphia, 2002, Churchill Livingstone.

57. Yard E: A comparison of high school sports injury surveillance data reporting by certified athletic trainers and coaches, *J Athl Train*, 44(6):645–52, 2009.

58. Zemper E: Epidemiology of athletic injuries. In McKeag D: *ACSM's primary care sports medicine*, Philadelphia, 2007, Lippincott, Williams & Wilkins.

59. Zinder S, et al.: National Athletic Trainers' Association Position Statement: Skin diseases, *Journal of Athletic Training* 45(4):411–28, 2010.

## ANNOTATED BIBLIOGRAPHY

Board of Certification. BOC facility principles, 2013, www.bocatc.org/imstories/resources/boc_facility_safety_1404af.pdf

*This document provides the means for secondary and postsecondary educational institutions and organizations to self-assess their policies, procedures, and facilities to ensure the safe, effective, and legal provision of athletic health care services.*

Harrelson G, Gardner G, Winterstein A: *Administrative topics in athletic training: Concepts to practice*, Thoroughfare, NJ, 2009, Slack Incorporated.

*Addresses important administrative issues and procedures as well as fundamental concepts, strategies, and techniques related to the management of all aspects of an athletic training health care delivery system.*

Karwowski W, Marras W: *Occupational ergonomics: engineering and administrative controls,* Boca Raton, FL, 2003, CRC Press.

*Focuses on prevention of work-related musculoskeletal disorders with an emphasis on engineering and administrative controls.*

Konin J: *The clinical athletic trainer,* Gaithersburg, MD, 1997, Slack.

A unique, practical book that specifically addresses the administration of a health care program for athletic trainers working in a
clinical setting.

Konin J, Frederick M: *Documentation for athletic training,* Thorofare,
NJ, 2011, Slack.

Presents the basic principles of medical documentation, various
styles of writing, legal considerations, documentation for reimbursement, and many types of written documentation, including
evaluations, injury reports, medical releases, and the like.

Mueller F, Cantu R: *Football fatalities and catastrophic injuries
1931–2008,* Durham, NC, 2011, Carolina Academic Press.

This text summarizes the epidemiologic data that has been collected on catastrophic injuries in football and other sports that
has been collected over the past 70+ years.

Occupational Safety and Health Administration: Ergonomics for the prevention of Musculoskeletal disorders, Washington, D.C., 2011, U.S.
Department of Labor.

Provides recommendations for industrial facilities to reduce the
number and severity of work-related musculoskeletal disorders.

Rankin J, Ingersoll C: *Athletic training management: concepts and applications,* St. Louis, 2006, McGraw-Hill.

Designed for upper-division undergraduate or graduate students
interested in all aspects of organization and administration of an
athletic training program.

Ray R, Konin J: *Management strategies in athletic training,* Champaign,
IL, 2011. Human Kinetics.

The first text that covered the principles of organization and
administration as they apply to many different employment settings in athletic training; contains many examples and case studies based on principles of administration presented in the text.

Wilson A, Boyling J: *Effective management of musculoskeletal injury: a
clinical ergonomics approach to prevention, treatment, and rehabilitation,* Philadelphia, 2002, Churchill Livingstone.

A practical guide designed to help clinicians understand the
workplace and lifestyle factors that contribute to musculoskeletal
injuries. Examines ergonomic causes as well as personal and psychosocial factors, in addition to discussing cumulative and
chronic types of injury.

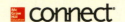

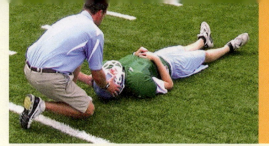
© William E. Prentice

**3**

# Legal Concerns and Insurance Issues

## ■ Objectives

*When you finish this chapter you should be able to*

- Analyze the legal considerations for the athletic trainer acting as a health care provider.
- Define the legal concepts of torts, negligence, and assumption of risk.
- Identify measures that the athletic trainer can take to minimize the chances of litigation.

- Explain product liability.
- Categorize the essential insurance requirements for the protection of the patient.
- Classify the types of insurance necessary to protect the athletic trainer who is acting as a health care provider.

## ■ Outline

## ■ Key Terms

liability
negligence
torts
nonfeasance
malfeasance
misfeasance
duty of care

sovereign immunity
Good Samaritan law
assumption of risk
health insurance
managed care
Affordable Care Act (ACA)

## ■ Connect Highlights   connect

*Visit connect.mcgraw-hill.com for further exercises to apply your knowledge:*

- Clinical application scenarios covering chances of litigation, legal considerations, and insurance
- Click-and-drag questions covering legal considerations and insurance nomenclature
- Multiple-choice questions covering legal concepts and considerations, litigation, and insurance
- Selection questions covering chances of litigation

# LEGAL CONCERNS FOR THE ATHLETIC TRAINER

Ours is a litigious society in which legal actions and subsequent lawsuits have become the rule rather than the exception.[35,43] Nowhere is this more true than in our health care system. Ironically, athletic trainers, like all health care providers, are constantly held accountable both for things they do and things they don't do when treating patients. The potential always exists that techniques and procedures athletic trainers use in providing health care will result in some legal action regarding issues of liability and negligence, regardless of the setting in which they practice.[33] **Liability** means being legally responsible for the harm one causes another person.[35] A great deal of care must be taken in following athletic training procedures to reduce the risk of being sued by an athlete and being found liable for negligence.[3,12,35,41]

## The Standard of Reasonable Care

**Negligence** is the failure to use reasonable care—care that persons would normally exercise to avoid injury to themselves or to others under similar circumstances.[14] The *standard of reasonable care* assumes that an individual is neither exceptionally skillful nor extraordinarily cautious but is a person of reasonable and ordinary prudence. Put another way, it is expected that an individual will be thoughtful and careful relative to the situation at hand and will exercise due care in its handling. In most cases in which someone has been sued for negligence, the actions of a hypothetical, reasonably prudent person are compared with the actions of the defendant to ascertain whether the course of action the defendant followed was in conformity with the judgment exercised by such a reasonably prudent person.[16] Essentially, an athletic trainer is held to a reasonable prudent professional standard, rather than a reasonably prudent person standard.

The standard of reasonable care requires that an athletic trainer act according to the standard of care of an individual with similar educational background or training.[16] An athletic trainer who is well educated in his or her field and who is certified and/or licensed must act in accordance with those qualifications.

## Torts

**Torts** are legal wrongs committed against the person or property of another.[34] All individuals are expected to conduct themselves without injuring others. When they do so, either intentionally or by negligence, they can be required by a court to pay money to the injured party ("damages"), so that ultimately the defendants need to "fix" their intentional or careless mistake by paying for the harm they cause. Punitive damages can "make them suffer," but those are only awarded for intentional torts.

A tort also serves as a deterrent by sending a message that people should expect to pay if they intentionally harm others.

Such wrongs may emanate from **nonfeasance** (also referred to as an *act of omission*), wherein the individual fails to perform a legal duty; from **malfeasance** (also referred to as an *act of commission*), wherein an individual commits an act that is not legally his or hers to perform; or from **misfeasance,** wherein an individual improperly does something that he or she has the legal right to do.[21] In any instance, if injury results, the person can be held liable. In the case of nonfeasance, an athletic trainer may fail to refer a seriously injured patient for the proper medical attention. In the case of malfeasance, the athletic trainer may perform a therapeutic treatment that violates the practice of another licensed health care professional and as a result serious medical complications develop. In a case of misfeasance, the athletic trainer may incorrectly administer a treatment technique procedure he or she has been trained to perform.

**Negligence** If an athletic trainer is sued, the complaint typically is for the tort of negligence. To establish negligence, an individual making the complaint must establish four things: (1) a **duty of care** existed between the person injured and the person responsible for that injury; (2) the defendant breached this duty by conduct that fell short of the standard of care; (3) the defendant caused the injury to occur; and (4) personal, property, or punitive damages resulted.[24] If the athletic trainer breaches a duty to exercise reasonable care, but there is no reasonable connection between the failure to use reasonable care and the injury suffered, the suit for negligence will not succeed.

An example of negligence is when an athletic trainer, through improper or careless handling of a therapeutic agent, seriously burns a patient. Another illustration, occurring all too often in sports, is one in which a coach or some other individual moves a possibly seriously injured athlete from the field of play to permit competition or practice to continue and does so either in an improper manner or before consulting those qualified to know the proper course of action. Should a serious or disabling injury result, the individual who made the decision may be found liable.[24]

Athletic trainers employed by an institution have a duty to provide athletic training care to individuals at that institution. An athletic trainer who is employed by the public schools or by a state-funded college or university may be protected by the legal doctrine of **sovereign immunity,** which essentially states that neither the government nor any individual who is employed by the government can be held liable for negligence. However, it should be made clear that the level of protection afforded by sovereign immunity may vary significantly from state to state.

A baseball batter was struck with a pitched ball directly in the orbit of the right eye and fell immediately to the ground. The athletic trainer ran to the player to examine the eye. There was some immediate swelling and discoloration around the orbit, but the eye appeared to be normal. The player insisted that he was fine and told the athletic trainer he could continue to bat. After the game the athletic trainer told the patient to go back to his room, put ice on his eye, and check in tomorrow. That night the baseball player began to hemorrhage into the anterior chamber of the eye and suffered irreparable damage to his eye. An ophthalmologist stated that if the patient's eye had been examined immediately after the injury, the bleeding could have been controlled and there would not have been any damage to his vision.

**?** If the patient brings a lawsuit against the athletic trainer, what must the patient prove if he is to win a judgment?

Clinical athletic trainers have a greater choice than institutional athletic trainers of whom they may choose to treat as a patient. Once the athletic trainer assumes the duty of caring for a patient, the athletic trainer has an obligation to make sure that appropriate care is given. It should be made clear that the athletic trainer, or any other person, is not obligated to provide first-aid care for an injured person outside his or her scope of employment. However, if the athletic trainer chooses to become involved as a caregiver for an injured person, he or she is expected to provide reasonable care consistent with his or her level of training. The **Good Samaritan law** has been enacted in most states to provide limited protection against legal liability to any individual who voluntarily chooses to provide first aid, should something go wrong. As long as the first-aid provider does not overstep the limits of his or her professional training and exercises what would be considered reasonable care in the situation, the provider will not be held liable. Good Samaritan laws vary tremendously from state to state, so it is important for athletic trainers to know the laws of their state.

A person possessing more training in a given field or area is expected to possess a correspondingly higher level of competence than is a student.[15] An individual will therefore be judged in terms of his or her performance in any situation in which legal liability may be assessed. It must be recognized that liability per se in all its various aspects is not assessed at the same level nationally, but varies in interpretation from state to state and from area to area. Athletic trainers therefore should know and acquire the level of competence expected in their particular area. In essence, negligence is conduct that results in the creation of an unreasonable risk of harm to others.[10]

## Statutes of Limitation

A *statute of limitation* sets a specific length of time that individuals may sue for damages from negligence.[39] The length of time to bring suit varies from state to state, but in general plaintiffs have between one and five years to file suit for negligence. The statute of limitations begins to run on a plaintiff's time to file a lawsuit for negligence either from the time of the negligent act or omission that gives rise to the suit or from the time of the discovery of an injury caused by the negligent act or omission. Some states permit an injured minor to file suit up to three years after the minor reaches the age of 18.[7] Therefore, an injured minor's cause of action for negligence against an athletic trainer remains valid for many years after the negligent act or omission occurred or after the discovery of an injury caused by the negligent act or omission.[7]

**?** How should the first-aid care provided by a certified athletic trainer working in a health club differ from the care that may be provided by a lay person?

3–2 Clinical Application Exercise

## Assumption of Risk

An athlete assumes the risk of participating in an activity when he or she knows of and understands the dangers of that activity and voluntarily chooses to be exposed to those dangers. An assumption of risk can be expressed in the form of a waiver signed by an athlete or his or her parents or guardian or can be implied from the conduct of an athlete under the circumstances of his or her participation in an activity.[7]

**Assumption of risk** may be asserted as a defense to a negligence suit. The athletic trainer bears the burden of proving that an individual assumed the risk. One way of proving this but not the only way is by producing the document signed by that individual or his or her parents or guardian or by proving that the risk of the activity was known, understood, and voluntarily accepted.[7]

Assumption of risk, however, is subject to many and varied interpretations by courts, especially when a minor is involved. Minors can assume risk, but the court will figure out whether it was reasonable based on the participant's age, intelligence, instructions provided, and other criteria. Although individuals participating in a sports program are considered to assume a normal risk, this assumption in no way excuses those in charge from exercising reasonable care and prudence in the conduct of such activities, or from foreseeing and taking precautionary measures against accident-provoking circumstances.[7,17] In general, courts have been fairly consistent in upholding assumption of risk releases of liability for adults unless there is evidence of fraud, misrepresentation, or duress.[8] The most important thing about assumption of risk and liability relative to the athletic trainer is not about whether the participant assumes the risk of participating, but whether the athletic trainer has fully informed him or her of the risks of treatment, return to play, and other risks.

## Reducing the Risk of Litigation

The athletic trainer can significantly decrease the risk of litigation by paying attention to a number of important guidelines:

1. Work to establish good personal relationships with athletes, parents, patients, clients, and coworkers.
2. Establish specific policies and guidelines for the operation of an athletic training facility or clinic, and maintain qualified and adequate supervision of the facility, its environs, facilities, and equipment at all times.
3. Develop, review annually, and carefully follow an emergency action plan.
4. Become familiar with the health status and medical history of the individuals under his or her care (see Chapter 2) so as to be aware of problems that could present a need for additional care or caution.
5. Keep factually accurate and timely records that document all injuries and rehabilitation steps, and set up a record retention policy that allows records to be kept and used in defense of litigation that may be brought by a patient. A record retention system needs to keep records long enough to defend against suits brought by patients after they reach the age of 18.
6. Document efforts to create a safe rehabilitation or training environment.
7. Have a detailed job description in writing.
8. Obtain, from parents or guardians when minors are involved, written consent for providing health care (see Chapter 2).
9. Maintain the confidentiality of medical records (see Chapter 2).
10. Exercise extreme caution in the administration, if allowed by law, of nonprescription medications; athletic trainers may not dispense prescription drugs.
11. Use only those therapeutic methods that he or she is qualified to use and that the law states may be used.
12. Do not use or permit the presence of faulty or hazardous equipment.
13. Work cooperatively with the coach and the team physician in the selection and use of sports protective equipment, and insist that the best equipment be obtained, properly fitted, and properly maintained.
14. Do not permit injured players to participate unless cleared by the team physician.
15. Develop an understanding with the coaches that an injured patient will not be allowed to reenter competition until, in the opinion of the team physician or the athletic trainer, he or she is psychologically and physically able. Athletic trainers should not allow themselves to be pressured to clear a patient until he or she is fully cleared by the physician.
16. Follow the express orders of the physician at all times.
17. Purchase professional liability insurance that provides adequate financial coverage, and be aware of the limitations of the policy.
18. Know the limitations of his or her expertise as well as the applicable state regulations and restrictions that limit the athletic trainer's scope of practice.
19. Use common sense in making decisions about a patient's health and safety.

In the case of an injury, the athletic trainer must use reasonable care to prevent additional injury until further medical care is obtained.[29] (See Chapter 12 for additional comments.)

## Product Liability

Product liability is the liability of any or all parties along the chain of commerce of any product for damage caused by that product.[19] This includes the manufacturer of component parts, an assembling manufacturer, the wholesaler, and the retail store owner. Products containing inherent defects that cause harm to a consumer of the product or to someone to whom the product was loaned or given are the subjects of product liability suits. Product liability claims can be based on negligence, strict liability, or breach of warranty of fitness depending on the circumstances upon which the claim is based. Many states have enacted comprehensive product liability statutes, and these statutory provisions can be very diverse. There is no federal product liability law.

Manufacturers of athletic and rehabilitation equipment have a duty to produce equipment that will not cause injury as long as it is used as intended.[23] If the product is not used correctly by the consumer, the manufacturer cannot be held liable. Manufacturers are strictly liable for defects in the design and production of equipment that produces injury. An athletic trainer must not alter the equipment in any way. To do so invalidates the manufacturer's warranty and places liability solely on the athletic trainer. An express warranty is the manufacturer's written statement that a product is safe. For example, warning labels on football helmets inform the player of possible dangers inherent in using the product. Individuals must read and sign a form indicating that they have read and understand the warning. The National Operating

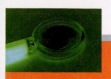

Committee on Standards for Athletic Equipment (NOCSAE) establishes minimum standards for football helmets that must be met to ensure their safety.

## INSURANCE CONSIDERATIONS

Because of the high cost of medical care, every athlete should be covered by appropriate insurance policies that maximize the benefits should injury occur.[20] **Health insurance** is a contract between an insurance company and a policyholder in which the insurance company agrees to reimburse a portion of the total medical bill after some deductible has been paid by the policyholder.[39] During the past 40 years, the insurance industry has undergone a significant evolutionary process. Health care reform initiated in the 1990s was focused on the concept of **managed care,** in which costs of a health care provider's medical care were closely dictated, monitored, and scrutinized by insurance carriers. Higher costs for medical care and a substantial increase in litigation relative to health care providers significantly increased the costs of health insurance.[20]

In 2010, the **Affordable Care Act (ACA)** was signed into law, and it represents a substantial regulatory overhaul of the system of health care in the United States. The Affordable Care Act includes comprehensive health insurance reforms designed to eliminate some of the worst practices of insurance companies and to essentially put consumers back in charge of their health care.[6] The ACA builds upon the existing managed care health insurance system by (1) making health insurance coverage more accessible and affordable, (2) improving the quality of health care, (3) establishing legal protections for consumers, and (4) providing mechanisms for consumers to choose the insurance that is the best fit for them individually. As of 2014, most Americans not covered by either an employer-sponsored health plan, or other public insurance programs, are required to have an approved private-insurance policy or pay a penalty.[44] *Focus Box 3–1* identifies the key features and benefits of the Affordable Care Act.

### Types of Insurance

The major types of insurance about which individuals concerned with athletic training and sports medicine should have some understanding are general health insurance, accident insurance, professional liability insurance, and catastrophic insurance, as well as insurance for errors and omissions. There is a need to protect adequately all who are concerned with health and safety. *Focus Box 3–2: "Common insurance terminology"* lists some of the more common insurance terms.

**General Health Insurance** Every person must have a *general health insurance* policy that covers illness, hospitalization, and emergency care. Some institutions offer primary insurance coverage in which all medical expenses are paid for by the institution. The institutions pay an extremely high premium for this type of coverage. Most institutions offer some type of *secondary insurance* coverage, which pays the remaining medical bills once the personal insurance company has made its payment. It will cover many

> Every person must have a general health insurance policy that covers illness, hospitalization, and emergency care.

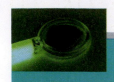

### Common insurance terminology[11]

*Allowable charge*: the maximum amount, according to the individual policy, that insurance will pay for each procedure or service performed.

*Beneficiary*: a person eligible to receive the benefits of a specific policy or program.

*Benefits*: services that an insurer, a government agency, or a health care plan offers to pay for an insured individual.

*Case management services*: the process in which the attending physician or agent coordinates the care given to a patient by other health care providers and/or community organizations.

*Claim*: a form sent to an insurance company, requesting payment for covered medical expenses; information includes the insured's name and address, procedure codes, diagnostic codes, charges, and date of service.

*Clean claim*: a filed claim with all the necessary information that may be immediately processed.

*Coinsurance*: also referred to as copayment; the insurer and the insured split the cost of health care at a specified percentage, usually either 80/20 or 70/30.

*Contract*: a legally binding agreement between an insurance company and a physician describing the duties of both parties.

*Copayment*: a provision in an insurance policy requiring the policyholder to pay a specified percentage of each medical claim.

*Customary fees*: the average fee charged for a specified service or procedure in a defined geographical area.

*Deductible*: the amount owed by the insured on a yearly basis before the insurance company will begin to pay for services rendered.

*Dependent*: a person legally eligible for benefits based on his or her relationship with the policyholder.

*Exclusions*: specified medical services, disorders, treatments, diseases, and durable medical equipment that are listed as uncovered or not reimbursable in an insurance policy.

*Explanation of benefits (EOB)*: an insurance report accompanying all claim payments that explains how the insurance company processed a claim.

*Fee schedule*: a comprehensive listing of the maximum payment amount that an insurance company will allow for specified medical procedures performed on a beneficiary of the plan.

*Gatekeeper*: the primary care physician assigned by the insurer who oversees the medical care rendered to a patient and initiates all specialty and ancillary services.

*Participating provider*: a health care provider who has entered into a contract with an insurance company to provide medical services to the beneficiaries of a plan; the provider agrees to accept the insurance company's approved fee and will only bill the patient for the deductible, the copayment, and uncovered services.

*Policyholder*: the person who takes out the medical insurance policy.

*Premium*: a periodic payment made to an insurance company by an individual policyholder.

*Third-party administrator*: an independent organization that collects premiums, pays claims, and provides administrative services within a health care plan.

*UCR allowable charge*: usual, customary, and reasonable charge that represents the maximum amount an insurance company will pay for a given service based on geographical averages.

---

additional charges such as deductibles, copays, or coverage limits the primary insurer does not pay for. For example, if an athlete is injured, many colleges or universities will submit the medical bill to the family's primary insurer for payment. The college or university will use a secondary insurance policy to cover any out-of-pocket expenses that the family would have paid. It is important to look closely into the athlete's family's primary insurer coverage to see exactly what is covered and what is not before an injury occurs. This is a time-consuming process, but it may eliminate many surprises that often arise with insurers.

Many people are covered under some type of *family health insurance* policy. However, the institution or corporation must make certain that personal health insurance is arranged for or purchased by individuals not covered under family policies.[36] A form letter directed to the parents of all minors should be completed and returned to the institution to make certain that appropriate coverage is provided (Figure 3–1). Some so-called comprehensive plans do not cover every health need. For example, they may cover physicians' care but not hospital charges. Many of these plans require large prepayments before the insurance takes effect. Supplemental policies, such as accident insurance and catastrophic insurance, are designed to take over where general health insurance stops.

**Accident Insurance** Besides general health insurance, low-cost *accident insurance* is available. It often covers accidents on school grounds while the student is in attendance or accidents that occur in the workplace. The purposes of this insurance are to protect against financial loss from medical and hospital bills, encourage an injured

## STUDENT-ATHLETE INSURANCE INFORMATION

Student's Full Name:______________________________ PID ____________

Date of Birth: ______/______/______ Sex: M_____ F_____ Sport: ______________________

UNC Hospital Medical Record Number (if first year, see attached instructions) ______________________

IS YOUR SON/DAUGHTER COVERED BY **HEALTH INSURANCE**? YES________ *NO________
Please complete insurance information below. Submit a copy of insurance card, **front & back**. *Make sure copy is* ***legible***.
*If you check no, please note all eligible students are required to have health insurance.

**Policyholder's Information (Required to obtain authorization)**

Insurance Company Name: ______________________________ State issued ____________

Policy Number ______________ Group # ______________ Type-HMO, PPO ________

Policyholder Name: ______________________________ Date of Birth: ______/______/______

Relationship to Student Athlete: ______________ Email of Policyholder ______________________

Home Address, City, State, Zip: ______________________________________________

Home Phone Number:______________ Cell Number ______________________

Policyholder's Employer: ______________________________ Phone: ____________

Address, City, State, Zip: ______________________________________________

Do you have **prescription drug coverage**? Yes_____ No_____
**If so, please complete plan information below and send a copy of the front and back of the Rx card.**

Rx Insurance Plan Name: ______________________________
ID # ______________________________
Rx Group # ______________________________
PCN # ______________________________
BIN # ______________________________
Pharmacy Health Desk # ______________________________
Do you have a separate Rx card? Yes_____ No_____

I give my permission to file a claim for medical services with the above health care insurer.

Parent's Signature:______________________ Date:______________________

FIGURE 3-1 Sample Student-Athlete Insurance Form
Source: Data from Campus Health Service, University of North Carolina.

An athletic trainer who recently became certified is planning on working summer camps for an area high school before he starts his full-time employment in the fall.

? What should the athletic trainer do to protect himself from liability?

patient to receive prompt medical care, encourage prompt reporting of injuries, and relieve an institution or a corporation of financial responsibility.[42]

General insurance may be limited; thus, accident insurance for a specific activity may be needed to provide additional protection.[4] This type of coverage is limited and does not require knowledge of fault, and the amount it pays is limited. For serious injuries requiring surgery and lengthy rehabilitation, accident insurance is usually not adequate. This inadequacy can put families with limited budgets into a financial bind. Of particular concern is insurance that does not adequately cover catastrophic injuries.

**Catastrophic Insurance** Although catastrophic injuries are relatively uncommon, when they do occur, the consequences to the individual, family, and institution, as well as to society, can be staggering.[36] In the past when available funds have been completely diminished, the family was forced to seek funding elsewhere, usually through a lawsuit. For example, in athletics, organizations such as the National Collegiate Athletic Association (NCAA)

During a state gymnastics meet, a gymnast fell off the uneven parallel bars and landed on her forearm. The athletic trainer suspected a fracture and decided an X-ray was needed. The gymnast's parents had general health insurance through a PPO, but because the gymnast was in severe pain, she was sent to the nearest emergency room to be treated. Unfortunately, the emergency facility was not on the list of preferred providers, and the insurance company denied the claim. The athletic trainer assured the parents that the meet organizers would take care of whatever medical costs were not covered by their insurance policy.

**?** Because the PPO denied the claim, what type of insurance policy should the meet organizers carry to cover the medical costs?

> Because of the amount of litigation for alleged negligence, all professionals should be fully protected by professional liability insurance.

and National Association of Intercollegiate Athletics (NAIA) provide plans for the athlete who requires a lifetime of extensive medical and rehabilitative care because of a permanent disability.[4] A program at the secondary-school level is offered to districts by the National Federation of State High School Associations (NFHS). These plans provide coverage for medical, rehabilitation, and transportation costs not covered by other insurance benefits.[36] Costs for catastrophic insurance are based on the number of sports and the number of hazardous sports offered by the institution.

**Professional Liability Insurance** Most employers have general liability insurance to protect against damages that may arise from injuries occurring on their property. Liability insurance covers claims of negligence on the part of individuals.[9] Its major concern is whether supervision was reasonable and if unreasonable risk of harm was perceived by the individual who was injured.[28]

Because of the amount of litigation based on alleged negligence, premiums have become almost prohibitive. Typically, a victim's lawsuit has taken a shotgun approach, suing the employer athletic trainer, physician, administrator, and company or school district. If a piece of equipment is involved, the product manufacturer is also sued.

All athletic trainers should carry *professional liability insurance* and must clearly understand the limits of its coverage. Liability insurance typically covers negligence in a civil case. If a criminal complaint is filed, however, liability insurance will not cover the athletic trainer.

To offset the shotgun approach of lawsuits and to cover what is not covered by a general liability policy, *errors and omissions liability insurance* has evolved. It is designed to cover school employees, officers, and the district against suits claiming malpractice, wrongful actions, errors and omissions, and acts of negligence.[39] Even when working in a program that has good liability coverage, each person within that program who works directly with students must have his or her own personal liability insurance.

# THIRD-PARTY REIMBURSEMENT

Third-party reimbursement is the primary mechanism of payment for medical services in the United States.[20] The policyholder's insurance company reimburses health care professionals for services performed. Medical insurance companies may provide group and individual coverage for employees and dependents.[20] Managed care involves a prearranged system for delivering health care that is designed to control costs while continuing to provide quality care. To cut payout costs, many insurance companies pay for preventive care (to reduce the need for hospitalization) and limit where the individual can go for care. A number of health care systems have been developed to contain costs.[22]

> Third-party reimbursement involves reimbursement by the policyholder's insurance company for services performed by health care professionals.

## Health Maintenance Organizations

Health maintenance organizations (HMOs) provide preventive measures and limit where the individual can receive care. Except in emergencies, permission must be obtained before the individual can go to another provider. HMOs generally pay 100 percent of the medical costs as long as care is rendered at an HMO facility. Many supplemental policies do not cover the medical costs that would normally be paid by the general policy. Therefore, an athlete treated outside the HMO may be ineligible for any insurance benefits. Many HMOs determine fees using a capitation system, which limits the amount that will be reimbursed for a specific service. It is essential that the athletic trainer understand the limits of and restrictions on coverage at his or her institution or company.

> **Third-party payers:**
> - HMO
> - PPO
> - POS
> - EPO
> - PHO
> - TPA
> - Medicare
> - Medicaid
> - Workers compensation
> - Indemnity plans
> - Capitation

## Preferred Provider Organizations

Preferred provider organizations (PPOs) provide discount health care but also limit where a person can go for treatment of an illness. The athletic trainer must be apprised in advance as to where the ill patient should be sent. Patients sent to a facility that is not on the approved list may be required to pay for care, whereas, if they are sent to a preferred facility, all costs are paid.[1] PPOs may provide added services, such as physical therapy, more easily and at no cost or at a much lower cost than would another insurance policy. PPOs pay on a fee-for-service basis.

## Point of Service Plan

The point of service (POS) plan is a combination of the HMO and PPO plans. It is based on an HMO structure, yet it allows members to go outside the HMO to obtain services. This flexibility is allowed only with certain conditions and under special circumstances.

## Exclusive Provider Organizations

Exclusive provider organizations (EPOs) are also a combination of the HMO and PPO plans. They are restrictive in the number and types of providers they have and consequently are more like an HMO. Most will not pay anything if you use out-of-network providers.

## Physician Hospital Organization

Physician hospital organizations (PHOs) involve a major hospital or hospital chain and its physicians. A PHO organization contracts directly with employers to provide services and/or contracts with a managed care organization.

## Third-Party Administrators

Third-party administrators (TPAs) are frequently used to administer services and to pay claims for self-insured group plans and thus function as pseudo insurance companies. They perform member services, such as enrollment and billing, and assist with controlling utilization without the financial risk.

## Medicare

Medicare is the federal health insurance program for the aged and disabled. Most people at retirement age qualify for Medicare benefits. There are four parts, or sections, to Medicare. Part A, the hospital portion, is normally premium-free at retirement to the beneficiary. Part B, the physician portion, has a monthly premium charge to the beneficiary.

Part C is a program that allows a person to choose among several types of health care plans, including medical savings accounts, managed care plans, and private fee-for-service plans.

Part D, a federal program to subsidize the costs of prescription drugs for Medicare beneficiaries, went into effect in 2006. Beneficiaries can either join a Prescription Drug Plan (PDP) for drug coverage only, or they can join a Medicare Advantage (MA) plan that covers both medical services and prescription drugs.

## Medicaid

Medicaid is a health insurance program for people with low incomes and limited resources. Medicaid is funded by both the federal government and individual states, with the states responsible for handling the administration of the program. Individual states administer Medicaid; thus, benefits vary by state.

## Workers Compensation

Workers compensation laws and benefits for injured workers are mandated by the states. Employers pay the premiums, and the claims are settled by workers compensation insurance carriers whose goal is to return injured workers to the workforce as soon as possible.

## Indemnity Plans

An indemnity plan is the most traditional form of billing for health care. It is a fee-for-service plan that allows the insured party to seek medical care without restrictions on utilization or cost. The provider charges the patient or a third-party payer for services provided. Charges are based on a set fee schedule.

## Capitation

Capitation is a form of reimbursement used by managed care providers in which members make a standard payment each month regardless of how much service is rendered to the member by the provider.

## Third-Party Reimbursement for Athletic Trainers

Athletic trainers have always been able to bill third-party payers for services rendered. For many years, most insurers were reluctant to reimburse the athletic trainer for the health care services provided. Throughout the 1990s and early 2000s, there was a significant increase in reimbursement from third-party payers for athletic trainers working in a variety of settings, including rehabilitation clinics, hospitals, physicians' offices, and college and university settings.[26] Most third-party payers view "licensed health care professionals" as the only reimbursable entities, and fortunately in most states this includes certified athletic trainers.

In 1995, NATA established the Reimbursement Advisory Group to monitor managed care changes and to help the athletic trainer secure a place as a health care provider. Specifically, this group was charged with developing a model for approaching third-party payers for the reimbursement of athletic training services, of educating athletic trainers

> An athletic trainer working in a clinic is seeking third-party reimbursement for athletic training services performed. The athletic trainer is experiencing difficulty obtaining reimbursement from certain payers because of uncertainty about the effectiveness of the treatment program.
>
> **?** What can the athletic trainer do to address the concerns of the third-party payers?

**3-6 Clinical Application Exercise**

on issues related to reimbursement, and, perhaps most important, of designing and implementing a data-based clinical outcomes study.[5] In 1996, NATA initiated the Athletic Training Outcomes Assessment project designed to present supporting data that measure the results of interventions involving athletic training procedures. This three-year study was designed to provide data that focused on functional outcomes, including assessing the patients' perceptions of their functional capabilities and their overall satisfaction with their treatment program; assessing the physical, emotional, and social well-being of patients; assessing health care cost effectiveness relative to time lost from activity due to injury; and assessing the number of treatments.[1] The results of this study were critical in securing reimbursement for athletic training services, because the majority of third-party payers currently require outcomes research when evaluating a contract.[25]

**Centers for Medicare & Medicaid Services (CMS) Ruling** In 2005, the Centers for Medicare & Medicaid Services (CMS) issued a decision that has had and will continue to have a crippling effect on the ability of athletic trainers to receive reimbursement for health care services.[40] The ruling stated that they would "no longer pay for therapy 'incident to' a physician's services unless the provider is a physical therapist, occupational therapist or speech/language pathologist." The U.S. Congress subsequently passed this ruling making it a federal law. Under this law, physicians are not able to bill Medicare for treatment provided by athletic trainers. Though not bound by this law, there is little doubt that the majority of third-party payers tend to follow the lead of Medicare and Medicaid when deciding who will be reimbursed for health care services provided. With passage of this law, it became clear that the federal government does not recognize athletic trainers as providers of rehabilitative services for Medicare patients, no matter what age.[40]

Certainly, this law directly and immediately affected reimbursement for athletic trainers working in clinics and hospitals or as an athletic trainer in physician practice. It has also caused many clinical athletic trainers who also work in secondary schools to lose their jobs. It is likely that the CMS law will also negatively impact future state and national legislative efforts on behalf of athletic trainers. Since that law was enacted, the NATA has continued to explore every means of legal recourse to have this law reversed or at least modified. In 2009, the Athletic Trainers' Equal Access to Medicare Act (bill HR 1137) was introduced in the United States House of Representatives. This act sought to ensure that Medicare beneficiaries would have better access to health care provided by state licensed, certified athletic trainers. Unfortunately, this bill did not make it out of the congressional committee level, and thus it never became a law. Certainly, securing third-party reimbursement for athletic training services must continue to be a priority, especially for the clinical athletic trainer.[37]

## Insurance Billing

The athletic trainer must routinely make certain that insurance claims are filed immediately and correctly.[38] Athletic trainers working in educational settings can facilitate this process by collecting insurance information on every individual at the beginning of the year. The athletic trainer must ensure that every individual is adequately covered by a reliable insurance company. Although extremely time consuming, the athletic trainer can save a lot of headaches by vetting individual athlete's insurance policies to make sure exactly what is covered by that particular policy and what is not. Letters should be drafted to the parents of all athletes, explaining the limits of the school insurance policy and what the parents must do to process a claim if injury does occur. Schools with secondary policies should stress that the parents must submit all bills to their insurance company before they submit the remainder to the school. In educational institutions, most claims will be filed with a single insurance company, which will pay for medical services provided by individual health care providers.

**Filing an Insurance Claim** In most cases, when filing an insurance claim for a patient seen in a clinic or hospital, individuals other than health care providers are employed to make certain that a patient has provided current insurance information.[13] The athletic trainer will likely not be the individual who is responsible for following up on insurance claims filed with third-party payers.

In other employment settings, filing claims becomes the responsibility of the athletic trainer. This task can be highly time-consuming, taking the athletic trainer away from his or her major role of working directly with the patient. Because of the intricacies and time involved with continuously updating policy information, filing claims, and following up on communications with patients, parents, doctors, and vendors, a staff person other than the athletic trainer should be assigned this responsibility.

When filing an insurance claim to submit for reimbursement, athletic trainers will find that most carriers accept a standard form labeled HCFA-1500/HCFA-1450 (Blue Cross Blue Shield uses Form UB-92). These forms must be completed in detail with as much information as possible. Experience dictates that the more accurately and thoroughly these forms are completed, the quicker and higher the rate of reimbursement. In some situations it may be necessary for the athletic trainer to request approval from insurance companies before treating patients.[37] For example, preauthorization from the insurance provider is usually required when ordering any type of imaging other than radiographs.

Athletic trainers working in the clinical setting should understand that the clinic must be able to collect reimbursement from third-party payers for services provided. Pre-authorization from the insurance provider is usually necessary when ordering any type of imaging other than radiographs.

Two types of billing codes must be used when submitting a claim on standard HCFA-1500 or UB-92 forms to

**?** When filing an insurance claim for rehabilitation services following injury, what can an athletic trainer do to improve the reimbursement rate as well as to speed up the process?

third-party payers: a *diagnostic code* and a *procedural code*.[18] A diagnostic code is required for all procedural billing, and they can be found in a book called the *International Statistical Classification of Diseases and Related Health Problems* (ICD-10-Clinical Modifications). This is a six-digit code that specifies the condition or injury that the athletic trainer or any other health care provider is treating.[32] For example, code S93.419 indicates that the patient has a sprain of the calcaneofibular ligament in the ankle.

The *Current Procedure Terminology Code* (CPT) was first developed by the American Medical Association in 1966. Each year, an annual publication designates changes corresponding to significant updates in medical technology and practice. The CPT code is used to identify specific medical procedures used in treating a patient.[32] Table 3–1 lists the current CPT codes most often used by the athletic trainer.

Athletic trainers should never release medical records to third-party payers unless written authorization has

A sports medicine clinic is considering hiring an athletic trainer. However, the clinic administrator is concerned that the athletic trainer cannot bill third-party payers for services provided.

**?** What does the administrator need to be told about third-party reimbursement for athletic training services?

### TABLE 3–1 Description of Billing Codes Used by Athletic Trainers

The following is a guide to procedure billing codes that may be used by athletic trainers when billing for athletic training services:

| Code | Description |
| --- | --- |
| 97005/97006 | Athletic trainer evaluation and reevaluation (per visit) |
| 97750 | Physical performance test (each 15 minutes) treatment charges |
| 97116 | Gait training (each 15 minutes) |
| 97110 | Therapeutic exercise (each 15 minutes) |
| 97112 | Neuromuscular reeducation (each 15 minutes) |
| 97530 | Therapeutic activities (each 15 minutes) |
| 97113 | Aquatic therapeutic exercise (each 15 minutes) |
| 97124 | Massage (each 15 minutes) |
| 97530 | Body mechanics training (each 15 minutes) |
| 97140 | Manual therapy (each 15 minutes) |
| 97504 | Orthotics fitting and training (each 15 minutes) |
| 97150 | Therapeutic procedures—group (each visit) |
| 97150 | Supervised exercise (each visit) |
| 11040 | Debridement (each visit) |
| 97139 | Wound care (each 15 minutes) |
| 97139 | Taping (each visit) |
| 95831 | Manual muscle testing—extremity/trunk |
| 95851 | Range of motion (ROM) measurements |
| 95852 | ROM measurements of hand, with or without comparison with normal side |
| 97545 | Work hardening/conditioning (initial 2 hours) |
| 97035 | Ultrasound (each 15 minutes) |
| 97035 | Phonophoresis (each 15 minutes) (must bill for ultrasound if billing for this service) |
| 97032 | Electrical stimulation (each 15 minutes) |
| 97033 | Iontophoresis (each 15 minutes) |
| 97032 | Constant electrical stimulation (each 15 minutes) |
| 97034 | Contrast baths (each 15 minutes) |
| 97014 | Electric stimulation (application to one or more areas) |
| 97022 | Whirlpool (application to one or more areas) |
| 97010 | Hot packs (application to one or more areas) |
| 97010 | Cold packs/ice massage (application to one or more areas) |
| 97012 | Traction, mechanical (not time-based) |
| 97016 | Compression pump (application to one or more areas) |

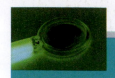

## FOCUS 3–3 Focus on Healthcare Administration and Professional Responsibilities

### Guidelines for documentation of patient records

When the athletic trainer is submitting a bill to a third-party payer for reimbursement for services provided, the following information should be included:

- The patient's updated medical history form
- The patient's most recent physical examination findings
- Initial evaluation of the patient by the athletic trainer (SOAP note format)
- Copies of notes to or from the referring physician
- Diagnostic test results
- An impression or diagnosis
- A prescription or other state-mandated documentation from a physician

- Established functional, measurable, and time-based treatment goals
- Documentation that the treatment plan and goals were discussed and understood by the patient or guardian
- The type, frequency, and number of treatments necessary to treat the problem
- Copies of daily treatment records
- Weekly progress notes
- Established prognosis for recovery

been obtained from the patient, according to HIPAA and FERPA guidelines.[27] (See Chapter 2.) It is also essential when billing for and receiving reimbursement that the athletic trainer keep meticulous, accurate, and detailed documentation of all procedures, charges submitted, and payments received for services.[2,38] *Focus Box 3–3*: "Guidelines for documentation of patient records" identifies criteria that should be routinely followed when billing for charges.

**National Provider Identifier (NPI)** All Athletic Trainers must obtain an NPI. The National Provider Identifier (NPI) is a government-issued identification number for individual health care providers and provider organizations (i.e., clinics, hospitals, group practices). Covered health care providers and all health plans and health care clearinghouses must use the NPIs in administrative and financial transactions, according to the Health Insurance Portability and Accountability Act (HIPAA). The NPI is a 10-digit numeric identifier. As of 2007, any health care provider who uses standard electronic transactions, such as electronic claims, eligibility verifications, claims status inquiries, and claim attachments, is required by federal law to include NPIs on electronic transactions. To apply for an NPI, go to https://NPPES.cms.hhs.gov.

## SUMMARY

- A great deal of care must be taken in following athletic training procedures that conform to the legal guidelines governing liability for negligence.
- Liability is the state of being legally responsible for the harm one causes another person. It assumes that an athletic trainer would act according to the standard of care of any individual with similar educational background and training.
- An athletic trainer who fails to use reasonable care—care that persons would normally exercise to avoid injury to themselves or to others under similar circumstances—may be found liable for negligence.
- Although athletes participating in a sports program are considered to assume a normal risk, this assumption in no way exempts those in charge from exercising reasonable care.

- Athletic trainers can significantly decrease the risk of litigation by making certain that they have done everything possible to provide a reasonable degree of care to the injured patient.
- The major types of insurance about which athletic trainers should have some understanding are general health insurance, accident insurance, professional liability insurance, catastrophic insurance, and insurance for errors and omissions.
- Third-party reimbursement is the primary mechanism of payment for medical services in the United States. A number of different health care systems have been developed to contain costs.
- It is essential that the athletic trainer ensure that insurance claims are filed immediately and correctly using appropriate forms and billing codes.

## WEB SITES

America's Health Insurance Plans: www.ahip.org
*The nation's most prominent trade association representing the private health care system. It is the nation's premier provider of self-study courses on health insurance and managed care.*

Duhaime & Co. Legal Dictionary: www.duhaime.org /dictionary
*This is a site that has put together an extensive list of legal terms with clear definitions and explanations.*

Legal Information Institute at Cornell: www.law.cornell .edu/wex/Sports_law

*Part of a series of legal information, this site specifically addresses law in sport but is rather technical. The relevant area to sports medicine is addressed in the area titled "Torts."*

Sports Lawyers Journal: www.law.tulane.edu/tlsjournals /slj/index.aspx
*Specialized academic and professional publication on legal aspects of sports.*

## SOLUTIONS TO CLINICAL APPLICATION EXERCISES

3–1 An athletic trainer who assumes the duty of caring for an athlete has an obligation to make sure that appropriate care is given. If the athletic trainer fails to provide an acceptable standard of care, there is a breach of duty on the part of the athletic trainer, and the athlete must then prove that this breach caused the injury or made the injury worse.

3–2 A person possessing more training in a given field or area is expected to possess a correspondingly higher level of competence than a layperson is. A certified athletic trainer will therefore be judged in terms of his or her performance in any situation in which legal liability may be assessed.

3–3 In personal injury cases, the individual would typically have between one and five years to file suit for negligence. The statute of limitations begins to run on a plaintiff's time to file a lawsuit for negligence either from the time of the negligent act or omission that gives rise to the suit or from the time of the discovery of an injury caused by the negligent act or omission.

3–4 The athletic trainer should purchase private professional liability insurance. In addition, the athletic trainer should keep proper records of injuries and keep those records in his or her possession.

3–5 Besides general health insurance, low-cost accident insurance often covers accidents on school grounds while the athlete is competing. The purposes of this insurance are to protect against financial loss from medical and hospital bills, encourage an injured athlete to receive prompt medical care, encourage prompt reporting of injuries, and relieve a school of financial responsibility.

3–6 The athletic trainer could initiate an outcomes research project designed to present supporting data that measure the results of interventions involving athletic training procedures. This research project would assess the athletes' perceptions of their functional capabilities and overall satisfaction with their treatment program, the cost-effectiveness of the health care relative to time lost from activity due to injury, and the number of treatments. The majority of third-party payers currently require outcomes research when evaluating a contract.

3–7 The athletic trainer should file an insurance claim for reimbursement, using the standard form labeled HCFA-1500. The form should be completed in detail with as much information as possible. The athletic trainer who completes these forms accurately and thoroughly probably experiences a quicker and higher rate of reimbursement.

3–8 It should be pointed out that athletic trainers can bill third-party payers for services rendered to a patient. Whether the insurance company will reimburse the athletic trainer for services is up to the individual third-party payer. With the approval of the uniform billing code for athletic training services, it is more likely that the athletic trainer will be successfully reimbursed for treating patients.

## REVIEW QUESTIONS AND CLASS ACTIVITIES

1. What are the athletic trainer's major legal concerns for negligence and for assumption of risk?
2. What measures can an athletic trainer take to minimize the chances of litigation, should an athlete be injured?
3. Invite an attorney who is familiar with sports litigation to class to discuss how athletic trainers can protect themselves from lawsuits.
4. Discuss what the athletic trainer must do to provide reasonable and prudent care in dealing with an injured patient.
5. Why is it necessary for an individual to have both general health insurance and accident insurance?
6. Briefly discuss the various methods of third-party reimbursement.
7. Why should an athletic trainer carry individual liability insurance?
8. What are the critical considerations for filing insurance claims?

## REFERENCES

1. Albolm M, Campbell D, Konin J: *Reimbursement for athletic trainers,* Thorofare, NJ, 2001, Slack.
2. Altman S: Legal aspects of crisis-management communication: What to communicate, *Athletic Therapy Today* 10(3):6, 2005.
3. Appenzeller H: *Safe at first: A guide to help sports administrators reduce their liability,* Chapel Hill, NC, 1999, Carolina Academic Press.
4. Belk J: *Health insurance today: A practical approach,* St. Louis, 2012, Elsevier.
5. Campbell D: Workshop on third-party reimbursement, *NATA News* 3:34, 1996.
6. Coffin R: Affordable Care Act. *Journal of Medical Practice Management* 28(5):317–19, 2013.
7. Cotten D: 2005. Are you safe? Courts in an increasing number of states are enforcing liability waivers signed by parents on behalf of minors, *Athletic Business* 29(3):66–68; 70–72, 2005.
8. Cotten D: Waivers and releases can protect against liability, *Fitness Management* 20(4):24, 2004.
9. Cotten D: What is covered by your liability insurance policy? A risk management essential, *Exercise Standard and Malpractice Reporter* 15(4):54, 2001.
10. Cozillio M: *Sports law: Cases and materials,* Durham, NC, 2007, Carolina Academic Press.

11. De Carlo M: Reimbursement for healthcare services. In Konin J: *Clinical athletic training,* Thorofare, NJ, 1997, Slack. Used with permission.
12. Eickhoff-Shemek J, Evans J: An investigation of law and legal liability content in masters academic programs in sports medicine and exercise science, *Journal of Legal Aspects of Sport* 10(3):172, 2000.
13. Flight M: *Law, liability, and ethics for medical office professionals,* Independence, KY, 2010, Cengage Learning.
14. Frenkel D: Medico-legal aspects in sport (abstract), *Exercise & Society Journal of Sport Science* (28):90, 2001.
15. Gallup E: *Law and the team physician,* Champaign, IL, 1995, Human Kinetics.
16. Gardiner S: *Sports law,* New York, 2012, Routledge.
17. Gardiner S, Gray J: Training regimes and medical treatment of elite sports athletes: Issues of legal liability. (Abstract) *Journal of Science & Medicine in Sport 7* (4 Supplement): 111, 2004.
18. Garrison S: Fundamentals of coding, payment and documentation: Understanding their role and impact in healthcare, Chicago, 2011, American Medical Association.
19. Gorman L: Product liability in sports medicine. *Athletic Therapy Today* 4(4):36, 1999.
20. Green M, Rowell J: *Understanding health insurance: A guide to billing and reimbursement,* Albany, 2010, Delmar.

21. Harris D: *Contemporary issues in healthcare law and ethics,* Chicago, 2007, Health Administration Press.
22. Health Insurance Association of America: *Fundamentals of health insurance,* Washington, DC, 1997, HIAA.
23. Henderson J: *Products liability: Problems and the consumer.* Canton, OH, 1995, Professional Reports Corporation.
24. Herbert D, Herbert W: *Legal aspects of preventive, rehabilitative and recreational exercise programs,* ed 4, Canton, OH, 2002, PRC.
25. Hertel J: Research training for clinicians: The crucial link between evidence-based practice and third-party reimbursement (editorial), *J Athl Train* 40(2):69, 2005.
26. Hunt V: Reimbursement efforts continue steady progress, *NATA News,* October 10–12, 2002.
27. Jones D: HIPAA: Friend or foe to athletic trainers? *Athletic Therapy Today* 8(2):17, 2003.
28. Jones R: Professional and general liability insurance: When and why you need it. *Sports Medicine Bulletin* 9(24):6, 2013.
29. Kane S, White R: Medical malpractice and the sports medicine clinician, *Clinical Orthopedics and Related Research,* 467(2):412–19, 2009.
30. McClean S: *Legal and ethical aspects of healthcare,* New York, 2009, Cambridge University Press.
31. Mitten M: Legal considerations in treating the injured athlete, *J Orthop Sports Phys Ther* 21(1):38, 1995.

32. Moisio M: *Guide to health insurance billing,* Clifton Park, NY, 2006, Thompson Delmar Learning.
33. Pozgar G: *Legal aspects of health care administration,* 2011, Jones & Bartlett.
34. Osborne B: Principles of liability for athletic trainers: Managing sport-related concussion, *Journal of Athletic Training* 36(3):316–21, 2001.
35. Quandt E: Legal liability in covering athletic events, *Sports Health: A Multidiciplinary Approach,* 1(1):84–90, 2009.
36. Rankin J: *Athletic training management: Concepts and applications,* New York, 2006, McGraw-Hill.
37. Ray R: Uniform billing code takes effect for ATCs, *NATA News,* Winter: 20, 2000.
38. Ray R: *Management strategies in athletic training,* Champaign, IL, 2011, Human Kinetics.
39. Rosenbaum S: *Law and the American health care system,* St. Paul, MN, 2012, West Academic-Foundation Press.
40. Rule change jeopardizes referrals to ATCs: *Physician Sportsmed* 33(7):10, 2005.
41. Sharp, L: *Sports law: A managerial approach,* Scottsdale, AZ, 2014, Holcomb Hathaway Publishers.
42. Vaughn E: *Fundamentals of risk and insurance,* New York, 2002, Wiley.
43. Wong G: *Essentials of sports law,* ed 4, Westport, CT, 2010, Greenwood Press
44. Yagoda L: *Affordable Care Act for dummies,* Hoboken, NJ, 2014, John Wiley & Sons.

## ANNOTATED BIBLIOGRAPHY

Albolm M, Campbell D, Konin J: *Reimbursement for athletic trainers,* Thorofare, NJ, 2001, Slack.

Presents a "how to" approach for filing claims, appealing denials, and approaching payers. Covers all current trends in health care reimbursement as well as future directions for reimbursement.

Appenzeller, H: *Youth sports and the law: A guide to legal issues,* Chapel Hill, NC, 2000, Carolina Academic Press.

Studies various court cases to understand the legal principles involved in sport participation. The objective of the book is to provide better and safer sporting experiences for today's children.

Appenzeller, H: *Risk management in sport: Issues and strategies,* Chapel Hill, NC, 2005, Carolina Academic Press.

Discusses risk management in sport law and industry. Topics include tort liability; medical, event, and facility issues; warnings, waivers, and informed consent; and youth sport and the law.

Champion, W: *Fundamentals of sports law,* St. Paul, MN, 2005, Thomson/West.

This introductory text lays out the basic ideas and legal documents important to attorneys, compliance officers, agents, athletic directors, and sports administrators.

Grayson, E: *Ethics, injury and the law in sports medicine,* New York, NY, 2000, Butterworth-Heinemann.

Provides an up-to-date review of the status of sports medicine and the law. Addresses the key legal and ethical issues in sports and exercise medicine. For practitioners and students preparing for sport and exercise medicine exams.

Green, M, Rowell, J: *Understanding health insurance: A guide to billing and reimbursement,* Albany, NY, 2010, Delmar.

Provides a comprehensive resource for dealing with issues related to insurance.

Moisio, M: *Guide to health insurance billing,* Clifton Park, NY, 2006, Thompson Delmar Learning.

All aspects of the billing process, from key terms to state and federal regulations, to guidelines for completing and submitting claims to health insurance programs.

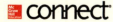

# PART II

# Risk Management

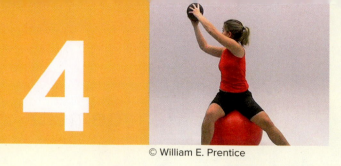

© William E. Prentice

# 4

# Fitness and Conditioning Techniques

## ■ Objectives

*When you finish this chapter you should be able to*

- Examine the roles of the athletic trainer and the strength and conditioning coach in getting an athlete fit.
- Identify the principles of conditioning.
- Defend the importance of the warm-up and cool-down periods.
- Evaluate the importance of strength and flexibility and cardiorespiratory endurance for both athletic performance and injury prevention.

- Analyze specific techniques and principles for improving cardiorespiratory endurance, muscular strength, and flexibility.
- Discuss fitness testing and identify specific tests to assess various fitness parameters.
- Apply the concept of periodization and identify the various training periods in each phase.

## ■ Key Terms

SAID principle
cardiorespiratory endurance
training effect
high-intensity
  interval training
muscular strength
power
muscular endurance
hypertrophy
atrophy
core
isometric exercise
concentric (positive)
  contraction
eccentric (negative)
  contraction

isotonic exercise
accommodating resistance
isokinetic exercise
circuit training
plyometric exercise
agonist
antagonist
autogenic inhibition
ballistic stretching
dynamic stretching
static stretching
proprioceptive neuromuscular
  facilitation (PNF)

## ■ Connect Highlights   connect®

*Visit connect.mcgraw-hill.com for further exercises to apply your knowledge:*

- Clinical application scenarios covering cardiorespiratory endurance, fitness training, conditioning and periodization
- Click-and-drag questions covering muscular endurance, cardiorespiratory fitness, and conditioning activities
- Multiple-choice questions covering warm-up, cool-down, muscular strength, roles of the athletic trainer in training athlete, and fitness testing
- Selection questions covering flexibility

Exercise is an essential factor in fitness conditioning, injury prevention, and injury rehabilitation. An athletic trainer working with an athletic population in secondary schools, in colleges and universities, or at the professional level is well aware that to compete successfully at a high level, the athlete must be fit. An athlete who is not fit is more likely to sustain an injury. The athletic trainer should recognize that improper conditioning is one of the primary contributing factors to sports injuries. It is essential that the athlete engage in *conditioning exercises* that can minimize the possibility of injury while maximizing performance.[55]

The basic principles of conditioning exercises also apply to techniques of therapeutic, rehabilitative, or reconditioning exercises that are specifically concerned with restoring normal body function following injury. Athletic trainers providing patient care in a clinic or hospital are more likely to apply these principles to reconditioning or rehabilitation of an injured patient. The term *therapeutic exercise* is perhaps most widely used to indicate exercises that are used in a rehabilitation program.

Regardless of whether the primary focus is making certain an athlete is fit or reconditioning an injured patient, the athletic trainer must understand the basic principles for improving cardiorespiratory endurance, muscle strength and endurance, and flexibility.

# THE RELATIONSHIP BETWEEN ATHLETIC TRAINERS AND STRENGTH AND CONDITIONING COACHES

The responsibility for making certain that an athlete is fit for competition depends on the personnel who are available to oversee this aspect of the athletic program. At the professional level and at most colleges and universities, a full-time strength and conditioning coach is employed to conduct both team and individual training sessions. Many, but not all, strength coaches are certified by the National Strength and Conditioning Association. If a strength coach is involved, it is essential that both the athletic trainers and the team coaches communicate freely and work in close cooperation with the strength coach to ensure that the athletes achieve an optimal level of fitness.

The specific role of the athletic trainer is to critically review the training and conditioning program designed by the strength and conditioning coach and to be extremely familiar with what is expected of the athletes on a daily basis. The athletic trainer should feel free to offer suggestions and make recommendations that are in the best interest of the athletes' health and well-being. If it becomes apparent that a particular exercise or a specific training session seems to be causing an inordinate number of injuries, the athletic trainer should inform the strength and conditioning coach of the problem, so that some alternative exercise can be substituted.

If an athlete is injured and is undergoing a rehabilitation program, it should be the athletic trainer's responsibility to communicate to the strength and conditioning coach how the conditioning program should be limited and/or modified. The athletic trainer must respect the role of the strength and conditioning coach in getting the athlete fit. However, the responsibility for rehabilitating an injured patient should belong to the athletic trainer.

In the majority of secondary-school settings, if a strength and conditioning coach is not available, the responsibility for ensuring that the athlete gets fit lies with the athletic trainer and the team coaches. In this situation, the athletic trainer very often assumes the role of a strength and conditioning coach in addition to his or her athletic training responsibilities. The athletic trainer frequently finds it necessary not only to design training and conditioning programs but also to oversee the weight room and to educate young, inexperienced athletes about getting themselves fit to compete. The athletic trainer must demand the cooperation of the team coaches in supervising the training and conditioning program.

# PRINCIPLES OF CONDITIONING

The following principles should be applied in all conditioning programs to minimize the likelihood of injury:

1. *Safety.* Make the conditioning environment safe. Take time to educate individuals regarding proper techniques, how they should feel during the workout, and when they should push harder or back off.[41]
2. *Warm-up/cool-down.* Take time to do an appropriate warm-up before engaging in any activity. Do not neglect the cool-down period after a training bout.
3. *Motivation.* Athletes are generally highly motivated to work hard because they want to be successful in their sport. Varying the training program and incorporating techniques of periodization can keep the program enjoyable rather than routine and boring. (See the discussion of periodization at the end of this chapter.)
4. *Overload.* To improve in any physiological component, the individual must work harder than he or she is accustomed to working. Logan and Wallis identified

the **SAID principle,** which directly relates to the principle of overload.[62] SAID is an acronym for specific adaptation to imposed demands. The SAID principle states that, *when the body is subjected to stresses and overloads of varying intensities, it will gradually adapt over time to overcome whatever demands are placed on it.* For example, in weight training, as you progressively add more weight, the muscle tends to adapt to this increase in resistance by increasing in size and efficiency. Although overload is a critical factor in conditioning, the stress must not be great enough to produce damage or injury before the body has had a chance to adjust specifically to the increased demands.

5. *Consistency.* An individual must engage in a conditioning program on a regularly scheduled basis if it is to be effective.

6. *Progression.* Increase the intensity of the conditioning program gradually and within the individual's ability to adapt to increasing workloads.

7. *Intensity.* Stress the intensity of the work rather than the quantity. Coaches and athletic trainers too often confuse working hard with working for long periods of time. They make the mistake of prolonging the workout rather than increasing tempo or workload. The tired athlete is prone to injury.

8. *Specificity.* Identify specific goals for the conditioning program. The program must be designed to address specific components of fitness (i.e., strength, flexibility, cardiorespiratory endurance) relative to the activity in which the individual is participating.

9. *Individuality.* The needs of different individuals vary considerably. The successful coach is one who recognizes these individual differences and adjusts or alters the conditioning program accordingly to best accommodate the individual.

10. *Minimal stress.* Expect that athletes will train as close to their physiological limits as they can. Push the athletes as far as possible, but consider other stressful aspects of their lives and allow them time to be away from the conditioning demands of their sport.

# WARM-UP AND COOL-DOWN
## Warm-Up

It is generally accepted that a period of warm-up exercises should take place before a training session begins, although a systematic review of the evidence-based literature reveals that there is insufficient evidence to endorse or discontinue a warm-up prior to exercise to prevent injuries, although the weight of the evidence favors a decreased risk of injury.[39] Nevertheless, most athletic trainers would agree empirically that a warm-up period is a precaution against unnecessary musculoskeletal injuries and possible muscle soreness.[28] Some evidence suggests that a good dynamic warm-up may also improve certain aspects of performance.[3,40,97]

The function of the warm-up is to prepare the body physiologically for some upcoming physical work.[27] The purpose is to gradually stimulate the cardiorespiratory system to a moderate degree to increase the blood flow to working skeletal muscles and increase muscle temperature.[103]

Moderate activity speeds up the metabolic processes that produce an increase in core body temperature. An increase in the temperature of skeletal muscle alters the mechanical properties of the muscle. The elasticity of the muscle (the length to which the muscle can be stretched) is increased, and the viscosity (the rate at which the muscle can change shape) is decreased, which means that the muscle changes in shape more rapidly.

A good warm-up routine should begin with 2 or 3 minutes of slow walking, light jogging, or cycling to increase metabolism and warm up the muscles. Breaking into a light sweat is a good indication that muscle temperature has increased. Although research has indicated that increasing core temperature is effective in reducing injuries, there is moderate to strong evidence that stretching during the warm-up does not reduce injury.[90] Empirically, many professionals feel that stretching should be a part of the warm-up, and they continue to recommend that flexibility exercises be included. Six to twelve minutes of dynamic stretching is recommended to improve flexibility.[83] Passive stretching, although not harmful, may not improve performance.[82]

**Dynamic Warm-Up** For many years, the accepted technique was to perform a light jog followed by some static stretching. A more contemporary approach to the warm-up is to use an active, or "dynamic," warm-up to prepare for physical activity. A dynamic warm-up involves continuous movement using hopping, skipping, and bounding activities with several different footwork drills and patterns. It enhances coordination and motor ability as it revs up the nervous system. It prepares the muscles and joints in a more activity-specific manner than static stretching. The dynamic warm-up forces individuals to focus and concentrate. It should include exercises that address all the major muscle groups. The entire dynamic warm-up can be done in as little as 5 minutes or as long as 20 minutes, depending on the goals, age, and fitness level of the group. *Focus Box 4–1:* "Dynamic warm-up routine" lists a series of activities that can be included in a dynamic warm-up. Activity should begin immediately following the warm-up routine.

The individual should not wait longer than 15 minutes to begin the main sports activity after the warm-up, although the effects may last up to about 45 minutes.[77]

> Warming up involves general body warming and warming specific body areas for the demands of the sport.

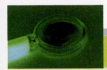

## FOCUS 4–1 Focus on Therapeutic Intervention

### Dynamic warm-up routine

Two sets of cones are spaced 10 to 20 yards apart. The individual performs the following dynamic exercises between the cones, then jogs back to the start.

1. Jog forward
2. Jog backward
3. Walking calf stretch
4. Walking hamstring stretch
5. Hand-assisted knee stretch to chest
6. Hand-assisted knee stretch to opposite shoulder
7. Hand-assisted walking adductor stretch
8. Lateral shuffle moving to the right followed by the left
9. Walking lateral lunge to the right followed by the left
10. Skipping with low knees
11. Walking lunge, arms extended overhead
12. Walking lunge with rotation to each side
13. Walking quadriceps stretch
14. Jogging butt kicks
15. Open the gate exercise
16. Close the gate exercise
17. Carioca to the right followed by the left
18. Power high knees skipping
19. Prancing
20. High knees running
21. Back pedaling butt kicks
22. Forward sprint

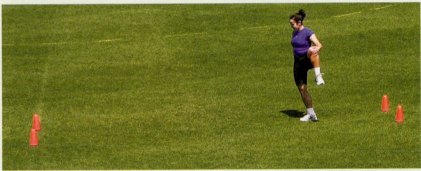
© William E. Prentice

## Cool-Down

Following a workout or training session, a cool-down period may be beneficial. The cool-down period enables the body to cool and return to a resting state. Such a period should last about 5 to 10 minutes. An example of a cool-down activity would be to have the individual jog and progressively decrease the pace to a walk to allow the metabolism to return to resting levels. This would be followed by stretching activities.

Although the warm-up period is common, the importance of a cool-down period afterward is often ignored. Again, experience and observation indicate that persons who stretch during the cool-down period tend to have fewer problems with muscle soreness after strenuous activity.[79]

A marathon runner comes into the sports medicine clinic, complaining of feeling tightness in her lower extremity during workouts. She states that she has a difficult time during her warm-up and cannot seem to "get loose" until her workout is almost complete. She feels that she is always on the verge of pulling a muscle.

❓ What should the athletic trainer recommend as a specific warm-up routine that this patient should consistently do before beginning her workout?

## CARDIORESPIRATORY ENDURANCE

**Cardiorespiratory endurance** is the ability to perform whole-body, large-muscle activities for extended periods of time. The cardiorespiratory system provides a means by which oxygen is supplied to the various tissues of the body.[44] For anyone who engages in exercise, cardiorespiratory endurance is critical both for performance and for preventing undue fatigue that may predispose the person to injury.

### Transport and Utilization of Oxygen

Basically, transport of oxygen throughout the body involves the coordinated function of four components: heart, lungs, blood vessels, and blood. The improvement of cardiorespiratory endurance through training occurs because of the increased capability of each of these four elements collectively to provide necessary oxygen to the working tissues. The greatest rate at which oxygen can be taken in and used during exercise is referred to as *maximum aerobic capacity* ($\dot{V}O_2$max).[34] The performance of

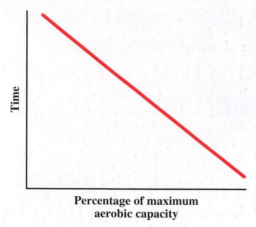

FIGURE 4–1   The greater the percentage of maximum aerobic capacity required during an activity, the less time the activity may be performed.

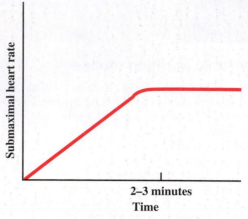

FIGURE 4–2   Two to three minutes are required for heart rate to plateau at a given workload.

any activity requires a certain rate of oxygen consumption that is about the same for all persons, depending on the level of fitness. Generally, the greater the rate or intensity of the performance of an activity, the greater the oxygen consumption. Each person has his or her own maximal rate of oxygen consumption. That person's ability to perform an activity or to fatigue is closely related to the amount of oxygen required by that activity and is limited by the person's maximal rate of oxygen consumption. The greater the percentage of maximum oxygen consumption required during an activity, the less time the activity may be sustained (Figure 4–1).[69]

The maximal rate at which oxygen can be used is a genetically determined characteristic; a person inherits a certain range of maximum aerobic capacity, and the more active that person is, the higher the existing maximum aerobic capacity will be in that range.[31] A conditioning program allows an individual to increase maximum aerobic capacity to its highest limit within that person's range. Maximum aerobic capacity is most often presented in terms of the volume of oxygen used relative to body weight per unit of time (ml/kg/min). A normal maximum aerobic capacity for most college-age athletes would fall in the range of 45 to 60 ml/kg/min.[92] A world-class male or female marathon runner may have a maximum aerobic capacity in the 70 to 80 ml/kg/min range.

Three factors determine the maximal rate at which oxygen can be used: external respiration involving the ventilatory process or pulmonary function; gas transport, which is accomplished by the cardiovascular system (i.e., the heart, blood vessels, and blood); and internal respiration, which involves the use of oxygen by the cells to produce energy. Of these three factors, the most limiting is generally the ability to transport oxygen through the system; thus, the cardiovascular system limits the overall rate of oxygen consumption.

A high maximum aerobic capacity within an individual's inherited range indicates that all three systems are working well.

## Effects on the Heart

The heart is the main pumping mechanism, circulating oxygenated blood throughout the body to the working tissues. As the body begins to exercise, the muscles use oxygen at a much higher rate, and the heart must pump more oxygenated blood to meet this increased demand. The heart is capable of adapting to this increased demand through several mechanisms. Heart rate shows a gradual adaptation to an increased workload by becoming more efficient and increasing proportionally to the intensity of the exercise. Heart rate will plateau at a given level after about 2 to 3 minutes (Figure 4–2). At rest, the heart beats about 70 times per minute. The maximal heart rate is different in everybody, but it can be estimated by multiplying the person's age in years by .70 and subtracting it from 208.

Monitoring heart rate is an indirect method of estimating oxygen consumption. In general, heart rate and oxygen consumption have a linear relationship, although at very low intensities and at high intensities this linear relationship breaks down (Figure 4–3).[36] During higher-intensity activities, maximal heart rate may be achieved before maximal oxygen consumption, which will continue to rise.[59] The greater the intensity of the exercise, the higher the heart rate. Because of these existing relationships, it should become apparent that the rate of oxygen consumption can be estimated by taking heart rate.[17]

A second mechanism by which the heart is able to adapt to increased demands during exercise is to increase the *stroke volume*—the volume of blood being pumped out with each beat.[17] The heart pumps out approximately 70 ml of blood per beat. Stroke volume can continue to increase only to the point at which there is simply not enough time between beats for the heart to

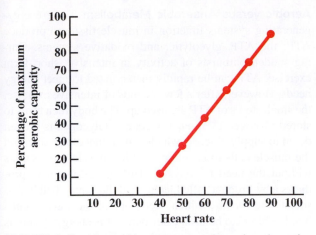

FIGURE 4–3   Maximal heart rate is achieved at about the same time as maximum aerobic capacity.

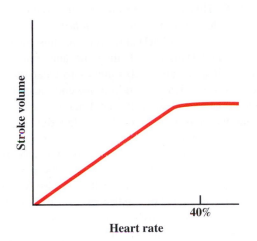

FIGURE 4–4   Stroke volume plateaus at 40 percent of maximal heart rate.

fill up. This point occurs at about 40 percent of maximal heart rate, and above this level increases in the volume of blood being pumped out per unit of time must be caused entirely by increases in heart rate (Figure 4–4).[66]

Stroke volume and heart rate together determine the volume of blood being pumped through the heart in a given unit of time. This is referred to as the *cardiac output,* which indicates how much blood the heart is capable of pumping in exactly 1 minute.[66] Approximately 5 L of blood are pumped through the heart during each minute at rest. Thus, cardiac output is the primary determinant of the maximal rate of oxygen consumption possible (Figure 4–5). During exercise, cardiac output increases to approximately four times that experienced during rest in the normal individual and may increase as much as six times in the elite endurance athlete.

A **training effect** occurs with regard to cardiac output of the heart—the stroke volume increases while exercise heart rate is reduced at a given standard exercise load. The heart becomes more efficient because it is capable of pumping more blood with each stroke. Because the heart

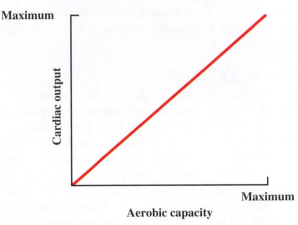

FIGURE 4–5   Cardiac output limits maximum aerobic capacity.

is a muscle, it will hypertrophy to some extent, but this hypertrophy is in no way a negative effect of training.

$$\text{Cardiac output} = \text{Increased stroke volume} \times \text{Decreased heart rate}$$

## Effects on Work Ability

Cardiorespiratory endurance plays a critical role in an individual's ability to resist fatigue. Fatigue is closely related to the percentage of maximum aerobic capacity that a particular workload demands.[17] Without sufficient oxygen, glycogen stores are quickly depleted. For example, Figure 4–6 presents two individuals, A and B. A has a maximum aerobic capacity of 50 ml/kg/min, whereas B has a maximum aerobic capacity of only 40 ml/kg/min. If A and B are both exercising at the same intensity, A will be working at a much lower percentage of maximum aerobic capacity than B. Consequently, A should be able to sustain his or her activity over a much longer period of time. Performance may be impaired if the ability to use oxygen efficiently is

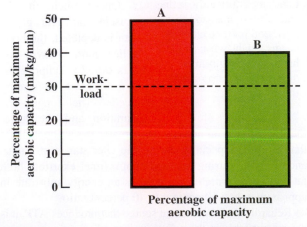

FIGURE 4–6   Person A should be able to work longer than Person B as a result of lower utilization of maximum aerobic capacity.

impaired. Thus, improvement of cardiorespiratory endurance should be an essential component of any conditioning program.

## The Energy Systems

Various sports activities involve specific demands for energy. For example, sprinting and jumping are high-energy activities, requiring a relatively large production of energy for a short time. Long-distance running and swimming, on the other hand, are mostly low-energy activities per unit of time, requiring energy production for a prolonged time. Other physical activities demand a blend of both high- and low-energy output. These various energy demands can be met by the different processes in which energy can be supplied to the skeletal muscles.

### ATP: The Immediate Energy Source
Energy is produced from the breakdown of nutrient foodstuffs.[66] This energy is used to produce *adenosine triphosphate (ATP)*, which is the ultimate usable form of energy for muscular activity. ATP is produced in the muscle tissue from blood glucose or glycogen. Glucose is derived from the breakdown of dietary carbohydrates. Glucose not needed immediately is stored as glycogen in the resting muscle and liver. Stored glycogen in the liver can later be converted back to glucose and transferred to the blood to meet the body's energy needs. Fats and proteins can also be metabolized to generate ATP.

Once much of the muscle and liver glycogen is depleted, the body relies more heavily on fats stored in adipose tissue to meet its energy needs. The longer the duration and the lower the intensity of an activity, the greater the amount of fat that is used, especially during the later stages of endurance events. During rest and submaximal exertion, both fat and carbohydrates are used as an energy substrate in approximately a 60 percent to 40 percent ratio.[66]

Regardless of the nutrient source that produces ATP, it is always available in the cell as an immediate energy source. When all available sources of ATP are depleted, more must be regenerated for muscular contraction to continue.

### Aerobic versus Anaerobic Metabolism
Three energy-generating systems function in muscle tissue to produce ATP: the ATP, glycolytic, and oxidative systems. During sudden outbursts of activity in intensive, short-term exercise, ATP can be rapidly metabolized to meet energy needs. However, after a few seconds of intensive exercise, the small stores of ATP are used up. The body then turns to stored glycogen as an energy source. Glycogen is broken down to supply glucose, which is then metabolized within the muscle cells to generate ATP for muscle contractions without the need for oxygen. This breakdown also produces a by-product called lactic acid that immediately dissociates to *lactate,* which seeps out of the muscle cells into the blood to be used elsewhere. This energy system is referred to as *anaerobic metabolism.*[85]

As exercise continues, the body has to rely on a more complex form of carbohydrate and fat metabolism to generate ATP. This energy system requires oxygen and is therefore referred to as *aerobic metabolism.* The aerobic system burns the lactate using oxygen, thus removing it and creating far more ATP than the anaerobic system. Normally, it takes about 20 minutes to clear the lactate from the system. Training to improve endurance helps an individual get rid of the lactic acid before it can build to the point where it contributes to muscle fatigue.[5]

In most activities, both aerobic and anaerobic systems function simultaneously.[66] The degree to which the two are involved is determined by the intensity and duration of the activity. If the intensity of the activity is such that sufficient oxygen can be supplied to meet the demands of working tissues, the activity is considered to be aerobic. Conversely, if the activity is of high enough intensity or the duration is such that there is insufficient oxygen available to meet energy demands, the activity becomes anaerobic. Consequently, an oxygen debt is incurred, which must be paid back during the recovery period. For example, short bursts of muscle contraction, as in running or swimming sprints, use predominantly the anaerobic system. However, endurance events depend a great deal on the aerobic system. Most activities use a combination of anaerobic and aerobic metabolism and all activities will initially utilize the anaerobic energy system (Table 4–1).

## Training Techniques for Improving Cardiorespiratory Endurance

Cardiorespiratory endurance may be improved through several different training techniques.[68] Largely, the amount of improvement possible will be determined by an individual's initial levels of cardiorespiratory endurance.

### Continuous Training
Continuous training involves four considerations:

- *Frequency* of the activity
- *Intensity* of the activity
- *Type* of activity
- *Time* of the activity

TABLE 4–1

## Comparison of Aerobic versus Anaerobic Activities

| | Mode | Relative Intensity | Performance | Frequency | Duration | Miscellaneous |
|---|---|---|---|---|---|---|
| Aerobic activities | Continuous, long-duration, sustained activities | Less intense | 50% to 85% of maximum range | At least three but not more than six times per week | 20 to 60 min | Less risk to sedentary or older individuals |
| Anaerobic activities | Explosive, short-duration, burst-type activities | More intense | 85% to 100% of maximum range | Three to four times per week | 10 sec to 2 min | Used in sport and team activities |

**Frequency** To see at least minimal improvement in cardiorespiratory endurance, it is necessary for the average person to engage in no fewer than three sessions per week.[5] If possible, an individual should aim for four or five sessions per week. A competitive athlete should be prepared to train as often as six times per week. Everyone should take at least one day per week off to allow for both psychological and physiological rest.

> A female soccer player has a grade 1 ankle sprain that is likely to keep her out of practice for about a week. She has worked extremely hard on her fitness levels and is concerned that not being able to run for an entire week will hurt her cardiorespiratory fitness.
>
> ❓ What types of activity should the athletic trainer recommend during her rehabilitation period that can help her maintain her existing level of cardiorespiratory endurance?

**Intensity of Activity** The intensity of the exercise is also a critical factor, although recommendations regarding training intensities vary. This is particularly true in the early stages of training, when the body is forced to make a lot of adjustments to increased workload demands.

**Determining Exercise Intensity by Monitoring Heart Rate** The objective of aerobic exercise is to elevate heart rate to a specified target rate and maintain it at that level during the entire workout. Because heart rate is directly related to the intensity of the exercise and to the rate of oxygen utilization, it becomes a relatively simple process to identify a specific workload (pace) that will make the heart rate plateau at the desired level.[35] By monitoring heart rate, athletes know whether the pace is too fast or too slow to get the heart rate into a target range.[85]

Heart rate can be increased or decreased by speeding up or slowing down the pace. As mentioned, heart rate increases proportionately with the intensity of the workload and will plateau after 2 to 3 minutes of activity. Thus, the athlete should be actively engaged in the workout for 2 to 3 minutes before measuring his or her pulse.

Several formulas allow you to identify a training *target heart rate*.[44,54] To calculate a specific target heart rate, you must first determine your maximum heart rate (MHR). Exact determination of MHR involves exercising an individual at a maximal level and monitoring the heart rate (HR) using an electrocardiogram. This is a difficult process outside of a laboratory. Maximum heart rate is related to age, and, as you get older, your MHR decreases. An approximate estimate of MHR for individuals of both genders would be:

$$HR_{max} = 208 - 0.7 \times Age$$

For a 20-year-old individual, maximum heart rate would be about 194 beats per minute ($208 - 0.7 \times 20$).

*Heart rate reserve* is used to determine upper and lower limits of the target heart rate range. Heart rate reserve (HRR) is the difference between resting heart rate $(HR_{rest})^*$ and maximum heart rate $(HR_{max})^*$.

$$HRR = HR_{max} - HR_{rest}$$

The greater the difference, the larger your heart rate reserve and the greater your range of potential training heart rate intensities. The *Karvonen equation* is used to calculate target heart rate at a given percentage of training intensity.[53]

To use the Karvonen equation, you need to know your HRR.

$$Target\ HR = HR_{rest} + \%\ of\ target\ intensity \times HRR$$

When using estimated $HR_{max}$ or/and $HR_{rest}$, the values are always predictions. So, in a 20-year-old with a calculated $HR_{max}$ of 194 and an $HR_{rest}$ of 70 beats per minute, the heart rate reserve is (124 ($194 - 70 = 124$)). For moderate-intensity activity, the heart should work in a range between the lower limit and an upper limit. The lower limit is calculated by taking 70 percent of the heart rate reserve and adding the resting heart rate, which would be 157 beats per minute ($(124 \times 0.7) + 70 = 157$). The upper limit is calculated by taking 79 percent of the heart rate reserve and adding the resting heart rate ($(124 \times 0.79) + 70 = 168$).

The American College of Sports Medicine (ACSM) recommends that young healthy individuals train at either

*True resting heart rate should be monitored with the subject lying down.

moderate intensity (70 to 79 percent of maximum heart rate) or vigorous intensity (greater than 80 percent of maximum heart rate) levels to improve cardiorespiratory endurance and reduce the risk for chronic disease.[5] Individuals who are less fit, have led a previously sedentary lifestyle, are overweight, have a history of risk factors for heart disease, are elderly, have arthritis, and who have special instructions from a physician should engage initially in low-intensity workouts. For those individuals, the important thing is for them to become active; if they are persistent they should gradually be able to increase the intensity of the activity.[5]

*Determining Exercise Intensity through Rating of Perceived Exertion* Rating of perceived exertion (RPE) can be used in addition to heart rate monitoring to indicate exercise intensity.[35] During exercise, individuals are asked to rate subjectively on a numerical scale from 6 to 20 exactly how they feel relative to their level of exertion (Table 4–2). More intense exercise that requires a higher level of oxygen consumption and energy expenditure is directly related to higher subjective ratings of perceived exertion. Over time, individuals can be taught to exercise at a specific RPE that relates directly to more objective measures of exercise intensity.

*Type of Activity* The type of activity used in continuous training must be aerobic.[17] Aerobic activities are those that elevate the heart rate and maintain it at that level for an extended time. Aerobic activities generally involve repetitive, whole-body, large-muscle movements performed over an extended time. Examples of aerobic activities are running, jogging, walking, cycling, swimming, rope skipping, stair-climbing, and cross-country skiing. The advantage of these aerobic activities as opposed to more intermittent activities, such as racquetball, squash, basketball, or tennis, is that aerobic activities are easy to regulate by either speeding up or slowing down the pace. Because

the given intensity of the workload elicits a given heart rate, these aerobic activities allow athletes to maintain heart rate at a specified or target level. Intermittent activities involve variable speeds and intensities that cause the heart rate to fluctuate considerably. Although these intermittent activities improve cardiorespiratory endurance, their intensity is much more difficult to monitor.

*Time (Duration) of Activity* For minimal improvement to occur, the ACSM recommends 20 to 60 minutes of workout/activity with the heart rate elevated to training levels.[5] Generally, the greater the duration of the workout, the greater the improvement in cardiorespiratory endurance. The competitive athlete should train for at least 45 minutes per session.

**High-Intensity Interval Training** Unlike continuous training, **high-intensity interval training** involves activities that are more intermittent. Interval training consists of alternating periods of relatively intense work and active recovery.[19] It allows for performance of much more work at a more intense workload over a longer period than does working continuously.[19] In continuous training, the athlete strives to work at an intensity of about 60 to 85 percent of maximum heart rate. Obviously, sustaining activity at the higher intensity over a 20-minute period is extremely difficult. The advantage of high-intensity interval training is that it allows work at the 80 percent or higher level for a short period followed by an active period of recovery during which the athlete may be working at only 30 to 45 percent of maximum heart rate. Thus, the intensity of the workout and its duration can be greater than with continuous training. High-intensity interval training has also been shown to improve cardiorespiratory fitness ($VO2_{max}$) in as little as 2 weeks.[94]

Most sports are intermittent, involving short bursts of intense activity followed by a sort of active recovery period (e.g., football, basketball, soccer, or tennis).[42] Training with the high-intensity interval training technique allows the athlete to be more sport specific during the workout. With high-intensity interval training, the overload principle is applied by making the training period much more intense. There are several important considerations in high-intensity interval training. The *training period* is the amount of time that continuous activity is actually being performed, and the *recovery period* is the time between training periods. A *set* is a group of combined training and recovery periods, and a *repetition* is the number of training/recovery periods per set. *Training time* or *distance* refers to the rate or distance of the training period. The training/recovery ratio indicates a time ratio for training versus recovery.

An example of high-intensity interval training is a soccer player running sprints. An interval workout would involve running ten 120-yard sprints in under 20 seconds each, with a 1-minute walking recovery period between each sprint. During this training session, the soccer player's heart rate will probably increase to 85 to 90 percent of maximum level during the sprint and will probably fall to the 35 to 45 percent level during the recovery period.

| TABLE 4–2 | Rating of Perceived Exertion |
|---|---|
| **Scale** | **Verbal Rating** |
| 6 | |
| 7 | Very, very light |
| 8 | |
| 9 | Very light |
| 10 | |
| 11 | Fairly light |
| 12 | |
| 13 | Somewhat hard |
| 14 | |
| 15 | Hard |
| 16 | |
| 17 | Very hard |
| 18 | |
| 19 | Very, very hard |
| 20 | |

**Fartlek Training** *Fartlek,* a training technique that is a type of cross-country running originated in Sweden. Fartlek literally means "speed play." It is similar to interval training in that the athlete must run for a specified period; however, specific pace and speed are not identified. The course for a fartlek workout should be a varied terrain with some level running, some uphill and downhill running, and some running through obstacles such as trees or rocks. The object is to put surges into a running workout, varying the length of the surges according to individual purposes. One big advantage of fartlek training is that because the pace and terrain are always changing, the training session is less regimented and allows for an effective alternative in the training routine. Most people who jog or walk around the community are really engaging in a fartlek-type workout.

Again, if fartlek training is going to improve cardiorespiratory endurance, it must elevate the heart rate to at least minimal training levels (60 to 85 percent). Fartlek may best be used as an off-season conditioning activity or as a change-of-pace activity to counteract the boredom of a training program that uses the same activity day after day.

## Equipment for Improving Cardiorespiratory Endurance

The extent and variety of fitness and exercise equipment available to the consumer are at times mind boggling (Figure 4–7). Prices of equipment can range from $2 for a jump rope to $60,000 for certain computer-driven isokinetic devices. It is certainly not necessary to purchase

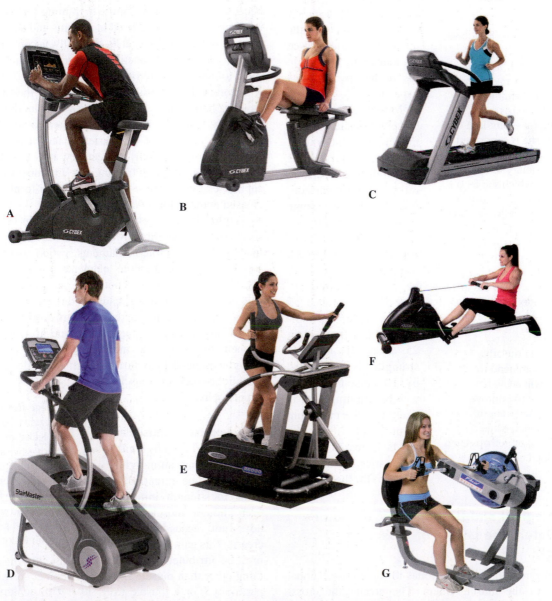

FIGURE 4–7   Fitness equipment. **(A)** Stationary bike. **(B)** Recumbent bike. **(C)** Treadmill. **(D)** Stair climber. **(E)** Elliptical exerciser. **(F)** Rowing machine. **(G)** Upper-extremity ergometer.
(a–c) Courtesy Cybex International; (d) Courtesy Stairmaster; (e) Courtesy Body-Solid, Inc; (f) Stamina Products, Inc.; (g) Courtesy First Degree Fitness

expensive exercise equipment to see good results. Many of the same physiological benefits can be achieved from using a $2 jump rope as from running on a $10,000 treadmill.

# THE IMPORTANCE OF MUSCULAR STRENGTH, ENDURANCE, AND POWER

The development of **muscular strength** is an essential component of a conditioning program for every athlete. Strength is the ability of a muscle to generate force against some resistance. Most movements in sports are explosive and must include elements of both strength and speed if they are to be effective. If a large amount of force is generated quickly, the movement can be referred to as a **power** movement. Without the ability to generate power, an athlete is limited in his or her performance capabilities.[77]

Muscular strength is closely associated with muscular endurance. **Muscular endurance** is the ability to perform repetitive muscular contractions against some resistance for an extended period of time. As muscular strength increases, there tends to be a corresponding increase in endurance.[59,99] For example, an individual can lift a weight 25 times. If muscular strength is increased by 10 percent through weight training, it is likely that the maximum number of repetitions will be increased because it is easier for the individual to lift the weight.

## Physiological and Biomechanical Factors That Determine Levels of Muscular Strength

Muscular strength is proportional to the cross-sectional diameter of the muscle fibers. The greater the cross-sectional diameter or the bigger a particular muscle, the stronger it is, and thus the more force it is capable of generating. The size of a muscle tends to increase in cross-sectional diameter with weight training. This increase in muscle size is referred to as **hypertrophy.**[51] Conversely, a decrease in the size of a muscle is referred to as **atrophy.**

**Size of the Muscle** Strength is a function of the number and diameter of muscle fibers composing a given muscle. The number of fibers is an inherited characteristic; thus, an individual with a large number of muscle fibers to begin with has the potential to hypertrophy to a much greater degree than does someone with relatively fewer fibers.[51]

**Explanations for Muscle Hypertrophy** A number of theories have been proposed to explain why a muscle hypertrophies in response to strength training.[66] Some evidence exists that the number of muscle fibers increases because fibers split in response to training.[37] However, this research has been conducted in animals and should not be generalized to humans. It is generally accepted that the number of fibers is genetically determined and does not seem to increase with training.

Another hypothesis is that because the muscle is working harder in weight training, more blood is required to supply that muscle with oxygen and other nutrients. Thus, the number of capillaries is increased. This hypothesis is only partially correct; few new capillaries are formed during strength training, but a number of dormant capillaries may become filled with blood to meet the increased demand for blood supply.

A third theory to explain this increase in muscle size seems the most credible. Muscle fibers are composed primarily of small protein filaments, called myofilaments, which are the contractile elements in muscle. These myofilaments increase in both size and number as a result of strength training, causing the individual muscle fibers themselves to increase in cross-sectional diameter.[37] This increase is particularly true in men, although women also see some increase in muscle size.[1] More research is needed to further clarify and determine the specific causes of muscle hypertrophy.

**Improved Neuromuscular Efficiency** Typically with weight training, an individual sees some remarkable gains in strength initially, even though muscle bulk does not necessarily increase. This gain in strength must be attributed to something other than muscle hypertrophy. For a muscle to contract, an impulse must be transmitted from the nervous system to the muscle.

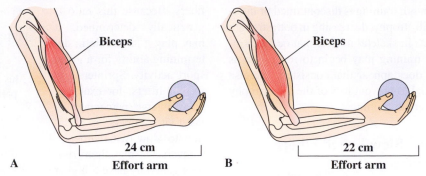

**A**      24 cm      **B**      22 cm

Effort arm      Effort arm

**FIGURE 4–8** The position of attachment of the muscle tendon on the arm can affect the ability of that muscle to generate force. Person B should be able to generate greater force than person A because the tendon attachment is closer to the resistance.

Each muscle fiber is innervated by a specific motor unit. By overloading a particular muscle, as in weight training, the muscle is forced to work efficiently. Efficiency is achieved by getting more motor units to fire, causing a stronger contraction of the muscle.[101] Consequently, it is not uncommon to see extremely rapid gains in strength when a weight-training program is first begun due to an improvement in neuromuscular function.[51]

**Other Physiological Adaptations to Resistance Exercise** In addition to muscle hypertrophy, there are a number of other physiological adaptations to resistance training.[85] The strength of noncontractile structures, including tendons and ligaments, is increased. The mineral content of bone is increased, making the bone stronger and more resistant to fracture. Maximal oxygen uptake is improved when resistance training is of sufficient intensity to elicit heart rates at or above training levels. Several enzymes important in aerobic and anaerobic metabolism also increase.[17,66]

**Biomechanical Factors** Strength in a given muscle is determined not only by the physical properties of the muscle itself but also by biomechanical factors that dictate how much force can be generated through a system of levers to an external object.[47] If we think of the elbow joint as one of these lever systems, we would have the biceps muscle producing flexion of this joint (Figure 4–8). The position of attachment of the biceps muscle on the lever arm—in this case, the forearm—will largely determine how much force this muscle is capable of generating.[43] If there are two persons, A and B, and person B has a biceps attachment that is farther from the center of the joint than is person A's, then person B should be able to lift heavier weights because the muscle force acts through a longer lever (moment) arm and thus can produce greater torque around the joint.

The length of a muscle determines the tension that can be generated.[47] By varying the length of a muscle,

different tensions may be produced. This *length-tension* relationship is illustrated in Figure 4–9. At position B in the curve, the interaction of the crossbridges between the actin and myosin myofilaments within the sarcomere is at a maximum. Setting a muscle at this length will produce the greatest amount of tension. At position A the muscle is shortened, and at position C the muscle is lengthened. In either case, the interaction between the actin and myosin myofilaments through the crossbridges is greatly reduced, and the muscle is not capable of generating significant tension.

**Overtraining** Overtraining can have a negative effect on the development of muscular strength. Overtraining can result in psychological breakdown (staleness) or physiological breakdown, which may involve musculoskeletal injury, fatigue, or sickness. Engaging in proper and efficient resistance training, eating a proper diet, and getting appropriate rest can minimize the potential negative effects of overtraining.

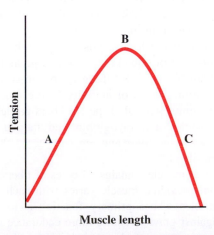

**FIGURE 4–9** Because of the length-tension relation in muscle, the greatest tension is developed at point B, with less tension developed at points A and C.

**Reversibility** If strength training is discontinued or interrupted, the muscle will atrophy, decreasing in both strength and mass. Adaptations in skeletal muscle that occur in response to resistance training may begin to reverse in as little as 48 hours. It does appear that consistent exercise of a muscle is essential to prevent loss of the hypertrophy that occurs due to strength training.

## Fast-Twitch versus Slow-Twitch Fibers and Muscular Endurance

Skeletal muscle fibers in a particular motor unit are either *slow-twitch* or *fast-twitch* fibers, each of which has distinctive metabolic and contractile capabilities. Slow-twitch (ST) fibers, also referred to as type I or slow oxidative (SO) fibers, are dense with capillaries and are rich in mitochondria and myoglobin, giving the muscle tissue its characteristic red color. They can carry more oxygen and thus are more resistant to fatigue than are fast-twitch fibers.[17] Slow-twitch fibers are associated primarily with long-duration, aerobic-type activities.[66]

> **Four basic types of muscle fibers:**
> - Slow-twitch, or type I
> - Fast-twitch type IIa
> - Fast-twitch type IIb
> - Fast-twitch type IIx

Fast-twitch (FT) fibers are referred to as type II or fast oxidative glycolytic (FOG) fibers. They are capable of producing quick, forceful contractions but have a tendency to fatigue more rapidly than do slow-twitch fibers. Fast-twitch fibers are useful in short-term, high-intensity activities, which mainly involve the anaerobic system. Fast-twitch fibers are capable of producing powerful contractions, whereas slow-twitch fibers produce a long-endurance type of force.

Fast-twitch fibers can be subdivided into three groups, although all three types are capable of rapid contraction. Type IIa fibers, like slow-twitch muscle fibers, are moderately resistant to fatigue. Type IIx, also known as fast glycolytic (FG) and occasionally type IId, are less dense in mitochondria and myoglobin than type IIa. This is the fastest muscle type in humans and it can contract more quickly and with a greater amount of force than type IIa. But these fibers can sustain only short, anaerobic bursts of acitivity before muscle contraction becomes painful. Type IIb fibers are less dense in mitochondria and myoglobin and fatigue rapidly. They are white in color and are considered the "true" fast-twitch fibers.[66]

Any given muscle contains all types of fibers, and the ratio in an individual muscle varies with each person.[17] Those muscles whose primary function is to maintain posture against gravity require more endurance and have a higher percentage of slow-twitch fibers. Muscles that produce powerful, rapid, explosive strength movements tend to have a much greater percentage of fast-twitch fibers. Because this ratio is genetically determined, it may play a large role in determining ability for a given sport activity. Sprinters and weight lifters, for example, have a large percentage of fast-twitch fibers in relation to slow-twitch fibers.[17] Conversely, marathon runners generally have a higher percentage of slow-twitch fibers.

The metabolic capabilities of both fast-twitch and slow-twitch fibers may be improved through specific strength and endurance training. It appears that there can be an almost complete change from slow-twitch to fast-twitch and from fast-twitch to slow-twitch fiber types in response to training.[66] Fibers that are in the process of transitioning from one fiber type to another share some properties of both type I and type II fibers and are referred to as "hybrid" fibers.

## Skeletal Muscle Contractions

Skeletal muscle is capable of three types of contraction: *isometric contraction, concentric contraction,* and *eccentric contraction.*[25] An isometric contraction occurs when the muscle contracts to increase tension but there is no change in the length of the muscle. Considerable force can be generated against some immovable resistance even though no movement occurs. In concentric contraction, the muscle shortens in length as a contraction is developed to overcome or move some resistance. In eccentric contraction, the resistance is greater than the muscular force being produced, and the muscle lengthens while continuing to contract. Concentric and eccentric contractions are both considered to be dynamic movements.[25]

> **Skeletal muscle is capable of three types of contraction:**
> - Isometric
> - Concentric
> - Eccentric

It is critical to understand that functional movements involve acceleration, deceleration, and stabilization in all three planes of motion simultaneously. Functional movements are controlled by neuromuscular mechanoreceptors located within the muscle.[25]

> A high-school shot-putter has been working intensely on weight training to improve his muscular power. In particular, he has been concentrating on lifting extremely heavy free weights, using a low number of repetitions (three sets of six to eight repetitions). Although his strength has improved significantly over the last several months, he is not seeing the same degree of improvement in his throws, even though his coach says that his technique is very good.
>
> **?** The athlete is frustrated with his performance and wants to know if there is anything else he can do in his training program that might enhance his performance.

## Techniques of Resistance Training

There are a number of techniques of resistance training for strength improvement, including functional strength-training exercises, core stability training, isometric exercise, progressive resistance exercise, isokinetic exercise, circuit training, calisthenic strengthening exercises, and plyometric exercise. Regardless of which of these techniques is used, one basic principle of training is extremely important. For a muscle to improve in strength, it must be forced to work at a higher level than it is accustomed to working. In other words, the muscle must be *overloaded.* Without overload, the muscle will be able to maintain strength as long as training is continued against a resistance the muscle is accustomed to. To most effectively build muscular strength, weight training requires a consistent, increasing effort against progressively increasing resistance.[32] If this principle of overload is applied, all eight conditioning techniques can produce improvement in muscular strength over a period of time.

**Functional Strength Training** For many years, the strength-training techniques in conditioning or rehabilitation programs have focused on isolated, single-plane exercises used to elicit muscle hypertrophy in a specific muscle. These exercises have a very low neuromuscular demand because they are performed primarily with the rest of the body artificially stabilized on stable pieces of equipment.[25] The central nervous system controls the ability to integrate the proprioceptive function of a number of individual muscles that must act collectively to produce a specific movement pattern that occurs in three planes of motion. If the body is designed to move in three planes of motion, then isolated training does little to improve functional ability. When strength training using isolated, single-plane, artificially stabilized exercises, the entire body is not being prepared to deal with the imposed demands of normal daily activities (walking up or down stairs, getting groceries out of the trunk, etc.).[25] Functional strength training provides a unique approach that may revolutionize the way the sports medicine community thinks about strength training.

To understand the approach to functional strength training, the athletic trainer must understand the concept of the *kinetic chain* and must realize that the entire kinetic chain is an integrated functional unit. The kinetic chain is composed of not only muscle, tendons, fasciae, and ligaments but also the articular system and the neural system. All of these systems function simultaneously as an integrated unit to allow for structural and functional efficiency. If any system within the kinetic chain is not working efficiently, the other systems are forced to adapt and compensate; this can lead to tissue overload, decreased performance, and predictable patterns of injury. The functional integration of the systems allows for optimal neuromuscular efficiency during functional activities.[16,25]

During functional movements, some muscles contract concentrically (shorten) to produce movement, others contract eccentrically (lengthen) to allow movement to occur, and still other muscles contract isometrically to create a stable base on which the functional movement occurs. These functional movements occur in three planes. Functional strength training uses integrated exercises designed to improve functional movement patterns in terms of not only increased strength and improved neuromuscular control but also high levels of stabilization strength and dynamic flexibility.[16]

Unlike traditional strength-training techniques, which use barbells, dumbbells, or exercise machines and single-plane exercises day after day, a primary principle of functional strength training is to make use of training variations to force constant neural adaptations instead of concentrating solely on morphological changes. Exercise variables that can be changed include the plane of motion, body position, base of support, upper- or lower-extremity symmetry, the type of balance modality, and the type of external resistance.[25] Table 4–3 lists these exercise training variables. Figure 4–10 provides examples of functional strengthening exercises.

**Core Stability Training** A core stabilization training program is designed to help an individual gain strength, neuromuscular control, power, and muscle endurance of the muscles in the lumbar spine, in the abdomen, and around the hips and pelvis.[87] These muscles are collectively referred to as the **core**.[26] The concept of core stability training is essential. A weak core is a fundamental problem of inefficient movements that lead to injury.[61] If the muscles in the extremities are strong and the core is weak, the force required for efficient movements cannot be produced. Core stability training should be an important component of all comprehensive strengthening programs.[18,30,74] Dynamic core stabilization programs and exercises are discussed in detail in Chapters 16 and 25. Figure 4–11 shows several examples of exercises that may be used to improve core stability.

**Isometric Exercise** An **isometric exercise** involves a muscle contraction in which the length of the muscle remains constant while tension develops toward a maximal force against an immovable resistance.[9] The muscle should generate a maximal force for 10 seconds at a time, and this contraction should be repeated 5 to 10 times per day. Isometric exercises are capable of increasing muscular strength; unfortunately, strength gains are relatively specific to the joint angle at which training is performed. At other angles, the strength curve drops off dramatically because of a lack of motor activity at that angle.

Another major disadvantage of isometric exercises is that they tend to produce a spike in systolic blood pressure, which can result in potentially life-threatening

| TABLE 4–3 | Exercise Training Variables | | | | | | |
|---|---|---|---|---|---|---|
| **Plane of Motion** | **Body Position** | **Base of Support** | **Upper-Extremity Symmetry** | **Lower-Extremity Symmetry** | **Balance Modality** | **External Resistance** |
| ▪ Sagittal<br>▪ Frontal<br>▪ Transverse<br>▪ Combination | ▪ Supine<br>▪ Prone<br>▪ Side-lying<br>▪ Sitting<br>▪ Kneeling<br>▪ Half kneeling<br>▪ Standing | ▪ Exercise bench<br>▪ Stability ball<br>▪ Balance modality<br>▪ Other | ▪ 2 arms<br>▪ Alternate arms<br>▪ 1 arm<br>▪ 1 arm w/ rotation | ▪ 2 legs<br>▪ Staggered stance<br>▪ 1 leg<br>▪ 2-leg unstable<br>▪ Staggered stance unstable<br>▪ 1-leg unstable | ▪ Floor<br>▪ Sport beam<br>▪ ½ foam roll<br>▪ Airex pad<br>▪ Dyna disc<br>▪ BOSU<br>▪ Proprio shoes<br>▪ Sand | ▪ Barbell<br>▪ Dumbbell<br>▪ Cable machines<br>▪ Tubing<br>▪ Medicine balls<br>▪ Power balls<br>▪ Bodyblade<br>▪ Other |

Source: Modified from National Academy of Sports Medicine, Phoenix, AZ.

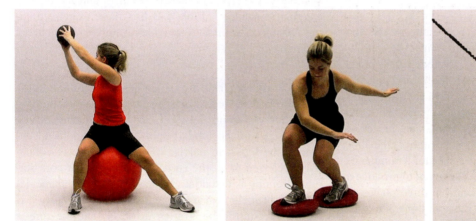

A

B

C

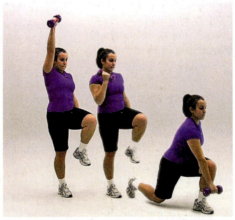

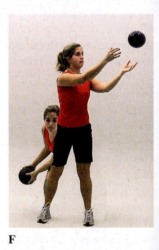

D

E

F

FIGURE 4–10   Functional strengthening exercises use simultaneous movements (concentric, eccentric, and isometric contractions) in three planes on both stable and unstable surfaces. **(A)** Stability ball diagonal rotations with weighted ball. **(B)** Tandem stance on Dyna disc with trunk rotation. **(C)** Standing diagonal rotations with cable or tubing reistance. **(D)** Weight-resisted multiplanar lunges. **(E)** Front lunge balance to one-arm press. **(F)** Weighted-ball double arm rotation toss from squat.

© William E. Prentice

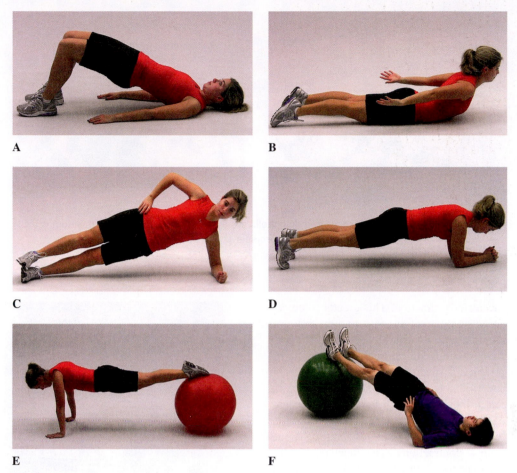

FIGURE 4–11   Core stability exercises.
**(A)** Bridging. **(B)** Prone cobra. **(C)** Side-lying isolated abdominal. **(D)** Human arrow.
**(E)** Stability ball push-up. **(F)** Hip-ups on stability ball.
© William E. Prentice

cardiovascular accidents.[77] This sharp increase in blood pressure results from an individual holding his or her breath and increasing intrathoracic pressure. Consequently, the blood pressure the heart experiences is increased significantly. This phenomenon has been referred to as the Valsalva effect. To avoid or minimize this increase in pressure, it is recommended that breathing be continued during the maximal contraction.

Isometric exercises are useful in the rehabilitation of certain injuries; this use is discussed in the rehabilitation sections in Chapters 18 through 26.

**Progressive Resistance Exercise** A third technique of resistance training is perhaps the most commonly used and the most popular technique for improving muscular strength. *Progressive resistance exercise (PRE)* strengthens muscles through a contraction that overcomes some fixed resistance produced by equipment, such as dumbbells, barbells, resistance tubing or bands, or various weight machines (Figure 4–12). Progressive resistance exercise uses

isotonic contractions that generate force while the muscle is changing in length.[32]

***Isotonic Contractions*** Isotonic contractions may be either concentric or eccentric. An individual who is performing a biceps curl offers a good example of an isotonic contraction. To lift the weight from the starting position, the biceps muscle must contract and shorten in length. This shortening contraction is referred to as a **concentric,** or **positive, contraction.** If the biceps muscle does not remain contracted when the weight is being lowered, gravity will cause the weight to simply fall back to the starting position. Thus, to control the weight as it is being lowered, the biceps muscle must continue to contract while gradually lengthening. A contraction in which the muscle is lengthening while still applying force is called an **eccentric,** or **negative, contraction.**[52]

***Eccentric Contractions versus Concentric Contractions*** It is possible to generate greater amounts of force against resistance with an eccentric contraction

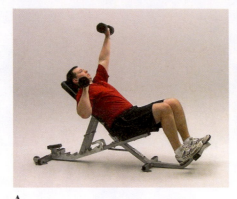

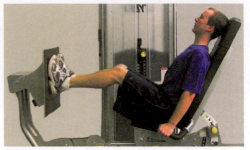

A                                          B

FIGURE 4–12  **(A)** Barbells and dumbbells are free weights that assist in developing isotonic strength. **(B)** Many machine exercise systems provide a variety of exercise possibilities.
© William E. Prentice

than with a concentric contraction. This greater force occurs because eccentric contractions require a much lower level of motor unit activity to achieve a certain force than do concentric contractions. Because fewer motor units are firing to produce a specific force, additional motor units may be recruited to generate increased force. In addition, oxygen utilization is much lower during eccentric exercise than during comparable concentric exercise. Thus, eccentric contractions are more resistant to fatigue than are concentric contractions. The mechanical efficiency of eccentric exercise may be several times higher than that of concentric exercise.[52]

Concentric contractions accelerate movement, whereas eccentric contractions decelerate motion. For example, the hamstrings must contract eccentrically to decelerate the angular velocity of the lower leg during running. Likewise, the external rotators in the rotator cuff muscles surrounding the shoulder contract eccentrically to decelerate the internally rotating humerus during throwing. Because of the excessive forces involved with these eccentric contractions, injury to the muscles is quite common. Thus, eccentric exercise must be routinely incorporated into the strength-training program to prevent injury to those muscles that act to decelerate movement.

***Free Weights versus Machine Weights***  Various types of exercise equipment can be used with progressive resistance exercise, including free weights (barbells and dumbbells) or exercise machines. Dumbbells and barbells require the use of iron plates of varying weights that can be changed easily by adding or subtracting equal amounts of weight to both sides of the bar. The exercise machines have a stack of weights that are lifted through a series of levers or pulleys. The stack of weights slides up and down on a pair of bars that restrict the movement to only one plane. Weight can be increased or decreased simply by changing the position of a weight key (Figure 4–13).

Both free weights and exercise machines have advantages and disadvantages. The exercise machines are

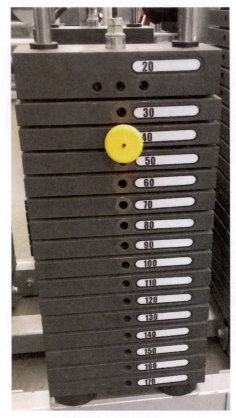

FIGURE 4–13  On most exercise machines the resistance can be easily changed by inserting a weight key into the weight stack at the desired weight level.
© William E. Prentice

relatively safe to use compared with free weights. It is also a simple process to increase or decrease the weight on exercise machines by moving a single weight key, although changes can generally be made only in increments of 10 or 15 pounds. The iron plates used with free weights must be added or removed from each side of the barbell or dumbbell.

Figure 4–14 shows examples of different isotonic strengthening exercises.

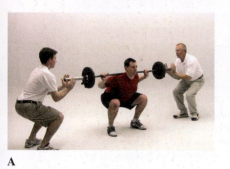

A

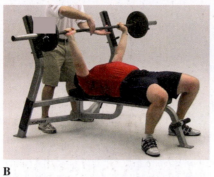

B

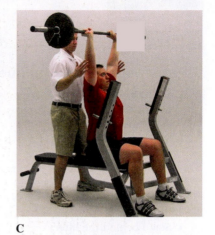

C

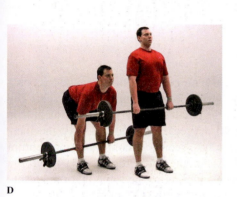

D

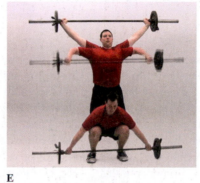

E

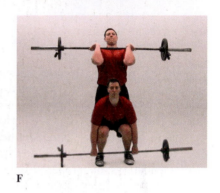

F

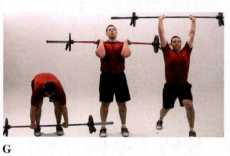

G

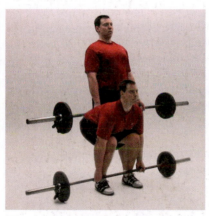

H

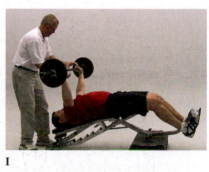

I

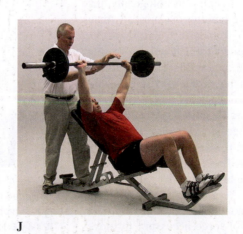

J

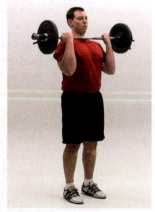

K

FIGURE 4–14  Examples of isotonic strengthening exercises using barbells, shown with appropriate spotting techniques where required. **(A)** Squat. **(B)** Bench press. **(C)** Military press. **(D)** Romanian dead lift. **(E)** Snatch. **(F)** Power clean. **(G)** Clean and jerk. **(H)** Dead lift. **(I)** Decline press. **(J)** Incline press. **(K)** Standing bicep curl.

© William E. Prentice

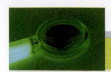
### Proper spotting techniques

- Make sure the lifter understands how to get out of the way of missed attempts, particularly with overhead techniques.
- Check to see that the lifter is in a safe, stable position.
- Communicate with the lifter to know how many reps are to be done, whether a liftoff is needed, and how much help the lifter wants in completing a rep.
- Stand behind the lifter.

- When spotting dumbbell exercises, spot as close to the dumbbells as possible above the elbow joint.
- If heavy weights exceed the limits of your ability to control the weight, use a second spotter.
- Make sure the lifter uses the proper grip.
- Make sure the lifter inhales and exhales during the lift.
- Make sure the lifter moves through a complete range of motion at the appropriate speed.
- Always be in a position to protect both the lifter and yourself from injury.

*Spotting for free weight exercises* When training with free weights, it is essential that the lifter have a partner who can assist in performing a particular exercise. This assistance is particularly critical when the weights to be lifted are extremely heavy. A *spotter* has three functions: to protect the lifter from injury, to make recommendations on proper lifting technique, and to help motivate the lifter. *Focus Box 4–2:* "Proper spotting techniques" provides some guidelines for correct spotting techniques.

*Isotonic Training* Regardless of which type of equipment is used, the same principles of **isotonic exercise** may be applied. In progressive resistance exercise, it is essential to incorporate both concentric and eccentric contractions. Research has clearly demonstrated that the muscle should be overloaded and fatigued both concentrically and eccentrically for the greatest strength improvement to occur.[59,66]

When an individual is weight training specifically to develop muscular strength, the concentric, or positive, portion of the exercise should require 1 to 2 seconds, and the eccentric, or negative, portion of the lift should require 2 to 4 seconds. The ratio of negative to positive should be approximately one to two. Physiologically, the muscle will fatigue much more rapidly concentrically than eccentrically.

Individuals who have weight trained with both free weights and machines realize the difference in the amount of weight that can be lifted. Unlike the machines, free weights have no restricted motion and can thus move in many different directions, depending on the forces applied. With free weights, an element of muscular control on the part of the lifter to prevent the weight from moving in any direction other than vertical will usually decrease the amount of weight that can be lifted.[48]

One problem often mentioned in relation to isotonic training is that the amount of force necessary to move

a weight through a range of motion changes according to the angle of pull of the contracting muscle. The amount of force is greatest when the angle of pull is approximately 90 degrees. In addition, once the inertia of the weight has been overcome and momentum has been established, the force required to move the resistance varies according to the force that the muscle can produce through the range of motion. Thus, it has been argued that a disadvantage of any type of isotonic exercise is that the force required to move the resistance is constantly changing throughout the range of movement.

Certain exercise machines are designed to minimize this change in resistance by using a cam system (Figure 4–15). The cam has been individually designed for each piece of equipment so that the resistance is variable throughout the movement. The cam system attempts to alter resistance so that the muscle can handle a greater load—at the points at which the joint angle or muscle length is at a mechanical disadvantage, the cam reduces the resistance to muscle movement. Whether this design does what it claims is

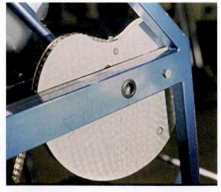

FIGURE 4–15 The cam system on the Nautilus equipment is designed to equalize the resistance throughout the full range of motion.

© William E. Prentice

debatable. This change in resistance at different points in the range is called **accommodating resistance,** or variable resistance.

**PRE Techniques** Perhaps the single most confusing aspect of progressive resistance exercise is the terminology used to describe specific programs. The following list of terms and their operational definitions may help clarify the confusion:

- Repetitions—the number of times a specific movement is repeated.
- Repetitions maximum (RM)—the maximum number of repetitions at a given weight.
- One repetition maximum (1 RM)—the maximum amount of weight that can be lifted one time.
- Set—a particular number of repetitions.
- Intensity—the amount of weight or resistance lifted.
- Recovery period—the rest interval between sets.
- Frequency—the number of times an exercise is done in 1 week.

A considerable amount of research has been done in the area of resistance training to determine optimal techniques in terms of the intensity or the amount of weight to be used, the number of repetitions, the number of sets, the recovery period, and the frequency of training. It is important to realize that there are many different effective techniques and training regimens. Regardless of specific techniques used, it is certain that to improve strength the muscle must be overloaded in a progressive manner.[15] This overload is the basis of progressive resistance exercise. The amount of weight used and the number of repetitions must be enough to make the muscle work at a higher intensity than it is used to working at. This overload is the single most critical factor in any strength-training program. The strength-training program must also be designed to meet the specific needs of the individual.

There is no such thing as an optimal strength-training program. Achieving total agreement on a program of resistance training—with specific recommendations about repetitions, sets, intensity, recovery time, and frequency—among researchers or other experts in resistance training is impossible. However, the following general recommendations will provide an effective resistance-training program.

In adults, for any given exercise, the amount of weight selected should be sufficient to allow six to eight repetitions maximum (RM) in each of three sets with a recovery period of 60 to 90 seconds between sets.[12] Initial selection of a starting weight may require some trial and error to achieve this six to eight RM range. If at least three sets of six repetitions cannot be completed, the weight is too heavy and should be reduced. If it is possible to do more than three sets of eight repetitions, the weight is too light and should be increased.[12] Progression to heavier weights is determined by the ability to perform at least eight RM in each of three sets. An increase of about 10 percent of the current weight being lifted should still allow at least six RM in each of three sets.[12]

Occasionally, athletes may be tested at 1 RM to determine the greatest amount of weight that can be lifted one time.[32] Extreme caution should be exercised when trying to determine 1 RM. Attention should be directed toward making sure the athlete has had ample opportunity to warm up and that the lifting technique is correct before attempting a maximum lift. Determining 1 RM should be done very gradually to minimize the chances of injuring the muscle.

A particular muscle or muscle group should be exercised consistently every other day.[12] Thus, the frequency of weight training should be at least three times per week but no more than four times per week. It is common for serious weight trainers to lift every day; however, they exercise different muscle groups on successive days. For example, Monday, Wednesday, and Friday may be used for upper-body muscles, whereas Tuesday, Thursday, and Saturday are used for lower-body muscles.

**Training for Muscular Strength versus Endurance** Muscular endurance is the ability to perform repeated muscle contractions against resistance for an extended period of time. Most weight-training experts believe that muscular strength and muscular endurance are closely related.[77] As one improves, the other tends to improve also.

When weight training for strength, use heavier weights with a lower number of repetitions. Conversely, endurance training uses relatively lighter weights with a greater number of repetitions.

Endurance training should consist of three sets of 10 to 15 repetitions, using the same criteria for weight selection, progression, and frequency as recommended for progressive resistance exercise.[9] Thus, suggested training regimens for muscular strength and endurance are similar in terms of sets and numbers of repetitions.[99] Persons who possess great levels of strength also tend to exhibit greater muscular endurance when asked to perform repeated contractions against resistance.

**Isokinetic Exercise** An **isokinetic exercise** involves a muscle contraction in which the length of the muscle is changing while the contraction is performed at a constant velocity.[76] In theory, maximal resistance is provided throughout the range of motion by the machine. The resistance provided by the machine will move only at some preset speed regardless of the force applied to it by the individual.[1] Thus, the key to isokinetic exercise is not the resistance, but the speed at which the resistance can be moved.[1,76]

Currently, only one isokinetic device is available commercially—Biodex (Figure 4–16). Isokinetic devices rely

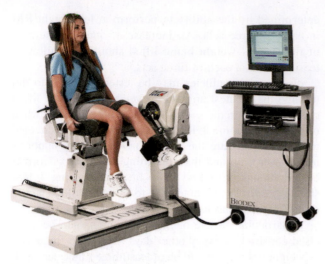

FIGURE 4-16 During isokinetic exercise, the speed of movement is constant regardless of the force applied by the athlete.

Photo courtesy of Biodex Medical Systems, Inc.

on hydraulic, pneumatic, or mechanical pressure systems to produce constant velocity of motion. Isokinetic devices are capable of resisting both concentric and eccentric contractions at a fixed speed to exercise a muscle.

A major disadvantage of an isokinetic unit is its cost. The unit comes with a computer and printing device and is used primarily as a diagnostic and rehabilitative tool in the treatment of various injuries.

Isokinetic devices are designed so that, regardless of the amount of force applied, the resistance can be moved only at a certain speed. That speed will be the same whether maximal force or only half the maximal force is applied. Consequently, when training isokinetically, it is absolutely necessary to exert as much force against the resistance as possible (maximal effort) for maximal strength gains to occur. This need for maximal effort is one of the major problems with an isokinetic strength-training program.

Anyone who has been involved in a weight-training program knows that on some days it is difficult to find the motivation to work out. Because isokinetic training does not require a maximal effort, it is easy to "cheat" and not go through the workout at a high level of intensity. In a progressive resistance exercise program, the individual knows how much weight has to be lifted with how many repetitions.[55] Thus, isokinetic training is often more effective if a partner system is used as a means of motivation toward a maximal effort.

When isokinetic training is done properly with a maximal effort, it is theoretically possible that maximal strength gains are best achieved through the isokinetic training method in which the velocity and force of the resistance are equal throughout the range of motion.[1] However, there is no conclusive evidence-based research to support this theory. Whether changing force capability is, in fact, a deterrent to improving the ability to generate force against some resistance is debatable.

In the athletic training setting, isokinetics are perhaps best used as a rehabilitative and diagnostic tool rather than as a conditioning device.[1]

**Circuit Training** **Circuit training** employs a series of exercise stations that consist of various combinations of weight training, flexibility, calisthenics, and brief aerobic exercises. Circuit training is used in the majority of fitness centers in corporate and health club settings. Circuits may be designed to accomplish many different training goals. With circuit training, the individual moves rapidly from one station to the next and performs whatever exercise is to be done at that station within a specified time period. A typical circuit consists of 8 to 12 stations, and the entire circuit is repeated three to five times.

Circuit training is definitely an effective technique for improving strength and flexibility. Certainly, if the pace or the time interval between stations is rapid and if workload is maintained at a high level of intensity with heart rate at or above target training levels, the cardiorespiratory system may benefit from this circuit. However, little research evidence exists to show that circuit training is effective in improving cardiorespiratory endurance. It should be, and is most often, used as a technique for developing and improving muscular strength and endurance.

**Bodyweight Strengthening Exercises** Bodyweight exercises are one of the more easily available means of developing strength. Isotonic movement exercises can be graded according to intensity by using gravity as an aid, by ruling gravity out, by moving against gravity, or by using the body or a body part as a resistance against gravity. Most bodyweight exercises require the individual to support the body or move the total body against the force of gravity. Push-ups are a good example of a vigorous antigravity free exercise. Bodyweight-like exercises are used in functional strength training, discussed earlier. To be considered maximally effective, the isotonic bodyweight exercises like all types of exercise, must be performed in an exacting manner and in full range of motion. In most cases, 10 or more repetitions are performed for each exercise and are repeated in sets of two or three.

Some free exercises use an isometric, or holding, phase instead of a full range of motion. Examples of these exercises are back extensions and sit-ups. When the exercise produces maximum muscle tension, it is held between 6 and 10 seconds and then repeated one to three times.

**Plyometric Exercise** **Plyometric exercise** is a technique that includes specific exercises that encompass a rapid stretch of a muscle eccentrically, followed immediately by a rapid concentric contraction of that muscle to facilitate and develop a forceful, explosive movement over a short period of time.[2,24] This effect requires that the time between eccentric contraction and concentric contraction be very short. It is theorized that this extra power is due to the muscle gaining potential energy. This energy dissipates rapidly, so the action must be quick. The process is frequently referred to as the *stretch-shortening* cycle and is the underlying mechanism of plyometric training. The greater the stretch put on the muscle from its resting length immediately before the concentric contraction, the greater the resistance the muscle can overcome. Plyometric exercises emphasize the speed of the eccentric phase.[23] The rate of the stretch is more critical than the magnitude of the stretch.

All movements involve repeated stretch-shortening cycles. Picture a jumping athlete preparing to transfer forward energy to upward energy. As the final step is taken before jumping, the loaded leg must stop the forward momentum and change it into an upward direction. As this happens, the muscle undergoes a lengthening eccentric contraction to decelerate the movement and prestretch the muscle. This prestretch energy is then immediately released in an equal and opposite reaction, thereby producing kinetic energy. The neuromuscular system must react quickly to produce the concentric shortening contraction to prevent falling and produce the upward change in direction. Consequently, specific functional exercises to emphasize this rapid change of direction must be used. Because plyometric exercises train specific movements in a biomechanically accurate manner, the muscles, tendons, and ligaments are all strengthened in a functional manner.

An advantage of plyometric exercises is that they can help develop eccentric control in dynamic movements.[80] Plyometric exercises involve hops, bounds, and depth jumping for the lower extremities and use medicine balls and other types of weighted equipment for the upper extremities (Figure 4–17). Depth jumping is an example of a plyometric exercise in which an individual jumps to the ground from a specified height and then quickly jumps again as soon as ground contact is made.[24] Plyometrics place a great deal of stress on the musculoskeletal system. The learning and perfection of specific jumping skills and other plyometric exercises must be technically correct and specific to the individual's age, activity, physical development, and skill development.[72]

## Strength Training for the Female

Strength training is critical for the female. Significant muscle hypertrophy in the female is dependent on the presence of the hormone testosterone. Testosterone is considered a male hormone, although all females possess some testosterone in their systems. Females with higher testosterone levels tend to have more masculine characteristics, such as increased facial and body hair, a deeper voice, and the potential to develop a little more muscle bulk.[66]

Both males and females experience initial rapid gains in strength due to an increase in neuromuscular efficiency, as discussed previously.[101] However, in the female, these rapid initial strength gains tend to plateau after 3 to 4 weeks. Minimal improvement in muscular strength will be realized during a continuing strength-training program because the muscle will not continue to hypertrophy to any significant degree.

Perhaps the most critical difference between males and females regarding physical performance is the ratio of strength to body weight. The reduced *strength-to-body-weight ratio* in females is the result of their higher percentage of body fat. The strength-to-body-weight ratio may be significantly improved through weight training by decreasing the percentage of body fat while increasing lean weight.[45]

## Strength Training in Prepubescents and Adolescents

The principles of resistance training discussed previously may be applied to younger individuals. A number of sociological questions regarding the advantages and disadvantages of younger—in particular, prepubescent—individuals engaging in rigorous strength-training programs emerge, however. From a physiological perspective, experts have for years debated the value of strength training in young individuals. Recently, a number of studies have indicated that, if properly supervised, prepubescents and adolescents can improve strength, power, endurance, balance, and proprioception; develop a positive body image; improve sport performance; and prevent injuries.[5,71] A prepubescent child can experience gains in levels of muscle strength without significant muscle hypertrophy.[41]

An athletic trainer supervising a conditioning program for a young athlete should certainly incorporate resistive exercise into the program. However, close supervision, proper instruction, and appropriate modification of progression and intensity based on the extent of physical maturation of the individual are critical to the effectiveness of the resistive exercises.[71] A functional strengthening program that uses calisthenic strengthening exercises with body weight as resistance should be encouraged.

## The Relationship between Strength and Flexibility

It is often said that strength training has a negative effect on flexibility.[86] For example, we tend to think of

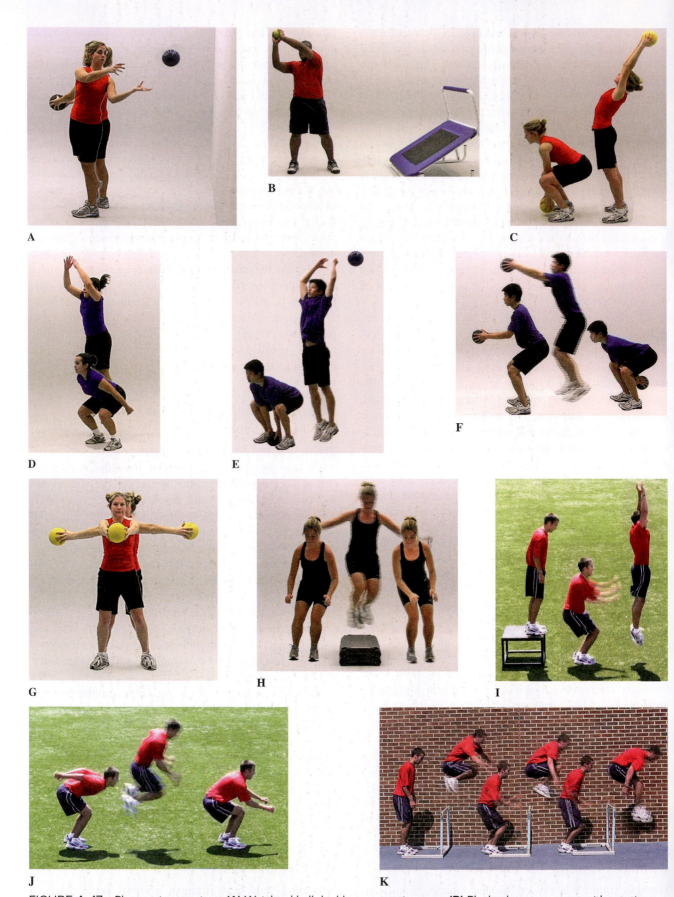

FIGURE 4–17    Plyometric exercises. **(A)** Weighted ball double-arm rotation toss. **(B)** Plyoback two-arm toss with rotation. **(C)** Weighted ball squat to stand extension. **(D)** Squat jumps. **(E)** Overhead weighted ball throw. **(F)** Weighted ball forward jump from squat. **(G)** Weighted ball standing rotations. **(H)** Double-leg lateral hop overs. **(I)** Depth jump to vertical jump. **(J)** Repeat two-leg standing long jump. **(K)** Three-hurdle jumps.

individuals who have highly developed muscles as having lost much of their ability to move freely through a full range of motion. Occasionally, an individual develops so much bulk that the physical size of the muscle prevents a normal range of motion. It is certainly true that strength training that is not properly done can impair movement; however, weight training, if done properly through a full range of motion, will not impair flexibility. Proper strength training probably improves dynamic flexibility and, if combined with a rigorous stretching program, can greatly enhance the powerful and coordinated movements that are essential for success in many athletic activities. In all cases, a heavy weight-training program should be accompanied by a strong flexibility program.

# IMPROVING AND MAINTAINING FLEXIBILITY

Flexibility is the ability to move a joint or series of joints smoothly and easily through a full range of motion.[4] Flexibility can be discussed in relation to movement involving only one joint, such as the knees, or movement involving a whole series of joints, such as the spinal vertebral joints, which must all move together to allow smooth bending or rotation of the trunk.

## The Importance of Flexibility

Maintaining a full, nonrestricted range of motion has long been recognized as essential to normal daily living. Lack of flexibility can also create uncoordinated or awkward movement patterns resulting from lost neuromuscular control.[13] In most individuals, functional activities require relatively "normal" amounts of flexibility. However, some sport activities, such as gymnastics, ballet, diving, and karate, require increased flexibility for superior performance (Figure 4–18).[6]

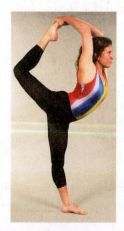

FIGURE 4–18   Good flexibility is essential to successful performance in many sport activities.
© William E. Prentice

Flexibility is generally seen as essential for improving performance in physical activities. However, a review of the evidence-based information in the literature looking at the relationship between flexibility and improved performance is at best conflicting and inconclusive.[90,96] Although many studies done over the years have suggested that stretching improves performance,[27,57,73] several recent studies have found that stretching causes decreases in performance parameters, such as strength, endurance, power, joint position sense, and reaction times.[11,38,56,65,67,89,93,102] The same can be said when examining the relationship between flexibility and the incidence of injury. Although it is generally accepted that good flexibility reduces the likelihood of injury, a true cause-effect relationship has not been clearly established in the literature.[7,8,22,73,102]

## Factors That Limit Flexibility

A number of factors may limit the ability of a joint to move through a full, unrestricted range of motion.

The *bony structure* may restrict the endpoint in the range. An elbow that has been fractured through the joint may deposit excess calcium in the joint space, causing the joint to lose its ability to fully extend. However, in many instances bony prominences stop movements at normal endpoints in the range.

Excessive *fat* may also limit the ability to move through a full range of motion. An athlete who has a large amount of fat on the abdomen may have severely restricted trunk flexion when asked to bend forward and touch the toes. The fat may act as a wedge between two lever arms, restricting movement wherever it is found.

*Skin* might also be responsible for limiting movement. For example, an athlete who has had some type of injury or surgery involving a tearing incision or laceration of the skin, particularly over a joint, will have inelastic scar tissue at that site. This scar tissue is incapable of stretching with joint movement.

*Muscles and their tendons,* along with their surrounding fascial sheaths, are most often responsible for limiting range of motion. An individual who performs stretching exercises to improve flexibility about a particular joint is attempting to take advantage of the highly elastic properties of a muscle. Over time, it is possible to increase the elasticity, or the length that a given muscle can be stretched.[81] Individuals who have a good deal of movement at a particular joint tend to have highly elastic and flexible muscles.

*Connective tissue* surrounding the joint, such as ligaments on the joint capsule, may be subject to contractures. Ligaments and joint capsules do have some elasticity; however, if a joint is immobilized for a period of time, these structures tend to lose some elasticity and shorten. This condition is most commonly seen after surgical repair of an unstable joint, but it can also result from long periods of inactivity.

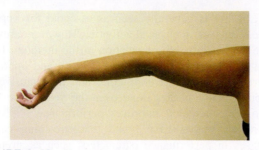

FIGURE 4–19    Excessive joint motion, or hypermobility, can predispose an individual to injury.

© William E. Prentice

*Neural tissue tightness* resulting from acute compression, chronic repetitive microtrauma, muscle imbalances, joint dysfunction, or poor posture can create morphological changes in neural tissues that may result in irritation, inflammation, and pain. Pain causes muscle guarding to protect inflamed and irritated neural structures, and this alters normal movement patterns. Over time neural fibrosis results, decreasing the elasticity of neural tissue and preventing normal movement of surrounding tissues.

It is also possible for an individual to have relatively slack ligaments and joint capsules. These individuals are generally referred to as being hypermobile. An example of hypermobility is an elbow or a knee that hyperextends beyond 180 degrees (Figure 4–19). Frequently, the instability associated with hypermobility presents as great a problem in movement as ligamentous or capsular contractures.

The elasticity of skin contractures caused by scarring, ligaments, joint capsules, and musculotendinous units can be improved to varying degrees over time through stretching. With the exception of bony structure, age, and gender, all the other factors that limit flexibility also may be altered to increase range of joint motion.

## Agonist versus Antagonist Muscles

Understanding flexibility requires defining the terms *agonist* and *antagonist*. Most joints in the body are capable of more than one movement. The knee joint, for example, is capable of flexion and extension. Contraction of the quadriceps group of muscles on the front of the thigh causes knee extension, whereas contraction of the hamstring muscles on the back of the thigh produces knee flexion.

To achieve knee extension, the quadriceps group contracts while the hamstring muscles relax and stretch. The muscle that contracts to produce a movement—in this case, the quadriceps—is referred to as the **agonist** muscle. The muscle being stretched in response to contraction of the agonist muscle is called the **antagonist** muscle. In knee extension, the antagonist muscle is the hamstring group. Some degree of balance in strength between agonist and antagonist muscle groups is necessary to produce normal, smooth, coordinated movement and to reduce the likelihood of muscle strain caused by muscular imbalance.[61]

## Active and Passive Range of Motion

*Active range of motion,* also called *dynamic flexibility,* is the degree to which a joint can be moved by a muscle contraction, usually through the midrange of movement.[98] Dynamic flexibility is not necessarily a good indicator of the stiffness or looseness of a joint because it applies to the ability to move a joint efficiently, with little resistance to motion.[88]

*Passive range of motion,* sometimes called *static flexibility,* is the degree to which a joint may be passively moved to the endpoints in the range of motion. No muscle contraction is involved to move a joint through a passive range.

When a muscle actively contracts, it produces a joint movement through a specific range of motion. However, if passive pressure is applied to an extremity, it is capable of moving farther in the range of motion. It is essential in sport activities that an extremity be capable of moving through a nonrestricted range of motion. For example, a hurdler who cannot fully extend the knee joint in a normal stride is at a considerable disadvantage because stride length and thus speed will be reduced significantly.

Passive range of motion is important for injury prevention. In many sports situations, a muscle is forced to stretch beyond its normal active limits. If the muscle does not have enough elasticity to compensate for this additional stretch, the musculotendinous unit will likely be injured.

## Mechanisms for Improving Flexibility

For many years the efficacy of stretching in improving range of motion has been theoretically attributed to neurophysiological phenomena involving the stretch reflex.[20] However, a more recent study that extensively reviewed the existing literature has suggested that improvements in range of motion resulting from stretching must be explained by mechanisms other than the stretch reflex.[22] Studies reviewed indicate that changes in the ability to tolerate stretch and/or the viscoelastic properties of the stretched muscle are possible mechanisms.

**Neurophysiological Basis of Stretching**   Every muscle in the body contains various types of mechanoreceptors that, when stimulated, inform the central nervous system of what is happening with that muscle. Two of these mechanoreceptors are important in the stretch

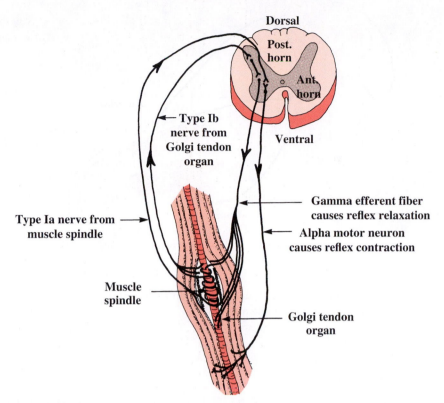

**FIGURE 4–20** Stretch reflex. The muscle spindle produces a reflex resistance to stretch, and the Golgi tendon organ causes a reflex relaxation of the muscle in response to stretch.

reflex: the *muscle spindle* and the *Golgi tendon organ* (Figure 4–20). Both types of receptors are sensitive to changes in muscle length. The Golgi tendon organs are also affected by changes in muscle tension.

When a muscle is stretched, both the muscle spindles and the Golgi tendon organs immediately begin sending sensory impulses to the spinal cord. Initially, impulses coming from the muscle spindles along type Ia nerve fibers to the spinal cord signal the central nervous system that the muscle is being stretched. Impulses return to the muscle from the spinal cord along alphamotor neurons, causing the muscle to reflexively contract, thus resisting the stretch.[64] The Golgi tendon organs respond to the change in length and the increase in tension by firing off sensory impulses that are carried to the spinal cord along type Ia nerve fibers. If the stretch of the muscle continues for an extended period of time (at least 6 seconds), impulses from the Golgi tendon organs begin to override muscle spindle impulses. The impulses from the Golgi tendon organs, unlike the signals from the muscle spindle, cause a reflex relaxation of the antagonist muscle. This reflex relaxation serves as a protective mechanism that will allow the muscle to stretch through relaxation without exceeding the extensibility limits, which could damage the muscle fibers.[10] This relaxation of the antagonist muscle during contractions is referred to as **autogenic inhibition.**

In any synergistic muscle group, a contraction of the agonist causes a reflex relaxation in the antagonist muscle, allowing it to stretch and protecting it from injury. This phenomenon is referred to as *reciprocal inhibition* (Figure 4–21).[90]

**The Effects of Stretching on the Physical and Mechanical Properties of Muscle** The neurophysiological mechanisms of both autogenic and reciprocal inhibition result in reflex relaxation with subsequent lengthening of a muscle. Thus, the mechanical properties of that muscle that physically allow lengthening to occur are dictated via neural input.

Both muscle and tendon are composed largely of noncontractile collagen and elastin fibers. Collagen enables a tissue to resist mechanical forces and deformation, whereas elastin composes highly elastic tissues that assist in recovery from deformation.[95]

Unlike tendon, muscle also has active contractile components, which are the actin and myosin myofilaments.

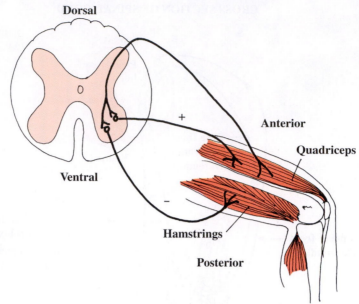

FIGURE 4–21   Reciprocal inhibition. A contraction of the agonist will produce relaxation in the antagonist.

Collectively, the contractile and noncontractile elements determine the muscle's capability of deforming and recovering from deformation.[60]

Both the contractile and the noncontractile components appear to resist deformation when a muscle is stretched or lengthened. The percentage of their individual contribution to resisting deformation depends on the degree to which the muscle is stretched or deformed and on the velocity of deformation. The noncontractile elements are primarily resistant to the degree of lengthening, while the contractile elements limit high-velocity deformation. The greater the stretch, the more the noncontractile components contribute.[95]

Lengthening of a muscle via stretching allows for viscoelastic and plastic changes to occur in the collagen and elastin fibers. The viscoelastic changes that allow slow deformation with imperfect recovery are not permanent. However, plastic changes, although difficult to achieve, result in residual or permanent change in length due to deformation created by long periods of stretching.

The greater the velocity of deformation, the greater the chance for exceeding that tissue's capability to undergo viscoelastic and plastic change.[60]

## Stretching Techniques

The maintenance of a full, nonrestricted range of motion has long been recognized as critical to injury prevention and as an essential component of a conditioning program.[8] The goal of any effective flexibility program should be to improve the range of motion at a given articulation by altering the extensibility of the

neuromusculotendinous structures that produce movement at that joint.[31,46] Exercises that stretch these neuromusculotendinous structures over several months increase the range of motion possible at a given joint.[86]

**Ballistic Stretching** **Ballistic stretching** involves a bouncing movement in which repetitive contractions of the agonist muscle are used to produce quick stretches of the antagonist muscle. The ballistic stretching technique, although apparently effective in improving range of motion, has been criticized in the past because increased range of motion is achieved through a series of jerks or pulls on the resistant muscle tissue.[4] The concern was that, if the forces generated by the jerks are greater than the tissues' extensibility, muscle injury may result.

**Dynamic Stretching** Certainly, successive, forceful contractions of the agonist muscle that result in stretching of the antagonist muscle may cause muscle soreness. For example, forcefully kicking a soccer ball 50 times may result in muscle soreness of the hamstrings (antagonist muscle) as a result of eccentric contraction of the hamstrings to control the

A construction worker has a history of multiple hamstring strains, usually when lifting and moving heavy wooden beams. He is very concerned that he is likely to reinjure his hamstring. He asks the athletic trainer overseeing a work hardening program if there is anything he should be doing to minimize the chances of reinjury.

**?** What recommendations should the athletic trainer make?

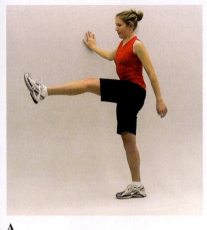
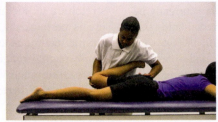
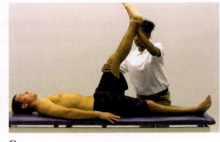

A                                B                                C

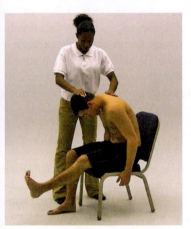
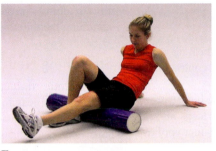

D                                E

FIGURE 4–22   Stretching techniques. **(A)** Dynamic stretch for hip flexors and extensors. **(B)** Static stretch for knee extensors. **(C)** Slow-reversal-hold-relax PNF techniques for hamstrings. **(D)** Slump-stretch for sciatic nerve. **(E)** Myofascial stretching for hamstrings.
© William E. Prentice

dynamic movement of the quadriceps (agonist muscle). Stretching that is controlled usually does not cause muscle soreness.[64] This is the difference between ballistic stretching and dynamic stretching. In fact, in the athletic population, **dynamic stretching** has become the stretching technique of choice. The argument has been that dynamic stretching exercises are more closely related to the types of activities that athletes engage in and should be considered more functional.[29,64] Thus, dynamic stretching exercises are routinely recommended for athletes prior to beginning an activity (Figure 4–22A).

**Static Stretching** The **static stretching** technique is a widely used and effective technique of stretching. This technique involves passively stretching a given antagonist muscle by placing it in a maximal position of stretch and holding it there for an extended time (Figure 4–22B). Recommendations for the optimal time for holding this stretched position vary from as short as 3 seconds to as long as 60 seconds.[63] Recent data indicate that 30 seconds

may be an optimal time to hold the stretch. The static stretch of each muscle should be repeated three or four times.[10]

Much research has been done comparing ballistic and static stretching techniques for the improvement of flexibility. It has been shown that both static and ballistic stretching are effective in increasing flexibility and that there is no significant difference between the two. However, static stretching offers less danger of exceeding the extensibility limits of the involved joints because the stretch is more controlled. Ballistic stretching is apt to cause muscle soreness, whereas static stretching generally does not and is commonly used in injury rehabilitation of sore or strained muscles.[4,58]

Static stretching is certainly a much safer stretching technique, especially for sedentary or untrained individuals. However, many physical activities involve dynamic movement. Thus, stretching as a warm-up for these types of activities should begin with static stretching followed by ballistic and dynamic stretching, which more closely resemble the dynamic activity.

**PNF Stretching Techniques** Proprioceptive neuro-muscular facilitation (PNF) techniques were first used by physical therapists for treating patients who had various types of neuromuscular paralysis.[78] More recently, PNF exercises have been used as a stretching technique for increasing flexibility.

A number of different PNF techniques are currently being used for stretching, including slow-reversal-hold-relax, contract-relax, and hold-relax techniques. All involve some combination of alternating contraction and relaxation of both agonist and antagonist muscles. All three techniques use a 10-second active push phase followed by a 10-second passive relax phase repeated three times for a total of 60 seconds.

Using a hamstring stretching technique as an example (Figure 4–22C), the slow-reversal-hold-relax technique would be done as follows:[78]

- With the patient lying supine with the knee extended and the ankle flexed to 90 degrees, the athletic trainer passively flexes the hip joint to the point at which there is slight discomfort in the muscle.
- At this point, the patient begins actively pushing against the athletic trainer's resistance by contracting the hamstring muscle.
- After actively pushing for 10 seconds, the hamstring muscles are relaxed and the agonist quadriceps muscle is actively contracted while the athletic trainer applies passive pressure to further stretch the antagonist hamstrings. This action should move the leg so that there is increased hip joint flexion.
- The relaxing phase lasts for 10 seconds, after which the patient again actively pushes against the athletic trainer's resistance, beginning at this new position of increased hip flexion.
- This push-relax sequence is repeated at least three times.

The contract-relax and hold-relax techniques are variations on the slow-reversal-hold-relax method. In the contract-relax method, the hamstrings are isotonically contracted so that the leg actually moves toward the floor during the push phase. The hold-relax method involves an isometric hamstring contraction against immovable resistance during the push phase. During the relax phase, both techniques involve the relaxation of hamstrings and quadriceps while the hamstrings are passively stretched. The same basic PNF technique can be used to stretch any muscle in the body. The PNF stretching techniques are perhaps best performed with a partner, although they may also be done using a wall as resistance (see Chapter 16).[78]

***Comparing Techniques*** Although all four stretching techniques have been demonstrated to improve flexibility, there is still considerable debate as to which technique produces the greatest increases in range of motion. In the past, the ballistic technique has not been recommended because of the potential for causing muscle soreness. However, most sport activities are dynamic in nature (e.g., kicking, running), and those activities use the stretch reflex to enhance performance.[29] In highly trained individuals, it is unlikely that dynamic stretching will result in muscle soreness. Static stretching is perhaps the most widely used technique. It is a simple technique and does not require a partner. A fully nonrestricted range of motion can be attained through static stretching over time.[33]

The PNF stretching techniques can produce dramatic increases in range of motion during one stretching session. Studies comparing static and PNF stretching suggest that PNF stretching can produce greater improvement in flexibility over an extended training period.[63,79,81] The major disadvantage of PNF stretching is that it requires a partner for stretching, although stretching with a partner may have some motivational advantages. *Focus Box 4–3:* "Guidelines and precautions for stretching" provides recommendations for various stretching techniques.

## Stretching Neural Structures

The athletic trainer should be able to differentiate between tightness in the musculotendinous unit and abnormal neural tension. When an individual performs both active and passive multiplanar movements, tension is created in the neural structures that exacerbates pain, limits range of motion, and increases radiating neural symptoms, including numbness and tingling. For example, the slump stretch position is used to detect an increase in nerve/root tension in the sciatic nerve and stretching should be done to assist in relieving tension (Figure 4–22D).

## Stretching Fascia

Tight fascia, the connective tissue that surrounds the musculotendinous unit, can significantly limit motion. Damage to the fascia due to injury, disease, or inflammation creates pain and motion restriction. Thus, it may be necessary to release tightness in the area of injury. Stretching of tight fascia can either be done manually or by using a firm foam roller (Figure 4–22E). Myofascial release as a treatment technique is discussed in detail in Chapter 16.

## Alternative Stretching Techniques

**The Pilates Method of Stretching** The Pilates method is a somewhat different approach to stretching for improving flexibility. This method has become extremely popular and widely used among personal fitness trainers and physical therapists. Pilates is an exercise technique devised by German-born Joseph Pilates, who established the first Pilates studio in the

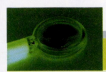

## FOCUS 4–3 Focus on Therapeutic Intervention

### Guidelines and precautions for stretching

The following guidelines and precautions should be incorporated into a sound stretching program:

- Warm up using a slow jog or fast walk before stretching vigorously.
- To increase flexibility, the muscle must be stretched within pain tolerances and tissue healing limitations to attain functional or normal range of motion.
- Stretch only to the point where you feel tightness or resistance to stretch or perhaps some discomfort. Stretching should not be painful.
- Increases in range of motion are specific to whatever joint is being stretched.
- Exercise caution when stretching muscles that surround painful joints. Pain is an indication that something is wrong and should not be ignored.
- Avoid overstretching the ligaments and capsules that surround joints, beyond their limits of extensibility.
- Exercise caution when stretching the lower back and neck. Exercises that compress the vertebrae and their disks may cause damage.

- Stretching from a seated position rather than a standing position takes stress off the low back and decreases the chances of back injury.
- Stretch those muscles that are tight and inflexible.
- Strengthen those muscles that are weak and loose.
- Be sure to continue normal breathing during a stretch. Do not hold your breath.
- Static, dynamic, and PNF techniques are most often recommended for individuals who want to improve their range of motion.
- Ballistic stretching should be done only by those who are already flexible or are accustomed to stretching and should be done only after static stretching.
- Stretching should be done at least three times per week to see minimal improvement. Stretching five or six times per week is recommended to see maximum results.

---

United States before World War II. The Pilates method is a conditioning program that improves muscle control, flexibility, coordination, strength, and tone. The basic principles of Pilates exercise are to make people more aware of their bodies as single, integrated units; to improve body alignment and breathing; and to increase efficiency of movement.[75] Unlike other exercise programs, the Pilates method does not require the repetition of exercises but instead consists of a sequence of carefully performed movements, some of which are carried out on specially designed equipment (Figures 4–23 and 4–24). Each exercise is designed to stretch and strengthen the muscles involved. There is a specific breathing pattern for each exercise to help direct energy to the areas being worked, while relaxing the rest of the body. The Pilates method works many of the deeper muscles together, improving coordination and balance, to achieve efficient and graceful movement. Instead of seeking an ideal or perfect body, the goal is for the practitioner to develop a healthy self-image through the attainment of better posture, proper coordination, and improved flexibility. This method concentrates on correcting body alignment, lengthening all the muscles of the body into a balanced whole, and building endurance and strength without putting undue stress on the lungs and heart.[75] Pilates instructors believe that problems such as soft-tissue injuries can cause bad posture, which can lead to pain and discomfort. Pilates exercises aim to correct this.

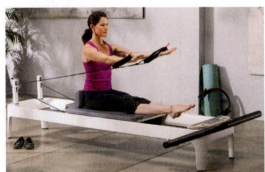

A

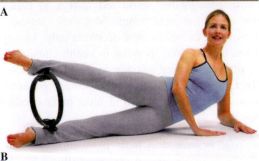

B

FIGURE 4–23  Pilates techniques using equipment. **(A)** Reformer. **(B)** Magic ring.

Photos courtesy Balanced Body

Normally, a beginner sees a Pilates instructor on a one-to-one basis for the first session. The instructor assesses the client's physical condition and asks the client about any problems and about the client's lifestyle.

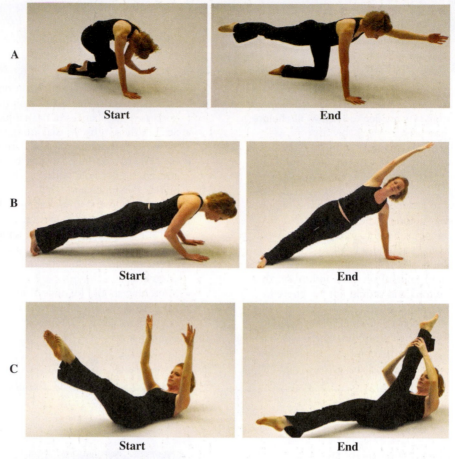

FIGURE 4–24   Pilates floor exercises.
**(A)** Alternating arm, opposite leg extensions. **(B)** Push-up to a side plank.
**(C)** Alternating legs scissors.
© William E. Prentice

The client is then shown a series of exercises that work joints and muscles through a range of motion appropriate for the client's needs. A class in a studio might involve working on specially designed equipment that primarily uses resistance against tensioned springs to isolate and develop specific muscle groups. Mat work classes involve a repertoire of exercises on a floor mat only. This type of class has become very popular in health clubs and gyms and is often compared to other forms of body conditioning. In fact, the Pilates mat exercises are generally less strenuous than mat exercises in most other conditioning classes.

**Yoga** Yoga originated in India approximately 6,000 years ago. Its basic philosophy is that most illness is related to poor mental attitudes, posture, and diet. Practitioners of yoga maintain that stress can be reduced through combined mental and physical approaches. Yoga can help an individual cope with stress-induced behaviors and conditions, such as overeating, hypertension, and smoking. Yoga's meditative aspects are believed to help alleviate psychosomatic illnesses. Yoga aims to unite the body and mind to reduce stress. For example, Dr. Chandra Patel, a

yoga expert, has found that persons who practice yoga can reduce their blood pressure indefinitely as long as they continue to practice yoga. Yoga consists of various body postures and breathing exercises. Hatha yoga uses a number of positions through which the practitioner may progress, beginning with the simplest and moving to the more complex (Figure 4–25).[84] The various positions are intended to increase mobility and flexibility. However, practitioners must use caution when performing yoga positions. Some can be dangerous, particularly for someone who is inexperienced in yoga technique.

Slow, deep, diaphragmatic breathing is an important part of yoga. Many people take shallow breaths; however, breathing deeply, fully expanding the chest when inhaling, helps lower blood pressure and heart rate.[84] Deep breathing has a calming effect on the body, and it increases production of endorphins.

## Measuring Range of Motion

Accurate measurement of the range of joint motion takes some practice on the part of the clinician. Various devices have been designed to accommodate variations in

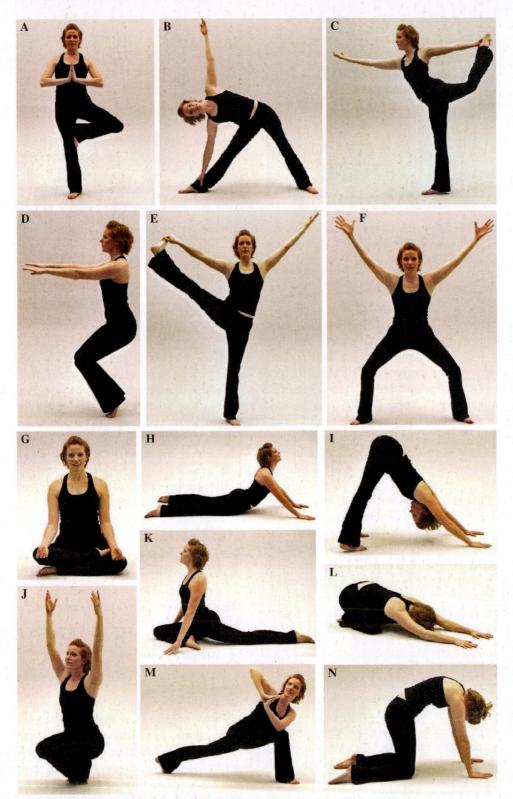

FIGURE 4–25   Yoga positions.
**(A)** Tree. **(B)** Triangle. **(C)** Dancer. **(D)** Chair. **(E)** Extended hand to big toe. **(F)** Big mountain.
**(G)** Lotus. **(H)** Cobra. **(I)** Downward facing dog. **(J)** Static squat. **(K)** Pigeon. **(L)** Child.
**(M)** Runner's lunge with twist. **(N)** Cat.
© William E. Prentice

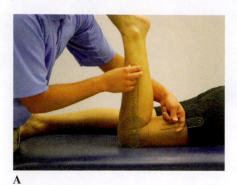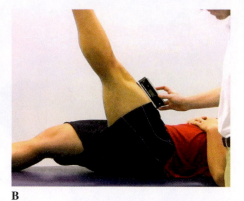

FIGURE 4–26 A goniometer can be used to measure joint angles and range of motion. **(A)** Universal goniometer. **(B)** Inclinometer.
© William E. Prentice

the size of the joints and the complexity of movements in articulations that involve more than one joint.[49] Of these devices, the simplest and most widely used is the *goniometer* (Figure 4–26A). A goniometer is a large protractor with measurements in degrees. By aligning the two arms parallel to the longitudinal axis of the two segments involved in motion about a specific joint, it is possible to obtain relatively accurate measures of range of movement. The goniometer has its place in a rehabilitation setting, where it is essential to assess improvement in joint flexibility for the purpose of modifying injury rehabilitation programs.[91]

Some clinics use an *inclinometer* instead of a goniometer. An inclinometer is a more precise measuring instrument with high reliability that has most often been used in research settings. However, inclinometers are affordable and can easily be used to accurately measure range of motion of all joints of the body, from complex movements of the spine to simpler movements of the large joints of the extremities, and the small joints of fingers and toes (Figure 4–26B).[91]

## FITNESS ASSESSMENT

Fitness testing provides the athletic trainer or strength and conditioning coach with information about the effectiveness of the conditioning program for an individual. Testing may be done in a pretest/posttest format to determine significant improvement from some baseline measure. Tests may be used to assess flexibility, muscular strength, endurance, power, cardiorespiratory endurance, speed, balance, or agility, depending on the stated goals of the training and conditioning program. A variety of established tests can be used to assess these parameters. *Focus Box 4–4: "Fitness testing"* lists various tests that can be administered, along with recommended references to consult for specific testing procedures and for in-depth testing directions.

## PERIODIZATION IN CONDITIONING

Serious athletes no longer engage only in preseason conditioning and in-season competition. Sports conditioning is a year-round endeavor. *Periodization* is an approach to conditioning that brings about peak performance while reducing injuries and overtraining in the athlete through a conditioning program that is followed throughout the various seasons.[93] Periodization takes into account that athletes have different conditioning needs during different seasons and modifies the program according to individual needs (Table 4–4).[50]

### Macrocycle

Periodization organizes the conditioning program into cycles. The complete training period, which could be a year, in the case of seasonal sports, or 4 years, for an Olympic athlete, is referred to as a *macrocycle*. With seasonal sports, the macrocycle can be divided into a preseason, an in-season, and an

> Sports conditioning often falls into three seasons: preseason, in-season, and off-season.

off-season. Throughout the course of the macrocycle, intensity, volume, and specificity of conditioning are altered, so that an athlete can achieve peak levels of fitness for competition. As competition approaches, conditioning sessions change gradually and progressively from high-volume, low-intensity, non–sport-specific activity to low-volume, high-intensity, sport-specific training.[100]

**Mesocycles** Within the macrocycle are a series of *mesocycles,* each of which may last for several weeks or even months. A mesocycle is further divided into *transition, preparatory,* and *competition* periods.[100]

**Transition Period** The transition period begins after the last competition and comprises the early part of the

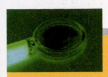

**Preparatory Period** The preparatory period occurs primarily during the off-season, when there are no upcoming competitions. The preparatory period has three phases: the hypertrophy/endurance phase, the strength phase, and the power phase.

During the hypertrophy/endurance phase, which occurs in the early part of the off-season, conditioning is at a low intensity with a high volume of repetitions, using activities that may or may not be directly related to a specific sport. The goal is to develop a base of endurance on which more intense conditioning can occur. This phase may last from several weeks to 2 months.

During the strength phase, which also occurs during the off-season, the intensity and volume progress to moderate levels. Weight-training activities should become more specific to the sport or event.

The third phase, or power phase, occurs in the preseason. The athlete trains at a high intensity at or near the level of competition. The volume of training is decreased so that full recovery is allowed between sessions.

**Competition Period** In certain cases, the competition period lasts for only a week or less. With seasonal sports, however, the competition period may last for several months. In general, this period involves high-intensity conditioning at a low volume. As conditioning volume decreases, an increased amount of time is spent on skill training or strategy sessions. During the competition period, it may be necessary to establish microcycles, which are periods lasting from 1 to 7 days. During a weekly microcycle, conditioning should be intense early in the week and should progress to moderate and finally to light training the day before a competition. The goal is to make sure that the athlete will be at peak levels of fitness and performance on days of competition.[14]

> **4–8 Clinical Application Exercise**
>
> Following the competitive season, a college football player took the months of December and January off from intense training. He played only basketball and occasionally rode an exercise bike, thus completing the transitional period of the macrocycle. It is now time for him to begin the preparatory phase of training.
>
> **?** What activities should he begin with, and how should these activities progress over the next several months?

### Cross Training

Cross training is an approach to training and conditioning for a specific sport that involves substituting alternative activities that have some carryover value to that sport. For example, a swimmer could engage in jogging, running, or aerobic exercise to maintain levels of cardiorespiratory conditioning. Cross training is particularly useful in both the transition and the early preparatory

off-season. The transition period is generally unstructured, and the athlete is encouraged to participate in sport activities on a recreational basis. The idea is to allow the athlete to escape both physically and psychologically from the rigor of a highly organized training regimen.

**TABLE 4–4  Periodization Training**

| Season | Period/Phase | Type of Training Activity |
|--------|--------------|---------------------------|
| Off-season | Transition period | Unstructured<br>Recreational |
| | Preparatory period<br>   Hypertrophy/endurance phase | Cross training<br>Low intensity<br>High volume<br>Non–sport specific |
| | Strength phase | Moderate intensity<br>Moderate volume<br>More sport specific |
| Preseason | Power phase | High intensity<br>Decreased volume<br>Sport specific |
| In-season | Competition period | High intensity<br>Low volume<br>Skill training<br>Strategy<br>Maintenance of strength and power gained during the off-season |

periods. It adds variety to the training regimen, thus keeping training during the off-season more interesting and exciting. However, although cross training can be effective in maintaining levels of cardiorespiratory endurance, it is not sport specific and thus should not be used during the preseason.

## SUMMARY

- Proper physical conditioning for sports participation should prepare the athlete for high-level performance while helping prevent injuries inherent to that sport.
- Physical conditioning must follow the SAID principle, which is an acronym for specific adaptation to imposed demands. Conditioning must work toward making the body as lean as possible, commensurate with the athlete's sport.
- A proper warm-up should precede conditioning, and a proper cool-down should follow. It takes at least 15 to 30 minutes of gradual warm-up to bring the body to a state of readiness for vigorous sports training and participation. Warming up consists of a general, unrelated activity followed by a specific, related activity.
- Cardiorespiratory endurance is the ability to perform whole-body, large-muscle activities repeatedly for long periods of time. Maximal oxygen consumption is the greatest determinant of the level of cardiorespiratory endurance. Most sport activities involve some combination of both aerobic and anaerobic metabolism.

Improvement of cardiorespiratory endurance may be accomplished through continuous, interval, or speed play training.
- Strength is the capacity to exert a force or the ability to perform work against a resistance. There are many ways to develop strength, including functional strength training; core stability training; and isometric, isotonic, and isokinetic muscle contraction. Isometric exercise generates heat energy by forcefully contracting the muscle in a stable position that produces no change in the length of the muscle. Isotonic exercise involves shortening and lengthening a muscle through a complete range of motion. Isokinetic exercise allows resisted movement through a full range at a specific velocity. Circuit training uses a series of exercise stations to improve strength and flexibility. Plyometric training uses a quick, eccentric contraction to facilitate a more explosive concentric contraction.
- Optimum flexibility is necessary for success in most sports. Too much flexibility can allow joint trauma to occur, and too little flexibility can result in muscle

tears or strains. Ballistic stretching exercises should be avoided. The safest means of increasing flexibility are dynamic stretching, static stretching, and the proprioceptive neuromuscular facilitation (PNF) technique, consisting of slow-reversal-hold-relax, contract-relax, and hold-relax methods.

- Year-round conditioning is essential in most sports to assist in preventing injuries. Periodization is an approach to conditioning that attempts to bring about peak performance while reducing injuries and overtraining in the athlete by developing a training and conditioning program to be followed throughout the various seasons.

## WEB SITES

National Academy of Sports Medicine: www.nasm.org
*Contains a wealth of information on fitness exercises and activities.*

National Strength and Conditioning Association: www.nsca.com
*This organization distributes a wealth of information relative to strength training and conditioning.*

Stretching and Flexibility: Everything you never wanted to know: www.bradapp.com/docs/rec/stretching/
*Prepared by Brad Appleton, detailed information on stretching and stretching techniques is presented, including normal ranges of motion, flexibility, how to stretch, the physiology of stretching, and the types of stretching including PNF.*

## SOLUTIONS TO CLINICAL APPLICATION EXERCISES

4–1  The warm-up should begin with a 5- to 7-minute slow jog, during which the athlete should break into a light sweat. At that point, she should engage in stretching (using either static or PNF techniques), concentrating on quadriceps, hamstrings, groin, and hip abductor muscles. Each specific stretch should be repeated four times, and the stretch should be held for 15 to 20 seconds. Once the workout begins, the athlete should gradually and moderately increase the intensity of her activity. She may also find it effective to stretch during the cool-down period after the workout.

4–2  Although athletes should make every effort to maintain existing levels of fitness during the rehabilitation period, to improve their fitness to competitive levels, athletes in any sport must practice or engage in that specific activity. The football player must begin a heavy strength-training program for the upper body immediately in the postseason and must continue to progressively return to heavy lifting with the lower extremities as soon as the healing process will allow. It is essential for this player to progressively increase the intensity and variety of conditioning drills that specifically relate to performance at his position.

4–3  Because this athlete suffers from a lower-extremity injury in which weight bearing is limited, alternative activities, such as swimming or riding a stationary exercise bike, should be incorporated into her rehabilitation program immediately. If the pressure on her ankle when riding an exercise bike is too painful, she may find it helpful initially to use a bike that incorporates upper-extremity exercise. The athletic trainer should recommend that this soccer player engage in a minimum of 30 minutes of continuous training as well as some higher-intensity interval training to maintain both aerobic and anaerobic fitness.

4–4  Weight training will not have a negative effect on flexibility as long as the lifting is done properly. Lifting the weight through a full range of motion will improve strength and simultaneously maintain range of motion. A female swimmer is not likely to bulk up to the point that muscle size affects range of motion. It is also important

to recommend that this athlete continue to incorporate active stretching into her training regimen.

4–5  The athletic trainer can discuss the rationale for strength and conditioning with the athlete. Helping the athlete understand why it is important to increase strength and endurance can increase her motivation. In addition to improving performance and efficiency, muscular endurance and strength are also critical in preventing athletic injuries. The athletic trainer should work with the coaches to provide a periodization program that will keep the athlete's interest and prevent atrophy from occurring.

4–6  The shot put, like many other dynamic movements in sports, requires not only great strength but also the ability to generate that strength rapidly. To develop muscular power, this athlete must engage in dynamic, explosive training techniques that will help him develop his ability. Power lifting techniques should be helpful. Plyometric exercises using weights for added resistance will help him improve his speed of muscular contraction against some resistive force.

4–7  The athletic trainer should recommend that the construction worker engage in a regular, consistent flexibility program using either static or PNF stretching techniques. Stretching should be done several times a day if possible. The worker should also be instructed to engage in full range of motion strength training for the hamstrings. The athletic trainer should also explain that when the construction worker feels tightness or discomfort during a training session, he should stop the activity immediately to avoid making a hamstring strain more severe.

4–8  During the early part of the preparatory period, training should be at a low intensity with a high volume of repetitions, using activities that may or may not be directly related to football. This phase may last from several weeks to 2 months. The intensity and volume of these activities should progress to moderate levels. Weight-training activities should eventually become more specific to football. Just before the preseason, the athlete should train at a high intensity, and the volume of training should decrease to allow full recovery between sessions.

## REVIEW QUESTIONS AND CLASS ACTIVITIES

1. In terms of injury prevention, list as many advantages as you can for conditioning.
2. How does the SAID principle relate to sports conditioning and injury prevention?
3. What is the value of proper warm-up and cool-down to sports injury prevention?
4. Critically observe how a variety of sports use warm-up and cool-down procedures.
5. Discuss the relationships among maximal oxygen consumption, heart rate, stroke volume, and cardiac output.
6. Differentiate between aerobic and anaerobic training methods.
7. How is continuous training different from interval training?
8. How may increasing strength decrease susceptibility to injury?
9. Compare different techniques of increasing strength. How may each technique be an advantage or a disadvantage to the athlete in terms of injury prevention?
10. Compare ways to increase flexibility and how they may decrease or increase the athlete's susceptibility to injury.
11. Why is year-round conditioning so important for injury prevention?

# REFERENCES

1. Alemany J: Comparison of acute responses to isotonic or isokinetic eccentric muscle action: Differential outcomes in skeletal muscle damage and implications for rehabilitation, *International Journal for Sports Medicine* 65(1):1–7, 2014.

2. Allerheiligen W: Speed development and plyometric training. In Baechle T, editor: *Essentials of strength training and conditioning,* Champaign, IL, 2008, Human Kinetics.

3. Allerheiligen W: Stretching and warm-up. In Baechle T, editor: *Essentials of strength training and conditioning,* Champaign, IL, 2008, Human Kinetics.

4. Alter M: *The science of flexibility,* Champaign, IL, 2004, Human Kinetics.

5. American College of Sports Medicine: *Guidelines for exercise testing and prescription,* Philadelphia, 2013, Lippincott, Williams and Wilkens.

6. Andersen J: Flexibility in performance: Foundational concepts and practical issues, *Athletic Therapy Today* 11(3):9, 2006.

7. Andersen J: Stretching before and after exercise: Effect on muscle soreness and injury risk, *J Athl Train* 40(3):218, 2005.

8. Armiger P: Preventing musculotendinous injuries: A focus on flexibility, *Athletic Therapy Today* 5(4):20, 2000.

9. Baker D: Generality vs. specificity: A comparison of dynamic and isometric measures of strength and speed-strength, *Eur J Appl Physiol* 68:350, 1994.

10. Bandy W: The effect of static stretch and dynamic range of motion training on the flexibility of the hamstring muscles, *J Orthop Sports Phys Ther* 27(4):295, 1998.

11. Behm D: Effect of acute static stretching on force, balance, reaction time, and movement time, *Med Sci Sports Exerc* 36(8):1397, 2004.

12. Berger R: *Conditioning for men,* Boston, 1973, Allyn & Bacon.

13. Blanke D: Flexibility. In Mellion M, editor: *Sports medicine secrets,* Philadelphia, 2002, Hanley & Belfus.

14. Bompa T: *Periodization: Theory and methodization of training,* Champaign, IL, 2010, Human Kinetics.

15. Bompa T: *Serious strength training,* Champaign, IL, 2012, Human Kinetics.

16. Boyle M: *Functional training for sports,* Champaign, IL, 2004, Human Kinetics.

17. Brooks G: *Exercise physiology: Human bioenergetics and its applications,* San Francisco, 2004, McGraw-Hill.

18. Brumitt J: *Core assessment and training,* Champaign, IL, 2010, Human Kinetics.

19. Buchheit M: High-intensity interval training, solutions to the programming puzzle, *Sports Medicine* 43(10):927–954, 2013.

20. Burke D: The theoretical basis of proprioceptive neuromuscular facilitation, *Strength Cond* 14(4):496, 2000.

21. Carter C: Training the child athlete: Physical fitness, health and injury, *British Journal of Sports Medicine* 45:880–885, 2011.

22. Chalmers G: Re-examination of the possible role of Golgi tendon organ and muscle spindle reflexes in proprioceptive neuromuscular facilitation muscle stretching, *Sports Biomechanics* 3(1):159, 2004.

23. Chimera N, Swanik K, Swanik C: Effects of plyometric training on muscle activation strategies and performance in female athletes, *J Athl Train* 39(1):24, 2004.

24. Chu D: Plyometrics in sports injury rehabilitation and training, *Athletic Therapy Today* 4(3):7, 1999.

25. Clark M: *NASM essentials of corrective exercise training,* Baltimore, MD: 2011, Lippincott, Williams & Wilkins.

26. Colston M: Core Stability, Part 1: Overview and the concept, *Athletic Therapy and Training,* 17(1):8–13, 2012.

27. Costa, P: Warm-up, stretching and cool-down strategies for combat sports, *Strength and Conditioning Journal* 33(6):71–79, 2011.

28. Cross K: Effects of a static stretching program on the incidence of lower extremity musculotendinous strains, *J Athl Train* 34(1):11, 1999.

29. Curtis N: Stretching and functional flexibility, *Athletic Therapy Today* 11(3):30, 2006.

30. Dale B: Principles of core stabilization for athletic populations, *Athletic Therapy Today* 10(4):13, 2005.

31. Decoster L: The effects of hamstring stretching on range of motion: A systematic literature review, *J Orthop Sports Phys Ther* 3(6):377, 2005.

32. DeLorme T: *Progressive resistance exercise,* New York, 1951, Appleton-Century-Crofts.

33. DePino G: Duration of maintained hamstring flexibility after cessation of an acute static stretching protocol, *J Athl Train* 35(1):56, 2000.

34. Enoksen E: The effect of high- vs. low-intensity training on aerobic capacity in well-trained male middle-distance runners, *Journal of Strength and Conditioning Research* 25(3):812–18, 2011.

35. Eston R. Perceived exertion: Recent advances and novel applications in children and adults, *Journal of Exercise Science and Fitness* 7(2):11–17, 2009.

36. Ferrar K: A systematic review and meta-analysis of submaximal exercise-based equations to predict maximal oxygen uptake in young people, *Pediatric Exercise Science* 26(3)342–57, 2014.

37. Fleck S: *Designing resistance training programs,* Champaign, IL, 2003, Human Kinetics.

38. Fowles J: Reduced strength after passive stretch of the human plantarflexors, *J App Physiol* 89(3):1179, 2000.

39. Fradkin A: Does warming up prevent injury in sport? The evidence from randomized controlled trials? *Journal of Science and Medicine in Sport* 9(3):214–20, 2006.

40. Fradkin A: Effects of warming up on physical performance: A systematic review with meta-analysis, *Journal of Strength and Conditioning Research* 24(1):140–48, 2010.

41. Gardner P: Youth strength training, *Athletic Therapy Today* 8(1):42, 2003.

42. Gist N: Sprint interval training effects on aerobic capacity: A systematic review and meta-analysis, *Sports Medicine* 44(2):269–79, 2014.

43. Goldberg L: *Strength ball training,* Champaign, IL, 2006, Human Kinetics.

44. Gormley S: Effect of intensity of aerobic training on $VO2_{max}$, *Medicine and Science in Sports and Exercise* 40(7):1336–43, 2008.

45. Gravelle B, Blessing D: Physiological adaptation in women concurrently training for strength and endurance, *J Strength Cond Res* 14(1):5, 2000.

46. Gribble P: Effects of static and hold-relax stretching on hamstring range of motion using the FlexAbility LE1000, *J Sport Rehabil* 8(3):195, 1999.

47. Harman E: The biomechanics of resistance exercise. In Baechle T, editor: *Essentials of strength training and conditioning,* Champaign, IL, 2008, Human Kinetics.

48. Hilbert S: Free weights versus machines, *Strength Cond* 21(6):66, 1999.

49. Holt L: Modifications to the standard sit-and-reach flexibility protocol, *J Athl Train* 34(1):43, 1999.

50. Issurin V: New horizons for the methodology and physiology of training periodization, *Sports Medicine* 40(3):189–206, 2010.

51. Jones T: Performance and neuromuscular adaptations following differing ratios of concurrent strength and endurance training, *Journal of Strength and Conditioning Research* 27(12):3342–51, 2013.

52. Kaminski T: Concentric versus enhanced eccentric hamstring strength training: Clinical implications, *J Athl Train* 33(3):216, 1998.

53. Karvonen M: The effects of training on heart rate: A longitudinal study, *Ann Med Exp Biol* 35:305, 1957.

54. Klinger T: Prescribing target heart rates without the use of a graded exercise test, *Clinical Exercise Physiology* 3(4):207, 2001.

55. Knight K: Isotonic contractions might be more effective than isokinetic contractions in developing muscle strength, *J Sport Rehabil* 10(2):124, 2001.

56. Kokkonen J: Acute stretching inhibits strength endurance, *Med Sci Sports Exerc* 35(5):11, 2001.

57. Kokkonen J: Chronic stretching improves sport specific skills, *Med Sci Sports Exerc* 29(5):67, 1997.

58. Kovacs M: The argument against static stretching before sport and physical activity, *Athletic Therapy Today* 11(3):6, 2006.

59. Kraemer W: *Strength training for sport,* Cambridge, MA, 2002, Blackwell Science.

60. Kubo K: Effect of stretching training on the viscoelastic properties of human tendon structures in vivo, *J App Physiol* 92(2):595, 2002.

61. Leetun D: Core stability measures as risk factors for lower extremity injury in athletes, *Med Sci Sports Exerc* 36(6):926, 2005.

62. Logan G: Recent findings in learning and performance. Paper presented at the Southern Section Meeting, California Association for Health, Physical Education, and Recreation, Pasadena, 1960.

63. Maddigan M: A comparison of assisted and unassisted proprioceptive neuromuscular facilitation techniques and static stretching, *Journal of Strength and Conditioning Research* 26(5):1238–44, 2012.

64. Mann D: Functional stretching: Implementing a dynamic stretching program, *Athletic Therapy Today* 6(3):10, 2001.

65. Marek S: Acute effects of static and proprioceptive neuromuscular facilitation stretching on muscle strength and power output, *J Athl Train* 40(2):94, 2005.

66. McArdle W: *Exercise physiology, energy, nutrition, and human performance,* Philadelphia, 2014, Lippincott, Williams and Wilkins.

67. McHugh M: To stretch or not to stretch: The role of stretching in injury prevention and performance, *Scandinavian Journal of Medicine and Science in Sports* 20(2):169–81, 2010.
68. McLaughlin J: Test of the classic model for predicting endurance running performance, *Medicine and Science in Sports and Exercise* 42(5):991–97, 2010.
69. Merce J: Analysis of peak oxygen consumption and heart rate during elliptical and treadmill exercise, *J Sport Rehabil* 10(1):48, 2001.
70. Middlesworth M: More than ergonomics: Warm-up and stretching key to injury prevention, *Athletic Therapy Today* 7(2):32, 2002.
71. Moreno A: The practicalities of adolescent resistance training, *Athletic Therapy Today* 8(3):26, 2003.
72. Moss R: Physics, plyometrics, and injury prevention, *Athletic Therapy Today* 7(2):44, 2002.
73. Nelson R: An update on flexibility. *Natl Strength Condit Assoc J* 27(1):10, 2005.
74. Okada T: Relationship between core stability, functional movement and performance, *Journal of Strength and Conditioning Research* 25(1):252–61, 2011.
75. Owsley A: An introduction to clinical Pilates. *Athletic Therapy Today* 10(4):19, 2005.
76. Parr J: Symptomatic and functional responses to concentric-eccentric isokinetic versus eccentric-only isotonic exercise, *J Athl Train,* 44(5): 462–68, 2009.
77. Prentice W: *Get fit stay fit,* ed 7, Philadelphia, 2015, F.A. Davis.
78. Prentice W: Proprioceptive neuromuscular facilitation techniques. In Prentice W, editor: *Rehabilitation techniques in sports medicine and athletic training,* Thorofare, NJ, 2015, Slack.
79. Puentedura E: Immediate effects of quantified hamstring stretching: Hold-relax proprioceptive neuromuscular facilitation versus static stretching, *Physical Therapy in Sport* 12(3):122–26, 2011.
80. Radcliffe J: *High-powered plyometrics,* Champaign, IL: 2015, Human Kinetics.
81. Rubley M: Flexibility retention 3 weeks after a 5-day training regime, *J Sport Rehabil* 10(2):105, 2001.
82. Ryan E: Do practical durations of stretching alter muscle strength. A dose-response study, *Medicine and Science in Sport and Exercise* 40(8):1529–37, 2008.
83. Ryan E: Acute effects of different volumes of dynamic stretching on vertical jump performance, flexibility and muscle endurance, *Clinical Physiology and Functional Imaging* 34(6):485–92, 2014.
84. Ryba T: The benefits of yoga for athletes: The body, *Athletic Therapy Today* 11(2):32, 2006.
85. Sartor F: Estimation of maximal oxygen uptake via submaximal exercise testing in sports, clinical, and home settings, *Sports Medicine* 43(9):865–73. 2015.
86. Schilling B: Stretching: Acute effects on strength and power performance, *Strength Cond* 22(1):44, 2000.
87. Sekendiz B: Effects of Swiss-ball core strength training on strength, endurance, flexibility and balance in sedentary women, *Journal of Strength and Conditioning Research* 24(11):3032–40, 2010.
88. Sexton P: The importance of flexibility for functional range of motion, *Athletic Therapy Today* 11(3):13, 2006.
89. Siatras T: Static and dynamic acute stretching effect on gymnasts' speed in vaulting, *Ped Ex Sci* 15:383, 2003.
90. Small K: A systematic review into the efficacy of static stretching as part of a warmup for the prevention of exercise-related injury, *Research in Sports Medicine* 16(3):213–31, 2008.
91. Soames R: *Joint motion: Clinical measurement and evaluation,* Philadelphia, 2002, Elsevier.
92. Swain D: Validation of a new method for estimating $VO2_{max}$ based on VO2 reserve, *Med Sci Sports Exerc* 36(8):1421, 2004.
93. Swanson J: Periodization for the multisport athlete, *Strength Cond* 26(4):50, 2004.
94. Talalian J: Two weeks of high-intensity aerobic interval training increases the capacity for fat oxidation during exercise in women, *Journal of Applied Physiology* 102(4): 1439–47, 2007.
95. Taylor D: Viscoelastic characteristics of muscle: Passive stretching versus muscular contractions, *Med Sci Sports Exerc* 29(12):1619, 1997.
96. Thacker S: The impact of stretching on sports injury risk: A systematic review of the literature, *Med Sci Sports Exerc* 36(3):371, 2004.
97. Thomas M: The functional warm-up, *Strength Cond* 22(2):51, 2000.
98. Van Hatten B: Passive versus active stretching, *Phys Ther* 85(1):80, 2005.
99. Walker M: Relationship between maximum strength and relative endurance for the empty-can exercise, *J Sport Rehabil* 12(1):31, 2003.
100. Wathen D: Periodization: Concepts and applications. In Baechle T, editor: *Essentials of strength training and conditioning,* Champaign, IL, 2008, Human Kinetics.
101. Wilkerson G: Neuromuscular changes in female collegiate athletes resulting from a plyometric jump training program, *J Athl Train* 39(1): 17, 2004.
102. Winters M: Passive versus active stretching of hip flexor muscles in subjects with limited hip extension: A randomized clinical trial, *Phys Ther* 84(9):800, 2004.
103. Zentz C: Warm up to perform up, *Athletic Therapy Today* 5(2):59, 2000.

# ANNOTATED BIBLIOGRAPHY

Adler S, Beckers D, Buck M: *PNF in practice: an illustrated guide,* New York, 2008, Springer.

*A heavily illustrated text that covers all aspects of PNF.*

Alter M: *The science of flexibility,* Champaign, IL, 2004, Human Kinetics.

*Explains the principles and techniques of stretching and details the anatomy and physiology of muscle and connective tissue. Includes guidelines for developing a flexibility program, illustrated stretching exercises, and warm-up drills.*

Anderson B: *Stretching,* Bolinas, CA, 2010, Shelter.

*An extremely comprehensive best-selling text on stretching exercises for the entire body.*

Baechle T, editor: *Essentials of strength training and conditioning,* Champaign, IL, 2008, Human Kinetics.

*A book from the National Strength Coaches Association that explains the science, theory, and practical application of various aspects of conditioning in a very concise, easily understood text.*

Bishop, J: *Fitness through aerobics,* Philadelphia, PA, 2010, Benjamin Cummings.

*This text uses the most up-to-date fitness and wellness information on aerobic dance exercise.*

Cardinale, M. Newton, R, *Strength and conditioning: Biological principles and practical applications,* Hoboken, NJ, 2011, John Wiley.

*This book provides good scientific and practical information in the field of strength and conditioning.*

Fleck, S, Kraemer, W, *Designing resistance training programs,* Champaign, IL, 2014, Human Kinetics.

*A clear, readable, state-of-the-art guide to developing individualized training programs for both athletes and fitness enthusiasts.*

Kovacs, M, *Dynamic stretching: The revolutionary new warm-up method to improve power, performance and range of motion.* Berkeley, CA, 2009, Ulysses Press.

*Teaches how to prepare your body for physical activity while simultaneously improving strength, power, speed, agility, and endurance.*

Leibenson, C. *Functional training handbook,* Baltimore, MD, 2014, Lippincott, Williams & Wilkins.

*This practical guide delivers clear, how-to information, an array of sport-specific guidelines, and key principles that foster lifelong health, mobility, and athletic development.*

National Strength and Conditioning Association, *Developing the core,* Champaign, IL, 2013, Human Kinetics.

*The National Strength and Conditioning Association (NSCA) brings you the authoritative resource on strengthening the core to maximize sport performance.*

Powers, S, Howley, E. *Exercise physiology: Theory and application to fitness and performance,* New York, 2011, McGraw-Hill.

*Written especially for exercise science and physical education students, this text provides a solid foundation in theory illuminated by application and performance models to increase understanding and to help students apply what they've learned in the classroom.*

Radcliffe, J, Farentinos, R, *High powered plyometrics*, Champaign, IL, 2015. Human Kinetics.

*Detailing plyometric exercises for a variety of sports, this guide explains how plyometrics work and how to incorporate plyometrics into a comprehensive strength- and power-training program.*

Prentice W: *Fitness and wellness for life,* ed 7, Dubuque, IA, 1999, WCB/McGraw-Hill.

*A comprehensive fitness text that covers all aspects of a training and conditioning program.*

Verstegen M, Williams P: *Core performance: the revolutionary workout program to transform your body and your life,* Mountain View, CA, 2005, Rodale Press.

*Concentrates primarily on core stabilization exercises to improve posture and improve performance in athletes.*

Wiksten D, Peters C: *The athletic trainer's guide to strength and endurance training,* Thorofare, NJ, 2000, Slack.

*Layout offers ease of reference, sport-specific programs, information on nutritional supplements, and illustrations on weight training and supplemental routines.*

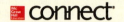

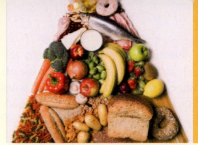

© Image Source/Glow Images

# 5

# Nutrition and Supplements

## ■ Objectives

*When you finish this chapter you should be able to*

- Distinguish the six classes of nutrients and describe their major functions.
- Explain the importance of good nutrition in enhancing performance and preventing injuries.
- Assess the advantages and disadvantages of dietary supplements.
- Discuss popular eating and drinking practices.
- Discuss the advantages and disadvantages of consuming a pre-event meal.

- Differentiate between body weight and body composition.
- Explain the principle of caloric balance and how to assess it.
- Assess body composition using skinfold calipers.
- Evaluate methods for losing and gaining weight.
- Recognize the signs of bulimia nervosa and anorexia nervosa.

## ■ Key Terms

amino acids

osteoporosis

lactase deficiency

anemia

glycemic index (GI)

glycogen supercompensation

obesity

adipose cell

body composition

## ■ Connect Highlights  connect®

*Visit connect.mcgraw-hill.com for further exercises to apply your knowledge:*

- Clinical application scenarios covering methods of losing and gaining weight, nutrition to enhance performance and prevent injury, dietary supplements, and caloric balance and how to assess it
- Click-and-drag questions covering vitamins, minerals, prevent meals, and body composition
- Multiple-choice questions covering nutrients, proper nutrition to enhance performance, dietary supplements, hydration, and eating disorders
- Selection questions covering nutrients and their major functions

The relation of nutrition, diet, and weight control to overall health and fitness should be an issue of critical importance to everyone. Individuals who practice sound nutritional habits reduce the likelihood of injury and illness by maintaining a higher standard of healthful living.[11] We know that eating a well-balanced diet can positively contribute to the development of strength, flexibility, and cardiorespiratory endurance.[66,81] Unfortunately, misconceptions, fads, and, in many cases, superstitions regarding nutrition have a significant impact on dietary habits.[48]

Many athletes associate successful performance with the consumption of special foods or supplements.[25] An athlete who is performing well may be reluctant to change dietary habits regardless of whether the diet is physiologically beneficial to overall health.[85] There is no question that the psychological aspect of allowing the athlete to eat whatever he or she is most comfortable with can greatly affect performance. The problem is that these eating habits tend to become accepted as beneficial and may become traditional when, in fact, they may be physiologically detrimental to athletic performance. Thus, many nutrition "experts" tend to disseminate nutritional information based on traditional rather than experimental information.[25] The athletic trainer must possess a strong knowledge of nutrition so that he or she may serve as an informational resource for the athlete.[10,46,66] **SoR:A** The athletic trainer should make an effort to establish a support team that includes a registered dietitian, sports nutritionist, or other health care professional with expertise in nutrition.[10] **SoR:A**

An athletic trainer working in the clinical, corporate, or industrial setting may be responsible for overseeing employee fitness or wellness programs. Providing direct nutritional counseling, organizing health fairs or workshops that focus on various aspects of nutrition, and serving as a resource in disseminating information related to diet and nutrition may all be part of the responsibilities of that position.

## NUTRITION BASICS

*Nutrition* is the science of the substances in food that are essential to life. Nutrients have three major functions: the growth, repair, and maintenance of all tissues; the regulation of body processes; and the production of energy.[22]

The nutrients are categorized into six major classes: *carbohydrates, fats* (often called *lipids*), *proteins, water, vitamins,* and *minerals.* Carbohydrates, proteins, and fats are referred to as the *macronutrients:* the absorbable components of food, from which energy is derived. Vitamins, minerals, and water are con-

> The six classes of nutrients are carbohydrates, fats, proteins, water, vitamins, and minerals.

sidered to be *micronutrients,* which are necessary for regulating normal body functions. They do not provide energy, but without sufficient quantities of micronutrients, the energy from macronutrients cannot be utilized. For example, certain vitamins are necessary for other vitamins to be absorbed. Most foods are actually mixtures of these nutrients. Some nutrients can be made by the body, but an *essential nutrient* must be supplied by the diet.[85] Not all substances in food are considered nutrients. There is no such thing as the perfect food; that is, no single natural food contains all the nutrients needed for health. A summary of current percentages and recommended percentages of calories from protein, carbohydrate, and fat is shown in Figure 5–1.

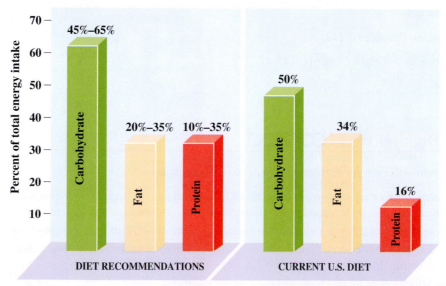

FIGURE 5–1 Comparison of calories from protein, carbohydrate, and fat.
(Based on 2015–2020 Dietary Guidelines)

It is recommended that the majority, about 45 to 65 percent, of the calories consumed be in the form of carbohydrates. Fat should account for between 20 to 35 percent of the total caloric intake. Only 10 to 35 percent of the caloric intake should be protein. For an athlete who requires additional energy during the course of a day, the extra calories consumed should be in the form of carbohydrates.[82]

Nutrient-dense foods are those that supply adequate amounts of vitamins and minerals in relation to their caloric value. The so-called junk foods provide excessive amounts of calories from fat and sugar in relation to vitamins and minerals and therefore are not nutrient dense. However, many people live on junk foods that displace more nutrient-dense foods from their diet.[67] This behavior is not healthful in the long run.[83]

Nutrient-dense foods supply adequate amounts of vitamins and minerals in relation to caloric value.

# ENERGY SOURCES

## Carbohydrates

Anyone who is physically active has increased energy needs. Carbohydrates are the body's most efficient source of energy and should be relied on to fill those needs.[50] Carbohydrate intake should account for 45 to 65 percent of total caloric intake. The following sections describe different forms of carbohydrates and their role in the production of energy and the maintenance of health.[13] It is important to understand that not all carbohydrates are digested and absorbed at the same rate.

**Sugars** Carbohydrates are classified as simple (sugars) or complex (starch and most forms of fiber). Sugars are further divided into monosaccharides and disaccharides. Monosaccharides, or single sugars, are found mostly in fruits, syrups, and honey. Glucose (blood sugar) is a monosaccharide. Milk sugar (lactose) and table sugar (sucrose) are combinations of two monosaccharides and are called disaccharides. Because sugar contributes little in the way of other nutrients, the amount of sugar eaten should account for no more than 100 calories a day for women and 150 calories a day for men.

Carbohydrates are sugars, starches, and fiber.

**Starches** Starches are complex carbohydrates. A starch is made up of long chains of glucose units. During the digestion process, the starch chain is broken down and the glucose units are free to be absorbed. Food sources of starch, such as rice, potatoes, and breads, often provide vitamins and minerals in addition to serving as the body's principal source of glucose. Many people believe that starchy foods contribute to obesity. However, most of these foods are eaten with fats from butter, margarine, sauces, and gravies that make the food more enjoyable but contribute an excess of calories.

The body cannot use starches and many sugars directly from food for energy. It must obtain the simple sugar glucose (blood sugar). During digestion and metabolism, starches and disaccharide sugars are broken down and converted to glucose. The glucose that is not needed for immediate energy is stored as glycogen in the liver and muscle cells. Glucose can be released from glycogen later if needed. The body, however, can store only a limited amount of glucose as glycogen. Any extra glucose is converted to body fat. When the body experiences an inadequate intake of dietary carbohydrate, it uses protein to make glucose, but the protein is then diverted from its own important functions. Therefore, a supply of glucose must be kept available to prevent the use of protein for energy. This is called the protein-sparing action of glucose.

Glycolysis is the process that breaks down glucose to produce energy.

**Fiber** Fiber forms the structural parts of plants and is not digested by humans. Fiber is not found in animal sources of food. There are two kinds of dietary fiber: soluble and insoluble. Soluble fiber includes gums and pectins; cellulose is the primary insoluble form. Sources of soluble fiber are oatmeal, legumes, and some fruits. Food sources of insoluble fiber include whole-grain breads and bran cereals.

Because it is not digested, fiber passes through the intestinal tract and adds bulk. Fiber aids normal elimination by reducing the amount of time required for wastes to move through the digestive tract, which is believed to reduce the risk of colon cancer. Also, increased fiber intake is thought to reduce the risk of coronary artery disease. Soluble forms of fiber bind to cholesterol passing through the digestive tract and prevent its absorption, which can reduce blood cholesterol levels. Foods rich in saturated fats (meats, in particular) often take the place of fiber-rich foods in the diet, thus increasing cholesterol absorption and formation. Consumption of adequate amounts of fiber has been associated with lowered incidences of obesity, constipation, colitis, appendicitis, and diabetes.

The recommended amount of fiber in the diet is approximately 25 grams per day for women and 38 grams per day for men.[77] Unfortunately, the average person consumes only 15 grams per day. Fiber intake should be increased by increasing the amount of whole-grain cereal products and fruits and vegetables in the diet rather than by using fiber supplements. However, excessive consumption of fiber may cause intestinal discomfort as well as increased losses of calcium and iron.

## Fats

Fats are an essential component of the diet. They are the most concentrated source of energy, providing more than twice the calories per gram when compared with carbohydrates or proteins. Fat is used as a primary source of energy. Some dietary fat is needed to make food more flavorful and for sources of the fat-soluble vitamins. Also, a minimal amount of fat is essential for normal growth and development.

Unfortunately, in the typical American diet, fat represents approximately 40 to 50 percent of the total caloric intake. This intake is believed to be too high and may contribute to the prevalence of obesity, certain cancers, and coronary artery disease. Intake should be limited to less than 20 to 35 percent of total calories.[83]

**Saturated versus Unsaturated Fat** Both plant and animal foods provide sources of dietary fat. About 95 percent of the fat consumed is in the form of triglyc-

> **Fats may be saturated or unsaturated.**

erides. Depending on their chemical nature, fatty acids may be saturated or unsaturated. The unsaturated fatty acids can be subdivided into monounsaturates and polyunsaturates. Therefore, the terms *saturated, monounsaturated,* and *polyunsaturated* are used to describe the chemical nature of the fat in foods. The triglycerides that make up food fats are usually mixtures of saturated and unsaturated fatty acids but are classified according to the type that predominates. In general, fats containing more unsaturated fatty acids are from plants and are liquid at room temperature. Saturated fatty acids are derived mainly from animal sources.

*Trans* fatty acids (*trans* fat) have physical properties generally resembling saturated fatty acids, and their presence tends to harden oils. *Trans* fats have been used in many cookies crackers, dairy products, meats, potato chips, most junk foods, and fast foods. *Trans* fatty acids increase the risk of heart disease by boosting levels of bad cholesterol. Because they are not essential and provide no known health benefit, there is no safe level of *trans* fatty acids in the blood, and people should eat as little of them as possible while consuming a nutritionally adequate diet. There is a substantial ongoing effort by the Food and Drug Administration to eliminate *trans* fats from the U.S. food supply.

**Other Fats** Phospholipids and sterols represent the remaining 5 percent of fats. One example of phospholipids is lecithin; cholesterol is the best known sterol. Cholesterol is consumed in animal foods; it is not supplied by plant sources of food. Generally, it is wise to avoid eating foods high in cholesterol. Although cholesterol is essential to many bodily functions, the body can manufacture cholesterol from carbohydrates, proteins, and especially saturated fat. Thus, there is little, if any, need to consume additional amounts of cholesterol in the diet. When low-density cholesterol (LDL) becomes too high, the risk of developing cardiovascular diseases also increases. Saturated fat can raise the amount of low-density lipoprotein (LDL) and the level of "bad" cholesterol, thus increasing the risk for heart disease. The American Heart Association recommends consuming less than 300 mg per day. Their guidelines also advise limiting saturated fats and *trans* fats, both of which can raise LDL cholesterol.[3]

One type of unsaturated fatty acid seems to serve as a protective mechanism against certain disease processes. The omega-3 fatty acids apparently have the capability of reducing the likelihood of heart disease, stroke, and hypertension. These fatty acids are found in cold-water fish.

## Proteins

Proteins make up the major structural components of the body. They are needed for the growth, maintenance, and repair of all body tissues. In addition, proteins are needed to make enzymes, many hormones, and antibodies that help fight infection. In general, the body prefers not to use much protein for energy; instead, it relies on fats and carbohydrates. Protein intake should be around 10 to 35 percent of total calories.

**Amino Acids** The basic units that make up proteins are smaller compounds called **amino acids.** Most of the body's proteins are made up of about 20 amino acids. Amino acids can be linked together in a wide variety of combinations, which is why there are so many different forms and uses of proteins. Most of the amino acids can be produced as needed in the body. The others cannot be made to any significant degree and therefore must be supplied by the diet. The amino acids obtained through food are referred to as the *essential amino acids*. The amount of protein and the levels of the individual essential amino acids are important for determining the quality of diet. A diet that contains large amounts of protein will not support growth, repair, and maintenance of tissues if the essential amino acids are not available in the proper proportions.[39]

Most of the proteins from animal foods contain all the essential amino acids that humans require and are called complete, or high-quality, proteins. Incomplete proteins—that is, proteins that do not contain all the essential amino acids—usually are from plant sources of food. Beans and legumes are a potential source of protein and iron for vegetarians.

> Proteins are made up of amino acids.

**Protein Sources and Need** Most people do not have difficulty meeting their protein needs because the typical diet is rich in protein. Athletes need more than the recommended daily allowance (RDA) of protein (1.2–2.0 g/kg/BW).[32] Many athletes consume more than twice the recommended amounts of protein. There is no advantage to consuming more protein, particularly in the form of protein supplements. If more protein is supplied than needed, the body must convert the excess to fat for storage. This conversion can create a situation in which excess water is removed from cells, leading to dehydration and possible damage to the kidneys or liver. Although this is not generally a concern in healthy adults.[62] Protein supplements may also create imbalances of the chemicals that make up proteins, the amino acids, which is not desirable. A condition of the bones, osteoporosis, has been linked to a diet that contains too much protein.[4]

Increased physical activity increases a person's need for energy, not necessarily for protein.[39] The increases in muscle mass that result from conditioning and training are associated with only a small increase in protein requirements, which can easily be met with the usual diet. Therefore, an athlete does not need protein supplements.

A company employee who regularly goes to the corporate fitness center complains to the athletic trainer that she constantly feels tired and lethargic, even though she thinks that she is eating well and getting a sufficient amount of sleep. A coworker has suggested that she begin taking vitamin supplements, which the coworker claims give her more energy and make her more resistant to fatigue. The employee asks the athletic trainer's advice about the kind of vitamins she needs to take.

**?** What facts should the athletic trainer explain about vitamin supplementation, and what recommendations should he or she make?

# REGULATOR NUTRIENTS

## Vitamins

Although vitamins are required in extremely small amounts when compared with water, proteins, carbohydrates, and fats, they perform essential functions, primarily as regulators of body processes.[13] Thirteen vitamins have specific roles in the body, many of which are still being explored. In the past, letters were assigned as names for vitamins. Today, most are known by their scientific names. Vitamins are classified into two groups: fat-soluble vitamins, which are dissolved in fats and stored in the body, and water-soluble vitamins, which are dissolved in watery solutions and are not stored. Table 5–1 lists the vitamins and indicates their primary functions.

**Fat-Soluble Vitamins** Vitamins A, D, E, and K are fat soluble. They are found in the fatty portions of foods and in oils. Because they are stored in the body's fat, it is possible to consume excess amounts, which can accumulate and lead to toxicity if the upper intake levels (ULs) are exceeded.

> Fat-soluble vitamins: A, D, E, and K.

**Water-Soluble Vitamins** The water-soluble vitamins are vitamin C, known as ascorbic acid, and the B-complex vitamins thiamin, riboflavin, niacin, $B_6$, folate, $B_{12}$, biotin, and pantothenic acid. Although vitamins are not metabolized for energy, thiamin, riboflavin, niacin, biotin, and pantothenic acid are used to regulate the metabolism of carbohydrates, proteins, and fats to obtain energy. Vitamin $B_6$ regulates the body's use of amino acids. Folate and vitamin $B_{12}$ are important in normal blood formation. Vitamin C is used for building bones and teeth, maintaining connective tissues, and strengthening the immune system. Unlike fat-soluble vitamins, water-soluble vitamins cannot be stored to any significant extent in the body and should be supplied in the diet each day.[50]

> Water-soluble vitamins: C, thiamin, riboflavin, niacin, $B_6$, $B_{12}$, folate, biotin, and pantothenic acid.

**Antioxidants** Certain nutrients, called antioxidants, may prevent premature aging, certain cancers, heart disease, and other health problems.[59] An antioxidant protects vital cell components from the destructive effects of certain agents, including oxygen. Vitamin C, vitamin E, and beta-carotene

> Antioxidants: vitamin C, vitamin E, and beta-carotene.

| TABLE 5–1 | Vitamins | | | |
|---|---|---|---|---|
| Vitamin | Major Function | Most Reliable Sources | Deficiency | Excess (toxicity) |
| **Fat-Soluable Vitamins** | | | | |
| A | Maintains skin and other cells that line the inside of the body, bone and tooth development, growth, vision in dim light | Liver, milk, egg yolk, deep green and yellow fruits and vegetables | Night blindness, dry skin, growth failure | Headaches, nausea, loss of hair, dry skin, diarrhea |
| D | Normal bone growth and development | Exposure to sunlight, fortified dairy products, eggs and fish liver oils | Rickets in children—defective bone formation leading to deformed bones | Appetite loss, weight loss, failure to grow |
| E | Prevents destruction of polyunsaturated fats caused by exposure to oxidizing agents, protects cell membranes from destruction | Vegetable oils, some in fruits and vegetables, whole grains | Breakage of red blood cells leading to anemia | Nausea and diarrhea, interferes with vitamin K absorption if vitamin D is also deficient, not as toxic as other fat-soluble vitamins |
| K | Production of blood-clotting substances | Green, leafy vegetables; normal bacteria that live in intestines | Increased bleeding time | |
| **Water-Soluble Vitamins** | | | | |
| Thiamin | Needed for release of energy from carbohydrates, fats, and proteins | Cereal products, pork, peas, dried beans | Lack of energy, nerve problems | |
| Riboflavin | Energy from carbohydrates, fats, and proteins | Milk, liver, fruits and vegetables, enriched breads and cereals | Dry skin, cracked lips | |
| Niacin | Energy from carbohydrates, fats, and proteins | Liver, meat, poultry, peanut butter, legumes, enriched breads and cereals | Skin problems, diarrhea, mental depression, eventually death (rarely occurs in U.S.) | Skin flushing, intestinal upset, nervousness, intestinal ulcers |
| $B_6$ | Metabolism of protein, production of hemoglobin | White meats, whole grains, liver, egg yolk, bananas | Poor growth, anemia | Severe loss of coordination from nerve damage |
| $B_{12}$ | Production of genetic material, maintains central nervous system | Foods of animal origin | Neurological problems, anemia | |
| Folate (folic acid) | Production of genetic material | Wheat germ; liver; yeast; mushrooms; green, leafy vegetables; fruits | Anemia | |
| C (ascorbic acid) | Formation and maintenance of connective tissue, tooth and bone formation, immune function | Fruits and vegetables | Scurvy (rare), swollen joints, bleeding gums, fatigue, bruising | Kidney stones, diarrhea |
| Pantothenic acid | Energy from carbohydrates, fats, proteins | Widely found in foods | Not observed in humans under normal conditions | |
| Biotin | Use of fats | Widely found in foods | Rare under normal conditions | |

are antioxidants. Beta-carotene is a plant pigment found in dark green, deep yellow, and orange fruits and vegetables. The body can convert beta-carotene to vitamin A. In the early 1980s, researchers reported that smokers who ate large quantities of fruits and vegetables rich in beta-carotene were less likely to develop lung cancer than were other smokers.[71] Since that time, more evidence has accumulated about the benefits of a diet rich in the antioxidant nutrients.[71]

Some experts believe that it is important to increase intake of antioxidants, even if it means taking supplements. Others are more cautious.[71] Excess beta-carotene pigments circulate throughout the body and may turn the skin yellow. However, the pigment is not believed to be toxic, like its nutrient cousin, vitamin A. On the other hand, increasing intake of vitamins C and E is not without some risk. Excess vitamin C is not well absorbed. The excess is irritating to the intestines and creates diarrhea. Although less toxic than vitamins A and D, too much vitamin E causes health problems. The issue of whether athletes need to use antioxidant supplements is controversial. Currently, there is limited scientific evidence to recommend antioxidant supplements to athletes or other physically active individuals.[57]

**Vitamin Deficiencies** The illness that results from a lack of any nutrient, especially those nutrients, such as vitamins, that are needed only in small amounts, is referred to as a deficiency disease.[13] Vitamin deficiency diseases are rare. Adequate amounts of the vitamins, as with other nutrients, can be obtained if a wide variety of foods are eaten. Vitamin supplements can cause toxic effects if large enough quantities are taken. Table 5–1 describes some of vitamins' toxicity problems.

## Minerals

More than 20 mineral elements have a role in body function and therefore must be supplied in the diet. The most essential minerals are listed in Table 5–2. Most minerals are stored in the body, especially in the liver and bones. Magnesium is needed in energy-supplying reactions; sodium and potassium are important for the transmission of nerve impulses. Iron plays a role in energy metabolism but is also combined with a protein to form hemoglobin,

| TABLE 5–2 | Minerals | | | |
|---|---|---|---|---|
| **Mineral** | **Major Role** | **Most Reliable Sources** | **Deficiency** | **Excess** |
| Calcium | Bone and tooth formation, blood clotting, muscle contraction, nerve function | Dairy products, calcium-enriched orange juice and bread | May lead to osteoporosis | Calcium deposits in soft tissues |
| Phosphorus | Skeletal development, tooth formation | Meats, dairy products, other protein-rich foods | Rarely seen | |
| Sodium | Maintenance of fluid balance | Salt (sodium chloride) added to foods and sodium-containing preservatives | | May contribute to the development of hypertension |
| Iron | Formation of hemoglobin; energy from carbohydrates, fats, and proteins | Liver and red meats, enriched breads and cereals | Iron-deficiency anemia | Can cause death in children from supplement overdose |
| Copper | Formation of hemoglobin | Liver, nuts, shellfish, cherries, mushrooms, whole-grain breads and cereals | Anemia | Nausea, vomiting |
| Zinc | Normal growth and development | Seafood, meats | Skin problems, delayed development, growth problems | Interferes with copper use, may decrease high-density lipoprotein levels |
| Iodine | Production of the hormone thyroxin | Iodized salt, seafood | Mental and growth retardation, lack of energy | |
| Fluorine | Strengthens bones and teeth | Fluoridated water | Teeth are less resistant to decay | Damage to tooth enamel |

the compound that transports oxygen in red blood cells. Calcium has many important functions: It is necessary for proper bone and teeth formation, blood clotting, and muscle contraction. In general, minerals have roles that are too numerous to detail. Eating a wide variety of foods is the best way to obtain the minerals needed in the proper concentrations.[55]

## Water

Water is the most essential of all the nutrients and should be the nutrient of greatest concern to the athlete.[15] It is the most abundant nutrient in the body, accounting for approximately 60 percent of the body weight, although this varies considerably (+/−10%) among individuals due to age and percent of body fat. Water is essential for all the chemical processes that occur in the body, and an adequate supply of water is necessary for energy production and the normal digestion of other nutrients. Although water does not supply any energy (calories), an adequate amount of water is needed for energy production in all cells. Water also takes part in digestion and maintenance of the proper environment inside and outside cells. Water is also necessary for temperature control and for the elimination of waste products of nutrient and body metabolism. Too little water leads to dehydration, and severe dehydration can lead to death. The Institute of Medicine determined that an adequate intake (AI) for men is roughly about 3 liters of total beverages a day and for women is about 2.2 liters of total beverages a day.

The body has a number of mechanisms designed to maintain body water at a near-normal level. Too little water leads to accumulation of solutes in the blood. These solutes signal the brain that the body is thirsty while signaling the kidneys to conserve water. Excessive water dilutes these solutes, which signals the brain to stop drinking and the kidneys to get rid of the excess water.

Water is the only nutrient that is of greater importance to the athlete than to those people who are more sedentary, especially when the athlete is engaging in prolonged exercise in a hot, humid environment.[36] Such a situation may cause excessive sweating and subsequent losses of large amounts of water. When the body burns carbohydrate and fat for energy, it produces a great deal of heat. During exercise, that heat is lost from the body primarily by sweating. Sweating is how the body uses water to keep itself from overheating. Restriction of water during this time results in dehydration. Symptoms of dehydration include fatigue, vomiting, nausea, exhaustion, fainting, and possibly death.

**Electrolyte Requirements** Electrolytes, including sodium, chloride, potassium, magnesium, and calcium, are electrically charged ions dissolved in body water. Among many other functions, electrolytes maintain the balance of water inside and outside the cell. In other words, electrolytes, especially sodium, are essential in helping the body rehydrate quickly.[2] Electrolyte replenishment may be needed when a person is not fit, suffers from extreme water loss, or has just completed an exercise period and is expected to perform at near-maximum effort within the next few hours. In most cases, electrolytes can be sufficiently replaced with a balanced diet, which can, if necessary, be salted slightly more than usual. Free access to water and sports drinks (ad libitum) before, during, and after activity should be the rule (see Chapter 6).[42] In some people, electrolyte losses can produce muscle cramping and intolerance to heat. Sweating results not only in body water loss but in some electrolyte loss as well.[53] Chapter 6 discusses fluid and electrolyte replacement in great detail.

> Electrolytes: sodium, chloride, potassium, magnesium, and calcium.

> Replacing fluid after heavy sweating is far more important than replacing electrolytes.

## NUTRIENT REQUIREMENTS AND RECOMMENDATIONS

A nutrient requirement is the amount of the nutrient that is needed to prevent the nutrient's deficiency disease. Nutrient needs vary among individuals within a population. A recommendation for a nutrient is different from the requirement for a nutrient. Scientists establish recommendations for nutrients and calories based on extensive scientific research and assessment of present dietary intakes.[85]

In the past, the *U.S. recommended dietary allowances (U.S. RDAs)* have served as the benchmark of nutritional adequacy in the United States. Over the past several years, new information has emerged about nutrient requirements that necessitated updating of the RDAs.[24] RDAs have been changed to *dietary reference intakes (DRIs),* which are established using an expanded concept that includes indicators of good health and the prevention of chronic disease, as well as possible adverse effects of overconsumption.[85] *Dietary reference intakes* is an umbrella term that encompasses sets of dietary recommendations that include not only recommended intakes (RDAs) intended to help individuals meet their daily nutritional requirements but also tolerable upper intake levels (ULs), which help individuals avoid harm from consuming too much of a nutrient; estimated average requirements (EARs), which are the average daily nutrient intake levels estimated to meet the requirements of half the healthy individuals in a particular age group; and AI, which is the recommended average daily intake level based on experimentally developed estimates of nutrient intake that are used when the RDA cannot be determined.[24]

# FOOD LABELS

Over the past 20 years, food labels have provided helpful nutritional information for consumers. In 1994, a new nutritional labeling format changed the look and importance of food product packaging. People were becoming concerned about the amount of fat, cholesterol, sodium, and fiber in the typical American diet, thus producing the drive for a more health-conscious label. Health educators believe that the new format has made it easier for consumers to make more informed, healthful food selections. In 2006, the U.S. Food and Drug Administration (FDA) mandated that trans fat be added to the label. In 2016, the FDA updated the "Nutrition Facts" label for packaged foods to reflect the latest scientific information to emphasize important elements, such as calories, serving sizes, and percentage of daily value, which are important in addressing current public health problems like obesity and heart disease.[21] Figure 5–2 shows the new, redesigned Nutrition Facts label approved by the FDA. The new label will be required on most packaged food by July 2018.

# MyPlate

The USDA's new food icon MyPlate, introduced in 2011, is the government's primary food group symbol, designed to help consumers adopt healthy eating habits consistent with the 2015 Dietary Guidelines for Americans.[77] (See Figure 5–3.) The intent is to help consumers think about building a healthy diet, which consists of fruit, vegetable, grain, protein, and dairy food groups.

# Nutrition Facts

8 servings per container

**Serving size**      **2/3 cup (55g)**

**Amount per serving**

## Calories    230

| | % Daily Value* |
|---|---|
| **Total Fat** 8g | **10%** |
| Saturated Fat 1g | **5%** |
| *Trans* Fat 0g | |
| **Cholesterol** 0mg | **0%** |
| **Sodium** 160mg | **7%** |
| **Total Carbohydrate** 37g | **13%** |
| Dietary Fiber 4g | **14%** |
| Total Sugars 12g | |
| Includes 10g Added Sugars | **20%** |
| **Protein** 3g | |
| Vitamin D 2mcg | 10% |
| Calcium 260mg | 20% |
| Iron 8mg | 45% |
| Potassium 235mg | 6% |

\* The % Daily Value (DV) tells you how much a nutrient in a serving of food contributes to a daily diet. 2,000 calories a day is used for general nutrition advice.

FIGURE 5–2  Food label indicating nutrition information per serving.

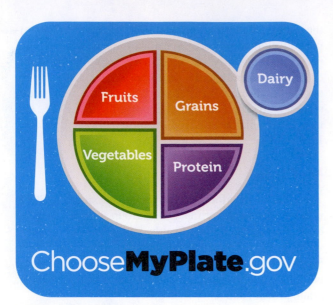

**FIGURE 5–3** MyPlate Icon.

Source: U.S. Department of Agriculture, U.S. Department of Health and Human Serivces, 2015.

A Web site, ChooseMyPlate.gov, provides practical information to several groups, including individual Americans, health professionals, nutrition educators, and the food industry, to help these consumers build healthier diets. Resources and tools for dietary assessment, nutrition education, and other user-friendly nutrition information can also be found on this Web site. Because the American population is experiencing epidemic rates of overweight and obesity, the hope is that the online resources and tools can empower people to make healthier food choices for themselves, their families, and their children. Hopefully, this approach will help to eliminate consumer frustration over what they report as contradictory nutrition information.

The newest 2015 to 2020 Dietary Guidelines for Americans form the basis of the federal government's nutrition education programs, federal nutrition assistance programs, and dietary advice provided by health and nutrition professionals. The guidelines and recommendations help professionals and the media understand and deliver relevant nutrition information to encourage healthy eating and help Americans make healthy choices for them and their families. *Focus Box 5–1* identifies the 2015 to 2020 Dietary Guidelines.

## DIETARY SUPPLEMENTS

Many people believe that exercise increases requirements for nutrients, such as proteins, vitamins, and minerals, and that it is possible and desirable to saturate the body with these nutrients.[17] There is no scientific basis for ingesting levels of these nutrients above DRI levels.[64] Exercise increases the need for energy, not for proteins, vitamins, and minerals.[13] Additionally, many athletes use nutritional supplements for performance enhancement.[61,69,80] But it is important to note that attempts to enhance performance should be based primarily on proper nutrition and permanent changes in the athlete's diet rather than relying on dietary supplementation. Thus, it is

> **Vitamin requirements do not increase during exercise.**

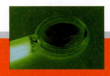

## FOCUS 5–1 Focus on Injury/Illness Prevention and Wellness Promotion

### 2015–2020 Dietary Guidelines for Americans*

*Guidelines*

1. ***Follow a healthy eating pattern across the lifespan.***

All food and beverage choices matter. Choose a healthy eating pattern at an appropriate calorie level to help achieve and maintain a healthy body weight, support nutrient adequacy, and reduce the risk of chronic disease.

2. ***Focus on variety, nutrient density, and amount.***

To meet nutrient needs within calorie limits, choose a variety of nutrient-dense foods across and within all food groups in recommended amounts.

3. ***Limit calories from added sugars and saturated fats and reduce sodium intake.***

Consume an eating pattern low in added sugars, saturated fats, and sodium. Cut back on foods and beverages higher in these components to amounts that fit within healthy eating patterns.

4. ***Shift to healthier food and beverage choices.***

Choose nutrient-dense foods and beverages across and within all food groups in place of less healthy choices. Consider cultural and personal preferences to make these shifts easier to accomplish and maintain.

5. ***Support healthy eating patterns for all.***

Everyone has a role in helping to create and support healthy eating patterns in multiple settings nationwide, from home to school to work to communities.

*From U.S. Department of Health and Human Services and U.S. Department of Agriculture. *2015–2020 Dietary Guidelines for Americans,* 8th ed., December 2015. Available at http://health.gov /dietaryguidelines/2015/guidelines/

essential that the athletic trainer not only become knowledgeable about the effects of nutrition on performance, but also rely on a registered dietitian or sports nutritionist to provide additional expertise.[13] **SoR:A** The athletes need to understand the level of regulation (or lack thereof) and should not assume a product is safe simply because it is sold over the counter. Dietary supplement manufacturers are not required to provide any evidence of product efficacy. Athletes must be aware that dietary supplement labels do not require third-party verification or truth in labeling.[13] **SoR:A** Athletic trainers should advise athletes that dietary supplements are not well regulated and may contain banned substances. Sport governing bodies should make the rules regarding banned substances and their philosophies regarding supplementation available to athletes.[13] **SoR:A** The athletic trainers should be aware of resources to identify products known to have adverse effects.[13] **SoR:C** (The use of various supplements for performance enhancement is discussed in Chapter 17.) NATA has published a position statement "Evaluation of Dietary Supplements for Performance Nutrition" (http://natajournals.org/doi/pdf/10.4085/1062-6050-48.1.16) that discusses the use of dietary supplements in athletes.

## Vitamin Supplements

Many individuals believe that taking large amounts of vitamin supplements can lead to superior health and performance.[85] A megadose of a nutrient supplement is essentially an overdose; the amount ingested far exceeds the DRI levels.[13] The rationale used for such excessive intakes is that if taking a pill that

> Since the majority of supplements are not regulated, these over-the-counter products may contain banned substances. Athletes should consult their athletic trainer or team physician prior to taking any supplement.

contains the DRI for each vitamin and mineral makes a person healthy, taking a pill that has 10 times the DRI should make that individual 10 times healthier.[55]

An example of a popular practice has been to take megadoses of vitamin C. Such doses do not prevent the common cold or slow aging. However, it has been shown that vitamin C reduces the duration and severity of colds. Given the low cost and safety of the vitamin, it may be worthwhile for common cold patients to test whether therapeutic vitamin C is beneficial for them on an individual basis.[31] Fruits, juices, and vegetables are reliable sources of vitamin C that also supply other vitamins and minerals.[55]

Vitamin E protects certain fatty acids in cell membranes from being damaged.[55] There is not much evidence to support the notion that this vitamin can extend life expectancy or enhance physical performance. Vitamin E does not enhance sexual ability, prevent graying hair, or cure muscular dystrophy. A person can obtain adequate amounts of vitamin E by consuming whole-grain products, vegetable oils, and nuts.

The B-complex vitamins that are involved in obtaining energy from carbohydrates, fats, and proteins are often abused by individuals who believe that vitamins provide energy. B-vitamins are found in lots of energy drinks; although the public often thinks it is the B-vitamins that give them the rush, in reality it is the caffeine. Any increased need for these nutrients is easily fulfilled when a person eats more nutritious foods while training.[80] If athletes do not increase their food consumption, they will lose weight because of their high level of caloric expenditure.

Vitamin D is essential for intestinal absorption of calcium. A deficiency has been linked to numerous disorders including osteoporosis and autoimmune diseases. Recently, vitamin D supplementation for athletes has become controversial as there is little current evidence that vitamin D supplementation in athletes who are not vitamin D deficient helps to improve performance. For athletes who are vitamin D deficient, it is recommended that serum vitamin D concentration be monitored by a health care professional and/or nutritionist to determine the need for supplementation.[57]

If an individual is not eating a well-balanced diet, taking a multiple vitamin once each day would be helpful and, in fact, is recommended by many physicians to make certain that minimum DRIs are met.

## Mineral Supplements

Obtaining adequate levels of certain minerals can be a problem for some people.[55] Calcium and iron intakes may be low for those who do not include dairy products, red meats, or enriched breads and cereals in their diet. The following sections explore some minerals that can be deficient in the diet and some suggestions for improving the quality of the diet so that supplements are not necessary.

**Calcium Supplements** Calcium is the most abundant mineral in the body. It is essential for bones and teeth as well as for muscle contraction and the conduction of nerve impulses. However, the importance of obtaining adequate calcium supplies throughout life has become more recognized. If calcium intake is too low to meet needs, the body can remove calcium from the bones. Over time, bones become weakened and appear porous on X-rays. These bones are brittle and often break spontaneously. This condition is called **osteoporosis** and is

A rowing athlete complains of feeling tired lately and more exhausted than usual after workouts. She also states that she has noticed many bruises on her legs and arms. The bruises randomly appear in different places all over her body. When asked about her diet, she mentions she eats two meals a day and it is food she grabs on the run. She cannot remember the last time she had a meal with vegetables or quality meat.

**?** What do you suspect might be wrong with her, and what is your suggested plan of action?

estimated to be eight times more common among women than men. It becomes a serious problem for women after menopause.[4] (See Chapter 29.)

The RDA for young adults (14 to 18 years) is 1,300 mg (an 8-ounce glass of milk contains about 300 mg of calcium). Unfortunately, about 25 percent of all females in the United States consume less than 300 mg of calcium per day, well below the RDA. High-protein diets and alcohol consumption also increase calcium excretion from the body. Exercise causes calcium to be retained in bones, so physical activity is beneficial. However, younger females who exercise to extremes, so that their normal hormonal balance is upset, are prone to develop premature osteoporosis.[4] Calcium supplementation, preferably as calcium carbonate or citrate rather than phosphate, may be advisable for females who have a family history of osteoporosis.

Milk products are the most reliable sources of calcium. Many people complain that milk and other dairy products upset their stomach. They may lack an enzyme, called lactase, that is needed to digest the milk sugar lactose. This condition is referred to as lactose intolerance, or **lactase deficiency**.[13] The undigested lactose enters the large intestine, where the bacteria that normally reside there use it for energy. The bacteria produce large quantities of intestinal gas, which causes discomfort and cramps. Many lactose-intolerant people also suffer from diarrhea. Fortunately, scientists have produced the missing enzyme, lactase. Lactase is available without prescription in forms that can be added to foods before eating or can be taken with meals.

**Iron Supplements** Iron deficiency is a common problem, especially for young females. Lack of iron can result in iron-deficiency **anemia** (see Chapter 29).[65] Iron is needed to properly form hemoglobin. With anemia, the oxygen-carrying ability of the red blood cells is reduced, so muscles cannot obtain enough oxygen to generate energy.[20] Anemia leaves a person feeling tired and weak. Obviously, an athlete cannot compete at peak level while suffering from an iron deficiency. Excess intake of iron can be toxic, however, and may result in constipation.

## Protein Supplements

Athletes often believe that more protein is needed to build bigger muscles.[39] It is true that athletes who are developing muscles in a conditioning program need a relatively small amount of extra protein. Many athletes, particularly those who are training with heavy weights or who are bodybuilders, routinely take protein supplements that are commercially produced and marketed.[39] It should be added that some supplements that claim to be muscle building can contain substances that are banned by different sport governing bodies. To build muscle, athletes should consume 1.2 to 1.7 grams per kilogram of body weight every day.[62] This range goes from slightly above to about double the protein RDA (0.8 gram per kilogram of desirable body weight).[18] Anyone eating a variety of foods, but especially protein-rich foods, can easily meet the higher amounts. Thus, athletes do not need protein supplements, because their diets typically exceed even the most generous protein recommendations. An active adult most likely requires 0.6 gram per pound, or 66 percent more than the DRI.[62]

## Creatine Supplements

Creatine is a naturally occurring organic compound synthesized by the kidneys, liver, and pancreas. Free creatine can also be obtained from ingesting meat and fish that contain approximately 5 grams per kilogram. Creatine has an integral role in energy metabolism.[73]

There are two main types of creatine: free creatine and phosphocreatine. Phosphocreatine is stored in skeletal muscle and is used during anaerobic activity to produce ATP, with the assistance of the enzyme creatine kinase. With creatine supplementation, phosphocreatine depletion is delayed and performance is enhanced through the maintenance of the normal metabolic pathways.[70]

The positive physiological functions of creatine include increasing the resynthesis of ATP, thus allowing for increased intensity in a workout; acting as a lactic acid buffer, thus prolonging maximal effort and improving exercise recovery time during maximum-intensity activities; stimulating protein synthesis; decreasing total cholesterol while improving the HDL-to-LDL ratio; decreasing total triglycerides; and increasing fat-free mass.[73] Oral supplementation with creatine may enhance muscular performance during high-intensity resistance exercise.[84] It has been suggested that creatine supplementation may reduce the incidence of muscle cramps.[27] Side effects of creatine supplementation include weight gain, due primarily to an increase in total body water,[58] gastrointestinal disturbances, and renal dysfunction. There are apparently no other known long-term side effects.

It has been suggested that an initial *loading phase* should consist of ingesting approximately 0.3 gram of creatine per kilogram of body weight per day.[63] The dosage should be split over four or five times per day, with approximately 16 ounces of water per dose. The loading phase lasts for 5 days. A loading phase is not necessarily required, however. It has been shown that ingesting creatine at a much lower dose of 3 grams per day increases total muscle creatine to the same values observed with 5 days of 20 grams per day; however, this takes approximately 30 days.[84] Thus, the high "loading" dose is unnecessary to realize an increase in muscle creatine content. After completing the loading phase, one should take a maintenance dosage every day equal to about 0.03 gram of creatine per kilogram of body weight for a month. Then a "wash-out" phase should last for 1 month, during which there is no supplementation.[84]

In August 2000, the NCAA Committee on Competitive Safeguards and Medical Aspects of Sports banned the distribution of all muscle-building substances, including creatine, by NCAA member institutions. However the use of creatine itself is not necessarily banned by other organizations.

## Herbal Supplements

The use of herbs as natural alternatives to drugs and medicines has clearly become a trend among American consumers. Most herbs, as edible plants, are safe to ingest as foods; as natural medicines, they are claimed to have few side effects, although occasionally a mild, allergic reaction may occur.[51] Those taking herbs should also be mindful of potential interactions.[43]

Herbs can offer the body nutrients that are reported to nourish the brain, glands, and hormones.[76] Unlike vitamins, which work best when taken with food, herbs do not need to be taken with other foods, because they provide their own digestive enzymes.[23]

Herbs in their whole form are not drugs. As medicine, herbs are essentially body balancers that work with the body's functions so that it can heal and regulate itself. Herbal formulas can be general for overall strength and nutrient support or specific to a particular ailment or condition.[38]

Hundreds of herbs are widely available at all quality levels. They are readily available at health food stores. However, unlike both food and medicine, no federal or governmental controls regulate the sale of herbs to ensure the quality of the products being sold.[23] The consumer of herbal products must exercise extreme caution.

*Focus Box 5–2:* "Commonly used herbs" lists the most popular and widely used herbal products sold in health food stores. Some additional potent and complex herbs,

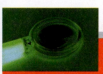

# FOCUS 5–2 Focus on Injury/Illness Prevention and Wellness Promotion

## Commonly used herbs

The indications for using these herbs have at least minimal scientific basis in the literature. However, there is a substantial lack of strong evidence-based support for their use.

**Cayenne (capsaicin)**–pain control; may cause stomach irritation.

**Cascara**–used as a laxative; can cause dehydration.

**Dong quai**–weak evidence that it can be used to treat abnormal heart rhythm, prevent accumulation of platelets in blood vessels, protect the liver, promote urination, act as a mild laxative, promote sleep, and fight infection.

**Echinacea**–promotes wound healing and strengthens the immune system.

**Feverfew**–weak evidence that it prevents and relieves migraine headaches, arthritis, and PMS.

**Garlic**–weak evidence that it can be effective in treating atherosclerosis by reducing total blood cholesterol and triglyceride levels and raising HDL levels; also for use in treating hypertension, diabetes, the common cold, tuberculosis, and intestinal parasites.

**Garcina cambagia**–used to promote loss of fat.

**Ginkgo biloba**–weak evidence for its use in treating dementia and Alzheimer's disease, memory impairment, eye problems, intermittent claudication, and tinnitus.

**Ginseng**–used to prevent Alzheimer's disease, cancer, depression, diabetes, chronic respiratory disease, menopausal symptoms, and stress; has been shown to enhance cardiovascular health by raising HDL while reducing total cholesterol levels, fertility/sexual performance, immune system function, mental performance and mood, and physical endurance.

**Green tea**–contains component EGCG; has traditionally been used to prevent or slow growth in a variety of cancers; not enough evidence to determine improvement in mental alertness, weight loss, lowering cholesterol levels, or protecting skin from sun damage.

**Guarana°**–used as a stimulant because it contains large amounts of caffeine; often in weight-loss products.

**Kava**–used to reduce anxiety and insomnia; increased risk of severe liver damage.

**Ma huang°(ephedrine)**–derived from the ephedra plant; has been used in China for medicinal purposes, including increased energy, appetite suppression, increased fat burning, and preservation of muscle tissue from breakdown; a central nervous system stimulant drug that was used in many diet pills; in 1995, the FDA revealed adverse reactions to ephedrine, such as heart attacks, strokes, paranoid psychosis, vomiting, fever, palpitations, convulsions, and comas; banned by the FDA in 2003.

**Mate**–central nervous system stimulant.

**Saw palmetto**–used to treat inflamed prostate; also used as a diuretic.

**Senna**–used as a laxative; can cause water and electrolyte loss.

**St. John's wort**–used as an antidepressant; also used to treat nervous disorders, depression, and seasonal affective disorder.

**Valerian**–used to treat insomnia, anxiety, and stress.

**Vohimbe**–used to increase libido and blood flow to sexual organs in the male.

°Banned by some athletic organizations and/or the FDA. However, all of these substances are readily available over the Internet.

such as capsicum, lobelia, sassafras, mandrake tansy, canada snake root, wormwood, woodruff, poke root, and rue, may be useful in small amounts and as catalysts but should not be used alone.

**Ephedrine** Ephedrine is a stimulant that has been used as an ingredient in diet pills, illegal recreational drugs, and legitimate over-the-counter medications to treat congestion and asthma.[57] Ephedrine is similar to an amphetamine. In December 2003, the FDA banned the use of ephedrine as a dietary supplement. For several years the FDA warned consumers about the potential dangers of using ephedrine. The NCAA, the National Football League, the National Basketball Association, minor league baseball, and the USOC have banned the use of ephedrine by their athletes. However, some companies continue to sell supplements that contain ephedrine or other stimulants despite the fact that these supplements have caused numerous problems. Ephedrine is known to produce the following adverse reactions: heart attack, stroke, tachycardia, paranoid psychosis, depression, convulsions, fever, coma, vomiting, palpitations, hypertension, and respiratory depression.[57]

## Glucose Supplements

Ingesting large quantities of glucose in the form of honey, candy bars, or pure sugar immediately before physical activity may have a significant impact on performance.[72] As carbohydrates are digested, large quantities of glucose enter the blood. This increase in blood sugar (glucose) levels stimulates the release of the hormone insulin. Insulin allows the cells to use the circulating glucose, so that blood glucose levels soon return to normal.[50] It was hypothesized that a decline in blood sugar levels was detrimental to performance and endurance. However, recent evidence indicates that the effect of eating large quantities of carbohydrates is beneficial rather than negative.[19,72]

Nevertheless, some athletes are sensitive to high-carbohydrate feedings and experience problems with increased levels of insulin. Also, some athletes cannot tolerate large amounts of the simple sugar fructose. For these individuals, too much fructose leads to intestinal upset and diarrhea. Athletes should test themselves with various high-carbohydrate foods to see whether they are affected (but not before a competitive event).[50]

# EATING AND DRINKING PRACTICES

## Caffeine Consumption

Caffeine is a central nervous system stimulant. Most people who consume caffeine in coffee, tea, or carbonated beverages are aware of its effect of increasing alertness

and decreasing fatigue. Chocolate contains compounds that are related to caffeine and have the same stimulating effects. However, large amounts of caffeine cause nervousness, irritability, increased heart rate, insomnia, and headaches.[50] Also, headaches are a withdrawal symptom experienced when a person tries to stop consuming caffeinated products.[50]

Although small amounts of caffeine do not appear to harm physical performance, cases of nausea and lightheadedness have been reported. Caffeine enhances the use of fat during endurance exercise, thus delaying the depletion of glycogen stores.[85] This delay would help endurance performance. Caffeine also helps make calcium more available to muscles during contraction, allowing the muscles to work more efficiently. Caffeine is no longer on the banned list for Olympic athletes, but it is still on the NCAA banned substances list. It should not be present in a drug test in levels greater than that resulting from drinking five or six cups of coffee.

**Energy Drinks** Over the last decade, consumption of energy drinks has increased dramatically, and there are now literally hundreds of energy drinks available to the consumer. Red Bull, Rockstar, AMP, Monster, and 5-hour Energy are just a few of the most common energy drinks. It must be clarified that energy drinks are different than sport drinks. Sports drinks contain no caffeine. Generally, the energy drinks contain caffeine in doses ranging anywhere from 50 mg to in excess of 500 mg, with the average between 70 and 80 mg per serving.[33] They are marketed for their performance-enhancing and stimulant drug effects. An obvious risk of caffeine intoxication exists when consuming a high amount of caffeine, which can cause adverse effects including nervousness, insomnia, headache, tachycardia (increased heart rate), and rarely seizure activity or occasionally death. Problems with caffeine dependence and withdrawal have also been reported.[33] Energy drinks also have a high concentration of carbohydrate, and most are carbonated.

There is currently little government regulation of energy drinks, including content labeling and health warnings. Because caffeine is a drug and not a nutrient, it is not listed on the nutrition facts panel. Of even greater concern is the combined use of caffeine and alcohol. Studies suggest that such combined use may increase the rate of alcohol-related injury.

## Alcohol Consumption

Alcohol use is prevalent among athletes at all levels. It appears that alcohol consumption is higher among athletes when compared to non-athlete peers.[13] The depressant effects of alcohol on the central nervous system include decreased physical coordination, slowed reaction times, and decreased mental alertness. Also, this drug increases the production of urine, resulting in body water losses (diuretic effect). Alcohol does provide energy for the body; each gram of pure alcohol (ethanol) supplies seven calories. However, sources of alcohol provide little other nutritional value with regard to vitamins, minerals, and proteins. Therefore, the use of alcoholic beverages by the athlete is strongly discouraged before, during, and after physical activity.

## Consumption of Organic, Natural, and Health Foods

Many people are concerned about the quality of the foods they eat—not just the nutritional value of the food but also its safety. Organic foods are grown without the use of synthetic fertilizers and pesticides. Those who advocate the use of organic farming methods claim that these foods are nutritionally superior and safer than the same products grown using chemicals, such as pesticides and synthetic fertilizers.[16]

All foods (except water) are organic; that is, they contain the element carbon. Organically produced foods are often more expensive than the same foods that have been produced by conventional means. There is no advantage to consuming organic food products. They are not more nutritious than foods produced by conventional methods. Nevertheless, for some people the psychological benefit of believing that they are doing something good for their bodies justifies the extra cost.

Natural foods have been subjected to little processing and contain no additives, such as preservatives or artificial flavors.[16] Processing can protect nutritional value. Preservatives save food that would otherwise spoil and have to be destroyed. Both organic and natural foods can be described as health foods.

## Vegetarianism

Vegetarianism is an alternative to the usual American diet. All vegetarians use plant foods to form the foundation of their diet; animal foods are either totally excluded or included in a variety of eating patterns.[26] People who choose to become vegetarians do so for economic, philosophical, religious, cultural, or health reasons. Vegetarianism is no longer considered to be a fad if it is practiced intelligently. However, the vegetarian diet may create deficiencies if nutrient needs are not carefully considered. Individuals who follow this eating pattern must plan their diet carefully so that their caloric needs are met.[26] The types of vegetarian dietary patterns are categorized as follows.

**Vegetarians:** total vegetarians, lactovegetarians, ovolactovegetarians, and semivegetarians.

- *Vegans:* Individuals who do not eat red meat, fish, poultry, eggs, or dairy products are vegans or true vegetarians. This diet has been found to be adequate for most adults if they give careful consideration to obtaining enough calories; sources of vitamin $B_{12}$; and the minerals calcium, zinc, and iron. It is not recommended for pregnant women, infants, or children because of the difficulty in consuming the quantity of plant foods necessary to meet the caloric and nutritional needs during these life stages.

- *Lactovegetarians:* Individuals who consume dairy products along with plant foods. Meat, fish, poultry, and eggs are excluded from the diet. Iron and zinc levels can be low in people who practice this form of vegetarianism.

- *Lacto-ovo-vegetarians:* People who consume both dairy products and eggs in their diet, along with plant foods. Meat, fish, and poultry are excluded. Again, iron could be a problem.

- *Ovo-vegetarians:* People who eat eggs but not dairy products.

- *Flextarians:* People who consume animal products but exclude red meats. Plant products still form an important part of the diet. This diet is usually adequate.

## Pre-Event Nutrition

The importance and content of the pre-event meal has been heatedly debated among coaches, athletic trainers, and athletes.[30] The trend has been to ignore logical thinking about what should be eaten before competition and to upholding the tradition of "rewarding" the athlete for hard work by serving foods that may hamper performance. For example, the traditional steak-and-eggs meal before football games is great for coaches and athletic trainers; however, the athlete gains nothing from this meal. The important point is that too often people are concerned primarily with the pre-event meal and fail to realize that the nutrients consumed over several days before competition are much more important than what is eaten 3 hours before an event. (See *Focus Box 5–3:* "The pregame meal.") The purpose of the pre-event meal should be to maximize carbohydrate stored in the muscles as well as blood glucose. It has been suggested that the athlete consume carbohydrates 3 to 4 hours before practice or competition.[30] But it has also been suggested that consuming carbohydrates immediately before competition causes an increased release of insulin, which increases the rate at which muscles burn carbohydrate, thus lowering blood glucose levels (hypoglycemia). Different carbohydrates are digested and absorbed at different rates. The **glycemic index (GI)** is a scale that indicates how much different types of carbohydrate effect blood glucose levels.[9] Consuming foods that have a low to medium GI prior to an event is recommended because they produce only small fluctuations in blood glucose and insulin levels and release energy more slowly over a longer time period. Ingesting carbohydrates that have a high GI within an hour of exercise may actually lower blood glucose. Figure 5–4 lists the glycemic index range for common foods.

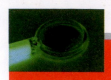

## The pregame meal

- Try to achieve the largest possible storage of carbohydrates (glycogen) in both resting muscle and the liver. This storage is particularly important for endurance activities but may also be beneficial for intense, short-duration exercise.
- A stomach that is full of food during contact sports is subject to injury. Therefore, the type of food eaten should allow the stomach to empty quickly. Carbohydrates are easier to digest than are fats or proteins. A meal that contains plenty of carbohydrates leaves the stomach and is digested faster than a fatty meal. It would be wise to replace the traditional steak-and-eggs pre-event meal with a low-fat one containing a small amount of pasta, tomato sauce, and bread.
- Foods should not cause irritation or upset to the gastrointestinal tract. Foods high in cellulose and other forms of fiber, such as whole-grain products, fruits, and vegetables, increase the need for defecation. Highly spiced foods and gas-forming foods (such as onions, baked beans, or peppers) must also be avoided because any type of disturbance in the gastrointestinal tract may be detrimental to performance. Carbonated beverages and chewing gum also contribute to the formation of gas.
- Liquids consumed should be easily absorbed and low in fat content and should not act as a laxative. Whole milk, coffee, and tea should be avoided. Water intake should be increased, particularly if the temperature is high.
- A meal should be eaten approximately 3 to 4 hours before the event or before exercising. This timing allows for adequate stomach emptying, but the individual will not feel hungry during activity.
- The athlete should not eat any food that he or she dislikes. Most important, the individual must feel psychologically satisfied by any pre-event meal. If not, performance may be impaired more by psychological factors than by physiological factors.

Additionally the foods selected should minimize gastrointestinal distress and should be foods that the individual athlete prefers. It is also critical to make certain that the athlete is appropriately hydrated.

**Low Glycemic Index (<55)**
**Most fruits—grapefruit, apples, oranges**
**Whole-grain cereals, breads, pasta**
**Nuts**
**Beans and legumes**
**Green leafy vegetables**
**Yogurt, milk**
**Medium Glycemic Index (56–69)**
**Sweet potato**
**Spaghetti**
**Basmati rice**
**Bagel**
**Macaroni and cheese**
**Raisins**
**Ice cream**
**High Glycemic Index (>70)**
**White bread**
**White rice**
**Corn flakes**
**Baked potato**
**Watermelon**
**Popcorn**
**Sports drinks**

FIGURE 5–4   Glycemic Index Food Recommendations for Pre-Event Meals.

Athletes should be encouraged to become conscious of their diets. However, no experimental evidence exists to indicate that performance may be enhanced by altering a diet that is basically sound. A nutritious diet may be achieved in many ways, and the diet that is optimal for one athlete may not be the best for another. In many instances, the individual is the best judge of what he or she should or should not eat in the pre-event meal or before exercising. It seems that a person's best guide is to eat whatever he or she is most comfortable with.

**Liquid Food Supplements** Liquid food supplements (e.g., Gatorade G Series Recover Shake, Sustagen) have been recommended as effective pre-event meals and are being used by secondary-school, college, university, and professional teams with some indications of success.[62] These supplements supply from 225 to 400 calories per average serving. Athletes who have used these supplements report elimination of the usual pregame symptoms of dry mouth, abdominal cramps, leg cramps, nervous defecation, and nausea.

Under ordinary conditions, it usually takes approximately 4 hours for a full meal to pass through the stomach and the small intestine. Pregame emotional tension often delays the emptying of the stomach; therefore, the undigested food mass remains in the stomach and upper bowel for a prolonged time, even up to or through the actual period of competition, and frequently results in nausea, vomiting, and cramps. This unabsorbed food mass is of no value to the athlete. Team physicians who have experimented with the liquid food supplements say that a major advantage of the supplements is that they clear both the stomach and the upper bowel before game time, thus making available the caloric energy that would otherwise still be in an unassimilated state. There is merit in the use of such food supplements for pregame meals.[62]

## Recommendations for Restoring Muscle Glycogen after Exercise

When the time period between exercise sessions is relatively short (less than 8 hours), the athlete should begin consuming carbohydrates to restore supplies of muscle glycogen as soon as possible after the workout to maximize recovery between sessions.[37] Ideally, the foods should have a high glycemic index. Given that complete muscle glycogen restoration takes at least 20 to 24 hours, athletes should not waste time. They should ingest approximately 0.45 to 0.55 grams of carbohydrate per pound of body weight for each of the first 4 hours after exercise or until they eat their next large meal. During this period, nutrient-rich carbohydrate foods, such as fruits and vegetables or a high-carbohydrate drink, are recommended.[37] Over a 24-hour period, carbohydrate intake should range from 2.3 grams to as much as 5.5 grams per pound of body weight, depending on the intensity of the activity.[37] Pasta, potatoes, oatmeal, and sports drinks are recommended. It has been suggested that adding a small amount of protein (15 to 25 grams) to a carbohydrate supplement enhances aerobic endurance performance above that which occurs with carbohydrate alone, and stimulates muscle protein synthesis and repair. Peanut butter and tuna are recommended as good sources of protein.

## Eating Fast Foods

Eating fast food is a way of life in American society.[67] Athletes, especially young athletes, have for the most part grown up as fast-food junkies. Furthermore, travel budgets and tight schedules dictate that fast food is a frequent choice for coaches on road trips.[66] Aside from occasional problems with food flavor, the biggest concern in consuming fast foods, as can be seen in Table 5–3, is that 40 to 50 percent of the calories consumed are from fats. To compound this problem, these already sizable meals are often "supersized" at a more affordable price for those who want maximum fat, salt, and calories in a single sitting.

On the positive side, most fast-food restaurants now offer healthy menu items such as whole-wheat breads and rolls, salad bars, and low-fat milk products. Nutrition information can be found at the point of purchase, on the Web site, or using an App for smartphones. *Focus Box 5–4:* "Tips for selecting fast foods" provides suggestions for eating more healthfully at fast-food restaurants.

## Low-Carbohydrate Diets

For many years, it was recommended that fat intake be limited as a means of controlling weight. More recently, the recommendation was to severely limit the intake of carbohydrate in the diet.[79] There are many versions of a low-carbohydrate diet, all of which recommend a strict reduction in the consumption of carbohydrates. Most "low-carb" diets replace carbohydrates with a high-fat and moderate-protein diet. The low-calorie and low-fat diets that have been recommended for years have failed to realize that dietary fat is not necessarily converted into body fat. However, carbohydrates are readily converted into fat. In a high-carbohydrate meal, the increased blood glucose stimulates insulin production by the pancreas. Insulin allows blood glucose to be used by the cells, but it also causes fat to be deposited, and it stimulates the brain to produce hunger signals. Thus, there is a tendency to eat more carbohydrates, and the cycle repeats. It has been shown that most overweight people became overweight due to a condition called *hyperinsulinemia*—elevated insulin levels in the blood. Restricting carbohydrate intake halts this cycle by decreasing insulin levels. Carbohydrate restriction also increases the levels of *glucagon*, which is a hormone that causes body fat to be burned and aids in removing cholesterol deposits in the arteries. Severely restricting carbohydrate intake puts the body into a state of ketosis, in which blood glucose levels stabilize, insulin level drops, and because the body is burning fat, fairly rapid weight loss occurs.[79] However, if an individual is an athlete or is physically active they need carbohydrates and should instead focus on making carbohydrates readily available to working muscles. This does not happen when consuming a low-carbohydrate diet.

## Glycogen Supercompensation (Carbohydrate Loading)

Because the quantity of glycogen stored in a muscle directly affects the endurance of that muscle, many athletes preparing for endurance events engage in a practice called glycogen super compensation also known as carbohydrate loading.[50] For endurance events, maximizing the amount of glycogen that can be stored, especially in muscles, may make the difference between finishing first or at the end of the pack. Athletes can increase glycogen supplies in muscle and liver by reducing the training program a few days before competing and by significantly increasing carbohydrate intake during the week before the event.[43] Several studies have investigated effects of endurance training, pre-event carbohydrate-loading protocols (that range from one to seven days pre-event), and supplementing carbohydrate during an endurance event. By reducing training before the competition, the athlete can eliminate any metabolic waste products that may hinder performance. The high-carbohydrate diet restores glycogen levels in muscle and the liver.

| | | Protein (g) | Carbohydrate (g) | Fat (g) | Calories from fat | Cholesterol (mg) | Sodium (mg) |
|---|---|---|---|---|---|---|---|
| **TABLE 5–3** | **Examples of Fast-Food Choices and Nutritional Value** | | | | | | |
| **Food** | **Calories** | | | | | | |
| *Hamburgers* | | | | | | | |
| McDonald's hamburger | 250 | 12 | 31 | 9 | 80 | 25 | 520 |
| Dairy Queen single hamburger w/cheese | 400 | 19 | 34 | 18 | 160 | 65 | 930 |
| Hardee's Original 1/3 Pound Thickburger | 860 | 35 | 52 | 58 | 540 | 105 | 1,630 |
| Wendy's double hamburger, white bun | 800 | 50 | 42 | 48 | — | 105 | 1,530 |
| McDonald's Big Mac | 540 | 25 | 45 | 29 | 260 | 75 | 1,040 |
| Burger King Whopper sandwich | 650 | 22 | 50 | 37 | 340 | 60 | 910 |
| In-n-Out cheeseburger with onion | 480 | 22 | 39 | 27 | 240 | 60 | 1,000 |
| *Chicken* | | | | | | | |
| Arby's crispy chicken sandwich | 540 | 27 | 48 | 27 | 240 | 55 | 990 |
| Burger King chicken sandwich | 660 | 28 | 48 | 40 | 360 | 75 | 1,170 |
| Dairy Queen chicken sandwich | 600 | 24 | 59 | 30 | 270 | 55 | 1,250 |
| Church's Crispy Nuggets (5 pieces) | 162 | 9 | 13 | 7 | 190 | 21 | 759 |
| Kentucky Fried Chicken Original Recipe Bites (6) | 200 | 22 | 7 | 9 | 80 | 60 | 660 |
| *Fish* | | | | | | | |
| Burger King Fish Filet Sandwich | 470 | 23 | 65 | 13 | 117 | 50 | 1,240 |
| Long John Silver's Fish | 470 | 18 | 48 | 23 | 207 | 45 | 1,210 |
| Bojangles Filet of Fish Sandwich | 335 | 23 | 25 | 16 | 144 | 61 | 645 |
| *Others* | | | | | | | |
| Hardee's Jumbo Chili Dog | 380 | 15 | 24 | 25 | 230 | 50 | 1,130 |
| Taco Bell Burrito Supreme | 390 | 17 | 52 | 13 | 120 | 30 | 1,090 |
| Arby's roast beef sandwich (regular) | 350 | 23 | 39 | 12 | 110 | 45 | 950 |
| Hardee's roast beef sandwich (regular) | 300 | 18 | 28 | 14 | 130 | 40 | 850 |
| *French fries* | | | | | | | |
| Arby's french fries | 400 | 7 | 74 | 29 | 260 | 0 | 1,200 |
| McDonald's french fries (medium) | 380 | 4 | 48 | 19 | 170 | 0 | 270 |
| Wendy's french fries (medium) | 420 | 5 | 55 | 21 | — | 0 | 460 |
| *Shakes* | | | | | | | |
| Dairy Queen (vanilla, medium) | 730 | 17 | 115 | 23 | 210 | 60 | 310 |
| McDonald's | | | | | | | |
|    Vanilla | 530 | 11 | 86 | 15 | 140 | 60 | 160 |
|    Chocolate | 560 | 12 | 91 | 16 | 150 | 60 | 240 |
|    Strawberry | 550 | 12 | 90 | 16 | 150 | 60 | 160 |
| *Soft drinks* | | | | | | | |
| Coca-Cola | 210 | — | 58 | — | — | — | 15 |
| Diet Coke | 0 | — | 0 | — | — | — | 30 |
| Sprite | 210 | — | 56 | — | — | — | 55 |
| Dr Pepper | 260 | — | 71 | — | — | — | 90 |
| Sprite Zero | 0 | — | 0 | — | — | — | 35 |
| Mountain Dew | 290 | — | 81 | — | — | — | 105 |
| Pepsi | 269 | — | 75 | — | — | — | 54 |
| Diet Pepsi | 0 | — | 0 | — | — | — | 65 |

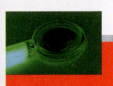

## FOCUS 5–4 Focus on Injury/Illness Prevention and Wellness Promotion

### Tips for selecting fast foods

- Limit deep-fried foods, such as fish and chicken sandwiches and chicken nuggets, which are often higher in fat than plain burgers are. If you are having fried chicken, remove some of the breading before eating.
- Order roast beef, turkey, or grilled chicken, where available, for a lower-fat alternative to most burgers.
- Choose a small order of fries with your meal rather than a large one, and request no salt. Add a small amount of salt yourself if desired. If you are ordering a deep-fat-fried sandwich or one that is made with cheese and sauce, skip the fries altogether and try a plain baked potato (add butter and salt sparingly) or a dinner roll instead of a biscuit, or try a side salad to accompany your meal.
- Choose regular sandwiches instead of "double," "jumbo," "deluxe," or "ultimate" sandwiches. And order plain types rather than those with the works, such as cheese, bacon, mayonnaise, and special

sauce. Pickles, mustard, ketchup, and other condiments are high in sodium. Choose lettuce, tomatoes, and onions.
- At the salad bar, load up on fresh greens, fruits, and vegetables. Be careful of salad dressings, added toppings, and creamy salads (potato salad, macaroni salad, coleslaw). These can quickly push calories and fat to the level of other menu items or higher.
- Many fast-food items contain large amounts of sodium from salt and other ingredients. Try to balance the rest of your day's sodium choices after a fast-food meal.
- Alternate water, low-fat milk, or skim milk with a soda or a shake.
- For dessert, or a sweet-on-the-run, choose low-fat frozen yogurt where available.
- Remember to balance your fast-food choices with your food selections for the whole day.

---

Glycogen supercompensation may be accomplished over a 6-day period divided into three phases. In phase 1 (days 1 and 2), training should be hard and dietary intake of carbohydrates restricted. During phase 2 (days 3 through 5), training is cut back and the individual eats plenty of carbohydrates. Studies have indicated that glycogen stores may be increased from 50 to 100 percent, theoretically enhancing endurance during a long-term event. Phase 3 (day 6) is the day of the event, during which a normal diet must be consumed.

Additional suggested carbohydrate-loading protocols focus on the benefits that can occur, without a glycogen-depletion period, in as little as one to three days, provided that training during loading days does not deplete already stored glycogen. A 3-day modified carbohydrate-loading regimen on days 1 and 2 involves tapered training with 10 to 12 grams of carbohydrate per kilogram of body weight. Day 3 is a rest day again with 10 to 12g CHO/kg/BW, prior to competition on day 4. It has been recommended that glycogen supercompensation not be done more than two or three times a year. Glycogen supercompensation is only of value in long-duration events that produce glycogen depletion, such as a marathon.[50]

### Fat Loading

Some endurance athletes have used fat loading in place of carbohydrate loading. Their intent was to have a better source of energy at their disposal. The deleterious effects of this procedure outweigh any benefits that may be derived. Associated with fat loading is cardiac protein and potassium depletion, causing arrhythmias and increased levels of serum cholesterol as a result of the ingestion of butter, cheese, cream, and marbled beef.

## BODY COMPOSITION AND WEIGHT CONTROL

Gain or loss of weight often poses a problem because an individual's ingrained eating habits are difficult to change.[27] The athletic trainer's inability to adequately supervise the athlete's meal program in terms of balance and quantity further complicates the problem. An intelligent and conscientious approach to weight control requires a team approach between the athlete, coach, athletic trainer and, if at all possible, a registered dietitian

---

A recreational runner has been training to run his first marathon. He feels good about his level of conditioning but wants to make certain that he does everything that he can do to maximize his performance. He is concerned about eating the right type of foods both before and during the marathon to help ensure that he does not become excessively fatigued.

**?** What recommendations should the athletic trainer make regarding glycogen supercompensation, the pre-event meal, and food consumption during the event?

or sports nutritionist.[75] The athletic trainer should be skilled and appropriately trained in the use of the various body composition assessment techniques and should periodically track an athlete's body composition to make certain that individual goals of that athlete are met.[76] Such understanding allows individuals to better discipline themselves as to the quantity and kinds of foods they should eat.[29]

## Body Composition

Desirable body weight is most often determined by consulting age-related height and weight charts, such as those published by life insurance companies. Unfortunately, these charts are inaccurate because they involve broad ranges and often fail to take individual body types into account. Health and performance, rather than body weight, may best be determined by body composition.[34]

*Body composition* refers to both the fat and nonfat components of the body. The portion of total body weight that is composed of fat tissue is referred to as the percentage of body fat. The total body weight that is composed of nonfat or lean tissue, which includes muscles, tendons, bones, and connective tissue, is referred to as lean body weight. Body composition measurements provide an accurate determination of precisely how much weight an individual may gain or lose.[50]

The average college-age female has between 20 and 25 percent body fat. The average college-age male has between 12 and 15 percent body fat. Male endurance athletes may get their fat percentage as low as 8 to 12 percent, and female endurance athletes may reach 10 to 18 percent. Body fat percentage should not go below 3 percent in males and 12 percent in females, because below these percentages the internal organs tend to lose their protective padding of essential fat, potentially subjecting them to injury.[7]

Being overweight and being obese are different conditions.[8] Being overweight implies having excess body weight relative to physical size and stature. Being overweight may not be a problem unless a person is also overfat, which means that the percentage of total body weight that is made up of fat is excessive. **Obesity** implies an excessive amount of body fat, much greater than what would be considered normal. Females with body fat above 30 percent and males with body fat above 20 percent are considered to be obese.[7]

Two factors determine the amount of fat in the body: the number of fat, or adipose, cells and the size of each adipose cell. Proliferation, or hyperplagia, of adipose cells begins at birth and continues to puberty. It is thought that after early adulthood the number of fat cells remains fixed, although some evidence suggests that the number of cells is not necessarily fixed.[50] Adipose cell size also increases gradually, or hypertrophies, to early adulthood and can increase or decrease as a function of caloric balance. In adults, weight loss or gain is primarily a function of the change in cell size, not cell number. Obese adults tend to exhibit a great deal of adipose cell hypertrophy.

The **adipose cell** stores triglyceride (a form of liquid fat). This liquid fat moves in and out of the cell according to the energy needs of the body, which are determined to some extent by activity type. The greatest amount of fat is used in activities of moderate intensity and long duration. The greater the amount of triglyceride contained in the adipose cell, the greater the amount of total body weight composed of fat. One pound of body fat is made up of approximately 3,500 calories stored as triglyceride within the adipose cell.

### Assessing Body Composition

Body composition assessments should be used to determine body weight and body composition goals that are safe for the athlete.[76] **SoR:B** Methods for assessing **body composition** most commonly used by athletic trainers are measurement of skinfold thickness;[12] hydrostatic, or underwater, weighing; DXA measurements; BOD POD measurements; measurement of electrical impedance; and, assessing body mass index. For all of these assessment techniques the athlete should be in a hydrated state.[76] **SoR:B**

**Skinfold Measurements** The method of measuring the thickness of skinfolds is based on the fact that about 50 percent of the fat in the body is contained in the subcutaneous fat layers and is closely related to total fat. The remainder of the fat in the body is found around organs and vessels and serves a shock-absorptive function. The skinfold technique measures the thickness of the subcutaneous fat layer with a skinfold caliper (Figure 5–5), at very specific locations, using a well-defined technique.[68] Its accuracy is relatively low; however, expertise in measurement is easily developed, and the time required for this technique is considerably less than for the others. It has been estimated that error in skinfold measurement is plus or minus 3 to 5 percent.[12]

Researchers have offered several different techniques for measuring body composition via skinfolds. A technique proposed by Jackson and Pollack,[34] which measures the thigh, triceps, suprailiac, abdomen, and chest skinfolds, is widely used.[50]

**Hydrostatic Weighing** Hydrostatic (underwater) weighing involves placing a subject in a specially designed underwater tank to determine body density. Fat tissue is

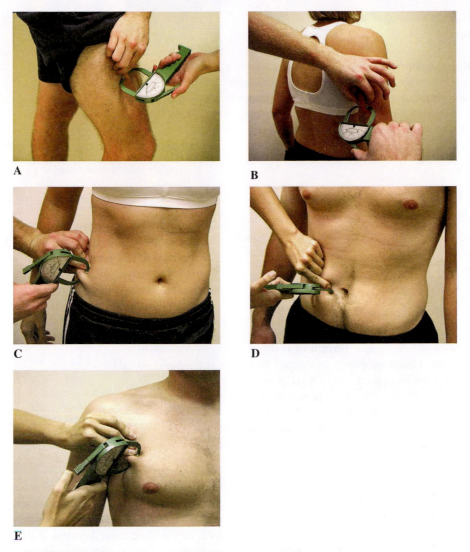

FIGURE 5–5    Sites and techniques for measuring body composition.
**(A)** Thigh. **(B)** Triceps. **(C)** Suprailiac. **(D)** Abdomen. **(E)** Chest.
© William E. Prentice

less dense than lean tissue. Therefore, the more body fat present, the more the body floats (buoyancy) and the less it weighs in water. Body composition is calculated by comparing the weight of the submerged individual with the weight before entering the tank. If done properly, this technique is very accurate. Unfortunately, the tank and equipment are expensive and generally not available to most athletic trainers. In addition, this technique has other drawbacks. It is time-consuming (especially for large groups), and subjects must exhale completely and hold their breath while under water. Many individuals have fears about this aspect of the technique.

**BOD POD**  The BOD POD Body Composition System uses the relationship between pressure and volume to derive the body volume of a subject seated in a fiberglass chamber. The principle is similar to hydrostatic weighing except, instead of using water to measure body volume,

the BOD POD uses air displacement to measure body volume.

**Bioelectrical Impedance**  This technique involves the measurement of resistance to the flow of electrical current through the body between selected points.[35] It is based on the principle that electricity will choose to flow through the tissue that offers the least resistance, or impedance. Fat is generally a poor conductor of electrical energy, whereas lean tissue is a fairly good conductor. Thus, the higher the percentage of body fat, the greater the resistance to the passage of electrical energy. Very simply, this method predicts the percent body fat by measuring bioelectrical impedance.[35] Bioelectrical impedance measures can be affected by levels of hydration; if the body is dehydrated, the measurement will tend to overestimate percent body fat relative to measurements taken when there is normal hydration.[35] The equipment available for taking these measurements is fairly expensive and generally includes computer software.

**Dual Energy X-ray Absorptiometry (DXA)** This new DXA technology is the most recent and the most accurate technique of assessing body composition, but it is fairly expensive, costing around $300 per test. The instrument uses total body X-ray technique to look at the density of the body and can then estimate the amount of lean and fat tissue.

## Determining Body Mass Index

A relatively easy way to determine the extent of overweight or obesity is to use a person's body weight and height measurements to calculate body mass index (BMI).[50] BMI is a ratio of body weight to height. This technique represents a method for measuring health risks from obesity using height/weight measurements. BMI might not be useful for athletes who have a high lean mass and low fat mass, making it appear that an athlete is overfat when in fact he or she has a low percent of body fat but high muscle mass. Health problems associated with excess body fat tend to be associated with a BMI of more than 25. A BMI of 25 to 30 indicates that a person is overweight. A BMI of 30 or more indicates a state of obesity.[50] *Focus Box 5–5:* "Determining body mass index" will help you calculate BMI.

## Assessing Caloric Balance

Changes in body weight are almost entirely the result of changes in caloric balance.[40]

Caloric balance =
Number of calories consumed – Number of calories expended

If more calories are consumed than expended, this positive caloric balance results in weight gain. Conversely, weight loss results from a negative caloric balance, in which more calories are expended than are consumed. Caloric balance may be calculated by maintaining accurate records of both the number of calories consumed in the diet and the number of calories expended for metabolic needs and in activities performed during the day.

**Caloric Consumption** Caloric balance is determined by the number of calories consumed regardless of whether the calories are contained in fat, carbohydrate, or protein. There are differences in the caloric content of these foodstuffs:

> Positive caloric balance leads to weight gain; negative caloric balance leads to weight loss.

Carbohydrate = 4 calories per gram

Protein = 4 calories per gram

Fat = 9 calories per gram

Alcohol = 7 calories per gram

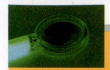

## FOCUS 5–5
## Focus on Examination, Assessment, and Diagnosis

### Determining body mass index

1. Weigh yourself to determine your body weight in pounds.
2. Divide your weight in pounds by 2.2 to determine kilograms.
3. Measure your height in inches.
4. Multiply your height in inches by 2.54 and divide by 100 to convert your height to meters.
5. Multiply your height in meters by your height in meters to get your height in meters squared.
6. Divide your weight in kilograms by your height in meters squared to determine your BMI.

1. _____ Divided by 2.2 = _____
   Weight (lbs)                  Weight (kg)
2. _____ Times 2.54 divided by 100 = _____
   Height (in)                           Height (m)
3. _____ Times _____ = _____
   Height (m)      Height (m)      Height (m²)
4. _____ Divided by _____ = _____
   Weight (kg)        Height (m²)     Body mass
                                      index

Estimations of caloric intake for college athletes range between 2,000 and 5,000 calories per day. Estimations of caloric expenditure range between 2,200 and 4,400 calories on average. Energy demands will be considerably higher in endurance-type athletes, who may require as many as 7,000 calories per day.[50]

**Caloric Expenditure** Calories may be expended by three processes: basal metabolism, work (any activity that requires more energy than sleeping), and excretion. When estimating caloric expenditure, it is first necessary to determine the amount of calories (energy) needed to support basal metabolism. This is the minimal amount of energy required to sustain the body's vital functions, such as respiration, heartbeat, circulation, and maintenance of body temperature during a 24-hour period. The basal metabolic rate (BMR) is the rate at which calories are spent for these maintenance activities. BMR is most accurately determined in a laboratory through a measurement process known as indirect calorimetry, which measures a person's oxygen uptake. Measurement of BMR using this procedure is generally done as soon as the subject awakes, in a quiet, warm environment, and after a 12-hour fast.

Once BMR has been determined, it is necessary to calculate the energy requirements of all physical activities done in a 24-hour period. This is the second component of energy needs, referred to as work. There is a wide variation in energy output for work. It is determined by the type, intensity, and duration of a physical activity. Body size is also a factor; heavier people expend more energy in an activity than do lighter people. Specific energy expenditures may be determined by consulting charts that predict the energy used in an activity based on (1) the time spent in each activity in minutes and (2) the metabolic costs of each activity in kilocalories per minute per pound (kcal/min/lb) of body weight.

## Methods of Weight Loss

An individual has several ways to go about losing weight: dieting, increasing the amount of physical exercise, or a combination of diet and exercise.

An ice hockey attackman has an excellent level of fitness and has superb skating ability and stick work. He is convinced that the only thing keeping him from moving to the next level is his low body weight. In recent years, he has engaged in more weight-training activities to improve his muscular endurance and, to a lesser extent, to increase his strength.

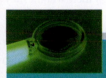 **?** What recommendations should the athletic trainer make for him to be successful in his weight-gaining efforts?

Weight loss through dieting alone is difficult, and in most cases dieting alone is an ineffective means of weight control. Long-term weight control through dieting alone is successful only 2 percent of the time.[13] About 35 to 45 percent of weight decrease due to dieting results from a loss of lean tissue. The minimum caloric intake should not go below 1,000 to 1,200 calories per day for a female and not below 1,200 to 1,400 calories per day for a male.[44]

Weight loss through exercise involves an 80 to 90 percent loss of fat tissue with almost no loss of lean tissue. Weight loss through exercise alone is almost as difficult as losing weight through dieting. However, exercise not only results in weight reduction but also may enhance cardiorespiratory endurance, improve strength, and increase flexibility.[7] For these reasons, exercise has some distinct advantages over dieting in any weight-loss program.

The most efficient method of decreasing the percentage of body weight that is fat is through some combination of diet and exercise.[76] A moderate caloric restriction combined with a moderate increase in caloric expenditure results in a negative caloric balance. This method is relatively fast and easy compared with either of the other methods because habits are being moderately changed.

In any weight-loss program, the goal should be to lose 1.5 to 2 pounds per week. Weight loss of more than 4 to 5 pounds per week may be attributed to dehydration as opposed to a loss of body fat.[7] A weight-loss program must emphasize the long-haul approach. It generally takes a long time to put on extra weight, and there is no reason to expect that true loss of excess body fat can be accomplished in a relatively short time. The American College of Sports Medicine has made specific recommendations for weight loss that are identified in *Focus Box 5–6:* "Key Recommendations for Weight Loss and Weight Maintenance."[1]

## Methods of Weight Gain

The aim of a weight-gaining program should be to increase lean body mass—that is, muscle as opposed to body fat. Muscle mass should be increased only by muscle work combined with an appropriate increase in dietary intake. Muscle mass cannot be increased by the intake of any special food or vitamin.[41]

## FOCUS 5–6 Focus on Healthcare Administration and Professional Responsibilities

### Key recommendations for weight loss and weight maintenance*

- Lose weight to lower blood pressure, total cholesterol, LDL-cholesterol, triglycerides, and blood glucose, and to raise low levels of HDL-cholesterol.
- Use the BMI to assess overweight and obesity and waist circumference measurement to assess abdominal fat content.
- The initial goal of weight-loss therapy should be to reduce current body weight by about 10 percent.
- The combination of a reduced-calorie diet and increased physical activity is recommended.
- Low-calorie diets with reduced fat and carbohydrates that create a deficit of 500 to 1,000 kcal/day will help achieve a weight loss of 1 to 2 pounds per week.

- Physical activity for 30 to 45 minutes, 3 to 5 days a week should be part of a comprehensive weight-loss therapy, and weight-control program
- Weight loss should be about 1 to 2 pounds per week for a period of 6 months.
- A weight-maintenance program should be a priority after the initial 6 months of weight-loss therapy.
- Weight maintenance should employ the combination of a low-calorie diet, increased physical activity, and behavior modification.

*Adapted from https://www.nhlbi.nih.gov/health/educational/lose_wt/recommen.htm

A tennis coach observes that one of her players has lost a significant amount of weight. Along with this loss of weight, the athlete's level of play has begun to decrease. The coach becomes seriously concerned when another player tells the coach that she thinks her room-mate was purposely throwing up after a team meal on a recent road trip. After briefly questioning the athlete about her eating habits, the coach asks the athletic trainer to become involved in dealing with this situation.

**?** How should the athletic trainer respond to this request?

The recommended rate of weight gain is approximately 1 to 2 pounds per week.[41] Each pound of lean body mass gained represents a positive caloric balance. This positive balance is an intake in excess of an expenditure of approximately 2,500 calories. One pound of fat represents the equivalent of 3,500 calories; lean body tissue contains less fat, more protein, and more water and represents approximately 2,500 calories. To gain 1 pound of muscle, an excess of approximately 2,500 calories is needed; to lose 1 pound of fat, approximately 3,500 calories in excess of intake must be expended in activities. Adding 500 to 1,000 calories daily to the usual diet will provide the energy needs of gaining 1 to 2 pounds per week and fuel the increased energy expenditure of the weight-training program. Weight training must be part of the weight-gaining program. Otherwise, the excess intake of energy will be converted to fat.[41]

# DISORDERED EATING

Disordered eating can be defined as a spectrum of abnormal eating behaviors, ranging from mild food restriction and occasional binge eating and purging to severe conditions of bulimia nervosa and anorexia nervosa. Disordered eating is a multifactorial disorder that includes social, familial, physiological, and psychological components. It appears that depression and difficulty expressing one's feelings develop in response to experiencing family conflict, lack of family cohesion, childhood physical and emotional abuse, and neglect. These factors may influence whether an individual develops a problem eating behavior as well as the severity of the disorder. Individuals who engage in disordered eating behaviors, as well as individuals at risk for developing these behaviors, may benefit from interventions that address adaptive ways to cope with depression.[49] In the athletic population, the incidence of disordered eating behaviors and pathological eating disorders is significantly higher than in the general population.[87] This relatively high incidence in athletes has been attributed to the athlete's attempt to control body weight or body composition in an effort to improve his or her performance. There is strong evidence that disordered eating, eating disorders, and amenorrhea occur more frequently in sports that emphasize leanness.[56] In addition to the emotional stress and social pressures characteristic of eating disorders, there are also serious physiological effects, which can compound one another and ultimately affect the athlete's overall health and performance. Athletes with disordered eating should be referred to a mental health practitioner for evaluation, diagnosis, and recommendations for treatment.[56] A brief physiological screening test (consisting of four measurements and a 14-item questionnaire) has been developed to detect eating disorders in female collegiate athletes.[6] Athletic trainers working with young athletes, particularly active females, should be educated about these disorders and work within their resources to develop strategies for prevention and management.[75,78] Links to the NATA position statement "Preventing, detecting and managing eating disorders in athletes" can be found at http://www.nata.org/sites/default/files/PreventingDetectingAndManagingDisorderedEating.pdf.

## Binge Eating

At some point in time just about everyone overeats, such as at Thanksgiving when you have seconds and even thirds of just about everything on the table. But if this overeating becomes a recurrent problem that a person usually does in secret with strong feelings of guilt or shame about not being able to control these episodes, this behavior may be considered a binge eating disorder. Individuals who have binge eating disorder will continue to eat when they are not hungry, or will eat so much they are uncomfortable or even nauseated. They simply cannot stop eating even though the urge to quit is there; they will often eat alone and try to eat very quickly in an attempt to hide their problem. People with a binge eating disorder become depressed and develop anxiety and seem to obsess about losing and/or gaining weight even though their weight may be normal. Binge eating disorders may occur in 5 percent of the population and are more likely to occur in females (60 percent) than in males (40 percent).[45]

To be officially classified as having a binge eating disorder, an individual worries about eating a larger amount of food at one time than a normal person would consume within a 2-hour period, often when he or she is bored or depressed. Binge eating episodes occur at least two times a week for 6 months.[45]

**Bulimia Nervosa** The bulimic person is commonly female, ranging in age from adolescence to middle age. It is estimated that 1 out of every 200 American girls, ages 12 to 18 years (1 to 2 percent of the population) will develop patterns of bulimia nervosa, anorexia nervosa, or both.[5] Certainly, bulimia can be found in males as well. The bulimic individual typically gorges herself with thousands of calories after a period of starvation and then purges herself through induced vomiting and further fasting or through the use of laxatives or diuretics. This secretive binge-eating–purging cycle may go on for years.

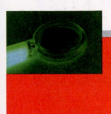

## FOCUS 5–7 Focus on Injury/Illness Prevention and Wellness Promotion

### Identifying the individual with an eating disorder

An individual with an eating disorder may display the following signs:

- Social isolation and withdrawal from friends and family
- A lack of confidence in athletic abilities
- Ritualistic eating behavior (e.g., organizing food on plate)
- An obsession with counting calories
- An obsession with constantly exercising, especially just before a meal
- An obsession with weighing self
- A constant overestimation of body size
- Patterns of leaving the table directly after eating to go into the restroom
- Problems related to eating disorders (e.g., malnutrition, menstrual irregularities, or chronic fatigue)
- A family history of eating disorders

Typically, the bulimic patient is white and belongs to a middle-class or upper-middle-class family. She is perfectionistic, obedient, overcompliant, highly motivated, successful academically, well liked by her peers, and a good athlete.[75] She most commonly participates in gymnastics, track, and dance. Male wrestlers and gymnasts may also develop bulimia nervosa. (See *Focus Box 5–7:* "Identifying the individual with an eating disorder.")

Binge-purge patterns of eating can cause stomach rupture, disruption of heart rhythm, and liver damage. Stomach acids brought up by vomiting cause tooth decay and chronically inflame the mucous lining of the mouth and throat.

It must be made clear that binge eating associated with an eating disorder is different from *overeating*. Everyone overeats from time to time, such as at parties or on holidays. This may occur due to stress but more often due to celebration of an event or because the food tastes great. Bingeing is a loss of control, such as when eating a couple of cookies turns into finishing the entire bag, then looking for ice cream or leftover pizza. The person cannot stop eating, then feels guilty and tries to purge by vomiting. The bulimic experiences this scenario repeatedly.

**Anorexia Nervosa** It has been estimated that 30 to 50 percent of all individuals diagnosed as having anorexia nervosa also develop some symptoms of bulimia nervosa. Anorexia nervosa is characterized by a distorted body image and a major concern about weight gain. As with bulimia nervosa, anorexia nervosa affects mostly females. It usually begins in adolescence and can be mild without major consequences or can become life threatening. As many as 15 to 21 percent of individuals diagnosed as anorexic ultimately die from this disorder. Despite being extremely thin, the individual sees herself as too fat. These individuals deny hunger and are hyperactive, engaging in abnormal amounts of exercise, such as aerobics or distance running.[74] In general, the anorexic individual is highly secretive, and the athletic trainer must be sensitive to eating problems. Early intervention is essential. Any individual with signs of bulimia nervosa or anorexia nervosa must be confronted in a kind, empathetic manner by the athletic trainer. Individuals with eating disorders must be referred for psychological or psychiatric treatment. Unfortunately, simply referring an anorexic person to a health education clinic is not usually effective. The key to the treatment of anorexia nervosa seems to be getting the patient to realize that a problem exists and that he or she could benefit from professional help. The individual must voluntarily accept such help if treatment is to be successful.[7]

**Anorexia Athletica** Anorexia athletica is a condition specific to athletes that is characterized by several of the features common to anorexia nervosa, but without the self-starvation practices. Athletes with anorexia athletica may exhibit a variety of signs, including disturbance of body image, a weight loss greater than 5 percent of body weight, gastrointestinal complaints, primary amenorrhea, menstrual dysfunction, absence of medical illness explaining the weight reduction, excessive fear of becoming obese, bingeing or purging, compulsive eating, and/or restriction of caloric intake.

**Female Athlete Triad Syndrome** Female athlete triad syndrome is a potentially fatal problem that involves a combination of an eating disorder (either bulimia or anorexia), amenorrhea, and osteoporosis (diminished bone density).[54,60] Severe undernutrition impairs reproductive and skeletal health and menstrual irregularities and low bone mineral density increase stress fracture risk.[56] The incidence of this syndrome is uncertain; however, some studies have suggested that eating disorders in female athletes may be as high as 62 percent in certain sports, with amenorrhea being common in at least 60 percent of female athletes.[32] However, the major risk of this syndrome is that the bone lost in osteoporosis may not be regained.[52]

Screening for this syndrome should occur at the preparticipation exam or annual health screening exam, and athletes with one component of the triad should be evaluated for the others.[56] Multidisciplinary treatment should include a physician (or other health care professional), a registered dietitian, and, for athletes with disordered eating or an eating disorder, a mental health practitioner.[56]

## SUMMARY

- The classes of nutrients are carbohydrates, fats, proteins, vitamins, minerals, and water. Carbohydrates, fats, and proteins provide the energy required for muscular work during activity and play a role in the function and maintenance of body tissues. Vitamins are substances in food that have no caloric value but are necessary to regulate body processes. Vitamins are either fat soluble (vitamins A, D, E, and K) or water soluble (B-complex vitamins and vitamin C). Minerals are necessary in most physiological functions of the body. Water is the most essential of all the nutrients and should be of great concern to anyone involved in physical activity.

- A nutritious diet consists of eating a variety of foods in amounts recommended in MyPlate. A diet that meets those recommended amounts does not require supplementation.

- Protein supplementation during weight training is not necessary if a nutritious diet is maintained. Many males and especially females may require calcium supplementation to prevent osteoporosis. It may be necessary to supplement the diet with extra iron to prevent iron-deficiency anemia.

- Organic or natural foods have no beneficial effect on performance. Vegetarian diets can provide all the essential nutrients if the diet is well thought out and properly prepared.

- The pre-event meal should be higher in carbohydrates, easily digested, eaten 3 to 4 hours before an event, and psychologically pleasing.

- Glycogen supercompensation involves maximizing resting stores of glucose in the muscles, blood, and liver before a competitive event.

- Body composition indicates the percentage of total body weight composed of fat tissue versus the percentage composed of lean tissue. The size and number of adipose cells determine percent body fat. Percent body fat can be assessed by measuring the thickness of the subcutaneous fat at specific areas of the body with a skinfold caliper.

- Changes in body weight are caused almost entirely by a change in caloric balance, which is a function of the number of calories taken in and the number of calories expended. Weight can be lost either by increasing caloric expenditure through exercise or by decreasing caloric intake. Diets generally do not work. The recommended technique for losing weight involves a combination of moderate calorie restriction and a moderate increase in physical exercise during the course of each day. Weight gain should be accomplished by increasing caloric intake and engaging in a weight-training program. It is possible to gain weight and lose fat, thus changing body composition. Muscle weighs more than fat.

- Anorexia nervosa is a disease in which a person suffers a pathological weight loss because of a psychological aversion to food and eating. Bulimia nervosa is an eating disorder that involves bingeing and subsequent purging. Anorexia athletica is similar to anorexia nervosa without starvation. Female athlete triad syndrome is a combination of an eating disorder, amenorrhea, and osteoporosis.

## WEB SITES

**National Athletic Trainers Association Position, Official, Consensus, and Support Statements**
*Evaluation of Dietary Supplements for Performance Nutrition* (February 2013) www.natajournals.org/doi/pdf/10.4085/1062-6050-48.1.16
*Safe Weight Loss and Maintenance Practices in Sport and Exercise* (2011)
www.nata.org/sites/default/files/JAT-46-3-16-turocy-322-336.pdf
*Preventing, Detecting, and Managing Disordered Eating in Athletes* (2008)
www.nata.org/sites/default/files/PreventingDetectingAndManagingDisorderedEating.pdf
*Fluid Replacement for Athletes* (2000)
http://www.nata.org/sites/default/files/FluidReplacementsForAthletes.pdf

Academy on Nutrition and Dietetics: www.eatright.org
*Provides informative nutritional tips as well as gateways to nutrition and related sites.*

American Heart Association: www.americanheart.org
*Complete with comprehensive nutrition guidelines, the American Heart Association is a great resource for health practitioners and laypersons.*

Center for Food Safety and Applied Nutrition—FDA: www.fda.gov/AboutFDA/CentersOffices/OfficeofFoods/CFSAN/default.htm
*Timely fact sheets and press releases are available from the Food and Drug Administration.*

Female Athlete Triad Coalition: www.femaleathletetriad.org
*Promotes optimal health and well-being for female athletes, active girls, and women.*

Fitness and Sports Nutrition http://fnic.nal.usda.gov/lifecycle-nutrition/fitness-and-sports-nutrition
*A variety of fitness and sports nutrition topics and resources from organizations and institutes that specialize in sports medicine and exercise science research.*

Food and Nutrition Information Center: www.fnic.nal
.usda.gov/
*This site is part of the information centers at the National Agricultural Library and offers access to information on healthy eating habits, food composition, and many additional resources.*

Gatorade Sports Science Institute: www.gssiweb.com
*This Web site provides information for coaches, athletic trainers, physicians, nutritionists, and others in the field of sports medicine, sports nutrition, and exercise science.*

MyPlate: www.choosemyplate.gov
*Government Web site designed to help consumers adopt healthy eating habits consistent with the 2010 Dietary Guidelines.*

National Eating Disorders Association: www
.nationaleatingdisorders.org
*Get answers to any questions about eating disorders and their prevention. If you have an eating disorder*

*(or know someone who has), NEDA has information that may help.*

National Institutes of Health Office of Dietary Supplements: www.ods.od.nih.gov
*Gives a current overview of individual vitamins, minerals, and other dietary supplements.*

SuperTracker: www.supertracker.usda.gov
*From the U.S. Department of Agriculture, get your personalized nutrition and physical activity plan, track your foods and physical activities to see how they stack up, and get tips and support to help you make healthier choices and plan ahead.*

U.S. Dietary Guidelines: www.health.gov/dietaryguidelines
*This site details the revised 2015 U.S. Dietary Guidelines for Americans.*

## SOLUTIONS TO CLINICAL APPLICATION EXERCISES

5–1 The important consideration for weight control is the total number of calories that are consumed relative to the total number of calories expended. It makes no difference whether the calories consumed are carbohydrates, fat, or protein. Fat contains more than twice the number of calories than either carbohydrates, or protein contains, so an athlete can eat significantly more food and still have about the same caloric intake if the diet is high in carbohydrates. This dancer should be told that it is also essential to consume at least some fat, which is necessary for the production of several enzymes and hormones.

5–2 For a person who is truly consuming anything close to a well-balanced diet, vitamin supplementation is generally not necessary. However, if taking a one-a-day type of vitamin supplement makes her feel better, there is no harm. Vitamins do not provide energy. Her tiredness could be related to a number of medical conditions (e.g., mononucleosis). An iron-deficiency anemia may be detected through a laboratory blood test. The athletic trainer should refer this individual to a physician for blood work.

5–3 This athlete should be referred to the team physician and nutritionist. From her history, the athletic trainer can assume she is not consuming enough iron by not eating meats or other nutritious foods. Iron is essential for hemoglobin formation and energy formation. In addition, since she is not eating vegetables in a well-balanced diet, she is not receiving an adequate amount of vitamin K, which is found in green, leafy vegetables. Vitamin K is important in blood coagulation.

5–4 A small amount of protein (slightly above to about double the protein DRI) is needed for developing muscles in a training program. However, an athlete can easily get these necessary higher amounts by eating a variety of foods, especially protein-rich foods. Thus, athletes do not need protein supplements, because their diets typically exceed protein recommendations.

5–5 The amount of glycogen that can be stored in the muscle and liver can be increased by reducing the training program a few days before competing and by significantly increasing carbohydrate intake during the week before the event. Nutrients consumed over several days before competition are much more important than what is eaten 3 hours before an event. The purpose of the pre-event meal should be to provide the competitor with sufficient nutrient energy and fluids for competition while taking into consideration the digestibility of the food. Glucose-rich drinks taken at regular intervals are beneficial for highly intense and prolonged events that severely deplete glycogen stores.

5–6 The athletic trainer should recommend that this athlete set a goal of 18 to 20 percent body fat. If the softball player needs to lose weight, she must consume fewer calories than she is burning off, and this is not something that can be achieved in a short period of time. It also must be explained that weight control is simply a matter of achieving caloric balance and making lifestyle changes in terms of eating and exercise habits to achieve caloric balance.

5–7 This athlete must understand the importance of adding lean tissue muscle mass rather than increasing his percentage of body fat. His caloric intake must be increased so that he is in a positive caloric balance of about 500 calories per day. Additional caloric intake should consist primarily of carbohydrates. Additional supplementation with protein is not necessary. It is absolutely essential that this athlete incorporate a weight-training program using heavy weights that will overload the muscle, forcing it to hypertrophy over a period of time.

5–8 Treating eating disorders is difficult even for health care professionals specifically trained to counsel these individuals. The athletic trainer should approach the individual, not with accusation but with support, showing concern about her weight loss and expressing a desire to help her secure appropriate counseling. Remember that the athlete must first be willing to admit that she has an eating disorder before treatment and counseling will be effective. Eliciting the support of close friends and family can help with treatment.

## REVIEW QUESTIONS AND CLASS ACTIVITIES

1. What is the value of good nutrition in terms of performance and injury prevention?
2. Ask coaches of different sports about the type of diet they recommend for their athletes and their rationale behind the diet.
3. Have a nutritionist talk to the class about food myths and fallacies.
4. Have each member of the class prepare a week's food diary; then compare it with other class members' diaries.
5. What are the daily dietary requirements, according to MyPlate? Should the requirements of the typical athlete's diet differ from those requirements? If so, in what ways?
6. Debate the value of vitamin and mineral supplements.
7. Describe the advantages and disadvantages of supplementing iron and calcium.
8. Is there some advantage to pre-event nutrition?

9. Are there advantages or disadvantages in a vegetarian diet for the athlete?
10. What is the current thinking on the value of creatine as a nutritional supplement?
11. What is the primary concern of using herbs?
12. Discuss the importance of monitoring body composition.
13. Explain the most effective technique for losing weight.
14. Contrast the signs and symptoms of bulimia nervosa and anorexia nervosa. If an athletic trainer is aware of an individual who may have an eating disorder, what should he or she do?

## REFERENCES

1. American Heart Association: 2013 ACC/AHA Guideline on the Treatment of Blood Cholesterol to Reduce Atherosclerotic Cardiovascular Risk in Adults, *Circulation* 129(25): S46–S48, 2014.
2. American College of Sports Medicine: The physiological and health effects of oral creatine supplementation, *Med Sci Sports Exerc* 32(3):706, 2000.
3. American College of Sports Medicine: Position stand on the appropriate intervention strategies for weight loss and prevention of weight regain for adults, *Med Sci Sports Exerc* 33(12):2145, 2001.
4. Anderson J: Nutrition and bone in physical activity and sport. In Wolinsky I, Hickson J, editors: *Nutrition in exercise and sport,* Boca Raton, FL, 1998, CRC Press.
5. Beals K: *Disordered eating among athletes: A comprehensive guide for health professionals* Champaign, IL, 2004, Human Kinetics.
6. Black D: Physiologic screening test for eating disorders/ disordered eating among female collegiate athletes, *J Athl Train* 38(4): 286, 2003.
7. Bonci C, et al.: National Athletic Trainers' Association position statement: Preventing, detecting and managing disordered eating in athletes, *J Athl Train* 43(1):80, 2008.
8. Brownell K: *Food and addiction: A comprehensive handbook*, New York, 2014, Oxford University Press.
9. Brukner P: Maximizing performance: Nutrition. In P. Brukner (ed.), *Clinical sports medicine,* ed 3, Sydney, Australia, 2010, McGraw-Hill.
10. Buell J, et al.: National Athletic Trainers Association position statement: Evaluation of dietary supplements for performance nutrition, *Journal of Athletic Training* 48(1):124–36, 2013.
11. Burke L: *Clinical sports nutrition,* Sydney, Australia, 2014, McGraw-Hill.
12. Brzycki M: What's the most accurate way to measure body composition? *Fitness Management* 20(2):45, 2004.
13. Byrd-Bredbenner C: *Perspectives in nutrition,* New York, 2008, McGraw-Hill.
14. Campbell B: Pre-exercise carbohydrate supplementation does not suppress rate of fatigue during resistance exercise in trained females, *Medicine and Science in Sport and Exercise* 44:596, 2012.
15. Casa D, et al.: National Athletic Trainers' Association position statement: Fluid replacement for athletes, *J Athl Train* 35(2):212, 2000.
16. Clark N: Organic foods, *American Fitness* 25(5):34, 2007.
17. Clark N: *Nancy Clark's sports nutrition guide book,* Champaign, IL, 2013, Human Kinetics.
18. Coleman E: Protein requirements for athletes, *Clinical Nutrition Insight* 38(9):1–3, 2012.
19. Coyle E: Highs and lows of carbohydrate diets, *Sports Science Exchange* 17(2):1, 2004.

20. Dubnov G: Prevalence of iron depletion and anemia in top-level basketball players, *Int J Sport Nutr Exerc Metab* 14(1):30, 2004.
21. Food and Drug Administration: Changes to the Nutrition Facts Label, 2016, U.S Department of Health and Human Services. http://www.fda.gov/Food/GuidanceRegulation/GuidanceDocumentsRegulatoryInformation/Labeling-Nutrition/ucm385663.htm
22. Friedman-Kester K: The function of functional foods, *Athletic Therapy Today* 7(3):46, 2002.
23. Friedman-Kester K: Herbal remedies are drugs, too! *Athletic Therapy Today* 7(4):40, 2002.
24. Friedman-Kester K: RDAs, RDIs—R U confused? *Athletic Therapy Today* 6(3):56, 2001.
25. Froiland K: Nutritional supplement use among college athletes and their sources of information, *Int J Sport Nutr Exerc Metab* 14(1):104, 2004.
26. Fuhrman J: Fueling the vegetarian athlete, *Current Sports Medicine Reports,* 9(4):233–41, 2010.
27. Gorinski R: In pursuit of the perfect body composition: Do dietary strategies make a difference? *Athletic Therapy Today* 6(6):54, 2001.
28. Greenwood M: Cramping and injury incidence in collegiate football players are reduced by creatine supplementation, *J Athl Train* 38(3):216–19, 2003.
29. Gutgesell M: Weight concerns, problem eating behaviors, and problem drinking behaviors in female college athletes, *J Athl Train* 38(1):62, 2003.
30. Hale C: The precompetition meal, *Athletic Therapy Today* 6(3):21, 2001.
31. Hemila H: Vitamin C for preventing and treating the common cold, *The Cochrane Library* DOI: 10.1002/14651858.CD000980.pub4, 2013.
32. Hostetter K: The need for qualified intervention for the female athlete triad syndrome patient, *Athletic Therapy and Training,* 15(3):29–33, 2010.
33. Hoyte C: The use of energy drinks, dietary supplements, and prescription medications by United States college students to enhance athletic performance, *Journal of Community Health* 38(3):575–80, 2013.
34. Jackson A: Generalized equations for predicting body density of women, *Med Sci Sports Exerc* 12:175, 1980.
35. Kemble D: Accuracy of bioelectrical impedence analyzers in college athletes: Does hydration matter? *Journal of Strength and Conditioning Research,* 24(1):1, 2010.
36. Kleiner S: Fluids for performance, *Athletic Therapy Today* 5(1):51, 2000.
37. Kleiner S: Postexercise-recovery nutrition, *Athletic Therapy Today* 6(2):40, 2001.
38. Kleiner S: Performance herbs. In S. Kleiner (ed.), *Power eating,* 2nd ed. Champaign, IL, 2013, Human Kinetics.
39. Kleiner S: Protein power, *Athletic Therapy Today* 7(1):24, 2002.
40. Kleiner S: Top-ten rules for healthy weight control, *Athletic Therapy Today* 7(2):38, 2002.

41. Litt A: Tactics for gaining weight. In Litt A, editor: *Fuel for young athletes,* Champaign, IL, 2004, Human Kinetics.
42. Lopez R: Exercise and hydration: Individualizing fluid replacement guidelines, *Strength and Conditioning Journal* 34(4):49–54, 2012.
43. Martin M: Drug-herb interactions: Are your athletes at risk? *Athletic Therapy Today* 10(1): 15, 2005.
44. Martinsen M: Preventing eating disorders among young elite athletes: A randomized controlled trial, *Medicine and Science in Sport and Exercise* 46(3):435–47, 2014.
45. Mason T: Profiles of binge eating: The interaction of depressive symptoms, eating styles, and body mass index, *Eating Disorders* 22(5):450–60, 2014.
46. Massad S, Headley S: Nutrition assessment: Considerations for athletes, *Athletic Therapy Today* 4(6):6, 1999.
47. Maughn R: Dietary supplements for athletes: Emerging trends and recurring themes, *Journal of Sport Sciences* 29(1): 56–57, 2011.
48. Maughn R: *Sports nutrition,* Malden, MA, 2002, Blackwell Scientific.
49. Mazzeo S, Espelage D: Association between childhood physical and emotional abuse and disordered eating behaviors in female undergraduates: An investigation of the mediating role of alexithymia and depression, *Journal of Counseling Psychology* 49(1):86, 2002.
50. McArdle W, Katch F, Katch V: *Sports and exercise nutrition,* Philadelphia, 2013, Lippincott, Williams and Wilkins.
51. McVicar J: *The complete herb book.* Westport, CT, 2008, Firefly Books.
52. Merrick M: Osteoporosis and the female athlete, *Athletic Therapy Today* 6(3):42, 2001.
53. Meyer N: Fueling for fitness: Food and fluid recommendations for before, during, and after exercise, *ACSM'S Health & Fitness Journal* 16(3):7–12, 2012.
54. Mountjoy M: The IOC consensus statement: Beyond the female athlete triad-relative energy deficiency in port, *British Journal of Sports Medicine* 48:491–97, 2014.
55. Mueller K: *The athlete's guide to sports supplements,* Champaign, IL, 2013, Human Kinetics.
56. Nattiv A, et al.: The female athlete triad, *Medicine and Science in Sport and Exercise* 39(10)1867–82, 2007.
57. Powers M: Ephedra and its application to sport performance: Another concern for the athletic trainer? *J Athl Train* 36(4):420, 2001.
58. Powers M: Creatine supplementation increases total body water without altering fluid distribution, *J Athl Train* 38(1):44, 2003.
59. Powers S: Antioxidant and vitamin D supplements for athletes: Sense or nonsense? *Journal of Sports Sciences,* 29 (1 Supplement): S47–S55, 2011.
60. Rauh M: Relationships among injury and disordered eating, menstrual dysfunction, and low bone mineral density in high school athletes: A prospective study, *J Athl Train* 45(3):243–52, 2010.

61. Ray T: What you need to know about performance-enhancing supplements, *Athletic Therapy Today* 11(2):56, 2006.

62. Reimers K: The role of liquid supplements in weight gain, *Strength Cond* 17(1):64, 1995.

63. Rodriguez N: Introduction of protein summit 2.0: Continued exploration of the impact of high-quality protein on optimal health, *American Journal of Clinical Nutrition* 101(6):1317S–195, 2015.

64. Rosenbloom C: Risky business: Dietary Supplement use by athletes, *Nutrition Today* 50(5):240–46, 2015.

65. Sandstrom G: Iron deficiency in adolescent female athletes—Is iron status affected by regular sporting activity? *Clinical Journal of Sports Medicine* 36(1):37–44, 2012.

66. Sawyer T, editor: *A guide to sport nutrition: For student-athletes, coaches, athletic trainers, and parents*, Champaign, IL, 2003, Sagamore.

67. Schlosser E: *Fast food nation: The dark side of the all-American meal*, New York, 2012, Harper Perennial.

68. Selkow N: Subcutaneous thigh fat assessment: A comparison of skinfold calipers and ultrasound imaging, *J Athl Train* 46(1):50–54, 2011.

69. Smith-Ryan A: *Sports nutrition and performance enhancing supplements*, Ronkonkoma, NY, 2013, Linus Learning.

70. Smith-Ryan A: The effect of creatine loading on neuromuscular fatigue in women, *Medicine and Science in Sport and Exercise*, 46(5)990–97, 2014.

71. Snyder M: *The antioxidant counter: A pocket guide to the revolutionary ORAC scale for choosing healthy foods*, Berkeley, 2011, Ulysses Press.

72. Spriet L: Nutritional strategies to influence adaptations to training, *Journal of Sports Sciences* 22(1):127, 2004.

73. Stout J: *Essentials of creatine in sports and health*, Clifton, NJ, 2010, Humana Press.

74. Sundgot-Borgen J: Eating disorders in athletes. In Sundgot-Borgen J, editor: *Nutrition in sport*, Oxford, England, 2000, Blackwell.

75. Turk J, Prentice W: Collegiate coaches' knowledge of eating disorders, *J Athl Train* 34(1): 19, 1999.

76. Turocey P, et al.: National Athletic Trainers Association position statement: Safe weight loss and maintenance practices in sport and exercise, *Journal of Athletic Training* 46(3):322–36, 2011.

77. U.S. Department of Health and Human Services and U.S. Department of Agriculture: *2015 – 2020 Dietary Guidelines for Americans*, 8th ed., 2015.

78. Vaughn J: Collegiate athletic trainers confidence in helping female athletes with eating disorders, *J Athl Train* 39(1):71, 2004.

79. Vinci D: Navigating the low-carb craze, *Athletic Therapy Today* 10(1):20, 2005.

80. Vinci D: Negotiating the maze of nutritional ergogenic aids, *Athletic Therapy Today* 8(2): 28, 2003.

81. Vinci D: The training room: Developing a sports-nutrition game plan, *Athletic Therapy Today* 7(5):52, 2002.

82. Vinci D: What's for lunch? *Athletic Therapy Today* 8(1):50, 2003.

83. Weil A: *Eating well for optimal health: The essential guide to food, diet and nutrition*, London, 2008, Sphere.

84. Wilder N: The effects of low-dose creatine supplementation versus creatine loading in collegiate football players, *J Athl Train* 36(2): 124, 2001.

85. Williams M: *Nutrition for health, fitness and sports*, Boston, 2009, McGraw-Hill.

86. Winterstein A, Storrs C: Herbal supplements: Considerations for the athletic trainer, *J Athl Train* 36(4):425, 2001.

87. Zawila L: The female, collegiate, cross-country runner: Nutritional knowledge and attitudes, *J Athl Train* 38(1):67, 2003.

# ANNOTATED BIBLIOGRAPHY

Clark N: *Sport nutrition guidebook: Eating to fuel your active lifestyle*, Champaign, IL, 2008, Human Kinetics.

*Provides real-life case studies of nutritional advice given to athletes; also provides recommendations for pregame meals.*

Dunford M, Doyle J: *Nutrition for sport and exercise*, Belmont, CA, 2014, Cengage Learning.

*Integrates nutrition and exercise physiology principles, emphasizing scientific reasoning and examining evidence for current nutritional recommendations.*

Fink H, Burgoon L, Mikesky A: *Practical applications in sports nutrition*, Sudbury, MA, 2009, Jones and Bartlett.

*Provides an introduction to sports nutrition including general nutrition concepts and a thorough explanation of athletic performance and consultation skills.*

Girard–Eberle S: *Endurance sports nutrition*, Champaign, IL, 2014, Human Kinetics.

*A guide for selecting the optimal foods, drinks, and supplements to train longer, recover more quickly, avoid injuries, and achieve performance goals in any endurance endeavor.*

Maughan R: *Sports nutrition*, IOC Medical Commission, 2014, Wiley Blackwell.

*A practical guide to eating for health and performance based on a consensus statement from the International Olympic Committee.*

Rosenbloom C, Coleman E: *Sports nutrition: A practice manual for professionals*, Chicago, IL, 2012, Academy of Nutrition & Dietetics.

*This book is a go-to source for specific evidence-based information on different sports nutrition topics.*

Smith-Ryan A, Jose, A: Sports nutrition and performance enhancing supplements, Ronkonkoma, NY, 2013, Linus Learning.

*A focused resource that provides the latest sports nutrition science, and refutes many positions held so dearly by the anti-supplement crowd.*

Williams M: *Nutrition for fitness and sport*, Boston, 2009, McGraw-Hill.

*Thorough coverage of the role nutrition plays in enhancing health, fitness, and sport performance. Current research and practical activities incorporated throughout.*

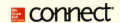

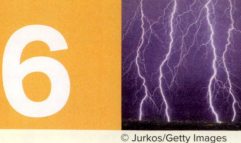
© Jurkos/Getty Images

# 6

# Environmental Considerations

## ■ Objectives

*When you finish this chapter you should be able to*

- Describe the physiology of hyperthermia.
- Recognize the clinical signs of heat stress and how they can be prevented.
- Identify the causes of hypothermia and the major cold disorders and how they can be prevented.
- Examine the problems that high altitude might present to the athlete, and explain how they can be managed.
- Review how an athlete should be protected from exposure to the sun.
- Describe precautions that should be taken in a lightning storm.
- List the problems that air pollution presents to the athlete and how they can be avoided.
- Discuss what effect circadian dysrhythmia can have on athletes and the best procedures for handling this problem.
- Compare the effect of synthetic versus natural turf on the incidence of injury.

## ■ Outline

## ■ Key Terms

hypothermia
hyponatremia
circadian dysrhythmia

hypothermia
acclimatization
SPF

## ■ Connect Highlights    connect

*Visit connect.mcgraw-hill.com for further exercises to apply your knowledge:*

- Clinical application scenarios covering physiology of hyperthermia, clinical signs of heat stress, high altitude management, circadian dysrhythmia, protection of exposure to the sun, precautions of inclement weather, and playing surfaces
- Click-and-drag questions covering heat conditions, clinical signs of heat stress and prevention, environmental conditions, and air quality
- Multiple-choice questions covering recognition and prevention of hyperthermia and heat illnesses, inclement weather, sun exposure, circadian dysrhythmia, and playing surfaces
- Selection questions covering hyponatremia, lightning safety, and prevention of heat illnesses

One of the primary responsibilities of the athletic trainer in preventing injuries is to make certain that the practice and playing environment is as safe as it can possibly be. Certainly no one has control over the weather. However, the potential dangers of having athletes engage in practices or competitions when adverse weather or environmental conditions exist cannot be ignored. Ignoring or minimizing the potential threat to the health and well-being of athletes who practice or compete under adverse environmental conditions can have serious legal consequences should a situation arise that results in injury to an athlete.

Environmental stress can adversely affect performance and in some instances can pose a serious health threat.[47] The environmental categories that are of concern to athletic trainers, particularly those involved in outdoor sports, are hyperthermia, hypothermia, altitude, exposure to the sun, lightning storms, air pollution, and circadian dysrhythmia (jet lag).

# HYPERTHERMIA

**Hyperthermia** is a condition in which, for one reason or another, body temperature is elevated. Over the years, hyperthermia has caused a number of deaths in athletes at the secondary-school, collegiate, and professional levels.[64]

It is vitally important that the athletic trainer and the coaching staff have knowledge about temperature and humidity factors to assist them in planning practice. The athletic trainer must clearly understand when environmental heat and humidity are at a dangerous level and must make recommendations to the coaches accordingly to prevent the occurrence of heat-related illnesses.[97,99] In addition, the athletic trainer must recognize and properly manage the clinical signs and symptoms of heat-related illnesses. It is the responsibility of the athletic trainer to educate relevant personnel, including coaches, administrators, security guards, EMS staff, and athletes, about preventing exertional heat-related illnesses and the policies and procedures that must be followed should they occur.[17,29] SoR:C

## Heat Stress

Regardless of the level of physical conditioning, athletes must take extreme caution when exercising in hot, humid weather. Prolonged exposure to extreme heat can result in heat illness.[17,29] Heat stress is preventable, but each year many athletes suffer illness and even death from a heat-related cause.[48] Anyone who engages in exercise in hot, humid environments is particularly vulnerable to heat stress.[33] Some athletes have medical conditions such as sickle-cell trait (see Chapter 29) which make them more susceptible to the dangers of exercising in hot humid conditions. Young athletes and elderly are particularly susceptible to heat stress.[122]

Although heat-related illnesses most often occur in hot, humid, sunny conditions, an individual training or competing in a cold environment may also be susceptible if he or she becomes dehydrated or if protective equipment does not allow heat dissipation through the sweating mechanism.[26]

The physiological processes in the body will continue to function only as long as body temperature is maintained within a normal range.[23] The maintenance of normal temperature in a hot environment depends on the body's ability to dissipate heat. Body temperature can be affected by five factors, described in the following sections.

**Metabolic Heat Production** Normal metabolic function results in the production and radiation of heat.[78] Consequently, metabolism always causes an increase in body heat that depends on the intensity of the physical activity. The higher the metabolic rate, the more heat produced.

| Heat can be gained or lost through: |
| --- |
| • Metabolic heat production |
| • Conductive heat exchange |
| • Convective heat exchange |
| • Radiant heat exchange |
| • Evaporative heat loss |

**Conductive Heat Exchange** Physical contact with other objects can result in either a heat loss or a heat gain. A football player competing on artificial turf on a sunny August afternoon experiences an increase in body temperature simply by standing on synthetic turf.

**Convective Heat Exchange** Convection occurs when a mass of either air or water moves around an individual. Body heat can be either lost or gained, depending on the temperature of the circulating medium. A cool breeze tends to cool the body by removing heat from the body surface. Conversely, if the temperature of the circulating air is higher than the temperature of the skin, body heat increases.

**Radiant Heat Exchange** Radiant heat from sunshine causes an increase in body temperature. Obviously, the effects of this radiation are much greater in the sunshine than in the shade.[45] On a cloudy day, the body also emits radiant heat energy; thus, radiation may result in either heat loss or heat gain. During exercise the body attempts to dissipate heat produced by metabolism by dilating superficial arterial and venous vessels, thus channeling blood to the superficial capillaries in the skin.

**Evaporative Heat Loss** Sweat glands in the skin allow water to be transported to the surface, where it evaporates, taking large quantities of heat with it. When the temperature and radiant heat of the environment become higher than body temperature, the loss of body heat becomes highly dependent on the process of sweat evaporation.

The rate of sweating is critical for an athlete to dissipate heat. A normal person can sweat off about 1 quart of water per hour for about 2 hours. However,

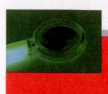

## FOCUS 6–1 Focus on Injury/Illness Prevention and Wellness Promotion

### Variations in sweat rates

Sweat rates can vary considerably from one athlete to another and are determined by a number of factors:

- Athlete's height and weight (heavier athletes sweat more)
- Degree of acclimatization (well-acclimated athletes sweat earlier and more)
- Fitness level (fit athletes sweat more)
- Hydration status (athletes who begin activity well hydrated sweat earlier)
- Environmental conditions
- Clothing
- Intensity and duration of activity
- Heredity

certain individuals can lose as much as 2 quarts of water (4 pounds) per hour.[88] *Focus Box 6–1:* "Variations in sweat rates" identifies the factors that influence sweat rates. Sweating does not cause heat loss. The sweat must evaporate for heat to be dissipated. But the air must be relatively free of water for evaporation to occur. Heat loss through evaporation is severely impaired when the relative humidity reaches 65 percent and virtually stops when the humidity reaches 75 percent.[78]

### Preventing Heat Illness

The athletic trainer should understand that heat illness is preventable if he or she exercises some common sense and caution.[18] Athletes should be encouraged to hydrate properly before, during, and after exercise, sleep at least 7 hours per night in a cool environment, eat a balanced diet, and allow 2 to 3 hours for food, fluids, electrolytes, and other nutrients to be digested and absorbed before the next practice to maximize recovery.[8,29] **SoR:C** An athlete can only perform at an optimal level when dehydration and hyperthermia are minimized by the ingestion of ample volumes of fluid during exercise and when commonsense precautions are used to keep cool.[5,89,122] (See *Focus Box 6–2:* "NATA recommendations for preventing heat illness." A link to the NATA position

| Prevention of hyperthermia: |
| --- |
| • Appropriate hydration |
| • Unrestricted fluid and electrolyte replacement |
| • Gradual acclimatization |
| • Identification of susceptible individuals |
| • Appropriate uniforms |
| • Weight records |
| • Monitoring of the heat index |

statement "Exertional heat illnesses" can be found at http://natajournals.org/doi/pdf/10.4085/1062-6050-50.9.07. The following factors should be considered when planning a training or competitive program that is likely to take place during hot weather.

**Hydration** Athletes should always begin activities in a well-hydrated state.[17,29,34] It is essential that the athlete be aware of the importance of ingesting sufficient fluids throughout the 24-hour period preceding exercise, to make certain that he or she is appropriately hydrated. Hydration status can be assessed by measuring body weight changes before and after exercise sessions, monitoring urine color and comparing with a color chart, measuring urine specific gravity (USG) using a refractometer (see Chapter 13), measuring urine volume, or using a combination of these factors.[29] Perhaps the easiest way to check this is to monitor the color of the urine. The urine should appear to be light yellow (the color of lemonade). If it is completely clear, this may indicate overhydration. Dark urine (the color of cider) indicates dehydration.

The hydration process should involve ingesting small quantities of fluid at regular intervals throughout the day rather than drinking a huge volume all at once.[66] It has been recommended that an athlete drink 17 to 20 fluid ounces of water or a sports drink 2 to 3 hours before exercise and drink another 7 to 10 fluid ounces of water or a sports drink 10 to 20 minutes before exercise.[89]

**Hyponatremia** It is possible for an athlete to overhydrate. **Hyponatremia** is a condition involving a fluid/electrolyte disorder that results in an abnormally low concentration of sodium in the blood.[29] It is most often caused by ingesting so much fluid before, during, and after exercise that the concentration of sodium is decreased.[110] It can also occur due from having too little sodium in the diet or in ingested fluids over a period

> **Hyponatremia occurs with low blood sodium levels.**

of prolonged exercise.[85] An individual with a high rate of sweating and a significant loss of sodium, who continues to ingest large quantities of fluid over a several-hour period of exercise (as in a marathon or triathlon), is particularly vulnerable to developing hyponatremia.[104] Hyponatremia can be avoided completely by making certain that fluid intake during exercise does not exceed fluid loss and that sodium intake is adequate.[85] The signs and symptoms of exertional hyponatremia are a progressively worsening headache; nausea and vomiting; swelling of the hands and feet; lethargy, apathy, or agitation; and low blood sodium (<130 mmol/L). Ultimately, a very low concentration of sodium can compromise the central nervous system, creating a life-threatening situation for the athlete.[38]

If the athletic trainer suspects hyponatremia and blood sodium levels cannot be determined on-site, measures to rehydrate the athlete should be delayed and the athlete

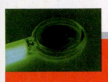

## NATA recommendations for preventing heat illness[29]

- Ensure that appropriate medical care is available.
- Conduct a thorough physician-supervised preparticipation exam to identify susceptible individuals.
- Acclimatize athletes over 7 to 14 days.
- Educate athletes and coaches regarding the prevention, recognition, and treatment of heat illnesses.
- Educate athletes to balance fluid intake with sweat and urine losses to maintain adequate hydration.
- Encourage athletes to sleep 6 to 8 hours per night in a cool environment.
- Monitor environmental conditions and develop guidelines for altering practice sessions based on those conditions.
- Provide an adequate supply of water or sports drinks to maintain hydration.

- Weigh high-risk athletes before and after practice to make certain they are not dehydrated.
- Minimize the amount of equipment and clothing worn in hot, humid conditions.
- Minimize warm-up time in hot, humid conditions.
- Allow athletes to practice in shaded areas and use cooling fans when possible.
- Have appropriate emergency equipment available (e.g., fluids, ice, immersion tank, rectal thermometer, telephone or two-way radio).

Source: Based on NATA Position Statement on Exertional Heat Illnesses, 2002. Binkley, H., Beckett, J., Casa, D., Kleiner, D., & Plummer, P. 2002. National Athletic Trainers' Association position statement: Exertional heat illnesses. *Journal of Athletic Training* 37(3):329–342.

should be transported immediately to a medical facility.[38] At the medical facility, the delivery of sodium, certain diuretics, or intravenous solutions may be necessary. A physician should clear the athlete before he or she is allowed to return to play.

**Dehydration** An athlete who does not replenish fluids is likely to become dehydrated. Whenever an individual is exercising, some dehydration will occur, because it is difficult to balance fluid loss through sweating with fluid intake. An individual is said to have mild dehydration when fluids lost are less than 2 percent of normal body weight.[29,115] SoR:B Even mild dehydration can impair cardiovascular and thermoregulatory response and can reduce the capacity for exercise and have a negative effect on performance.[34,89] Individuals who have a body mass loss of more than 2 percent are becoming dehydrated may exhibit any or all of the following symptoms and signs: thirst, dry mouth, headache, dizziness, irritability, lethargy, excessive fatigue, and possibly cramps. Obviously, an athlete who is dehydrated needs to replace fluids and should be moved to a cool environment. The athlete should rehydrate with a sports drink that contains carbohydrates and electrolytes (particularly sodium and potassium) and should not return to full activity until he or she is symptom free and has returned to normal body weight.[42] It is important to note that fluid replacement should not exceed fluid loss. Again, individuals can determine when they have reached an

> Mild dehydration is the loss of less than 2 percent of body weight.

> Fluid intake should equal fluid loss.

appropriate level of hydration by monitoring the color of their urine.

**Fluid and Electrolyte Replacement** During hot weather, it is essential that athletes continually replace fluids lost through evaporation by drinking large quantities of water or other beverages throughout the day to remain in a state of euhydration.[29,53,73,78,116] SoR:B It should also be mentioned that eating foods high in fluid content such as fruits and vegetables can also help with fluid replacement. Consuming these foods and adding salt to the meal, soup, or broth, and/or a salty snack increases the fluid retention during the rehydration process.[108] The average adult doing minimal physical activity requires at least 2.5 liters, or about 10 glasses, of water a day. A normal sweat-loss rate for a person during an hour of exercise ranges between 0.8 and 3 liters, with an average of 1.5 liters per hour. Because water is so vital, the healthy body carefully manages its internal water levels.[109] When body weight drops by 1 to 2 percent (1.5 to 3 pounds in a 150-pound individual), he or she begins to feel thirsty.[89] Drinking water and other beverages eventually returns the internal water levels to normal. However, if thirst signals are ignored and body water continues to decrease, dehydration results. People who are dehydrated cannot generate enough energy, and they feel weak. Dehydration is more likely to occur when an individual is outdoors and is sweating heavily while engaging in some strenuous activity. To prevent dehydration, an athlete should make sure to replace the lost water by drinking plenty of fluids and not relying on thirst as a signal that it's time to have a drink. By the time thirst develops, the body is already slightly dehydrated. Many people ignore their thirst, or if they do heed it, they don't drink enough, especially during physical activity. Most people replace only about 50 percent of the water they lose through sweating.[89] For this reason, athletes should consciously consume fluids before, during, and after practice and competition.[67]

Athletes must have unlimited access to fluids. There is no acceptable reason for allowing or causing an athlete to become hypohydrated.[92] Failure to permit ad libitum access to fluids not only undermine an athlete's performance but also may predispose the athlete to unnecessary heat illnesses (Figure 6–1).

A number of adverse physiological and potentially pathological effects can be caused by hypohydration, including reduced muscular strength and endurance, decreased blood and plasma volume, altered cardiac function, impaired thermoregulation, decreased kidney function, reduced glycogen stores, and loss of electrolytes.[21,92] Athletes who are taking creatine or using carbohydrate gels for energy must make certain to consume sufficient fluids to stay appropriately hydrated.[6,119]

It has been shown that replacing lost fluids with an appropriately formulated sports drink is more effective than using water alone.[89] Research has shown that because of the flavor, an athlete is likely to drink more sports drinks than plain water. In addition, sports drinks replace both the fluids and the electrolytes that are lost in sweat, and they provide energy in the form of carbohydrates to the working muscles. Water is a good thirst quencher, but it is not a good rehydrator because it actually "turns off" thirst before the body is completely rehydrated. Water also "turns on" the kidneys prematurely, so an individual loses fluid in the form of urine more quickly than when he or she is drinking a sports drink.

> Sports drinks are more effective than water for fluid replacement.

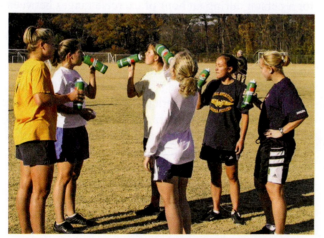

FIGURE 6–1    Athletes must have unlimited access to fluids, especially in hot weather.
© William E. Prentice

The small amount of sodium in sports drinks allows the body to hold on to the fluid consumed rather than losing it through urine.[89]

Not all sports drinks are the same. How a sports drink is formulated dictates how well it works to provide rapid rehydration and energy. The optimal level of carbohydrate is 14 grams per 8 ounces of water (6 percent carbohydrate) for the quickest fluid absorption.[42] Sports drinks or even carbohydrate gels with greater than 6 percent carbohydrate, as well as sports drinks with too little carbohydrate, are absorbed more slowly. For this reason, appropriately formulated sports drinks should be used without diluting to maximize their rate of absorption. Most sports drinks contain no carbonation or artificial preservatives, so they are satisfying during exercise and cause no stomach bloating. Also, most sports drinks contain a minimal number of calories.

It has been clearly established that sports drinks are effective for enhancing long-term endurance exercise.[17,34,109] It has also been suggested that sports drinks are effective for improving performance during both endurance activities and short-term, high-intensity activities, such as soccer, basketball, and tennis, that last from 30 minutes to an hour.[42] *Focus Box 6–3:* "Recommendations for fluid replacement" provides some suggestions for using sports drinks. A link to the NATA position statement on "Fluid replacement for athletes" can be found at https://www.nata.org/sites/default/files/fluidreplacementsforathletes.pdf.[34]

**Gradual Acclimatization** Gradual acclimatization is critical in avoiding heat stress. The first 2 to 3 weeks of preseason present the greatest risk of exertional heat illnesses, particularly in equipment-intensive sports.[29] Acclimatization should involve not only becoming accustomed to heat but also becoming acclimatized to exercising in hot temperatures.[62] A good preseason conditioning program, started well before the advent of the competitive season and carefully graded as to intensity, is recommended.[33] Progressive exposure should occur over a 7- to 14-day period.[29] **SoR:B** During the first 5 or 6 days, an 80 percent acclimatization can be achieved on the basis of a 2-hour practice period in the morning and a 2-hour practice period in the afternoon. Each practice period should be broken down into 20 minutes of work alternated with 20 minutes of rest in the shade. Equipment restrictions may help the athlete become gradually acclimated. Special considerations and modifications may be necessary for those wearing protective equipment during periods of high environmental stress.[29] **SoR:B** *Focus Box 6–4:* "NCAA-mandated guidelines for acclimatization in preseason football practices" shows how the NCAA mandates the use of equipment in preseason football. A link to the NATA consensus statement "Preseason heat acclimatization guidelines for high school athletes" can be found at www.nata.org/health-issues/heat-acclimatization.

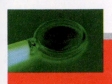

## Recommendations for fluid replacement*

- Athletes should begin all exercise sessions well hydrated[115] (determined by light yellow color of urine).
- A hydration protocol for fluid replacement should be established.
- To ensure proper hydration, the athlete should consume 17 to 20 ounces of water or a sports drink 2 to 3 hours before exercise and then 7 to 10 ounces 10 to 20 minutes before exercise.
- Fluid replacement beverages should be easily accessible during activity and should be consumed at a minimal rate of 7 to 10 ounces every 10 to 20 minutes.
- During activity, the athlete should consume the maximal amount of fluid that can be tolerated, but it is important that fluid intake does not exceed fluid loss.
- A cool, flavored beverage at refrigerator temperature is recommended.[22]

- The addition of proper amounts of carbohydrates and electrolytes to a fluid replacement solution is recommended for exercise events that last longer than 50 minutes or are intense.
- For vigorous exercise lasting less than 1 hour, the addition of carbohydrates and electrolytes does enhance physical performance.
- A 6 percent carbohydrate solution appears to be optimal (14 grams of carbohydrate per 8-ounce serving). A concentration greater than 8 percent slows gastric emptying.
- Adding a modest amount of sodium (0.3 to 0.7 gram per liter) is acceptable to stimulate thirst and increase fluid intake.

*Based on recommendations from the National Athletic Trainers' Association,[34] American College of Sports Medicine,[1] and Gatorade Sport Science Institute.[89]

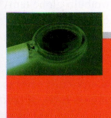

# FOCUS 6–4 Focus on Injury/Illness Prevention and Wellness Promotion

## NCAA-mandated guidelines for acclimatization in preseason football practices[92]

Equipment guidelines for preseason participation impact only days 1–5 of the acclimatization period.

Days 1–2: Single 3-hour practice *or* single 2-hour practice and single 1-hour field session; only helmets may be worn.

Days 3–4: Single 3-hour practice *or* single 2-hour practice and single 1-hour field session; only helmets and shoulder pads may be worn.

Day 5: Single 3-hour practice *or* single 2-hour practice and single 1-hour field session; full equipment may be worn.

After Day 5: One day between days with multiple practices. Less than 5 hours total practice time. Walk-through less than 2 hours.

Source: Based on National Collegiate Athletic Association (NCAA): *NCAA sports medicine handbook 2013–2014.* Indianapolis, IN: 2013, NCAA.

**Identifying Susceptible Individuals** Initially, it is essential to conduct a thorough, physician-supervised, preparticipation medical screening before the season starts to identify those athletes who may be predisposed to heat illness on the basis of risk factors and those who have a history of exertional heat illness.[17,29] **SoR:C** Athletes who are currently sick with a viral infection, have a fever, or have a serious skin rash are more susceptible to heat illnesses and should not participate until the condition is resolved.[29] **SoR:B** Athletes with a large muscle mass are particularly prone to heat illness.[33] Body build must be considered when determining individual susceptibility to heat stress. Overweight individuals may have as much as 18 percent greater heat production than underweight individuals, because metabolic heat is produced proportionately to surface area. It has been found that heat illness victims tend to be overweight. Death from heatstroke increases at a ratio of approximately four to one as body weight increases.[31]

Women are apparently more physiologically efficient at body temperature regulation than are men. Although women possess as many heat-activated sweat glands as men do, they sweat less and manifest a higher heart rate when working in heat.[78] Although slight differences exist, the same precautionary measures apply to both genders.

Other individuals who are susceptible to heat stress include the young, the elderly, those with relatively poor fitness levels, those with a history of heat illness, and anyone with a febrile condition.[92] A link to the NATA official statement "Youth football and heat related illness" can be found at https://www.nata.org/sites/default/files/heatrelatedillness.pdf.

**Heat Index**
**Temperature (°F)**

| Relative humidity (%) | 80 | 82 | 84 | 86 | 88 | 90 | 92 | 94 | 96 | 98 | 100 | 102 | 104 | 106 | 108 | 110 |
|---|---|---|---|---|---|---|---|---|---|---|---|---|---|---|---|---|
| 40 | 80 | 81 | 83 | 85 | 88 | 91 | 94 | 97 | 101 | 105 | 109 | 114 | 119 | 124 | 130 | 136 |
| 45 | 80 | 82 | 84 | 87 | 89 | 93 | 96 | 100 | 104 | 109 | 114 | 119 | 124 | 130 | 137 | |
| 50 | 81 | 83 | 85 | 88 | 91 | 95 | 99 | 103 | 108 | 113 | 118 | 124 | 131 | 137 | | |
| 55 | 81 | 84 | 86 | 89 | 93 | 97 | 101 | 106 | 112 | 117 | 124 | 130 | 137 | | | |
| 60 | 82 | 84 | 88 | 91 | 95 | 100 | 105 | 110 | 116 | 123 | 129 | 137 | | | | |
| 65 | 82 | 85 | 89 | 93 | 98 | 103 | 108 | 114 | 121 | 128 | 136 | | | | | |
| 70 | 83 | 86 | 90 | 95 | 100 | 105 | 112 | 119 | 126 | 134 | | | | | | |
| 75 | 84 | 88 | 92 | 97 | 103 | 109 | 116 | 124 | 132 | | | | | | | |
| 80 | 84 | 89 | 94 | 100 | 106 | 113 | 121 | 129 | | | | | | | | |
| 85 | 85 | 90 | 96 | 102 | 110 | 117 | 126 | 135 | | | | | | | | |
| 90 | 86 | 91 | 98 | 105 | 113 | 122 | 131 | | | | | | | | | |
| 95 | 86 | 93 | 100 | 108 | 117 | 127 | | | | | | | | | | |
| 100 | 87 | 95 | 103 | 112 | 121 | 132 | | | | | | | | | | |

**Likelihood of Heat Disorders with Prolonged Exposure or Strenuous Activity**

☐ **Caution** ☐ **Extreme caution** ☐ **Danger** ☐ **Extreme danger**

FIGURE 6–2    Heat Index.
Courtesy of the National Weather Service and National Oceanic and Atmospheric Administration.

**Selecting Appropriate Uniforms** Uniforms should be selected on the basis of temperature and humidity. Initial practices should be conducted in short-sleeved T-shirts, shorts, and socks, and athletes should be moved gradually into short-sleeved net jerseys, lightweight pants, and socks as acclimatization proceeds. All early-season practices and games should be conducted in lightweight uniforms with short-sleeved net jerseys and socks. The use of dark-colored clothing or uniforms should be discouraged. Rubberized suits should never be used.[92]

**Maintaining Weight Records** Careful weight records of all players must be kept. Weights should be measured both before and after practice for at least the first 2 weeks of practice or as long as hot, humid conditions persist. If a sudden increase in temperature or humidity occurs during the season, weight should be recorded again for a period of time. A loss of greater than 2 percent of body weight indicates that the athlete is severely dehydrated and should be held out of practice until normal body weight has returned.[29,122] SoR:B A weight gain during a practice or event may indicate that the athlete is overdrinking and should limit fluid intake and consume salty foods prior to the next weight in.[58]

**Monitoring the Heat Index** The athletic trainer must exercise common sense when overseeing the health care of athletes who are training or competing in the heat. Obviously, when the combination of heat, humidity, and bright sunshine is present, extra caution is warranted (Figure 6–2). A preseason heat acclimatization policy should be developed for organized sports and event

guidelines formulated for hot, humid weather conditions based on the type of activity and the wetbulb globe temperature index (WBGT).[31] SoR:B The universal WBGT index provides the athletic trainer with an objective means for determining necessary precautions for practice and competition in hot weather.[20] A digital psychrometer is used to determine the index and incorporates several different temperature measurements (Figure 6–3). A dry bulb temperature (DBT) is recorded from a standard mercury thermometer. A wet bulb temperature (WBT) uses

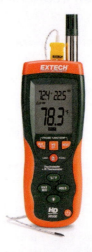

FIGURE 6–3    Digital psychrometer. Used to determine the WBGT heat index.
Courtesy ExTech

a wet wick or piece of gauze wrapped around the end of a thermometer. A globe temperature (GT) measures the sun's radiation and has a black metal casing around the end of the thermometer. Once the three measurements have been taken, the following formula is used to calculate the WBGT index:

$$WBGT = [0.1 \times DBT] + [0.7 \times WBT] + [GT \times 0.2]$$

If only web bulb and dry bulb temperatures are taken, the WBGT index is calculated using the following modified formula:

$$WBGT = [0.3 \times DBT] + [0.7 \times WBT]$$

Using this formula yields a universally accepted WBGT index (Table 6–1), on which recommendations on work periods, rest periods and fluid replacement relative to outdoor activity are based. Rest breaks should be in the shade or in a cooling zone and should allow enough time for all athletes to consume fluids. Players should be permitted to remove equipment (e.g., helmets) during rest periods.[29] **SoR:B** Table 6–2 is a modification of the WBGT index that indicates activity restrictions for outdoor physical conditioning in hot weather.

Newer psychrometers use digital sensors. Recording the temperature requires about 90 seconds.

| TABLE 6–1 | Universal WBGT Index Fluid Replacement Recommendations | | | | | | |
|---|---|---|---|---|---|---|---|
| | | Easy Work | | Moderate Work | | Hard Work | |
| Heat Category | WBGT °F | Work/Rest* | Water per Hour | Work/Rest* | Water per Hour | Work/Rest* | Water per Hour |
| 1 | 78–81.9 | No limit | 1/2 qt | No limit | 3/4 qt | 40/20 min | 3/4 qt |
| 2 | 82–84.9 | No limit | 1/2 qt | 50/10 min | 3/4 qt | 30/30 min | 1 qt |
| 3 | 85–87.9 | No limit | 3/4 qt | 40/20 min | 3/4 qt | 30/30 min | 1 qt |
| 4 | 88–89.9 | No limit | 3/4 qt | 30/30 min | 3/4 qt | 20/40 min | 1 qt |
| 5 | ≥90 | 50/10 min | 1 qt | 20/40 min | 1 qt | 10/50 min | 1 qt |

*Rest means minimal physical activity (sitting or standing) and should be accomplished in the shade if possible.

| TABLE 6–2 | Activity Restrictions for Outdoor Physical Conditioning in Hot Weather | |
|---|---|---|
| WBGT* (° F) | Flag Color† | Precautionary Actions‡ |
| <80° F | **White** | No precautions necessary |
| 80°–85° F | Green | Take at least 15 minutes of breaks each hour if working or exercising in direct sunlight |
| 85°–88° F | Yellow | Take at least 30 minutes of breaks each hour if working or exercising in direct sunlight |
| 88°–90° F | Red | Take at least 40 minutes of breaks each hour if working or exercising in direct sunlight |
| >90° F | **Black** | Take at least 45 minutes of breaks each hour if working or exercising in direct sunlight |

From The National Weather Service, National Oceanic and Atmospheric Administration (NOAA), U.S. Department of Commerce.

*WGBT is wet bulb globe temperature.
Calculation of WBGT: $0.7\ T_{wb} + 0.2\ T_{bg} + 0.1\ T_{db}$, where $T_{wb}$ is wet bulb temperature; $T_{bg}$ is black globe temperature; $T_{db}$ is dry bulb temperature.
†Flag color indicates a warning flag, which is placed in a location visible from a practice field, that is used to notify everyone using that facility what the conditions are and the restrictions that should be applied.
‡Guidelines assume that athletes are wearing summer-weight clothing and that all activities are constantly supervised by an athletic trainer to assure early detection of problems. When equipment must be worn, as in football, please use guidelines one step below. For example, if WBGT is 86° F (yellow), then use the guidelines for red.

A digital psychrometer is relatively inexpensive and easy to use.

## Recognizing and Managing Heat Illnesses

In 2015, an updated and revised NATA Position Statement "Exertional Heat Illnesses" was released (http://natajournals.org/doi/pdf/10.4085/1062-6050-50.9.07).[29] Exercising in a hot, humid environment can cause various forms of heat illness, including heat rash, heat syncope, exercise-associated muscle (heat) cramps, exertional heat exhaustion, and exertional heatstroke.[6,10,12,68,95] Appropriate medical care must be available, and all personnel must be familiar with prevention, recognition, and treatment of exertional heat illness.[96] Certified athletic trainers have the authority to restrict an athlete from participating if exertional heat illness is suspected.[32] **SoR:C**

**Heat Rash** Heat rash, also called prickly heat, is a benign condition associated with a red, raised rash accompanied by sensations of prickling and tingling during sweating. It usually occurs when the skin is continuously wet with unevaporated sweat. The rash is generally localized to areas of the body that are covered with clothing. Continually toweling the body can help prevent the rash from developing.[41]

**Heat Syncope** Heat syncope, or heat collapse, is associated with rapid physical fatigue during overexposure to heat. It is usually caused by standing in heat for long periods or by not being accustomed to exercising in the heat. It is caused by peripheral vasodilation of superficial vessels, hypotension, or a pooling of blood in the extremities, which results in dizziness, nausea, and fainting (loss of consciousness). Heat syncope is quickly relieved by laying the athlete down in a cool environment, elevating the lower extremities, and replacing fluids.[17] **SoR:B**

**Exercise-Associated Muscle (Heat) Cramps** Exercise-associated muscle (heat) cramps are extremely painful muscle cramps that occur during or after exercise most commonly in the calf and abdomen, although any muscle can be involved (Table 6–3).[35] Other symptoms may include pain, dehydration, thirst, sweating, or fatigue.[107] **SoR:C**

The occurrence of heat cramps has been traditionally attributed to excessive loss of water and depletion of electrolytes or ions (sodium, chloride, potassium, magnesium, and calcium). Profuse sweating involving losses of large amounts of water and small quantities of these ions was hypothesized to interfere with the concentration of these elements within the body resulting in painful muscle contractions and cramps.[65] More recent evidence suggests that cramping may more likely be due to altered neuromuscular control that occurs with muscle overload and fatigue rather than a fluid and/or electrolyte imbalance.[61,102] Muscle cramps appear to occur most often in those muscle groups under high demand during the activity.[61] Muscle fatigue alters neuromuscular control by increasing muscle spindle activity while decreasing Golgi tendon organ activity, thereby facilitating a reflex contraction or cramp of the muscle.[102]

Currently there are no well-designed randomized, controlled studies that have identified effective prevention measures for exercise-associated muscle cramps.[29] Although ingestion of fluids and electrolytes may not necessarily prevent muscle cramps, it is certainly critical in preventing other exertional heat illnesses.[10,16] Avoiding fatigue and overexertion during exercise may reduce the likelihood of altered neuromuscular control.[15,107] The most current recommendation for immediate treatment of exercise-associated muscle cramps is ingestion of fluids, preferably a sports drink, and mild, prolonged stretching with ice massage of the muscle in cramp.[15] **SoR:B** An athlete who experiences muscle cramps may have difficulty returning to practice or competition for the remainder of the day, because cramping is likely to reoccur with physical exertion.[74] **SoR:B**

**Exertional Heat Exhaustion** Exertional heat exhaustion is a more moderate form of heat illness that occurs from environmental heat stress and strenuous physical exercise. In exertional heat exhaustion, an athlete becomes de-

> Exertional heat exhaustion results from dehydration.

hydrated to the point that he or she is unable to sustain adequate cardiac output and thus cannot continue intense exercise. Mild hyperthermia is characteristic of heat exhaustion, with a rectal temperature of less than 105°F and no evidence of central nervous system

> Measuring rectal temperature is critical to differentiate heat exhaustion from heatstroke.

(CNS) dysfunction.[55] The assessment of rectal temperature is the clinical gold standard for obtaining core body temperature of patients with exertional heat illnesses.[27] **SoR:A** Obtaining an accurate rectal temperature measurement is essential for the athletic trainer to differentiate between heat exhaustion and heatstroke.[29] **SoR:A** Rectal temperature is core temperature. Measuring temperature at any other site with any other type of thermometer will not provide a sufficiently accurate reading.[55,77] See *Focus Box 6–5:* "Measuring rectal temperature" for a description of the procedure. An athlete who is experiencing heat exhaustion shows signs and symptoms of dehydration and/or electrolyte depletion, including pale skin; profuse sweating; stomach cramps with nausea, vomiting, or diarrhea; headache; persistent muscle cramps; and dizziness with loss of coordination.[17]

An athlete who has exertional heat exhaustion must be immediately removed from play and taken to a shaded or air-conditioned area. Excess clothing or equipment should be removed, and the athlete should lie down with his or her legs elevated.[29] **SoR:C** Cooling efforts

| TABLE 6–3 | Heat Disorders | | | |
|---|---|---|---|---|
| **Disorder** | **Cause** | **Clinical Features and Diagnosis** | **Prevention** | **Treatment** |
| Heat syncope | Rapid physical fatigue during overexposure to heat | Pooling of blood in extremities, leading to dizziness, fainting, and nausea | Gradually acclimatize to exercising in a hot, humid environment | Lying down in a cool environment, replenishing fluids |
| Exercise-associated muscle (heat) cramps | Hard work in heat, sweating heavily, imbalance between water and electrolytes (sodium) | Muscle twitching and cramps, usually after midday; occurs in arms, legs, and abdomen | Acclimatize athlete properly; provide large quantities of fluids; increase intake of calcium, sodium, and potassium slightly | Ingesting large amounts of salty fluid, mild stretching, ice massage of affected muscle |
| Exertional heat exhaustion | Prolonged sweating leading to dehydration and an inability to sustain adequate cardiac output | Excessive thirst, dry tongue and mouth, weight loss, fatigue, weakness, incoordination, mental dullness, low urine volume, slightly elevated body temperature, high serum protein and sodium, reduced swelling | Supply adequate fluids; provide adequate rest and opportunity for cooling | Bed rest in cool room, IV fluids if drinking is impaired; increase fluid intake to 6 to 8 L/day; sponge with cool water; keep records of body weight and fluid balance; provide semiliquid food until salination is normal |
| Exertional heatstroke | Thermoregulatory failure of sudden onset | Abrupt onset; CNS abnormalities, including headache, vertigo, and fatigue; flushed skin; relatively less sweating than seen with heat exhaustion; rapidly increasing pulse rate that may reach 160 to 180; increased respiration; blood pressure seldom rises; rapid rise in temperature to 104°F (40°C); athlete feels as if he or she is burning up; diarrhea, vomiting; can lead to permanent brain damage; circulatory collapse may produce death | Ensure proper acclimatization and proper hydration; educate those supervising activities conducted in the heat; adapt activities to the environment; screen participants with history of heat illness for malignant hyperthermia | Take immediate emergency measures to reduce temperature below 102°F within 30 minutes of collapse (e.g., immersion in ice-water bath or sponge cool water and air fan over body, massage limbs); remove to hospital as soon as possible |

Source: Modified from Berkow, R: *The Merck manual of diagnosis and therapy,* ed. 14, Rahway, NJ: Merck & Co, 1982.

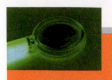

## Measuring rectal temperature

Monitoring temperature with a thermometer inserted into the rectum is the most exact way of determining core temperature. Normal rectal temperature is 99.6°F (37.5°C).

- When using a glass thermometer shake the thermometer down to below the 97.8°F mark (36.18°C).
- Cover the tip of the glass thermometer or a flexible digital thermometer with lubricating or petroleum jelly.

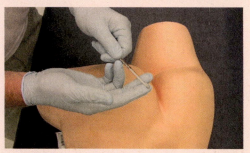

© William E. Prentice

- Place the athlete on his or her stomach with one leg flexed.
- Spread the buttocks and gently insert the thermometer 3 to 4 inches (8 to 10 cm) into the rectum. Never force it. Hold the buttocks together to keep the thermometer in place.
- If using a flexible digital thermometer tape can be used to secure it in place.

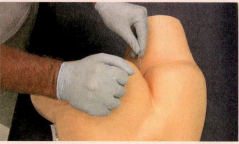

© William E. Prentice

- Do not release your grip on a glass thermometer.
- Leave the thermometer in place for 3 minutes.
- To read the temperature on a glass thermometer, slowly turn the thermometer until you can see the line of mercury.
- Wash the thermometer carefully in soap and warm water after each use. Store in a safe place.

intravenous fluid replacement should be initiated by a physician. Same-day return to activity is not recommended and should be avoided.[8] **SoR:C** The athletic trainer should continually monitor heart rate, blood pressure, and core temperature. If rapid improvement is not observed, the athlete must be transported to an emergency facility. Exertional heat exhaustion, if not properly managed, can progress to exertional heatstroke. Before returning to play, the athlete must be completely rehydrated and should be cleared by a physician.

**Exertional Heatstroke** Unlike heat cramps and exertional heat exhaustion, exertional heatstroke is a serious, life-threatening emergency (Table 6–3).[35,75] It is the most severe form of heat illness and is induced by strenuous physical exercise and increased environmental heat stress. It is characterized by CNS dysfunction and potential tissue damage resulting from a significantly elevated body temperature.[30] As body temperature rises, extreme circulatory and metabolic stresses can produce damage and severe physiological dysfunction, which can ultimately result in death.[52]

Heatstroke can occur suddenly and without warning.[75] The specific cause of heatstroke is unknown. It is clinically characterized by sudden collapse with CNS dysfunction, such as altered consciousness, seizures, confusion, emotional instability, irrational behavior, or decreased mental acuity. Measured rectal or gastrointestinal temperature is 105°F or higher.[29] **SoR:B** Additionally, the victim is flushed and has hot skin, with sweating about 75 percent of the time, although about 25 percent of the cases have less sweating than would be seen with heat exhaustion.

A wrestler collapses during a match and exhibits signs of profuse sweating, pale skin, mildly elevated temperature (102° F), dizziness, hyperventilation, and rapid pulse. When questioned by the athletic trainer, the wrestler indicates that earlier in the day he took diuretic medication to facilitate water loss in an effort to help him make weight.

**?** What type of heat illness is the athlete experiencing, and what does the athletic trainer need to do to manage this situation appropriately?

A high-school football team is doing conditioning outside. The temperature is 80°F with 85 percent humidity. The players have their helmets on and are running 100-yard sprints. One player looks like he is becoming fatigued and slightly disoriented. Thirty yards into the sprint, the athlete collapses.

**?** What is the immediate course of action to treat this athlete? What is wrong with the athlete?

**Heatstroke is a life-threatening emergency.**

should continue until rectal temperature has lowered to 102°F. Rehydration should begin immediately with water or a sports drink as long as the athlete is not nauseated or vomiting. If the athlete cannot take fluids orally,

Other symptoms include shallow, fast breathing; a rapid, strong pulse; nausea, vomiting, or diarrhea; headache, dizziness, or weakness; decreased blood pressure; and dehydration.[29] **SoR:A** The heatstroke victim experiences a breakdown of the thermoregulatory mechanism due to excessively high body temperature, and the body loses the ability to dissipate heat through sweating.[86]

The possibility of death from heatstroke can be significantly reduced if the victim's body temperature is lowered to 102°F or less within 30 minutes after collapse.[3,29] **SoR:B** The longer that the body temperature is elevated to 105°F or higher, the higher the mortality rate.[29] **SoR:B** Thus, the key to managing this condition is aggressive and immediate whole-body cooling.[79,80] After determining rectal temperature and assessing airway, breathing, and circulation, **immediately immerse the athlete in a cold water bath** (35–58°F) up to their neck, and then remove equipment and clothing.[82] **SoR:B**[28,39,56,102] **SoR:B** If it is not possible to immerse the athlete in cold water, sponge him or her down with cool water and fan with a towel.[111] Also ice bags may be placed at the neck, and over other major arterial vessels.[114] **SoR:B** Call the rescue squad. It is imperative that the victim be transported to a hospital as quickly as possible. However, it is recommended that the victim be cooled down first until the temperature is lowered to 102°F and then transported if on-site rapid cooling and adequate medical supervision are available.[53,76] **SoR:B** If rescue squad transport is delayed, it may be necessary to transport the victim in whatever vehicle happens to be available. Following exertional heatstroke, the athlete should avoid exercise until asymptomatic and gradually return to full practice after being cleared by a physician.

Patients with exertional heat stroke who are immediately cooled can be sent home on the same day. They may be able to resume modified activity within 1 month with a physician's clearance. However, if immediate treatment is delayed longer than 30 minutes, patients may experience residual complications for months or years after the event.[29] **SoR:C**

In all cases, after a 7- to 21-day rest period and physician clearance, the patient can begin a progression of physical activity, in a temperate environment, with equipment added gradually. The ability to progress depends largely on whether the patient experiences any negative symptoms with training.[80] **SoR:C**

***Malignant Hyperthermia*** Malignant hyperthermia is a rare, genetically inherited muscle disorder that causes hypersensitivity to anesthesia and extreme exercise in hot environments.[23] It is characterized by muscle breakdown.[69] This disorder causes muscle temperatures to increase faster than core temperature, and its symptoms are similar to those of heatstroke. The athlete complains of muscle pain after exercise, and rectal temperature remains elevated for 10 to 15 minutes after exercise. During this period, muscle tissue is destroyed and products of muscle breakdown may damage the kidneys and cause acute renal failure.[87] The condition may be fatal if not treated immediately. Muscle biopsy is necessary for diagnosis. Athletes with malignant hyperthermia should be disqualified from competing in hot, humid environments.[69]

***Acute Exertional Rhabdomyolysis*** Acute exertional rhabdomyolysis is a syndrome characterized by sudden catabolic destruction and degeneration of skeletal muscle accompanied by leakage of myoglobin (muscle protein) and muscle enzymes into the vascular system.[11] It can occur in healthy individuals during intense exercise in extremely hot and humid environmental conditions. It can result in the gradual onset of muscle weakness, swelling, and pain and the presence of darkened urine and renal dysfunction; in severe cases, the individual experiences sudden collapse, renal failure, and death. Rhabdomyolysis has been associated with individuals with sickle-cell trait.[23] If rhabdomyolysis is suspected, the athlete should be referred to a physician immediately.

## Clinical Indications and Treatment

*Focus Box 6–6:* "Environmental conduct of sports, particularly football" lists the clinical symptoms of the various hyperthermia conditions and the indications for treatment. Although the Focus Box calls particular attention to some of the procedures for football, the precautions in general apply to all sports. Because of the specialized equipment worn by the players, football requires special consideration. Many football uniforms are heat traps, compounding the environmental heat problem, which is not true of lighter uniforms.[10]

## Guidelines for Athletes Who Intentionally Lose Weight

Wrestlers or other athletes who purposely dehydrate themselves as a means of making weight are predisposing themselves to heat-related illness and may, in fact, be creating a potentially life-threatening situation. Weight loss to make a predetermined weight limit should not be accomplished through dehydration. The process must be gradual over a period of several weeks, or even months, and should result from a reduction in the percentage of body fat relative to lean body mass. The NCAA and many state high-school federations have established guidelines for weight loss and set policies for how and when a wrestler can weigh in officially.[90]

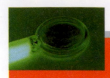

## Environmental conduct of sports, particularly football

I. General warning
   A. Most adverse reactions to environmental heat and humidity occur during the first few days of training.
   B. It is necessary to become thoroughly acclimatized to heat to successfully compete in hot or humid environments.
   C. Occurrence of a heat injury indicates poor supervision of the sports program.

II. Athletes who are most susceptible to heat injury
   A. Individuals unaccustomed to working in the heat
   B. Overweight individuals, particularly large linemen
   C. Eager athletes who constantly compete at capacity
   D. Ill athletes who have an infection, a fever, or a gastrointestinal disturbance
   E. Athletes who receive immunization injections and subsequently develop temperature elevations

III. Prevention of heat injury
   A. Take a complete medical history and provide a physical examination.
      1. Include a history of previous heat illnesses or fainting in the heat.
      2. Include an inquiry about sweating and peripheral vascular defects.
   B. Evaluate general physical condition and type and duration of training activities for previous month.
      1. Extent of work in the heat
      2. General training activities
   C. Measure temperature and humidity on the practice or playing fields (WBGT index).
      1. Make measurements before and during training or competitive sessions.
      2. Adjust activity level to environmental conditions.
         a. Decrease activity if hot or humid.
         b. Eliminate unnecessary clothing when hot or humid.
   D. Acclimatize athletes to heat gradually.
      1. Acclimatization to heat requires work in the heat.
         a. Use recommended type and variety of warm-weather workouts for preseason training.
         b. Provide graduated training program for first 7 to 14 days and on other abnormally hot or humid days.
      2. Adequate rest intervals and fluid replacement should be provided during the acclimatization period.
   E. Monitor body weight loss during activity in the heat.
      1. Body fluid should be replaced as it is lost.
         a. Allow additional fluid as desired by players.
         b. Provide salt on training tables (no salt tablets should be taken).
         c. Weigh athletes each day before and after training or competition.
            (1) Treat athlete who loses excessive weight each day.
            (2) Treat well-conditioned athlete who continues to lose weight for several days.
   F. Monitor clothing and uniforms.
      1. Provide lightweight clothing that is loose-fitting at the neck, waist, and sleeves; use shorts and T-shirt at beginning of training.
      2. Avoid excessive padding and taping.
      3. Avoid the use of long stockings, long sleeves, double jerseys, and other excess clothing.
      4. Avoid the use of rubberized clothing or sweatsuits.
      5. Provide clean clothing daily–all items.
   G. Provide rest periods to dissipate accumulated body heat.
      1. Rest athletes in cool, shaded area with some air movement.
      2. Avoid hot brick walls and hot benches.
      3. Instruct athletes to loosen or remove jerseys or other garments.
      4. Provide fluids during the rest period.
      5. Remove helmets or other headgear.

IV. Trouble signs: Stop activity!

| Headache | Visual | Unsteadiness | Diarrhea | Weak, rapid | Faintness |
| Nausea | disturbance | Collapse | Cramps | pulse | Chill |
| Mental slowness | Fatigue | Unconsciousness | Seizures | Pallor | Cyanotic |
| Incoherence | Weakness | Vomiting | Rigidity | Flush | appearance |

Source: Data from ER Buskirk and WC Grasley, Human Performance Laboratory, The Athletic Institute, The Pennsylvania State University.

# HYPOTHERMIA

## Cold Stress

Cold weather is a frequent adjunct to many outdoor sports in which the sport itself does not require heavy, protective clothing; consequently, the weather becomes a pertinent factor in injury susceptibility.[83] In most instances, the activity itself enables the athlete to increase the metabolic rate sufficiently to function physically in a normal manner and dissipate the resulting heat and perspiration through the usual physiological mechanisms.[19] An athlete may fail to warm up sufficiently or may become chilled because of relative inactivity for varying periods of time demanded by the sport, during either competition or training; consequently, the athlete is exceedingly prone to injury.[24] Low temperatures alone can pose some problems, but when such temperatures are further accentuated by wind, the chill factor becomes critical (Figure 6–4).[83] For example, a runner proceeding at a pace of 10 mph directly into a wind of 5 mph creates a chill factor equivalent to a 15 mph headwind.

A third factor, dampness or wetness, further increases the risk of hypothermia. Air at a temperature of 50°F is relatively comfortable, but water at the same temperature is intolerable. The combination of cold, wind, and dampness creates an environment that easily predisposes the athlete to hypothermia.[105]

> Low temperatures accentuated by wind and dampness can pose major problems for athletes.

Sixty-five percent of the heat produced by the body is lost through radiation. This loss occurs most often from the warm, vascular areas of the head and neck, which may account for as much as 50 percent of total heat loss.[91] Twenty percent of heat loss is through evaporation, of which two-thirds is through the skin and one-third is through the respiratory tract.[19]

As an athlete's muscular fatigue builds up during strenuous physical activity in cold weather, the rate of exercise begins to drop and may reach a level at which the body heat loss to the environment exceeds the metabolic heat production, resulting in definite impairment of neuromuscular responses and exhaustion.[19] A relatively small drop in body core temperature can induce shivering sufficient to materially affect an athlete's neuromuscular coordination. Shivering ceases below a body temperature of 85°F to 90°F (29.4°C to 32.2°C). Death is imminent if the core temperature drops to between 77°F and 85°F (25°C and 29°C).

## Prevention

Prevention should begin with identifying those athletes through medical history who have risk factors that could potentially predispose them to injuries related to cold exposure.[24] SoR:C Athletes and coaches should be educated to recognize and treat cold injury and the risks associated with activity in cold environments.[36] SoR:C Develop event and practice guidelines that include recommendations for managing athletes who are participating in cold, windy, and wet conditions.[24] SoR:C

Apparel for competitors must be geared to the weather.[7] The functions of such apparel are to provide a semitropical microclimate for the body and to prevent chilling. Several fabrics available on the market are waterproof and windproof but permit the passage of heat and allow sweat to evaporate. The clothing should not restrict movement, should be as lightweight as possible, and should consist of material that will permit the free passage of sweat and body heat that would otherwise accumulate on the skin or the clothing and provide a chilling factor when activity ceases. An individual should routinely dress in thin

> Dress in thin layers of clothing that can be added and removed.

### Temperature (°F)

| Wind (mph) \ Calm | 40 | 35 | 30 | 25 | 20 | 15 | 10 | 5 | 0 | −5 | −10 | −15 | −20 | −25 | −30 | −35 | −40 | −45 |
|---|---|---|---|---|---|---|---|---|---|---|---|---|---|---|---|---|---|---|
| 5 | 36 | 31 | 25 | 19 | 13 | 7 | 1 | −5 | −11 | −16 | −22 | −28 | −34 | −40 | −46 | −52 | −57 | −63 |
| 10 | 34 | 27 | 21 | 15 | 9 | 3 | −4 | −10 | −16 | −22 | −28 | −35 | −41 | −47 | −53 | −59 | −66 | −72 |
| 15 | 32 | 25 | 19 | 13 | 6 | 0 | −7 | −13 | −19 | −26 | −32 | −39 | −45 | −51 | −58 | −64 | −71 | −77 |
| 20 | 30 | 24 | 17 | 11 | 4 | −2 | −9 | −15 | −22 | −29 | −35 | −42 | −48 | −55 | −61 | −68 | −74 | −81 |
| 25 | 29 | 23 | 16 | 9 | 3 | −4 | −11 | −17 | −24 | −31 | −37 | −44 | −51 | −58 | −64 | −71 | −78 | −84 |
| 30 | 28 | 22 | 15 | 8 | 1 | −5 | −12 | −19 | −26 | −33 | −39 | −46 | −53 | −60 | −67 | −73 | −80 | −87 |
| 35 | 28 | 21 | 14 | 7 | 0 | −7 | −14 | −21 | −27 | −34 | −41 | −48 | −55 | −62 | −69 | −76 | −82 | −89 |
| 40 | 27 | 20 | 13 | 6 | −1 | −8 | −15 | −22 | −29 | −36 | −43 | −50 | −57 | −64 | −71 | −78 | −84 | −91 |
| 45 | 26 | 19 | 12 | 5 | −2 | −9 | −16 | −23 | −30 | −37 | −44 | −51 | −58 | −65 | −72 | −79 | −86 | −93 |
| 50 | 26 | 19 | 12 | 4 | −3 | −10 | −17 | −24 | −31 | −38 | −45 | −52 | −60 | −67 | −74 | −81 | −88 | −95 |
| 55 | 25 | 18 | 11 | 4 | −3 | −11 | −18 | −25 | −32 | −39 | −46 | −54 | −61 | −68 | −75 | −82 | −89 | −97 |
| 60 | 25 | 17 | 10 | 3 | −4 | −11 | −19 | −26 | −33 | −40 | −48 | −55 | −62 | −69 | −76 | −84 | −91 | −98 |

Frostbite times: ▮ 30 minutes  ▮ 10 minutes  ▮ 5 minutes

**FIGURE 6–4** Low temperatures can pose serious problems for the athlete, but wind chill can be a critical factor.
Courtesy of the National Weather Service and National Oceanic and Atmospheric Administration

layers of clothing that can easily be added or removed as the temperature decreases or increases.[91] Continuous adjustment of these layers will reduce sweating and the likelihood that clothing will become damp or wet. Again, wetness or dampness plays a critical role in the development of hypothermia. To prevent chilling, athletes should wear warm-up suits before exercising, during activity breaks or rest periods, and at the termination of exercise. A hat should also be worn to limit heat loss from the head. Activity in cold, wet, and windy weather poses some problems because such weather reduces the insulating value of clothing; consequently, the individual may be unable to achieve energy levels equal to the subsequent body heat losses. Runners who wish to continue outdoor work in cold weather should use lightweight insulating clothing and, if breathing cold air seems distressful, should use ski goggles and a ski face mask or should cover the mouth and nose with a free-hanging cloth.[7]

Inadequate clothing, improper warm-up, and a high chill factor form a triad that can lead to musculoskeletal injury, chilblains, frostbite, or the minor respiratory disorders associated with lower tissue temperatures.[2] For work or sports in temperatures below 32°F (0°C), it is advisable to add a layer of protective clothing for every 5 mph of wind.[91]

As is true in a hot environment, athletes exercising in a cold environment need to replace fluids. Dehydration causes reduced blood volume, which means less fluid is available for warming the tissues.[24,78,82] **SoR:C** Athletes performing in a cold environment should be weighed before and after practice, especially in the first 2 weeks of the season.[36] Severe overexposure to a cold climate occurs less often than hyperthermia does in a warm climate; however, it is still a major risk of winter sports, long-distance running in cold weather, and swimming in cold water.[7]

## Mild Hypothermia

The signs and symptoms of hypothermia include vigorous shivering, increased blood pressure, fine motor skill impairment, lethargy, apathy, and mild amnesia. In mild hypothermia, rectal temperature will be between 98.66°F and 95.6°F.[24] **SoR:A**

Treatment of mild hypothermia involves moving the individual to a warm dry environment, removing wet or damp clothing, and using blankets for rewarming. When rewarming, apply heat only to the trunk and other areas of heat transfer, including the axilla, chest wall, and groin. Massaging the extremities could cause *afterdrop* in which cool blood from the extremities cools the core leading to a drop in core temperature. Provide warm, nonalcoholic fluids and foods containing 6 percent to 8 percent carbohydrates to help sustain shivering.[24,60,81] **SoR:C**

## Moderate/Severe Hypothermia

The signs and symptoms of moderate and severe hypothermia, which may include cessation of shivering, very cold skin upon palpation, and depressed vital signs progressing to impaired mental function, slurred speech, unconsciousness, gross motor skill impairment, and arrhythmia in severe hypothermia. In moderate hypothermia rectal temperature will be between 90.6°F and 95.6°F, or below 90.6°F (32.6°C) for severe hypothermia.[24,44,81] **SoR:A**

Treatment is the same as for mild hypothermia, except the patient may require CPR and transport to a medical care facility.[24] **SoR:C**

## Common Cold Injuries

Local cooling of the body can result in tissue damage ranging from superficial to deep. Exposure to a damp, freezing cold can cause frost nip. In contrast, exposure to dry temperatures well below freezing more commonly produces a deep, freezing type of frostbite.[36]

Below-freezing temperatures may cause ice crystals to form between or

> **Cold injuries in sports:**
> - Frost nip
> - Chilbain
> - Frostbite

within the cells and may eventually destroy the cells. Local capillaries can be injured, blood clots may form, and blood may be shunted away from the injury site to ensure the survival of the nonaffected tissue.[19]

**Frost Nip** Frost nip affects the ears, nose, cheeks, chin, fingers, and toes. It commonly occurs when there is a high wind, severe cold, or both. The skin initially appears very firm, with cold, painless areas that may peel or blister in 24 to 72 hours. Affected areas can be treated early by firm, sustained pressure of the hand (without rubbing), by blowing hot breath on the spot, or if the injury is to the fingertips, by placing them in the armpits.

**Chilblain** *Chilblain* results from prolonged and constant exposure to cold for more than 60 minutes with the temperature at 50°F or less. In time, there is skin redness, swelling, tingling, and pain in the toes and fingers.[113] **SoR:A** Treatment involves removing wet or constrictive clothing and covering with warm, loose, dry clothing or blankets. Do not disturb blisters, apply friction massage, apply creams or lotions, or use high levels of heat. Continually monitor the affected area for return of circulation and sensation.[113] **SoR:C** This adverse response is caused by problems of peripheral circulation and can be avoided by preventing further cold exposure.

**Superficial Frostbite** *Superficial frostbite* involves only the skin and subcutaneous tissue. Symptoms include edema, redness or mottled gray skin appearance, stiffness, and transient tingling or burning.[24] **SoR:A** Palpating the injured area will reveal a sense of hardness but with yielding of the underlying deeper tissue structures. When rewarming, by immersing the area in warm water (98°F to 104°F), the superficial frostbite will at first feel numb, then will sting and burn. Once rewarming has begun, it is recommended that affected tissue not be allowed to refreeze, as tissue necrosis can result.[24] **SoR:C**. Avoid a friction massage of the affected area. Later the area may produce blisters, which should be left intact.[19]

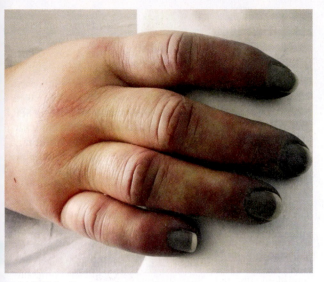

FIGURE 6–5   Frostbite on fingertips.
© William E. Prentice

**Deep Frostbite** *Deep frostbite* is a serious injury, in which tissues are frozen. This medical emergency requires immediate hospitalization.[64] As with frost nip and superficial frostbite, the tissue is initially cold, hard, pale or white, and numb.[24] **SoR:A** Gradual rewarming is required, including hot drinks, heating pads, or hot water bottles. The affected tissue should be immersed in a warm water bath (98°F to 104°F). During rewarming, the tissue becomes blotchy red, swollen, and extremely painful. As with superficial frostbite do not use friction massage, leave blisters intact, and avoid the use of alcohol. Later the injury may develop necrosis causing a loss of tissue (Figure 6–5). A link to the NATA position statement "Environmental cold injuries" can be found at www.nata.org/sites/default/files/EnvironmentalColdInjuries.pdf.

# ALTITUDE SICKNESS

Most athletic events are not conducted at extreme altitudes. For example, Mexico City's elevation, which is 7,600 feet (2,316 m), is considered moderate, yet at this height there is a 7 percent to 8 percent decrease in

> **Most athletic events are not conducted at high altitudes.**

maximum oxygen uptake.[59] This loss in maximum oxygen uptake represents a 4 percent to 8 percent deterioration in an athlete's performance in endurance events, depending on the duration of effort and lack of wind resistance.[71] Often, the athlete's body compensates for this decrease in maximum oxygen uptake with corresponding tachycardia.[59] When the body is suddenly without its usual oxygen supply, hyperventilation can occur. Many of these responses result from the athlete having fewer red blood cells than necessary to adequately capture the available oxygen in the air.[59]

## Adaptation to Altitude

A major factor in altitude adaptation is the problem of oxygen deficiency. With a reduction in barometric pressure, the partial pressure of oxygen in inspired air is also low. Under these circumstances, the existing circulating red blood cells become less saturated, depriving tissue of needed oxygen.[71]

An individual's adaptation to high altitude depends on whether he or she is a native, resident, or visitor to the area. Natives of areas with high altitudes (e.g., the Andes and Nepal) have a larger chest capacity, more alveoli, more capillaries that transport blood to tissue, and a higher red blood cell level. In contrast, the resident or the individual who stays at a high altitude for months or years makes a partial adaptation. His or her later adaptation includes the conservation of glucose, an increased number of mitochondria (the sources of energy in a cell), and increased formation of hemoglobin. In the visitor or the person who is in an early stage of adaptation to high altitude, a number of responses represent a physiological struggle. The responses include increased breathing, increased heart action, increased hemoglobin in circulating blood, increased blood alkalinity, and increased myoglobin, as well as changes in the distribution of blood flow and cell enzyme activity. Dehydration has also been linked to altitude sickness.[71]

There are many uncertainties about when to have an athlete go to an area of high altitude to train and compete.[78] Some experts believe that having the athlete arrive 2 to 3 weeks before competition provides the best adjustment period, whereas others believe that, for psychological as well as physiological reasons, 3 days before competition is enough time.[59] This shorter adjustment period allows for the recovery of the acid-base balance in the blood but does not provide enough time for the athlete to achieve a significant adjustment in blood volume and maximum cardiac output.[71]

## Altitude Illnesses

Athletic trainers must understand that some of their athletes may become ill when suddenly subjected to high altitudes.[50] These illnesses include acute mountain sickness, high altitude pulmonary edema (HAPE), high altitude cerebral edema (HACE), and an adverse reaction to the sickle-cell trait.

**Acute Mountain Sickness** One out of three individuals who go from a low to a moderate altitude of 7,000 to 8,000 feet (2,133 to 2,438 m) experience mild to moderate symptoms of acute mountain sickness.[13] Symptoms include headache, nausea, vomiting, sleep disturbance, and dyspnea, which may last up to 3 days.[50] These symptoms have been attributed to a tissue disruption in the brain that affects the sodium and potassium balance. This imbalance can cause excess fluid retention within the cells and the subsequent occurrence of abnormal pressure.[50]

**High Altitude Pulmonary Edema (HAPE)** At an altitude of 9,000 to 10,000 feet (2,743 to 3,048 m), high altitude pulmonary edema (HAPE) may occur. Characteristically, lungs at this altitude will accumulate a small amount of fluid within the alveolar walls.[71] In most individuals, this fluid is absorbed in a few days, but in some it continues to collect and forms pulmonary edema. Symptoms of high altitude pulmonary edema are dyspnea, cough, headache, weakness, and unconsciousness.[71] The treatment of choice is to move the athlete to a lower altitude as soon as possible and give oxygen. The condition rapidly resolves once the athlete is at a lower altitude.[50]

**High Altitude Cerebral Edema (HACE)** High altitude cerebral edema (HACE), usually in conjunction with HAPE, is a life-threatening condition that can lead to coma or death. It occurs in about 1 percent of people adjusting to altitudes above 9,000 feet (2,743 m). HACE is likely the result of increased cerebral edema caused by increased cerebral blood flow due to the increased permeability of cerebral endothelium when exposed to hypoxia. Increased cerebral blood flow results in increased intracranial pressure, which is responsible for many of the clinical manifestations of HACE. Symptoms consist of a severe headache that may precede mental dysfunction (hallucinations, bizarre behavior, and coma) and neurological abnormalities (loss of coordination, paralysis, and cerebellar signs). Descent to lower altitudes may save those afflicted with HACE.[13]

**Sickle-Cell Trait Reaction** Approximately 8 percent to 10 percent of African Americans (approximately 2 million persons) have the sickle-cell trait. In most, the trait is benign. It relates to an abnormality of the structure of the red blood cells and their hemoglobin content.[71] When the abnormal hemoglobin molecules become deoxygenated as a result of exercise at a high altitude, the cells tend to clump together. This process causes an abnormal sickle shape in the red blood cell, which can be destroyed easily. This condition can cause an enlarged spleen, which has been known to rupture at high altitudes (see Chapter 29).[71] The NATA consensus statement on "Sickle Cell Trait and the Athlete" can be found at www.nata.org/sites/default /files/SickleCellTraitAndTheAthlete.pdf.

# OVEREXPOSURE TO SUN

Athletes, along with coaches, athletic trainers, and other support staff, frequently spend a great deal of time outdoors in direct sunlight. Precautions to protect these individuals from overexposure to ultraviolet light by applying sunscreens are often totally ignored.[101]

## Long-Term Effects on Skin

The most serious effects of long-term exposure to ultraviolet light are premature aging of the skin and skin cancer.[46] Lightly pigmented individuals are more susceptible to these maladies. Premature aging of the skin is characterized by dryness, cracking, and a decrease in the elasticity of the skin. Skin cancer is the most common malignant tumor found in humans and has been epidemiologically and clinically associated with exposure to ultraviolet radiation. Damage to DNA is suspected as the cause of skin cancer, but the exact cause is unknown. The major types of skin cancer are basal cell carcinoma, squamous cell carcinoma, and malignant melanoma. Fortunately, the rate of cure exceeds 95 percent with early detection and treatment.[46,112]

## Sunscreens

Sunscreens applied to the skin can help prevent many of the damaging effects of ultraviolet radiation. A sunscreen's effectiveness in absorbing the sunburn-inducing radiation is expressed as the sun protection factor (**SPF**). An SPF of 6 indicates that an athlete can be exposed to ultraviolet light six times longer than without a sunscreen before the skin begins to turn red. Higher numbers provide longer periods of protection. However, athletes who have a family or personal history of skin cancer may experience significant damage to the skin even when wearing an SPF-15 sunscreen. Therefore, these individuals should wear an SPF-30 sunscreen.

Sunscreen should be worn regularly by athletes, coaches, and athletic trainers who spend time outside, particularly if they have a fair complexion, light hair, blue eyes, or skin that burns easily.[45] People with dark complexions should also wear sunscreens to prevent sun damage.[46]

Sun exposure causes a premature aging of the skin (wrinkling, freckling, prominent blood vessels, coarsening of skin texture), induces the formation of precancerous growths, and increases the risk of developing basal and squamous cell skin cancers. Because 60 to 80 percent of lifetime sun exposure is often obtained by age 20, everyone over 6 months of age should use sunscreens.

Sunscreens are needed most between the months of March and November but should be used year-round.

A track athlete is competing in a day-long outdoor track meet. She is extremely concerned about getting sunburned and has liberally applied sunscreen with an SPF of 30 during the early morning. It is a hot, sunny day, and she is sweating heavily. She is worried that her sunscreen has worn off and asks the athletic trainer for more sunscreen. The athletic trainer hands her sunscreen with an SPF of 15 and she complains that it is not strong enough to protect her.

**?** What can the athletic trainer tell the athlete to assure her that she will be well protected by the sunscreen she has been given?

They are needed most between the hours of 10 A.M. and 4 P.M. and should be applied 15 to 30 minutes before sun exposure. Although clothing and hats provide some protection from the sun, they are not a substitute for sunscreens (a typical white cotton T-shirt provides an SPF of only 5). Reflected sunlight from water, sand, and snow may effectively increase sun exposure and the risk of burning.

# LIGHTNING SAFETY

Research indicates that lightning is the number two cause of death by weather phenomena, accounting for 110 deaths per year.[72] As a result of the danger associated with electrical storms to athletes and staff who practice and compete outdoors, the NATA has established a position statement "Lightning safety for athletics and recreation" (www.nata.org/sites/default/files/2013_lightning-position-statement.pdf) with guidelines for athletic trainers.[117] Each institution should develop a specific emergency action plan for each venue to be implemented in case of a lightning storm.[117] SoR:C The EAP should include establishing a chain of command to determine who should monitor both the weather forecast and changing weather of a threatening nature and to determine who makes the decision to remove from, and ultimately to return a team to, the practice field, based on preestablished criteria.[14,117] SoR:C A specific lightning safety plan for large-scale events and venues should be established as part of the emergency action plan.[93] SoR:C Thunderstorms pose a hazard to not only spectators and sports participants but also to emergency care personnel. These individuals must ensure their own personal safety before venturing into the venue to provide aid.[117] SoR:A

If you hear thunder or see lightning, you are in immediate danger and should seek a protective shelter in an indoor facility at once.[117] SoR:A An indoor facility, which is a fully enclosed building with wiring and plumbing, such as a school, field house, library, or home, should be identified for each venue to serve as a safe place from lightning.[14,117] SoR:A However, if an indoor facility is not available, fully enclosed metal vehicles, such as school buses, cars, and vans, are also safe locations for evacuation.[14,117] SoR:A If none of these is available, the following guidelines are recommended. Avoid standing near large trees, flagpoles, or light poles.[14,37,117] SoR:A Additional unsafe locations include most places termed *shelters,* such as nonmetal picnic, park, sun, bus, and rain shelters and storage sheds.[14,37,117] SoR:A Open areas such as tents, dugouts, refreshment stands, gazebos, screened porches, press boxes, and open garages are unsafe.[14,37,117] SoR:A People inside a building should not use plumbing, showers, sinks, locker rooms, indoor pools, appliances, or electronics during an electrical storm.[14,117] SoR:A

The most dangerous storms give little or no warning; thunder and lightning are not heard or seen.[14] Lightning is always accompanied by thunder, although 20 to 40 percent of thunder cannot be heard because of atmospheric disturbances. If thunder can be heard, lightning is close enough to be a potential danger and everyone should move to a safe location.[94] SoR:A The misconception that it is possible to see lightning coming and have time to act before it strikes could prove to be fatal. In reality, the lightning that we see flashing is actually the return stroke flashing upward from the ground to the cloud, not downward. When you see the lightning strike, it has already hit.[98]

> The most dangerous storms give little or no warning.

The athletic trainer should establish a reliable means of monitoring local weather, which may mean contracting with a local weather service that can provide immediate notification via a smartphone of potential threatening weather.[117] SoR:C The athletic trainer should consider using the National Weather Service or subscribing to a commercial, real-time lightning detection service that has been independently and objectively verified.[14,43,117] SoR:C The National Weather Service may issue a *watch* when the risk of a hazardous weather event is significantly increased, but its presence, location, or timing is unclear; the purpose is to provide enough time to set plans in motion. A *warning* is issued when hazardous weather (i.e., conditions posing a threat to life or property) is occurring, is imminent, or has a very high probability of occurring. Decisions regarding suspending play should be based on the recommendation from the National Weather Service or commercial lightning detection service.[117]

Specific criteria and guidelines should be developed both for suspending play and resuming activity in the emergency action plan.[14,117] SoR:C The athletic trainer should watch the sky to look for approaching storms that have not yet been observed that may produce lightning and be prepared to suspend or postpone activities if a thunderstorm appears imminent.[14,72,117] SoR:A Individuals in charge of outdoor events have an obligation to warn participants of imminent lightning danger.[57] SoR:C Time must be allowed for all individuals to leave an outdoor facility and be inside the previously identified safe locations after being warned that an approaching thunderstorm known to be producing lightning is within 5.75 miles.[14,117] SoR:C Anyone who feels they are in danger from impending

A lacrosse team is practicing on a remote field with no indoor facility in close proximity. The weather is rapidly worsening, with the sky becoming dark and the wind blowing harder. Twenty minutes are left in the practice session, and the coach is hoping to finish practice before it begins to rain. Suddenly, there is a bolt of lightning and an immediate burst of thunder.

? How should the athletic trainer manage this extremely dangerous situation?

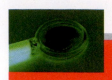
## Lightning safety[117]

Establish a comprehensive emergency action plan for every outdoor venue:

1. Establish a chain of command for making decisions during lightning storms.
2. Use a reliable means of monitoring the weather.
3. Identify locations safe from the lightning hazard.
4. Establish specific criteria to suspend and resume activity.
5. Have the necessary equipment readily available to provide emergency care should a lightning strike occur.
6. Promote lightning safety slogans.

---

lightning should have the right to vacate an unsafe area without fear of repercussion or penalty.[117] **SoR:C**

The rule for resuming activity is very clear. Activities should be suspended until 30 minutes after the last strike of lightning is seen (or it is at least 5.75 miles away) and after the last sound of thunder is heard. This 30-minute clock must be restarted for each lightning flash within 5.75 miles and each time thunder is heard.[14,117] **SoR:A**

*Focus Box 6–7:* "Lightning safety" identifies guidelines that should be followed during an electrical storm. A link to the NATA position statement "Lightning safety for athletics and recreation" can be found at www.nata.org /sites/default/files/2013_lightning-position-statement.pdf.

### Lightning Detectors

A lightning detector is a handheld unit that detects lightning by sensing the electromagnetic field generated by the strike to detect the presence and the distance of lightning/ thunderstorm activity occurring within a 40-mile distance (Figure 6–6). It allows you to know the level of activity of the storm, and it determines whether the storm is moving toward, away from, or stationary to your position. When the lightning detector detects a lightning strike, it emits an audible warning tone and lights the range indicator, allowing

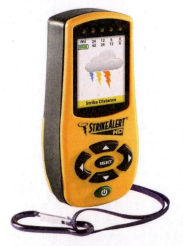

**FIGURE 6–6**    Portable handheld lightning detector.
Courtesy Outdoors Technologies, Colorado Springs, CO

you to see the distance to the last, closest detected lightning strike. If the lightning detector flashes in the 0–6 range, this is generally considered to be a threatening environmental condition, and all activity should immediately be moved to an indoor shelter. Lightning detectors are extremely reliable, as the readings are instantaneous. Often priced under $200, they are thus an inexpensive alternative to contracting with a weather service to provide information on potentially dangerous weather conditions over a pager system.

## AIR POLLUTION

Air pollution is a significant problem everywhere in the United States but particularly in urban areas with large industries and heavy automobile traffic. Because athletes are outside for long periods of time during training or competition, they may be

> Air pollution is a major problem in urban areas with large industries and heavy automobile traffic.

more susceptible to the effects of air pollution than is a sedentary individual who remains indoors.[84] There are two types of pollution: photochemical haze and smog. Photochemical haze consists of nitrogen dioxide and stagnant air that are acted on by sunlight to produce ozone.[100] Smog is produced by the combination of carbon monoxide, sulfur dioxide, and particulate matter that emanates from the combustion of a fossil fuel, such as coal.

### Ozone

Ozone is formed by the action of sunlight on carbon-based chemicals known as hydrocarbons, acting in combination with nitrogen dioxide.[47] It is the main component of the air pollution referred to as smog. Hydrocarbons are emitted by motor vehicles, oil and chemical storage facilities, and industrial sources, such as gas stations, dry cleaners, and degreasing operations. Ozone is at its highest level when higher temperatures and the increased amount of sunlight during the summer combine with stagnant atmospheric conditions.

When individuals are engaged in physical tasks requiring minimal effort, an increase in ozone in the air does not usually reduce functional capacity in normal work output. However, when individuals increase their work output (e.g., during exercise), their work capacity is decreased. The athlete may experience shortness of breath, coughing, chest tightness, pain during deep breathing, nausea, eye irritation, fatigue, lung irritation, and a lowered resistance to lung infections.[4] Over a period of time, individuals may to some degree become desensitized to ozone. Asthmatics are at greater risk when ozone levels increase.

## Nitrogen Dioxide

Nitrogen dioxide is produced from combustive processes, such as in automobiles, power plants, home heaters, and gas stoves. Nitrogen dioxide is a light brown gas that is a component of urban haze. It plays an important role in the atmospheric reactions that generate ozone and acid rain. Nitrogen dioxide can irritate the lungs and lower resistance to respiratory infections, such as influenza, and may cause increased incidences of acute respiratory disease in children.[100]

## Sulfur Dioxide

Sulfur dioxide ($SO_2$) is a colorless gas that is a component of burning coal or petroleum. As an air contaminant, it causes an increased resistance to air movement into and out of the lungs, a decreased ability of the lungs to rid themselves of foreign matter, shortness of breath, coughing, fatigue, and increased susceptibility to lung diseases. Sulfur dioxide causes an adverse effect mostly on asthmatics and other sensitive individuals. Nose breathing lessens the effects of sulfur dioxide because the nasal mucosa acts as a sulfur dioxide scrubber.[84]

## Carbon Monoxide

Carbon monoxide (CO) is a colorless, odorless gas. In general, it reduces hemoglobin's ability to transport oxygen and restricts the release of oxygen to the tissue. Besides interfering with performance during exercise, carbon monoxide exposure interferes with various psychomotor, behavioral, and attention-related activities.[84]

> Carbon monoxide (CO) reduces hemoglobin's ability to transport and release oxygen in the body.

## Particulate Matter

Particulate matter is a type of air pollution that consists of solids in the atmosphere, such as dirt, soil dust, pollens, molds, ashes, soot, and aerosols, that have been found to present a serious danger to health. Particulate pollution comes from such diverse sources as factory smokestacks, vehicle exhaust, wood burning, mining, construction, and agriculture. Fine particles, less than 2.5 microns in diameter, are easily inhaled into the lungs, where they can be absorbed into the bloodstream or remain embedded for long periods of time.[4] Exposure to particulate air pollution can trigger asthma attacks and cause wheezing, coughing, and respiratory irritation in individuals who have chronic obstructive pulmonary disease (COPD), including emphysema and bronchitis.[100]

## Prevention

To avoid problems created by air pollution, the athlete must stop or significantly decrease physical activity during periods of high pollution. If activity is conducted, it should be performed when commuter traffic has lessened and when ambient temperature has lowered. Ozone levels rise during dawn, peak at midday, and are much reduced after the late-afternoon rush hour. Running should be avoided on roads containing a concentration of auto emissions and carbon monoxide.[84] Table 6–4 provides guidelines for activity based on the air quality index for ozone.

| TABLE 6–4 | Air Quality Guide for Ozone* | |
|---|---|---|
| **Air Quality** | **Air Quality Index** | **Protect Your Health** |
| Good | 0–50 | No health impacts are expected when air quality is in this range. |
| Moderate | 51–100 | Unusually sensitive people should consider limiting prolonged outdoor exertion. |
| Unhealthy for sensitive groups | 101–150 | Active children and adults and people with respiratory disease, such as asthma, should limit prolonged outdoor exertion. |
| Unhealthy | 151–200 | Active children and adults and people with respiratory disease, such as asthma, should avoid prolonged outdoor exertion; everyone else, especially children, should limit prolonged outdoor exertion. |
| Very unhealthy (alert) | 201–300 | Active children and adults and people with respiratory disease, such as asthma, should avoid all outdoor exertion; everyone else, especially children, should limit outdoor exertion. |

*Modified from United States Environmental Protection Agency, Air and Radiation, EPA-456/F-99-002, Washington, DC, 20460, 1999.

# CIRCADIAN DYSRHYTHMIA (JET LAG)

Jet power makes it possible to travel thousands of miles in just a few hours. Athletes and athletic teams are quickly transported from one end of the country to the other and to foreign lands. For some athletes, such travel induces a particular physiological stress, resulting in a syndrome that is identified as **circadian dysrhythmia** and that reflects a desynchronization of the athlete's biological and biophysical time clock.[118]

The term *circadian* (from the Latin *circa dies,* "about a day") implies a period of time of approximately 24 hours. The body maintains many cyclical mechanisms (circadian rhythms) that follow a pattern (e.g., the daily rise and fall of body temperature or the tidal ebb and flow of the cortical steroid secretion, which produces other effects on the metabolic system that are in themselves cyclical). Body mechanisms adapt at varying rates to time changes. Some adjust immediately (e.g., protein metabolism), whereas others take time (e.g., the rise and fall of body temperature, which takes approximately 8 days to adjust). Other body mechanisms, such as the adrenal hormones, which regulate metabolism and other body functions, may take as long as 3 weeks to adjust. Even intellectual proficiency, or the ability to think clearly, is cyclical.

The term *jet lag* refers to the physical and mental effects caused by traveling rapidly across several time zones.[118] It results from the disruption of both circadian rhythms and the sleep-wake cycle. As the length of travel increases over several time zones, the effects of jet lag become more profound.[63]

Disruption of circadian rhythms has been shown to cause fatigue, headache, problems with the digestive system, and changes in blood pressure, heart rate, hormonal release, endocrine secretions, and bowel habits.[54] Any of these changes may have a negative effect on athletic performance and may predispose the athlete to injury.[118]

Younger individuals adjust more rapidly to time zone changes than do older people, although the differences are not great. The stress induced in jet travel occurs only when flying either east or west at high speed. Travel north or south has no effect on the body unless several time zones are crossed in an east or west progression. There is 30 to 50 percent faster adaptation in individuals flying westward than in individuals flying eastward.[54] In fact, flying from the west to the east has been demonstrated to decrease performance.[103] The changes in time zones, illumination, and environment prove somewhat disruptive to the human physiological mechanisms, particularly when a person flies through five or more time zones, as occurs in some international travel.[54] Some people are more susceptible to the syndrome than are others, but the symptoms can be sufficiently disruptive to interfere with an athlete's ability to perform maximally in a competitive event.[118] In some cases, an athlete becomes ill for a short period of time, with severe headache, blurred vision, dizziness, insomnia, or extreme fatigue. The negative effects of jet lag can be reduced by paying attention to the guidelines in *Focus Box 6–8:* "Minimizing the effects of jet lag."

---

---

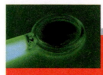

## FOCUS 6–8 Focus on Injury/Illness Prevention and Wellness Promotion

### Minimizing the effects of jet lag

- Depart for a trip well rested.
- Preadjust circadian rhythms by getting up and going to bed 1 hour later for each time zone crossed when traveling west and 1 hour earlier for each time zone crossed when traveling east.
- When traveling west, eat light meals early and heavy meals late in the day. When traveling east, eat a heavy meal earlier in the day.[103]
- Drink plenty of fluids to avoid dehydration, which occurs because of dry, high-altitude, low-humidity cabin air.
- Consume caffeine in coffee, tea, or soda when traveling west. Avoid caffeine when traveling east.[103]

(Caffeine is only a mild diuretic and causes no greater increase in urine output than drinking water.[54])

- Exercise or training should be done later in the day if traveling west and earlier in the day if traveling east.
- Reset watches according to the new time zone after boarding the plane.
- If traveling west, get as much sunlight as possible on arrival.
- On arrival, immediately adopt the local time schedule for training, eating, and sleeping. Forget about what time it is where you came from.
- Avoid using alcohol before, during, and after travel.

---

# SYNTHETIC TURF

Synthetic turf was first used in the Houston Astrodome in 1966 and was first marketed under the trade name AstroTurf. The artificial surface was said to be more durable, offer greater consistency, require less maintenance, be more "playable" during inclement weather, and offer greater performance characteristics, such as increased speed and resiliency. Since the late 1960s, a number of companies have manufactured synthetic surfaces that are variations of AstroTurf. Today synthetic surfaces have a relatively new option in "resilient infill turf," which its manufacturers claim is more similar to natural grass and considerably less expensive than other types of synthetic turf.[121] It is made of polyethylene and polypropylene yarns that sit on a base of sand, crumbled rubber pellets, or a combination of both. The consumer can choose from a number of artificial turf products, including AstroTurf, Nexturf, FieldTurf, AstroPlay, Omniturf, EasyTurf, SyntheticTurf, Sof-Step 200, SprlnTurf, and Avery SportsTurf.[106]

> A collegiate athletic director is trying to make a decision about replacing a natural grass playing field with a new synthetic playing surface. He asks the athletic trainer to provide him with recommendations relative to the incidence of injury on natural grass versus synthetic turf.
>
> **?** What can the athletic trainer tell him?

There has been an ongoing debate over the advantages and disadvantages of synthetic surfaces compared with natural surfaces.[120] From an injury perspective, the evidence in the literature is not conclusive to indicate that a synthetic surface is more likely to cause injury than a natural surface.[40,49,70,120,121] Empirically, most athletes, coaches, and athletic trainers agree that injuries are more likely to occur on synthetic surfaces than on natural grass, and most of these individuals would rather practice and play on natural grass. In recent years, the trend in many colleges, universities, and professional arenas has been to move away from synthetic surfaces, replacing them with natural grass. New hybrid grasses are now available that are more durable.

It has been argued that synthetic surfaces lose their inherent shock absorption capability as they age.[49] It has been demonstrated that training injuries are more likely to occur if training always occurs on artificial turf.[40] Higher speeds are said to be possible on artificial surfaces; thus, injuries involving collision can be more severe because of increased force on impact.[121] A shoe that does not "stick" to the artificial surface but still provides solid footing will significantly reduce the likelihood of injury.[121]

Two injuries that seem to occur more frequently in athletes competing on an artificial surface are abrasions and turf toe (a hyperextension of the great toe). The incidence of abrasions can be greatly reduced by wearing pads on the elbows and knees. Turf toe is less likely to occur if the shoe has a stiff, firm sole.

## SUMMARY

- Environmental stress can adversely affect an athlete's performance and pose a serious health problem.
- Hyperthermia is one of sport's major concerns. In times of high temperatures and humidity, athletes should always exercise caution. The key to preventing heat-related illness is rehydration, acclimatization, and common sense. Losing 2 percent or more of body weight due to fluid loss could pose a health problem.
- Cold weather requires athletes to wear the correct apparel and to warm up properly before engaging in sports activities. The wind chill factor must always be considered when performing. As is true in a hot environment, athletes in cold conditions must ingest adequate fluids. Extreme cold exposure can cause conditions such as frost nip, chilblains, and frostbite.
- An athlete going from a low to a high altitude in a short time may encounter problems with performance and may experience some health problems. Researchers are unsure about how much time it takes for adaptation to occur and about when to take the athlete

to the higher altitude, especially for an endurance event. Many athletic trainers believe that 3 days at the higher altitude provides enough time for adaptation to occur. Others believe that a much longer time period is needed. An athlete who experiences a serious illness because of his or her presence at a particular altitude must be returned to a lower altitude as soon as possible.

- Air pollution can be a major decrement to performance and can cause illness. Increased ozone levels can cause respiratory distress, nausea, eye irritation, and fatigue. Sulfur dioxide, a colorless gas, can also cause physical reactions in some athletes and can be a serious problem for asthmatics. Carbon monoxide, a colorless and odorless gas, reduces hemoglobin's ability to use oxygen and, as a result, adversely affects performance.
- Travel through time zones can place a serious physiological stress on the athlete. This stress is called circadian dysrhythmia, or jet lag. This disruption of biological rhythm can adversely affect performance and may even produce health problems. The athletic trainer

must pay careful attention to helping the athlete acclimatize to time-zone shifting.

- There is inconclusive evidence that the incidence of injury on artificial surfaces is higher than on natural surfaces, although most coaches, athletes, and athletic trainers seem to prefer practicing and playing on natural grass. Two frequently seen injuries that occur on artificial turf are abrasions and turf toe.

## WEB SITES

**National Athletic Trainers Association Position, Official, Consensus and Support Statements**

*Lightning Safety for Athletics and Recreation (2013)*
www.nata.org/sites/default/files/2013_lightning-position-statement.pdf

*Environmental Cold Injuries (2008)*
www.nata.org/sites/default/files/EnvironmentalColdInjuries.pdf

*Exertional Heat Illnesses (2002)*
www.nata.org/sites/default/files/ExternalHeatIllnesses.pdf

*Fluid Replacement for Athletes (2000)*
www.nata.org/sites/default/files/FluidReplacementsForAthletes.pdf

*Youth Football and Heat Related Illness (2005)*
www.nata.org/sites/default/files/HeatRelatedIllness.pdf

*Preseason Heat Acclimatization Guideline for Secondary School Athletics (2009)*
natajournals.org/doi/pdf/10.4085/1062-6050-44.3.332

*Inter-Association Task Force on Exertional Heat Illnesses (2003)*
www.nata.org/sites/default/files/inter-association-task-force-exertional-heat-illness.pdf

A hypothermia treatment technology Web site: www.hypothermia-ca.com

American Lung Association: www.lung.org
*The American Lung Association site looks at outdoor air pollution and its effects on the lungs.*

FEMA: Extreme Heat Fact Sheet: www.fema.gov/media-library/assets/documents/12364

*Doing too much on a hot day, spending too much time in the sun, or staying too long in an overheated place can cause heat-related illnesses.*

Gatorade Sport Science Institute: www.gssiweb.com
*This site provides the most up-to-date recommendations for fluid replacement and preventing heat illnesses.*

National Lightning Safety Institute (NLSI): www.lightningsafety.com
*The National Lightning Safety Institute provides consulting, education, training, and expert witnesses relating to lightning hazard mitigation.*

National Weather Service: www.lightningsafety.noaa.gov

WebMD Health: Heat Illness (Heat Exhaustion, Heatstroke, Heat Cramps): www.webmd.com/fitness-exercise/heat-exhaustion
*Prolonged or intense exposure to hot temperatures can cause heat-related illnesses, such as heat exhaustion, heat cramps, and heatstroke (also known as sunstroke).*

OA Guide to Hypothermia & Cold Weather Injuries: www.princeton.edu/~oa/safety/hypocold.shtml

OnHealth: Heat Illness (Heat Exhaustion, Heatstroke, Heat Cramps): www.webmd.com/first-aid/understanding-heat-related-illness-basics
*Prolonged or intense exposure to hot temperatures can cause heat-related illnesses, such as heat exhaustion, heat cramps, and heatstroke (also known as sunstroke).*

Sports Turf Managers Association: www.stma.org

## SOLUTIONS TO CLINICAL APPLICATION EXERCISES

6–1 The wrestler is experiencing heat exhaustion, which results from inadequate fluid replacement or dehydration. If conscious, the athlete should be forced to drink large quantities of water. By far the most rapid method of fluid replacement is for a physician to use an IV (fluids administered intravenously). It is desirable, but not necessary, to move the athlete to a cooler environment. The athlete should be counseled about the dangers of using diuretic medication.

6–2 The athletic trainer may suspect that the athlete is experiencing heatstroke. The course of action includes checking the athlete's vitals (airway, breathing, circulation) and activating the emergency action plan. Remove his helmet and as much excess clothing as is appropriate. The first priority is to cool the individual down as quickly as possible by immersing him in a cold-water tub. Continuously monitor his vital signs until the rescue squad arrives. The athlete's core temperature should be around 100°F before he is removed from the cold tub. If a cold tub is not available, use cold packs or cold-water spray. Move the athlete into the shade or to a cooler environment, if possible.

6–3 The athletic trainer should explain to the coach that heat-related illnesses are, for the most part, preventable. The athletes should come into preseason practice at least partially acclimatized to working in a hot, humid environment and during the first week of practice should become fully acclimatized. Temperature and humidity readings should be monitored, and practice should be modified according to conditions. Practice uniforms should maximize evaporation and minimize heat absorption to the greatest extent possible. Weight records should be maintained to identify individuals who are becoming dehydrated. Most important, the athletes must keep themselves hydrated by constantly drinking large quantities of water both during and between practice sessions.

6–4 The safest recommendation would be for the athlete to travel to Colorado 2 to 3 weeks before the event. If this arrival time is not practical, she should be in Colorado for at least 3 days before her first event.

6–5 The sun protection factor (SPF) indicates the sunscreen's effectiveness in absorbing the sunburn-inducing radiation. An SPF of 15 indicates that an athlete can be exposed to ultraviolet light 15 times longer than without a sunscreen before the skin will begin to turn red. Therefore, the athlete needs to understand that a higher SPF does not indicate a greater degree of protection. She must simply apply the sunscreen with an SPF of 15 twice as often as would be necessary with a sunscreen with an SPF of 30.

6–6 As soon as lightning is observed, the athletic trainer should immediately end practice and get the athletes under cover. If an indoor facility is not available, automobiles are a relatively safe alternative. The athletes should avoid standing under large trees or telephone poles.

6–7 Most important, the athletes should leave for the trip well rested. The day before leaving, the athletes should go to bed and get up 3 hours earlier than normal. Athletes should reset their watches according to the new time zone once they board the plane. During the trip they should drink plenty of fluids to prevent dehydration, but they should avoid caffeine. Their largest meal should be eaten earlier in the day. On arrival, athletes should immediately adopt the local time schedule for training, eating, and sleeping, and they should get as much sunlight as possible. Training sessions should be done earlier in the day.

6–8 The athletic trainer should inform the athletic director that the trend seems to be moving toward natural grass fields. The research data collected over the years have not clearly indicated that there is a difference in injury rates between natural grass and synthetic turf. However, it does seem that most athletes, coaches, and athletic trainers prefer natural turf. It should also be stressed that the newer synthetic surfaces are more like natural grass and may warrant additional investigation.

## REVIEW QUESTIONS AND CLASS ACTIVITIES

1. How do temperature and humidity cause heat illnesses?
2. What steps should be taken to prevent heat illnesses?
3. Describe the symptoms and signs of the most common heat illnesses.
4. How is heat lost from the body to produce hypothermia?
5. What should an athlete do to prevent heat loss?
6. Identify the physiological basis for the body's susceptibility to a cold disorder.
7. Describe the symptoms and signs of the major cold disorders affecting athletes.
8. How should athletes protect themselves from the effects of ultraviolet radiation from the sun?
9. What precautions can be taken to minimize the possibility of injury during an electrical storm?
10. What concerns should an athletic trainer have when athletes are to perform an endurance sport at high altitudes?
11. What altitude illnesses might be expected among some athletes, and how should those illnesses be managed?
12. What adverse effects could high air concentrations of ozone, nitrogen dioxide, sulfur dioxide, carbon monoxide, and particulate matter have on the athlete? How should they be dealt with?
13. How can the adverse effects of circadian dysrhythmia be avoided or lessened?
14. What are two common injuries in athletes who compete on artificial turf?

## REFERENCES

1. American College of Sports Medicine: Position stand on exercise and fluid replacement, *Med Sci Sports Exerc* 28(17):377–90, 1996.
2. American College of Sports Medicine: Position stand: Prevention of cold injuries during exercise. *Medicine and Science in Sports and Exercise* 38(11):2012–29, 2006.
3. Adams W: The timing of exertional heat stroke survival starts prior to collapse, *Med Sci Sports Exercise* 14(4):273–74, 2015.
4. American Lung Association, www.lungusa.org.
5. Armstrong L: Caffeine, body fluid electrolyte balance, and exercise performance, *Int J Sport Nutr* 12(2):189, 2002.
6. Armstrong L: Exertional heat illness during training and competition, *Med Sci Sport Exer* 39(3):556–72, 2007.
7. Armstrong L: Heat and cold illnesses during distance running, *Med Sci Sports Exerc* 28(12):377–90, 1996.
8. Armstrong L: Nutritional strategies for football: Counteracting heat, cold, high altitude, and jet lag, *Journal of Sports Sciences* 24(7):723, 2006.
9. Armstrong L: Return to exercise training after heat exhaustion, *J Sport Rehabil* 16(3):182–89, 2007.
10. Armstrong L: The American football uniform: Uncompensable heat stress and hyperthermic exhaustion, *J Athl Train* 45(2):117–27, 2010.
11. Baxter R: Diagnosis and treatment of acute exertional rhabdomyolysis, *J Ortho Sports Phys Ther* 33(3):124, 2003.
12. Becker J: Heat-related illness, *American Family Physician* 83(11):1325–30, 2011.
13. Bellis F: Acute mountain sickness: An unexpected management problem, *British Journal of Sports Medicine* 36(2):147, 2002.

14. Bennett B: Lightning safety guidelines. In Klossner D, ed: *National collegiate athletic association sports medicine handbook*, Overland Park, KS, 2011, National Collegiate Athletic Association.
15. Bergeron M: Muscle cramps during exercise—is it fatigue or electrolyte deficit? *Curr Sports Med Rep* 7(4):S50–S55, 2008.
16. Bergeron M: Reducing sports heat illness risk, *Pediatrics in Review* 34(6):270–79, 2012.
17. Binkley H, et al.: National Athletic Trainers' Association position statement: Exertional heat illnesses, *J Athl Train* 37(3):329, 2002.
18. Broman D: The implementation of a protocol for the prevention and management of exertional heat illness in sport, *British Journal of Sports Medicine* 48(7):573, 2014.
19. Brukner P: Exercise in the cold. In Brukner P, ed: *Clinical sports medicine,* ed 4, Sydney, Australia, 2011, McGraw-Hill.
20. Budd G: Wet-bulb globe temperature (WBGT)—its history and its limitations, *Journal of Science and Medicine in Sports* 11(1):20–32, 2008.
21. Bunn J: Hydration and performance. In Campbell W, *Sports nutrition: Enhancing athletic performance*, New York, 2013, CRC Press.
22. Burdon C: Influence of beverage temperature on palatability and fluid ingestion during endurance exercise: A systematic review, *International Journal of Sport Nutrition and Exercise Metabolism* 22(3):199–211, 2012.
23. Capacchione J: The relationship between exertional heat illness, exertional rhabdomyolysis, and malignant hyperthermia, *Anesthesia and Analgesia* 109(4):1065–69, 2009.

24. Cappaert T: National Athletic Trainers' Association position statement: Environmental cold injuries, *J Athl Train* 43(4):640, 2008.
25. Carter III, R: Exertional heat illness and hyponatremia: An epidemiological perspective. *Current Sports Medicine Reports* 7(4): S20, 2008.
26. Carlson M: Exercising in the cold, *ACSM's Health & Fitness Journal* 16(1):8–12, 2012.
27. Casa D, et al.: Validity of devices that assess body temperature during outdoor exercise in the heat, *J Athl Train* 42(3):333–42, 2007.
28. Casa D: Cold water immersion: The gold standard for exertional heatstroke treatment, *Exer & Sport Sci Rev,* 35(3):141–49, 2007.
29. Casa D, et al.: National Athletic Trainers' Association position statement: Exertional heat illness, *Journal of Athletic Training* 50(9):986–1000, 2015.
30. Casa D: Exertional heat stroke: New concepts regarding cause and care, *Current Sports Medicine Reports* 11(3):115–23, 2012.
31. Casa D, et al.: Inter-Association Task Force on preventing sudden death in secondary school athletics programs: Best-practices recommendations, *Journal of Athletic Training* 48(4):546–53, 2013.
32. Casa D, et al.: National Athletic Trainers' Association position statement: Preventing sudden death in sports, *J Athl Train* 47(1):96–118, 2012.
33. Casa D: Preseason heat-acclimatization guidelines for secondary school athletes, *Journal of Athletic Training* 44(3):332–33, 2009.
34. Casa D, et al.: National Athletic Trainers' Association position statement: Fluid replacement for athletes, *J Athl Train* 35(2):212, 2000.

35. Casey E: Heat emergencies, *Athletic Therapy Today* 11(3):44, 2006.

36. Castillani J: Health and performance challenges during sports training and competition in cold weather, *British Journal of Sports Medicine* 46(11):788–91, 2012.

37. Cherington M: Lightning injuries in sports: Situations to avoid, *Sports Med* 31(4):301–8, 2001.

38. Cleary M: Exertional hyponatremia: Considerations for athletic trainers, *Athletic Therapy Today* 10(4):61, 2005.

39. Clements J: Ice-water immersion and cold-water immersion provide similar cooling rates in runners with exercise-induced hyperthermia, *J Athl Train* 37(2):146, 2002.

40. Conklin A: Grass gets greener: Division 1-A football programs are gradually switching from synthetic turf to grass—and the reasons behind the shift may surprise you, *Sports Med Update* 15(1):11, 2000.

41. Coris E: Heat illness in athletes: The dangerous combination of heat, humidity and exercise, *Sports Med* 34(1):9, 2004.

42. Coyle E: Fluid and fuel intake during exercise, *Journal of Sports Sciences* 22(1):39, 2004.

43. Cummins K: An overview of lightning location systems: History, techniques, and data uses, with an in-depth look at the U.S. NLDN, *IEEE Trans Electromagnet Compat* 51(3):499–518, 2009.

44. Danzl D: Accidental hypothermia. In Marx J, *Rosen's emergency medicine: Concepts and clinical practice*, vol 3, St. Louis, MO, 2006, Mosby.

45. Davis J: Sun and active patients: Preventing cumulative skin damage, *Physician Sportsmed* 28(7):79, 2000.

46. Davis M: Ultraviolet therapy. In Prentice, W, ed: *Therapeutic modalities in sports medicine,* St. Louis, 2003, McGraw-Hill.

47. DeFranco M: Environmental issues for team physicians, *American Journal of Sports Medicine* 36(11):26–33, 2008 .

48. Dotan F: Temperature regulation and elite young athletes, *Medicine and Sport Science* 56(1):126–49, 2011.

49. Dragoo J: The effect of playing surface on injury rate: A review of the current literature, *Sports Medicine* 40(11):981–90, 2010.

50. Eichner R: Acute mountain sickness: New research on causes, coping, *Sports Med Digest* 25(11):121, 2003.

51. Eichner R: Heat cramps in sports, *Current Sports Medicine Reports* 7(4):178–79, 2008.

52. Eichner R: Toward ending fatal heat stroke in football players, *J Athl Train* 45(2):105–6, 2010.

53. Fawcett C: Fluid-electrolyte replacement, *J Athl Train* 41(S):59, 2006.

54. Forbes S: Circadian disruption and remedial interventions: Effects and interventions for jet lag for athletic peak performance, *Sports Medicine* 42(3):185–208, 2012, Mar 1.

55. Gagnon D: Aural canal, esophageal, and rectal temperatures during exertional heat stress and the subsequent recovery period, *J Athl Train* 45(2):157–63, 2010.

56. Gagnon D: Cold-water immersion and the treatment of hyperthermia: Using 38. 6°C as a safe rectal temperature cooling limit, *J Athl Train* 45(5):439–44, 2010.

57. Gratz J: Lightning safety and large stadiums, *Bull Am Meteorol Soc* 87(9):1187–94, 2006.

58. Hew-Butler T, et al.: Statement of the Second International Exercise-Associated Hyponatremia Consensus Development Conference, New Zealand, 2007, *Clin J Sport Med* 18(2):111–21, 2008.

59. Hoffman J: Exercise at altitude. In Hoffman J, ed: *Physiological aspects of sport training and performance,* Champaign, IL, 2002, Human Kinetics.

60. Hoffman, J: Exercise in the cold. In Hoffman J, ed: *Physiological aspects of sport training and performance*, Champaign, IL, 2014, Human Kinetics.

61. Hoffman M: Muscle cramping during a 161-km ultramarathon: Comparison of characteristics of those with and without cramping, *Sports Medicine Open* 1(1):24, 2015.

62. Inter-association task force on exertional heat illnesses consensus statement, *NATA News* 6:24, 2003.

63. Johnson R: *Travel fitness,* Champaign, IL, 1995, Human Kinetics.

64. Jones C: Emergency management of cold-induced injuries, *Emergency Medicine* 43(1):6–10, 2011.

65. Jung A: Influence of hydration and electrolyte supplementation on incidence and time to onset of exercise-associated muscle cramps, *J Athl Train* 40(2):71, 2005.

66. Kay D: Fluid ingestion and exercise hyperthermia: Implications for performance, thermoregulation, metabolism, and development of fatigue, *Journal of Sports Sciences* 18(2):71, 2000.

67. Kerksick C: Fluid needs of athletes. In Taylor L, *Nutritional guidelines for athletic performance*, New York, 2012, CRC Press.

68. Kleiner D: A new exertional heat illness scale, *Athletic Therapy Today* 7(6):65, 2002.

69. Kozack J: Malignant hyperthermia, *Phys Ther* 81:945, 2001.

70. Lemack L: The artificial turf debate, *Sports Med Update* 15(1):14, 2000.

71. Levine B: Exercise at high altitudes. In Torg J, Shephard R, eds: *Current therapy in sports medicine,* St. Louis, 1995, Mosby.

72. Lightning safety awareness statement, American Meteorological Society, http://www.ametsoc.org/policy/lightningpolicy_2002.htm

73. Lopez R: Exercise and hydration: Individualizing fluid replacement guidelines, *Journal of Strength and Conditioning Research* 34(4):49–54, 2012.

74. Maquirriain J: The athlete with muscular cramps: Clinical approach. *J Am Acad Orthop Surg* 15(7):425–31, 2007.

75. Mazerolle S: Current knowledge, attitudes, and practices of certified athletic trainers regarding recognition and treatment of exertional heat stroke, *J Athl Train* 45(2):170–80, 2010.

76. Mazerolle S: Evidence-based medicine and the recognition and treatment of exertional heat stroke, Part II: A perspective from the clinical athletic trainer, *J Athl Train* 46(5):533–42, 2011.

77. Mazerolle S: Is oral temperature an accurate measurement of deep body temperature? A systematic review, *J Athl Train* 46(5):566–73, 2011.

78. McArdle W: *Exercise physiology,* Philadelphia, 2010, Lea & Febiger.

79. McDermott B: Acute whole-body cooling for exercise-induced hyperthermia: A systematic review, *J Athl Train* 44(1):84–93, 2009.

80. McDermott B: Recovery and return to activity following exertional heat stroke: Considerations for the sports medicine staff, *J Sport Rehabil* 16(3):163–81, 2007.

81. McMahon J: Cold weather issues in sideline and event management, *Current Sports Medicine Reports* 11(3):135–41, 2012.

82. Miller K: Cold-water immersion for hyperthermic humans wearing American football uniforms, *J Athl Train* 50(8):792–99, 2015.

83. Miller T: Preparing for cold weather exercise, *NSCA's Performance Training Journal* 3(1):19, 2004.

84. Mittleman M: Air pollution, exercise, and cardiovascular risk, *New England Journal of Medicine*, 357:1147–49, 2007.

85. Montain S: Exercise-associated hyponatremia: Quantitative analysis to understand the aetiology, *British Journal of Sports Medicine* 40(2):98, 2006.

86. Moss R: Another look at sudden death and exertional hyperthermia, *Athletic Therapy Today* 7(3):44, 2002.

87. Muldoon S: Is there a link between malignant hyperthermia and exertional heat illness? *Exerc Sport Sci Rev* 32(4):174, 2004.

88. Murray B: Fluid replacement: The American College of Sports Medicine position stand, *Sports Science Exchange* 9(4):1, 1996.

89. Murray R: Guidelines for fluid replacement during exercise, *Australian Journal of Nutrition and Dietetics* 53(4 suppl):S17, 1996.

90. *NCAA sports medicine handbook, 2014–2015,* Indianapolis, 2015, National Collegiate Athletic Association.

91. Nimmo M: Exercise in the cold, *Journal of Sports Sciences* 22(10):886, 2004.

92. National Collegiate Athletic Association (NCAA): *NCAA sports medicine handbook 2013–2014,* Indianapolis, IN, 2013, NCAA.

93. National Oceanic Atmospheric Administration: Lightning safety: large venues. http://www.weather.gov/os/lightning/more.htm, 2012.

94. National Weather Service: Lightning fact page. http://www.lightningsafety.noaa.gov/statistics.htm, 2012.

95. Nichols A: Heat-related illness in sports and exercise, *Current Reviews in Musculoskeletal Medicine* 7(4):355–65, 2014.

96. Noakes T: A modern classification of the exercise-related heat illnesses, *Journal of Science and Medicine in Sport* 11(1):33–39, 2008.

97. Noonan B: Heat- and cold-induced injuries in athletes: Evaluation and management, *Journal of the American Academy of Orthopaedic Surgeons* 20(12):74, 2012.

98. Oglesbee S: Lightning strikes, *Journal of Emergency Medical Services* 39(5):44–49, 2014.

99. Parker J: Contemporary issues of heat illness, *Sport Journal* 14(1):1, 2011.

100. Peden D: Air pollutants, exercise, and risk of developing asthma in children, *Clinic J Sports Med* 13(1):62, 2003.

101. Peterson J: 10 nice-to-know facts about being in the sun, *ACSM's Health and Fitness Journal* 12(4):48, 2008.

102. Proulx C: Effect of water temperature on cooling efficiency during hyperthermia in humans, *J App Physiol* 94(4):1317, 2003.

103. Reilly T: How can traveling athletes deal with jet lag? *Kinesiology* 41(2):128–35, 2009.

104. Rosner M: Exercise-associated hyponatremia. In Simon E, *Hyponatremia*, New York, 2013, Springer.

105. Rush S: Winter exercise, *ACSM's Health and Fitness Journal* 5(6):23, 2001.

106. Scholand G: Straight talk: Researching synthetic turf suppliers, *Athletic Management* 17(3):59, 2005.

107. Schwellnus M: Cause of exercise associated muscle cramps (EAMC)—altered neuromuscular control, dehydration or electrolyte depletion? *Br J Sports Med*, 43(6):401–8, 2009.

108. Sharp R: Role of whole foods in promoting hydration after exercise in humans, *Journal of the American College of Nutrition* 26(5):592S–596S, 2007.

109. Sherriffs S: Hydration in sport and exercise: Water, sports drinks and other drinks, *Nutrition Bulletin* 34(4):374–79, 2009.

110. Siegel A: Hydration and its disorders: New understandings, new treatments, *AMAA Journal* 19(1):13, 2006.

111. Smith J: Cooling methods used in the treatment of exertional heat illness, *British Journal of Sports Medicine* 39(8):503, 2005.

112. Taylor K: Ultraviolet radiation: Recognizing hidden potential for injury, *Athletic Therapy and Training* 15(3):75–80, 2010.

113. Thomas J: Non-freezing cold injury. In Pandolf K: *4,* Falls Church, VA, 2002, Office of the Surgeon General, US Army.

114. Tyler C: Cooling the neck region during exercise in the heat, *J Athl Train* 46(1):61–8, 2011.

115. Volpe S: Estimation of prepractice hydration status of National Collegiate Athletic Association Division I Athletes, *J Athl Train* 44(6):624–29, 2009.

116. Wallace C: Fluid replacement and dehydration. In *NFHS Sports Medicine Handbook,* Indianapolis, 2011, NFHS.

117. Walsh K, et al.: National Athletic Trainers' Association position statement: Lightning safety for athletics and recreation, *Journal of Athletic Training* 48(2):258–70, 2013.

118. Waterhouse J: Identifying some determinants of "jet lag" and its symptoms: A study of athletes and other travelers, *British Journal of Sports Medicine* 36(1):54, 2006.

119. Watson G: Creatine use and exercise heat tolerance in dehydrated men, *J Athl Train* 41(1):18, 2006.

120. Williams S: A review of football injuries on third- and fourth-generation artificial turfs compared with natural turf, *Sports Medicine* 41(11):903–23, 2011.

121. Wright J: Playing field issues in sports medicine, *Current Sports Medicine Issues* 9(3):129–33, 2010.

122. Yeargin S: Thermoregulatory responses and hydration practices in heat-acclimatized adolescents during preseason high school football, *J Athl Train* 45(2):136–46, 2010.

## ANNOTATED BIBLIOGRAPHY

Armstrong LE: *Performing in extreme environments: Training and working in intense heat, frigid cold, under water, high altitude, air pollution,* Champaign, IL, 2000, Human Kinetics.

*Looks at exercise as it is affected by a variety of environmental conditions.*

Giesbrecht G, Wikerson J: *Hypothermia, frostbite and other cold injuries: Prevention, recognition and treatment,* Seattle, 2006, Mountaineers Books.

*A comprehensive guide to recognizing, preventing, and treating hypothermia and other cold injuries.*

Graver D, Armstrong L: *Exertional heat illness,* Champaign, IL, 2003, Human Kinetics.

*Focuses on all aspects of heat illness and is a good resource for the athletic trainer.*

Klossner D, ed: *NCAA sports medicine handbook 2011–2012,* Indianapolis, IN, National Collegiate Athletic Association.

*Contains guidelines and recommendations for preventing heat illness, hypohydration, and cold stress, and for lightning safety.*

Maughan R, Murray R: *Sports drinks: Basic science and practical aspects,* Boca Raton, FL, 2001, CRC Press.

*Provides a review of current knowledge on issues relating to the formulation of sports drinks and the physiological responses to their ingestion during physical activity.*

Pollard A, Murdoch D: *High altitude medicine handbook,* Abbington, England, 2003, Radcliffe Medical Press.

*A compilation of pertinent information on almost every aspect of health and illness at altitudes higher than 2,500 meters.*

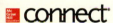

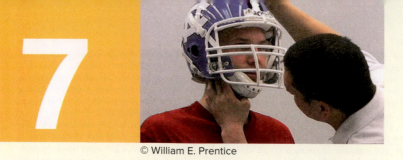
© William E. Prentice

# 7

# Protective Equipment

## ■ Objectives

*When you finish this chapter you should be able to*

- Fit selected protective equipment properly (e.g., football helmets, shoulder pads, and running shoes).
- Differentiate between good and bad features of selected protective devices.
- Contrast the advantages and disadvantages of customized versus off-the-shelf foot and ankle protective devices.

- Rate the protective value of various materials used in sports to make pads and orthotic devices.
- List the steps in making a customized foam pad with a thermomoldable shell.

## ■ Outline

## ■ Key Terms

pronators                                                                supinators

## ■ Connect Highlights    connect

*Visit connect.mcgraw-hill.com for further exercises to apply your knowledge:*

- Clinical application scenarios covering the use and application of protective equipment and the construction of pads and orthotic devices
- Click-and-drag questions covering fitting protective equipment, construction and application of protective devices
- Multiple-choice questions covering prophylactic bracing, construction of protective pads, and knowledge and application of protective equipment
- Selection questions covering anatomy of the shoe

One of the main responsibilities of the athletic trainer is to try to minimize the likelihood of injury or reinjury. A number of factors either singly or collectively can contribute to the incidence of injury. Certainly, the selection, fitting, and maintenance of protective equipment are critical not only in injury prevention but also in injury rehabilitation. Regardless of whether the athletic trainer works at the secondary-school, collegiate, or professional level or in a clinical, hospital, corporate, or industrial setting, it is essential that the athletic trainer have some knowledge about the types of protective equipment available for a particular activity and how that equipment should best be fitted and maintained to reduce the possibility of injury.[59]

This protection is particularly important in direct-collision sports, such as football, hockey, and lacrosse, but it can also be important in indirect-contact sports, such as basketball and soccer. When protective sports equipment is selected and purchased, a significant commitment is made to safeguard athletes' health and welfare.

During the rehabilitation period following injury, the athletic trainer must be knowledgeable about the types of protective rehabilitation equipment available and about how that equipment should be utilized to facilitate the recovery process.

## SAFETY STANDARDS FOR SPORTS EQUIPMENT AND FACILITIES

There is serious concern about the standards for protective sports equipment, particularly material durability standards. These concerns include who should set the standards, the mass production of equipment, equipment testing methods, and requirements for wearing protective equipment. Standards are also needed for protective equipment maintenance, repair, and replacement. Too often, old, worn-out, and ill-fitting equipment is passed down from the varsity players to the younger and often less experienced players, compounding their risk of injury.[63] It is critical for those responsible for purchasing athletic equipment to be less concerned with the color, look, and style of a piece of equipment and more concerned with its ability to prevent injury.[65] Many national organizations are addressing these issues. Engineering, chemistry, biomechanics, anatomy, physiology, physics, computer science, and other related disciplines are applied to solve problems inherent in safety standardization of sports equipment and facilities.

> Old, worn-out, poorly fitted equipment should never be passed down to younger, less experienced players because it compounds their chances for injury.

*Focus Box 7–1:* "Equipment regulatory agencies" lists agencies that regulate protective sports equipment.

## LEGAL CONCERNS IN USING PROTECTIVE EQUIPMENT

As with other aspects of sports participation, litigation related to the use of protective equipment is increasing. Both manufacturers and those who purchase sports equipment must foresee all possible uses and misuses of the equipment and must warn the user of any potential risks inherent in using or misusing that equipment.

If an injury occurs as a result of an individual using a piece of equipment that is determined to be defective or inadequate for its intended purpose, the manufacturer is considered liable. If a piece of protective equipment is modified in any way by an athlete, a coach, or an athletic trainer (e.g., removing some pads from inside a football helmet), the liability on the part of the manufacturer is voided, and the individual who modified the equipment becomes liable. *The best way for an athletic trainer to avoid litigation is to follow exactly the manufacturer's instructions for using and maintaining protective equipment.*

If an athletic trainer modifies a piece of equipment and an individual wearing that equipment is injured, it is likely that any lawsuit would involve both the athletic trainer individually and the employing institution or company. This becomes a case of tort (described in Chapter 3) in which the injured person must show that the athletic trainer was negligent in his or her decision to alter a piece of equipment and that the negligence resulted in injury. The athletic trainer would then be legally liable for that action. (See *Focus Box 7–2:* "Guidelines for selecting, purchasing, and fitting protective gear and sports equipment to help minimize liability.")

## EQUIPMENT RECONDITIONING AND RECERTIFICATION

The National Operating Committee on Standards for Athletic Equipment (NOCSAE) is an organization that has established voluntary test standards to reduce head injuries by establishing minimum safety requirements for football helmets/face masks; baseball/softball batting helmets, baseballs and softballs; and lacrosse helmets/face masks.[54] These standards have been adopted by various regulatory bodies for sports, including the NCAA and the National Federation of State High School Associations (NFHS). Factors such as the type of helmet and the amount and intensity of usage determine the condition of each helmet over a period of time. The NOCSAE helmet standard is not a warranty, but simply a statement that a particular helmet model met the requirements of performance tests when it was

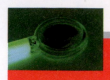

## Equipment regulatory agencies

American Society for Testing Materials
100 Barr Harbor Drive
PO Box C700
West Conshohocken, PA 19428-2959
(877) 909-2786
www.astm.org

Athletic Equipment Managers Association
c/o Sam Trusner
207 E. Bodman
Bement, IL 61813
(217) 678-1004
www.equipmentmanagers.org

Canadian Standards Association
178 Rexdale Boulevard
Toronto, ON
Canada
M9W 1R3
(416) 747-4000
www.csagroup.org

Hockey Equipment Certification Counsel
PO Box 4871134
US RT 9, Suite 4
Schroon Lake, NY 12870
(518) 532-7459
www.hecc.net

National Athletic Trainers Association
1620 Valwood Parkway
Carrollton, TX 75006
(214) 637-6282
www.nata.org

National Collegiate Athletic Association
700 W. Washington Street
Indianapolis, IN 46206-6222
(317) 917-6222
www.ncaa.org

National Association of Intercollegiate Athletics
1200 Grand Blvd.
Kansas City, MO 64106
(816) 595-8000
www.naia.org

National Federation of State High School Athletic Associations
690 W. Washington Street
Indianapolis, IN 46204
(317) 972-6900
www.nfhs.org

National Operating Committee on Standards for Athletic Equipment
11020 King Street, Suite 215
Overland Park, KS 66210
(913) 888-1340
www.nocsae.org

Sporting Goods Manufacturers Association
8505 Fenton Street, Suite 211
Silver Springs, MD 20910
(301) 495-6321
www.sgma.com

US Consumer Product Safety Commission
4330 East-West Highway
Bethesda, MD 20814
(301) 504-7923
www.cpsc.gov

manufactured or reconditioned. NOCSAE does recommend that the consumer adhere to a program of periodically having used helmets reconditioned and recertified. Because of the difference in the amount and intensity of usage on each helmet, the consumer should use discretion regarding the frequency with which certain helmets are to be reconditioned and recertified. Helmets that regularly undergo the reconditioning and recertification process can meet standard performance requirements for many seasons, depending on the model and usage. *Focus Box 7–3:* "Guidelines for purchasing and reconditioning helmets" provides some guidelines.

## USING OFF-THE-SHELF VERSUS CUSTOM PROTECTIVE EQUIPMENT

"Off-the-shelf" equipment is premade and packaged by the manufacturer and when taken out of the package may be used immediately without modification. Examples of off-the-shelf equipment are neoprene sleeves, sorbethane shoe inserts, and protective ankle braces. Custom equipment is constructed according to the individual characteristics of the athlete. Using off-the-shelf items may cause problems with sizing and

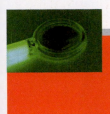

## FOCUS 7–2 Focus on Injury/Illness Prevention and Wellness Promotion

### Guidelines for selecting, purchasing, and fitting protective gear and sports equipment to help minimize liability

- Buy sports equipment from reputable manufacturers.
- Buy the safest equipment that resources permit.
- Make sure that all equipment is assembled correctly.
- Ensure that the person who assembles equipment is competent to do so and follows the manufacturer's instructions to the letter.
- Maintain all equipment properly, according to the manufacturer's guidelines.
- Use equipment only for the purpose for which it was designed.
- If an athlete is wearing some type of immobilization device (e.g., cast, brace), make certain that this does not violate the rules of that sport.
- Warn individuals who use the equipment about all possible risks that using the equipment could entail.
- Use great caution in constructing or customizing of any piece of equipment.
- Do not use defective equipment.
- Routinely inspect all equipment for defects and render all defective equipment unusable.

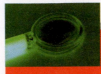

## FOCUS 7–3 Focus on Injury/Illness Prevention and Wellness Promotion

### Guidelines for purchasing and reconditioning helmets

- Purchase only NOCSAE-approved helmets.
- Purchase helmets for the appropriate skill level. For example, do not purchase youth helmets for high-school football.
- Assign a code number to each helmet purchased, and record the date of purchase.
- Fit helmets according to manufacturer's recommendations.
- Recheck helmets for proper fit during the season.
- Review written warranty information and comply with manufacturer's requirement(s) for cleaning/reconditioning/recertification.
- Replace or repair broken or damaged helmets before returning to service.
- Develop a written accounting of player use, inspections, reconditioning, recertification, and disposal of each helmet.
- Clean helmets and other equipment according to manufacturer's recommendations on a regular schedule during the season and at the end of the season prior to off-season storage in order to avoid infections.
- Recertify/recondition each football helmet according to manufacturer's warranty.
- Recertify/recondition helmets every 2 years using a certified NOCSAE-approved vendor if no warranty exists or after the warranty expires.

An athletic training student must acquire a basic understanding of protective sports equipment.

**?** What competencies relative to protective sports equipment must an athletic training student have?

exact fit. In contrast, a custom piece of equipment can be specifically sized and made to fit the protective and support needs of the individual. Generally, custom equipment is more expensive than off-the-shelf equipment. This increased cost may be attributed to the time that is necessary for an athletic trainer, a physical therapist, an orthotist, or an ortho tech to evaluate, construct, fit, and adjust a custom piece of equipment.

## HEAD PROTECTION

Direct-collision sports, such as football and hockey, require special protective equipment, especially for the head.[24] Football and ice hockey provide frequent opportunities for body contact but hockey players generally move faster and therefore create greater impact forces. Besides direct head contact, hockey has the added injury elements of swinging sticks and fast-moving pucks. Other sports using fast-moving projectiles are baseball, with its pitched ball and swinging bat; field hockey; lacrosse; and track and field, with the javelin, discus, and shot, which can also produce serious head injuries.[24]

### Football Helmets

NOCSAE has developed standards for football helmet certification.[54] An approved helmet must protect against concussive forces that may injure the brain. Collisions that cause concussions are usually with another player or the turf.[49]

> **Football helmets must be NOCSAE certified.**

Schools must provide the athlete with quality equipment, especially football helmets. All helmets must have NOCSAE[54] certification. However, a helmet that is certified is not necessarily completely fail-safe.[48] It is the responsibility of the athletic trainer to enforce the standard use of NOCASE-certified football helmets and to educate athletes, coaches, and parents that even though helmets help to prevent head injuries such as skull fractures, they do not significantly reduce the risk of concussions.[11,49] **SoR:B**

To make this danger especially clear, NOCSAE has adopted the following recommended warning to be placed on all football helmets:

> WARNING: NO HELMET CAN PREVENT ALL HEAD OR ANY NECK INJURIES A PLAYER MIGHT RECEIVE WHILE PARTICIPATING IN FOOTBALL. DO NOT USE THIS HELMET TO BUTT, RAM OR SPEAR AN OPPOSING PLAYER. THIS IS IN VIOLATION OF THE FOOTBALL RULES AND SUCH USE CAN RESULT IN SEVERE HEAD OR NECK INJURIES, PARALYSIS OR DEATH TO YOU AND POSSIBLE INJURY TO YOUR OPPONENT.[54]

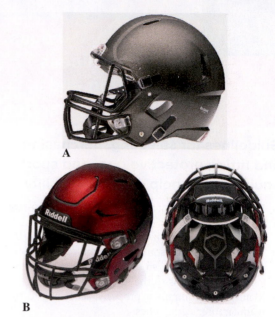

FIGURE 7–1 Examples of air-filled helmets. **(A)** Riddell Revolution Speed. **(B)** Riddell SpeedFlex. Courtesy Riddell.

Each player's helmet must have this visible, exterior warning label or a similar one ensuring that players have been made aware of the risks involved in the game of American football. The warning label must be attached to each helmet by both the manufacturer and the reconditioner.[54] It is important to have each player read this warning, after which it is read aloud by the equipment manager. The athlete then should sign a statement agreeing that he or she understands this warning.

A link to the NATA position statement "Head down contact and spearing in tackle football" can be found at www.nata.org/sites/default/files/HeadDownContact-AndSpearingInTackleFB.pdf. A variety of football helmets are available on the market (Figure 7–1), although the number of companies producing these helmets has decreased significantly over the years. This decrease in the number of helmet manufacturers can be attributed primarily to the number of lawsuits and liability cases that have forced many companies out of business.

The lightweight Revolution Speed helmet from Riddell extends the protective shell to the jaw area to provide protection to the side of the head and the jaw as well as improved front-to-back fit and stability.[55] The face guard system is designed to isolate the attachment points of the face guard from the shell, thus reducing jarring to the player from low-level impacts to the face guard (Figure 7–1A).

The latest in helmet technology attempts to minimize the impact forces transmitted to the athlete's head by having a shell that flexes at specific points to reduce and dissipate the forces. The Riddell SpeedFlex also incorporates a system of five accelerometers (sensors) that measure forces and the direction of an impact to the helmet and transmits that information to a computer that warns an athletic trainer whenever an athlete sustains a significant impact to the head (Figure 7–1B).

**Fitting a Football Helmet** When fitting a football helmet, closely follow the manufacturer's directions for a proper fit (Figure 7–2). (See *Focus Box 7–4:* "Proper football helmet fit.") The football helmet must be routinely checked for proper fit, especially in the first few days that it is worn. A check for snugness should be made by inserting a credit card between the head and the liner. Fit is proper when the credit card is resisted firmly when moved back and forth. If a team that travels to a different altitude and air pressure uses air bladder helmets, the helmet fit must be routinely rechecked.

Chin straps are also important in maintaining the proper head and helmet relationship. Three basic types of chin straps are in use today: a two-snap, a four-snap, and a six-snap strap. Many coaches prefer the four-snap chin strap because it keeps the helmet from tilting forward and backward. The chin strap should always be locked so that it cannot be released by a hard external force to the helmet.

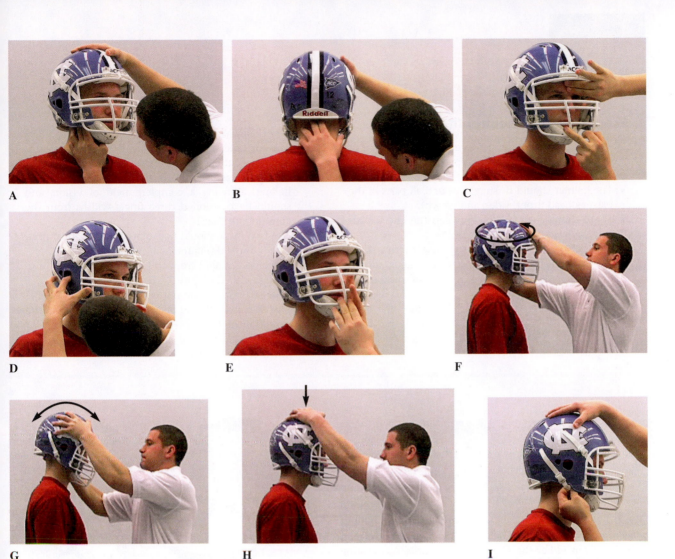

FIGURE 7–2   Properly fitting a football helmet. **(A)** Check snugness of cheek pads. **(B)** Helmet should cover base of skull. **(C)** Two finger widths above eyes. **(D)** Ear holes line up. **(E)** Three finger widths from face mask. **(F, G, H)** Helmet should not shift on head. **(I)** Check chin straps.

© William E. Prentice

Jaw pads are also essential to keep the helmet from rocking laterally. They should fit snugly against the player's cheekbones. Certification of a helmet's ability to withstand the forces of the game is of no avail if the helmet is not properly fitted or maintained. Loop straps can be used to fix the face mask to the helmet. These can be easily cut to remove the face mask should there be an injury that requires CPR or spinal injury. Various quick release face mask attachment systems have also been developed for use in securing the face mask to the helmet. While these systems have been designed to facilitate face mask removal in an emergency, athletic trainers should gain familiarity with these new systems and the obstacles they may present.[64,67]

## Ice Hockey Helmets

Like football helmets, ice hockey helmets have been upgraded and standardized.[39] Blows to the head in ice hockey, in contrast to football, are usually singular rather than multiple. An ice hockey helmet must withstand not only high-velocity impacts (e.g., being hit with a stick or a puck, which produces low mass and high velocity) but also the high-mass–low-velocity forces produced by running into the boards or falling on the ice.[50] In each instance, the hockey helmet, like the football helmet, must be able to disperse the impact over a large surface area

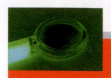

### Proper football helmet fit

After measuring the circumference of the head 1 inch above the eyebrow and selecting the appropriate helmet size:

- First, the air bladder should be inflated.
- The helmet should fit snugly around all parts of the player's head (front, sides, and crown).
- There should be no gaps between the cheek pads and the head or face (Figure 7-2A).
- The helmet should cover the base of the skull. The pads placed at the back of the neck should be snug, but not to the extent of discomfort (Figure 7-2B).
- The helmet should not come down over the eyes. It should sit (front edge) ¾ of an inch, or about two finger widths, above the player's eyebrows (Figure 7-2C).

- The ear holes should be aligned with the external opening in the ear canal (Figure 7-2D).
- The face mask should be attached securely to the helmet, allowing a complete field of vision, and should be positioned three finger-widths from the chin (Figure 7-2E).
- The face mask should not rotate when manual pressure is applied (Figure 7-2F).
- It should not shift front to back when manual pressure is applied (Figure 7-2G).
- It should not bottom out on impact (Figure 7-2H ).
- The chin strap should be an equal distance from the center of the helmet (Figure 7-2I).
- Straps must keep the helmet from moving up and down or side to side.

---

> Ice hockey helmets must withstand the high-velocity impact from a stick or puck and the low-velocity forces from falling or hitting a board.

through a firm exterior shell and, at the same time, be able to decelerate forces that act on the head through a proper energy-absorbing liner. It is essential for all hockey players to wear protective helmets that carry the stamp of approval from either the Canadian Standards Association (CSA) (Figure 7–3) or the Hockey Equipment Certification Council (HECC). *Focus Box 7–5*: "Properly fitting the ice hockey helmet" offers some tips.

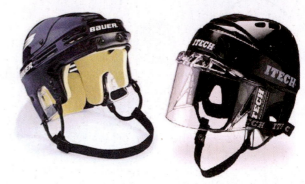

FIGURE 7–3   Ice hockey helmets.
Courtesy Sports Authority

### Baseball/Softball Batting Helmets

Like ice hockey helmets, the baseball/softball batting helmet must withstand high-velocity impacts.[24] Unlike football and ice hockey, baseball and softball have not produced a great deal of data on batting helmets. It has

been suggested, however, that baseball and softball helmets do little to adequately dissipate the energy of the ball during impact[28] (Figure 7–4). A possible solution is to add external padding or to improve the helmet's

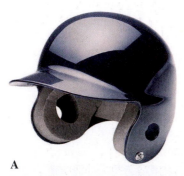

A

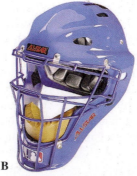

B

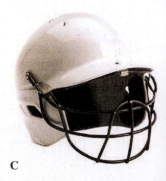

C

FIGURE 7–4   There is some question about how well baseball batting helmets protect against high-velocity impacts. **(A)** Batter's helmet. **(B)** Catcher's helmet and mask. **(C)** Batter's face mask and face shield.
Courtesy Sports Authority

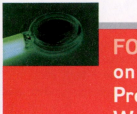

## FOCUS 7–5 Focus on Injury/Illness Prevention and Wellness Promotion

### Properly fitting the ice hockey helmet[50]

- The helmet should be comfortably snug at the forehead, top, back, and sides of the head.
- The helmet should not shift or wobble on the head–this will reduce protection and comfort and could also be distracting during play.
- The chin strap should be adjusted, so that it gently contacts the chin when the mouth is closed.
- The helmet should fit flat and snug on the head above the eyebrows without tilting forward or back.
- If the helmet is loose or not properly fastened, it loses its protective qualities.
- The bottom of a full cage face mask should rest gently on the chin when properly fitted.

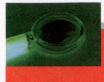

## FOCUS 7–6 Focus on Injury/Illness Prevention and Wellness Promotion

### Guidelines for fitting a cycling helmet

- The helmet should be level on the head.
- If it is not level, adjust the fit, using the extra foam fitting pads on the inside to provide contact with the head all the way around.
- With a "one size fits all" model with a fitting ring, adjust the fit by tightening the ring if needed.
- Adjust the rear (nape) straps, then the front straps, to position the Y fitting where the straps come together just under the ear. (It may be necessary to slide the straps across the top of the helmet to get them even on both sides.)
- Next, adjust the chin strap so that it is comfortably snug.
- Next adjust the rear stabilizer if the helmet has one.
- Shake your head around violently.
- Push under the front edge and push up and back. If the helmet moves more than an inch or so from level, tighten the straps so that the helmet is level and feels solid but comfortable on the head.

suspension. The use of a helmet with an ear flap can afford some additional protection to the batter. Each runner and on-deck batter is required to wear a baseball or softball helmet that carries the NOCSAE stamp, which is similar to the warning on football helmets.

## Cycling Helmets

Unlike the other helmets discussed, cycling helmets are designed to protect the head during one impact. Football, hockey, and baseball helmets are more durable and can survive repeated impacts.[49] Helmet use in high-velocity sports such as cycling has been shown to protect against traumatic head and facial injury.[11] **SoR:A** Many states require the use of cycling helmets, especially by adolescents (Figure 7–5). *Focus Box 7–6:* "Guidelines for fitting a cycling helmet" outlines fitting procedures.

## Lacrosse Helmets

Helmets are required equipment for all male lacrosse players. Women's lacrosse requires only a protective eye guard.

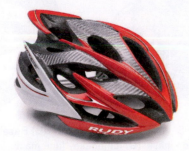

**FIGURE 7–5** Cycling helmet.
Courtesy Rudy Project North America

Lacrosse helmets are made of a hard plastic with a wire mesh cage, or face mask, to protect the front of the face (Figure 7–6). The face mask must have a center bar running from the top to the bottom. The helmet is designed to absorb repeated impact from a hard, high-velocity projectile. Helmets come in a variety of sizes and are usually measured in inches. Lacrosse helmets use a four-point buckling system both to ensure that they stay on and to allow for a better fit. Goalie helmets add a throat protector.[17]

## Soccer Headgear

Several companies have marketed headgear for soccer players to reduce concussions and other head injuries that occur from heading a soccer ball.[12] The headgear is essentially a headband with a piece of foam in the front that is about 1½ to 2 inches (3.8 to 5 cm) wide. To date there is one study that demonstrates that headgear is effective in reducing the risk of concussions or other head injuries.[25] Interestingly, some have identified increases in head accelerations during heading while wearing soccer headgear.[68,70] Furthermore, conflicting evidence exists regarding the effectiveness of soccer headgear to reduce impact responses associated with heading a soccer ball.[12,75] While some evidence suggests that a soccer player may become concussed after heading a soccer ball, it is far more likely that the soccer player will get a concussion by hitting his or her head on another player.[21]

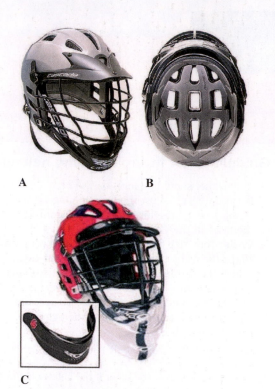

FIGURE 7–6  **(A)** Men's lacrosse helmet. **(B)** Inside padding. **(C)** Goalie helmet with throat protector.

Courtesy Sports Authority

## FACE PROTECTION

Devices that provide face protection fall into five categories: full face guards, throat protection, mouth guards, ear guards, and eye protection devices.

### Full Face Guards

Face guards are used in a variety of sports to protect against flying or carried objects during a collision with another player (Figure 7–7).[33] Since the adoption of face

guards and mouth guards for use in football, the incidence of facial injuries (e.g., lacerations, nose fractures, eye injuries) has dramatically decreased. However, the number of concussions and, to some extent, neck injuries has increased because the head is more often used to make initial contact.[15] The catcher in baseball, the goalie in hockey, and the lacrosse player should all be adequately protected against facial injuries, particularly lacerations and fractures (Figure 7–8).

A variety of face masks and bars are available to the player, depending on the position played and the degree of protection needed.[33] In football, no face guard should have less than two bars. Proper mounting of the face mask and bars is imperative for maximum safety. All mountings should be made in such a way that the bar attachments are flush with the helmet. A 3-inch (7.62 cm) space should exist between the top of the face guard and the lower edge of the helmet. No helmet should be drilled more than one time on each side, and this drilling must be done by a factory-authorized reconditioner. Attachment of a bar or face mask not specifically designed for the helmet can invalidate the manufacturer's warranty.

Ice hockey face masks have been shown to reduce the incidence of facial injuries.[3,47] In secondary school and collegiate hockey, face masks are required not just for the goalie but for all players. Helmets should be equipped with commercial plastic-coated wire mask guards or full

| Face protection |
|---|
| • Face guards |
| • Throat protection devices |
| • Mouth guards |
| • Ear guards |
| • Eye protection devices |

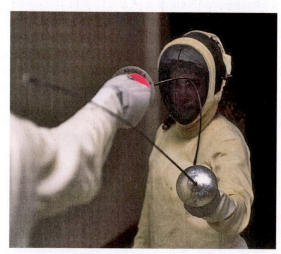

FIGURE 7–7  Sports such as fencing require complete face protection.

© William E. Prentice

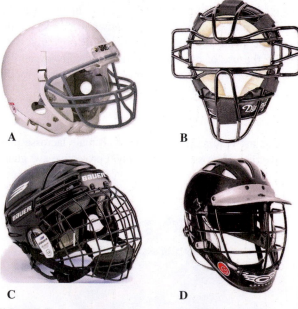

FIGURE 7–8  **(A)** Football face mask. **(B)** Baseball catcher's face mask. **(C)** Ice hockey face mask. **(D)** Lacrosse face mask.

Courtesy Sports Authority

face shields, which must meet standards set by the Hockey Equipment Certification Council (HECC) and the American Society for Testing Materials (ASTM). The openings in the guard must be small enough to prevent a hockey stick from entering. Plastic guards, such as polycarbonate face shields, have been approved by the HECC, the ASTM, and the CSA Committee on Hockey Protective Equipment. The rule also requires that goalkeepers wear commercial throat protectors in addition to face protectors. The National Federation of High School Associations (NFHS) rule is similar to the NCAA rule that requires players to wear face guards.

## Throat (Laryngotracheal) Protection

A laryngotracheal injury, though relatively uncommon, can be fatal.[49] Baseball catchers, lacrosse goalies, and ice hockey goalies are most at risk. Throat protection should be mandatory for these sports. Throat protectors may be built into the helmet or they can be attached separately (Figure 7–9).

## Mouth Guards

The majority of dental traumas can be prevented if the athlete wears a correctly fitted, customized intraoral mouth guard (Figure 7–10).[43,46,58] Consistent evidence to support the use of mouth guards for reducing or minimizing concussion

is not available. However, substantial evidence demonstrates that a properly fitted mouth guard reduces dental injuries.[11,51] **SoR:B** Mouth guards also minimize lacerations to the lips and cheeks and fractures to the mandible. The mouth protector should give the athlete proper and tight fit, comfort, unrestricted breathing, and unimpeded speech during competition. A loose mouth guard will soon be ejected onto the ground or left unused in the locker room.[2] The athlete's air passages should not be obstructed in any way. It is best when the mouth guard is retained on the upper jaw and projects backward only as far as the last molar, thus permitting speech. Maximum protection is afforded when the mouth guard is composed of a flexible, resilient material and is formed to fit to the teeth and upper jaw.[18]

> A properly fitted mouth guard protects the teeth, absorbs blows to the chin, and can prevent concussion.

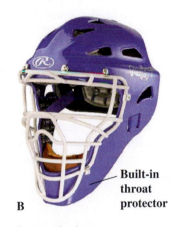
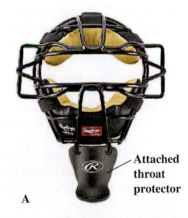

**A** — Attached throat protector

**B** — Built-in throat protector

FIGURE 7–9 A throat protector can be attached to **(A)** the catcher's face mask in baseball and softball or **(B)** a goalie mask in lacrosse and ice hockey.
Courtesy Sports Authority

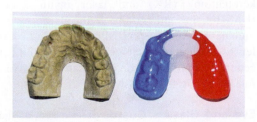
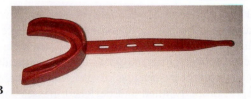

**A**

**B**

FIGURE 7–10 Mouth guards. **(A)** Custom-fit from a mold and **(B)** heat moldable.
© William E. Prentice

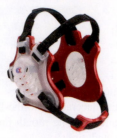

FIGURE 7–11   Wrestling headgear is worn primarily for the purpose of protecting the ears.
Courtesy Cliff Keen Athletic

Cutting down mouth guards to cover only the front teeth should never be permitted. This invalidates the manufacturer's warranty against dental injuries, and a cut-down mouth guard can become dislodged and lead to an obstructed airway.

The three types of mouth guards generally used in sports are the stock variety, the commercial mouth guard formed after submersion in boiling water, and the custom-fabricated type, which is formed over a mold made from an impression of the athlete's maxillary arch.[18,58,78]

Many secondary schools and colleges require that mouth guards be worn at all times during participation. For example, the NCAA football rules mandate that all players wear a properly manufactured mouth guard. A time-out is charged to a team if a player fails to wear the mouth guard.[36] To assist enforcement, official mouth guards are required to be in a highly visible color.

## Ear Guards

With the exception of wrestling, water polo, and boxing, most contact sports do not make a special practice of protecting the ears. All these sports can cause irritation of the ears to the point that permanent deformity can ensue. To avoid this problem, ear guards should be worn routinely (Figure 7–11).

## Eye Protection Devices

The National Society to Prevent Blindness estimates that the highest percentage of eye injuries are sports- or play-related. Most injuries are from blunt trauma. Protective devices must be sport specific.[39]

**Glasses**   For the individual who must wear corrective lenses, glasses can be both a blessing and a nuisance. They may slip on sweat, get bent when hit, fog from perspiration, detract from peripheral vision, and be difficult to wear with protective headgear. Even with all these disadvantages, properly fitted and designed glasses can provide adequate protection and withstand the rigors of the sport.

Athletes should wear polycarbonate lenses, which are virtually unbreakable.[73] These are the newest type of lenses available, and they are the safest. If the athlete has glass lenses, they must be case-hardened to prevent them from splintering on impact. When a case-hardened lens breaks, it crumbles, eliminating the sharp edges that may penetrate the eye. The cost of this process is relatively low. The only disadvantages are that the glasses are heavier than average and may be scratched more easily than regular glasses.[40] Another possible sports advantage of glass-lensed glasses is that they can be created so the lenses become color-tinted when exposed to ultraviolet rays from the sun and then return to a clear state when removed from the sun's rays. These lenses are known as photochromic lenses.

**Contact Lenses**   The individual who can wear contact lenses without discomfort can avoid many of the inconveniences of glasses. The greatest advantage to contact lenses is probably the fact that they "become a part of the eye" and move with it.

Contact lenses come mainly in two types: the corneal type, which covers just the iris of the eye, and the scleral type, which covers the entire front of the eye, including the white. Peripheral vision as well as astigmatism and corneal waviness are improved through the use of contact lenses. Unlike glasses, contact lenses do not normally cloud during temperature changes. They also can be tinted to reduce glare. For example, yellow lenses can be used against ice glare and blue ones against glare from snow. Some serious disadvantages of wearing contact lenses are the possibility of corneal irritation caused by dust getting under the lens and the possibility of a lens becoming dislodged during body contact. In addition, only certain individuals can wear contacts with comfort, and some individuals are unable to ever wear them because of certain eye idiosyncrasies. Athletes currently prefer the soft, hydrophilic lenses to the hard type. Adjustment time for the soft lenses is shorter than for the hard, they can be more easily replaced, and they are more adaptable to the sports environment. Disposable lenses and lenses that can be worn for an extended period are also available. In the last few years, the cost of contact lenses has dropped significantly.

The advent of two eye surgery procedures, radial kerotectomy (RK) and laser insitu keratomileusis (LASIK), has potentially reduced the need for individuals to wear vision-correcting glasses or contact lenses. Although relatively expensive, the LASIK procedure has proven to be a safe and effective technique for correcting faulty vision.

**Eye and Glasses Guards**   It is essential that athletes take special precautions to protect their eyes, especially in sports that use fast-moving projectiles and implements, such as handball and racquetball (Figure 7–12).[40] Besides

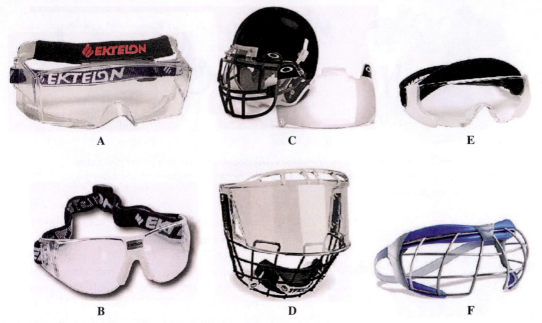

FIGURE 7–12  **(A & B)** Athletes playing sports that involve small, fast projectiles should wear closed eye guards. **(C)** Polycarbonate shield for a football helmet. **(D)** Shield for an ice hockey face mask. **(E)** Field hockey goggle. **(F)** Lacrosse goggle.

Courtesy Sports Authority

> **Eye protection must be worn by all athletes who play sports that use fast-moving projectiles.**

the more obvious sports of ice hockey, lacrosse, and baseball, the racquet sports can also cause serious eye injury. Athletes not wearing glasses should wear closed eye guards to protect the orbital cavity. Athletes who normally wear glasses with plastic or case-hardened lenses are to some degree already protected against eye injury from an implement or a projectile; however, greater safety is afforded by the polycarbonate frame that surrounds and fits over the athlete's glasses. The protection that the guard affords is excellent, but it hinders vision in some planes. Polycarbonate eye shields can be attached to football face masks, hockey helmets, and baseball and softball helmets.

## NECK PROTECTION

Experts in cervical injuries consider the major value of commercial and customized cervical collars to be mostly a reminder to the athlete to be cautious rather than to provide a definitive restriction (see Figure 7–16C).[29]

## TRUNK AND THORAX PROTECTION

Trunk and thorax protection is essential in many contact and collision sports. Sports such as football, ice hockey, baseball, and lacrosse use extensive body protection. Areas that are most exposed to impact forces must be properly covered with some material that offers protection against soft-tissue compression. Of particular concern are the external genitalia and the exposed bony protuberances of the body that have insufficient soft tissue for protection, such as shoulders, ribs, and spine (Figure 7–13).

As discussed earlier, the problem that arises in wearing protective equipment is that, although it is armor against injury to the athlete wearing it, it can also serve as a weapon against all opponents. Standards must become more stringent in determining what equipment is absolutely necessary for body protection and at the same time is not itself a source of trauma. Proper fit and proper maintenance of equipment are essential.

### Football Shoulder Pads

Two general types of shoulder pads are available: cantilevered and noncantilevered (Figure 7–14). A cantilever is a strap that extends from the front to the back of the shoulder pads that causes the shoulder pads to arch above the tip of the shoulder, thus dispersing pressure onto the pads rather than on the shoulder. The player who uses the shoulder a great deal in blocking and tackling requires the bulkier, cantilevered type, whereas a quarterback, receiver, or youth football player might prefer to use the noncantilevered pads, which don't restrict shoulder motion as much as the cantilevered pads. Over the years, the shoulder pad's front and rear panels have been extended along with

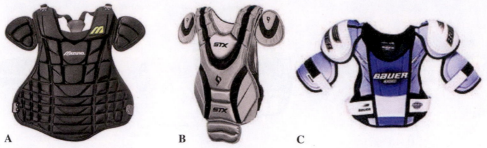

FIGURE 7–13   Chest and thorax protectors. **(A)** Baseball catcher's chest protector. **(B)** Lacrosse goalie chest protector. **(C)** Ice hockey thorax protector and shoulder pads.
Courtesy Sports Authority

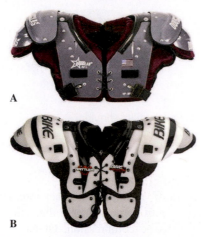

FIGURE 7–14   Shoulder pads protect both the shoulder and thorax. **(A)** Noncantilevered pads. **(B)** Cantilevered pads.
Courtesy Sports Authority

the cantilever. *Focus Box 7–7:* "Rules for fitting football shoulder pads" summarizes fitting guidelines (Figure 7–15).

Some athletic trainers use a combination of football and ice hockey shoulder pads to prevent injuries high on the upper arm and shoulder. A pair of supplemental shoulder pads are placed under the football pads (Figure 7–16 A&B). The deltoid cap of the hockey pad is connected to the main body of the hockey pad by an adjustable lace. The distal end of the deltoid cap is held in place by a Velcro strap. The chest pad is adjustable to ensure proper fit for any size athlete. The football shoulder pads are placed over the hockey pads. The athletic trainer should observe for a proper fit. Larger football pads may be needed. A neck collar can be attached to the shoulder pads and has been shown to be effective in minimizing neck movement (Figure 7–16C).[29]

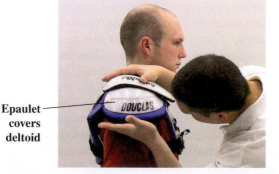
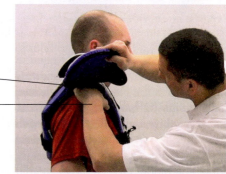

FIGURE 7–15   Fitting the shoulder pads.
© William E. Prentice

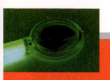

# FOCUS 7–7  Focus on Injury/Illness Prevention and Wellness Promotion

## Rules for fitting football shoulder pads

- The width of the shoulder is measured to determine the proper size of pad.
- The inside shoulder pad should cover the tip of the shoulder in a direct line with the lateral aspect of the shoulder.
- The epaulets and cups should cover the deltoid muscle and allow movements required by the athlete's position.
- The neck opening must allow the athlete to raise the arm overhead, but not allow the pad to slide back and forth.

- If a split-clavicle shoulder pad is used, the channel for the top of the shoulder must be in the proper position.
- Straps underneath the arm must hold the pads firmly in place, but not so they constrict soft tissue. A collar and drop-down pads may be added to provide more protection.
- After fitting, make sure the pads don't shift when the athlete puts on the jersey.

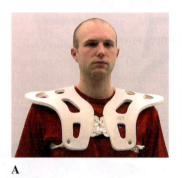
**A**

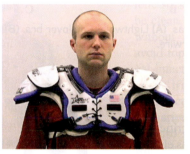
**B**

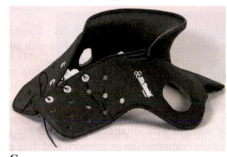
**C**

FIGURE 7–16  **(A & B)** Customized foam is placed on the underside of the shoulder pad to provide additional protection to the acromioclavicular joint or clavicle. **(C)** A cowboy collar can be attached to the shoulder pad.
© William E. Prentice

## Sports Bras

Manufacturers have made significant efforts to develop athletic support bras for women who participate in all types of physical activity. In the past, the primary concern was for breast protection against external forces that could cause bruising. Most sports bras are now designed to minimize excessive vertical and horizontal movements of the breasts that occur with running and jumping.[57]

To be effective, a bra should hold the breasts to the chest and prevent stretching of the ligaments of Cooper, which causes premature sagging (Figure 7–17). Metal

> To be effective, a bra should hold the breasts tightly to the chest.

parts (snaps, fasteners, underwire support) rub and abrade the skin and should be avoided. Shoulder straps should be at least 1 inch (2.5 cm) wide for comfort. Nonsupport bras lack sufficient padding, and seams over nipples compound the rubbing of the bra on the nipple, which can lead to irritation.[13]

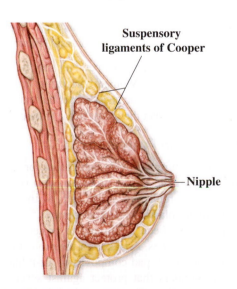

FIGURE 7–17  Stretching of ligaments of Cooper causes premature sagging.

Chapter Seven ■ Protective Equipment  **197**

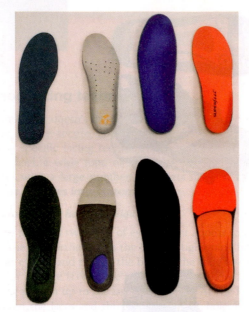

FIGURE 7–24   Commercially manufactured orthotic devices. Top view and bottom view of four different sets of orthotics.

© William E. Prentice

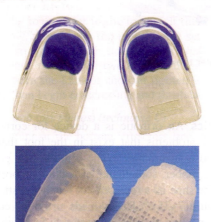

FIGURE 7–25   Different styles of heel cups.

© William E. Prentice

more often, has the advantage of saving time. Off-the-shelf pads are

manufactured for almost every type of common structural foot condition, ranging from corns and bunions to fallen arches and pronated feet. Off-the-shelf foot pads are commonly used before more customized orthotic devices are made. These products offer a compromise to the custom-made foot orthotics by providing some biomechanical control.[37] Indiscriminate use of these aids, however, may intensify the pathological condition or cause the athlete to delay seeing the team physician or team podiatrist for evaluation.[31]

For the most part, foot devices are fabricated and customized from a variety of materials such as foam, felt, plaster, aluminum, and spring steel (see the section "Construction of Protective and Supportive Devices" later in this chapter).

## Ankle Braces

Ankle stabilizers, either alone or in combination with ankle taping, are becoming increasingly popular (Figure 7–26).[9,32,52,77] There has been significant debate regarding the efficacy of ankle supports in the prevention of ankle sprains.[30,35] Most studies indicate that bracing is effective in reducing ankle injury,[26,71] but other studies have shown no effects[8,34] or even negative effects.[8,30] Bracing probably has little or no effect on performance; any change in performance is due to the athlete's perception of support and comfort.[61] When compared with ankle taping, these devices do not loosen significantly during exercise.[22] A study that

A basketball player with a history of ankle sprains needs support during practice.

**?** Which type of ankle support is cost efficient and most reliable: tape or commercial supports?

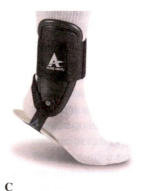

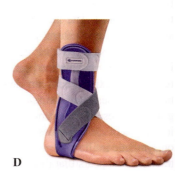

FIGURE 7–26   Commercial ankle supports for an injured ankle. **(A)** Lace-up brace. **(B)** Lace-up with straps brace. **(C)** Rigid support brace. **(D)** Rigid support with stabilizing straps.

(a) Courtesy McDavid; (b–c) Courtesy Active Ankle; (d) Courtesy Bauerfeind

collectively analyzed the data from 19 studies of the effects of different types of ankle support on ankle motion before and after activity showed significantly greater frontal-plane ankle-motion restriction after exercise for a semirigid stirrup brace design than for taping or a lace-up-type brace.[22] Several studies have documented a beneficial effect of semirigid ankle bracing on sprain incidence, whereas others comparing the effects of taping and a lace-up brace on sprain incidence support the superiority of bracing for injury prevention.[20,30,41,74] Recent studies have focused on the proprioceptive effects and how ankle braces influence balance, postural sway, and joint position sense.[35,74,79]

## Shin and Lower Leg

The shin and lower leg are particularly vulnerable to being kicked, especially in soccer, or hit with a stick in field hockey. The anterior surface of the tibia is exposed, lacking any soft-tissue protection. Contusion to the anterior surface of the tibia can result in swelling and significant pain. Contusion of the exposed muscle either lateral or medial to the tibia can result in compartment syndromes (see Chapter 19). Shin guards should be used to protect the anterior shin from direct blows. For maximum protection, the shin guards should extend from just below the tibial tubercle proximally to just above the malleoli distally (Figure 7–27).

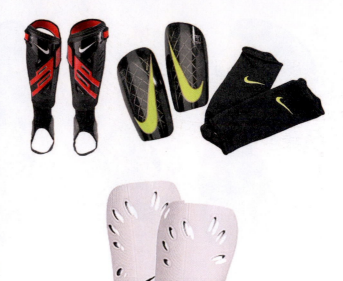

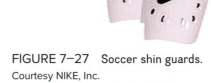

FIGURE 7–27   Soccer shin guards.
Courtesy NIKE, Inc.

## Thigh and Upper Leg

Thigh and upper-leg protection is widely used in collision sports, such as hockey, football, and soccer. Generally, pads slip into ready-made pockets in the uniform (Figure 7–28A). In some instances, customized pads should be constructed and held in place with tape or an elastic wrap. Neoprene sleeves can be used for support following strain to the hamstring, groin, or quadriceps muscles (Figure 7–28B).

## Knee Supports and Protective Devices

**Knee Pads**  Elastic knee pads or guards are extremely valuable in sports in which the athlete falls or receives a

direct blow to the anterior aspect of the knee. An elastic sleeve containing a resilient pad may help dissipate an anterior striking force and reduce contusions but fails to protect the knee against lateral, medial, or twisting forces that result in stress to the ligaments.

**Knee Braces**  Because of the high incidence of injury to the knee joint, manufacturers have designed a host of different knee braces for a variety of purposes.[11] *Protective knee braces* are used prophylactically to prevent injuries to the medial collateral ligament in contact sports such as football (Figure 7–29).[60] Although these protective braces have been widely used in the past, the American

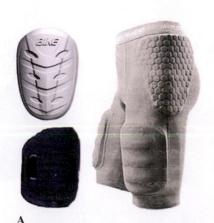

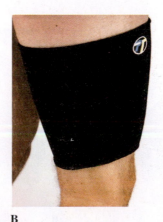

A                                                B

FIGURE 7–28   **(A)** Protective thigh pads. **(B)** Neoprene thigh sleeve.
(a) Courtesy Sports Authority; (b) Courtesy Pro-Tec Athletics

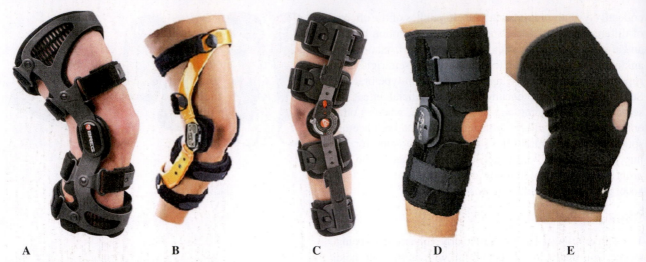

| A | B | C | D | E |

FIGURE 7–29 Knee braces. **(A)** Prophylactic knee brace. **(B)** Functional brace. **(C)** Rehabilitative brace. **(D)** Neoprene with medial support brace. **(E)** Neoprene brace.

(a, c) © 2014 Breg, Inc.; (b, d) Courtesy DJO Global; (e) Courtesy NIKE, Inc.

Orthopedic Society for Sports Medicine has expressed concern about their efficacy in reducing injuries to the collateral ligaments.[53] Several studies have actually shown an increase in the incidence of injuries to the medial collateral ligament in athletes wearing these braces.[60] Others have shown a positive influence on joint position sense[4] but little or no effect on performance.[19]

*Rehabilitative braces* are widely used following surgical repair or reconstruction of the knee joint to allow for controlled progressive immobilization (Figure 7–29C).[6] These braces have hinges that can be easily adjusted to allow range of motion to be progressively increased.

*Functional knee braces* may be worn both during and following the rehabilitative period to provide support during functional activities (Figure 7–29B).[14,16,62] Functional braces can be purchased ready made or can be custom made.[72] Some physicians strongly recommend that their patients consistently[51] wear these braces during physical activity, whereas others do not feel that they are necessary.[13,76]

*Neoprene braces with medial and lateral supports* may be used by individuals who have sustained injury to the collateral ligaments and feel that they need extra support medially and laterally[69] (Figure 7–29B).

A variety of *neoprene sleeves* may also be used to provide some support for patellofemoral conditions (Figure 7–29E).[19]

## ELBOW, WRIST, AND HAND PROTECTION

As with the lower extremity, the upper extremity requires protection from injury and prevention of further injury after trauma. Although the elbow joint is less commonly injured than the ankle, knee, or shoulder, it is still vulnerable to instability, contusion, and muscle strain. A variety of off-the-shelf protective neoprene sleeves and pads and hinged adjustable rehabilitative braces can offer protection to the elbow (Figure 7–30).

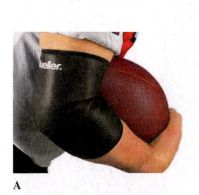 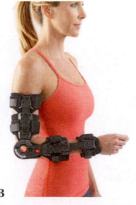 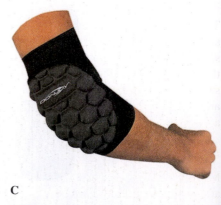

| A | B | C |

FIGURE 7–30 **(A)** Neoprene elbow sleeve. **(B)** Hinged rehabilitative elbow brace. **(C)** Elbow pad.

(a) Courtesy Mueller Sports Medicine; (b) © 2014 Breg, Inc.; (c) Courtesy DJO Global

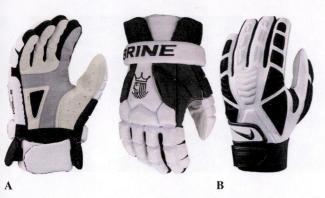

**A**　　　　　　　　　　　　**B**

FIGURE 7–31　The hand is an often neglected area of the body in sports. **(A)** Lacrosse gloves. **(B)** Football lineman's glove. (a) Courtesy Warrior Sports; (b) Courtesy NIKE, Inc.

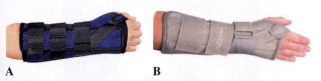

**A**　　　　　　　　　　**B**

FIGURE 7–32　Wrist and hand braces and immobilizers. Courtesy DJO Global

In sports medicine, injuries to the wrist, hand, and fingers are occasionally trivialized and considered insignificant. But injuries to the distal aspect of the upper extremity can be functionally disabling, especially in those sports that involve throwing and catching.[27] In both contact and noncontact sport activities, the wrist, hand, and particularly the fingers are susceptible to fracture, dislocation, ligament sprains, and muscle strains.[27] Protective gloves are essential in preventing injuries in sports such as lacrosse and ice hockey (Figure 7–31). It is also common to use both off-the-shelf and custom-molded splints both for support and for immobilization of an injury (Figure 7–32).

# CONSTRUCTION OF PROTECTIVE AND SUPPORTIVE DEVICES

The athletic trainer should be able to design and construct protective and supportive devices when necessary. Certainly, the athletic trainer must understand the theoretical basis for constructing protective pads and supports. However, the ability to construct an effective and appropriate protective device is more of an art than a science.

## Custom Pad and Orthotic Materials

Many materials are available to the athletic trainer attempting to protect or support an injured area. In general, these materials can be divided into soft and hard materials.

**Soft Materials** The primary soft-material media found in athletic training rooms are gauze padding, cotton, adhesive felt or adhesive sponge rubber felt, and an assortment of foam rubber.

*Gauze padding* is less versatile than other pad materials. It is assembled in varying thicknesses and can be used as an absorbent or protective pad.

*Cotton* is a cheap and widely used material that has the ability to absorb, to hold emollients, and to offer a mild padding effect.

*Adhesive felt (moleskin)* or *sponge rubber* material contains an adhesive mass on one side, thus combining a cushioning effect with the ability to be held in place by the adhesive mass. It is a versatile material that is useful on all body parts (Figure 7–33A).

*Felt* is a material composed of matted wool fibers pressed into varying thicknesses that range from ¼ to 1 inch (0.6 to 2.5 cm) (Figure 7–33B). Its benefit lies in its comfortable, semiresilient surface, which gives a firmer pressure than most sponge rubbers. Because felt absorbs perspiration, it clings to the skin, and it has less tendency to move than sponge rubber does. Because of its absorbent qualities, felt should be replaced daily. Currently, it is most often used as support and protection for a variety of foot conditions.

*Foams* are currently the materials most often used for providing injury protection in sports. They come in many different thicknesses and densities (Figure 7–33C). They are usually resilient, nonabsorbent, and able to protect the body against compressive forces. Some foams are open celled, whereas others are closed celled (Figure 7–34). The closed-cell type is preferable in sports because it rebounds to its original shape quickly. Foams can be easily worked through cutting, shaping, and faceting. Some foams are thermomoldable; when heated, they become highly pliant and easy to shape. When cooled, they retain the shape in which they were formed. A new class of foams is composed of viscoelastic polymers. Sorbothane is one example. This foam has a high energy-absorbing quality, but it also has a high density, making it heavy (Figure 7–33D). Used in inner soles in sports shoes, foam helps prevent blisters and effectively absorbs anterior/posterior and medial/lateral ground reaction forces. Foams generally range from ⅛ to ½ inch (0.3 to 1.25 cm) in thickness.

**Nonyielding Materials** A number of hard, nonyielding materials are used in athletic training for making protective shells and splints.

***Thermomoldable Plastics*** Plastic materials are widely used in sports medicine for customized orthotics. They can brace, splint, and shield a body area. They can provide casting for a fracture; support for a foot defect; or a firm, nonyielding surface to protect a severe contusion. Plastics used for these purposes differ

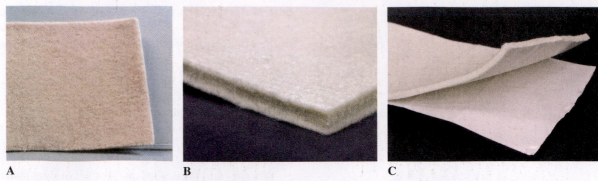

**FIGURE 7–33** Soft Materials. **(A)** Adhesive moleskin. **(B)** Orthopedic felt. **(C)** Adhesive foam.
© William E. Prentice

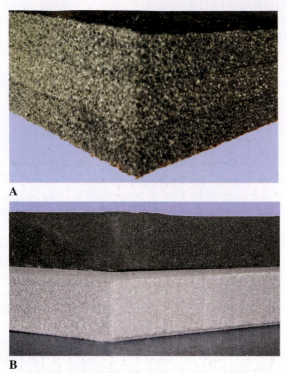

**FIGURE 7–34** Foam padding. **(A)** Open-celled foam.
**(B)** Closed-cell foam.
© William E. Prentice

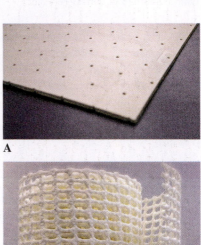

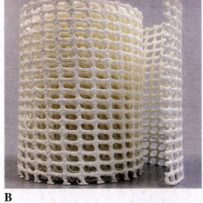

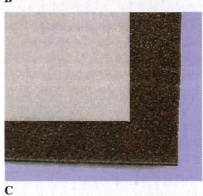

**FIGURE 7–35** Thermomoldable plastics. **(A)** Orthoplast.
**(B)** X-Lite. **(C)** Plastazote and Aliplast sheets.
© William E. Prentice

in their chemical composition and reaction to heat. The two categories are heat-forming plastics and heat-plastic foams.

Heat-forming plastics are of the low-temperature variety and are the most popular in athletic training. When heated to 140°F to 180°F (60°C to 82.2°C), depending on the material, the plastic can be accurately molded to a body part. Orthoplast and X-Lite (synthetic rubber thermoplast) are popular types (Figure 7–35A&B).

> Heat-forming plastics of the low-temperature variety are the most popular in athletic training.

Heat-plastic foams are plastics that have differences in density as a result of the addition of liquids, gas, or crystals. They are commonly used as shoe orthotic inserts and other body padding. Plastazote and Aliplast

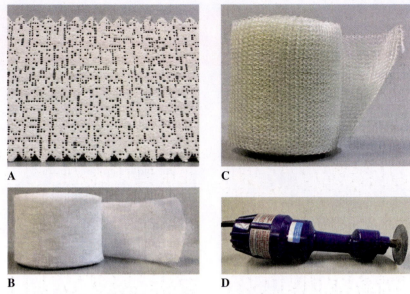

FIGURE 7–36   Casting materials and saw. **(A)** Plaster roll.
**(B)** Cast padding roll. **(C)** Fiberglass roll. **(D)** Cast saw.
© William E. Prentice

(polyethylene foams) are two commonly used products (Figure 7–35C).

Usually, the plastic is heated until soft and malleable. It is then molded into the desired shape and allowed to cool, thereby retaining its shape. Various pads and other materials can also be fastened in place. The rules and regulations of various sport activities may place limitations on the use of rigid thermomoldable plastics.

**Casting Materials** Applying plaster casts to injured body areas has long been a practice in sports medicine. The material of choice is fiberglass, which uses resin and a catalytic converter, plus water, to produce hardening. Besides casts, this material makes effective shells for splints and protective pads. Once hardened, the fiberglass is trimmed to shape with a cast saw (Figure 7–36).

**Tools Used for Customizing** Many different tools are needed to work with the various materials used to customize protective equipment. These tools include adhesives, adhesive tape, heat sources, shaping tools, and fastening material.

**Adhesives** A number of adhesives are used in constructing custom protective equipment. Many cements and glues join plastic to plastic or join other combinations of materials.

**Adhesive Tape** Adhesive tape is a major tool in holding various materials in place. Linen and elastic tape can hold pads to a rigid backing or to adhesive felt (moleskin) and can be used to protect against sharp edges (see Chapter 8).

**Heat Sources** To form thermomoldable plastics, a heat source must be available. Three sources are commonly found in training rooms: the commercial moist heat unit, a hot air gun or hair dryer, and a convection oven with a temperature control. The usual desired temperature is 160°F (71°C) or higher.

**Shaping Tools** Commonly, the tools required to shape custom devices are heavy-duty scissors, sharp-blade knives, and cast saws.

**Fastening Material** Once formed, customized protective equipment often must be secured in place. Fastening this equipment requires the availability of a great variety of materials. For example, if something is to be held securely, Velcro can be used when a device must be continually put on and removed. Leather can be cut and riveted in place to form hinge straps with buckles attached. Various types of laces can be laced through eyelets to hold something in place. Tools that allow for this type of construction include a portable drill, a hole punch, and an ice pick.

**Customized Hard-Shell Pads** A hard-shell pad is often required for an athlete who has an injury, such as a painful contusion (bruise), that must be completely protected from further injury. *Focus Box 7–10:*

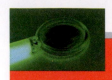

# FOCUS 7–10 Focus on Injury/Illness Prevention and Wellness Promotion

## How to construct a hard-shell pad

1. Select proper material and tools, which might include the following:
   a. Thermomoldable plastic sheet (Orthoplast, Hexalite)
   b. Scissors
   c. Felt material
2. Palpate and mark the margins of the tender area that needs protection.
3. Cut a felt piece to fit in the area of tenderness.
4. Heat plastic until malleable.
5. Place heated plastic over felt and wrap in place with an elastic wrap.

6. When cooled, remove elastic wrap and felt pad.
7. Trim shell to desired shape; a protective shell has now been made to provide a "bubble" relief.
8. If needed, add a softer inner layer of foam to distribute and lessen force further.
   a. Cut a doughnut-type hole in softer foam material the same size as the injury site.
   b. Cut foam the same shape as the hard shell.
   c. Use tape or an adhesive to affix the foam to the shell.

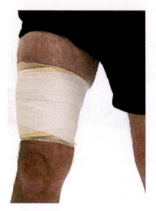

FIGURE 7–37   Hard-shell pad wrapped on the thigh.
© William E. Prentice

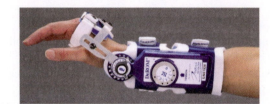

FIGURE 7–38   Dynamic splint for the hand and fingers.
Courtesy DeRoyal

"How to construct a hard-shell pad" provides the procedures needed to customize such a pad (Figure 7–37).

**Dynamic Splints** Occasionally, it is necessary to fabricate and apply a dynamic splint in treating injuries to the hand and fingers (Figure 7–38). Most often, an occupational therapist would make a dynamic splint; however, the athletic trainer is certainly capable of designing such a splint. A dynamic splint is used to provide long-duration tension on a healing structure (usually a tendon) so that it can return to normal function. Dynamic splints use a combination of thermoplastic material, Velcro, and pieces of rubber band or elastic to provide dynamic assistance.

## SUMMARY

- The proper selection and proper fitting of protective equipment are essential in the prevention and rehabilitation of many sports injuries. Because of the number of current litigations, sports equipment standards regarding the durability of the material and the fit and wear requirements of the equipment are of serious concern. Manufacturers must foresee all possible uses and misuses of their equipment and warn the user of any potential risks.

- Athletic trainers must be concerned about head protection in many collision and contact sports. The football helmet must be used only for its intended purpose and not as a weapon. To avoid unwarranted litigation, a warning label must be placed on the outside of the helmet indicating that the helmet is not fail-safe and must be used as intended. Properly fitting the helmet is of critical importance.

- Face protection is important in sports that have fast-moving projectiles, use implements that are in close proximity to other athletes, and facilitate body collisions. Protecting teeth and eyes is of particular significance. The customized mouth guard, fitted to individual requirements, provides the best protection for the teeth and protects against concussions. Eyes must be protected against projectiles and sports implements. The safest eye guard for the athlete wearing contact lenses or glasses is the closed type that completely protects the orbital cavity.
- Many sports require protection of various parts of the athlete's body. American football players, ice hockey players, and baseball catchers are examples of players who require body protection. Commonly, the protection is for the shoulders, chest, thighs, ribs, hips, buttocks, groin, genitalia (male athletes), and breasts (female athletes).

- Footwear is essential to prevent injuries. Socks must be clean, without holes, and made of appropriate materials. Shoes must be suited to the sport and must be properly fitted. The wide part of the foot must match the wide part of the shoe. If the shoe has cleats, they must be positioned at the metatarsophalangeal joints.
- Currently, there are many off-the-shelf pieces of specialized protective equipment on the market. They may be designed to support ankles, knees, or other body parts. In addition to stock equipment, athletic trainers often construct customized equipment out of a variety of materials to pad injuries or support feet. Professionals such as athletic trainers, orthopedists, podiatrists, physical therapists, and orthotists may devise orthopedic footwear and orthotic devices to improve the biomechanics of the athlete's foot.

## WEB SITES

Douglas Protective Equipment: www.douglaspads.com
*Manufacturer and distributor of football, hockey, and baseball protective padding.*

National Operating Committee on Standards for Athletic Equipment: www.nocsae.org

Protective Eyewear for Young Athletes: www.kidsource.com/kidsource/content/eyewear.html
*A joint statement of the American Academy of Pediatrics and American Academy of Ophthalmology.*

Riddell: www.riddell.com
*Riddell is an equipment manufacturing company, and this site gives information about the safety of the*

*products they sell and the necessary standards for safety equipment.*

Road Runner Sports: www.roadrunnersports.com
*Provides good information for fitting shoes, sports bras, and running apparel.*

The Training Room: www.thetrainingroom.com
*Sports orthopedic braces, orthotics, protective sports equipment, and athletic injury treatment.*

## SOLUTIONS TO CLINICAL APPLICATION EXERCISES

7–1 The athletic training student must acquire the following protective equipment competencies:
  - Identify good-quality and poor-quality commercial protective equipment.
  - Properly fit commercial protective equipment.
  - Construct protective and supportive devices.

7–2 The athletic trainer should initiate the following steps:
  1. Call a team meeting in which he or she fully explains the risks entailed in the use and fitting of the equipment.
  2. Report and repair any defective pieces of equipment immediately.
  3. Send out a letter to each parent or guardian, explaining equipment limitations. This letter must be signed and returned to the athletic trainer.
  4. Call a meeting of parents, team members, and coaches in which he or she further explains equipment limitations.

7–3 The athletic trainer explains that the helmet cannot prevent serious neck injuries. Striking an opponent with any part of the helmet or face mask can place abnormal stress on cervical structures. Most severe neck injuries occur from striking an opponent with the top of the helmet; this action is known as axial loading.

7–4 Mouth guards serve several important purposes in preventing injury in athletics, especially contact sports, such as ice hockey. Mouth guards help prevent or minimize lacerations, fractures, and possibly reduce the incidence of cerebral concussions. For a mouth guard to work effectively, proper fit is essential and must not interfere with breathing or speech. A custom-fabricated mouth guard is produced from a mold of each athlete, causing the fit to be more precise. If the fit is improved, athletes are more likely to wear their mouth guards.

7–5 The athletic trainer provides the following advice:
  - Shoes should be purchased to fit the larger foot.
  - The athlete should wear athletic socks when fitting shoes.
  - Shoes should be purchased at the end of the day.
  - Shoes should feel snug but comfortable when the athlete jumps up and down and performs cutting motions.
  - Shoe length and width should allow full toe function.
  - The wide part of the foot should match the wide part of the shoe.
  - The shoe should bend at its widest part.
  - Each foot should be measured from the heel to the end of the largest toe.

7–6 A verified commercial ankle support provides more consistent support for a longer period of time and is more cost efficient.

7–7 To construct a hard-shell protective thigh pad, the athletic trainer follows these steps:
1. Mark the area on the athlete to be protected.
2. Cut a foam piece to cover the injury temporarily.
3. Heat thermomoldable plastic and place over the foam piece to form a bubble.
4. Cut a plastic sheet to form to the athlete's thigh.
5. Create a doughnut-shaped foam lining to surround the injury.
6. Secure the foam doughnut to the plastic piece.
7. Secure the pad in place with elastic wrap.

## REVIEW QUESTIONS AND CLASS ACTIVITIES

1. What are the legal responsibilities of the athletic trainer in terms of protective equipment?
2. Invite an attorney to class to discuss product liability and its impact on the athletic trainer.
3. What are the various sports with high risk factors that require protective equipment?
4. How can the athletic trainer select and use safety equipment to decrease the possibility of sports injuries and litigation?
5. Why is continual inspection and/or replacement of used equipment important?
6. What are the standards for fitting football helmets? Are there standards for any other helmets?
7. Invite your school equipment manager to class to demonstrate all the protective equipment and how to fit it to the athlete.
8. Why are mouth guards important, and what are the advantages of custom-made mouth guards over the stock type?
9. What are the advantages and disadvantages of glasses and contact lenses in athletic competition?
10. How do you fit shoulder pads for the different-sized players and their positions?
11. Why is breast protection necessary? Which types of sports bras are available and what should the athlete look for when purchasing one?
12. How do you properly fit shoes? What type of shoes should you use for the various sports and the different floor and field surfaces?

## REFERENCES

1. AAPSM Running shoes recommendations: *American Academy of Podiatric Sports Medicine Newsletter* 2, May 2006.
2. Amis T: Influence of intra-oral maxillary sports mouthguards on the airflow dynamics of oral breathing, *Med Sci Sports Exerc* 32(2):284, 2000.
3. Apslund C: Facial protection and head injuries in ice hockey: A systematic review, *Br J Sports Med* 43:993–99, 2009.
4. Baltaci G, et al.: The effect of prophylactic knee bracing on performance: Balance, proprioception, coordination, and muscular power, *Knee Surgery, Sports Traumatology Arthroscopy,* 19(10)1722–28, 2011.
5. Benson B: Is protective equipment useful in preventing concussion? A systematic review of the literature, *Br J Sports Med* 43(Suppl I):i56–i67, 2009.
6. Beynnon B: The effect of bracing on proprioception of knees with anterior cruciate ligament injury, *J Ortho Sports Phys Ther* 32(1):32, 2002.
7. Bone S: If the shoe fits …, *Athletic Therapy Today* 6(6):52, 2001.
8. Bot S, Verhagen EALM, van Mechelen W: The effect of ankle bracing and taping on performance: A review of the literature, *International Sports Medicine Journal I* 4(5): 171, 2003.
9. Boyce S: Management of ankle sprains: A randomised controlled trial of the treatment of inversion injuries using an elastic support bandage or an Aircast ankle brace, *Br J Sports Med* 39(2):91, 2005.
10. Bridge M: Knee bracing in sports medicine: A review, *Techniques in Knee Surgery* 7(4):251–60, 2008.
11. Broglio S, et al.: National Athletic Trainers' Association position statement: Management of Sport Concussion, *Journal of Athletic Training* 49(2):245–65, 2014.
12. Broglio S: The efficacy of soccer headgear, *J Athl Train* 38(3):220–24, 2003.
13. Brown N: An investigation into breast support and sports bra use in female runner, *Journal of Sport Sciences* 32(9):801–9, 2014.
14. Campbell B: Temporal influences of functional knee bracing on torque production of the lower extremity, *J Sport Rehabil* 15(3):216, 2006.
15. Cantu R: Brain injury-related fatalities in American football, 1945–1999. *Neurosurgery* 52(4):846–53, 2003.
16. Carlson L: Use of functional knee braces after ACL reconstruction, *Athletic Therapy Today* 7(3):48, 2002.
17. Caswell S: Lacrosse helmet designs and the effects of impact forces, *J Athl Train* 37(2):164, 2002.
18. Chalmers D: Mouthguards: Protection for the mouth in the Rugby Union, *Sports Med* (5): 339–49, 1998.
19. Chew K: Current evidence and clinical applications of therapeutic knee braces, *Am J Phys Med Rehabil* 86: 678–86, 2007.
20. Clanto T: Ankle sprains, ankle instability and syndesmosis injuries. In Porter D, ed: *Baxter's the foot and ankle in sport*, New York, 2007, Mosby.
21. Comstock R: An evidence-based discussion of heading the ball and concussions in high school soccer, *JAMA Pediatr* 169(9):830–37, 2015.
22. Cordova M: Influence and support on joint range of motion before and after exercise: A meta-analysis, *J Orthop Sports Phys Ther* 30(7):170, 2000.
23. In Crabtree P, ed: Design and manufacture of customized orthotics for sporting applications, *The Engineering of Sport* 1(3):309–17, 2008.
24. Daneshvar D: Helmets and mouth guards: The role of personal equipment in preventing sport-elated concussions, *Clinics in Sports Medicine* 30(1):145–63, 2011.
25. Delaney J: The effect of protective headgear on head injuries and concussions in adolescent football (soccer) players, *Br J Sports Med* 42:110–15, 2008.
26. Dizon J: A systematic review on the effectiveness of external ankle supports in the prevention of inversion ankle sprains among elite and recreational players, *Journal of Science and Medicine in Sport* 13(3):306–17, 2010.
27. Downing N: Orthopedic injuries to the hand and wrist. In Hutson M, ed: *Sports Injuries,* New York, 2011, Oxford University Press.
28. Goldsmith W: Performance of baseball headgear, *Am J Sports Med* 10(1)31–37, 1982.
29. Gorden J: Effects of football collars on cervical hyperextension and lateral flexion, *J Athl Train* 38(3):209–15, 2003.
30. Gribble P: Bracing does not improve dynamic stability in chronic ankle instability subjects, *Physical Therapy in Sports* 11(1):3–7, 2010.
31. Gross M: The impact of custom semirigid foot orthotics on pain and disability for individuals with plantar fasciitis, *J Orthop Sports Phys Ther* 32(4):149, 2002.
32. Gross M: The role of ankle bracing for prevention of ankle sprain injuries, *J Orthop Sports Phys Ther* 33(10):572, 2003.
33. Halstead P: Performance testing updates in head, face, and eye protection, *J Athl Train* 36(3):322, 2001.
34. Hartsell H: Effects of bracing on isokinetic torque for the chronically unstable ankle, *J Sport Rehabil* 8(2):83, 1999.
35. Hartsell H: The effects of external bracing on joint position sense awareness for the chronically unstable ankle, *J Sport Rehabil* 9(4): 279, 2000.
36. Hawn K, Visser M, Sexton P: Enforcement of mouthguard use and athlete compliance in National Collegiate Athletic Association men's collegiate ice hockey competition, *J Athl Train* 37(2):204, 2002.
37. Hertel J. Effect of foot orthotics on quadriceps and gluteus medius electromyographic activity during selected exercises. *Arch Phys Med Rehabil* 86:26–30, 2005.

38. Hilgers M: Current trends in athletic shoe design, *Athletic Therapy Today* 14(6):23–26, 2009.

39. Hootman J: Use of protective eyewear among children participating in sports: National data and prevention implications (Abstract), *J Athl Train* 40(2 Suppl):S-71, 2005.

40. International Federation of Medicine: Position statement: Eye injuries and eye protection in sports, *Athletic Therapy Today* 4(5):6, 1999.

41. Kemler E: A systematic review on the treatment of acute ankle sprain: Brace versus other functional treatment types, *Sports Medicine* 41(3):185–97, 2011.

42. Kolger G: Biomechanics of longitudinal arch support mechanisms in foot orthoses and their effects on plantar aponeurosis strain, *Clin Biomech* 11(5):243–52, 1996.

43. Knapik J: Mouthguards in sport activities: History, physical properties and injury prevention effectiveness, *Sports Medicine* 37(2):117–44, 2007.

44. Kunde S: Relationship between running shoe fit and perceptual, biomechanical and mechanical parameters. *Footwear Science* 1(Suppl.1):19–20, 2009.

45. Labella C: Effect of mouth guards on dental injuries and concussions in college basketball, *Med Sci Sports Exerc* 34(1):41, 2002.

46. Lahti H: Dental injuries in ice hockey games and training, *Med Sci Sports Exerc* 34(3):400, 2002.

47. LaPrade R: The effect of mandatory use of face masks on facial lacerations and head and neck injuries in hockey. *Am J Sports Med* 23(6):773–75, 1995.

48. Levy M: Birth and evolution of the football helmet, *Neurosurg* 55:656–62, 2004.

49. Lord J: Protective athletic equipment. In RB Birrer and FG O'Connor, eds: *Sports Medicine for the Primary Care Physician,* ed 3, Boca Raton, FL, 2004, CRC Press.

50. McLeod T: Proper fit and maintenance of ice-hockey helmets, *Athletic Therapy Today* 10(6):54, 2005.

51. Mihalik J: Effectiveness of mouthguards in reducing neurocognitive deficits following sport-related concussion, *Dental Traumatology* 23(1):14–20, 2007.

52. Miller J: Dynamic analysis of custom fitted functional knee braces: EMG and brace migration during physical activity, *J Sport Rehabil* 8(2):109, 1999.

53. Mogolov R: Ankle brace improvements pay off for athletes, *Training & Conditioning* 17(7):48, 2007.

54. Najibi S: The use of knee braces, part 1: Prophylactic knee braces in contact sports, *Am J Sports Med* 33(4):602, 2005.

55. National Operating Committee on Standards for Athletic Equipment: *NOCSAE. Standard performance specifications for newly manufactured/recertified helmets.* Overland Park, KS, 2015, NOCASE.

56. New Revolution helmet being put to the test for improved safety on the field, *Sports Medicine Alert* 8(7):55, 2002.

57. Nigg B: Shoe inserts and orthotics for sport and physical activities, *Med Sci Sports Exerc* 31 (7 Suppl.):S421, 1999.

58. Page K: Breast motion and sports brassiere design: Implications for future research, *Sports Med* 27(4):205, 1999.

59. Patrick D: Scale of protection and the various types of sports mouthguard, *Br J Sports Med* 39(5):278, 2005.

60. Peterson L: Sports and protective equipment. In Peterson L, ed: *Sports injuries: Their prevention and treatment,* ed 3, Champaign, IL, 2001, Human Kinetics.

61. Pietrosimone B: A systemic review of prophylactic braces in the prevention of knee ligament injuries in college football players, *Journal of Athletic Training* 43(4):409–14, 2008.

62. Putnam A: Impact of ankle bracing on skill performance in recreational soccer players, *Phys Med Rehabil* 4(8)574–79, 2012.

63. Queen R: A comparison of cleat types during two football-specific tasks on Field-Turf, *British Journal of Sports Medicine* 42(4):278–84, 2008.

64. Rishiraj N: Effect of functional knee brace on acceleration, agility, leg power, and speed performance in healthy athletes, *Br J Sports Medicine* 45(15):1230–37, 2011.

65. Scibek J: Successful removal of football helmet face-mask clips after 1 season of use. *J Athl Train* 47(4)428–34, 2012.

66. Steinbach P: Armor for all. With player safety paramount, the purchasing of football equipment must ensure adequate supply and proper fit of helmets, shoes and everything in between, *Athletic Business* 26(8):96, 2002.

67. Swanik C: Orthotics in sports medicine, *Athletic Therapy Today* 5(1):5, 2000.

68. Swartz E: Emergency face-mask removal effectiveness: A comparison of traditional and nontraditional football helmet face-mask attachment systems, *J Athl Train* 45(6):560–69, 2010.

69. Tierney R: Sex differences in head acceleration during heading while wearing soccer headgear, *J Athl Train* 43(6):578–84, 2008.

70. Tiggelen D: The effects of a neoprene knee sleeve on subjects with a poor versus good joint position sense subjected to an isokinetic fatigue protocol, *Clinical Journal of Sports Medicine* 18(3):259–65, 2008.

71. Tobianski N: Soccer headgear increases peak acceleration of the head during purposeful heading (Abstract), *J Athl Train* 40(2 Suppl):S-82, 2005.

72. Ubell M: The effect of ankle braces on the prevention of dynamic forced ankle inversion, *Am J Sports Med* 31(6):935, 2003.

73. Vandertuin J: The role of functional knee braces in managing ACL injuries, *Athletic Therapy Today* 9(2):58, 2004.

74. Wannop, J: Footwear traction and lower extremity non-contact injury, *Medicine and Science in Sports and Exercise* 45(11):2137–43, 2013.

75. Wilkerson G: Biomechanical and neuromuscular effects of ankle taping and bracing, *J Athl Train* 37(4):436, 2002.

76. Withnall C: Effectiveness of headgear in football, *Br J Sports Med* 39(Suppl 1):40, 2005.

77. Wojtys E: Functional knee braces—the 25-year controversy. In Chan KM, ed: *Controversies in orthopedic sports medicine,* Champaign, IL, 2002, Human Kinetics.

78. Yaggie J: A comparative analysis of selected ankle orthoses during functional tasks, *Sport Rehabil* 10(3):174, 2001.

79. Yunker C: Evaluating the perceived preventative qualities associated with two different types of mouthguards (Abstract), *J Athl Train* 39 (2 Suppl):S-52, 2004.

80. Zinder S: Ankle bracing and the neuromuscular factors influencing joint stiffness, *J Athl Train* 44(4):363–69, 2009.

## ANNOTATED BIBLIOGRAPHY

Hunter S, Dolan M, Davis M: *Foot orthotics in therapy and sport,* Champaign, Ill, 1995, Human Kinetics.

*A detailed look at the fabrication of orthotic devices.*

Nicholas JA, Hirshman EB, editors: *The upper extremity in sports medicine,* St. Louis, MO, 1995, Mosby.

*Includes a chapter on protective equipment for the shoulder, elbow, wrist, and hand.*

Street S, Runkle D: *Athletic protective equipment: care, selection and fitting,* Boston, MA, 2001, McGraw-Hill.

*An overview of available athletic equipment and its usage. A resource for athletic trainers, coaches, and physical education teachers.*

Werd, M: *Athletic footwear and Orthoses in sports medicine,* New York, 2010, Springer.

*A concise manual for sports medicine specialists who want to effectively prescribe footwear and orthotics for the athlete.*

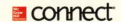

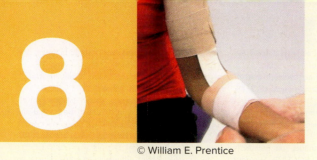
© William E. Prentice

# Wrapping and Taping

## ■ Objectives

*When you finish this chapter you should be able to*

- Discuss how the athletic trainer should approach using taping and wrapping techniques in clinical practice.
- Demonstrate the ability to apply elastic wraps to provide support, limit range of motion, or hold a protective pad in place for an injured body part.
- Identify the properties of elastic and nonelastic adhesive tape.

- Explain the process of applying and removing adhesive tape.
- Demonstrate the correct techniques for applying common taping procedures.
- Explain how Kinesio taping can be used in treating an injured patient.

## ■ Outline

## ■ Key Terms

wrap                              spica
dressing

## ■ Connect Highlights

*Visit connect.mcgraw-hill.com for further exercises to apply your knowledge:*

- Clinical application scenarios covering applying and removal of adhesive tape, correct techniques for applying common taping procedures, application of protective padding, application of taping and wrapping, using taping and wrapping techniques in clinical practice
- Click-and-drag questions covering process of applying and removing adhesive tape
- Multiple-choice questions covering use and application of taping and wrapping in clinical practice, application of protective padding, properties of elastic and nonelastic adhesive tape, common taping procedures, and Kinesio taping
- Video identification of various taping techniques

W rapping and taping techniques are used routinely by athletic trainers. They have been used to accomplish a variety of specific objectives, including the following:[5,19]

- Providing compression to minimize swelling in the initial management of injury
- Reducing the chances of injury by applying tape prophylactically before an injury occurs
- Providing additional support to an injured structure

Correctly and effectively applying a wrap or a "tape job" to a specific body part is a skill that has traditionally been left to the athletic trainer. It is true that athletic trainers have been instructed in and generally become highly proficient at applying a variety of wrapping and taping techniques to accomplish the objectives listed. Certainly, wrapping and taping skills are not difficult. They can be mastered by anyone willing to spend time practicing and learning what works best in a given situation. Of course, certain taping and wrapping techniques are more advanced and should be used only by those with some advanced experience. However, to be most effective in applying taping and wrapping techniques, the athletic trainer must have a sound background in and an understanding of anatomy and biomechanical function.

A review of the evidence-based support for using taping indicates that good research has shown the limited effectiveness of taping.[1,10] However, there are a number of studies that have demonstrated post-activity restraint of excessive ankle motion.[10,12,37] Although it is still widely used for a variety of reasons, the athletic training profession has advanced beyond simply applying a specific taping technique for every injury. In some specific instances, braces have been shown to be more effective alternatives to taping.[10,23,46]

Certainly, the taping techniques presented in this chapter are not intended to be an all-inclusive list. Applying tape to an injured body part involves an understanding of the science involved and mastery of the skill and techniques of applying a taping technique. Certainly, there is a "best" method that can be identified through systematic analysis. Athletic trainers utilize countless variations on basic taping techniques. Some of the techniques presented in this chapter, such as using cloth ankle wraps, triangular bandages, and open basket weave taping, have, to some extent, fallen out of favor in clinical practice in many settings. These techniques have been replaced by slings, shoulder and ankle braces, and compression wraps that some consider to be better and more effective. However, many clinicians continue to make use of these techniques because they have sound theoretical applicability and, for that reason, they are included in this chapter.

# WRAPPING

A **wrap** may be used to hold a **dressing** in place over an open wound, to secure a compressive or protective pad in place over an injured area, or to provide support or limit range of motion for an injured body part. A wrap may consist of roller gauze, a cloth ankle wrap or triangular bandage, or, most commonly in athletic training, an elastic wrap.

## Elastic Wrap Use

The *elastic wrap* is widely used by athletic trainers because of its elasticity, which allows it to conform easily to the contour of different body parts. If applied correctly it exerts consistent, even pressure.

The width and length of the elastic wrap may vary according to the body part to be wrapped. The sizes most frequently used are the 2-inch (5 cm) width by 6-yard (5.5 m) length for hand, finger, toe, and head wraps; the 3-inch (7.5 cm) width or 4-inch (10 cm) width by 10-yard (9 m) length for the extremities; and the 4-inch (10 cm) or 6-inch (15 cm) width by 10-yard (9 m) length for thigh, groin, and trunk. Double-length elastic wraps are useful when wrapping large body parts or areas. For ease and convenience in the application of the elastic wrap, the material is first rolled into a cylinder. When a wrap is selected, it should be a single piece that is free from wrinkles, seams, and any other imperfections that may cause skin irritation.[18]

If applied correctly by the clinician, a *cohesive elastic wrap* exerts constant, even pressure. It is lightweight and contours easily to the body part. The wrap is composed

> Wrinkles or seams in roller wraps may irritate skin.

of two layers of nonwoven rayon, which are separated by strands of spandex material. The cohesive elastic wrap is coated with a substance that makes the material adhere to itself, eliminating the need for metal clips or adhesive tape to hold it in place, as is required

> To apply a roller wrap, hold it in the preferred hand with the loose end extending from the bottom of the roll.

with standard elastic wraps. Athletic trainers sometimes use cohesive elastic wraps for "speed taping."

**Application** Application of the elastic wrap must be executed in a specific manner to maximize its effectiveness. When an elastic wrap is about to be placed on a body part, the roll should be held in the preferred hand, with the loose end extending from the bottom of the roll. The loose end is placed on the injured area and held in position by the other hand (Figure 8–1). The wrap cylinder is then unrolled and passed around

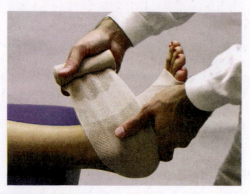

**FIGURE 8–1** Elastic wraps should be applied with firm, even pressure.

© William E. Prentice

the injured area. As the hand pulls the material from the roll, it also controls wrap tension and guides the wrap in the proper direction. To anchor and stabilize the wrap, a number of turns, one on top of the other, are made. Circling a body part requires the athletic trainer to alternate the wrap roll from one hand to the other and back again.

To provide maximum benefit, an elastic wrap should be applied firmly but not too tightly to encourage fluid to flow through the lymphatic system using gradually increasing tension from distal to proximal. Excessive pressure can hinder the normal blood flow within the part. The following points should be considered when using the elastic wrap:

1. A body part should be wrapped with surrounding muscles contracted to ensure unhampered movement or circulation.
2. It is better to use a large number of turns with moderate tension than a limited number of turns applied too tightly.
3. Each turn of the wrap should be overlapped by at least one-half of the overlying wrap to prevent the separation of the material while the individual is engaged in activity. Separation of the wrap turns tends to pinch and irritate the skin and leaves a space where edema can collect.
4. When limbs are wrapped, fingers and toes should be checked often for signs of circulation impairment. Abnormally cold or blue-colored (cyanotic) phalanges are signs of excessive wrap pressure.

The usual application of elastic wraps consists of several circular wraps directly overlying each other. Whenever possible, application begins distally at the smallest circumference of a

> **Begin application of wraps at the smallest part of the limb.**

limb and is then moved proximally. Wrists and ankles are the usual sites for beginning application of wraps of the limbs. Wraps are applied to these areas in the following manner:

1. The loose end of the elastic wrap is laid obliquely on the anterior aspect of the wrist or ankle and held in this position. The roll is then carried posteriorly under and completely around the limb and back to the starting point.
2. The triangular portion of the uncovered oblique end is folded over the second turn.
3. The folded triangle is covered by a third turn, which finishes a secure anchor.

After an elastic wrap has been applied, it is held in place by a locking technique. The method most often used to finish a wrap is to firmly tie or pin the wrap or place

> **Check circulation after applying an elastic wrap.**

adhesive tape over several overlying turns. Anytime an athletic trainer applies an elastic wrap to the athlete, the athletic trainer must always check for decreased circulation and blueness of the extremity as well as for a blood capillary refill.

The elastic wrap can be removed either by unwrapping or by carefully cutting with scissors. Whatever method of wrap removal is used, the athletic trainer must take precautions to avoid additional injury.

## Elastic Wrap Techniques

**Ankle Spica** The ankle and foot **spica** wrap (Figure 8–2) is primarily used for compression of acute injuries and for holding a compressive pad in place. On the ankle, a felt compressive horseshoe-shaped pad is commonly used for focal compression following acute injury (see Figure 19–25).

**Materials Needed** Depending on the size of the ankle and foot, a 3-inch (7.5 cm) wrap is used.

**Position of the Patient** The patient sits with his or her ankle and foot extended over the edge of a table, with the ankle at 90 degrees.

**Procedure**
1. Place an anchor around the foot near the metatarsal arch.
2. Bring the elastic wrap across the instep and around the heel, and return to the starting point.

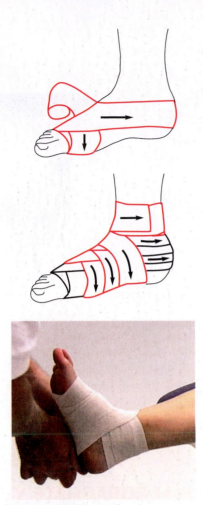

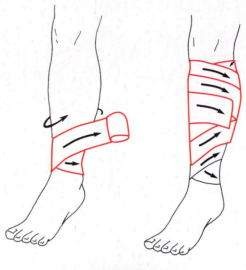

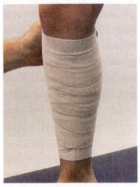

FIGURE 8–2 Ankle and foot spica.

Photo: © William E. Prentice

FIGURE 8–3 Spiral wrap.

Photo: © William E. Prentice

3. Repeat the procedure several times, with each succeeding revolution progressing upward on the foot and the ankle.

4. Overlap each spica over the preceding layer by approximately one-half.

5. In cases with considerable swelling, the athletic trainer may want to completely cover the heel, even though there is not typically that much swelling in that area.

**Spiral Wrap** The spiral wrap (Figure 8–3) is used for covering a large area of a cylindrical part.

**Materials Needed** Depending on the size of the area, a 3-inch (7.5 cm) or 4-inch (10 cm) wrap is required.

**Position of the Patient** If the wrap is for the lower limb, the patient bears weight on the opposite leg.

### Procedure

1. Anchor the elastic spiral wrap at the smallest distal circumference of the limb, and wrap proximally in a spiral against gravity.

2. To prevent the wrap from slipping down on a moving extremity, fold two pieces of tape lengthwise and place

them on the wrap at either side of the limb, or spray tape adherent on the injured area.

3. After the wrap is anchored, carry it upward in consecutive spiral turns, each overlapping the other by at least ½ inch (1.25 cm).

4. Terminate the wrap by locking it with circular turns, and then firmly secure the wrap with tape.

**Hip Spica** The following procedure is used to support a hip adductor strain (Figure 8–4).

**Materials Needed** One roll of double-length 6-inch (15 cm) elastic wrap and a roll of 1½-inch (3.8 cm) adhesive tape.

**Position of the Patient** The patient stands on a table and places his or her weight on the uninjured leg. The affected limb is relaxed and internally rotated.

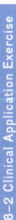

A dancer strains his right groin while performing a ballet lift

? Which elastic wrap should the athletic trainer apply when the dancer returns to dancing? Why?

8–2 Clinical Application Exercise

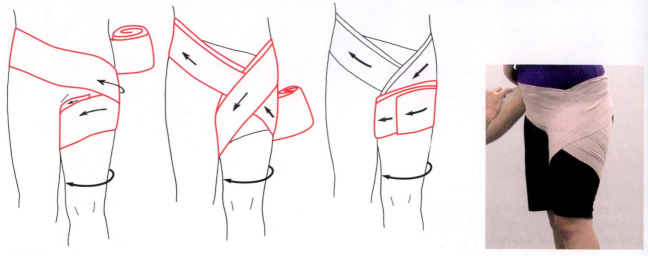

FIGURE 8–4   Hip spica using elastic wrap for hip adductor support (thigh internally rotated).
Photo: © William E. Prentice

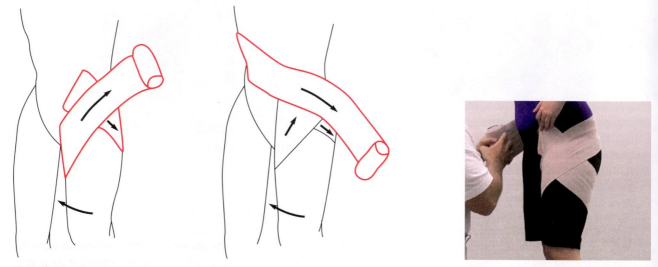

FIGURE 8–5   Hip spica using elastic wrap for hip flexion support (thigh slightly flexed). Pull up into hip flexion.
Photo: © William E. Prentice

## Procedure

1. Start the end of the elastic wrap at the upper part of the inner aspect of the thigh, and carry it posteriorly around the thigh. Then bring it across the lower abdomen and over the crest of the ilium on the opposite side of the body.
2. Continue the wrap around the back, repeating the same pattern and securing the wrap end with 1½-inch (3.8 cm) adhesive tape.

Variations of this method can be seen in Figure 8–5 (to support injured hip flexors) and Figure 8–6 (to support the hip extensors).

**Shoulder Spica**   The shoulder spica (Figure 8–7) is used mainly to hold a protective pad in place or to limit shoulder flexion or abduction.

**Materials Needed**   One roll of double-length 4-inch (10 cm) to 6-inch (15 cm) elastic wrap, 1½-inch (3.8 cm) adhesive tape, and padding for axilla.

**Position of the Patient**   The patient stands with his or her side toward the athletic trainer.

## Procedure

1. Pad the axilla well using either foam heel and lace pads or gauze pads to prevent skin irritation and constriction of blood vessels.
2. Anchor the wrap by one turn around the affected upper arm.
3. After anchoring the wrap around the arm on the injured side, carry the wrap around the back under the unaffected arm and across the chest to the injured shoulder.

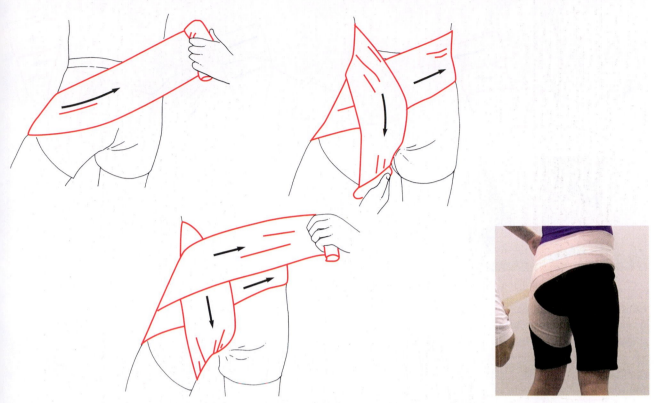

FIGURE 8–6   Hip spica using elastic wrap for hip extensor support (thigh extended and externally rotated).
Photo: © William E. Prentice

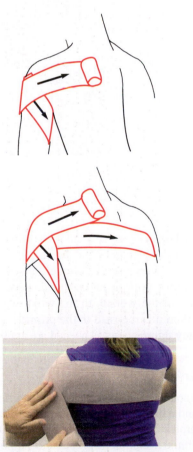

FIGURE 8–7   Shoulder spica using an elastic wrap.
Photo: © William E. Prentice

4. Encircle the affected arm again by the wrap, which continues around the back. Every figure-eight pattern moves progressively upward with an overlap of at least half of the previous underlying wrap.

**Elbow Figure-Eight Wrap**   The elbow figure-eight wrap (Figure 8–8) can be used to secure a dressing in the antecubital fossa or to restrain full extension in hyperextension injuries. When it is reversed, it can be used on the posterior aspect of the elbow.

***Materials Needed***   One 3-inch (7.5 cm) elastic wrap and 1½-inch (3.8 cm) adhesive tape.

***Position of the Patient***
The patient flexes his or her elbow between 45 and 90 degrees, depending on the restriction of movement required. The fist should be clenched.

***Procedure***
1. Anchor the wrap by encircling the lower arm.
2. Bring the roll obliquely upward over the posterior aspect of the elbow.

A wrestler sustains a left shoulder point injury. The athletic trainer cuts a sponge rubber doughnut to protect the shoulder from further injury.

? How is the doughnut held in place?

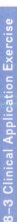
8–3 Clinical Application Exercise

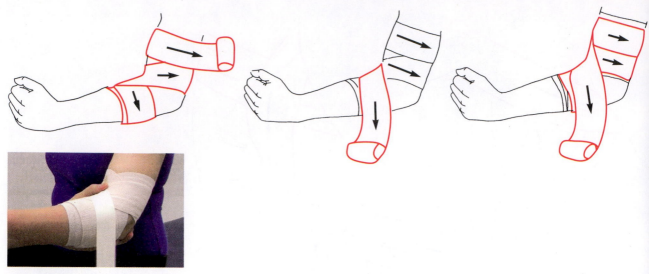

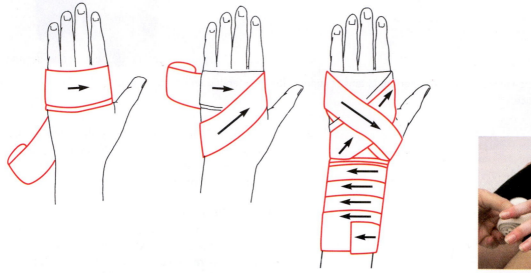

FIGURE 8–8   Elastic elbow figure-eight wrap (fist clenched).
Photo: © William E. Prentice

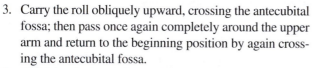

FIGURE 8–9   Hand and wrist figure-eight wrap.
Photo: © William E. Prentice

3. Carry the roll obliquely upward, crossing the antecubital fossa; then pass once again completely around the upper arm and return to the beginning position by again crossing the antecubital fossa.

4. Continue the procedure as described, but for every new sequence move upward toward the elbow one-half the width of the underlying wrap.

**Hand and Wrist Figure-Eight Wrap**   A figure-eight wrap (Figure 8–9) can be used for mild wrist and hand support and for holding dressings in place.

***Materials Needed***   One 2-inch (5 cm) elastic wrap and ½-inch (1.25 cm) tape.

***Position of the Patient***   The patient positions his or her elbow at a 45-degree angle. The fingers should be slightly spread.

***Procedure***
1. The anchor is executed with one or two turns of the wrap around the palm of the hand.
2. The roll is then carried obliquely across the anterior or posterior portion of the hand, depending on the position of the wound, to the wrist, which it circles once; then it is returned to the primary anchor.
3. As many figure eights as needed are applied.

## Cloth Ankle Wrap

Because tape is so expensive, the ankle wrap is an inexpensive and expedient technique that provides a minimal level of protection to the ankle (Figure 8–10). Due to an increase in the use of ankle braces and supports, the cloth ankle wrap is used infrequently in an athletic training setting.

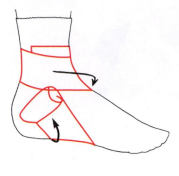

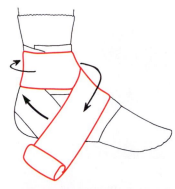

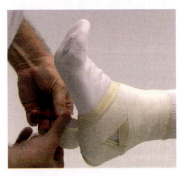

FIGURE 8–10   Ankle wrap.
Photo: © William E. Prentice

**Materials Needed**   Each wrap should be 2 inches (5 cm) wide and 108 inches (270 cm) long to ensure complete coverage and protection. The purpose of this wrap is to give mild support against lateral and medial motion of the ankle. It is applied over a sock.

**Position of the Patient**   The patient sits on a table, extending the lower leg off the table, with the ankle flexed to 90 degrees.

**Procedure**
1. Anchor the wrap just above the malleoli. Circle around the ankle, moving over the top of the foot straight downward over the medial arch.
2. From the arch, move the wrap under the foot, coming up on the lateral side and then angling the wrap upward to go around the back of the ankle just above the heel.
3. Move the wrap over the top of the foot, then straight down on the lateral side toward the bottom of the foot;

then go under the foot, angling upward on the medial side toward the back of the ankle just above the heel.
4. Go around the back of the ankle toward the top of the foot, thus completing one series of the wrap.
5. Complete a second and perhaps a third series with the remaining wrap.
6. For additional support apply two heel locks with 1½-inch (3.8 cm) adhesive tape over the ankle wrap.

## Triangular Bandages

Triangular bandages, usually made of cotton cloth, are primarily used as first-aid devices.[18] They are valuable in emergency bandaging because they are easy and quick to apply. The principal use of the triangular bandage in athletic training is to create an arm sling. There are two basic kinds of slings, the cervical arm sling and the shoulder arm sling, and each has a specific purpose.

> Triangular bandages can be applied easily and quickly.

**Cervical Arm Sling**   The cervical arm sling (Figure 8–11) is designed to support the forearm, wrist, and hand. A triangular bandage is placed around the neck and under the bent arm that is to be supported.

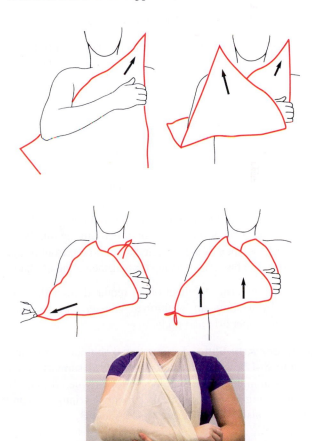

FIGURE 8–11   Cervical arm sling.
Photo: © William E. Prentice

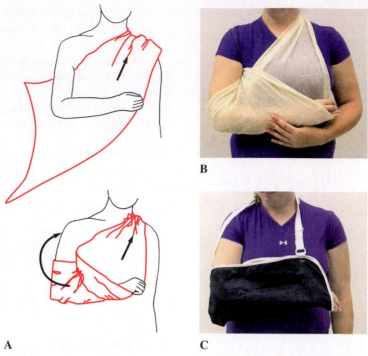

**FIGURE 8–12** **(A)** Shoulder arm sling. **(B)** Triangular bandage. **(C)** Sling.
© William E. Prentice

***Materials Needed*** One triangular bandage.

***Position of the Patient*** The patient stands with the affected arm bent at approximately a 70-degree angle.

***Procedure***
1. Position the triangular bandage under the injured arm, with the apex facing the elbow.
2. Carry the end of the triangle nearest the body over the shoulder of the uninjured arm. Allow the other end to hang down loosely.
3. Pull the loose end over the shoulder of the injured side.
4. Tie the two ends of the wrap in a square knot behind the neck. For the sake of comfort, the knot should be on either side of the neck, not directly in the middle.
5. Bring the apex of the triangle around to the front of the elbow and fasten by twisting the end, then tying in a knot.

If greater arm stabilization is required than that afforded by a sling, an additional wrap can be swathed about the upper arm and body.

**Shoulder Arm Sling** A commercial shoulder arm sling (Figure 8–12C) is suggested for forearm support when there is an injury to the shoulder girdle or when the cervical arm sling is irritating to the patient. A triangular bandage may also be used (Figure 8–12A and B).

***Materials Needed*** One triangular bandage and one safety pin.

***Position of the Patient*** The patient stands with his or her injured arm bent at approximately a 70-degree angle.

***Procedure***
1. Place the upper end of the shoulder sling over the uninjured shoulder side.
2. Bring the lower end of the triangle over the forearm, and draw it between the upper arm and the body, swinging it around the patient's back and then upward to meet the other end, where a square knot is tied.
3. Bring the apex end of the triangle around to the front of the elbow and fasten with a safety pin.

**Sling and Swathe** The sling and swathe combination is designed to stabilize the arm securely in cases of shoulder dislocation or fracture (Figure 8–13). First apply a cervical arm sling as previously described. Then stabilize the arm against the chest by wrapping a 6-inch (15.2 cm) elastic wrap completely around the torso. This is referred to as a swathe wrap. A commercial sling may also be used to create a sling and swathe.

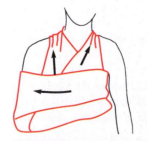 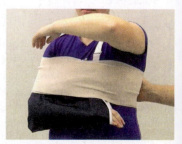

**FIGURE 8–13** Sling and swathe.
Photo: © William E. Prentice

# NONELASTIC AND ELASTIC ADHESIVE TAPING

Historically, taping has been an important part of athletic training. In recent years, it is fair to say that some research has raised questions about long-held ideas about the effectiveness of taping.[20,24,27,32,39] But it is certainly true that effectiveness of taping is largely determined by both the method that is used and the skill of the clinician who applies it. The psychological effect of taping is currently unknown.

## Nonelastic Adhesive Tape

Nonelastic adhesive tape has great adaptability because of its uniform adhesive mass, adhering qualities, and lightness, and because of the relative strength of the backing materials.[24] All these qualities are of value in holding wound dressings in place and in supporting and protecting injured areas. This tape comes in a variety of sizes; widths of ½, 1, 1½, and 2 inches (1.25, 2.5, 3.8, and 5 cm) are commonly used in sports medicine (Figure 8–14). When linen tape is purchased, factors such as cost, grade of backing, quality of adhesive mass, and properties of unwinding should be considered.

An athlete falls and sustains a dislocated right shoulder.

**?** How should the athlete be transported safely to the hospital?

**Tape Grade** Adhesive tape (usually white) is most often graded according to the number of longitudinal and vertical fibers per inch of backing material.[4] The heavier and more costly backing contains 85 or more longitudinal fibers and 65 vertical fibers per square inch. The lighter, less expensive grade has 65 or fewer longitudinal fibers and 45 vertical fibers.

When purchasing linen tape, consider:
- Grade of backing
- Quality of adhesive mass
- Winding tension

**Adhesive Mass** As a result of improvements in adhesive mass, certain essentials should be expected from tape. It should adhere readily when applied and should maintain this adherence in the presence of profuse perspiration and activity. Besides sticking well, the mass must contain as few skin irritants as possible and must be able to be removed easily without leaving a mass residue or pulling away the superficial skin.

**Winding Tension** The winding tension of a tape roll is important to the athletic trainer. The demands of sport activity place a unique demand on the unwinding quality of tape; if tape is to be applied for protection and support, there must be even and constant unwinding tension. In most cases, a proper wind needs little additional tension to provide sufficient tightness.

## Elastic Adhesive Tape

Elastic adhesive tape is often used in combination with nonelastic adhesive tape. Because of its conforming qualities, elastic tape is used for small, angular body parts, such as the feet, wrist, hands, and fingers. It is also used when circling a soft tissue muscle group that expands with contraction or engorges with blood during activity. As with nonelastic adhesive tape, elastic tape comes in a variety of widths (1-, 2-, 3-, and 4-inch [2.5, 5, 7.5, and 10 cm]) (Figure 8–15).

## Tape Storage

Tape should be stored in a cool place to avoid damaging the pliability of the tape fabric as well as affecting the adhesive qualities.

Store tape in a cool place, and stack it flat.

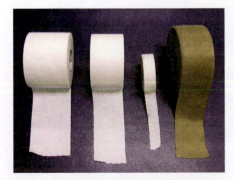

FIGURE 8–14  Nonelastic adhesive tape: 2", 1½", ½" (5 cm, 3.8 cm, 1.25 cm), and Leukotape.
© William E. Prentice

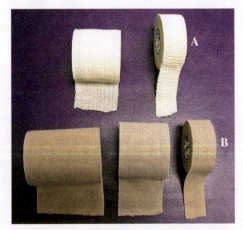

FIGURE 8–15  Elastic adhesive tape. **(A)** 2" (5 cm) and 1" (2.5 cm) light wrap tape. **(B)** 3" (7.5 cm), 2", and 1" elastic tape.
© William E. Prentice

The boxes of tape should be stacked so that the tape rests on its flat top or bottom to avoid distortion.

## Using Adhesive Tape

**Preparation for Taping** The athletic trainer must pay special attention when applying tape directly to the skin.[31] A list of supplies needed for proper taping appears in *Focus Box 8–1:* "Taping supplies." Perspiration, oil, and dirt prevent tape from adhering to the skin. Whenever tape is used, ideally the skin surface should be cleaned with soap and water to remove all dirt and oil. Also, hair should be shaved to prevent additional irritation when the tape is removed (Figure 8–16A). A quick-drying tape adherent spray can be used to help the tape adhere to the skin, although it is not absolutely necessary (Figure 8–16B). Also, at certain points, such as over bony prominences, the tape can produce friction blisters. Extra foam pads (heel and lace pads) with a small amount of lubricant can help minimize the occurrence of blisters (Figure 8–16C). Taping directly on skin provides maximum immediate support. However, applying tape day after day can lead to skin irritation. A roll of foam underwrap is thin, porous, extremely lightweight, and resilient, and it easily conforms to the contours of the

> Ideally, skin should be oil free and hair should be shaved before tape is applied.

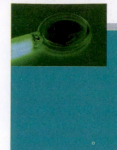

## FOCUS 8–1 Focus on Healthcare Administration and Professional Responsibilities

### Taping supplies

1. Razor–hair removal
2. Adhesive spray–tape adherent
3. Underwrap material–skin protection
4. Heel and lace pads
5. White nonelastic adhesive tape (½-inch, 1-inch, 1½-inch, and 2-inch [1.25 cm, 2.5 cm, 3.8 cm, and 5 cm])
6. Elastic adhesive tape (1-inch, 2-inch, and 3-inch [2.5 cm, 5 cm, and 7.5 cm])
7. Felt and foam padding material
8. Tape scissors
9. Tape cutters
10. Elastic wraps (2-inch, 3-inch, 4-inch, and 6-inch [5 cm, 7.5 cm, 10 cm, and 15 cm])
11. Double-length wraps

part to be taped and protects the skin to some degree. Underwrap should be applied only one layer thick (Figure 8–16D).[21] The underwrap should be anchored both proximally and distally (Figure 8–16E).

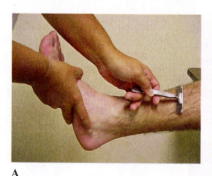

A

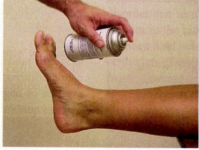

B

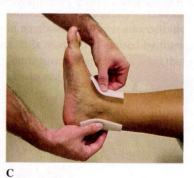

C

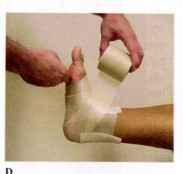

D

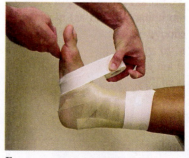

E

FIGURE 8–16   Taping preparation.
**(A)** Shaving. **(B)** Applying tape adherent. **(C)** Placing heel and lace pads. **(D)** Applying one layer of underwrap. **(E)** Applying anchor strips.
© William E. Prentice

**Rules for Tape Application** The following are a few of the important rules to be observed in the use of adhesive tape. In practice the athletic trainer will identify others.

1. *If the part to be taped is a joint, place it in the position in which it is to be stabilized.* If the part is musculature, make the necessary allowance for contraction and expansion.
2. *Overlap the tape at least half the width of the tape below.* Unless tape is overlapped sufficiently, the active athlete will separate it, exposing the underlying skin to irritation and allowing a space in which edema can occur.
3. *Avoid continuous taping with nonelastic adhesive tape.* Tape continuously wrapped around a part may cause constriction. Make one turn at a time and tear each encirclement to overlap the starting end by approximately 1 inch (2.5 cm).
4. *Keep the tape roll in the hand whenever possible.* By learning to keep the tape roll in the hand, seldom putting it down, and by learning to tear the tape, an athletic trainer can develop taping speed and accuracy.
5. *Smooth and mold the tape as it is laid on the skin.* To save additional time, smooth and mold tape strips to the body part as they are put in place; this is done by stroking the top with the fingers, palms, and heels of both hands.
6. *Allow tape to fit the natural contour of the skin.* Each strip of tape must be placed with a particular purpose in mind. Linen-backed tape is not sufficiently elastic to conform to surface irregularities, which requires precise control of the angles at which the longitudinal fibers of the tape are oriented during application. Failing to allow this fit creates wrinkles and gaps that can result in skin irritations.
7. *Start taping with an anchor piece and finish by applying a lock strip.* Commence taping, if possible, by sticking the tape to an anchor piece that encircles the part. This placement affords a good medium for the stabilization of succeeding tape strips, so that they will not be affected by the movement of the part.
8. *Where maximum support is desired, tape directly over skin.* In cases of sensitive skin, prewrap may be used as a tape base. With prewrap, some movement can be expected between the skin and the base.[3]
9. *Do not apply tape if skin is hot or cold from a therapeutic treatment.*

**Selecting Proper Tape Width** The correct tape width depends on the area to be covered. The more acute the angles, the narrower the tape must be to fit the many contours. For example, the fingers and toes usually require ½- or 1-inch (1.25 or 2.5 cm) tape; the ankles require 1½-inch (3.8 cm) tape; and the larger skin areas, such as thighs and back, can accommodate 2- to 3-inch (5 to 7.5 cm) tape with ease.

NOTE: Supportive tape improperly applied can aggravate an existing injury or can disrupt the mechanics of a body part, causing an initial injury to occur.

**Tearing Tape** Athletic trainers use various techniques to tear tape (Figure 8–17). The tearing method should permit the operator to keep the tape roll in hand most of the time.[39] The following is a suggested procedure:

> To tear tape, move hands quickly in opposite directions.

1. Hold the tape roll in the preferred hand with the middle finger hooked through the center of the tape roll and the thumb pressing its outer edge.
2. With the other hand, grasp the loose end between the thumb and index finger.
3. With both hands in place, pull both ends of the tape so that it is tight. Next, make a quick, scissorslike move to tear the tape. In tearing tape, one hand moves away from the body and the other hand moves toward the body. Remember, do not try to bend or twist the tape to tear it.

When tearing is properly executed, the torn edges of the nonelastic adhesive tape are relatively straight,

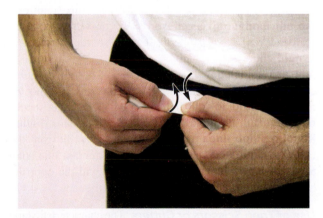
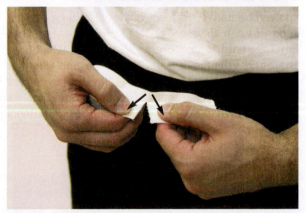

FIGURE 8–17 Technique for tearing adhesive tape.
© William E. Prentice

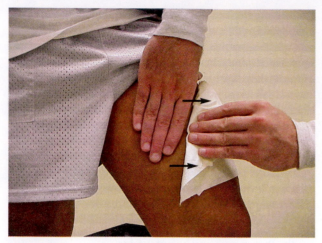

FIGURE 8–18   Removing tape by pulling in a direct line with the body.

© William E. Prentice

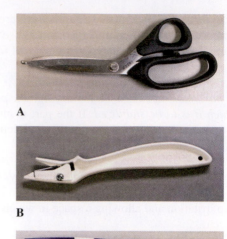

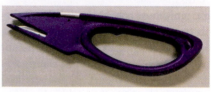

C

FIGURE 8–19   **(A)** Tape scissors. **(B)** Zip-cut tape cutter. **(C)** Shark tape cutter.

© William E. Prentice

without curves, twists, or loose threads sticking out. Once the first thread is torn, the rest of the tape tears easily. Learning to tear tape effectively from many different positions is essential for speed and efficiency. Many tapes other than the linen-backed type cannot be torn manually but require a knife, scissors, or razor blade.

**Removing Adhesive Tape** Tape usually can be removed from the skin by hand, by tape scissors or tape cutters, or by chemical solvents.[1]

> Peel the skin from the tape, not the tape from the skin.

*Manual Removal* When pulling tape from the body, be careful not to tear or irritate the skin. Tape must not be ripped off in an outward direction from the skin but should be pulled in a direct line with the grain of the hairs (Figure 8–18). Remember to remove the skin carefully from the tape and not to peel the tape from the skin. Use one hand to gently pull the tape in one direction, and the opposite hand to gently press the skin away from the tape.

*Use of Tape Scissors or Cutters* The characteristic tape scissors or cutters have a blunt nose that slips underneath the tape smoothly without gouging the skin (Figure 8–19). Take care to avoid cutting the tape too near the site of the injury, so that the scissors do not aggravate the condition. Cut on the uninjured side. A general rule of thumb is to start at the superior aspect of the joint and move inferiorly.

## COMMON TAPING PROCEDURES

### The Arch

**Arch Technique No. 1: With Arch Support** Taping can provide support to a depressed or flat arch (Figure 8–20). NOTE: The longitudinal arch should be lifted. CAUTION: When applying tape around the forefoot, be aware that the metatarsals must have room to spread when bearing weight.

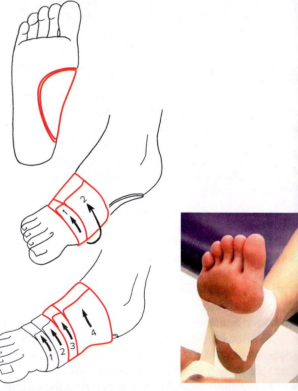

FIGURE 8–20   Arch taping technique no. 1, including an arch support and circular tape strips.

Photo: © William E. Prentice

*Materials Needed* One roll of 1½-inch (3.8 cm) adhesive tape, tape adherent, and a ⅛- or ¼-inch (0.3 or 0.6 cm) adhesive foam rubber pad or adhesive felt pad, cut to fit the longitudinal arch.

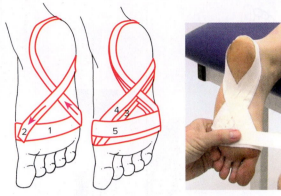

FIGURE 8–21   Arch taping technique no. 2 (X taping).

Photo: © William E. Prentice

**Site Preparation**  Clean foot of dirt and oil; if hairy, shave dorsum of foot. Spray area with tape adherent.

**Position of the Patient**  The patient is seated on the table with the foot that is to be taped extending approximately 6 inches (15 cm) over the edge of the table. To ensure proper position, allow the foot to hang in a relaxed position.

**Procedure**

1.  Place a series of strips of tape directly around the arch, pulling the arch up. If added support is required, add an arch support. The first strip should go just above the metatarsal arch (1).
2.  Each successive strip overlaps the preceding piece about half the width of the tape (2 through 4).

CAUTION: Avoid putting on so many strips of tape that range of motion is limited.

**Arch Technique No. 2: The X for the Longitudinal Arch**  Use the figure-eight method for taping the longitudinal arch (Figure 8–21).

**Materials Needed**  One roll of 1-inch (2.5 cm) adhesive tape and tape adherent.

**Site Preparation**  Same as for arch technique no. 1.

**Position of the Patient**  The patient lies face down on the table with the affected foot extending approximately 6 inches (15 cm) over the edge of the table. To ensure proper position, allow the foot to hang in a relaxed position.

**Procedure**

1.  Lightly place an anchor strip around the ball of the foot, making certain not to restrict toe range of motion (1).
2.  Start tape strip 2 from the lateral edge of the anchor. Move it upward at an acute angle, cross the center of the longitudinal arch, encircle the heel, and descend. Then cross the arch again and end at the medial aspect of the anchor (2). Repeat three or four times (3 and 4).
3.  Lock the taped Xs with a single piece of tape placed around the ball of foot (5).

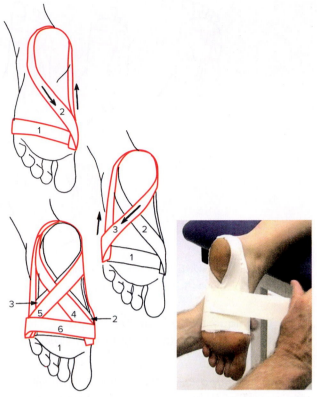

FIGURE 8–22   Teardrop arch taping technique no. 3 with double X and forefoot support.

Photo: © William E. Prentice

After all the X strips are applied, an option is to cover the entire arch with 1½-inch (3.8 cm) circular adhesive tape strips.

**Arch Technique No. 3: The X Teardrop Arch and Forefoot Support**  As its name implies, this taping supports the longitudinal arch and the forefoot (Figure 8–22).

**Materials Needed**  One roll of 1-inch (2.5 cm) adhesive tape and tape adherent.

**Position of the Patient**  The patient lies face down on the table with the foot to be taped extending approximately 6 inches (15 cm) over the edge of the table.

**Procedure**

1.  Place an anchor strip around the ball of the foot (1).
2.  Start tape strip 2 on the side of the foot, beginning at the base of the great toe. Take the tape around the heel, crossing the arch and returning to the starting point (2).
3.  The pattern of the third strip of tape is the same as the second strip except that it is started on the little toe side of the foot (3). Repeat two or three times (4 and 5).
4.  Lock the series of strips by placing tape around or just proximal to the ball joint (6).

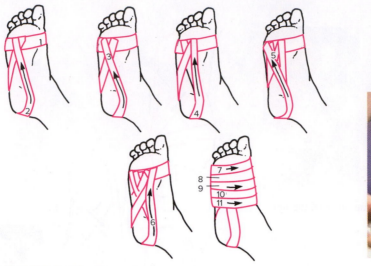

FIGURE 8–23   Fan arch taping technique.
Photo: © William E. Prentice

**Arch Technique No. 4: Fan Arch Support** The fan arch technique supports the entire plantar aspect of the foot (Figure 8–23).

*Materials Needed* One roll of 1-inch (2.5 cm) adhesive tape, one roll of 1½-inch (3.8 cm) adhesive tape, and tape adherent.

*Position of Patient* The patient is sitting on the table with the foot to be taped extending approximately 6 inches (15 cm) over the edge of the table.

*Procedure*
1. Using the 1-inch (2.5 cm) adhesive tape, place an anchor strip around the ball of the foot (1).
2. Starting at the third metatarsal head, take the tape around the heel from the lateral side and meet the strip where it began (2 and 3).
3. Start the next strip near the second metatarsal head and finish it on the fourth metatarsal head (4).
4. Begin the last strip on the fourth metatarsal head and finish it on the fifth metatarsal head (5). The technique, when completed, forms a fan-shaped pattern covering the metatarsal region (6).
5. Lock strips using 1½-inch (3.8 cm) adhesive tape and encircling the complete arch (7 through 11).

**LowDye Technique** The LowDye technique is an excellent method for managing a depressed or flattened medial longitudinal arch, foot pronation, arch strains, and plantar fasciitis[14,17,44] (Figure 8–24).

*Materials Needed* One roll of 1-inch (2.5 cm) adhesive tape, one roll of 1½-inch (3.8 cm) adhesive tape, and moleskin.

*Position of the Patient* The patient sits with the foot in a neutral position with the great toe and medial aspect of the foot in plantar flexion.

*Procedure*
1. Grasp the forefoot with the thumb under the distal 2 to 5 metatarsal heads, pushing slightly upward, with the tips of the second and third fingers pushing downward on the first metatarsal head. Apply two or three 1-inch (2.5 cm) adhesive tape strips laterally, starting from the distal head of the fifth metatarsal bone (1 through 3). Keep these lateral strips below the outer malleolus.
2. Secure the lateral tape strips by circling the forefoot with four 1½-inch (3.8 cm) adhesive tape strips (4 through 7). Start at the lateral dorsum of the foot, circle under the plantar aspect, and finish at the medial dorsum of the foot.

A waitress is seen in the clinic with a severe right foot pronation with a fallen medial longitudinal arch. She is subject to arch strains.

**?** What taping technique is designed for this situation?

## The Toes

**Sprained Great Toe** This procedure is used for taping a sprained great toe (Figure 8–25).

*Materials Needed* One roll of 1-inch (2.5 cm) adhesive tape and tape adherent and one roll of ½-inch (1.25 cm) tape.

*Site Preparation* Clean foot of dirt and oil, shave hair from toes, and spray area with tape adherent.

*Position of the Patient* The patient assumes a sitting position.

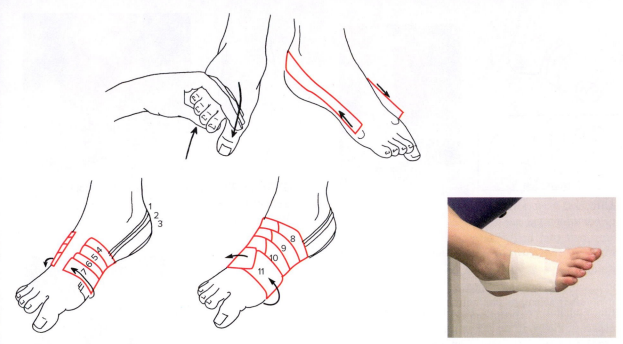

FIGURE 8–24  LowDye taping technique.
Photo: © William E. Prentice

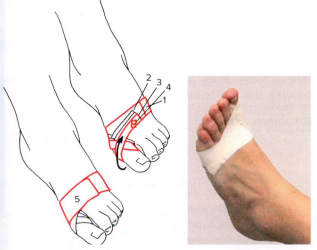

FIGURE 8–25  Taping for a sprained great toe.
Photo: © William E. Prentice

### Procedure

1. Use an anchor strip just proximal to metatarsal heads (1).
2. The greatest support is given to the joint by a half-figure-eight taping (2 through 4). Start the series at an acute angle on the top of the foot and swing down between the great and first toes, first encircling the great toe and then coming up, over, and across the starting point. Repeat this process, starting each series separately.
3. After the required number of half-figure-eight strips are in position, place a 1½-inch adhesive tape lock piece around the ball of the foot (5).

### Hallux Valgus

**Materials Needed**  One roll of 1-inch (2.5 cm) adhesive tape, tape adherent, and ¼-inch (0.6 cm) sponge rubber or felt (Figure 8–26).

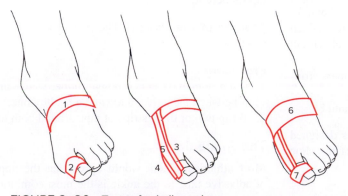

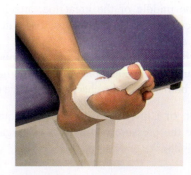

FIGURE 8–26  Taping for hallux valgus.
Photo: © William E. Prentice

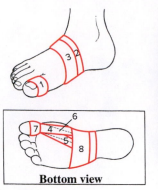
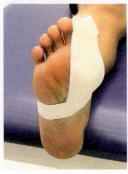
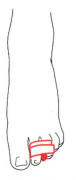

**Bottom view**

FIGURE 8–27   Turf toe taping.
Photo: © William E. Prentice

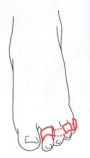
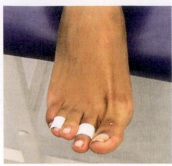

FIGURE 8–28   Hammer, or clawed, toe taping.
Photo: © William E. Prentice

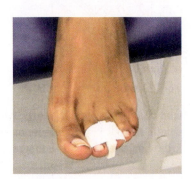

FIGURE 8–29   Fractured toe taping.
Photo: © William E. Prentice

***Position of the Patient*** The patient assumes a sitting position.

***Procedure***
1. Place anchor strips to encircle the midfoot and distal aspect of the great toe (1 and 2).
2. Place two or three strips on the medial aspect of the great toe to hold the toe in proper alignment (3 through 5).
3. Lock the ends of the strips with tape (6 and 7).
4. Cut a ¼-inch sponge rubber to form a wedge between the great and second toes.

**Turf Toe** Turf toe taping is designed to prevent excessive hyperextension of the metatarsophalangeal joint (Figure 8–27).

***Materials Needed*** One roll of 1½-inch (3.8 cm) adhesive tape, one roll of 1-inch (2.5 cm) adhesive tape, and tape adherent.

***Site Preparation*** Shave hair off the top of the forefoot and great toe. Spray the area with tape adherent.

***Position of the Patient*** The great toe is in a neutral position.

***Procedure***
1. Apply a 1-inch (2.5 cm) adhesive tape strip around the great toe. Using 1½-inch (3.8 cm) (1) adhesive tape, apply two arch anchors to the mid-arch area (2 and 3).
2. On the middle of the great toe, attach three 1-inch (2.5 cm) adhesive tape strips to create a checkrein (4, 5, and 6).
3. Attach the checkrein to the arch anchor tapes, strip-crossing the metatarsophalangeal joint line.
4. Lock both ends of the checkrein in place (7 and 8).

**Hammer, or Clawed Toes** This technique is designed to reduce the pressure of the bent toes against the shoe (Figure 8–28).[35]

***Materials Needed*** One roll of ½- or 1-inch (1.25 or 2.5 cm) adhesive tape and tape adherent.

***Position of the Patient*** The patient sits on the table with the affected leg extended over the edge.

***Procedure***
1. Tape one affected toe; then lace under the adjacent toe and over the next toe.
2. Tape can be attached to the next toe or can be continued and attached to the fifth toe.

**Fractured Toes** This technique splints the fractured toe with a nonfractured one (Figure 8–29).

***Materials Needed*** One roll of ½- or 1-inch (1.25 or 2.5 cm) adhesive tape, ⅛-inch (0.3 cm) sponge rubber, and tape adherent.

***Position of the Patient*** The patient assumes a sitting position.

***Procedure***
1. Cut a ⅛-inch (0.3 cm) sponge rubber wedge and place it between the affected toe and a healthy one.
2. Wrap two or three strips of tape around both toes.

## The Ankle Joint

Most athletic trainers would agree that the application of adhesive tape to the ankle is the most commonly used taping technique. Both athletic trainers and patients have maintained that, if applied appropriately, taping provides

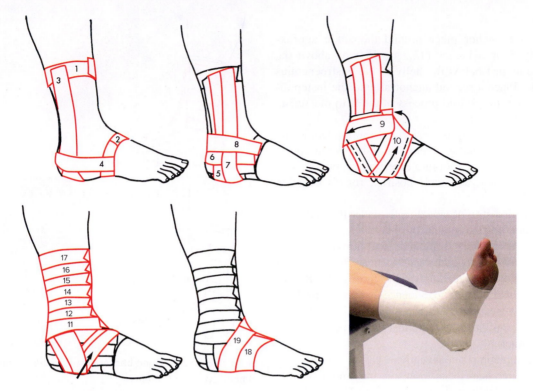

FIGURE 8–30   Closed basket weave ankle taping.

Photo: © William E. Prentice

comfort and support, with little interference with normal ankle function. A review of the evidence-based research has questioned the effectiveness of ankle taping in reducing the incidence of ankle sprain, and a number of studies have evaluated the extent to which adhesive tape provides a mechanical restraint to excessive ankle motion.[15,25,28,33,34] Studies also describe various tape-application techniques for the ankle and explain the benefits that may be derived from ankle taping.[9,31,42,46] A few studies have indicated that ankle taping loses its initial level of resistance to motion during exercise, but a majority of studies have demonstrated that the restraining effect on extreme ankle motion is not eliminated by prolonged activity.[36,37,46] Using underwrap under adhesive tape has been reported to extend the effectiveness of tape application in controlling motion longer than if the tape is applied directly to the skin.[12,21] However, it has not been explained how this happens.

As indicated in Chapter 7, a variety of ankle braces are used as alternatives to ankle taping. Some studies comparing the mechanical effects of various commercially available braces and taping have found comparable levels of postexercise motion limitation for taping and bracing.[8,10,28,46] But the majority have concluded that ankle bracing is superior to taping, based on less increase in ankle motion following exercise.[23,34,38] Despite this ongoing controversy of the relative effectiveness of taping ankles, it remains a clinical technique widely utilized by athletic trainers.

**Closed Basket Weave (Gibney) Technique** The closed basket weave, or Gibney, technique offers strong tape support and is primarily used in athletic training for newly sprained or chronically unstable ankles (Figure 8–30).

**Materials Needed** One roll of 1½-inch (3.8 cm) adhesive tape, underwrap, and tape adherent.

**Site Preparation** Ankle taping applied directly to the athlete's skin affords the greatest support; however, when it is applied and removed daily, skin irritation will occur. To avoid this problem, apply an underwrap material. Before taping, follow these procedures:

1. Clean the foot and ankle thoroughly.
2. Shave all the hair off the foot and ankle.
3. Apply a coating of tape adherent to protect the skin and offer an adhering base.
4. Apply a gauze pad coated with friction-reducing material, such as skin lube or Vasoline over the instep and to the back of the heel.
5. If underwrap is used, apply a single layer. The tape anchors extend beyond the underwrap and adhere directly to the skin.
6. Do not apply tape if skin is cold or hot from a therapeutic treatment.

**Position of the Patient** The patient sits on the table with the leg extended and the foot at a 90-degree angle.

## Procedure

1. Place one anchor piece around the ankle approximately 5 or 6 inches (12.5 or 15 cm) above the malleolus just below the belly of the gastrocnemius muscle. Place a second anchor around the instep directly over the styloid process of the fifth metatarsal (1 and 2).

2. Apply the first strip posteriorly to the malleolus and attach it to the ankle anchor (3). NOTE: When applying strips, pull the foot into eversion for an inversion sprain and into a neutral position for an eversion sprain.

3. Start the first strip of tape directly under the malleolus and attach it to the foot anchor (4).

4. Place three vertical strips and three horizontal strips on the ankle, with each piece of tape overlapping at least half of the preceding strip (5 through 8). It must be added that there is no evidence that a superior level of effectiveness has been achieved by alternating the application of strips of tape that are perpendicular to one another.

5. After completing the conventional basket weave, apply two or three heel locks to ensure maximum stability (9 and 10). Additional support is given by a heel lock. Starting high on the instep, bring the tape along the ankle at a slight angle, hooking the heel, leading under the arch, then coming up on the opposite side, and finishing at the starting point. Tear the tape to complete half of the heel lock (9). Repeat on the opposite side of the ankle (10).

6. After applying the basket weave series, continue the Gibney strips up the ankle, thus giving circular support (11 through 17).

7. For arch support, apply two or three circular strips laterally to medially (18 and 19).

**Open Basket Weave** This modification of the closed basket weave, or Gibney, technique is used with acute ankle injuries and is designed to control swelling without restricting circulation. Taping in this pattern may be used immediately after an acute sprain in conjunction with an elastic wrap and cold applications (Figure 8–31). A U-shaped, or "horseshoe," felt pad can be used for focal compression to assist in controlling swelling (see Figure 19–25). The specific technique for controlling swelling is discussed in detail in Chapter 12.

***Materials Needed*** One roll of 1½-inch (3.8 cm) adhesive tape and tape adherent.

***Position of the Patient*** The patient sits on the table with the leg extended and the foot held at a 90-degree angle.

### Procedure

1. Steps 1 through 4 and the first eight strips of tape applied are the same as described for the closed basket weave technique (see Figure 8–30).

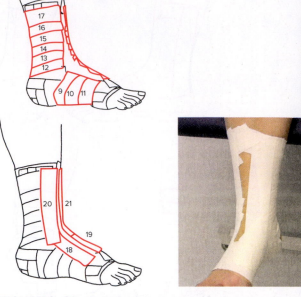

FIGURE 8–31   Open basket weave ankle taping.
Photo: © William E. Prentice

2. Leave a 1- to 1½-inch (1.5 to 3.8 cm) gap between the two ends of strips 11 through 17, exposing the anterior surface of the ankle (Figure 8–31).

3. Lock the gap between the Gibney ends with either one or two pieces of tape running on either side of the instep (18 through 21). NOTE: Application of a 3- or 4-inch (7.5 or 10 cm) elastic wrap over the open basket weave affords added control of swelling. Apply the elastic wrap distal to proximal to prevent swelling from moving into the toes.

**Continuous Elastic Tape Technique** This technique provides a fast alternative to other taping methods for the ankle (Figure 8–32).[31]

***Materials Needed*** One roll of 1½-inch (3.8 cm) adhesive tape, one roll of 2-inch (5 cm) elastic tape, tape adherent, and underwrap.

**Position of the Patient** The patient sits on the table, with the leg extended and the foot at a 90-degree angle.

### Procedure

1. Place one anchor strip around the ankle approximately 5 to 6 inches (12.5 cm to 15 cm) above the malleolus (1).

2. Apply three strips, covering the malleolli (2 through 4).

A cross-country runner steps in a hole and suffers a lateral sprain to the right ankle.

❓ What taping technique should be selected initially to provide ankle joint support while still allowing for swelling?

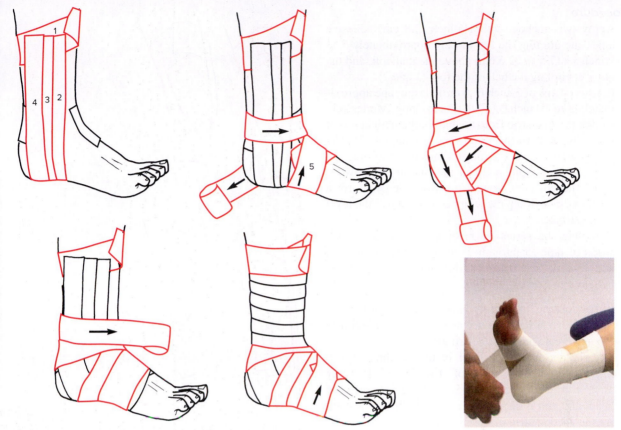

**FIGURE 8–32**  Continuous elastic tape technique for the ankle.
Photo: © William E. Prentice

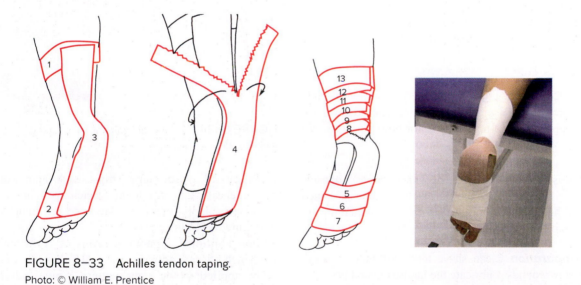

**FIGURE 8–33**  Achilles tendon taping.
Photo: © William E. Prentice

3. Start the stretch tape in a medial-to-lateral direction above the malleoli and continue, using two heel locks, one in each direction (5).

4. After completing the heel lock, begin distally and finish proximally by closing the vertical strips.

## The Lower Leg

**Achilles Tendon**  Achilles tendon taping is designed to prevent the Achilles tendon from overstretching (Figure 8–33).

***Materials Needed***  One roll of 3-inch (7.5 cm) elastic tape, one roll of 1½-inch (3.8 cm) adhesive tape, and tape adherent.

***Site Preparation***  Clean and shave the area, spray with tape adherent, and apply underwrap to the lower one-third of the calf.

***Position of the Patient***  The patient kneels or lies face down with the affected foot hanging relaxed over the edge of the table.

### Procedure

1. Apply two anchors with 1½-inch (3.8 cm) adhesive tape, one circling the leg loosely approximately 7 to 9 inches (17.5 to 22.5 cm) above the malleoli, and the other encircling the ball of the foot (1 and 2).
2. Cut two strips of 3-inch (7.5 cm) elastic tape approximately 8 to 10 inches (20 to 25 cm) long. Moderately stretch the first strip from the ball of the patient's foot along its plantar aspect up to the leg anchor (3). The second elastic strip (4) follows the course of the first, but cut it and split it down the middle lengthwise. Wrap the cut ends around the lower leg to form a lock. CAUTION: Keep the wrapped ends above the level of the strain.
3. Complete the series by placing two or three lock strips of tape (5 through 7) loosely around the arch and five or six strips (8 through 13) around the patient's lower leg.

Note that locking too tightly around the lower leg and foot tends to restrict the normal action of the Achilles tendon and create more tissue irritation.

A variation on this method is to use three 2-inch (5 cm) elastic strips in place of strips 3 and 4. Apply the first strip at the plantar surface of the first metatarsal head, and end it on the lateral side of the leg anchor. Apply the second strip at the plantar surface of the fifth metatarsal head, and end it on the medial side of the leg anchor. Center the third strip between the other two strips, and end it at the posterior aspect of the calf. Lock the strips with anchors of 3-inch (7.5 cm) elastic tape around the forefoot and lower calf.[2]

## The Knee

**Medial Collateral Ligament** Like patients with ankle instabilities, patients with unstable knees should never use tape and bracing as a replacement for proper exercise rehabilitation (Figure 8–34).[41]

***Materials Needed*** One roll of 2-inch (5 cm) adhesive tape, one roll of 3-inch (7.5 cm) elastic tape, a 1-inch (2.5 cm) heel lift, lubricant, gauze pad, tape adherent, and underwrap.

***Site Preparation*** Clean, shave, and dry skin to be taped. Cover skin wounds. Lubricate the hamstring and popliteal areas and apply tape adherent.

***Position of the Patient*** The patient stands on a 3-foot (90 cm) table, with the injured knee held in a moderately relaxed position by a 1-inch (2.5 cm) heel lift. Completely remove the hair from an area 6 inches (15 cm) above to 6 inches (15 cm) below the patella.

### Procedure

1. Lightly encircle the thigh and leg at the hairline with a 3-inch (7.5 cm) elastic tape anchor strip (1 and 2).

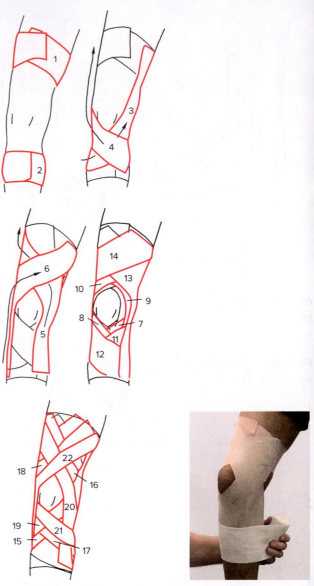

FIGURE 8–34   Collateral ligament knee taping.
Photo: © William E. Prentice

2. Precut 12 elastic tape strips, each approximately 9 inches (22.5 cm) long. Stretching them to their utmost, apply them to the knee as indicated in Figure 8–34 (3 through 14).
3. For additional support, a series of eight strips of 2-inch (5 cm) adhesive tape (15 through 22) may be applied in the same pattern. Some individuals find it advantageous to complete a knee taping by wrapping with an elastic wrap, thus providing an added precaution against the tape coming loose due to perspiration.

NOTE: Tape must not constrict the patella.

**Rotary Taping for Instability of an Injured Knee**
The rotary taping method has been used to provide the knee with support when it is unstable from injury to the medial collateral and anterior cruciate ligaments (Figure 8–35).

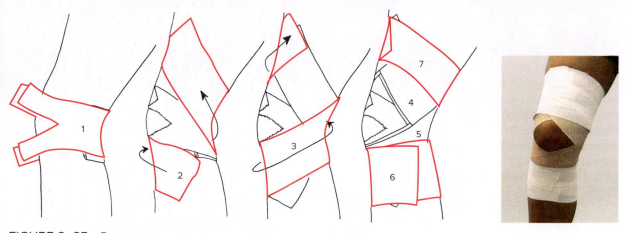

FIGURE 8–35    Rotary taping.
Photo: © William E. Prentice

**Materials Needed**  One roll of 3-inch (7.5 cm) elastic tape, tape adherent, 4-inch (10 cm) gauze pad, lubricant, scissors, and underwrap.

**Position of the Patient**  The patient stands on the table, with the affected knee flexed 15 degrees.

**Procedure**
1. Cut a 10-inch (25 cm) piece of 3-inch (7.5 cm) elastic tape with both the ends snipped. Place the gauze pad in the center of the 10-inch (25 cm) piece of elastic tape, to limit skin irritation and protect the popliteal nerves and blood vessels.
2. Put the gauze with the elastic tape backing on the popliteal fossa of the athlete's knee. Stretch both ends of the tape to the fullest extent and tear them. Place the divided ends firmly around the patella and interlock them (1).
3. Starting at a midpoint on the gastrocnemius muscle, spiral a 3-inch (7.5 cm) elastic tape strip to the front of the leg, then behind, crossing the popliteal fossa, and around the thigh, finishing anteriorly (2).
4. Repeat procedure 3 on the opposite side (3).
5. Apply two or four additional spiral strips for added strength (4 and 5).
6. Once they are in place, lock the spiral strips with two strips around the thigh and two around the calf (6 and 7).
NOTE: Tracing the spiral pattern with adhesive tape yields more rigidity.

**Hyperextension**  Hyperextension taping is designed to prevent the knee from hyperextending and may be used for a strained hamstring muscle or for slackened cruciate ligaments (Figure 8–36).

**Materials Needed**  One roll of 2½-inch (6.25 cm) tape or 2-inch (5 cm) elastic tape, cotton or a 4-inch (10 cm) gauze pad, tape adherent, underwrap, and a 2-inch (5 cm) heel lift.

**Position of the Patient**  Completely shave the patient's leg, including the area above midthigh and below midcalf. The patient stands on a 3-foot (90 cm) table with the injured knee flexed by a 2-inch (5 cm) heel lift.

**Procedure**
1. Place four anchor strips at the hairlines, two around the thigh and two around the leg (1 through 4). The strips should be loose enough to allow for muscle expansion during exercise.
2. Place a gauze pad at the popliteal space to protect the popliteal nerves and blood vessels from constriction by the tape.
3. Start the supporting tape strips by forming an X over the popliteal space (5 and 6).
4. Cross the tape with two more strips, and place one up the middle of the leg (7 through 9).
5. Complete the technique by applying four or five locking strips around the thigh and calf (10 through 18).
6. Apply an additional series of cross-strips if the athlete is heavily muscled. Lock the additional supporting strips in place with two or three strips around the thigh and leg.

**Patellofemoral Taping (McConnell Technique)**  Patellofemoral orientation may be corrected to some degree by using tape.[22,40] The clinician evaluates four components of patellar orientation: glide, tilt, rotation, and anteroposterior (AP) orientation.[22]

The glide component is a side-to-side movement of the patella in the groove. The tilt component is the

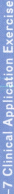

8-7 Clinical Application Exercise

A female basketball player complains of a chronic dull ache in her right patella.

**?** What taping technique can be used to correct this problem?

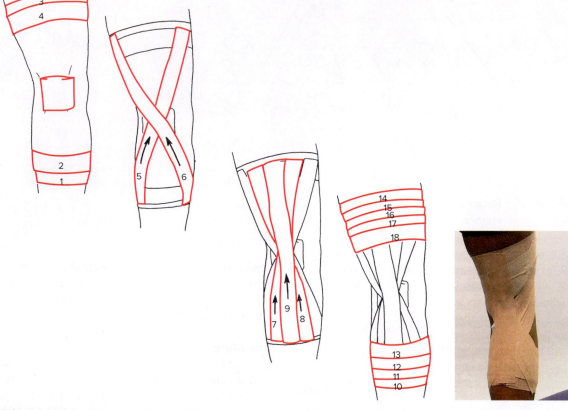

FIGURE 8–36  Hyperextension taping.
Photo: © William E. Prentice

height of the lateral patellar border relative to the medial border. Patellar rotation is determined by looking for deviation of the long axis of the patella from the long axis of the femur. Anteroposterior alignment evaluates whether the inferior pole of the patella is tilted either anteriorly or posteriorly relative to the superior pole. Correction of patellar position and tracking is accomplished by passive taping of the patella in a more biomechanically correct position.[45,48] In addition to correcting the orientation of the patella, the tape provides a prolonged, gentle stretch to soft-tissue structure that affects patellar movement.[13,22,49]

**Materials Needed** Two special types of extremely sticky tape are required. Fixomull and Leuko Sportape are manufactured by Biersdorf Australia, Ltd.

**Site Preparation** Clean and shave, and apply tape adherent.

**Position of the Patient** The patient is sitting with the knee fully extended.

**Procedure**

1. Extend two strips of Fixomull from the lateral femoral condyle just posterior to the medial femoral condyle around the front of the knee. This tape is used as a base to which the other tape may be adhered. Leuko

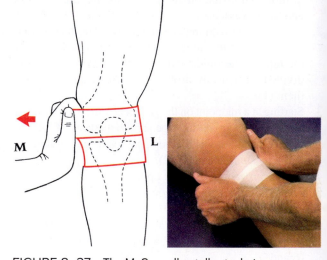

FIGURE 8–37  The McConnell patellar technique uses a base to which additional tape is adhered.
Photo: © William E. Prentice

Sportape is used from this point on to correct patellar alignment (Figure 8–37).

2. To correct a lateral glide, attach a short strip of tape one thumb's width from the lateral patellar border, pushing the patella medially in the frontal plane. Crease the skin between the lateral patellar border and the medial femoral condyle, and secure the tape on the medial side of the joint (Figure 8–38).

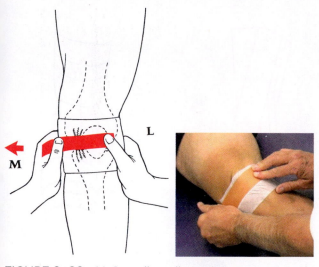

FIGURE 8–38   McConnell patellar technique to correct a lateral glide.
Photo: © William E. Prentice

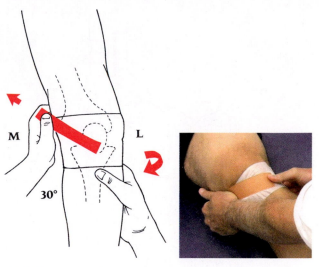

FIGURE 8–40   McConnell patellar technique to correct external rotation of the inferior pole.
Photo: © William E. Prentice

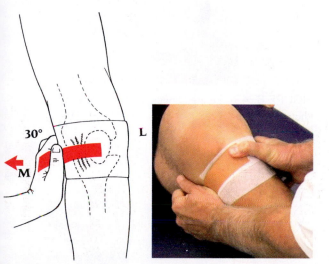

FIGURE 8–39   McConnell patellar technique to correct a lateral tilt.
Photo: © William E. Prentice

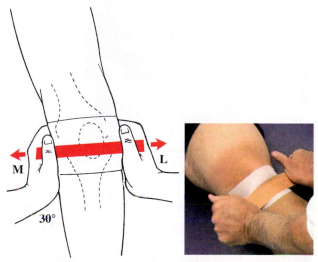

FIGURE 8–41   McConnell patellar technique to correct AP alignment with a superior tilt.
Photo: © William E. Prentice

3. To correct a lateral tilt, flex the knee to 30 degrees, adhere a short strip of tape beginning at the middle of the patella, and pull medially to lift the lateral border. Again, crease the skin underneath and adhere it to the medial side of the knee (Figure 8–39).

4. To correct an external rotation of the inferior pole relative to the superior pole, adhere a strip of tape to the middle of the inferior pole, pulling upward and medially while internally rotating the patella with the free hand. The tape is attached to the medial side of the knee (Figure 8–40).

5. For correcting AP alignment in which there is a superior tilt, take a 6-inch piece of tape, place the middle of the strip over the lower one-half of the patella, and attach it equally on both sides to lift the superior pole (Figure 8–41).

6. Once patellar taping is completed, the patient should be instructed to wear the tape all day during all activities.

The patient should periodically tighten the strips as they loosen.

NOTE: The McConnell technique for treating patellofemoral pain also stresses the importance of more symmetrical loading of the patella through reeducation and strengthening of the vastus medialis, although the efficacy of this technique is questionable.[7,22] Patellar taping may also enhance proprioception in the knee joint.[26]

## The Elbow

**Elbow Restriction**   Taping the elbow prevents hyperextension (Figure 8–42).[43]

**Materials Needed**   One roll of 1½-inch (3.8 cm) adhesive tape, tape adherent, and 2-inch (5 cm) elastic tape.

**Site Preparation**   Clean and shave area, and apply adherent.

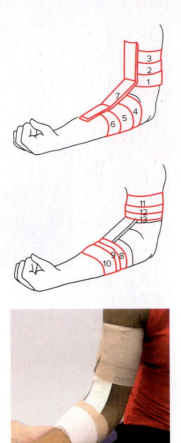

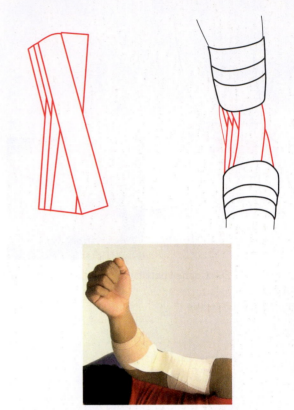

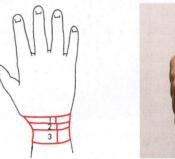

FIGURE 8–42   Elbow restriction taping.
Photo: © William E. Prentice

FIGURE 8–43   Fanned checkrein technique.
Photo: © William E. Prentice

FIGURE 8–44   Wrist taping technique no. 1.
Photo: © William E. Prentice

**Position of the Patient** The patient has the affected elbow flexed at 90 degrees.

**Procedure**

1. Apply three anchor strips loosely around the upper arm, using 2-inch (5 cm) elastic tape (1 through 3).
2. Apply three anchor strips around the upper forearm, using 2-inch (5 cm) elastic tape (4, 5, and 6).
3. Construct a checkrein by cutting a 10-inch (25 cm) and a 4-inch (10 cm) strip of tape and placing the 4-inch (10 cm) strip against the center of the 10-inch (25 cm) strip, blanking out that portion. Place the checkrein so that it spans the two anchor strips, with the blanked-out side facing downward. Leave the checkrein extended 1 to 2 inches past the anchor strips on both ends. This allows anchoring of the checkreins with circular strips to secure against slippage (7).
4. Place five additional 10-inch (25 cm) strips of tape over the basic checkrein.
5. Finish the procedure by securing the checkrein with three lock strips on each end (8 through 13). A figure-eight elastic wrap applied over the taping will prevent the tape from slipping because of perspiration.

NOTE: A variation of this method is to fan the checkreins, dispersing the force over a wider area (Figure 8–43).

## The Wrist and Hand

**Wrist Taping Technique No. 1** This wrist taping technique is designed for mild wrist strains and sprains (Figure 8–44).

**Materials Needed** One roll of 1-inch (2.5 cm) adhesive tape and tape adherent.

**Position of the Patient** The patient stands with the affected hand flexed toward the injured direction.

A volleyball player attempts to block a ball and reports that her elbow "bent backwards."

**?** What taping technique can be used to prevent this incident from reoccurring?

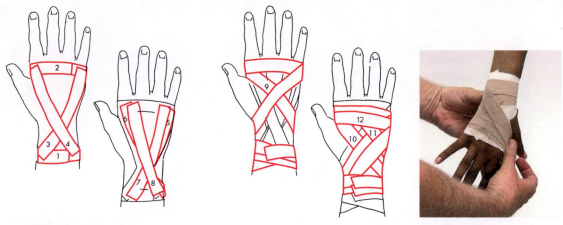

FIGURE 8–45   Wrist taping technique no. 2.
Photo: © William E. Prentice

The fingers may either be spread or the fist clenched to increase the breadth of the wrist for the protection of nerves and blood vessels.

### Procedure

1. Starting at the base of the wrist, bring a strip of 1-inch (2.5 cm) adhesive tape around both sides of the wrist (1).
2. In the same pattern, with each strip overlapping the preceding one by at least half its width, lay two additional strips in place (2 and 3).

**Wrist Taping Technique No. 2**  This wrist taping technique stabilizes and protects badly injured wrists (Figure 8–45).

***Materials Needed***  One roll of 1-inch (2.5 cm) adhesive tape and tape adherent.

***Position of the Patient***  The patient stands with the affected hand flexed toward the injured side and the fingers moderately spread to increase the breadth of the wrist for the protection of nerves and blood vessels.

### Procedure

1. Apply one anchor strip around the wrist approximately 3 inches (7.5 cm) from the hand (1); wrap another anchor strip around the spread hand (2).
2. With the wrist bent toward the side of the injury, run a strip of tape from the anchor strip near the little finger obliquely across the wrist joint to the wrist anchor strip. Run another strip from the anchor strip and the index finger side across the wrist joint to the wrist anchor. This forms a crisscross over the wrist joint (3 and 4). Apply a series of four or five crisscrosses, depending on the extent of splinting needed (5 through 8).
3. Apply two or three series of figure-eight tapings over the crisscross taping (9 through 11). Starting by encircling the wrist once, carry a strip over the back of the

hand obliquely upward across the back of the hand to where the figure eight started. Repeat this procedure to ensure a strong, stabilizing taping (12).

**Bruised Hand**  The following method is used to tape a bruised hand (Figure 8–46).

***Materials Needed***  One roll of 1-inch (2.5 cm) adhesive tape, one roll of ½-inch (1.25 cm) adhesive tape, ¼-inch (0.6 cm) thick sponge rubber pad, and tape adherent.

***Position of the Patient***  The fingers are spread moderately.

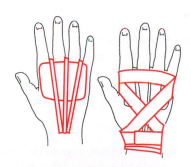

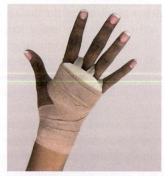

FIGURE 8–46   Bruised hand taping.
Photo: © William E. Prentice

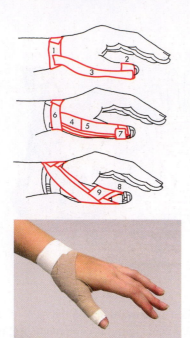

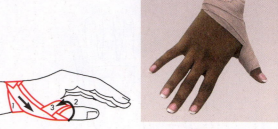

FIGURE 8–48   Thumb spica.
Photo: © William E. Prentice

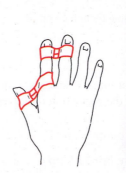

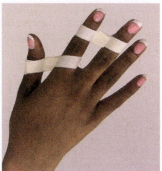

FIGURE 8–47   Sprained thumb taping.
Photo: © William E. Prentice

FIGURE 8–49   Finger and thumb checkreins.
Photo: © William E. Prentice

### Procedure

1. Lay the protective pad over the bruise and hold it in place with three strips of ½-inch (1.25 cm) tape laced through the webbing of the fingers.
2. Apply a basic figure-eight wrap made of 1-inch (2.5 cm) elastic tape.

**Sprained Thumb**   Sprained thumb taping is designed to give protection to the joint as well as support to the thumb (Figure 8–47).[11]

***Materials Needed***   One roll each of 1-inch (2.5 cm) adhesive tape and elastic tape and tape adherent.

***Position of the Patient***   The patient should hold the injured thumb in a relaxed, neutral position.

### Procedure

1. Place an anchor strip loosely around the wrist and another around the distal end of the thumb (1 and 2).
2. From the anchor at the tip of the thumb to the anchor around the wrist, apply four splint strips in a series on the side of greater injury (dorsal or palmar side) (3 through 5). They may be locked in place either with one lock strip around the wrist and one encircling the tip of the thumb (6 and 7) or simply with the thumb spica.
3. Add three thumb spicas. Start the first spica on the ulnar side at the wrist; carry it across the wrist; cross the strip and continue around the thumb; finish at the starting point. Each of the subsequent spica strips should overlap the preceding strip by at least ⅔-inch (1.7 cm) and adduct the thumb toward the web space (8 and 9).

The thumb spica with tape provides an excellent means of protection during recovery from an injury (Figure 8–48).

***Finger and Thumb Checkreins***   The sprained finger or thumb may require the additional protection afforded by a restraining checkrein (Figure 8–49).[11]

***Materials Needed***   One roll of 1-inch (2.5 cm) adhesive tape.

***Position of the Patient***   The patient spreads the injured fingers widely but within a range that is free of pain.

### Procedure

1. Bring a strip of ½-inch (1.25 cm) adhesive tape around the middle phalanx of the injured finger over to the adjacent finger and around it also. The tape left between the two fingers, which are spread apart, is called the checkrein.
2. Add strength with a lock strip around the center of the checkrein.

## KINESIO TAPING

Kinesio taping is a technique developed in Japan and widely used in Europe and Asia. It has become popular in the United States despite the fact that there is no research-based evidence that supports its effectiveness.[32,47] Kinesio tape differs from adhesive tape in that it is elastic and can be stretched to 140 percent of its original length before being applied to the skin, thus providing a constant tension (shear) force to the skin over which it is applied.[16] Although adhesive tape is structurally supportive, Kinesio tape is said to be therapeutic, activating neurological and circulatory systems with movement.[29] It is used both immediately following injury and during the rehabilitation process. Kinesio taping is used for edema reduction, pain management, and inhibition and facilitation of motor activity.[16]

Several mechanisms have been proposed through which Kinesio tape works, including improving circulation of blood and lymph by eliminating tissue fluid or bleeding beneath the skin; correcting muscle function by strengthening weakened muscles; decreasing pain through neurological suppression; and repositioning subluxed joints by relieving abnormal muscle tension.[29] It has also been suggested that the Kinesio tape stimulates cutaneous mechanoreceptors by applying pressure and stretching the skin, thus enhancing proprioception through increased cutaneous feedback, which signals information relative to joint movement or joint position.[30] Again, there is no evidence to date to support these claims.

The basic principle of Kinesio taping is to apply the tape from one end of a muscle to the other, with very little to no stretch on the tape from origin to insertion for muscle support and from insertion to origin during rehabilitation.[15] The muscle is placed on gentle functional stretch with application of the tape at approximately 10 percent of its resting static length.[16] Because the latex-free, 100 percent cotton fabric with body heat–activated adhesive Kinesio tape is air permeable and water resistant, it can be worn continuously for 3 to 4 days before a new application is required.[29] Kinesio tape can be purchased in rolls of 1-inch (2.5 cm), 1½-inch (3.8 cm), 2-inch (5 cm), and 3-inch (7.5 cm) widths. The tape comes in a variety of colors, although there is no physical or chemical difference between the colors.

Athletic trainers are familiar and comfortable with taping techniques that provide stability and support. The therapeutic techniques of Kinesio taping are not difficult. Figures 8–50 through 8–53 provide some common examples of Kinesio taping techniques.

## Kinesio Taping Techniques

### Plantar Fasciitis

***Materials Needed*** One roll of 1-inch (2.5 cm) Kinesio tape and one roll of 3-inch (7.5 cm) Kinesio tape.

***Position of the Patient*** The patient lies prone with the foot extending off the edge of the treatment table, with foot dorsiflexed and the toes extended (Figure 8–50).

***Procedure***
1. Place the base of 1-inch (2.5 cm) tape over heel with moderate stretch.

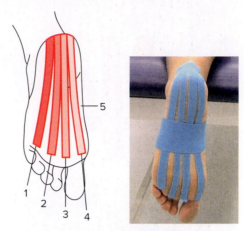

FIGURE 8–50  Kinesio taping for planter fasciitis.
Photo: © William E. Prentice

2. Extend four pieces of 1-inch (2.5 cm) tape over bottom of foot to the metatarsal heads while extending toes to stretch plantar fascia. Use a moderate to strong stretch (1 through 4).
3. Place one end of a 3-inch (7.5 cm) strip over the shaft of the fifth metatarsal. With the foot relaxed, extend tape over arch toward the medial side of the foot, adding moderate stretch (5).

### Patellofemoral Pain

***Materials Needed*** One roll of 2-inch (5 cm) Kinesio tape.

***Position of the Patient*** The patient sits with the leg extended (Figure 8–51).

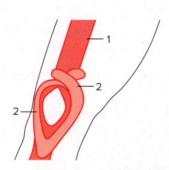

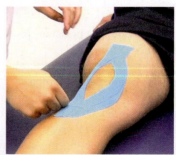

FIGURE 8–51  Kinesio taping technique for patellofemoral pain.
Photo: © William E. Prentice

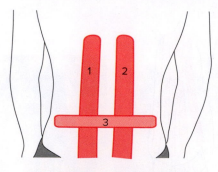

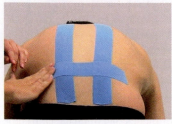

FIGURE 8–52   Kinesio taping for low back strain.
Photo: © William E. Prentice

### Procedure

1. Split a piece of 2-inch (5 cm) tape 10 inches (25 cm) long halfway. Position the anchor of the tape on the front of the thigh so that the Y-shape split is at the top of the patella (1).
2. Wrap tails downward around the patella, with very little or no stretch.
3. Split a piece of 2-inch (2.5 cm) tape 6 inches (15 cm) long halfway. Place the base of the second Y-shape tape slightly below the knee, and wrap tails upward around the patella, with very little or no stretch (2).

### Low Back Strain

***Materials Needed*** One roll of 3-inch (7.5 cm) Kinesio tape.

***Position of the Patient*** The patient is standing (Figure 8–52).

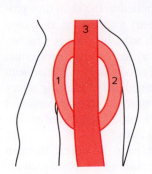
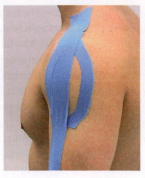

FIGURE 8–53   Kinesio taping for shoulder instability.
Photo: © William E. Prentice

### Procedure

1. Bend forward to stretch the back muscles. Apply two 3-inch (7.5 cm) strips beginning at the level of the waist, and extend up and along each side of the spine, adding very light stretch (1 and 2).
2. With the patient still bending forward, add light to moderate stretch and place the center of a 3-inch (7.5 cm) strip of tape over the strained area (3).

### Shoulder Instability

***Materials Needed*** One roll of 1-inch (2.5 cm) Kinesio tape and one roll of 2-inch (5 cm) Kinesio tape.

***Position of the Patient*** The patient is standing, arm hanging at side (Figure 8–53).

### Procedure

1. Using two pieces of 1-inch (2.5 cm) tape, place base of Y-shape strip below the insertion of the deltoid muscle. Extend both sides of the tape to wrap around the deltoid muscle, with no added stretch (1 and 2).
2. Abduct the shoulder to 90 degrees, and apply one strip of 2-inch (5 cm) tape over the tip of the shoulder, with little to no stretch, extending from the base of the neck to halfway down the upper arm (3).

## SUMMARY

- Elastic wraps provide compression, provide support, and reduce chances of injury.
- Elastic wraps must be applied uniformly, firmly but not so tightly as to impede circulation.
- Historically, taping has been an important aspect of athletic training. However, there are limited evidence-based studies that support its use.
- For supporting and protecting musculoskeletal injuries, two types of tape are currently used—nonelastic white adhesive and elastic adhesive.
- An adherent may be applied, followed by an underwrap material, if need be, to help avoid skin irritation.

- When tape is applied, it must be done in a manner that provides the least amount of irritation and the maximum support.
- For all tape applications, the correct materials must be used, the patient must be in an appropriate position, and the proper procedures must be carefully followed.
- Kinesio taping is used for therapeutic purposes both immediately following injury and during rehabilitation. Despite its popularity, it is no more effective than other techniques of elastic taping in the management or prevention of sports injuries.

## WEB SITES

Cramer First Aider:
   www.cramersportsmed.com/first-aider.html

Cramer Sports Medicine: www.cramersportsmed.com

Johnson & Johnson: www.jnj.com

Kinesio Taping Association: www.kinesiotaping.com

Mueller Sports Medicine—Retail Tape and Wrap:
   www.muellersportsmed.com/sports-medicine-product
   /athletic-tapes-wraps.html

Properties of Athletic Tape: www.bloodandbones.com
   /tape.html

## SOLUTIONS TO CLINICAL APPLICATION EXERCISES

8–1   First the ankle should be shaved. Then a tape adherent spray should be applied. Heel and lace pads with a small amount of lubricant should be applied over bony prominences. One layer of underwrap can be applied. Tape should be applied with even pressure, leaving no gaps.

8–2   The athletic trainer should apply a 6-inch (15 cm) elastic wrap as a hip adductor restraint. This technique is designed to prevent the groin from being overstretched and the hip adductors reinjured.

8–3   The athletic trainer should apply tape and a 4-inch (10 cm) double-length elastic shoulder spica to hold the doughnut in place.

8–4   The athletic trainer should apply a sling and swathe combination. This combination stabilizes the shoulder joint and upper arm.

8–5   The LowDye technique is designed to assist in the management of foot pronation and fallen medial longitudinal arch, which predisposes the patient to arch strain.

8–6   Initially, for a sprained ankle, the athletic trainer should select the open basket weave taping technique. This technique in conjunction with focal compression and cold application can also control swelling.

8–7   The McConnell taping technique can be employed to correct a lateral patellar glide.

8–8   The elbow restriction taping will help prevent elbow hyperextension.

## REVIEW QUESTIONS AND CLASS ACTIVITIES

1. What are some common types of wraps used in sports medicine today?
2. Observe the athletic trainer when he or she is dressing wounds in the training clinic.
3. Demonstrate the proper use of elastic wraps.
4. What types of tape are available? What is the purpose of each type? What qualities should you look for in selecting tape?
5. How should you prepare an area to be taped?
6. How should you tear tape?
7. How should you remove tape from an area? Demonstrate the various methods and cutters that can be used to remove tape.
8. Bring the different types of tape to class. Discuss their uses and the qualities to look for in purchasing tape. Have the class practice tearing tape and preparing an area for taping.
9. Take each joint or body part and demonstrate the common taping procedures used to give support to that area. Have the students pair up and practice these tapings on each other. Discuss the advantages and disadvantages of using tape as a supportive device.
10. How is Kinesio taping different from applying regular adhesive tape?

## REFERENCES

1. Abell B: *Taping and wrapping made simple*, Philadelphia, PA, 2009, Lippincott, Williams & Wilkins.
2. Alt W, Lohrer H, Gollhofer A: Functional properties of adhesive ankle taping: Neuromuscular and mechanical effects before and after exercise, *Foot and Ankle International* 20(4):238, 1999.
3. Benefit of ankle taping is short-lived with or without prewrap, *Sports Med Digest* 19(1):130, 1997.
4. Bragg RW, Macmahon JM, Overom EK: Failure and fatigue characteristics of adhesive athletic tape, *Med Sci Sports Exerc* 34(3):403, 2002.
5. Briggs J: Bandaging, strapping and taping. In Briggs J, editor: *Sports therapy: Theoretical and practical thoughts and considerations*, Chichester, UK, 2001 Corpus.
6. Callaghan M, Selfe J, Bagley P: The effects of patellar taping on knee joint proprioception, *J Athl Train* 37(1):19, 2002.
7. Camera J: The effect of patellar taping on some landing characteristics during counter movement jumps in healthy subjects, *Journal of Sport Science and Medicine* 10(1):707–11, 2011.
8. Cecchinato A, Bernier J, Cucina I: Effectiveness of ankle tape and ankle brace on joint position sense in subjects with unilateral functionally unstable ankle (Abstract), *J Athl Train* 40(2 Suppl):S-108, 2005.
9. Clay K: The impact of ankle taping upon range of movement and lower-limb balance before and after dynamic exercise. In Reilly

T: *Contemporary sport, leisure and ergonomics*, 2009, Taylor & Francis.
10. Cordova M, Ingersoll C, Palmieri R: Efficacy of prophylactic ankle support: An experimental perspective, *J Athl Train* 37(4):446, 2002.
11. Deivert R: Functional thumb taping procedure, *J Athl Train* 29(4):357, 1994.
12. Eils, E: The main function of ankle braces is to control the joint position before landing. *Foot Ankle Int.* 24(3):263–268, 2003.
13. Ernst GP, Kawaguchi J, Saliba E: Effect of patellar taping on knee kinetics of patients with patellofemoral pain syndrome, *J Orthop Sports Phys Ther* 29(11):661, 1999.
14. Franettovich M: Initial neuromotor and postural effects of augmented low-dye taping do not change after continued use, *Athletic Training and Sports Healthcare* 3(1):21–28, 2011.
15. Grindstaff T: Kinesiotaping technique for patellar tendinopathy, *Athletic Training & Sports Health Care* 2(3):98–99, 2010.
16. Halseth T, McChesney J, DeBeliso M: The effects of Kinesio taping on proprioception at the ankle, *Journal of Sports Science & Medicine* 3(1):1, 2004.
17. Holmes C, Wilcox D, Fletcher J: Effect of a modified, low-dye medial longitudinal arch taping procedure on the subtalar joint neutral position before and after, light exercise, *J Orthpo Sports Phys Ther* 32(5):305–309, 2002.

18. Karren K, Limmer D, Mistovich J, Hafen B: *First aid for colleges and universities*, San Francisco, CA, 2011, Benjamin-Cummings.
19. Knight KL: Taping, wrapping, bracing, and padding. In Knight KL, editor: *Assessing clinical proficiencies in athletic training: A modular approach*, ed 3, Champaign, IL, 2001, Human Kinetics.
20. Magnes, S: Taping and bracing for pelvic and hip injuries. In Seidenberg P: *The hip and pelvis in sports medicine and primary care*, New York, 2010, Springer.
21. Manfroy PP, Ashton-Miller JA, Wojtys EM: The effect of exercise, prewrap, and athletic tape on the maximal active and passive ankle resistance to ankle-inversion, *Am J Sports Med* 25(2):156, 1997.
22. McConnell J: A novel approach to pain relief pre-therapeutic exercise, *Journal of Science and Medicine in Sport* 3(3):325, 2000.
23. Merrick MA: Do ankle bracing and taping work? *Athletic Therapy Today* 5(6):40, 2000.
24. Metcalfe RC, Schlabach GA, Looney MA, et al.: A comparison of moleskin tape, linen tape, and lace-up brace on joint restriction and movement performance, *J Athl Train* 32(2):136, 1997.
25. Mickel T: Prophylactic bracing versus taping for the prevention of ankle sprains in high school athletes: A prospective, randomized trial, *Journal of Foot and Ankle Surgery* 45(6): 360–65, 2006.

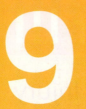

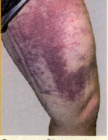

Courtesy Christopher
R. Bartlett

# 9

# Mechanisms and Characteristics of Musculoskeletal and Nerve Trauma

## ■ Objectives

*When you finish this chapter you should be able to*

- Analyze the mechanical properties of tissue based on the stress–strain curve model.
- Discuss the five types of tissue loads that can produce stress and strain.
- Examine the anatomical characteristics of the musculotendinous unit, synovial joint, bone, and nerve.

- Evaluate how mechanical loads applied to the musculotendinous unit, synovial joint, bone, and nerve produce injury in these structures.
- Identify and differentiate various injuries to the musculotendinous unit, synovial joint, bone, and nerve tissue.

## ■ Outline

## ■ Key Terms

| | | |
|---|---|---|
| trauma | muscle guarding | diastasis |
| load | clonic | dislocation |
| stiffness | tonic | subluxation |
| stress | muscle soreness | osteoarthritis |
| strain | tendinitis | bursitis |
| deformation | tendon | bursae |
| elasticity | crepitus | osteoblasts |
| yield point | tendinosis | osteoclasts |
| plastic | tenosynovitis | closed fracture |
| creep | contusion | open fracture |
| mechanical failure | ecchymosis | neuropraxia |
| muscle strain | myositis ossificans | neuritis |
| muscle cramps | synovial joints | referred pain |

## ■ Connect Highlights    connect

*Visit connect.mcgraw-hill.com for further exercises to apply your knowledge:*

- Clinical application scenarios covering the stress–strain curve model, anatomical characteristics, mechanical and tissue loads that produce injury, and identification of various injuries
- Click-and-drag questions covering the stress–strain curve, anatomical characteristics, mechanical and tissue loads, and various injuries sustained
- Multiple-choice questions covering the stress–strain curve, anatomical characteristics, mechanical and tissue loads, and various injuries sustained

The ability to recognize a specific injury to musculoskeletal and nerve structures and understand those mechanical factors that produce injuries or trauma is essential for the athletic trainer.[11] **Trauma** is defined as a physical injury or wound that is produced by an external or internal force.[3] This chapter provides the foundation for the identification, understanding, and management of injuries to be discussed throughout this text. It examines mechanical forces and tissue characteristics of injuries and the classification of these injuries.

# MECHANICAL INJURY

Newtonian physics maintains that force or mechanical energy is that which changes the state of rest or uniform motion of matter. When a force applied to any part of the body results in a harmful disturbance in function and or structure, a mechanical injury is said to have been sustained.[41] Injuries are caused by external forces directed on the body that result in internal alteration in anatomical structures that are of sufficient magnitude to cause damage or destruction to that tissue.[33] How the various tissues respond to the application of an external load is determined in large part by the mechanical properties of that tissue.

> The stress-strain curve represents the relationship between various tissue properties when a ligament is stretched.
>
> **?** How does external stress lead to an ankle sprain in a patient who steps awkwardly off a curb?

## Tissue Properties

Tissue properties are described according to mechanical terminology, and their relative relationships may best be illustrated by the stress–strain curve (Figure 9–1). A **load** is an external force acting on tissues that causes internal reactions within the tissues. **Stiffness** is the relative ability of a tissue to resist a particular load. The greater the stiffness, the greater the magnitude of load it can withstand. The internal resistance of the tissues to an external load is called a **stress.** The extent of the deformation of tissue when it is loaded is referred to as **strain.** The internal strain placed on the tissues from that stress results in **deformation** of those tissues. However, human tissue has **elasticity,** a *property* that allows a tissue to return to normal following deformation. When tissue is deformed to the extent that it no longer reacts elastically, the **yield point** has been reached. Beyond the yield point, some deformation persists after the load is removed and this results in permanent or **plastic** changes to the tissues. **Creep** is the deformation in the shape and/or properties of a tissue that occurs with the application of a constant load over time. When the ability of the tissue to withstand stress and strain is exceeded, **mechanical failure** of the tissue ultimately occurs, manifesting itself in injury to that tissue. Depending on the amount of deformation tissues can withstand prior to mechanical failure, they can be classified as being *ductile* or *brittle*. Ductile tissues can deform significantly before failing and consequently have a longer plastic area. Brittle tissues can deform very little before failure.[29,35]

## Tissue Loading

Five types of tissue loading can produce stress and strain: compression, tension, shearing, bending, and torsion.[17]

**Compression** Compression is produced by external loads applied toward one another on opposite surfaces in opposite directions (Figure 9–2A). Compression shortens and widens a structure. When the force can no longer be absorbed by the tissues, injury occurs. Constant compression over a period of time can also cause injury. Arthritic

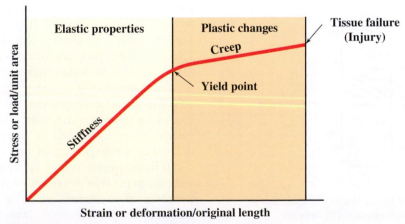

FIGURE 9–1   Stress–strain curve.

changes in cartilage, fractures, and contusions are commonly caused by compression forces.

**Tension** Tension is the force that pulls or stretches tissue (Figure 9–2B). Tension is generated in response to equal and opposite external loads that pull a structure apart. The structure elongates and tensile stress and strain result. Muscle strains and ligament sprains both occur due to increased tension.

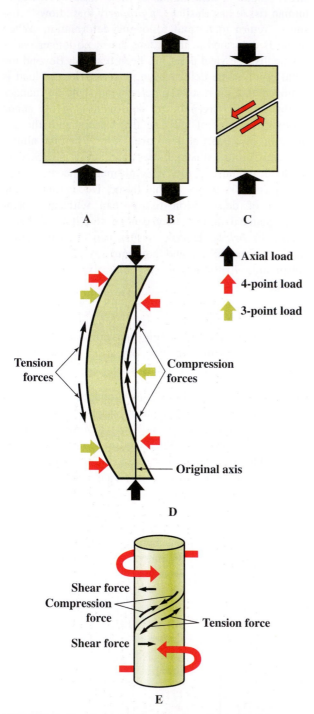

FIGURE 9–2    Types of tissue loading that can cause stress and strain. **(A)** Compression. **(B)** Tension. **(C)** Shearing. **(D)** Bending. **(E)** Torsion.

**Shearing** Shearing occurs when equal but not directly opposite loads are applied to opposing surfaces, forcing those surfaces to move in parallel directions relative to one another (Figure 9–2C). Injury occurs once shearing has exceeded the inherent strength of a tissue. Shearing stress can result in skin injuries such as blisters or abrasions or in vertebral disk injuries.

**Bending** Bending can occur in one of the following ways: when two force pairs act at opposite ends of a structure (4-point); when three forces cause bending (3-point); or when an already bowed structure is axially loaded (Figure 9–2D).[41] Regardless of the mechanism, the original axis is maintained while the convex side of the structure is elongated and subject to tension forces and the concave side is shortened and subject to compression forces. Shear forces also occur along the original axis. Bending of the long bones can result in fractures.

> **Tissue stresses:**
> - Compression
> - Tension
> - Shearing
> - Bending
> - Torsion

**Torsion** Torsion loads caused by twisting in opposite directions from the opposite ends of a structure cause shear stress over the entire cross section of that structure (Figure 9–2E). Maximal shear occurs in planes that are perpendicular and parallel to the applied loads, and maximal tension and compression occur in diagonal planes. Therefore, torsion could result in spiral fractures at an oblique angle in the long bones.

## Traumatic versus Overuse Injuries

No matter how much attention is directed toward the general principles of injury prevention, the nature of participation in physical activity dictates that sooner or later injury will occur. Traditionally, injuries have been classified as either acute or chronic.[25] Some health care professionals have argued that these terms are confusing. All injuries are acute—something initiates the injury process.[25] If the acute injury doesn't heal properly, at some point it becomes chronic. Exactly when that transition occurs is debatable. Debating how to define these terms precisely serves no useful purpose. It is perhaps less confusing to classify injuries according to the primary mechanism that causes an injury or condition. Generally, injuries are caused either by trauma or by overuse. Trauma was defined at the beginning of this chapter. Injuries that result from overuse can be either chronic, which occur with the repetitive dynamics of running, throwing, or jumping, or recurrent, which are traumatic injuries that occur multiple times.[25] Table 9–1 summarizes the general injury classifications and the types of tissue

| TABLE 9-1 | Classification and Load Characteristics of Injuries | |
|---|---|---|
| **Injury** | **Classification** | **Load** |
| Muscle strain | Traumatic | Tension/torsion/shearing |
| Muscle cramp | Overuse | Tension/compression |
| Muscle soreness | Overuse | Tension |
| Tendinitis/tendinosis | Overuse | Tension |
| Tenosynovitis | Overuse | Tension |
| Myofascial trigger point | Overuse/traumatic | Tension |
| Contusion | Traumatic | Compression |
| Ligament sprain | Traumatic | Tension/torsion/bending |
| Dislocation/subluxations | Traumatic | Tension/torsion/shearing |
| Osteoarthritis | Overuse | Compression/shearing/torsion |
| Bursitis | Overuse/traumatic | Compression/shearing |
| Capsulitis/synovitis | Overuse | Tension/compression/shearing/torsion |
| Bone fracture | Traumatic | Tension/compression/shearing/torsion/bending |
| Stress fracture | Overuse | Tension/compression/shearing/torsion/bending |
| Epiphyseal injury | Traumatic/overuse | Tension/compression/shearing/torsion/bending |
| Apophyseal injury | Traumatic/overuse | Tension/compression/shearing/torsion/bending |
| Neuropraxia | Traumatic | Compression/shearing |
| Neuritis | Overuse | Compression/tension/shearing |

loading that produce injury for the more common injuries that the athletic trainer is likely to see.

# MUSCULOTENDINOUS UNIT INJURIES

## Anatomical Characteristics

The musculotendinous unit consists of the muscle, the tendon, and the fascia that surrounds the muscle. Muscles are composed of contractile cells, or fibers, that produce movement. Muscle fibers possess the ability to contract as well as the properties of irritability, conductivity, and elasticity. There are three types of muscles in the body—smooth, cardiac, and striated. Of primary concern for athletic trainers are conditions that affect striated, or skeletal, muscles. Within the muscle fiber cell is a semifluid substance called sarcoplasm (cytoplasm). Myofibrils are surrounded by the endomysium, fiber bundles are surrounded by the perimysium, and the entire muscle is covered by the epimysium (Figure 9–3). The epimysium, perimysium, and endomysium may be combined with the fibrous tendon. The fibrous wrapping of a muscle may become a flat sheet of connective tissue (aponeurosis) that attaches to other muscles. Tendons have a high mechanical strength, good flexibility, and an optimal level of elasticity to perform their role.[38] Occasionally, they will pull away from a bone, a bone will fracture, or a muscle will tear before tendons and aponeuroses are injured. Skeletal muscles are generally well vascularized. Arteries, veins, lymph vessels, and bundles of nerve fibers spread into the perimysium. A complex capillary network goes throughout

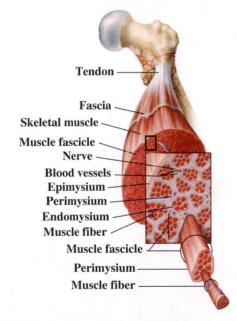

Tendon

Fascia
Skeletal muscle
Muscle fascicle
Nerve
Blood vessels
Epimysium
Perimysium
Endomysium
Muscle fiber
Muscle fascicle
Perimysium
Muscle fiber

FIGURE 9–3   Connective tissue associated with skeletal muscle.

the endomysium, coming into direct contact with the muscle fibers.[37]

## Muscle Strains

The muscle is composed of separate fibers that are capable of simultaneous contraction when stimulated by the central nervous system. Each muscle is attached to bone at both ends by strong, relatively inelastic tendons that cross over joints.

If a muscle is overstretched by tension or forced to contract against too much resistance, separation or tearing of the muscle fibers occurs. This damage is referred to as a **muscle strain** (Figure 9–4).[1] Muscle strains, like ligament sprains, are subject to various classification systems. The following is a simple system of strain classification:

- *Grade 1 strain.* Some muscle fibers have been stretched or actually torn. There is some tenderness and pain on active motion. Movement is painful, but full range of motion is usually possible.
- *Grade 2 strain.* A number of muscle fibers have been torn, and active contraction of the muscle is extremely painful. Usually, a depression, or divot, can be felt somewhere in the muscle belly at the place at which the muscle fibers have been torn. Some swelling may occur because of increased capillary permeability. Bleeding creates a hematoma that causes discoloration and ecchymosis although it does not occur immediately. Range of motion is decreased due to pain.
- *Grade 3 strain.* A complete rupture of a muscle has occurred in the area of the muscle belly at the point at which muscle becomes tendon or at the tendinous attachment to the bone. There is significant impairment to or perhaps total loss of movement due to disruption of nerve fibers. Initially, pain is intense but quickly diminishes because of complete unloading of the muscle.

Muscle strains can occur in any muscle and usually result from some uncoordinated activity between muscle groups.[1] Grade 3 strains are most common in the biceps tendon of the upper arm and in the Achilles heel cord in the back of the calf. Tears may occur at either the proximal or distal bicep insertions or in the musculotendinous junction.[38] Grade 3 strains involving large tendons that produce great amounts of force must be surgically repaired. Smaller musculotendinous ruptures, such as those that occur in the fingers, may heal by immobilization with a splint.

Regardless of the severity of the strain, the time required for rehabilitation is lengthy.[5] In many instances, muscle strains are incapacitating, making rehabilitation time for a muscle strain even longer than for a ligament sprain. Incapacitating muscle strains occur most frequently in the large, force-producing hamstring and quadriceps muscles of the lower extremity. The treatment of hamstring strains requires a healing period of 6 to 8 weeks and a considerable amount of patience. Trying to return to activity too soon often causes reinjury to the area of the muscle that has been strained, and the healing process must begin again.

## Muscle Cramps

**Muscle cramps** are extremely painful involuntary muscle contractions that occur most commonly in the calf, hamstrings, quadriceps, or abdomen, although any muscle can be involved.[14] Muscle cramps are thought to occur most often in those muscle groups that are overloaded and fatigued during high demand activities due to altered neuromuscular control rather than due to fluid and/or electrolyte imbalance as previously hypothesized.[39] Muscle fatigue alters neuromuscular control by increasing muscle spindle activity while decreasing Golgi tendon organ activity thus facilitating a reflex contraction or cramp of the muscle (see Chapter 6).[2]

## Muscle Guarding

Following injury, the muscles that surround the injured area contract to, in effect, splint that area, thus minimizing pain by limiting movement. Quite often this "splinting" is incorrectly referred to as a muscle spasm. The terms *spasm* and *spasticity* are more correctly associated with increased tone or contractions of muscle that occur because of some upper motor neuron lesion in the brain. Thus, **muscle guarding** is a more appropriate term for the involuntary muscle contractions that occur in response to pain following musculoskeletal injury.[28]

## Muscle Spasms

A muscle spasm is an involuntary muscle contraction that results in increased tension and shortening of that muscle or a group of muscles which interferes with voluntary movement. It occurs suddenly, is often painful and may be a consequence of neurological damage or disease. The two types of spasms are the **clonic** type, with alternating involuntary muscular

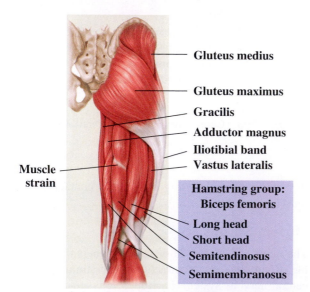

**FIGURE 9–4** A muscle strain results in tearing or separation of fibers.

Gluteus medius
Gluteus maximus
Gracilis
Adductor magnus
Iliotibial band
Vastus lateralis
Muscle strain
Hamstring group:
Biceps femoris
Long head
Short head
Semitendinosus
Semimembranosus

contraction and relaxation in quick succession, and the **tonic** type, with rigid muscle contraction that lasts a period of time. Muscle spasms may lead to a muscle strain.[10]

The term *spasticity* refers to a condition in which there is an abnormal increase in muscle stiffness and muscle tone that results in an involuntary inability to control those muscles. Spasticity is often caused by lesions affecting upper motor neurons (nerve pathways) from the central nervous system (including the brain and/or spinal cord) to the muscles. Spasticity occurs with conditions such as cerebral palsy, multiple sclerosis, traumatic brain injury, stroke, and spinal cord injury.

## Muscle Soreness

Overexertion in strenuous muscular exercise often results in muscular pain. All active people at one time or another have experienced **muscle soreness,** usually resulting from some physical activity to which they are unaccustomed. The older a person gets, the more easily muscle soreness seems to develop.

There are two types of muscle soreness. The first type of muscle pain is *acute-onset muscle soreness,* which accompanies fatigue. It is transient and occurs during and immediately after exercise. The second type involves delayed muscle *soreness* that appears approximately 12 hours after injury. This *delayed-onset muscle soreness (DOMS)* becomes most intense after twenty-four to 48 hours and then gradually subsides, so that the muscle becomes symptom free after 3 or 4 days.[8] DOMS is described as a syndrome of delayed muscle pain leading to increased muscle tension, swelling, and stiffness and to resistance to stretching.[9]

DOMS has several possible causes. It may occur from very small tears in the muscle tissue, which seems to be more likely with eccentric or isometric contractions. It may also occur because of disruption of the connective tissue that holds muscle tendon fibers together.[8]

Muscle soreness may be prevented by beginning exercise at a moderate level and gradually progressing the intensity of the exercise over time. Treatment of muscle soreness usually also involves static or PNF stretching activity.

> The two major types of muscle soreness associated with severe exercise are acute- and delayed-onset muscle soreness (DOMS).

## Tendon Injuries

The tendon contains wavy, parallel, collagenous fibers that are organized in bundles surrounded by a gelatinous material that decreases friction. A tendon attaches a muscle to a bone and concentrates a pulling force in a limited area. Tendons can produce and maintain a pull from 8,700 to 18,000 pounds per square inch.[40] When a tendon is loaded by tension, the wavy, collagenous fibers straighten in the direction of the load; when the tension is released, the collagen returns to its original shape. In tendons, collagen fibers will break if their physiological limits have been reached. A breaking point occurs after a 6 percent to 8 percent increase in length.[32] Because a tendon is usually double the strength of the muscle it serves, tears commonly occur at the muscle belly, musculotendinous junction, or bony attachment.[6] Clinically, however, a constant abnormal tension on tendons increases elongation by the infiltration of fibroblasts, which will cause more collagenous tissue to be produced. Repeated microtraumas can evolve into chronic muscle strain that resorbs collagen fibers and eventually weakens the tendon.[40] Collagen resorption occurs in the period of immobilization of a part. During resorption, collagenous tissues are weakened and susceptible to injury; therefore, a gradually paced conditioning program and early mobilization in the rehabilitation process are necessary.

## Tendinopathy/Tendinitis/Tendinosis

Of all the overuse problems associated with activity, chronic overuse injuries involving a tendon are the most common.[42] The term *tendinopathy* is the term that is most often used to refer to both *tendinitis,* which is an inflammation of the tendon, and *tendinosis,* which refers to microtears and degeneration of a tendon.[24] The suffix *-opathy* does not imply any specific type of pathology. Any term ending in the suffix *-itis* means inflammation is present.

> The suffix *-itis* means inflammation of.

Tendinitis means inflammation of a tendon. During muscle activity, a tendon must move or slide on other structures around it whenever the muscle contracts. If a particular movement is performed repeatedly, the tendon can become irritated and inflamed.[32] This inflammation is manifested by pain on movement, swelling, possibly some warmth, and usually crepitus.[87] *Crepitus* is a crackling feeling or sound. It is usually caused by the tendon's tendency to stick to the surrounding structure while it slides back and forth. This sticking is caused primarily by the chemical products of inflammation that accumulate on the irritated tendon.[24] The

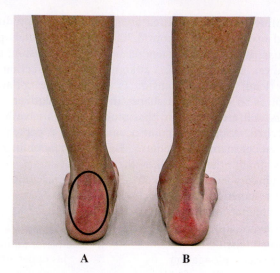

FIGURE 9–5 Tendinitis is an inflammation of the tendon. (**A**) Inflamed. (**B**) Normal.

© William E. Prentice

key to the treatment of tendinitis is rest. If the repetitive motion causing irritation to the tendon is eliminated, the inflammatory process will allow the tendon to heal. Unfortunately, athletes find it difficult to totally stop activity and rest for 2 or more weeks while the tendinitis subsides. The patient should substitute some form of activity, such as bicycling or swimming, to maintain present fitness levels while avoiding continued irritation of the inflamed tendon. In runners, tendinitis most commonly occurs in the Achilles tendon in the back of the lower leg (Figure 9–5). In swimmers, it often occurs in the muscle tendons of the shoulder joint. However, tendinitis can flare up in any activity in which overuse and repetitive movements occur.

If repetitive overuse continues and the inflamed or irritated tendon fails to heal, the tendon may begin to degenerate. The primary concern shifts from tendon inflammation to tendon degeneration, a condition referred to as *tendinosis*.[32] The suffix *-osis* means there is chronic degeneration without inflammation. *Most of the chronic problems that we have with tendons are correctly referred to as tendinosis.*[24] The symptoms are somewhat similar to tendinitis but there is no inflammation. The affected tendons are usually painful when moved or touched. The tendon sheaths may be visibly swollen with stiffness and restricted motion. Sometimes a tender lump appears. Tendinosis is more common in

middle or old age as the tendons become more susceptible to injury.[48] However, younger people who exercise vigorously as well as people who perform repetitive tasks are also susceptible. The key to treating tendinosis is engaging in exercises to strengthen the tendon and consistently stretching the tendon.

### Tenosynovitis

**Tenosynovitis** is very similar to tendinitis in that the muscle tendons are involved in inflammation. However, many tendons are subject to an increased amount of friction because of the tightness of the space through which they must move. In these areas of high friction, tendons are usually surrounded by synovial sheaths that reduce friction on movement. If the tendon sliding through a synovial sheath is subjected to overuse, inflammation is likely to occur. As with tendinitis, the inflammatory process produces by-products that are "sticky" and tend to cause the sliding tendon to adhere to the synovial sheath surrounding it.[4]

Tenosynovitis occurs most commonly in the long flexor tendons of the fingers as they cross over the wrist joint and in the biceps tendon around the shoulder joint. Treatment for tenosynovitis is the same as for tendinitis. Because both conditions involve inflammation, antiinflammatory drugs may be helpful in chronic cases.[4]

### Myofascial Trigger Points

A *myofascial trigger point* is a discreet, hypersensitive nodule within a taut band of skeletal muscle and/or fascia.[26] Palpation of this nodule reveals an area of harder-than-normal consistency. Trigger points are classified as being latent or active, depending on their clinical characteristics. A *latent trigger point* does not cause spontaneous pain but may restrict movement or cause muscle weakness. The individual presenting with muscle restrictions or weakness may become aware of pain originating from a latent trigger point only when pressure is applied directly over the point. An *active trigger point* causes pain at rest. Firm pressure applied over the point usually elicits a "jump sign," with the patient crying out, wincing, or withdrawing from the stimulus. It is tender to palpation with a referred pain pattern that is similar to the patient's pain complaint. This referred pain is not felt at the site of the trigger point origin but rather at a remote point. The pain is often described as spreading or radiating. Referred pain is an important characteristic of a trigger point. It differentiates a trigger point from a tender point, which is associated with pain at the site of palpation only. Trigger points are palpable within muscles as cordlike bands within a sharply circumscribed area of extreme tenderness. They are found most commonly in the muscles involved in postural support.[24] Acute trauma or repetitive microtrauma may lead to the development of stress on muscle fibers and the formation of trigger points.

## Contusions

A **contusion** is another word for a bruise. The mechanism that produces a contusion is familiar. A blow from some external object causes soft tissues (e.g., muscle, tendon, skin, fat) to be compressed against hard bone underneath (Figure 9–6). If the blow is hard enough, capillaries are torn, which allows bleeding into the tissues. Minor bleeding often causes **ecchymosis,** a bluish-purple discoloration of the skin that persists for several days. The contusion may be very sore to the touch, and, if damage has occurred to muscle, pain may be experienced on active movement. In most cases the pain ceases within a few days and discoloration usually disappears in a few weeks.[16]

The major problem with contusions occurs in an area that is subjected to repeated blows. If the same area—or, more specifically, a muscle—is bruised over and over again, small calcium deposits may begin to accumulate in the injured area. These pieces of calcium may be found between several fibers in the muscle belly, or calcium may build up to form a spur, which projects from the underlying bone. These calcium formations may significantly impair movement and are referred to as **myositis ossificans.**[1]

The key to preventing the occurrence of myositis ossificans from repeated contusions is to protect the injured area with padding. If the area is properly protected after the first contusion, myositis may never develop. Protection and rest may allow the calcium to be reabsorbed, eliminating any need for surgery.

The two areas that seem to be the most vulnerable to repeated contusions during physical activity are the quadriceps muscle group on the front of the thigh and the biceps muscle on the front of the upper arm. The formation of myositis ossificans in these or any other areas may be detected by X-rays.

### Atrophy and Contracture

Two complications of muscle and tendon conditions are atrophy and contracture. Muscle atrophy is the wasting away of muscle tissue. Its main causes are immobilization of a body part, inactivity, and loss of nerve innervation. A second complication is muscle contracture, an abnormal shortening of muscle tissue in which there is a great deal of resistance to passive stretch. A contracture is associated with a joint that, because of muscle injury, has developed unyielding and resisting scar tissue.

## SYNOVIAL JOINT INJURIES

### Anatomical Characteristics

Most of the joints in the body are **synovial joints** (Figure 9–7). All synovial joints are composed of two or more bones that articulate with one another to allow motion in one or more places.[37] The articulating surfaces of the bone are lined with a very thin, smooth, cartilaginous covering called *hyaline,* or *articular,* cartilage. All joints are entirely surrounded by a thick, ligamentous *joint capsule.* The inner surface of this joint capsule is lined by a very thin *synovial membrane* that is highly vascularized and innervated. The synovial membrane produces *synovial fluid,* which provides lubrication, shock absorption, and nutrition of the joint. The articular capsule, ligaments, outer aspects of the synovial membrane, and fat pads of the synovial joint are well supplied with nerves. The inner aspect of the synovial membrane, cartilage, and articular disks (menisci), if present, have nerves as well. The nerve receptors, called *mechanoreceptors,* provide information about the relative position of the joint and are found in the fibrous capsule and ligaments.

Some joints contain a thick *fibrocartilage* called a meniscus. The knee joint, for example, contains two wedge-shaped *menisci* that deepen the articulation and provide shock absorption in that joint. Finally, the main

A football player who plays wide receiver sustains repeated blows to his left quadriceps muscle.

**?** What type of injury could be sustained from repeated compressive forces to the quadriceps muscle?

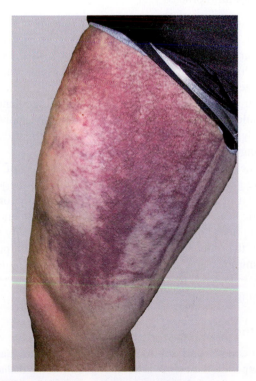

FIGURE 9–6  A contusion occurs when soft tissues are compressed between bone and some external force.

Courtesy Christopher R. Bartlett

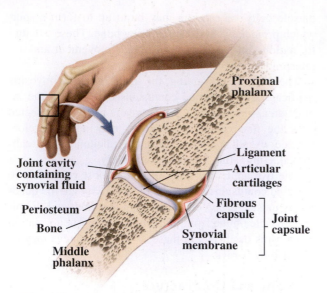

FIGURE 9–7    General anatomy of a synovial joint.

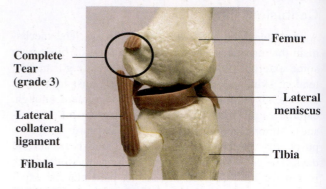

FIGURE 9–8    Grade 3 ligament sprain in the knee joint.
© William E. Prentice

structural support and joint stability are provided by the *ligaments,* which may be either thickened portions of a joint capsule or totally separate bands. Ligaments are composed of dense connective tissue arranged in parallel bundles of collagen composed of rows of fibroblasts. Although bundles are arranged in parallel, not all collagen fibers are arranged in parallel. Ligaments and tendons are very similar in structure. However, ligaments are usually more flattened than tendons, and collagen fibers in ligaments are more compact. The anatomical positioning of the ligaments determines in part what motions a joint can make.[37]

## Ligament Sprains

If stress is applied to a joint that forces motion beyond its normal limits or planes of movement, injury to the ligament is likely (Figure 9–8). The severity of damage to the ligament is classified in many different ways; however, the most commonly used system involves three grades (degrees) of ligament sprain:

- *Grade 1 sprain.* There is some stretching and separation of the ligament fibers, with minimal instability of the joint. Mild to moderate pain, localized swelling, and joint stiffness should be expected.
- *Grade 2 sprain.* There is some tearing and separation of the ligament fibers, with moderate instability of the joint. Moderate to severe pain, swelling, and joint stiffness should be expected.
- *Grade 3 sprain.* There is total tearing of the ligament, which leads to instability of the joint. A grade 3 sprain can result in a subluxation. Initially, severe pain may be present, followed by little or no pain as a result of total disruption of nerve fibers. Swelling may be great, and the joint tends to become very stiff

some hours after the injury. In some cases, a grade 3 sprain with marked instability requires surgical repair. Frequently, the force producing the ligament injury is so great that other ligaments or structures surrounding the joint may also be injured. Rehabilitation of grade 3 sprains involving surgery is a long-term process.

A basketball player steps on another player's foot and sustains a lateral ankle injury.

**?** What forces are applied, and what type of injury has been incurred?

Effusion of blood and synovial fluid into the joint cavity during a sprain produces joint swelling, local temperature increase, pain or point tenderness, and skin discoloration (ecchymosis). Ligaments and capsules, like tendons, can experience forces that completely rupture or produce an avulsion fracture. Ligaments and capsules heal slowly because of a relatively poor blood supply; however, their nerves are plentiful, often producing a great deal of pain when injured.[7]

The greatest problem in the rehabilitation of grade 1 and grade 2 sprains is restoring stability to the joint.[13] Once a ligament has been stretched or partially torn, inelastic scar tissue forms, preventing the ligament from regaining its original tension. To restore stability to the joint, the other structures surrounding that joint, primarily muscles and their tendons, must be strengthened. The increased muscle tension provided by strength training can improve stability of the injured joint.

## Dislocations and Subluxations

Dislocations and subluxations both result in **diastasis,** or separation of two articulating bones. A **dislocation** occurs when at least one bone in a joint (articulation) is forced completely out of its normal and proper alignment and must be manually or surgically put back into

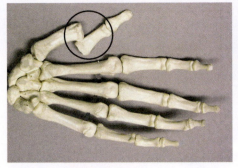 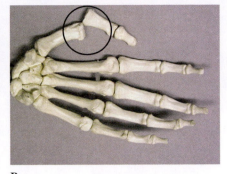

A                                                          B

FIGURE 9–9   A joint that is forced beyond its anatomical limits can become **(A)** completely dislocated or luxated or **(B)** subluxated.
© William E. Prentice

place or reduced. Dislocations most commonly occur in the shoulder joint, elbow, and fingers, but they can occur wherever two bones articulate (Figure 9–9A). A **subluxation** is like a dislocation except that a bone comes partially out of its normal articulation but then goes right back into place.[1] Subluxations most commonly occur in the shoulder joint and, in females, in the knee cap (patella) (Figure 9–9B).

In dislocations, deformity is almost always apparent; however, it may be obscured by heavy musculature, making it important for the examiner to routinely palpate, or feel, the injured site to determine the loss of normal contour. Comparison of the injured side with the uninjured side often reveals asymmetry.

Dislocations or subluxations will likely result in a rupture of the stabilizing ligaments and tendons surrounding the joint. Occasionally, an avulsion fracture occurs, in which an attached tendon or ligament pulls a small piece of bone away from the rest of the bone. In other cases, the force may separate growth plates (epiphysis) or cause a complete fracture of a long bone. These possibilities indicate the importance of administering complete and thorough medical attention to first-time dislocations. It has often been said, "Once a dislocation, always a dislocation." In most cases this statement is true because, once a joint has been either subluxated or completely dislocated, the connective tissues that bind and hold it in its correct alignment are stretched to such an extent that the joint is extremely vulnerable to subsequent dislocations.

A first-time dislocation should always be considered and treated as a possible fracture. Once it has been ascertained that the injury is a dislocation, a physician should be consulted for further evaluation. However, before the patient is taken to the physician, the injury should be properly splinted and supported to prevent any further damage.

**Dislocations should not be reduced immediately, regardless of where they occur.**[1] The athlete should get an X-ray to rule out fractures or other problems before reduction. Inappropriate techniques of reduction may only exacerbate the problem. Return to activity after dislocation or subluxation is largely dependent on the degree of soft-tissue damage.

## Osteoarthritis

Any mechanical system wears out with time. The joints in the body are mechanical systems, and wear and tear, even from normal activity, is inevitable.[23] The most common result of this wear and tear, a degeneration of the articular, or hyaline, cartilage, is referred to as **osteoarthritis**.[43] The cartilage may be worn away to the point of exposing, eroding, and polishing the underlying bone (Figure 9–10).

Any process that changes the mechanics of the joint eventually leads to degeneration of that joint. Degeneration is a result of repeated trauma to the joint and to the tendons, ligaments, and fasciae surrounding the joint. Such injuries may be caused by a direct blow or fall, by the pressure of carrying or lifting heavy loads, or by repeated trauma to the joint, as in running or cycling.[27]

Osteoarthritis most often affects the weight-bearing joints: the knees, hips, and lumbar spine. Also affected are the shoulders and cervical spine. Although many other joints may show pathological degenerative change, clinically the disease only occasionally produces symptoms in them. Any joint that is subjected to acute or chronic trauma may develop osteoarthritis.[42]

The symptoms of osteoarthritis are relatively local in character. Osteoarthritis may be localized to one side of the joint or may be generalized about the joint. One of the most distinctive symptoms is pain, which is brought about by friction that occurs with use and which is relieved by rest. Stiffness is a common complaint that occurs with rest and is quickly loosened with activity. This symptom is prominent upon rising in the morning. Joints may also show localized tenderness, creaking, or grating that may be heard and felt.[27] Clinical studies indicate that glucosamine sulfate is a safe and relatively effective treatment for osteoarthritis. However, no

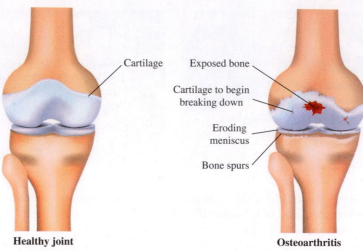

Healthy joint

Osteoarthritis

Cartilage

Exposed bone

Cartilage to begin
breaking down

Eroding
meniscus

Bone spurs

FIGURE 9–10   Osteoarthritis involves a degeneration of
hyaline cartilage, exposing underlying bone.

evidence to date supports or refutes a carryover effect to the athletic population and the injuries that occur in sport.[23,43]

## Bursitis

**Bursitis** most often occurs around joints, where there is friction between tendon and bone, skin and bone, or muscle and other muscles. Without some mechanism of protection in these high-friction areas, chronic irritation would exist (Figure 9–11).

**Bursae** are pieces of synovial membrane that contain a small amount of fluid (synovial fluid).[37] Just as oil lubricates a hinge, these small pieces of synovium permit motion of these structures without friction.

If excessive movement or perhaps some acute trauma occurs around the bursae, they become irritated and inflamed and begin producing large amounts of synovial fluid.[30] The longer the irritation continues or the more severe the acute trauma, the more fluid is produced. As fluid continues to accumulate in the limited space available, pressure increases, causing pain in the area. Bursitis can be an extremely painful condition that may severely restrict movement, especially if it occurs around a joint. Synovial fluid continues to be produced

until the movement or trauma producing the irritation is eliminated.

Occasionally, a bursa or synovial sheath completely surrounds a tendon, allowing more freedom of movement in a tight area. Irritation of this synovial sheath may restrict tendon motion. All joints are surrounded by many bursae. The three bursae that are most commonly irritated as a result of various types of physical activity are the subacromial bursa in the shoulder joint under the distal clavicle and acromion process; the olecranon bursa on the tip of the elbow; and the prepatellar bursa on the front surface of the patella. All three of these bursae produce large amounts of synovial fluid, affecting motion at their respective joints.

## Capsulitis and Synovitis

After repeated joint sprains or microtraumas, a chronic inflammatory condition called capsulitis may occur.[30] Usually associated with capsulitis is synovitis. Synovitis also occurs acutely, but a chronic condition can arise with repeated joint injury or with joint injury that is improperly managed. Chronic synovitis involves active joint congestion with edema. As with the synovial lining of the bursa, the synovium of a joint can undergo degenerative tissue changes. The synovium becomes irregularly thickened, exudation occurs, and a

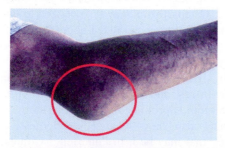

FIGURE 9–11   Elbow bursitis.
Courtesy James Gallaspy

A wrestler complains of pain, swelling, and warmth around the knee that always seem to be worse after practice.

**?** What should an athletic trainer suspect is wrong with the knee, and how should it be treated?

fibrous underlying tissue is present. Several movements may be restricted, and there may be joint noises, such as grinding or creaking.

# BONE INJURIES

## Anatomical Characteristics

Bone is a specialized type of dense connective tissue consisting of bone cells (osteocytes) that are fixed in a matrix, which consists of an intercellular material. The outer surface of a bone is composed of compact tissue, and the inner aspect is composed of a more porous tissue known as *cancellous bone*, also called *trabecular* or *spongy* bone (Figure 9–12). Compact tissue is tunneled by a marrow cavity. Throughout the bone run countless branching canals (haversian canals), which contain blood vessels and lymphatic vessels. On the outside of a bone is a tissue covering, the *periosteum*, which contains the blood supply to the bone.[37]

Bones perform five basic functions: body support, organ protection, movement (through joints and levers), calcium storage, and formation of blood cells (hematopoiesis).

Bones are classified according to their shapes. Classifications include bones that are flat, irregular, short, and long. Flat bones are in the skull, the ribs, and the scapulae; irregular bones are in the vertebral column and the skull. Short bones are primarily in the wrist and the ankle. Long bones consist of the humerus, ulna, femur, tibia, fibula, and phalanges.

Flat, irregular, and short bones have the same inner cancellous bone with an overlying layer of compact bone. A few irregular and flat bones (e.g., the vertebrae and the sternum) have some space in the cancellous bone that is filled with red marrow and sesamoid bones.

The gross structures of bone include the diaphysis, epiphysis, articular cartilage, periosteum, medullary (marrow) cavity, and endosteum. The diaphysis is the main shaft of the long bone. It is hollow and cylindrical and is covered by compact bone. The epiphysis is located at the ends of long bones. It is bulbous in shape, providing space for the muscle attachments. The epiphysis is composed primarily of cancellous bone, giving it a spongelike appearance. As discussed previously, the ends of long bones have a layer of hyaline cartilage that covers the joint surfaces of the epiphysis. This cartilage provides protection during movement and cushions jars and blows to the joint. A dense, white, fibrous membrane, the periosteum, covers long bones except at joint surfaces. Many fibers, called Sharpey's fibers, emanate from the periosteum and penetrate the underlying bone. Interlacing with the periosteum are fibers from the muscle tendons. Throughout the periosteum on its inner layer exist countless blood vessels and osteoblasts (bone-forming cells). The blood vessels provide nutrition to the bone, and the osteoblasts provide bone growth and repair. The medullar cavity, a hollow tube in the long bone diaphysis, contains a yellow, fatty marrow in adults. Lining the medullar cavity is the endosteum.[37]

**Bone Growth** Bone ossification occurs from the synthesis of bone's organic matrix by osteoblasts, followed immediately by the calcification of this matrix.

The epiphyseal growth plate is a cartilaginous disk located near the end of each long bone. The growth of the long bones depends on these plates. Ossification in long bones begins in the diaphysis and in both epiphyses. It proceeds from the diaphysis toward each epiphysis and from each epiphysis toward the diaphysis. The growth plate has layers of cartilage cells in different stages of maturity, with immature cells at one end and mature ones at the other end. As the cartilage cells mature, immature osteoblasts replace them later to produce solid bone.

Epiphyseal growth plates are often less resistant to deforming forces than are ligaments of nearby joints or the outer shaft of the long bones; therefore, severe twisting or a blow to an arm or a leg can result in growth disruption. Injury can prematurely close the growth plate, causing a loss of length in the bone.

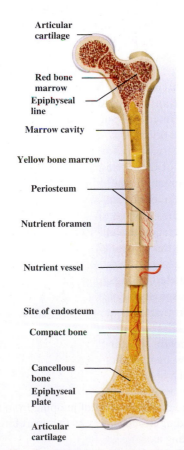

Articular cartilage
Red bone marrow
Epiphyseal line
Marrow cavity
Yellow bone marrow
Periosteum
Nutrient foramen
Nutrient vessel
Site of endosteum
Compact bone
Cancellous bone
Epiphyseal plate
Articular cartilage

FIGURE 9–12   Anatomical characteristics of bone (longitudinal section).

Growth plate dislocation can also cause deformity of the long bone.[20]

Bone diameter may increase as a result of the combined action of **osteoblasts** and **osteoclasts.** Osteoblasts build new bone on the outside of the bone; at the same time, osteoclasts increase the medullary cavity by breaking down bony tissue. Once a bone has reached its full size, there occurs a balance of bone formation and bone destruction, or osteogenesis and resorption, respectively. This process of balance may be disrupted by factors in sports conditioning or participation. These factors may cause greater osteogenesis than resorption. Conversely, resorption may exceed osteogenesis in situations in which the patient is out of shape but overtrains. On the other hand, women whose estrogen is decreased as a result of training may experience bone loss (see Chapter 29).[32] In general, bone loss begins to exceed bone gain by age thirty-five to forty. Gradually, bone is lost in the endosteal surfaces and then is gained on the outer surfaces. As the thickness of long bones decreases, they are less able to resist the forces of compression. This process also leads to increased bone porosity, known as osteoporosis.

Like other structures in the human body, bones are morphologically, biochemically, and biomechanically sensitive to both stress and stress deprivation. Therefore, bone's functional adaptation follows Wolff's law;[44] that is, every change in the form and function of a bone, or in its function alone, is followed by certain definite changes in its internal architecture.

## Bone Fractures

Fractures generally can be classified as either closed or open. A **closed fracture** is one in which there is little or no movement or displacement of the broken bones. Conversely, in an **open fracture** (Figure 9–13) there is enough displacement of the fractured ends that the bone actually breaks through surrounding tissues, including the skin (Figure 9–13). An open fracture increases the possibility of infection. Both types of fracture can be serious if not managed properly.[19] Signs and symptoms of a fracture include obvious deformity, point tenderness, swelling, and pain on active and passive movement. There may also be crepitus (popping or a grating sound on movement). The only definitive technique for determining if a fracture exists is to have it X-rayed.

## General Fracture Classifications

Fractures can result from direct trauma; in other words, the bone breaks directly at the site where a force is applied. A fracture that occurs some distance from where force is applied is called an indirect fracture. A sudden, violent muscle contraction or repetitive abnormal stress to a bone can also cause a

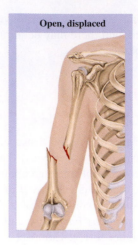

**Open, displaced**

FIGURE 9–13   In an open, displaced fracture, the end of the bone penetrates through the soft tissue creating an open wound.

fracture. The most common bone fractures can be classified as follows (Figure 9–14):[18]

*Greenstick fracture.* Greenstick fractures are incomplete breaks in bones that have not completely ossified, such as the bones of adolescents. This injury occurs most frequently in the convex bone surface, while the concave surface remains intact. The name is derived from the similarity of the fracture to the break in a green twig taken from a tree.

*Comminuted fracture.* Comminuted fractures consist of three or more fragments at the fracture site. This injury could be caused by a hard blow or a fall in an awkward position. These fractures impose a difficult healing situation because of the displacement of the bone fragments. Soft tissues are often interposed between the fragments, causing incomplete healing. Such cases may need surgical intervention.

An alpine skier catches his right ski tip and severely twists his lower leg.

**?** What type of serious injury could be created by this mechanism?

*Linear fracture.* Linear fractures are those in which the bone splits along its length. They are often the result of jumping from a height and landing in such a way as to impart force or stress to the long axis.

*Transverse fracture.* Transverse fractures occur in a straight line, more or less at right angles to the bone

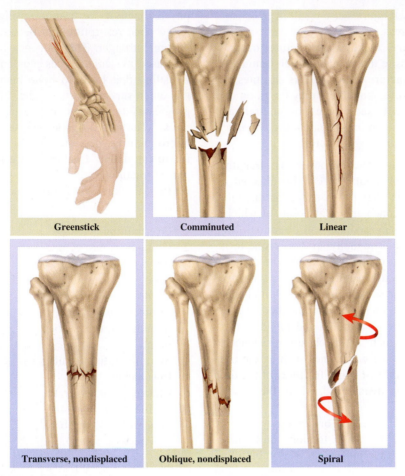

| Greenstick | Comminuted | Linear |
| Transverse, nondisplaced | Oblique, nondisplaced | Spiral |

FIGURE 9–14  Common classifications of bone fractures.

shaft. A direct outside blow usually causes this injury.

*Oblique fracture.* Oblique fractures are similar to spiral fractures. Oblique fractures occur when one end of the bone receives sudden torsion or twisting while the other end is fixed.

*Spiral fracture.* Spiral fractures have an S-shaped separation. They are common in football and skiing, sports in which the foot is firmly planted when the body is suddenly rotated in an opposing direction.

## Specific Fracture Types

*Impacted fracture.* Impacted fractures can result from a fall from a height, which causes a long bone to receive, directly on its long axis, a force of such magnitude that the osseous tissue is compressed. This stress telescopes one part of the bone on the other. Impacted fractures require immediate splinting by the athletic trainer and traction by the physician to ensure a normal length of the injured limb.

Other, less common fractures include the following:

*Avulsion fracture.* An avulsion fracture is the separation of a bone fragment from its cortex at an attachment of a ligament or tendon. This fracture usually occurs as a result of a sudden, powerful twist or stretch of a body part. A ligamentous avulsion can occur, for example, when a sudden eversion of the foot causes the deltoid ligament to avulse bone away from the medial malleolus. A tendinous avulsion can occur when an athlete falls forward while suddenly bending a knee, which causes a patellar fracture. The stretch of the patellar tendon pulls a portion of the inferior patellar pole apart.

*Blowout fracture.* Blowout fractures occur to the wall of the eye orbit as a result of a blow to the eye.

*Serrated fracture.* Serrated fractures, in which the two bony fragments have a sawtooth, sharp-edged fracture line, are usually caused by a direct blow. Because of the sharp and jagged bone edges, extensive internal damage, such as the severance of vital blood vessels and nerves, often occurs.

*Depressed fracture.* Depressed fractures occur most often in flat bones, such as those found in the skull. They are caused by falling and striking the head on a hard, immovable surface or by being hit with a hard object. Such injuries also result in gross pathology of soft areas.

*Contrecoup fracture.* Contrecoup fractures occur on the side opposite the point at which trauma was initiated. Fracture of the skull is, at times, a contrecoup fracture. An athlete may be hit on one side of the head with such force that the brain and internal structures compress against the opposite side of the skull, causing a fracture.

Many factors of bone structure affect its strength.[18] Anatomical strength or weakness can be affected by a bone's shape and its changes in shape or direction. Stress forces become concentrated at points at which a long bone suddenly changes shape and direction. Long bones that change shape gradually are less prone to injury than are those that change suddenly. The clavicle, for example, is prone to fracture because it changes from round to flat at the same point at which it changes direction. A hollow cylinder is one of the strongest structures for resisting both bending and torsion, stronger than a solid rod, which has much less resistance to such forces.[18] This may be why bones such as the tibia are primarily cylinders. Most spiral fractures of the tibia occur at its middle and distal third, where the bone is most solid.

Long bones can be stressed or forced to fail by compression, tension, bending, torsion, and shearing.[18] These forces, either singly or in combination, can cause a variety of fractures. For example, spiral fractures are caused by torsion, whereas oblique fractures are caused by the combined forces of axial compression, bending, and torsion. Transverse fractures occur because of bending (Figure 9–14). Because of its elastic properties, bone will bend slightly. However, bone is generally brittle and is a poor shock absorber because of its mineral content. This brittleness increases under tension forces more than under compression forces.

## Stress Fractures

Stress fractures have been variously called march, fatigue, and spontaneous fractures, although *stress fracture* is the most commonly used term. The exact cause of this fracture is not known, but there are a number of likely possibilities: an overload caused by muscle contraction, amenorrhea, an altered stress distribution in the bone accompanying muscle fatigue, a change in the ground reaction force (such as movement from a wood surface to a grass surface), or the performance of a rhythmically repetitive stress that leads up to a vibratory summation point, which appears to be the most likely cause.[36] Rhythmic muscle action performed over a period of time at a subthreshold level causes the stress-bearing capacity of the bone to be exceeded, hence, a stress fracture. A bone may become vulnerable to fracture during the first few weeks of intense physical activity or training. Weight-bearing bones undergo bone resorption and become weaker before they become stronger. The sequence of events results from increased muscular forces plus an increased rate of remodeling that leads to bone resorption, weakening of the outer surface of the bone, and rarefaction, which progresses to produce increasingly more severe fractures.[36] The four progressively severe fractures are focal microfractures, periosteal or endosteal response (stress fractures), linear fractures (stress fractures), and displaced fractures.

Typical causes of stress fractures in sports are as follows:

1. Overtraining
2. Going back into competition too soon after an injury or illness
3. Going from one event to other without proper training in the second event
4. Starting initial training too quickly
5. Changing habits or the environment (e.g., running surfaces, the bank of a track, or shoes)

Susceptibility to fracture can also be increased by a variety of postural and foot conditions. Flatfeet, a short first metatarsal bone, or a hypermobile metatarsal region can predispose an athlete to stress fractures (see Chapter 18).

Early detection of the stress fracture may be difficult. Stress fractures always must be suspected in susceptible body areas that fail to respond to usual management. Until there is a reaction in the bone, which may take several weeks, X-ray examination may fail to reveal any change.[34] Although nonspecific, a bone scan can provide early indications in a given area (Figure 9–15).

The signs of a stress fracture are swelling, focal tenderness, and pain. In the early stages of the fracture, the athlete complains of pain when active but not at rest. Later, the pain is constant and becomes more intense at night. Percussion, by light tapping on the bone at a site other than the suspected fracture, will produce pain at the fracture site.[34]

A long jumper experiences a sudden, sharp pain in the region of the left ischial tuberosity during a jump.

**?** What injuries are possible through this mechanism?

A young woman training for a marathon is complaining of pain in the lower leg. She consults with her physician, who determines that she has a stress fracture. She is confused about how a stress fracture is different from a normal fracture.

**?** How should the athletic trainer explain the difference between the two, and what is the course of management?

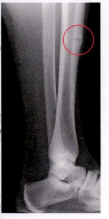
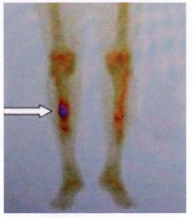

A                B

FIGURE 9–15   **(A)** X-ray and **(B)** bone scan of tibial stress fracture.

The most common sites of stress fracture are the tibia, fibula, metatarsal shaft, calcaneus, femur, pars interarticularis of the lumbar vertebrae, ribs, and humerus.

The management of stress fractures varies with the individual, injury site, and extent of injury. Stress fractures that occur on the compression side of bone heal more rapidly and are managed more easily compared with those on the tension side. Stress fractures on the tension side can rapidly produce a complete fracture.[18]

## Epiphyseal Conditions

Three types of epiphyseal growth site injuries can be sustained by children and adolescents performing sports activities. They are injury to the epiphyseal growth plate, physis articular epiphyseal injuries, and apophyseal injuries.[21] The most prevalent age range for these injuries is from 10 to 16 years.

Epiphyseal growth plate injuries (Figure 9–16) have been classified by Salter-Harris into five types as follows:[2,22]

> A musculoskeletal injury to a child or an adolescent should always be considered to involve a possible epiphyseal condition.

- Type I—complete separation of the physis in relation to the metaphysis without fracture to the bone
- Type II—separation of the growth plate and a small portion of the metaphysis
- Type III—fracture of the physis
- Type IV—fracture of a portion of the physis and metaphysis
- Type V—no displacement of the physis, but the crushing force can cause a growth deformity

**Apophyseal Injuries**  The young, physically immature athlete is particularly prone to apophyseal injuries.[12] The apophyses are traction epiphyses, in contrast to the pressure epiphyses of the long bones. These apophyses serve as origins, or insertions, for muscles on growing bone that provide bone shape but not length. Common apophyseal avulsion conditions found in sports are Severs disease and Osgood-Schlatter disease[12] (see Chapter 20).

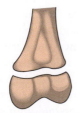
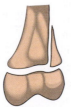
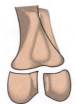

Type I—Separation of the physis       Type II—Fracture–separation of growth plate and small part of metaphysis       Type III—Fracture–part of physis

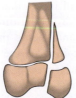
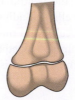

Type IV—Fracture–physis and metaphysis       Type V—Crushing of physis with no displacement–may cause premature closure

FIGURE 9–16   Salter-Harris classification of long bone epiphyseal injuries in children.

## Osteochondrosis

Osteochondrosis is a category of conditions of which the causes are not well understood. In general, the term refers to degenerative changes in the ossification centers of the epiphyses of bones, especially during periods of rapid growth in children.[12] Synonyms for this condition are as follows: if it is located in a point such as the knee, *osteochondritis dissecans* and, if located at a tubercle or tuberosity, *apophysitis.* Apophyseal conditions are discussed in the section on bone trauma in this chapter.

One suggested cause of osteochondrosis is aseptic necrosis, in which circulation to the epiphysis has been disrupted. Another suggestion is that trauma causes particles of the articular cartilage to fracture, eventually resulting in fissures that penetrate to the subchondral bone. If trauma to a joint occurs, pieces of cartilage may be dislodged, which can cause joint locking, swelling, and pain. If the condition occurs in an apophysis, there may be an avulsion fracture and fragmentation of the epiphysis along with pain, swelling, and disability.

## NERVE TRAUMA

A number of abnormal nerve responses can be attributed to athletic participation or injury. The most frequent type of nerve injury is neuropraxia produced by a direct trauma. A laceration can cut nerves, causing complications in healing of the injury. Fractures and dislocation can avulse or abnormally compress nerves.

### Anatomical Characteristics

Nerve tissue provides sensitivity and communication from the central nervous system (brain and spinal cord) to the muscles, sensory organs, various systems, and the periphery. The basic nerve cell is the neuron (Figure 9–17). The neuron cell body contains a large nucleus and branched extensions called dendrites, which respond to neurotransmitter substances released from other nerve cells. From each nerve cell arises a single axon, which conducts the nerve impulses. Large axons found in peripheral nerves are enclosed in neurilemmal sheaths composed of Schwann cells and satellite cells, which are tightly wound around the axon. In the central nervous system, various types of neuroglial cells, including astrocytes, oligodendrocytes, ependymal cells, and microglia, function collectively to bind neurons together and provide a supportive framework for the nervous tissue.[35]

### Nerve Injuries

Nerve injuries, as with injuries to other tissues in the body, can be traumatic or overuse. Trauma directly affecting nerves can produce a variety of sensory responses, including hypoesthesia (diminished sense of feeling), hyperesthesia (increased sense of feelings such as pain or touch), and paresthesia (numbness, prickling, or tingling, which may occur from a direct blow to or stretch of an area).[15] For example, a sudden nerve stretch or pinch can produce both a sharp or burning pain that radiates down a limb and muscle weakness. In **neuropraxia,** there is an interruption in conduction of the impulse down the nerve fiber. This is the mildest form of nerve injury. Neuropraxia is brought about by compression or relatively mild, blunt blows close to the nerve. It results in a temporary loss of function, which is reversible within hours to months of the injury (on average, 6 to 8 weeks). There is frequently greater involvement of motor than sensory function.[15] **Neuritis,** a chronic nerve problem, can be caused by a variety of forces that usually have been repeated or continued for a long time. Symptoms of neuritis can range from minor nerve problems to paralysis. More serious injuries involve the crushing of a nerve or complete division (severing). This type of injury may produce a lifelong physical disability, such as paraplegia or quadriplegia, and should therefore not be overlooked in any circumstance.

Specialized tissue, such as nerve cells, cannot regenerate once the nerve cell dies. In an injured peripheral nerve, however, the nerve fiber can regenerate

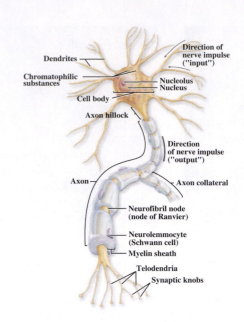

FIGURE 9–17   Basic anatomy of a neuron.

An 11-year-old soccer player fell on an outstretched hand during practice. There is obvious deformity in her right wrist.

**?** What is a possible complication with a fracture in this wrist?

significantly if the injury does not affect the cell body. For regeneration to occur, an optimal environment for healing must exist.

Regeneration is slow, at a rate of only 3 to 4 mm per day. Damaged nerves within the central nervous system regenerate very poorly compared with nerves in the peripheral nervous system.[15]

Pain that is felt at a point of the body other than its actual origin is known as **referred pain.** Another potential cause of referred pain is a trigger point, which occurs in the muscular system but refers pain to some other distant body part.

# BODY MECHANICS AND INJURY SUSCEPTIBILITY

If one carefully studies the mechanical structure of the human body, it is amazing that humans can move so effectively in the upright posture. Not only must the body overcome constant gravitational force, but it also must be manipulated through space by a complex system of somewhat inefficient levers, fueled by a machinery that operates at an efficiency level of approximately 30 percent. The bony levers that move the body must overcome considerable resistance in the form of inertia and muscle viscosity and in most instances must work at an extremely unfavorable angle of pull. All these factors mitigate the effectiveness of lever action to the extent that most movement is achieved at an efficiency level of less than 25 percent.

When determining the mechanical reasons for injuries to the musculoskeletal system, many factors can be identified. Hereditary, congenital, or acquired defects may predispose an athlete to a specific type of injury. Anomalies in anatomical structure or in body build (somatotype) may make an individual prone to injuries. The habitually incorrect application of skill is a common cause of overuse injuries.

## Microtrauma and Overuse Syndrome

Injuries as a result of abnormal and repetitive stress and microtraumas fall into a class with certain identifiable syndromes. Such stress injuries frequently result in either limitation or curtailment of performance. Most of these injuries are directly related to the dynamics of running, throwing, or jumping. The injuries may result from constant and repetitive stresses placed on bones, joints, or soft tissues; from forcing a joint into an extreme range of motion; or from prolonged strenuous activity. Some of the injuries falling into this category may be relatively minor; still, they can be disabling. Among injuries classified as repetitive stress and microtrauma are Achilles tendinitis; shinsplints; stress fractures, particularly of the fibula and second and fifth metatarsal bones; Osgood-Schlatter disease; runner's and jumper's knee; patellar chondromalacia; apophyseal avulsion, especially in the lower extremities of young, growing individuals; and intertarsal neuroma.

## Postural Deviations

Postural deviations are often an underlying cause of injuries. Postural malalignment may be the result of unilateral muscle and soft-tissue asymmetries or bony asymmetries. As a result, the individual engages in poor mechanics of movement (pathomechanics). Many activities are unilateral, thus leading to asymmetries in body development. The resulting imbalance is manifested by a postural deviation as the body seeks to reestablish itself in relation to its center of gravity. Often, such deviations are a primary cause of injury. For example, a consistent pattern of knee injury may be related to asymmetries within the pelvis and the legs (short-leg syndrome). Unfortunately, not much in the form of remedial work is usually performed. As a result, an injury often becomes chronic—sometimes to the point that participation in activity must be halted. When possible, the athletic trainer should seek to ameliorate or eliminate faulty postural conditions through therapeutic exercise. A number of postural conditions offer genuine hazards to athletes by making them exceedingly prone to specific injuries.[21] Some of the more important are discussed in the chapters on foot and leg anomalies, spinal anomalies, and various stress syndromes.

# SUMMARY

- "When a force applied to any part of the body results in a harmful disturbance in function or structure, a mechanical injury is said to have been sustained."[17] Mechanical terminology is used to describe tissue properties. Examples of this terminology are *load, stiffness, stress, strain, deformation, elastic, plastic, yield point,* and *tissue failure.*
- The five primary stresses leading to tissue trauma are compression, tension, shearing, bending, and torsion. Bending strain can produce a torque on a bone followed by injury. A torsion, or twisting, load can produce a spiral fracture along the long axis of a bone.
- Skeletal muscle trauma can involve any aspect of the musculotendinous unit. Forces that injure muscles are compression, tension, and shearing. Injuries to the musculotendinous unit include strains, cramps, muscle guarding, spasm, soreness, tendonosis/tendinitis/tendinopathy,

tenosynovitis, myofacial trigger points, contusions, and atrophy.

- Injuries to the synovial joints are common. Anatomically, synovial joints have relative strengths or weaknesses based on their ligamentous or capsular type and their muscle arrangements. Forces that can injure synovial joints are tension, compression, torsion, and shearing. Sprains involve injury to ligaments or the joint capsule. A grade 3 sprain may cause ligament rupture or an avulsion fracture. Synovial joint injuries include dislocation or subluxation, osteoarthritis, bursitis, and capsulitis and synovitis. Two major chronic synovial joint conditions are osteochondrosis and traumatic arthritis.
- Because of their shape, long bones are anatomically susceptible to fractures caused by changes in direction of the force applied to them. Mechanical forces that cause injury are compression, tension, bending, torsion, and shearing. Bending and torsional forces are forms of tension. Types of fractures include avulsion, blowout, comminuted, depressed, greenstick, impacted, longitudinal, oblique, serrated, spiral, transverse, and contrecoup. Stress fractures are commonly the result of overload to a given bone area. Three major epiphyseal injuries occur to the growth plate, the articular cartilage, and the apophysis.
- Nerve trauma can be produced by overstretching or compression. The sudden stretch of a nerve can cause a burning sensation. A variety of traumas to nerves can produce acute pain or a chronic pain, such as neuritis.
- Any individual with faulty body mechanics has an increased potential for injury.

## SOLUTIONS TO CLINICAL APPLICATION EXERCISES

9–1  An external tension load causes internal strain and deformation to the ligament. When the ligament can no longer respond elastically, the yield point has been exceeded and a ligament sprain occurs.

9–2  The football player has sustained a tension force to the long head of the biceps tendon, which caused a rupture or severe strain.

9–3  The mechanism of this elbow injury is repeated tension to the extensor tendons attached to the lateral epicondyle, causing microtraumas. Stress to this area can be reduced by increasing the grip circumference and flattening the backhand stroke.

9–4  Repeated contusion of any muscle may lead to the development of myositis ossificans. The key to treating myositis ossificans is prevention. An initial contusion to any muscle should be immediately protected with padding to prevent reinjury.

9–5  In stepping on another player's foot, the basketball player produces an abnormal ankle torsion and lateral ankle tension, stretching and tearing ligaments.

9–6  The athletic trainer should suspect that the wrestler has developed bursitis from constantly kneeling on the mat. Inflammation may best be treated by rest, ice, antiinflammatory medication, and protective padding of the knee.

9–7  Catching the ski tip produces a torsional force that could cause a boot-top spiral fracture.

9–8  During the jump, a powerful stretch of the biceps femoris could cause a serious strain or an avulsion fracture in the region of the ischial tuberosity.

9–9  A stress fracture is not an actual break of the bone; it is simply an irritation of the bone. Treatment of a stress fracture requires about 2 to 4 weeks of rest. However, the athletic trainer should point out that a stress fracture can become a true fracture if it is not rested; if that happens, 4 to 6 weeks of immobilization in a cast is necessary. Thus, it is critical that this athlete rest for the required amount of time.

9–10  An epiphyseal condition, such as an epiphyseal growth plate fracture, can occur in children and adolescents and needs to be considered with any musculoskeletal injury. These injuries can impair growth and further skeletal development.

## REVIEW QUESTIONS AND CLASS ACTIVITIES

1. Discuss the stress–strain curve and its associated tissue properties.
2. Differentiate among muscle strains, muscle cramps, muscle guarding, and muscle soreness.
3. How does a damaged nerve heal?
4. What are myofascial trigger points, where are they most likely to occur, and what are the signs and symptoms?
5. What is myositis ossificans and how can it be prevented?
6. How are tendinitis, tenosynovitis, and bursitis related to one another? Explain how osteoarthritis develops.
7. What structures are found at a joint? What are their functions?
8. Describe the injuries occurring to synovial joint structures.
9. Differentiate between a subluxation and a dislocation.
10. How do the three grades of ligament sprains differ?
11. Describe various types of fractures and the mechanisms that cause fractures to occur.
12. How does a stress fracture differ from a regular fracture?
13. Describe the most common epiphyseal conditions.
14. What are the relationships of postural deviations to injuries?
15. Discuss the concept of pathomechanics as it relates to microtraumas and overuse syndromes.
16. What forces injure muscle tissue?
17. Describe all types of muscle tendinous injuries.

18. What mechanical forces traumatize the musculotendinous unit and the synovial joint? How are the forces similar to one another, and how are they different?
19. What forces gradually weaken tendons and ligaments?
20. Contrast two synovial joint injuries.

21. List the structural characteristics that make a long bone susceptible to fracture.
22. What mechanical forces cause fracture of a bone?
23. How do stress fractures probably occur?

# REFERENCES

1. Blavelt CT, Nelson FRT: *A manual of orthopaedic terminology,* ed 8, Philadelphia, 2014, Elsevier.
2. Breulick K: Significant and serious dehydration does not affect skeletal muscle cramp threshold frequency, *British Journal of Sports Medicine* 47(11):710–14, 2013.
3. Browner B: *Skeletal trauma: Basic science, management, and reconstruction,* Philadelphia, 2014, WB Saunders.
4. Brukner P, Khan K: Sports injuries. In Brukner P, editor: *Clinical sports medicine,* ed 3, Sydney, 2011, McGraw-Hill.
5. Buckwalter J: 2005. Musculoskeletal tissue healing. In Weinstein S: *Turek's Orthopedics: Principles and their application.* Baltimore, Lippincott, Williams and Wilkins.
6. Butterwick DJ: Recognition of complete muscle or tendon ruptures, *Athletic Therapy Today* 7(l):43, 2002.
7. Cailliet R: *Medical orthopedics: Conservative management of musculoskeletal injuries,* Chicago, 2004, AMA Press.
8. Cheung K: Delayed onset muscle soreness: Treatment strategies and performance factors, *Sports Medicine* 33(2):145–64, 2003.
9. Cleary M, Kimura I, Sitler M: Temporal pattern of the repeated bout effect of eccentric exercise on delayed-onset muscle soreness, *J Athl Train* 37(1):32, 2002.
10. Delee J, Drez D, Miller M: *Delee and Drez's orthopaedic sports medicine: Principles and practice,* Philadelphia, 2014, WB Saunders.
11. Delforge G: *Musculoskeletal trauma: Implications for sports injury management,* Champaign, IL, 2003, Human Kinetics.
12. DiFiori JP: Overuse injuries in young athletes: An overview, *Athletic Therapy Today* 7(6): 25, 2002.
13. Drake D: Sports and performing arts medicine for traumatic injuries in sports, *Arch Phys Med Rehabil* 85(3 Suppl):S67, 2004.
14. Dumke CL: Muscle cramps are not all created equal, *Athletic Therapy Today* (3):42, 2003.
15. Feinberg J, Spielholz N: *Peripheral nerve injuries in the athlete,* Champaign, IL, 2003, Human Kinetics.
16. Gallaspie J, May D: *Signs and symptoms of athletic injuries,* St. Louis, 1996, McGraw-Hill.
17. Gomez M: *Biomechanics of soft-tissue injury,* Tuscon, AZ, 2011, Lawyers & Judges.
18. Gonza ER: Biomechanics of long bone injuries. In Gonza ER, Harrington IJ, editors: *Biomechanics of musculoskeletal injury,* Baltimore, 2008, Williams and Wilkins.
19. Hoppenfeld S, Murthy V, Taylor K: *Treatment and rehabilitation of fractures,* Philadelphia, 2000, Lippincott Williams and Wilkins.
20. Hunt T, Amato H: Epiphyseal-plate fracture in an adolescent athlete, *Athletic Therapy Today* 8(1):34, 2003.
21. Hutson M: *Sports injuries: Recognition and management,* ed 3, Oxford, England, 2001, Oxford University Press.
22. Jacobs D: Salter-Harris Type III fracture in a high school football player, *Athletic Therapy Today* 14(6):238, 2009.
23. James C, Uhl T: A review of articular cartilage pathology and the use of glucosamine sulfate, *J Athl Train* 36(4):413, 2001.
24. Khan K: Overuse tendinosis, not tendinitis. Part 1: a new paradigm for a difficult clinical problem. *Phys Sports Med* 28(5):38–43, 47–48, 2000.
25. Knight K: More precise classification of orthopedic injury types and treatment will improve patient care, *J Athl Train* 43(2):117–18, 2008.
26. Lavell E: Myofascial trigger points, *Anesthesiology Clinics* 25(4):841–51, 2007.
27. Levine D: Running and the development of osteoarthritis, part II: Human studies, *Athletic Therapy Today* 8(1):2, 2003.
28. Maehlum S: *Clinical guide to sports injuries,* Champaign, IL, 2004, Human Kinetics.
29. Martin R: *Skeletal tissue mechanics,* New York, 2015, Springer-Verlag.
30. Merrick M: Secondary injury after musculoskeletal trauma: A review and update, *J Athl Train* 37(2):209, 2002.
31. Miller K: Exercise-associated muscle cramps causes, treatment and prevention, *Sports Health* 2(4):279–83, 2010.
32. Molina F: The physiologic basis of tendinopathy development, *Athletic Therapy and Training* 16(6):5–8, 2011.
33. Norkin C: *Joint structure and function: A comprehensive analysis,* Philadelphia, 2011, F.A. Davis.
34. Patel D: Stress fractures: Diagnosis, treatment, and prevention, *American Family Physician* 83(1):39–46, 2011.
35. Porth CM: *Pathophysiology: Concepts of altered health states,* ed 8, Philadelphia, 2013, Lippincott, Williams and Wilkins.
36. Romani W, Gieck J, Perrin D: Mechanisms and management of stress fractures in physically active persons, *J Athl Train* 37(3): 306, 2002.
37. Saladin K: *Anatomy and physiology: Unity of function* New York, 2014, McGraw-Hill.
38. Sharma P: Tendon injury and tendinopathy: Healing and repair, *Journal of Bone & Joint Surgery* 87A(1):187–202, 2005.
39. Schwellnus M: Cause of exercise associated muscle cramps (EAMC)—altered neuromuscular control, dehydration or electrolyte depletion? *Br J Sports Med* 4(6):401–8, 2009.
40. Weintraub W: *Tendon and ligament healing: A new approach to sports and overuse injury,* Herndon, VA, 2003, Paradigm.
41. Whiting W: Biomechanics of musculoskeletal injury, Champaign, IL, 2008, Human Kinetics.
42. Wilder R, Sethi S: Overuse injuries: Tendinopathies, stress fractures, compartment syndrome, and shin splints, *Clin Sports Med* 23(1): 55, 2004.
43. Wilson TC: Articular-cartilage lesions of the knee and osteoarthritis in athletes: An overview, *Athletic Therapy Today* 8(1):20, 2003.
44. Wolff J: *Das geset der transformation der knockan,* Berlin, 1892, Hirschwald.

# ANNOTATED BIBLIOGRAPHY

Blavelt CT, Nelson RRT: *A manual of orthopaedic terminology,* ed 8, Philadelphia, 2014, Elsevier.

*A resource book for all individuals who need to identify medical words or their acronyms.*

Berry, D: *Athletic and Orthopedic Injury Assessment: A Case Study Approach,* 2010 Holcomb Hathaway.

*Case studies in this book use injury assessment examples to help readers link theory and clinical practice with the goal of becoming competent clinicians.*

Dandy D, Edwards D: *Essential orthopaedics and trauma,* St. Louis, MO, 2009, Elsevier.

*Presents essential core information for students and emphasizes common conditions and current orthopedic practice.*

Delforge G: *Musculoskeletal trauma: implications for sport injury management,* Champaign, IL, 2003, Human Kinetics.

*Focuses on the therapeutic management of sport-related soft-tissue injuries, fractures, and proprioceptive/sensorimotor impairments.*

Griffith HW, Pederson M: *Complete guide to sports injuries: how to treat fractures, bruises, sprains, dislocations, and head injuries,* New York, 2004, Penguin.

*Tells readers how to treat, avoid, and rehabilitate nearly 200 of the most common sports injuries, including fractures, bruises, sprains, strains, dislocations, and head injuries.*

Kjaer, M: *Textbook of sports medicine: basic science and clinical aspects of sports injury and physical activity,* Oxford, UK, 2003, Blackwell Science.

*Provides capsule summaries of the history, diagnosis, and treatment of orthopedic problems that respond to nonsurgical intervention in this primer for clinicians. Brief yet detailed entries explain the causes and treatment of impairments of the musculoskeletal system.*

Maehlum S: *Clinical guide to sports injuries,* Champaign, IL, 2015, Human Kinetics.

*Covers each step of the injury management process, beginning with the patient's presentation.*

Norris C: *Sports injuries: diagnosis and management,* Philadelphia, 2004, Elsevier.

*An overview of musculoskeletal injuries that are unique to sports and exercise.*

Peacinn M, Bojanic I: *Overuse injuries of musculoskeletal system,* Boca Raton, FL, 2003, CRC Press.

*A comprehensive text describing overuse injuries of the tendon, tendon sheath, bursae, muscle, muscle-tendon function, cartilage, and nerve.*

Szendroi, M: 2010. *Color Atlas of Clinical Orthopedics,* New York, Springer.

*This book is composed of a vast number of pictures presenting the clinical symptoms of the various orthopedic conditions. An in-depth overview of the characteristic clinical features of orthopedic conditions.*

Weintraub W: *Tendon and ligament healing: a new approach to sports and overuse injury,* Herndon, VA, 2003, Paradigm.

*Gives readers a clear understanding of the dynamic nature of tendons and ligaments from an excellent review of their structure, function, mechanics, injury, and healing processes.*

Williams JGP: *Color atlas of injury in sport,* Chicago, 1993, Mosby.

*An excellent visual guide to the area of sports injuries that covers the nature and incidence of sport injury, types of tissue damage, and regional injuries caused by a variety of sports activities.*

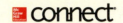

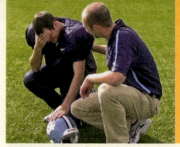
© William E. Prentice

# 10

# Tissue Response to Injury

## ■ Objectives

*When you finish this chapter you should be able to*

- Contrast the three phases of the healing process.
- Classify the physiological events that must take place during each phase of healing.
- Identify those factors that may impede the healing process.
- Discuss treatment techniques for modifying soft tissue healing, including using anti-inflammatory medications, therapeutic modalities, exercise rehabilitation, and platelet-rich plasma injections.
- Discuss the healing process relative to various soft-tissue structures, including cartilage, ligament, muscle, tendon, and nerve.

- Describe the healing process as it occurs in bone.
- Formulate a management plan for treating acute fractures.
- Define pain and discuss the various types of pain.
- Understand the neurophysiology of pain.
- Differentiate among the three mechanisms of pain control.
- Examine the various techniques for assessing pain.

## ■ Outline

## ■ Key Terms

margination
leukocytes
diapedesis
exudate
neutrophils
phagocytes
vasoconstriction
macrophages
lymphocytes
fibroblasts
fibroplasia

collagen
proteoglycans
glycosaminoglycans
microtears
macrotears
NSAIDs
prolotherapy
platelet-rich plasma (PRP)
avascular necrosis
trigger points
nociceptors

## ■ Connect Highlights    ▪ connect

*Visit connect.mcgraw-hill.com for further exercises to apply your knowledge:*

- Clinical application scenarios covering physiological events that occur during healing, healing process in bone, and assessment of pain
- Click-and-drag questions covering tissue response to injury, inflammatory response, and soft-tissue healing
- Multiple-choice questions covering healing process, management of acute injuries, techniques and mechanisms for assessing pain, and factors that impede healing
- Selection questions covering factors that impede healing and treatment of inflammation

# THE HEALING PROCESS

It is essential for the athletic trainer to possess an in-depth understanding of the healing process. The healing process consists of three phases: the inflammatory response phase, the fibroblastic repair phase, and the maturation-remodeling phase. The athletic trainer should recognize both the sequence and the time frames for these phases of healing and realize that certain physiological events must occur during each of the phases. Anything that an athletic trainer does that interferes with this healing process will likely slow the return to full activity. The healing process must have an opportunity to accomplish what it is supposed to. At best, the goal of the athletic trainer should be to try to create an environment that is conducive to the healing process. There is little that can be done to speed up the process physiologically, but there are many things that may be done during rehabilitation to impede healing. Although the phases of healing are often discussed as three separate entities, the healing process is a continuum. Phases of the healing process overlap one another and have no definitive beginning or end points (Figure 10–1).

## Inflammatory Response Phase

Once a tissue is injured, the process of healing begins immediately (Figure 10–2A).[17,44] The destruction of tissue produces direct injury to the cells of the various soft tissues.[45] Cellular injury results in altered metabolism and the liberation of chemical mediators that initiate the inflammatory response (Figure 10–3). It is characterized symptomatically by redness (*rubor*), swelling (*tumor*), tenderness and pain (*dolor*), increased temperature (*calor*), and loss of function (*functio laesa*).[38] *This initial inflammatory response is critical to the entire healing process. If this response does not accomplish what it is supposed to, or if it does not subside, normal healing cannot take place.*[15]

**Chemical Mediators** The events in the inflammatory response are initiated by a series of interactions involving several chemical mediators.[16] Some of these chemical mediators are derived from the invading organism, some are released by the damaged tissue, others are generated by several plasma enzyme systems, and still others are products of various white blood cells participating in the inflammatory response. Three chemical mediators, *histamine, leukotrienes, prostaglandins,* and *cytokines,* are important in limiting the amount of exudate, and thus swelling, after injury.[3] Histamine, released from the injured mast cells, causes vasodilation and increased cell permeability, owing to a swelling of endothelial cells and then separation between the cells. Leukotrienes and prostaglandins are responsible for **margination,** in which **leukocytes** (neutrophils and macrophages) adhere along the cell walls (Figure 10–2B). They also increase cell permeability locally, thus affecting the passage of fluid, proteins, and neutrophils through cell walls via **diapedesis** to form **exudate** in the extravascular spaces. Therefore, vasodilation and active hyperemia are important in exudate (plasma) formation and in supplying **neutrophils** to the injured area. As swelling continues and the extravascular pressure increases, the vascular flow to and the lymphatic flow from the area are decreased. The amount of swelling that occurs is directly related to the extent of vascular permeability and vessel damage. Cytokines—in particular, chemokines and interleukin, are the primary regulators of leukocyte traffic and help attract **phagocytes** to the site of inflammation.[16] Responding to the presence of chemokines, neutrophils and macrophages migrate to the site of inflammation within a few hours. Neutrophils peak at about 6 hours and macrophages peak between 12 and 24 hours.

**Vascular Reaction** The vascular reaction is controlled by chemical mediators and involves vascular spasm, the formation of a platelet plug, blood coagulation, and the

---

**10–1 Clinical Application Exercise**

A volleyball player has sprained her ankle just 2 days prior to the beginning of the conference tournament. The athlete, her parents, and her coach are extremely concerned that she is going to miss the tournament and want to know if anything can be done to help her get well more quickly.

**?** What can the athletic trainer tell this patient about the healing process?

---

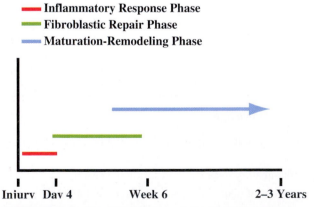

**Inflammatory Response Phase**
**Fibroblastic Repair Phase**
**Maturation-Remodeling Phase**

| Injury | Day 4 | Week 6 | 2–3 Years |

FIGURE 10–1 The three phases of the healing process fall along a continuum.

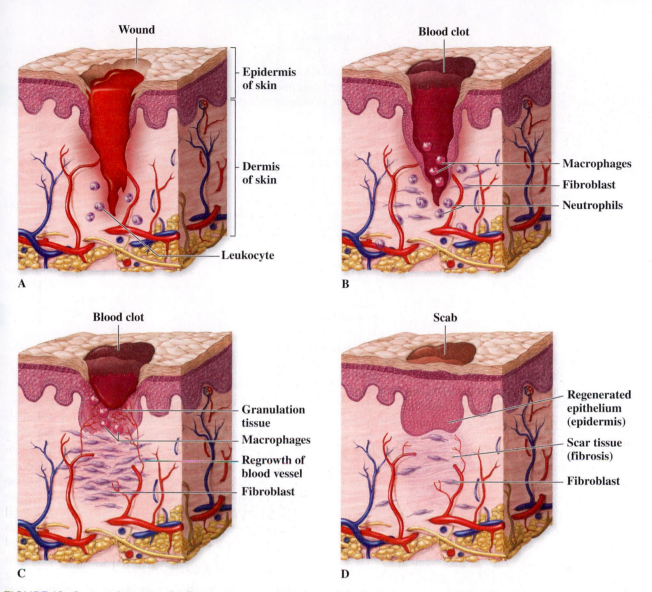

**Wound**

- Epidermis of skin
- Dermis of skin
- Leukocyte

**A**

**Blood clot**

- Macrophages
- Fibroblast
- Neutrophils

**B**

**Blood clot**

- Granulation tissue
- Macrophages
- Regrowth of blood vessel
- Fibroblast

**C**

**Scab**

- Regenerated epithelium (epidermis)
- Scar tissue (fibrosis)
- Fibroblast

**D**

FIGURE 10–2   Initial injury and inflammatory response phase of the healing process. **(A)** Cut blood vessels bleed into the wound. **(B)** Blood clot forms, and leukocytes clean the wound. **(C)** Blood vessels regrow, and granulation tissue forms in the fibroblastic repair phase of the healing process. **(D)** Epithelium regenerates, and connective tissue fibrosis occurs in the maturation-remodeling phase of the healing process.

growth of fibrous tissue.[22] The immediate vascular response to tissue damage is **vasoconstriction** of the vascular walls in the vessels leading away from the site of injury that lasts for approximately 5 to 10 minutes. This vasoconstriction presses the opposing endothelial wall linings together to produce a local anemia that is rapidly replaced by hyperemia of the area due to vasodilation. This increase in blood flow is transitory and gives way to slowing of the flow in the dilated vessels, thus enabling the leukocytes to slow down and adhere to the vascular endothelium. Eventually, there is stagnation and stasis.[23] The initial effusion of blood and plasma lasts for 24 to 36 hours.

**Function of Platelets** Platelets do not normally adhere to the vascular wall. However, injury to a vessel disrupts the endothelium and exposes the collagen fibers. Platelets adhere to the collagen fibers to create a sticky matrix on the vascular wall, to which additional platelets and leukocytes adhere, eventually forming a plug. These plugs obstruct local lymphatic fluid drainage and thus localize the injury response.[15]

**Formation of a Clot** The initial event that precipitates clot formation is the conversion of *fibrinogen* to *fibrin*. This transformation occurs because of a cascading effect beginning

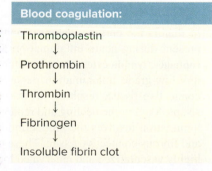

**Blood coagulation:**

Thromboplastin
↓
Prothrombin
↓
Thrombin
↓
Fibrinogen
↓
Insoluble fibrin clot

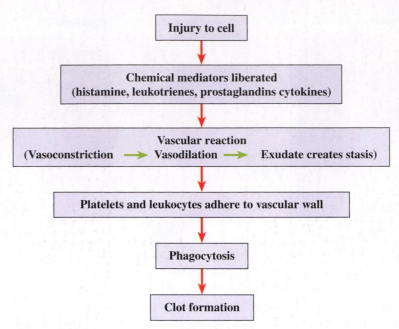

FIGURE 10–3 Inflammatory response sequence.

with the release of a protein molecule called *thromboplastin* from the damaged cell. Thromboplastin causes *prothrombin* to be changed into *thrombin* which in turn causes the conversion of fibrinogen into a very sticky fibrin clot that shuts off blood supply to the injured area.[52] Clot formation begins around 12 hours after injury and is completed within 48 hours.

As a result of a combination of these factors, the injured area becomes walled off during the inflammatory stage of healing. The leukocytes phagocytize most of the foreign debris toward the end of the inflammatory phase, setting the stage for the fibroblastic phase. This initial inflammatory response lasts for approximately 2 to 4 days after initial injury.

**Chronic Inflammation** A distinction must be made between the acute inflammatory response as previously described and chronic inflammation.[47] Chronic inflammation occurs when the acute inflammatory response does not respond sufficiently to eliminate the injuring agent and restore tissue to its normal physiological state. Thus, only low concentrations of the chemical mediators are present. The neutrophils that are normally present during acute inflammation are replaced by **macrophages, lymphocytes, fibroblasts,** and plasma cells.[47] As this low-grade inflammation persists, damage occurs to connective tissue, resulting in tissue necrosis and fibrosis, prolonging the healing and repair process. Chronic inflammation involves the production of granulation tissue and fibrous connective tissue. These cells accumulate in a highly vascularized and innervated loose connective tissue

> Chronic inflammation occurs from repeated acute microtraumas and overuse.

matrix in the area of injury.[47] The specific mechanisms that cause an insufficient acute inflammatory response are unknown, but they appear to be related to situations that involve overuse or overload with cumulative microtrauma to a particular structure.[15,23] There is no specific time frame in which the acute inflammation transitions to chronic inflammation. It does appear that chronic inflammation is resistant to both physical and pharmacological treatments.[18]

## Fibroblastic Repair Phase

During the fibroblastic repair phase of healing, proliferative and regenerative activity leading to scar formation and repair of the injured tissue follows the vascular and exudative phenomena of inflammation (see Figure 10–2C).[22] The period of scar formation, referred to as **fibroplasia,** begins within the first few days after injury and may last for as long as 4 to 6 weeks. During this period, many of the signs and symptoms associated with the inflammatory response subside. The patient may still indicate some tenderness to touch and will usually complain of pain when particular movements stress the injured structure. As scar formation progresses, complaints of tenderness or pain gradually disappear.[44]

During this phase, the growth of endothelial capillary buds into the wound is stimulated by a lack of oxygen, after which the wound is capable of healing aerobically. Along with increased oxygen delivery comes an increase in blood flow, which delivers nutrients essential for tissue regeneration in the area.[3]

The formation of a delicate connective tissue called *granulation tissue* occurs with the breakdown of the fibrin clot. Granulation tissue consists of fibroblasts, **collagen,** and capillaries. It appears as a reddish, granular mass of connective tissue that fills in the gaps during the healing process.

| Granulation tissue: |
| --- |
| • Fibroblasts |
| • Collagen |
| • Capillaries |

| Extracellular matrix: |
| --- |
| • Collagen |
| • Elastin |
| • Ground substance |
| • Proteoglycans |
| • Glycosaminoglycans |

As the capillaries continue to grow into the area, fibroblasts accumulate at the wound site, arranging themselves parallel to the capillaries. Fibroblastic cells begin to synthesize an *extracellular matrix* that contains protein fibers of *collagen* and *elastin,* a *ground substance* that consists of nonfibrous proteins called **proteoglycans, glycosaminoglycans,** and fluid. On about the sixth or seventh day, fibroblasts also begin producing collagen fibers that are deposited in a random fashion throughout the forming scar. There are at least 16 types of collagen, but 80 to 90 percent of the collagen in the body consists of Types I, II, and III. Type I collagen is found in skin, fasciae, tendon, bone, ligaments, cartilage, and interstitial tissues; Type II can be found in hyaline cartilage and vertebral disks; and Type III is found in skin, smooth muscle, nerves, and blood vessels. Type III collagen has less tensile strength than does Type I and tends to be found more in the fibroblastic repair phase.[37] As the collagen continues to proliferate, the tensile strength of the wound rapidly increases in proportion to the rate of collagen synthesis. As the tensile strength increases, the number of fibroblasts diminishes to signal the beginning of the maturation phase.

This normal sequence of events in the repair phase leads to the formation of minimal scar tissue. Occasionally, a persistent inflammatory response and continued release of inflammatory products promotes extended fibroplasia and excessive fibrogenesis that can lead to irreversible tissue damage.[12] Fibrosis can occur in synovial structures, as with adhesive capsulitis in the shoulder; in extraarticular tissues, such as tendons and ligaments; in bursae; or in muscle.

## Maturation-Remodeling Phase

The maturation-remodeling phase of healing is a long-term process (Figure 10–2D). This phase features a realignment or remodeling of the collagen fibers that make up scar tissue according to the tensile forces to which that scar is subjected. It involves a decrease in Type III collagen fibers and an increase in Type I fibers.[12] Ongoing breakdown and synthesis of collagen occur with a steady increase in the tensile strength of the scar matrix as well as a decrease in capillaries in that scar. With increased stress and strain, the collagen fibers realign in a position of maximum efficiency parallel to the lines of tension. The tissue gradually assumes normal appearance and function, although a scar is rarely as strong as the normal uninjured tissue. Usually, by the end of approximately 3 weeks, a firm, strong, contracted, nonvascular scar exists. The maturation phase of healing may require several years to be complete.

**The Role of Progressive Controlled Mobility during the Healing Process** Wolff's law states that bone and soft tissue will respond to the physical demands placed on them, causing them to remodel or realign along lines of tensile force.[37] Therefore, it is critical that injured structures be exposed to progressively increasing loads throughout the rehabilitative process.[25]

Controlled mobilization is superior to immobilization for scar formation, revascularization, muscle regeneration, and reorientation of muscle fibers and tensile properties in animal models.[29] However, a brief period of immobilization of the injured tissue during the inflammatory response phase is recommended and will likely facilitate the process of healing by controlling inflammation, thus reducing clinical symptoms. As healing progresses to the repair phase, controlled activity directed toward return to normal flexibility and strength should be combined with protective support or bracing.[17] Generally, clinical signs and symptoms disappear at the end of this phase.

As the remodeling phase begins, aggressive active range of motion and strengthening exercises should be incorporated to facilitate tissue remodeling and realignment.[48] To a great extent, pain dictates the rate of progression. With initial injury, pain is intense and tends to decrease and eventually subside altogether as healing progresses. Any exacerbation of pain, swelling, or other clinical symptoms during or after a particular exercise or activity indicates that the load is too great for the level of tissue repair or remodeling. The athletic trainer must be aware of the time required for the healing process and realize that being overly aggressive can interfere with that process.

## Factors That Impede Healing

**Extent of Injury** The nature or amount of the inflammatory response is determined by the extent of the tissue injury. **Microtears** of soft tissue involve only minor damage and are most often associated with overuse. **Macrotears** involve significantly greater destruction of soft tissue and result in clinical symptoms and functional alterations. Macrotears are generally caused by acute trauma.[16]

**Edema** The increased pressure caused by swelling retards the healing process, causes separation of tissues, inhibits neuromuscular control, produces reflexive neurological changes, and impedes nutrition in the injured part. Edema is best controlled and managed during the initial first-aid management period, as described previously.[32]

**Hemorrhage** Bleeding occurs with even the smallest amount of damage to the capillaries. Bleeding produces the same negative effects on healing as does the accumulation of edema, and its presence produces additional tissue damage and thus exacerbation of the injury.[52]

**Poor Vascular Supply** Injuries to tissues with a poor vascular supply heal poorly and slowly. This response is likely related to a failure in the initial delivery of phagocytic cells and fibroblasts necessary for scar formation.[52]

**Separation of Tissue** Mechanical separation of tissue can significantly affect the course of healing. A wound that has smooth edges that are in good apposition will tend to heal by *primary intention* with minimal scarring. Conversely, a wound that has jagged, separated edges must heal by *secondary intention,* with granulation tissue filling the defect and excessive scarring.[9,52]

**Muscle Spasm** Muscle spasm causes traction on the torn tissue, separates the two ends, and prevents approximation. Local and generalized ischemia may result from spasm.

**Atrophy** Wasting away of muscle tissue begins immediately with injury. Strengthening and early mobilization of the injured structure retard atrophy.[9]

**Corticosteroids** The use of corticosteroids in the treatment of inflammation is controversial. Steroid use in the early stages of healing has been demonstrated to inhibit fibroplasia, capillary proliferation, collagen synthesis, and increases in tensile strength of the healing scar. Their use in the later stages of healing and with chronic inflammation is debatable.[16]

**Keloids and Hypertrophic Scars** Keloids occur when the rate of collagen production exceeds the rate of collagen breakdown during the maturation phase of healing. This process leads to hypertrophy of scar tissue, particularly around the periphery of the wound.

**Infection** The presence of bacteria in the wound can delay healing and cause excessive granulation tissue, and frequently causes large, deformed scars.[16]

**Humidity, Climate, and Oxygen Tension** Humidity significantly influences the process of epithelization. Occlusive dressings stimulate the epithelium to migrate twice as fast without crust or scab formation. The formation of a scab occurs with dehydration of the wound and traps wound drainage, which promotes infection. Keeping the wound moist allows the necrotic debris to more easily go to the surface and be shed.

Oxygen tension relates to the neovascularization of the wound, which translates into optimal saturation and maximal tensile strength development. Circulation to the wound can be affected by ischemia, venous stasis, hematomas, and vessel trauma.

**Health, Age, and Nutrition** The elastic qualities of the skin decrease with aging. Degenerative diseases, such as diabetes and arteriosclerosis, also become a concern for older patients and may affect wound healing.[43] Nutrition is important for wound healing. In particular, vitamins C (collagen synthesis and immune system), K (clotting), and A (immune system); zinc for the enzyme systems; and amino acids play critical roles in the healing process.[28] Meeting the Dietary Recommended Intake (DRI) for vitamins is sufficient for wound healing.

# SOFT-TISSUE HEALING

## Cell Structure and Function

All organisms, from the simplest to the most complex, are composed of cells (Figure 10–4). The properties of a specific soft tissue of the body are derived from the structure and function of the cells. Individual cells contain a *nucleus* surrounded by *cytoplasm* and are enclosed by a *cell membrane* that selectively allows substances to enter and leave the cell. The nucleus contains *chromosomes*, which consist of DNA and protein. The functional and structural elements within the cell are called *organelles* and include *mitochondria, ribosomes, endoplasmic reticulum, centrioles, Golgi apparatusus,* and *microtubules.*[37]

All the tissues of the body can be defined as soft tissue except for bone. The human body has four types of soft tissue: epithelial tissue, which consists of the skin and the lining of vessels and many organs; connective tissue, which consists of tendons, ligaments, cartilage, fat, and blood vessels; muscle, which can be skeletal (striated), cardiac, or smooth; and nervous tissue, which consists of the brain, spinal cord, and nerves.[37]

Soft tissue can undergo adaptations as a result of healing and of the rehabilitative process following injury.[13] Soft-tissue adaptations include the following:

- Metaplasia—conversion of one kind of tissue into a form that is not normal for that tissue.
- Dysplasia—abnormal development of tissue.
- Hyperplasia—excessive proliferation of normal cells in the normal tissue arrangement.
- Atrophy—a decrease in the size of tissue due to cell death and resorption or decreased cell proliferation.
- Hypertrophy—an increase in the size of a tissue without necessarily increasing the number of cells.

## Cartilage Healing

Cartilage has a relatively limited healing capacity.[30] When chondrocytes are destroyed and the matrix is disrupted, the course of healing is variable, depending on whether damage is to cartilage alone or also to subchondral bone.[46] Injuries to articular cartilage alone fail to elicit clot formation or a cellular response. For the most part, the chondrocytes adjacent to the injury are the only cells that show any signs of proliferation and synthesis of matrix. Thus, the defect fails to heal, although the extent of the damage tends to remain the same.[19]

If subchondral bone is also affected, inflammatory cells enter the damaged area and formulate granulation tissue. In this case, the healing process proceeds normally, with differentiation of granulation tissue cells into chondrocytes occurring in about 2 weeks.[19] By approximately 2 months, normal collagen has been formed.[8]

## Ligament Healing

The healing process in the sprained ligament follows a course of repair similar to that of other vascular tissues.[41] Immediately after injury and for approximately 72 hours, there is a loss of blood from damaged vessels and an attraction of inflammatory cells into the injured area. If a ligament is sprained outside of a joint capsule (extraarticular ligament), bleeding occurs in a subcutaneous space. If an intraarticular ligament is injured, bleeding occurs inside the joint capsule until either clotting occurs or the pressure becomes so great that bleeding ceases.[10]

During the next 6 weeks, vascular proliferation with new capillary growth begins to occur, along with fibroblastic activity, resulting in the formation of a fibrin clot.[27] It is essential that the torn ends of the ligament be reconnected by bridging of this clot. A synthesis

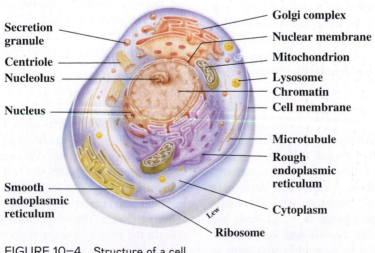

Secretion granule

Centriole

Nucleolus

Nucleus

Smooth endoplasmic reticulum

Golgi complex

Nuclear membrane

Mitochondrion

Lysosome

Chromatin

Cell membrane

Microtubule

Rough endoplasmic reticulum

Cytoplasm

Ribosome

FIGURE 10–4    Structure of a cell.

of collagen and a ground substance of proteoglycan in an intracellular matrix contributes to the proliferation of the scar that bridges the torn ends of the ligament. Initially, this scar is soft and viscous, but eventually it becomes more elastic. Collagen fibers are arranged in a random woven pattern with little organization. Gradually, there is a decrease in fibroblastic activity, a decrease in vascularity, and a maximum increase in the collagen density of the scar.[41] Failure to produce enough scar and failure to reconnect the ligament to the appropriate location on a bone are the two reasons ligaments are likely to fail.

Over the next several months, the scar continues to mature, with the realignment of collagen occurring in response to progressive stresses and strains.[27] The maturation of the scar may require as long as 12 months to complete.[3] The exact length of time required for maturation depends on mechanical factors, such as apposition of torn ends and length of immobilization.[51]

**Factors Affecting Ligament Healing** Surgically repaired extraarticular ligaments have healed with decreased scar formation and are generally stronger than unrepaired ligaments initially, although this strength advantage may not be maintained as time progresses.[10] Nonrepaired ligaments heal by fibrous scarring, effectively lengthening the ligament and producing some degree of joint instability. With intraarticular ligament tears, the presence of synovial fluid dilutes the hematoma, thus preventing the formation of a fibrin clot and spontaneous healing.[51]

Several studies have shown that actively exercised ligaments are stronger than those that are immobilized. Ligaments that are immobilized for several weeks after injury tend to decrease in tensile strength and exhibit weakening of the insertion of the ligament to bone.[41] Thus, it is important to minimize periods of immobilization and progressively stress the injured ligaments while exercising caution relative to biomechanical considerations for specific ligaments.[21]

It is not likely that the inherent stability of the joint provided by the ligament before injury will be regained. Thus, to restore stability to the joint, the structures that surround that joint, primarily muscles and their tendons, must be strengthened. The increased muscle tension provided by strength training can improve the stability of the injured joint.[25]

## Muscle Healing

Injuries to muscle tissue involve processes of healing and repair similar to those of other tissues. Initially, there will be hemorrhage and edema followed almost immediately by phagocytosis to clear debris. Within a few days, there is a proliferation of ground substance, and fibroblasts begin producing a gel-type matrix that surrounds the connective tissue, leading to fibrosis and scarring. At the same time, myoblastic cells (satellite cells) form in the area of injury, which eventually leads to the regeneration of new myofibrils. Thus, the regeneration of both connective tissue and muscle tissue has begun.[25]

Collagen fibers undergo maturation and orient themselves along lines of tensile force according to Wolff's law. Active contraction of the muscle is critical in regaining normal tensile strength.[25,50]

Regardless of the severity of the strain, the time required for rehabilitation is fairly lengthy. In many instances, rehabilitation time for a muscle strain is longer than for a ligament sprain. These incapacitating muscle strains occur most often in the large, force-producing hamstring and quadriceps muscles of the lower extremity. The treatment of hamstring strains requires a healing period of at least 6 to 8 weeks and a considerable amount of patience. Trying to return to activity too soon often causes reinjury to the area of the musculotendinous unit that has been strained, and the healing process must begin again.

## Tendon Healing

Unlike most soft-tissue healing, tendon injuries pose a problem.[4,17] The injured tendon requires dense fibrous union of the separated ends and both extensibility and flexibility at the site of attachment.[33] Thus, an abundance of collagen is required to achieve good tensile strength. Unfortunately, collagen synthesis can become excessive, resulting in fibrosis, in which adhesions form in surrounding tissues and interfere with the gliding that is essential for smooth motion.[36] Fortunately, over a period of time the scar tissue of the surrounding tissues becomes elongated in its structure because of a breakdown in the cross-links between fibrin units and thus allows the necessary gliding motion. A tendon injury that occurs where the tendon is surrounded by a synovial sheath can be potentially devastating.[49]

A typical time frame for tendon healing would be that during the second week the healing tendon adheres to the surrounding tissue to form a single mass.[29] During the third week, the tendon separates to varying degrees from the surrounding tissues. However, the tensile strength is not sufficient to permit a strong pull on the tendon for at least 4 to 5 weeks, the danger being that a strong contraction can pull the tendon ends apart.[24,35,42]

## Nerve Healing

Specialized tissue, such as nerve cells, cannot regenerate once the nerve cell dies. In an injured peripheral nerve, however, the nerve fiber can regenerate significantly if the injury does not affect the cell body.[37] The proximity of the axonal injury to the cell body can significantly affect the time required for healing. The closer an injury is to the cell body, the more difficult the regenerative process. In the case of a severed nerve, surgical intervention can markedly enhance regeneration.

For regeneration to occur, an optimal environment for healing must exist.[5] When a nerve is cut, several degenerative changes occur that interfere with the neural pathways (Figure 10–5). Within the first 3 to 5 days, the portion of the axon distal to the cut begins to degenerate and breaks into irregular segments. There is also a concomitant increase in metabolism and protein production by the nerve cell body to facilitate the regenerative process. The neuron in the cell body contains the genetic material and produces the chemicals necessary to maintain the axon. These substances cannot be transmitted to the distal part of the axon, and eventually there will be complete degeneration.[37]

In addition, the myelin portion of the Schwann cells around the degenerating axon also degenerates, and the myelin is phagocytized. The Schwann cells divide, forming a column of cells in place of the axon. If the cut ends of the axon contact this column of Schwann cells, the chances are good that an axon will eventually reinnervate distal structures. If the proximal end of the axon does not make contact with the column of Schwann cells, reinnervation will not occur.[37]

The axon proximal to the cut has minimal degeneration initially and then begins the regenerative process with growth from the proximal axon. Bulbous enlargements and several axon sprouts form at the end of the proximal axon. Within about two weeks, these sprouts grow across the scar that has developed in the area of the cut and enter the column of Schwann cells. Only one of these sprouts will form the new axon, while the others will degenerate. Once the axon grows through the Schwann cell columns, remaining Schwann cells proliferate along the length of the degenerating fiber and the neurolemmocytes form new myelin around the growing axon, which will eventually reinnervate distal structures.[20]

Regeneration is slow, at a rate of only 3 to 4 millimeters per day. Axon regeneration can be obstructed by scar formation due to excessive fibroplasia. Damaged nerves within the central nervous system regenerate very poorly compared with nerves in the peripheral nervous system. Central nervous system axons lack connective tissue sheaths, and the myelin-producing Schwann cells fail to proliferate.[7]

## Modifying Soft-Tissue Healing

The healing process is unique in each patient. In addition, different tissues vary in their ability to regenerate. For example, cartilage regenerates to some degree from the perichondrium, striated muscle is limited in its regeneration, and peripheral nerve fibers can regenerate only if their damaged ends are opposed. Usually, connective tissue will readily regenerate, but, as is true of all tissue, this possibility is dependent on the availability of nutrients.

Age and general nutrition can play a role in healing. Older patients may be more delayed in healing than are younger patients. In a patient with a poor nutritional status, injuries may heal more slowly than normal.

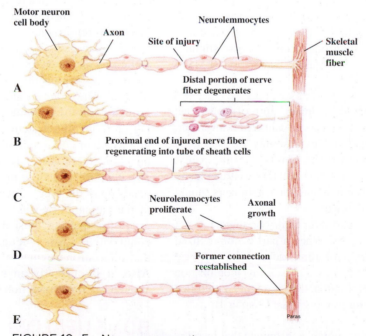

FIGURE 10–5   Neuron regeneration.
(A) If a neuron is severed through a myelinated axon, the proximal portion may survive, but (B) the distal portion will degenerate through phagocytosis. (C & D) The myelin layer provides a pathway for regeneration of the axon. (E) Innervation is restored.

Patients with certain organic disorders may heal slowly. For example, blood conditions such as anemia and diabetes often inhibit the healing process because of markedly impaired collagen deposition. Many of the current treatment approaches are designed to enhance the healing process. Current treatments are anti-inflammatory medications, therapeutic modalities, exercise rehabilitation, and prolotherapy.

**Anti-inflammatory Medications** It is a common practice for a physician to routinely prescribe nonsteroidal anti-inflammatory drugs (**NSAIDs**) for patients who have sustained an injury.[18] These medications are certainly effective in minimizing the pain and swelling associated with inflammation and may enhance a return to full activity. However, there are some concerns that the use of NSAIDs acutely following injury may actually interfere with inflammation, thus delaying the healing process. The use of NSAIDs is further discussed in Chapter 17.

**Therapeutic Modalities** Both cold and heat are used for different conditions. In general, heat facilitates an acute inflammatory response and cold slows the inflammatory response.[32]

A number of electrical modalities are used for the treatment of inflammation stemming from sports injuries. These procedures involve penetrating heat devices, such as shortwave and ultrasound therapy, and electrical stimulation, including transcutaneous electrical nerve stimulation (TENS) and electrical muscle stimulation (EMS)[32] (see Chapter 15).

**Exercise Rehabilitation** A major aim of soft-tissue rehabilitation through exercise is pain-free movement, full-strength power, and full extensibility of associated muscles. The ligamentous tissue, if related to the injury, should become pain free and have full tensile strength and full range of motion. The dynamic joint stabilizers should regain full strength and power.[18]

Immobilization of a part after injury or surgery is not always good for all injuries. When a part is immobilized over an extended period of time, adverse biochemical changes occur in collagenous tissue. Early mobilization used in exercise rehabilitation that is highly controlled may enhance the healing process[19] (see Chapter 16).

**Prolotherapy** Prolotherapy is a technique that involves injection of an irritant, nonpharmacological solution (e.g., dextrose, phenol, glycerine, lidocaine) into soft tissue for the purpose of increasing the inflammatory response, thus enhancing the healing process.[39] It is also referred to in the literature as proliferation therapy, proliferative injection therapy, and regenerative injection therapy. Prolotherapy has been used primarily to facilitate strengthening of weakened connective tissue (i.e., tendons and ligaments) and to reduce pain although it has also been used in treating a variety of other musculoskeletal conditions.[39] Injections are typically repeated every 3 to 6 weeks until no longer necessary. There is currently limited evidence in the literature to support the use of prolotherapy, although a number of randomized clinical trials are looking at this technique. Consequently, third-party payers are reluctant to reimburse for this therapeutic treatment.

***Platelet-Rich Plasma (PRP) Injections*** **Platelet-rich plasma (PRP)** injections are a type of prolotherapy that uses the patient's own platelets to promote the natural healing of a variety of musculoskeletal conditions such as tendinosis, tendinitis, ligament sprains, muscle strains, injuries to fibrocartilage, osteoarthritis, and wound healing.[6,31] To prepare a PRP injection, a small amount of the patient's own blood is drawn into a vial. The blood is then spun in a centrifuge to separate the blood into its various components: plasma, platelets and white blood cells, and red blood cells. The red blood cells are drained away, and the concentrated platelets, white cells, and some plasma are centrifuged again to separate the platelet-rich plasma from the platelet-poor plasma; then an anticoagulant is added to prevent early platelet clotting. The PRP is then injected into and around the injured tissues.[34] The concentrated platelets release bioactive proteins that include growth factors and signaling proteins that stimulate wound healing and tissue repair. Growth factors are peptides secreted by many different tissues (including platelets) that activate intracellular pathways responsible for growth, differentiation, and development of cells. Specific growth factors are responsible for healing in musculoskeletal tissues.[6] The concentrated platelets can increase the growth factors by as much as eightfold.[31] The signaling proteins attract stem cells that multiply and function to repair and rebuild damaged tissue. Following an injection, there is usually an increase in pain for 5 to 10 days. The number of injections that are necessary depends upon the type of condition, severity, and the age of the patient.[34] Because this is a relatively new technique for treating musculoskeletal injuries, there are comparatively few randomized controlled trial studies that offer strong evidence supporting its effectiveness. Also, it is currently an expensive treatment, costing about $1,000 per injection.

# BONE HEALING

Healing of injured bone tissue is similar to soft-tissue healing in that all phases of the healing process may be identified, although bone regeneration capabilities are somewhat limited. However, the functional elements of healing differ significantly from those of soft tissue. The tensile strength of the scar is the single most critical factor in soft-tissue healing, whereas bone has to contend with a number of additional forces, including torsion, bending, and compression.[26] Trauma to bone may vary from contusions of the periosteum to closed, nondisplaced fractures to severely displaced open fractures that also involve significant soft-tissue damage. When a fracture occurs, blood vessels in the bone and the periosteum are damaged, resulting in bleeding and subsequent clot formation (Figure 10–6). Hemorrhaging from the marrow is contained by the periosteum and the surrounding soft tissue in the region of the fracture. In about one week, fibroblasts have begun laying down a fibrous collagen network. The fibrin strands within the clot serve as the framework for proliferating vessels. *Chondroblast* cells begin producing fibrocartilage, creating a *callus* between the broken bones. At first, the callus is soft and firm because it is composed primarily of collagenous fibrin. The callus becomes firm and more rubbery as cartilage begins to predominate. Bone-producing cells called osteoblasts begin to proliferate and enter the callus, forming cancellous bone trabeculae, which eventually replace the cartilage. Finally, the callus crystallizes into bone, at which point remodeling of the bone begins. The callus can be divided into two portions, the external callus located around the periosteum on the outside of the fracture and the internal callus found between the bone fragments. The size of the callus is proportional both to the damage and to the amount of irritation to the fracture site during the healing process. Also during this time, osteoclasts begin to appear in the area to resorb bone fragments and clean up debris.[26,37]

The remodeling process is similar to the growth process of bone in that the fibrous cartilage is gradually replaced by fibrous bone and then by more structurally efficient lamellar bone. Remodeling involves an ongoing process during which osteoblasts lay down new bone and osteoclasts remove and break down bone according to the forces placed on the healing bone.[26] Wolff's law maintains that a bone will adapt to mechanical stresses and strains by changing size, shape, and structure. Therefore, once the cast is removed, the bone must be subjected to normal stresses and strains, so that tensile strength may be regained before the healing process is complete.[2]

The time required for bone healing is variable and based on a number of factors, such as the severity of the fracture, site of the fracture, extensiveness of the trauma, and age of the patient.[2] Normal periods of immobilization range from as short as three weeks for the small bones in the hands and feet to as long as eight weeks for the long bones of the upper and lower extremities. In some instances—for example, the four small toes—immobilization may not be required for healing. The healing process is certainly not complete when the splint or cast is removed. Osteoblastic and osteoclastic activity may continue for 2 to 3 years after severe fractures.

**Management of Acute Fractures** In the treatment of acute fractures, the bones commonly must be immobilized completely until X-ray studies reveal that the hard callus has been formed. It is up to the physician to know the various types of fractures and the best form of immobilization for each fracture.[26] Fractures can keep a patient from activity for several weeks or months, depending on the nature,

**10–6 Clinical Application Exercise**

A field hockey player falls and sustains an acute fracture of the left humerus.

? What are the healing events typical of this acute bone fracture?

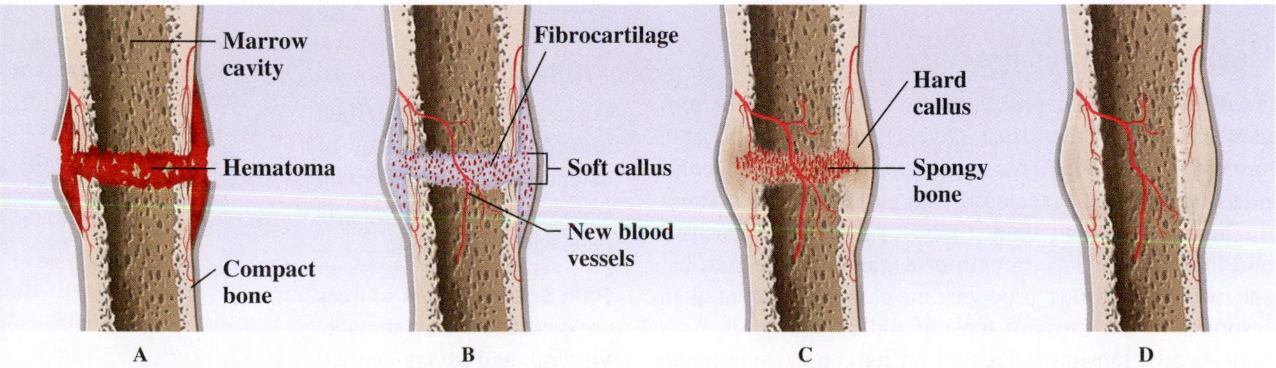


FIGURE 10–6 The healing of a fracture. **(A)** Blood vessels are broken at the fracture line; the blood clots and forms a fracture hematoma. **(B)** Blood vessels grow into the fracture and a fibrocartilage soft callus forms. **(C)** The fibrocartilage becomes ossified and forms a bony callus made of spongy bone. **(D)** Osteoclasts remove excess tissue from the bony callus and the bone eventually resembles its original appearance.

extent, and site of the fracture. During this period, certain conditions can seriously interfere with the healing process:[2,26,37]

- If there is a *poor blood supply to the fractured area* and one of the parts of the fractured bone is not properly supplied by the blood, that part will die and union or healing of the fracture will not take place. This condition is known as **avascular necrosis** and often occurs in the head of the femur, the navicular bone in the wrist, the talus in the ankle, and isolated bone fragments. The condition is relatively rare among vital, healthy, young patients except in the navicular bone of the wrist.

- *Poor immobilization of the fracture site,* resulting from poor casting by the physician and permitting motion between the bone parts, may not only prevent proper union but also, in the event that union does transpire, cause deformity to develop.
- *Infection* can materially interfere with the normal healing process, particularly in the case of a compound fracture, which offers an ideal situation for the development of a severe streptococcal or staphylococcal infection. The increased use of antibiotics has considerably reduced the prevalence of these infections coincidental with or immediately after a fracture. The closed fracture is not immune to contamination because infections within the body or poor blood supply can render it susceptible. If the fracture site becomes and remains infected, the infection can interfere with the proper union of the bone.
- Soft tissues that become positioned between the severed ends of the bone—such as muscle, connective tissue, or other soft tissue immediately adjacent to the fracture—can prevent proper bone union, often necessitating surgical intervention.

## Healing of Stress Fractures

As discussed in Chapter 9, stress fractures may be created by cyclic forces that adversely load a bone at a susceptible site. Fractures may be the result of axial compression or tension created by the pull of muscles. Stress on ligamentous and bony tissue can be either positive and increase relative strength or negative and lead to tissue weakness. Bone produces an electrical potential in response to the stress of tension and compression. As a bone bends, tension is created on its convex side along with a positive electrical charge; conversely, on the concave or compressional side, a negative electrical charge is created. Torsional forces produce tension circumferentially. Constant tension caused by axial compression or stress by muscular activity can result in an increase in bone resorption and, subsequently, a microfracture. In other words, if the osteoclastic activity is greater than the osteoblastic activity, the bone becomes increasingly susceptible to stress fractures.[14]

Like the healing of acute fractures, the healing of stress fractures involves restoring a balance of osteoclastic and osteoblastic activity. Achieving this balance requires recognition of the situation as early as possible. Stress fractures that go unhealed will eventually develop into complete cortical fractures that may, over a period of time, become displaced. A decrease in activity and the elimination of other factors in training that cause stress will allow the bone to remodel and to develop the ability to withstand stress.[14]

## PAIN

Pain can be defined as "an unpleasant sensory and emotional experience associated with actual or potential tissue damage, or described in terms of such damage."[1] Pain is a subjective sensation with more than one dimension and an abundance of descriptors of its qualities and characteristics. Pain is composed of a variety of human discomforts, rather than being a single entity. The perception of pain can be subjectively modified by past experiences and expectations. Much of what is done to treat patients' pain is to change their perceptions of pain. Certainly, reducing pain is an essential part of treatment. The athletic trainer's goal is to control acute pain by encouraging the body to heal through exercise designed to progressively increase functional capacity and to return the patient to full activity as swiftly and safely as possible.

## Types of Pain

Pain can be described according to a number of categories, such as pain sources, acute versus chronic pain, and referred pain.[12]

**Pain Sources** Pain sources are cutaneous, deep somatic, visceral, and psychogenic.[11] Cutaneous pain is usually sharp, bright, and burning and can have a fast or slow onset. Deep somatic pain

A cross-country runner sustains a stress fracture of her left tibia. Her left leg is ¾ inch shorter than her right leg.

**?** What is a possible cause of this injury?

A butterfly swimmer has been experiencing low back pain for more than 6 months. The pain is described as aching and throbbing.

**?** What type of pain is this athlete experiencing?

stems from structures such as tendons, muscles, joints, periosteum, and blood vessels. Visceral pain originates from internal organs. Visceral pain is diffused at first and later may be localized, as in appendicitis. In psychogenic pain, the individual feels pain but the cause is emotional rather than physical.[12]

**Acute versus Chronic Pain** Acute pain lasts less than 6 months. Tissue damage occurs and serves as a warning to the patient. Chronic pain, on the other hand, has a duration longer than 6 months. The International Association for the Study of Pain describes chronic pain as that which continues beyond the usual normal healing time.[8]

**Referred Pain** Referred pain occurs away from the actual site of irritation. This pain has been called an error in perception. Each referred pain site must also be considered unique to each individual. Symptoms and signs vary according to the nerve fibers affected. Response may be motor, sensory, or both. Four types of referred pain are myofascial, sclerotomic, myotomic, and dermatomic pain.

*Myofascial Pain* As discussed in Chapter 9, **trigger points** are small, hyperirritable areas within a muscle in which nerve impulses bombard the central nervous system and are expressed as a referred pain. Acute and chronic musculoskeletal pain can be caused by myofascial trigger points.[12] Such pain sites have variously been described as fibrositis, myositis, myalgia, myofasciitis, and muscular strain.

An active trigger point is hyperirritable and causes an obvious complaint. Pain radiating from an active trigger point does not follow a usual area of distribution, such as sclerotomes, dermatomes, or peripheral nerves. The trigger point pain area is called the reference zone, which can be close to the point of irritation or a considerable distance from it.[12]

*Sclerotomic, Myotomic, and Dermatomic Pain* Deep pain may originate from sclerotomic, myotomic, or dermatomic nerve irritation or injury.[11] A sclerotome is an area of bone or fascia that is supplied by a single nerve root. Myotomes are muscles supplied by a single nerve root. Dermatomes also are in an area of skin supplied by a single nerve root.

Sclerotomic pain is deep, aching, and poorly localized pain. Sclerotomic pain impulses can be projected to regions in the brain such as the hypothalamus, limbic system, and reticular formation and can cause depression, anxiety, fear, or anger. Autonomic changes, such as changes in vasomotor tone, blood pressure, and sweating, may also occur.

Dermatomic pain, in contrast to sclerotomic pain, is sharp and well localized. Unlike sclerotomic pain, dermatomic pain projects mainly to the thalamus and is relayed directly to the cortex, skipping autonomic and affective responses.

## Nociceptors and Neural Transmission

Pain receptors known as **nociceptors,** or free nerve endings, are sensitive to mechanical, thermal, and chemical stimuli.[11] They are commonly found in skin, periosteum surrounding bone, teeth, meninges, and some organs.

*Afferent* nerve fibers transmit impulses from the nociceptors toward the spinal cord, while *efferent* nerve fibers, such as motor neurons, transmit impulses from the spinal cord toward the periphery. First-order, or primary, afferents transmit impulses from a nociceptor to the dorsal horn of the spinal cord. There are four types of first-order neurons: Aα, Aβ, Aδ, and C. Aα and Aβ fibers are characterized as large-diameter afferents and Aδ and C fibers as small-diameter afferents. Aδ and C fibers transmit sensations of pain and temperature. Aδ neurons originate from nociceptors located in skin and transmit "fast pain," while C neurons originate from both superficial tissue (skin) and deeper tissue (ligaments and muscle) and transmit "slow pain."[12]

Second-order afferent fibers carry sensory messages from the dorsal horn to the brain and are categorized as nociceptive specific. Second-order afferents receive input from Aβ, Aδ, and C fibers. Second-order afferents serve relatively large, overlapping receptor fields. Nociceptive-specific second-order afferents respond exclusively to noxious stimulation and receive input only from Aδ and C fibers. All of second order neurons synapse prior to reaching the sensory cortex. A large portion of these fibers terminate in the thalamus with most others terminating in the periaqueductal gray region of the midbrain or at cell clusters within the reticular formation. Third-order neurons carry information from these areas to the sensory cortex, where the input is integrated, interpreted, and acted upon.

## Facilitators and Inhibitors of Synaptic Transmission

For information to pass between neurons, a transmitter substance must be released from one neuron terminal, enter the synaptic cleft, and attach to a receptor site on the next neuron. This occurs primarily due to chemicals called *neurotransmitters.* However, it has been shown that several compounds that are not true neurotransmitters can facilitate or inhibit synaptic activity. These include *serotonin,* which is active in descending pathways; *norepinephrine,* which inhibits pain transmission between first- and second-order neurons; *substance P,* which is active in small-diameter primary afferent neurons; *enkephalins,* found in descending pathways; and *β-endorphin,* found in the central nervous system.[40]

**Neurotransmitters:**

- Serotonin
- Norepinephrine
- Substance P
- Enkephalins
- β-endorphin

## Mechanisms of Pain Control

The neurophysiological mechanisms of pain control have not been fully explained. To date, three models of pain control have been proposed: the gate control theory, descending pathway pain control, and the release of β-endorphin. It is likely that some as-yet-unexplained combination of these three models is responsible for pain modulation.[1]

**Gate Control Theory**  Sensory information coming from cutaneous receptors in the skin is carried along afferent Aβ nerve fibers to the substantia gelatinosa in the dorsal horn of the spinal cord (Figure 10–7). Likewise, pain messages from the nociceptors are carried along the Aδ and C afferent fibers and enter the dorsal horn. Increased neural activity in Aβ afferent pathways triggers a release of enkephalin from *enkephalin interneurons* found in the dorsal horn thus inhibiting transmission in the Aδ and C fiber afferent pathways effectively "closing the gate" to the transmission of pain information to second-order neurons. Consequently, pain information is not transmitted and never reaches sensory centers in the brain. The gate control theory of pain control occurs at the spinal cord level.[12]

**Descending Pathway Pain Control**  Stimulation of descending pathways in the spinal cord may also inhibit pain impulses carried along the Aδ and C afferent fibers (Figure 10–8). It is theorized that previous experiences, emotional influences, sensory perception, and other factors influence the transmission of pain messages and thus the perception of pain. The information coming from higher centers in the brain stimulates a release of serotonin from the *periaqueductal gray* (PAG) matter of the midbrain and the raphe nucleus which travels along efferent descending pathways in the spinal cord. Serotonin enters the dorsal horn where it activates the release of

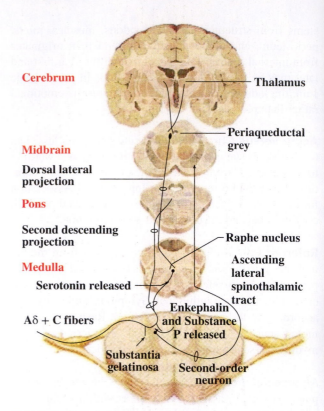

FIGURE 10–8  Descending pathway pain control. Influence from the thalamus stimulates the periaqueductal grey, the raphe nucleus, and the pons to inhibit the transmission of pain impulses through the ascending tracts.

the neurotransmitters enkephalin and substance P, which together block or inhibit the synaptic transmission of impulses from the Aδ and C afferent fibers to second-order afferent neurons.[12]

**Release of β-Endorphin**  It has been shown that noxious (painful) stimulation of nociceptors resulting in the transmission of pain information along Aδ and C afferents can stimulate the release of an endogenous opiate-like chemical called β-endorphin from the hypothalamus and anterior pituitary and dynorphin from the periaqueductal grey and the raphe nucleus (Figure 10–9). β-endorphin is endogenous to the central nervous system and is known to have strong analgesic effects. The exact mechanisms by which β-endorphin produces these potent analgesic effects are unclear. Acupuncture, acupressure, and point stimulation using electrical currents are all techniques that may stimulate the release of β-endorphin and dynorphin.[12]

## Pain Assessment

Pain is a complex phenomenon that is difficult to evaluate and quantify because it is subjective. Thus, obtaining an accurate and standardized assessment of pain is problematic. A number of validated assessment tools are available that allow the athletic trainer to develop a pain profile by identifying the type of pain a patient is experiencing, quantifying the intensity of pain, evaluating the effect of the

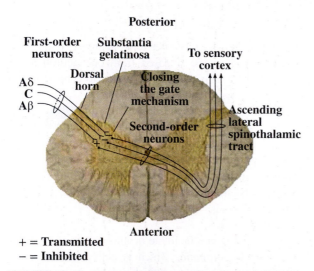

+ = Transmitted
− = Inhibited

FIGURE 10–7  Gate control theory. Sensory information carried on Aβ fibers "closes the gate" to pain information carried on Aδ and C fibers in the substantia gelatinosa, preventing the transmission of pain to sensory centers in the cortex.

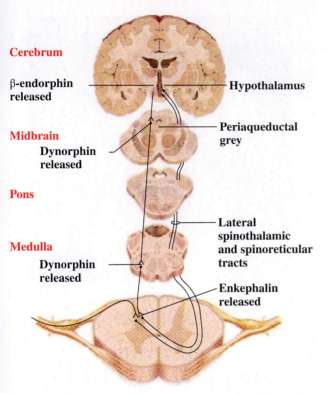

**Cerebrum**

β-endorphin released

Hypothalamus

**Midbrain**

Dynorphin released

Periaqueductal grey

**Pons**

**Medulla**

Dynorphin released

Lateral spinothalamic and spinoreticular tracts

Enkephalin released

FIGURE 10–9 β-endorphin released from the hypothalamus and dynorphin released from the periaqueductal grey and the medulla.

pain experience on a patient's level of functioning, and assessing the psychosocial impact of pain.

Pain measurement tools include simple *unidimensional scales* or *multidimensional questionnaires.* Pain measurement should include both the time frame and the clinical context of the pain. With unidimensional scales, individuals with acute pain are usually asked to describe their pain "right now" and may be asked about the average intensity over a fixed period to provide information on the course of the pain. Examples of commonly used unidimensional scales are verbal rating scales, the numeric rating scale, and the visual analog scale. Multidimensional pain assessment tools are more comprehensive pain assessments that require the determination of the quality of the pain and its effect on mood and function. They are used mainly to quantify these aspects of pain, and they take longer to administer than the unidimensional scales. The McGill Pain Questionnaire is an example of a multidimensional pain assessment tool.

**Visual Analog Scales** Visual analog scales are quick and simple tests that consist of a line, usually 2½ inches (10 cm) in length, the extremes of which are taken to represent the limits of the pain experience. The patient simply places a mark on that line based on the perceived level of pain. Scales can be completed daily or more often (Figure 10–10).

**Pain Charts** *Pain charts* can be used to establish spatial properties of pain. These two-dimensional graphic

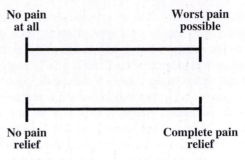

No pain at all                    Worst pain possible

No pain relief                    Complete pain relief

FIGURE 10–10   Visual analog scales.

portrayals are completed by the patient to assess the location of pain and a number of subjective components. Simple line drawings of the body in several postural positions are presented to the patient. On these drawings, the patient draws or colors in areas that correspond to his or her pain experience. Different colors are used for different sensations—for example, blue for aching pain, yellow for numbness or tingling, red for burning pain, and green for cramping pain. Descriptions can be added to the form to enhance the communication value. The form could be completed daily.

**McGill Pain Questionnaire** The *McGill Pain Questionnaire (MPQ)* is a tool with 78 words that describes the intensity and nature of pain. These words are grouped into 20 sets that are divided into four categories representing dimensions of the pain experience including sensory, affective, evaluative, and miscellaneous. Patients are asked to circle only the one word that best describes their current pain word in a set. While completion of the MPQ may take only 20 minutes, it is often frustrating for patients who do not speak English well. The MPQ is commonly administered to patients with low back pain. When administered every 2 to 4 weeks, it demonstrates changes in status very clearly.

**Activity Pain Indicators Profile** The Activity Pain Indicators Profile is a 64-question self-report tool used to assess functional impairment associated with pain. It measures the frequency of certain behaviors, such as housework, recreation, and social activities, that produce pain.

**Numeric Rating Scale** The numeric rating scale is the most common acute pain profile used in sports medicine. The patient is asked to verbally rate pain on a scale from 1 to 10, with 10 representing the worst pain he or she has experienced or can imagine. Usually, the scale is administered verbally before and after treatment. When treatments provide pain relief, questions are asked about the extent and duration of the relief.

## Treating Pain

An athletic trainer can approach pain management using a variety of treatment options, including therapeutic modalities and medications.

**Therapeutic Modalities** Many therapeutic modalities can provide pain relief.[32] There is not one best therapeutic agent for pain control. The athletic trainer must select the therapeutic agent that is most appropriate for each athlete, based on the athletic trainer's knowledge of the modalities and professional judgment (see Chapter 15). In no situation should the athletic trainer apply a therapeutic agent without first developing a clear rationale for the treatment. The therapeutic modalities used to control pain do little to promote tissue healing. They should be used to relieve acute pain following injury or surgery or to control pain and other symptoms, such as swelling, to promote progressive exercise. The athletic trainer should not lose sight of the effects of the modalities or the importance of progressive exercise in restoring the athlete's functional ability.

The athletic trainer can make use of the gate control mechanism of pain control by using superficial heat or cold, electrical stimulating currents, massage, and counterirritants to stimulate the large-diameter Aα and Aβ efferent nerve fibers. Noxious stimulation of acupuncture and trigger points using either electrical stimulating currents or deep acupressure massage techniques can mediate the release of β-endorphin and dynorphin.[12]

**Medications** A physician may choose to prescribe oral or injectable medications in treating a patient. The most commonly used medications are classified as analgesics, anti-inflammatory agents, or both.[10] The athletic trainer should become familiar with these drugs and note whether the patient is taking any medications (see Chapter 17). It is also important to work with the referring physician or a pharmacist to make sure that the patient takes the medications appropriately.

## Psychological Aspect of Pain

Pain, especially chronic pain, is a subjective psychological phenomenon.[40] When painful injuries are treated, the total patient must be considered, not just the pain or condition. Even in the most well-adjusted person, pain creates emotional changes. Constant pain often causes self-centeredness and an increased sense of dependency. Chapter 11 discusses in great detail the psychosocial aspects of dealing with injury and managing pain.

Patients vary in their pain thresholds (Figure 10–11). Some can tolerate enormous pain, whereas others find mild pain almost unbearable. Pain is perceived as being worse at night because persons are alone, more

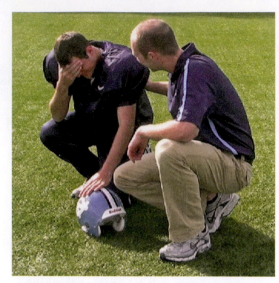

FIGURE 10–11 Coping with pain in sports is as much psychological as it is physical.
© William E. Prentice

aware of themselves, and devoid of external diversions. Personality differences can also cause differences in pain toleration. For example, patients who are anxious, dependent, and immature have less tolerance for pain than those who are relaxed and emotionally in control.

A number of theories about how pain is produced and perceived by the brain have been advanced. Only in the last few decades has science demonstrated that pain is both a psychological and a physiological phenomenon and is therefore unique to each individual.[4,40] Sports activities demonstrate this fact clearly. Through conditioning, an athlete learns to endure the pain of rigorous activity and to block the sensations of a minor injury. It is perhaps most critical for the athletic trainer to recognize that all pain is very real to the patient.

A gymnast is receiving electrical stimulation for chronic low back pain.

**?** What is the purpose of administering electrical stimulation for the chronic pain?

## SUMMARY

- The three phases of the healing process are the inflammatory response phase, the fibroblastic repair phase, and the maturation-remodeling phase, which occur in sequence but overlap one another in a continuum.
- During the inflammatory response phase, debris is phagocytized (cleaned up). The fibroblastic repair phase involves the deposition of collagen fibers to

form a firm scar. During the maturation-remodeling phase, collagen is realigned along lines of tensile force and the tissue gradually assumes normal appearance and function.
- Factors that may impede the healing process include the extent of the injury, edema, hemorrhage, poor vascular supply, separation of tissue, muscle spasm,

atrophy, corticosteroids, keloids and hypertrophic scars, infection, climate and oxygen tension, health, age, and nutrition.

- Treatment techniques that can be used to modify soft-tissue healing include anti-inflammatory medications, therapeutic modalities, exercise rehabilitation, and platelet-rich plasma injections.
- The healing of soft tissues, including cartilage, ligament, muscle, and nerve, follows a similar course. Unlike the other tissues, nerve has the capability of regenerating.

- Bone healing following fracture involves increased activity of osteoblastic cells and osteoclastic cells.
- Pain is a response to a noxious stimulus that is subjectively modified by past experiences and expectations.
- Pain is classified as either acute or chronic and can exhibit many different patterns.
- Three models of pain control are the gate control theory, descending pathway pain control, and the release of β-endorphin from higher centers of the brain.
- Pain perception may be influenced by a variety of cognitive processes mediated by the higher brain centers.

## WEB SITES

American Academy of Pain Management:
www.aapainmanage.org

American Pain Society: www.ampainsoc.org
World Union of Wound Healing Societies:
www.wuwhs.org

## SOLUTIONS TO CLINICAL APPLICATION EXERCISES

10–1 Little can be done to speed up the healing process physiologically. This athlete must realize that certain physiological events must occur during each phase of the healing process. Any interference with this healing process during a rehabilitation program will likely slow return to full activity. The healing process must have an opportunity to accomplish what it is supposed to.

10–2 Immobilization during the inflammatory process may be beneficial; however, controlled mobilization helps the tissue decrease atrophy and enhance the healing process. Controlled mobilization allows the athlete to perform progressive strengthening exercises in a timely manner.

10–3 Initially, a transitory vasoconstriction with the start of blood coagulation of the broken blood vessels occurs. Dilation of the vessels in the region of injury follows, along with the activation of chemical mediators via key cells.

10–4 A grade 2 lateral ankle sprain implies that the joint capsule and ligaments are partially torn. At 3 weeks, the injury has been

cleaned of debris and is undergoing the process of secondary healing. Granulation tissue fills the torn areas, and fibroblasts are beginning to form scar tissue.

10–5 In its acute phase, the injury was not allowed to heal properly. As a result, the injury became chronic, with a proliferation of scar tissue, lymphocytes, plasma cells, and macrophages.

10–6 Uncomplicated acute bone healing goes through five stages: hematoma formation, cellular proliferation, callus formation, ossification, and remodeling.

10–7 Because it is shorter, the left leg has the greater stress during running. This stress creates increased tension on the tibia's concave side, causing an increase in osteoclastic activity.

10–8 The pain is considered to be chronic, deep somatic pain stemming from the low back muscles. It is conducted primarily by the C-type nerve fibers.

10–9 The purpose is to stimulate the large, rapidly conducting nerve fibers to inhibit the smaller and slower nerves that carry pain impulses.

## REVIEW QUESTIONS AND CLASS ACTIVITIES

1. What are the three phases of healing, and what are the approximate time frames for each of these three phases?
2. What are the physiological events associated with the inflammatory response phase of the healing process?
3. How can you differentiate between acute and chronic inflammation?
4. How is collagen laid down in the area of injury during the fibroblastic repair phase of healing?
5. Explain Wolff's law and the importance of controlled mobility during the maturation-remodeling phase of healing.
6. What are some of the factors that can have a negative impact on the healing process?
7. Discuss treatment techniques for modifying soft-tissue healing, including anti-inflammatory medications, therapeutic modalities, exercise rehabilitation, and platelet-rich plasma injections.

8. Compare and contrast the course of healing in cartilage, ligaments, muscle, and nerve.
9. What is a basic definition of pain?
10. What are the different types of pain?
11. What are the characteristics of the various sensory receptors?
12. How does the nervous system relay information about painful stimuli?
13. Describe how the gate control mechanism of pain modulation may be used to modulate pain.
14. How does descending pathway pain control modulate pain?
15. What are the opiate-like substances, and how do they modulate pain?
16. What are the assessment scales available to help the athletic trainer determine the extent of pain perception?
17. How can pain perception be modified by cognitive factors?

# REFERENCES

1. Aronson PA: Pain theories: A review for application in athletic training and therapy, *Athletic Therapy Today* 7(4):8, 2002.
2. Bailon-Plaza A: Beneficial effects of moderate, early loading and adverse effects of delayed or excessive loading on bone healing, *Journal of Biomechanics* 36(8):1069, 2003.
3. Barrientos S: Growth factors and cytokines in wound healing, *Wound Repair and Regeneration*, 16(5):585–602, 2008.
4. Battery L: Inflammation in overuse tendon injuries, *Sports Medicine and Arthroscopy Reviews*, 19(3):213–17, 2011.
5. Black K: Perpheral afferent nerve regeneration. In Lephart S, Fu F, editors: *Proprioception and neuromuscular control in joint stability*, Champaign, IL, 2000, Human Kinetics.
6. Borrione P: Platelet-rich plasma in muscle healing, *American Journal of Physical Medicine and Rehabilitation*, 89(1):854, 2010.
7. Campbell W: Evaluation on management of peripheral nerve injury, *Clinical Neurophysiology*, 119(9):1951–65, 2008.
8. Casey C: Transition from acute to chronic pain and disability: A model including cognitive, affective and trauma factors, *Pain*, 134(2):69–79, 2008.
9. Clark B: In vivo alterations in skeletal muscle form and function after disuse atrophy, *Medicine and Science in Sport and Exercise*, 2009.
10. Creighton A: Basic science of ligament healing: Medial collateral ligament healing with and without treatment, *Sports Med Arthroscopy Review* 13(3):145, 2005.
11. Deleo J: Basic science of pain, *Bone Joint Surg* 88(s):58, 2006.
12. Denegar CR, Prentice W: Managing pain with therapeutic modalities. In Prentice WE, editor: *Therapeutic modalities in rehabilitation*, ed 4, New York, 2017, McGraw-Hill.
13. Diegelmann R: Wound healing: An overview of acute, fibrotic, and delayed healing, *Frontiers in Bioscience*, (2):283–89, 2004.
14. Ferry A: Stress fractures in athletes, *Physician and Sports Medicine*, 38(2):109–18, 2010.
15. Gallin J: *Inflammation: Basic principles and clinical correlates*, Baltimore, MD, 1999, Lippincott Williams & Wilkins.
16. Hildebrand K: The basics of soft tissue healing and general factors that influence such healing, *Sports Med Arthroscopy Review* 13(3):136, 2005.
17. Hill C: Rehabilitation of soft tissue and musculoskeletal injury. In O'Young B: *Physical medicine and rehabilitation secrets*, Philadelphia, PA, 2007, Hanley-Belfus.
18. Hubbel S: Tissue injury and healing: Using medications, modalities, and exercise to maximize recovery. In Bushbacher R, ed: *Sports medicine and rehabilitation: A sport specific approach*, Philadelphia, PA, 2008, Elsevier Health Services.
19. Irrgang J: Rehabilitation following surgical procedures to address articular cartilage lesions in the knee, *J Orthop Sports Phys Ther* 28(4): 232, 1998.
20. Isaacs J: Treatmnt of acute peripheral nerve injuries: Current concepts, *Journal of Hand Surgery*, 35(3):491–97, 2010.
21. Kocher M: Ligament healing and augmentation. In *Proceedings, National Athletic Trainers' Association, 10th annual meeting and clinical symposia*, Champaign, IL, 1999, Human Kinetics.
22. Ley K: *Physiology of inflammation*, Bethesda, MD, 2001, American Physiological Society.
23. Li J: Pathophysiology of acute wound healing, *Clinics in Dermatology*, 25(1):9–18, 1997.
24. Maffulli N: Basic science of tendons, *Sports Med Arthroscopy Review* 8(1):1, 2000.
25. Malone T, Garrett W, Zachewski J: Muscle: Deformation, injury and repair. In Zachazewski J, Magee D, Quillen W, eds: *Athletic injuries and rehabilitation*, Philadelphia, PA, 1996, WB Saunders.
26. Marsell R: The biology of fracture healing, *Injury*, 42(6):551–55, 2011.
27. Molloy T: The roles of growth factors in tendon and ligament healing, *Sports Med* 33(5):381, 2003.
28. Murdoch S: Managing the inflammatory response through nutritional supplements, *Athletic Therapy Today* 6(5):46, 2001.
29. Murrell G: The effects of immobilization and exercise on tendon healing, *Journal of Science and Medicine in Sport* 2(1 Supplement):40, 1999.
30. Musahl V: Cartilage injuries. In Ranawat A: *Musculoskeletal examination of the hip and knee*, Thorofare, NJ, 2011, Slack.
31. Paoloni J: Platelet-rich plasma treatment for ligament and tendon injuries, *Clinical Journal of Sports Medicine*, 21(1):37–45, 2011.
32. Prentice WE: *Therapeutic modalities in rehabilitation*, ed 4, New York, 2011, McGraw-Hill.
33. Rees J: Management of tendinopathy, *American Journal of Sports Medicine*, 37(9):1855–67, 2009.
34. Redler L: Platelet-rich plasma therapy: An systematic literature review and evidence for clinical use, *Physician and SportsMedicine* 39(1):42–51, 2011.
35. Sandrey M: Acute and chronic tendon injuries: Factors affecting the healing response and treatment, *J Sport Rehabil* 12(1):70, 2003.
36. Sandrey MA: Effects of acute and chronic pathomechanics on the normal histology and biomechanics of tendons: A review, *J Sport Rehabil* 9(4):339, 2000.
37. Seeley R: *Seeley's anatomy and physiology*, St. Louis, 2013, McGraw-Hill.
38. Serhan C: *Fundamentals of inflammation*, Cambridge, UK, 2010, Cambridge University Press.
39. Shah R: Utilization of prolotherapy for facilitation of ligament and tendon healing, *Athletic Therapy Today*, 15(6):25, 2010.
40. Shelemay K: *Pain and its transformations: The interface of biology and culture*, Boston, MA, 2007, Harvard University Press.
41. Steiner D: Pathophysiology of ligament injuries. In Comfort P: *Sports rehabilitation and injury prevention*, New York, 2010, John Wiley & Sons.
42. Taylor M: Treating chronic tendon injuries, *Athletic Therapy Today* 5(6):50, 2000.
43. Thompson L: Skeletal muscle adaptations with age, inactivity, and therapeutic exercise, *J Orthop Sports Phys Ther* 32(2):2002.
44. Velnar T: The wound healing process: An overview of the cellular and molecular mechanisms, *Journal of International Medical Research*, 37(5):1528–42, 2009.
45. Volgas D: *A manual of soft tissue management in orthopedic trauma*, New York, 2012, Thieme.
46. Walker J: Pathomechanics and classification of cartilage lesions, facilitation of repair, *J Orthop Sports Phys Ther* 28(4):216, 1998.
47. Ward P: Acute inflammation and chronic inflammation. In Serhan C: *Fundamentals of inflammation*, Cambridge, UK, 2010, Cambridge University Press.
48. Warren G, Ingalls C, Lowe D: What mechanisms contribute to the strength loss that occurs during and in the recovery from skeletal muscle injury? *J Orthop Sports Phys Ther* 32(2):2002.
49. Weintraub W: *Tendon and ligament healing: A new approach to sports and overuse injury*, Brookline , MA, 2005, Paradigm.
50. Westerblad H: Skeletal muscle: Energy metabolism, fiber types fatigue and adaptability, *Experimental Cell Research*, 316(18):3093–99, 2010.
51. Woo S: Basic science of ligament healing: anterior cruciate ligament graft biomechanics and knee kinematics, *Sports Med Arthroscopy Review* 13(3):161, 2005.
52. Young, A: The physiology of wound healing, *Surgery*, 29(10):475–79, 2011.

# ANNOTATED BIBLIOGRAPHY

Damjanov I, editor: *Anderson's pathology*, ed 10, Philadelphia, PA, 1996, Elsevier Science.

*A major pathology text that discusses inflammation and healing in depth.*

McCulloch J: *Wound healing:* Evidence-based management, Philadelphia, PA, 2010, Davis.

*An excellent discussion of factors influencing wound healing, evaluation, and methods of treatment.*

Melzack R, Wall P: *Handbook of pain management*, Philadelphia, PA, 2003, Elsevier.

*A summary of current knowledge of pain states and their management for all health care professionals involved in the diagnosis and treatment of patients with a wide variety of acute and chronic pain problems.*

Porth CM: *Pathophysiology: Concepts of altered health states*, ed 9, Philadelphia, PA, 2013, Lippincott, Williams & Wilkins.

*An in-depth text on the physiology of altered health; contains an excellent discussion on inflammation, healing, and pain.*

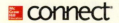

# PART IV

# Management Skills

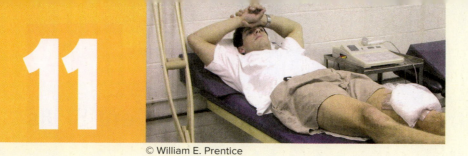

© William E. Prentice

# 11

# Psychosocial Intervention for Sports Injuries and Illnesses

## ■ Objectives

*When you finish this chapter you should be able to*

- Analyze the patient's psychological response to injury.
- Recognize the importance of social support for the injured athlete.
- Explain the relationship of stress and overtraining to the risk of injury.
- Describe the role of the athletic trainer as a counselor to the injured athlete.

- Identify the psychological factors important to rehabilitating the injured athlete.
- Compare and contrast the psychological skills training techniques that are used to manage the psychological aspects of injury.
- Recognize the different mental disorders and the appropriate referral and treatment techniques.

## ■ Outline

## ■ Key Terms

stressor
anxiety

catecholamine

## ■ Connect Highlights    McGraw-Hill Education **connect**

*Visit connect.mcgraw-hill.com for further exercises to apply your knowledge:*

- Clinical application scenarios covering psychological response to injury, social support, relationship of stress and overtraining, athletic trainer as a counselor, psychological factors in rehabilitation, psychological skills training techniques, and mental disorders
- Click-and-drag questions covering psychological response to injury, and the athletic trainer as a counselor
- Multiple-choice questions covering social support, relationship of stress and overtraining, psychological factors important in rehabilitation, psychological skills training techniques, and mental disorders

ertainly, the injured or ill patient experiences physical disability. But for many individuals, the psychological consequences of injury can be as debilitating as the physical injuries.[47] These psychological and sociological reactions, combined with the physical injury itself, can have an adverse impact on the injured athlete's successful return to competition. All of those involved with the health care of an injured patient must understand how the psyche, especially feelings and emotions, enters into that individual's reactions to injury or illness and ultimately how it affects the rehabilitation process (Figure 11–1).[17,35] The athletic trainer must also be aware of the cultural factors of an injured patient that may come into play during the rehabilitative process, and must be sensitive to those concerns on the part of the patient.[14]

Each individual reacts to injury and illness in a very personal way and makes unique adaptations to these challenges.[7] Some individuals view an injury or illness as devastating; others take such a setback in stride.[25] Some have problems with emotional control after sustaining an injury or illness. The athletic trainer must be aware that returning an injured patient to full, all-out competition requires that individual to be completely ready psychologically as well as physically.[14] Success in sports performance requires fundamental skills, such as speed, attention, concentration, stress management, and the ability to perform cognitive strategies.

Some individuals have a tendency to sustain injuries, whereas others under similar circumstances can stay injury free.[28] Countless physical and psychosocial factors can interact to predispose a person to injury as well as influence the effectiveness of the rehabilitation process.[61] No one personality type can be associated with accident-proneness. However, individuals who are risk takers seem to be more prone to injury. These individuals have a higher competition anxiety, demonstrate sensation-seeking behaviors, and have a high motivation for success, but they lack the appropriate coping skills to address these stressors.[28]

## THE PSYCHOLOGICAL RESPONSE TO INJURY

Not all patients deal with injury in the same manner.[7] One person may view an injury as disastrous; another may view it as an opportunity to show courage; a third may embrace the injury to avoid embarrassment over poor performance, to provide an escape from a losing team, or to discourage a domineering parent.[25]

Some factors are common among patients who are adjusting to injury and rehabilitation. The severity of the injury usually determines the length of rehabilitation.[25] Generally, injuries are classified as short-term (less than 4 weeks), long-term (more than 4 weeks), chronic (recurring), or terminating (career-ending). Regardless of the severity of the injury and the corresponding length of time required for rehabilitation, the injured athlete has to deal with a variety of emotions that may occur during three reactive phases of the injury and rehabilitation process (Figure 11–2). These reactive phases are reaction to injury, reaction to rehabilitation, and reaction to return to competition or career termination.[25] Not all individuals have all of these reactions, nor do all reactions fall precisely into the suggested sequence. Some psychologists have applied five stages of psychological reaction to injury. Based on Kübler-Ross's classic model of reactions to death and dying, which includes *denial, anger, bargaining, depression,* and *acceptance* (Figure 11–3).[32] Although this model is commonly considered to be applicable to terminal illnesses or death, it is generally not considered to be applicable to less significant injuries such as those that occur in sport. An alternative cognitive appraisal model has been proposed that focuses more on injured athletes' personal and situational factors and how these influence their cognitive appraisal of the injury situation.[61] It focuses on their interpretation of the injury rather than on the actual severity of the injury. Cognitive appraisal is what determines the athlete's emotional response (e.g., anger, depression, tension) and behavioral response (i.e., adherence to rehabilitation). These cognitive, emotional, and behavioral responses are interdependent and collectively influence recovery outcome. Other factors that can influence reactions to injury and rehabilitation are the athlete's coping skills, history of injury, social support, and personality traits.[31]

| Reactive phases: |
| --- |
| • Reaction to injury |
| • Reaction to rehabilitation |
| • Reaction to return |

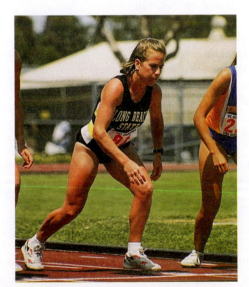

FIGURE 11–1 Sports participation can cause the athlete to experience either negative or positive stress.
© William E. Prentice

| Length of rehabilitation | Reaction to injury | Reaction to rehabilitation | Reaction to return |
|---|---|---|---|
| Short (<4 weeks) | Shock  Relief | Impatience  Optimism | Eagerness  Anticipation |
| Long (>4 weeks) | Fear  Anger | Loss of vigor  Irrational thoughts  Alienation | Acknowledgment |
| Chronic (recurring) | Anger  Frustration | Dependence or independence  Apprehension | Confidence or skepticism |
| Terminating (career-ending) | Isolation  Grief process | Loss of athletic identity | Closure and renewal |

FIGURE 11–2   Progressive reactions of athletes based on severity of injury and length of rehabilitation.

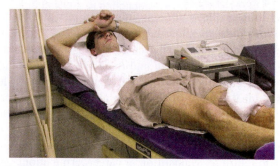

FIGURE 11–3   A sports injury can create psychological reactions characteristic of a sudden loss.

© William E. Prentice

With any type of injury, but particularly with those that require a lengthy period of rehabilitation, athletes whose whole life tends to revolve around a sport may have to make major adjustments in how they perceive themselves and may have to come to terms with how they are perceived by others.[50] Therefore, many athletes have difficulty controlling their emotions when they sustain an injury.

> Injury might mean major changes in the way an athlete behaves socially.

# THE ATHLETE AND THE SOCIOLOGICAL RESPONSE TO INJURY

Following injury, particularly one that requires long-term rehabilitation, all patients and especially athletes may have problems adjusting socially and may feel alienated from the rest of the team.[23] Athletes with an injury that requires weeks or months of rehabilitation before they can return to competition often feel that the coaches have ceased to care, that teammates have no time to spend with them, that friends are no longer around, and that their social life consists of time put into rehabilitation. Some athletes feel that they have received little support from coaches and teammates.[25,62]

Injured athletes may understand that the coach cares but has no expertise in injury management and must be concerned with getting the team ready without them. The athletic trainer has no expertise in coaching but is primarily interested in rehabilitating injuries. Injured athletes may feel unable to maintain or regain normal relationships with teammates.[57] The injured athlete is a reminder that injury can happen, and teammates may pull away from that constant reminder. Friendships based on athletic identification are now compromised because the athletic identification is gone; friends and team members may relate to injured athletes only in terms of what they did yesterday or as injured teammates, not as individuals. Injured athletes no longer feel the team camaraderie that provided a sense of belonging or importance. Athletes who can remain involved with the team, however, feel less isolated

> Patients who are injured must deal with both the physiological and the psychological aspects of injury.
>
> ? What stages of psychological reaction does the patient typically go through following injury?

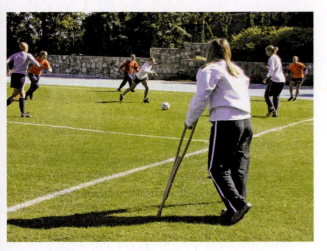

**FIGURE 11-4** It is important to make sure that injured athletes still feel that they are part of the team.
© William E. Prentice

and less guilty about not being able to help the team (Figure 11–4).[25]

## The Athlete's Need for Social Support

The loss of social support can be lessened by the organization of support groups or similar injury groups or by mentoring by athletes who have completed rehabilitation successfully.[18] After injury, athletes need the support of teammates to prevent feelings of negative self-worth and loss of identity. Support groups need to stress the importance of the athlete as a person as well as a team member.[30]

A supporting relationship between the athlete and the athletic trainer is critical to successful rehabilitation.[55] Establishing this relationship may be difficult. Injured athletes often question many aspects of the rehabilitation procedure. They question the doctor's diagnosis; they question the athletic trainer for working them too much and the coach for not paying attention to them. They wonder whether they are thought of as malingerers. They doubt that the athletic trainer, coach, or teammates know how important competition is to them.[25]

> A patient is just beginning a rehabilitation program following injury.
>
> ❓ What specific things can the athletic trainer do to provide social support to that patient?

Toward the end of rehabilitation, the athlete should begin sport-specific drills during practice time with his or her athletic team. The athlete then begins to reenter the team culture and is not isolated from the team environment.[65] Thus, the athlete puts more effort into functional, sport-specific situations that are generally less boring. In so doing, the athlete gains a more realistic appreciation of the skills needed to attain preinjury performance levels. Athletes can more easily tolerate the rehabilitation routine if they can see some carryover to their sport.[25]

## The Athletic Trainer's Role in Providing Social Support

The athletic trainer is often the first person an athlete interacts with after injury. When an athlete is injured and becomes a patient, he or she should get the perception that the athletic trainer cares for him or her as a person and not just as a part of the team.[29] His or her perception of the athletic trainer makes a difference in terms of recovery time and effort.[42] First the patient has to respect the athletic trainer as a person before he or she can trust the athletic trainer in the rehabilitative setting. Successful communication between the athletic trainer and the patient is essential for effective rehabilitation.[5] Taking an interest in athletes before injuries occur enables the athletic trainer to know their personalities and work with them to help build their confidence.[25]

**Be a Good Listener** Active listening is one of the athletic trainer's most important skills. The athletic trainer must learn to listen to the patient beyond the complaining and listen for fear, anger, dejection, or anxiety. With *fear,* the patient may be wondering what the injury means in terms of function and the consequences of the injury on peer relationships. *Anger* is often a feeling of being victimized by the injury and the unfairness of it— "of all people, why did this have to happen to me?". In dejection, the patient may be in low spirits, experiencing feelings of inadequacy, or lack of energy. With *anxiety,* the patient may wonder how he or she can survive the injury and what will happen if he or she cannot return to full competition.[45]

**Find Out What the Problem Is** During an injury evaluation, the athletic trainer should allow the patient to provide as much input about the injury as possible. Paraphrasing or restating the information to the patient will be invaluable to the athletic trainer who is unsure of the mechanism of injury or its results. Statements such as "I see" or "Go ahead" or simply silence allow patients to fully express themselves. One of the most important bits of information can be the question the athletic trainer poses at the end of gathering subjective information—"What else have I not asked you?" or "What else do I need to know about this injury?" Then the athletic trainer should give the patient input in the decision of how the rehabilitation will proceed.

**Be Aware of Body Language** Body language is important. The athletic trainer who continues to work on paperwork while talking to the patient is sending a message that he or she does not care. The athletic trainer needs to be concerned and should make eye contact with the patient and show a genuine interest in his or her problems. This will go a long way toward gaining the patient's confidence and respect.[25]

**Project a Caring Image** It is important for the athletic trainer to consider the patient as an individual instead of as an injury. If the injury is the only consideration, the athletic trainer is caring for the patient superficially, and the patient's attitude will project this.

The relationship between the athletic trainer and the patient should be a personal one. When the athletic trainer treats the patient as an equal, the relationship improves, and it helps the patient accept responsibility for his or her own rehabilitation. With injury, athletes lose control over their physical efforts. They have gone from practicing or competing 3 to 4 hours a day to no activity. They experience a temporary lifestyle change, and their feelings will affect the success or failure of the rehabilitation process. The athletic trainer must establish rapport and show a sense of genuine concern and caring for the patient.

Neglecting injured patients or giving them the perception that they are outcasts can also contribute to injury and reinjury. Athletic trainers who foster this attitude are communicating to patients that they have no self-worth if they are injured. Some athletic trainers go so far as to prevent injured patients from having contact with the team until they are ready to return, or they belittle the patient in front of his or her peers, believing that this will make the patient want to get back to competition quicker. This tactic may work with some patients who have minor injuries, but it may cause major adjustment difficulties for patients who suffer severe injuries.[25]

**Explain the Injury to the Patient** The athletic trainer is often the person who effectively explains the injury to the patient (Figure 11–5). The athletic trainer should take care to explain the situation to the patient

in understandable terms, avoiding the use of excessive medical terminology. The athletic trainer should avoid making false promises to make the patient feel better. In most cases, providing the patient with the simplest explanation acceptable is best. Athletes must be satisfied with the explanation of their injury. Disseminating injury information that is appropriate to a patient's emotional and intellectual level can be a challenge. The rate and degree of acceptance is not the same in all patients. The severity of the injury is important, but the patient's perception of that severity is what matters in the rehabilitation process.[25] Thus, the physiological must be interrelated with the psychological.

**Manage the Stress of Injury** The amount of stress associated with playing a sport and the meaning the sport has to the injured patient can impact the patient's compliance with rehabilitation.[22] The patient will have a more successful rehabilitation when he or she is fully engaged in it, much as an athlete will have a more successful sports career when he or she is interested and involved in the sport. Stress can be a deterrent to engaging in rehabilitation. Several techniques the athletic trainer can use, such as relaxation, imagery, cognitive restructuring, and thought stopping (discussed later in this chapter), may lessen a patient's stressful reaction to injury. Often a change in a patient's perception of his or her injury and rehabilitation can affect their outcome.[25]

**Help the Athlete Return to Competition** Returning to competition is another area in which the athletic trainer can help the injured patient. Often, the patient's perception is that he or she is ready to return and is not being allowed to or that he or she is being forced to return before being ready. The athletic trainer can help the patient make a decision based on facts, not clouded by emotions.

The athletic trainer can be of great help when an injured patient is unable or unwilling to continue to participate in his or her sport. Frequently, the athlete's identity is intertwined with the sport.[30] The transition into a completely different culture can be a stressful, frustrating, and traumatic experience for an injured patient.[25]

# PREDICTORS OF INJURY

## The Injury-Prone Athlete

Some athletes seem to have a pattern of injury, whereas others in exactly the same position with the same physical makeup are injury free.[32] It has been suggested that some psychological traits may predispose an athlete to repeated injury. No single personality type has been recognized as injury prone. However, the person who likes to take risks often seems injury prone.[30] Other types of athletes who may be

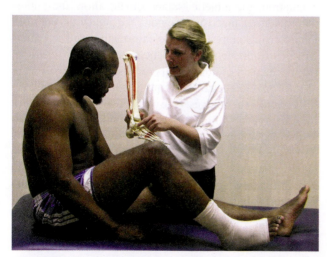

FIGURE 11–5 Educating the athlete about his or her injury is a major goal in the rehabilitation process.
© William E. Prentice

> Many injury-prone athletes are risk takers.

predisposed to injury are reserved, detached, or tender-minded players[19] and apprehensive, overprotective, or easily distracted players.[10] These individuals usually also lack the ability to cope with the stress associated with the risks and their consequences. Some other factors may also contribute to the likelihood of injury, such as trying to reduce anxiety by being more aggressive or continuing to play while injured because of fear of failure or guilt over unobtainable or unrealistic goals.[1,30]

Some athletes seem to get injured more often than others.

**?** What factors should the athletic trainer look for that might make the possibility of injury more likely in certain athletes?

## Stress and the Risk of Injury

A **stressor** is not something that an athlete can do to his or her body, but it is something that the brain tells the athlete is happening.[48] When change occurs, the brain interprets that change and tells the body how to react to it. Stress does not always imply a morbid change—it could also be associated with intense pleasure.[48] Stress is caused or triggered by stressors that may be physical, social, or psychological and that may be negative or positive in nature. Positive beneficial stress is referred to as *eustress,* whereas the term *distress* describes detrimental responses or negative stressors. Often, there is a fine line between eustress and distress. Sometimes the difference between eustress and distress is only a matter of interpretation; a stressor can be interpreted as either a threat or a challenge.

A number of studies on adverse stress have shown a relationship between life events or personal losses and physical injury among athletes who engage in high-intensity sports.[19,64] The stress-injury model proposes that athletes with a history of many stressors and personality characteristics that heighten the stress response will be more likely to feel that they are in a stressful situation and thus will manifest greater physiological activation and attentional disruptions. This stress response causes an increased risk of injury.[64] Negative stress tends to decrease the athlete's attentional focus and create muscle tension, which may lead to a reduction in flexibility, problems in coordination, and an overall decrease in movement efficiency. A loss of attentional focus can cause the athlete to miss important cues.[64]

All living organisms are endowed with the ability to cope effectively with stressful situations. Without stress, there would be very little constructive activity or positive change.[22]

**Sports participation is both a physical and an emotional stressor.**

Negative stress can contribute to poor health, whereas positive stress can enhance growth and development. A healthy life must have a balance of stress; too little stress causes a "rusting out," and too much can cause burnout.[32]

Every day athletes place their bodies in stressful situations. Their bodies undergo numerous "flight-or-fight" reactions to avoid injury or other physically and emotionally threatening situations.

**Physical Response to Stress** Many stress responses are apparent when athletes adjust to a physical injury and/or undergo a program of rehabilitation.[15]

Stress is a psychosomatic phenomenon. Injury can be a major stressor. Hormonal responses are reflected by an increase in the secretion of cortisol. Negative stress can produce fear and anxiety. Initially, in an acute reaction to a negative stress situation, secretions from the adrenal gland sharply increase, creating the well-known flight-or-fight response. With adrenaline in the bloodstream, pupils dilate, hearing becomes more acute, muscles become more responsive, and blood pressure increases to facilitate the absorption of oxygen. In addition to these responses, respiration and heart rate increase to further prepare the body for action.

In general, stress can be acute and chronic. During acute stress, the threat is immediate and the response is instantaneous. Physiologically, the primary reaction in the acute stage is produced by the release of epinephrine and norepinephrine from the adrenal medulla. Chronic stress persists over time and leads to an increase of blood corticoids from the adrenal cortex.

An athlete who is taken out of a sport because of an injury or illness reacts in a personal way. The athlete who has trained diligently, has looked forward to a successful season, and is suddenly thwarted in that goal by an injury or illness can be emotionally devastated.

At the time of injury or illness, the patient may normally fear the experience of pain or possible disability. The patient may feel a sense of anxiety about suddenly becoming disabled and being unable to continue sport participation.[48] An injury or illness is a stressor that results from an external or internal sensory stimulus. Coping with the stressor depends on the patient's cognitive appraisal.

**Emotional Response to Stress** Sports are stressors to the athlete. An athlete often walks a fine line between reaching and maintaining peak performance and

Most athletic trainers do not have academic training as counselors or psychologists.

**?** If an injured patient is not responding psychologically to the efforts of the athletic trainer to rehabilitate and return that individual to full activity, what options does the athletic trainer have for referring this patient for additional help?

11–4 Clinical Application Exercise

overtraining. Besides performance concerns, many peripheral stressors can be imposed on the athlete, such as unreasonable expectations by the athlete, the coaches, or the parents. Worries that stem from school, work, and family can also be major causes of emotional stress.

The athletic trainer is often the first person to notice that an athlete is stressed emotionally. The athlete whose performance is declining and whose personality is changing may need a conditioning program that is less demanding. Conferring with the athlete might reveal emotional and physical problems that need to be dealt with by a counselor, psychologist, or physician.

Injury prevention is both psychological and physiological. The athlete who enters a contest while angry, frustrated, or discouraged or while experiencing some other disturbing emotional state is more prone to injury than is the one who is better adjusted emotionally. The angry player, for example, wants to vent that anger in some way and therefore often loses perspective on desirable and approved conduct. In the grip of emotion, skill and coordination are sacrificed, resulting in an injury that otherwise would have been avoided.

Although athletic trainers are typically not educated as professional counselors or psychologists, they must nevertheless be concerned about the feelings of the athletes they work with.[51] No one can work closely with human beings without becoming involved with their emotions and, at times, their personal problems. The athletic trainer is usually a caring person and, as such, is placed in numerous daily situations in which close interpersonal relationships are important. The athletic trainer must have appropriate communication skills to confront an athlete's fears, frustrations, and daily crises and to refer individuals with serious emotional problems to the proper professionals.

> The athletic trainer must have some counseling skills.

The team physician, like the coach and the athletic trainer, plays an integral part in helping the athlete who is overly stressed. Many psychophysiological responses thought to be emotional are, in fact, caused by some undetected physical dysfunction. Therefore, referral to a physician, sport psychologist, clinical psychologist, or psychiatrist should be routine. (See *Focus Box 11–6:* "Keys to recognition and referral of student-athletes with psychological concerns.")

## Overtraining

Overtraining occurs because of an imbalance between a physical load placed on an athlete and his or her coping capacity.[2] Both physiological and psychological factors underlie overtraining. Overtraining can lead to staleness and eventual burnout.

**Staleness** There are countless reasons some athletes become "stale." The athlete could be training too hard and long without proper rest. Seasons can be long and practices can become repetitious and boring. Staleness is often attributed to emotional problems stemming from daily worries, fears, and anxieties. **Anxiety** is one of the most common mental and emotional stress producers. It is a vague fear, a sense of apprehension, and restlessness.[9] Typically, the anxious athlete is unable to describe the problem. The athlete feels inadequate in a certain situation but is unable to say why. Heart palpitations, shortness of breath, sweaty palms, a constricted throat, and headaches may accompany anxiety. Children who are pushed too hard by parents may acquire a number of psychological problems. They may even fail purposely in their sport just to rid themselves of the painful stress of achieving. A coach who acts as a drill sergeant—one who continually gives negative reinforcements—will likely cause athletes to develop symptoms of overstress. Athletes are more prone to staleness if the rewards of their efforts are minimal. A losing season commonly causes many athletes to become stale.

*Symptoms of Staleness* Staleness is evidenced by a wide variety of symptoms: a deterioration in the usual standard of performance, chronic fatigue, apathy, loss of appetite, indigestion, weight loss, and an inability to sleep or rest properly.[19] Many athletes will exhibit higher blood pressure or an increased pulse rate, both at rest and during activity, as well as increased **catecholamine** release. All these signs indicate adrenal exhaustion. Stale athletes become irritable and restless, have to force themselves to practice, and exhibit signs of boredom about everything connected with the activity (see *Focus Box 11–1:* "Recognizing signs and symptoms of staleness in athletes").[26]

Athletes who show signs of staleness also increase their potential for both acute and overuse injuries and infections.[30] Stress fractures and tendinitis are typical injuries that can occur with overtraining.

Overtraining must be recognized early and dealt with immediately.[60] The athlete should take a short break from training or decrease the workload by performing less work but with the same intensity.[60] When the athlete shows signs of a full recovery, a gradual return to the same workload can be initiated. Competition must be stopped. An abrupt cessation of training, however, can produce a serious physiological and psychological condition known as sudden exercise abstinence syndrome (see *Focus Box 11–2:* "Sudden exercise abstinence syndrome").

**Burnout** Burnout is a syndrome related to physical and emotional exhaustion that leads to a negative self-concept, negative job or sport attitudes, and loss of concern for the feelings of others.[12] Burnout stems from overwork and can

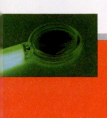

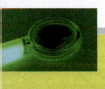

affect both the athlete and the athletic trainer. Athletes are often pulled in many directions trying to satisfy the demands of school, friends, family, and maybe a job in addition to their sport.

Burnout can be detrimental to an athlete's general health.[12] Symptoms include frequent headaches, gastrointestinal disturbances, sleeplessness, and chronic fatigue. Athletes suffering from burnout may also experience feelings of depersonalization, increased emotional exhaustion, a reduced sense of accomplishment, cynicism, and a depressed mood.[61]

## REACTING TO ATHLETES WITH INJURIES

Even though athletic trainers are proficient in the areas of injury prevention, injury rehabilitation, and nutrition, they are not usually academically trained counselors.[37] To meet other psychological needs of the athlete, the athletic trainer may need to refer the athlete to a sport psychologist or to a counselor or clinical psychologist if a sport psychologist is not available.[11,46]

No matter what reaction the injured athlete displays, the athletic trainer should respond to the patient as a person, not as an injury. An injured patient can be difficult to be around, especially in the early stages of a serious injury. The injury may suddenly force the patient to be dependent and helpless.[26] The patient may regress to childlike behavior, crying or displacing anger toward the person administering first aid. Table 11–1 provides some suggestions on rendering emotional first aid. During this time, comfort, care, and communication should be given freely.[41]

Those involved with health care for the injured patient must be honest, supportive, and respectful of the patient during the time of disability. They need to understand the patient at a deeper level and how he or she is coping with this stressful event.[63] A number of questions should be answered. Does the doctor-patient relationship contain confidence, trust, and optimism?[30] Does the patient fear that a pending surgery will be more painful or will make him or her unable to continue in the sport?[41] How long is the recovery? What is the possibility of reinjury?[41] Is forced retirement possible? If so, how well will the patient adjust? What are the athlete's attitudes toward rehabilitation?

### The Catastrophic Injury

A permanent functional disability is a catastrophic injury. Intervention must be directed toward the psychological impact of the trauma and the patient's ability to cope during medical treatment.[43] A catastrophic injury profoundly affects all aspects of a person's functioning. The athletic trainer must arrange for the patient to see a psychologist or a psychiatrist to make certain that the patient is

**TABLE 11–1** Emotional First Aid

| Type of Emotional Reaction | Outward Signs | Athletic Trainer's Reactions | |
|---|---|---|---|
| | | **Yes** | **No** |
| **Normal** | Weakness, trembling<br>Nausea, vomiting<br>Perspiration<br>Diarrhea<br>Fear, anxiety<br>Heart pounding | Be calm and reassuring | Avoid pity |
| **Overreaction** | Excessive talking<br>Argumentativeness<br>Inappropriate joke telling<br>Hyperactivity | Allow athlete to vent emotions | Avoid telling athlete he or she is acting abnormally |
| **Underreaction** | Depression; sitting or standing numbly<br>Little or no talking<br>Lack of emotion<br>Confusion<br>Failure to respond to questions | Be empathetic; encourage talking to express feelings | Avoid being abrupt; avoid pity |

receiving the best possible care.[56] The athletic trainer should also be cognizant of the effects of such an injury on other team members.

### The Psychological Effects of Injury on the Athletic Trainer

The relationships that an athletic trainer develops with a particular athlete or group of athletes are often very special. Athletic trainers tend to be very caring individuals and when one of those athletes is injured it is likely that the athletic trainer will be psychologically and emotionally affected by that injury as well. It is essential that the athletic trainer make decisions regarding care and management of that injury based on professional training and knowledge of the most appropriate course of action, given the circumstances and severity of the injury. The athletic trainer needs to make sure that emotional attachment to the injured athlete does not cloud or otherwise influence his or her decisions. The athletic trainer must be prepared to deal with significant injuries, to people he or she cares about, that may be psychologically disturbing or catastrophic. An athletic trainer must deal with the injured athlete and situation at hand and worry about how the injury has affected him or her personally at a later time. While the athletic trainer must be strong and confident in managing the initial injury, he or she may need to seek counseling to deal with the impact of that injury on his or her own emotional and psychological state.

# PSYCHOLOGICAL FACTORS IN THE REHABILITATION PROCESS

A successful program of rehabilitation takes the patient's psyche into consideration. Successful treatment that involves therapeutic modalities and exercise rehabilitation depends on rapport, cooperation, and education.[26]

*Rapport* is a relationship of mutual trust and understanding. Patients must thoroughly trust their athletic trainers or therapists to achieve maximum rehabilitation, and they must believe that their best interests are being considered at all times.[26]

> **The psychology of sports rehabilitation must include establishing**
> - Rapport
> - Cooperation
> - Education

A highly motivated athlete begrudges every moment spent out of action and can become somewhat difficult to handle if the rehabilitative process moves slowly.[8] Often, the patient blames the physician or the athletic trainer for not doing all that he or she can. To avoid this situation, the patient must learn early in the rehabilitative process that healing is a cooperative undertaking with the patient, physician, and athletic trainer acting as a team, working toward the same end—the return to full function as soon as physically and physiologically possible. To create this atmosphere, the patient must feel free to vent frustrations, to ask questions, and to expect clear answers about any aspect of the rehabilitative process. The patient must feel

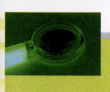

### Educating the injured patient about the rehabilitation process

1. Describe the injury clearly, using anatomy charts or other visual aids. The athlete must fully understand the nature of his or her injury and its prognosis (expected outcome), based on similar cases. A false hope for a fast comeback should not be engendered if a full recovery is doubtful.
2. Explain how the healing process occurs and estimate the time needed for such healing.
3. Describe in detail the consequences of not following proper procedures.
4. Describe an overall rehabilitative plan, including progressive steps or phases within the plan.
5. Explain each physical modality or exercise, how it works, and its purpose.
6. Make the athlete aware that recovery depends as much on his or her attitude toward the rehabilitative process as on what therapy is being given. A positive attitude leads to a conscientious and persistent effort to speed recovery.
7. Realize that the athlete needs to see immediate results.[14]
8. Plan rehabilitation around the athlete's schedule.[14]
9. Ensure that the rehabilitation facility is convenient to the athlete.
10. Monitor the athlete regularly.

a major responsibility to come into the athletic training clinic on time and not skip appointments. He or she must be motivated to perform all exercises correctly and all home exercises regularly.[6]

Many injured athletes lack patience. Nevertheless, patience and desire are necessary adjuncts in securing a reasonable rate of recovery.[23]

To ensure maximum positive responses from the patient in all aspects of rehabilitation, he or she must receive continual education. All education must be provided in layman's language and at a level appropriate for the patient's background and education. *Focus Box 11–3: "Educating the injured patient about the rehabilitation process"* is a list of educational matters that athletic trainers and therapists must address carefully.

## Psychological Approaches during the Phases of Rehabilitation

The rehabilitation process incorporates both therapeutic modalities and exercise rehabilitation. During each phase of rehabilitation, the athletic trainer or therapist must address the patient's specific psychological issues.[66]

**Immediate Postinjury Period** The immediate postinjury period is a time of fear and denial for the patient, who often has severe pain and disability. Emotional first aid must be administered.[68] The physician must give an accurate diagnosis and a full explanation of that diagnosis to the patient and family members. As much as possible, the patient needs to know the course of treatment, the prognosis, and the planned goals. The patient must know from the beginning that he or she is an integral part of rehabilitation.

> A patient has been rehabilitating a surgically repaired knee for 6 months. Physically, she is capable of returning to activity but seems very hesitant to engage in an activity where there is potential contact.
>
> **?** Should the athletic trainer push her back into activity despite her apprehension?
>
> **11–5 Clinical Application Exercise**

**Early Postoperative Period** When surgery is performed, the injured athlete becomes a disabled patient. Each phase of the healing process and the purpose of each treatment procedure should be explained to the patient. The patient should be encouraged to maintain aerobic conditioning by exercising the noninjured body parts.

**Advanced Postoperative, or Rehabilitation, Period** While the patient rehabilitates the injured body part, he or she should continue to condition unaffected body regions both aerobically and anaerobically. The patient must feel that he or she is in control and can make choices. The patient's confidence is increased by small successes. Milestones must be kept realistic, and positive verbal reinforcement must be given by the coach, peers, and sports medicine team.[68]

This period places greater emphasis on movement patterns that mimic a specific sport. Injured athletes need reassurance that they will be able to return to their sport and once again achieve success. Their fear of failure and anxiety should be dealt with by positive reinforcement.[63]

**Return to Full Activity** Many patients return to participation physically ready but psychologically ill prepared.[43] Although few patients will admit it, they return to participation feeling anxious about getting hurt again. This feeling may, in some ways, be a self-fulfilling prophecy. In other words, anxiety can lead to muscle tension, which in turn can lead to disruption of normal coordination, thus producing conditions that are favorable for reinjury or for injury to another body part.[43]

The athletic trainer allows the patient to regain full performance by progressing in small increments.[24] Return might include, first, performing all the necessary skills away from the team. This action may be followed by engaging in a highly controlled small-group practice and then attempting participation in full-team noncontact practice. The patient should be encouraged to express freely any anxiety that he or she may feel and to engage in full contact only when anxiety is at a minimum.

The use of scales developed specifically for the purpose of assessing the athlete's readiness to return to competitive activity can be helpful to both the athletic trainer, the physician, and the coach who must make that decision.[16]

## Goal Setting as a Motivator for Compliance during Rehabilitation

Goal setting has been shown to be an effective motivator for compliance to the rehabilitation of an athletic injury, as well as for reaching goals in a general sport setting.[59] Athletes have set goals since their first competition, usually starting at an early age. They have set goals to run faster, jump higher, shoot straighter, throw longer, hit harder, and so on. These goals have all had one thing in common: They were not achieved with one burst of effort but resulted from meeting many short-term goals before achieving the long-term goal.[59]

> Establishing progressive, attainable goals is essential in rehabilitation.

In any rehabilitation setting, patients need to know exactly what the goal is and have a sense that they can meet it.[59] For example, telling a patient that, by a certain day, he or she should be bearing partial weight with crutches is neither specific nor measurable. It is more effective to say that, by achieving a certain range of motion and strength level, the foot can be placed on the ground with weight bearing and that the measurement of success is that the partial weight bearing is without pain. The goal must be a challenge but one that the patient can reach with reasonable rehabilitation effort.[2] Goals that are easily reached have no reward in success. Goals must be personal and internally satisfying, not goals imposed on the patient by the athletic trainer. Setting goals needs to be a joint venture between the patient and the athletic trainer to be successful.[14] **The injured patient has to take responsibility for the progress of the injury and be responsible for doing the necessary rehabilitation.**[7]

Goal setting incorporates a multitude of other motivating factors that intuitively appear to increase the odds of compliance by reducing the stress associated with injury rehabilitation. These buffers incorporated within the goal-setting paradigm include positive reinforcement when goals are met, time management for incorporating goals into a lifestyle, a feeling of social support when goals are set with the athletic trainer, and feelings of increased self-efficacy when goals are achieved. Goals are easily understood by athletes, are concrete concepts, are active events, and are a natural part of their sport.[59] Goals can be set daily for a sense of accomplishment, weekly for a sense of progress, and monthly or yearly for long-term achievement.

# PSYCHOLOGICAL SKILLS TRAINING TECHNIQUES

Psychological skills training techniques have long been used to enhance sports skills.[39] Many of these techniques are appropriate for injured athletes in the process of healing and rehabilitating a serious injury or illness.[39]

Athletic trainers can help injured athletes to respond positively to their injuries via specific psychological skills training techniques.[67] It should be noted that serious emotional instabilities must be referred to a professional psychologist.[52] Some techniques that are available are quieting the anxious mind, mental and emotional assessment, pain control, and healing approaches.

## Techniques for Reducing Tension and Anxiety

Fear and anxiety are always present to some degree in a serious sports injury or illness. Fear of pain, loss of control, and unknown consequences of disability can create physical and emotional tensions. Two techniques that the athlete can learn to deal with anxiety and tension are meditation and progressive relaxation.

**Meditation** Meditators focus on a constant mental stimulus, such as a phrase, a sound, or a single word repeated silently or audibly, or they gaze steadily at some object. The passive attitude of meditation takes a "don't work at it" approach. As thoughts come into the consciousness, they are

> In general, athletes are highly motivated individuals.
>
> **?** What can the athletic trainer do to motivate an injured patient to be compliant with the rehabilitation program?

> An athlete who has experienced several different injuries throughout the season is anxious about performing at his usual level.
>
> **?** What can the athletic trainer recommend to help the patient relax before a game?

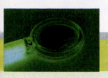
### The meditation technique

*Quieting the body*

The person sits comfortably in a position that maintains a straight back; the head is erect and the hands are placed loosely on each leg or on the arm of a chair, with both feet firmly planted on the floor. To ensure a relaxed state, the meditator should mentally relax each body part, starting at the feet. If a great deal of tension is present, Jacobson's relaxation exercise might be appropriate, or several deep breaths are taken in and exhaled slowly and completely, allowing the body to settle more and more into a relaxed state after each emptying of the lungs.

*The meditative technique*

Once the person is in a quiet environment and fully physically relaxed, the meditative process can begin. With each exhalation, the person emits a repetitive self-talk of a short word, such as *one* or *peace*. The word is repeated for 10 to 20 minutes. Such words as *peace* and *relaxed* are excellent relaxers; however, Benson[3] has suggested that the word *one* produces the same physiological responses as any other word. If extraneous thoughts occur, the person just returns to the meditation process.

*After meditating*

After repeating the special word, the person comes back to physical reality slowly and gently. As awareness increases, physical activity should also increase. Moving too quickly or standing up suddenly might produce lightheadedness or dizziness.

---

quietly turned away, and the individual returns to the focus of attention. The meditator takes a comfortable position and relaxes the various major body areas. To effectively conduct a meditation session, a quiet environment is essential. Normally, the eyes are closed unless the meditator is focusing on some external object (see *Focus Box 11–4: "The meditation technique"*).

**Progressive Relaxation** Progressive muscle relaxation is a commonly used technique for relaxation.[27] It can be considered intense training in the awareness of tension and tension's release. Progressive relaxation may be practiced in a reclining position or while seated in a chair. Each muscle group is tensed from 5 to 7 seconds, then relaxed for 20 to 30 seconds. In most cases, one repetition of the procedure is sufficient; however, if tension remains in the area, repeated contraction and relaxation is permitted. The sequence of tensing and releasing is systematically applied to the following body areas: the dominant hand and forearm; dominant upper arm; nondominant hand and forearm; nondominant upper arm; forehead; eyes and nose; cheeks and mouth; neck and throat; chest; back; respiratory muscles; abdomen; dominant upper leg, calf, and foot; and nondominant upper leg, calf, and foot. Throughout the session, a number of expressions for relaxing may be used: "Let the tension dissolve. Let go of the tension. I am bringing my muscles to zero. Let the tension flow out of my body."

After the individual has become aware of the tension in the body, the contraction is gradually decreased until little remains. At this point, the individual focuses on one area and mentally wills the tension to decrease to zero, or complete relaxation.

Jacobson's progressive relaxation normally takes longer than the time allowed in a typical session or than the individual would want to spend.[27] A short form can be developed that, although not as satisfactory, helps the individual become better aware of the body. The essence of Jacobson's method is to recognize and consciously release muscular tension.

> **An athlete has a chronic back injury.**
>
> ❓ How can the athletic trainer help the athlete deal with the chronic pain?

> **11–9 Clinical Application Exercise**
>
> A collegiate gymnast suffers a season-ending shoulder injury. She expresses concern about gaining weight due to the lack of exercise.
>
> ❓ How should the athletic trainer deal with this situation? What tools should he or she use?

### Techniques for Cognitive Restructuring

Some injured athletes practice irrational thinking and negative self-talk. This habit can hinder the treatment progress. An important approach to negative thoughts is cognitive restructuring.[22] Two successful methods to thought restructuring are refuting irrational thoughts and thought stopping.[26]

**Refuting Irrational Thoughts** This method is designed to deal with a person's internal dialogue. Psychologist

Albert Ellis developed a system to change irrational ideas and beliefs.[26] His system is called rational emotive therapy. The basic premise is that actual events do not create emotions; rather, it is the self-talk after the event that does. In other words, irrational self-talk causes anxiety, anger, and depression.

Individuals who are under severe stress should explore their self-talk. Following are two examples:

1. *Facts and events:* A tennis player, after surgical repair of her shoulder, is impatient about the speed of recovery. Emotions of anger and depression are present.
   *Negative self-talk:*
   "I was stupid to get hurt."
   "Why me? Why did I have to get hurt?"
   "I have never been laid up before. It's not fair!"
   *Positive self-talk:*
   "I was hurt and now I am doing my best to get well."
   "Every day I am getting better."
   "The athletic trainers are doing their best for me."

2. *Facts and events:* A football player blows a knee out and requires surgery. Emotions of anger and denial are present.
   *Negative self-talk:*
   "I was blindsided and no penalty was called."
   "I could have avoided such a serious injury if the coaches coached better."
   *Positive self-talk:*
   "I am hurt, but because of my good fitness level I will recover quickly."
   "I plan to do everything I am told to recover quickly."

**Thought Stopping** Thought stopping is an excellent cognitive technique for helping the athlete overcome worries and doubts. The anxious athlete, especially one who is hurt, will often repeat negative, unproductive, and unrealistic statements during self-talk, such as "I am no good to anyone now that I am hurt" or "Everyone on the team is going to pass me by while I am recovering." Thought stopping consists of focusing on the undesired thoughts and stopping them with the command "stop" or a loud noise. After the thought interruption, a positive statement is inserted, such as "My shoulder is healing and I'll play as well as or maybe better than before."[23]

## Imagery

Imagery is the use of the senses to create or re-create an experience in the mind.[13] Visual images used in the rehabilitation process include visual rehearsal, emotive imagery rehearsal, and body rehearsal.[36] Visual rehearsal uses both coping and mastery rehearsal. In coping rehearsal, athletes visually rehearse problems they feel may stand in the way of their return to competition. They then rehearse how they will overcome these

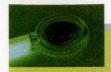

### Healing images

*Treatment modalities*

- Ultrasound increases circulation, bringing healthy new tissue to the area.
- Cold application inhibits pain.

*Exercise rehabilitation*

- Muscle fibers increase in size and become stronger.
- Joint range of motion increases, so joints become fully functional.

*Medications*

- Antiinflammatories decrease inflammation and swelling.
- Pain medication inhibits pain.

problems.[36] Mastery rehearsal aids in gaining the confidence and motivational skills necessary. Athletes visualize their successful return to competition, beginning with early practice drills and continuing on to the game situation.

Emotive rehearsal aids the injured athlete in gaining confidence and security by visualizing scenes relating to the positive feelings of enthusiasm, confidence, and pride—in other words, the emotional rewards of praise and success from participating well in competition.[10] Body rehearsal empirically helps patients in the healing process. It is suggested that patients visualize their bodies healing internally both during the rehabilitation procedures and throughout their daily activities.[50] To do this, patients have to have a good understanding of the injury and of the type of healing occurring during the rehabilitation process.[38]

Care should be taken to explain the healing and rehabilitative process clearly but not overwhelm patients with so much information that they become intimidated and fearful.[53] Educate patients only to the amount of knowledge they require (see *Focus Box 11–5: "Healing images"*).

## Techniques for Coping with Pain

The injured patient can be taught relatively simple techniques to inhibit pain.[1] At no time should pain be completely inhibited because pain is a protective mechanism. The patient can reduce pain in three ways: reducing muscle tension, diverting attention away from the pain, and changing the pain sensation to another sensation.

**Reducing Muscle Tension** The pain response can be associated with general muscular tension stemming from anxiety or from the pain-spasm-pain cycle of the injury. In both of these situations, muscle tension increases the sensation of pain. Conversely, relaxation methods that reduce muscle tension can also decrease the awareness of pain. Both the Benson[4] and the Jacobson[27] techniques of stress reduction can be advantageous in pain reduction.

**Diverting Attention** A positive method for decreasing pain perception is to divert attention from the injury.[28] The athletic trainer should engage the patient in mental problem solving, such as adding or subtracting a column of numbers or counting spots on the floor. The patient can also divert pain by fantasizing about pleasant activities, such as sunbathing at the beach, sailing, or skiing.

**Altering the Pain Sensation** Imagination is one of the most powerful forces available to human beings. Negative imagination can be a major cause of illness, stress, and muscular tension, whereas positive imagination can produce wellness and counteract stress.

Through imagination, the patient can alter pain sensation to another sensation.[28] For example, immersing a body part in ice-cold water can change the pain to a sensation of cold dampness. The patient can visualize that the injured part is relaxed and comfortable instead of painful. Imagining a peaceful scene at a pleasant spot, such as the beach or mountains, can both relax the athlete and divert attention from the pain.

# MENTAL DISORDERS

A mental illness is any disorder that affects the mind or behavior. The *Diagnostic and Statistical Manual of Mental Disorders* defines a mental disorder as "a syndrome characterized by clinically significant disturbances in an individual's cognition, emotional regulation, or behavior that reflects a dysfunction in the psychological, biological, or developmental process underlying mental functioning." They are "usually associated with significant distress or disability in social, occupational, or other important activities." Mental disorders are common in our society. It has been estimated that one in every four to five youths in the United States will experience impairment during his or her lifetime as a result of some mental health disorder.[34]

> An athlete goes to the athletic trainer concerned about her recent changes in mood. She says she feels positive and upbeat one minute but the next minute feels sad and apprehensive.
>
> ❓ What mood disorder might the athlete have, and how should this condition be managed?

If one considers the number of student-athletes in colleges and universities, as well as secondary and middle schools, the likelihood is high that there will be a significant number of athletes who experience one or more psychological concerns. Thus, it is critical that the athletic trainer work with school and athletic administrators and other health care providers to develop a plan to identify student-athletes with psychological concerns and most importantly facilitate an effective referral system to institutional or community-based mental health care professionals that may include physicians, psychiatrists, clinical psychologists, school counselors, nurses, or social workers for evaluation and treatment.[40,44,52] **SoR:B**

In 2015, an interassociation task force developed the consensus statement "Interassociation recommendations for developing a plan to recognize and refer student athletes with psychological concerns at the secondary school level: A consensus statement" http://natajournals.org/doi/pdf/10.4085/1062-6050-50.3.03. *Focus Box 11–6* discusses "Keys to recognition and referral of student-athletes with psychological concerns." In the past, mental disorders were generally classified as being either *neuroses* or *psychoses*.[20] A neurosis was thought to be an unpleasant mental symptom in a person who has intact reality testing. Symptoms of neurotic behavior included anxiousness, depression, or obsession with a solid base in reality. A psychosis was described as a disturbance in which there was a disintegration in personality and loss of contact with reality, characterized by delusions and hallucinations.[54] Mental illnesses are no longer classified as neuroses or psychoses. Instead, some 300 different mental problems have been identified.[20]

## Mood Disorders

Mood swings ranging from happiness to sadness are normal. However, a mood swing is pathological when it disrupts normal behavior, is prolonged, and is accompanied by physical symptoms (such as sleep disturbances or appetite disturbances).

| Mood disorders: |
| :--- |
| • Depression |
| • Seasonal affective disorder |

**Depression** *Depression* (unipolar) is a disease in which an individual experiences helplessness and misery, loss of energy, excessive guilt, diminished ability to think, changes in eating and sleeping habits, and recurrent thoughts of hurting themselves, suicide, or death.[3] One in five people suffer from some form of depression. In *bipolar depression* (formerly called manic depression), an individual goes from exaggerated feelings of happiness and great energy to extreme states of depression.[43] Treatment must be individualized and might include psychotherapy and antidepressant medication.

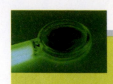

# FOCUS 11–6 Focus on Therapeutic Intervention

## Keys to recognition and referral of student-athletes with psychological conerns

- Recognize situations that may create stress
- Recognize symptoms of depression
- Recognize symptoms of anxiety
- Recognize signs that may be of concern based on psychological response to:
  - injury or loss of playing time or career
  - concussion
  - substance or alcohol abuse
  - ADHD
  - eating disorder
  - bullying or hazing
- Identify other behaviors to monitor

## Reasons for referral for psychological concerns

- The athletic trainer, school nurse, school counselor, team physician, or coach identifies potential psychological concerns for a student-athlete based on:
  - mental health history
  - present psychological status
  - preparticipation physical examination
  - the student-athlete's answers to follow-up questions
- Any evidence that the student-athlete has thoughts or feelings or shows signs of suicide
- Any concerns that the psychological state of a student-athlete may pose a threat that endangers the health and safety of others

*Developed from Neal, T, et al.: Inter-association recommendations for developing a plan to recognize and refer student-athletes with psychological concerns at the secondary school level: An executive summary of a consensus statement, *Journal of Athletic Training* 48(5):716–20, 2013.

**Seasonal Affective Disorder** Seasonal affective disorder (SAD) is characterized by mental depression related to a certain season of the year.[43] SAD is most likely to occur during the winter months due to a decrease in the amount of sunlight. The symptoms include fatigue, diminished concentration, and daytime drowsiness. It usually occurs in adults and is four times more common in women than in men. SAD is commonly treated with light therapy, stress management, antidepressants, and exercise.

## Anxiety Disorders

Anxiety disorders contribute to about 20 percent of all medical conditions among Americans seeking medical care.[20] Everyone occasionally experiences anxiety. Anxiety can cause a number of physiological responses, including sweating, increased heart rate, increased blood pressure, stomach discomfort, chills, dry mouth, difficulty concentrating, irritability, and sleep disturbances. Anxiety is abnormal when it begins to interfere with emotional well-being or normal daily functioning. *General anxiety* consists of persistent or unrealistic worrying that lasts for 6 months or longer.

**Panic Attacks** A *panic attack* is an unexpected and unprovoked emotionally intense experience of terror and fear. The physiological responses are similar to those of someone who fears he or she is in a life-threatening situation. Panic attacks occur in about 30 percent of young adults, are most likely to occur at night, and tend to run in families. Behavioral modification and medications that suppress fear are helpful in controlling panic attacks.[43]

> **Anxiety disorders:**
> - Panic attacks
> - Phobias

**Phobias** A *phobia* is a persistent and irrational fear of a specific situation, activity, or object that creates an intense desire to avoid the feared stimulus.[43] Some common phobias are fear of social situations, fear of height, fear of closed spaces, and fear of flying. Symptoms include increased heart rate, difficulty breathing, sweating, and dizziness. Treatments include behavioral modification, antidepressant or antianxiety medications, and systematic desensitization, a therapeutic technique in which the patient gradually confronts the source of the fear.

## Personality Disorders

All of us have individual personality traits that make us who we are. A personality disorder is a pathological disturbance in cognition, affect, interpersonal functioning, or impulse control.[20] Usually, the personality disorder is of long duration and can be traced to some event or circumstance occurring in adolescence. Treatment may involve psychotherapy and the use of psychopharmacological drugs.

> **Personality disorders:**
> - Paranoia
> - Obsessive-compulsive disorder
> - Posttraumatic stress disorder

**Paranoia** *Paranoia* is having unrealistic and unfounded suspicions about specific people or things.[54] Paranoid individuals are constantly on guard and cannot be convinced that their suspicions are not correct. Over time, resentment and anger develop toward a specific person or object. Paranoid individuals are often forced to seek medical care.

**Obsessive-Compulsive Disorder** *Obsessive-compulsive disorder* is characterized by a combination of emotional and behavioral symptoms. The symptoms of obsessive behavior are recurrent, inappropriate thoughts, feelings, impulses, or images arising from within that a person cannot eliminate by ignoring or neutralizing through other actions, even though they realize that they are wrong.[43] Compulsive behavior involves engaging in unreasonable repetitive acts, such as washing hands or counting in response to obsessive thoughts. This behavior interferes with normal daily functioning. Behavioral psychotherapy that attempts to restructure the environment to minimize the tendency to act compulsively, in addition to appropriate medication, is helpful.[1]

**Posttraumatic Stress Disorder** Individuals who suffer a psychologically traumatic event, such as a personal assault or abuse, a sexual assault or harassment, or a plane crash, may reexperience this event through nightmares or an exaggerated startle response.[20] They may experience a numbing of general responsiveness, insomnia, and increased aggression. This disorder may persist for decades. Group therapy with others who have had similar experiences seems to be beneficial.

**11–11 Clinical Application Exercise**

A patient was in a car accident in which a close friend was seriously injured. He has had difficulty sleeping and is beginning to have nightmares, which further compound his insomnia.

**?** What might the athletic trainer suspect is affecting this individual?

## SUMMARY

- The injured or ill patient experiences not only physical disability but also major psychological reactions. Sport can be a major psychophysiological stressor.
- The athlete who sustains a serious injury may experience psychological characteristics of sudden loss, including denial, anger, bargaining, depression, and acceptance. Injury can cause the athlete to have physical, emotional, social, and self-concept reactions.
- Some athletes, because of personality factors, experience an inordinate number of injuries and illnesses. Anxiety, low self-esteem, and poor discipline may cause an athlete to be accident-prone.
- Overtraining and staleness result in a physical load being placed on the athlete's ability to cope. Athletes who are pushed or who push themselves too hard may experience burnout. These conditions generate a higher incidence of overuse injuries.

- At all times, the injured or ill athlete must be treated as a person, not as an injury. Health care providers should offer comfort, care, and good communication.
- The rehabilitation process requires mutual trust, understanding, and cooperation. Rehabilitation must be an educational process. Education is carried out through each phase of rehabilitation. Health care personnel may encounter athletes who overcomply or comply poorly.
- Many psychological skills training aids can help the injured athlete through the rehabilitation process to reenter competition. Some of these aids are systematic desensitization, mental and emotional assessment, refuting irrational thoughts, and thought stopping.
- A mental illness is any disorder that affects the mind or behavior. The athletic trainer should recognize when a potential problem exists and refer the patient to an appropriate psychiatrist, psychologist, or counselor.

## WEB SITES

**National Athletic Trainers Association Consensus Statements**
*Interassociation Recommendations for Developing a Plan to Recognize and Refer Student-Athletes with Psychological Concerns at the Secondary School Level: A Consensus Statement (March 2015): http://natajournals.org/doi /pdf/10.4085/1062-6050-50.3.03*

Association for the Advancement of Applied Sport Psychology: www.appliedsportpsych.org
*Emphasis on the role of psychological factors in sport and exercise.*

Exercise and Sport Psychology: www.apadivisions .org/division-47/index.aspx

*This site belongs to the sports and exercise division of the American Psychological Association.*

Mind Games: Applied Sport Psychology for Every Athlete: www.drrelax.com
*This is a new, Web-based system of individualized psychological training.*

North American Society for Psychology of Sport and Physical Activity: www.naspspa.com

Sport Psychology for Athletes: www.drrelax.com /baseball.htm
*Discuss the use of psychological training and preparation.*

# SOLUTIONS TO CLINICAL APPLICATION EXERCISES

11–1 The athletic trainer can be a good listener, find out what the problem is, be aware of his or her body language, project a caring image, explain the injury to the patient, help manage the stress of injury, and prepare the athlete physically and psychologically to return to competition.

11–2 Many patients experience five stages of psychological reaction, beginning with denial that they are injured, followed by anger, bargaining, depression, and finally acceptance.

11–3 The athletic trainer should look for athletes who have personality characteristics that make them more prone to injury, athletes who are under stress, and athletes who are overtraining and exhibiting signs of staleness and/or burnout.

11–4 If the athletic trainer needs help with the psychological aspects of a rehabilitation program, the patient can be referred to a physician, a sport psychologist, a clinical psychologist, a psychiatrist, a school guidance counselor, or a social worker.

11–5 The athletic trainer must appreciate that, even though she is physically ready to return, she is not psychologically prepared and has not yet realized that she can compete physically. The athletic trainer should have her engage in practice activities that will progressively expose her to more chance of physical risk until she is totally confident that she is ready to return.

11–6 Athletes tend to be goal-oriented individuals. They are used to having goals set for them and striving to meet them. The athletic trainer can motivate the athlete by setting an ultimate goal and devising a series of short-term goals that should be met sequentially to achieve the long-term goal.

11–7 The athletic trainer should recommend and lead the athlete through meditation and/or progressive relaxation techniques in a quiet environment that will allow the athlete to relax mentally and focus on his abilities to perform at a high level.

11–8 The patient can be taught to inhibit pain by reducing tension and stress using the Benson and Jacobson techniques; by diverting attention from the chronic pain by engaging in problem solving; or by imagining or visualizing pleasant thoughts.

11–9 It is likely that the emotional distress caused by the accident is triggering posttraumatic stress disorder. Group therapy with others who have had similar experiences may be helpful.

# REVIEW QUESTIONS AND CLASS ACTIVITIES

1. What is the importance of psychology to sports injuries?
2. How does stress relate to athlete injuries and illnesses?
3. Discuss the psychology of loss in sports injuries.
4. Describe the physical, emotional, social, and self-concept factors in sports injuries.
5. As an athletic trainer, how would you psychologically assist the athlete who is about to undergo major knee surgery?
6. Discuss overtraining, staleness, and overuse injuries.
7. What actions would you take with an athlete who is stale?
8. Psychologically, how should an athletic trainer react to serious injury immediately after injury and during the disability?
9. Psychologically, what makes for a successful rehabilitation climate?
10. Discuss psychological problems common to the rehabilitation process and possible ways of intervening.
11. What psychological skills training techniques might be employed to assist the athlete who is fearful and anxious?
12. Practice teaching psychological skills training techniques.

# REFERENCES

1. Albinson C, Petrie T: Cognitive appraisals, stress, and coping: Preinjury and postinjury factors influencing psychological adjustment to sport injury, *J Sport Rehabil* 12(4):306, 2003.
2. Armstrong N: The elite young athlete. *Med Sport Sci.* 56(1):97–105, 2011.
3. Baum A: Suicide in athletes: A review and commentary, *Clinics in Sports Medicine*, 24(4): 853–69, 2005.
4. Benson HH: *Beyond the relaxation response,* New York, 2000, Harper Torch.
5. Bone J, Fry M: The influence of injured athletes' perceptions of social support from ATCs on their beliefs about rehabilitation, *J Sport Rehabil* 15(2):156, 2006.
6. Brewer B: Adherence to sport injury rehabilitation. In Hanrahan, S: *Routledge handbook of applied sport psychology* New York, 2010, Taylor & Francis.
7. Brewer B: Developmental differences in psychological aspects of sport-injury rehabilitation, *J Athl Train* 38(2):152, 2003.
8. Brinkman R: The motivational climate in the rehabilitation setting, *Athletic Therapy Today*, 15(2):44–46, 2010.
9. Cassidy C: Understanding sport-injury anxiety, *Athletic Therapy Today* 11(4):57, 2006.
10. Coote D, Tenenbaum G: Can emotive imagery aid in tolerating exertion efficiently? *J Sports Med Phys Fitness* 38(4):344, 1998.
11. Cramer-Roh JL, Perna FM: Psychology/counseling: A universal competency in athletic training, *J Athl Train* 35(4):458, 2000.
12. Cresswell S, Eklund R: The athlete burnout syndrome: Possible early signs, *Journal of Science and Medicine in Sport* 7(4):481, 2004.
13. Driediger M: Imagery use by injured athletes: A qualitative analysis, *Journal of Sport Sciences*, 24(3):261–72, 2007.
14. Fisher L, Wrisberg C: What athletic training students want to know about sport psychology, *Athletic Therapy Today* 11(3):32, 2006.
15. Ford I, Gordon S: Guidelines for using sport psychology in rehabilitation, *Athletic Therapy Today* 3(2):41, 1998.
16. Glazer D: Development and preliminary validation of the injury-psychological readiness to return to sport (I-PRRS) scale, *J Athl Train*, 44(2):185–89, 2009.
17. Gourlay L: Recognizing psychological disorders, part 1: Overview, *Athletic Therapy and Training*, 15(6):15–18, 2010.
18. Granquist M: Development of a measure of rehabilitation adherence for athletic training, *Journal of Sport Rehabilitation*, 19:249–67, 2010.
19. Gunnoe A, Horodyski ML, Tennant K: The effect of life events on incidence of injury in high school football players, *J Athl Train* 36(2):150, 2001.
20. Hales D: *An invitation to health,* Boston, MA, 2014, Cengage Learning.
21. Hamson-Utley J: Athletic trainers' and physical therapists' perceptions of the effectiveness of psychological skills within sport injury rehabilitation programs, *J Athl Train*, 43(3):258–64, 2008.
22. Hanley C: Stress-management interventions for female athletes: Relaxation and cognitive restructuring, *International Journal of Sport Psychology* 35(2):109, 2004.
23. Harris L: Development of the injured collegiate athlete, *J Athl Train* 38(1):75, 2003.
24. Hayden L: The role of athletic trainers in helping coaches to facilitate return to play, *Athletic Therapy and Training*, 16(1):24–26, 2011.
25. Hedgpeth EB, Gieck JJ: Considerations for rehabilitation of the injured athlete. In Prentice WE, editor: *Rehabilitation techniques in sports medicine and athletic training*, ed 6, Thorofare, NJ: 2015, Slack.
26. Horn TS: *Advances in sport psychology*, ed 3, Champaign, IL, 2008, Human Kinetics.
27. Jacobson E: *Progressive relaxation: A physiological & clinical investigation of muscular states & their significance in psychology and medical practice*, Chicago, 1974, University of Chicago Press.
28. Johnson U: Athletes experiences of psychosocial risk factors preceding injury, *Qualitative Research in Sport, Exercise, Health*, 3(1): 99–115, 2011.
29. Johnston L, Carroll D: Coping, social support, and injury changes over time and the effects of pain and exercise involvement, *J Sport Rehabil* 9(4):291, 2000.
30. Johnston L, Carroll D: The provision of social support to injured athletes: A qualitative analysis, *J Sport Rehabil* 7(4):267, 1998.

31. Kolt GS: Doing sport psychology with injured athletes. In Andersen MB, editor: *Sport Psychology in Practice,* Champaign, IL, 2005, Human Kinetics.

32. Kübler-Ross E: *On death and dying.: What the dying have to teach doctors, nurses, clergy, and their own families,* New York, 2014, Scribner.

33. Marra J: Assessment of certified athletic trainers' levels of cultural competence in the delivery of health care, *J Athl Train,* 45(4):380–85, 2010.

34. Merikangas, K: Lifetime prevalence of mental disorders in US adolescents: Results from the National Comorbidity Survey Replication—Adolescent Supplement (NCS-A), *Journal of the American Academy of Child and Adolescent Psychiatry* 49(10):980–89, 2010.

35. Mihalik J: Recognition of psychological conditions in adolescent athletes, *Athletic Therapy Today* 9(3):54, 2004.

36. Milne M, Hall C, Forwell L: Self-efficacy, imagery use, and adherence to rehabilitation by injured athletes, *J Sport Rehabil* 14(2):150, 2005.

37. Misasi S, Redmond C, Kemler D: Counseling skills and the athletic therapist, *Athletic Therapy Today* 3(1):35, 1998.

38. Monsma E: Keeping your head in the game: Sport-specific imagery and anxiety among injured athletes, *J Athl Train,* 44(4):410–17, 2009.

39. Naylor A: The role of mental training in injury prevention, *Athletic Therapy Today,* 14(2):27–29, 2009.

40. Neal, T., et al: Interassociation recommendations for developing a plan to recognize and refer student-athletes with psychological concerns at the secondary school level: An executive summary of a consensus statement, *Journal of Athletic Training* 48(5):716–20, 2013.

41. Newcomer R, Perna F: Features of posttraumatic distress among adolescent athletes, *J Athl Train* 38(2):163, 2003.

42. Newsom J, Knight P, Balnave R: Use of mental imagery to limit strength loss after immobilization, *J Sport Rehabil* 12(3):249, 2003.

43. Payne W, Hahn D: *Understanding your health,* New York, 2012, McGraw-Hill.

44. Reardon C: Sport psychiatry: A systematic review of diagnosis and medical treatment of mental illness in athletes, *Sports Medicine,* 40(11):961–80, 2010.

45. Robbins JE, Rosenfeld LB: Athletes' perceptions of social support provided by their head coach, assistant coach, and athletic trainer, pre-injury and during rehabilitation, *Journal of Sport Behavior* 24(3):277, 2001.

46. Rock JA, Jones MV: A preliminary investigation into the use of counseling skills in support of rehabilitation from sport injury, *J Sport Rehabil* 11(4):284, 2002.

47. Schwenz SJ: Psychology of injury and rehabilitation, *Athletic Therapy Today* 6(1):44, 2001.

48. Selye H: *Stress without distress,* New York, 1974, Lippincott.

49. Sharon P, et al.: Academic preparation of athletic trainers as counselors, *J Athl Train* 31(1):39–43, 1996.

50. Shell D, Ferrante AP: Recognition of adjustment disorders in college athletes: A case study, *Cl J Sports Med* 6(1):60–62, 1996.

51. Shelley G, Trowbridge C, Detling N: Practical counseling skills for athletic therapists, *Athletic Therapy Today* 8(2):57, 2003.

52. Smith R: Recognition, management, and referral of the injured athlete with psychological problems, *Athletic Therapy Today* 3(1):14, 1998.

53. Sordoni C, Hall C, Forwell L: The use of imagery by athletes during injury rehabilitation, *J Sport Rehabil* 9(4):329, 2000.

54. *Taber's cyclopedic medical dictionary,* Philadelphia, 2013, F.A. Davis.

55. Udry E: Staying connected: Optimizing social support for injured athletes, *Athletic Therapy Today* 7(3):42, 2002.

56. Van Raalte J: Referring clients to other professionals. In Andersen M: *Routledge handbook of applied sport psychology,* New York, 2013, Taylor & Francis.

57. Vela L: Transient disablement in the physically active with musculoskeletal injuries, part I: A descriptive model, *J Athl Train,* 45(6):615–29, 2010.

58. Walsh, A: The relaxation response: A strategy to address stress, *Athletic Therapy and Training,* 16(2):20–23, 2011.

59. Wayda V, Armenth-Brothers F, Boyce B: Goal setting: A key to injury rehabilitation, *Athletic Therapy Today* 3(1):21, 1998.

60. Weinberg R, Gould D; Burnout and overtraining. In Gould D, editor: *Foundations of sport and exercise psychology,* ed 5, Champaign, IL, 2014, Human Kinetics.

61. Weiss-Bjornstal M: An integrated model of response to sport injury: Psychological and sociological dynamics, *Journal of applied Sports Psychology* 10:46–69, 1998.

62. Wiese-Bjornstal D: Psychology and socioculture affect injury risk, response, and recovery in high-intensity athletes: A consensus statement, *Scandinavian Journal of Medicine and Science in Sports,* 20(2):103–11, 2010.

63. Williams A: Social support and sport injury, *Athletic Therapy Today,* 15(4):46, 2010.

64. Williams, J, Andersen, M: Psychosocial antecedents of sport injury: Review and critique of the stress and injury model, *Journal of Applied Sport Psychology* 10(1):5–25, 1998.

65. Wrisberg C: Recommendations for successfully integrating sport psychology into athletic therapy, *Athletic Therapy Today* 11(2):60, 2006.

66. Wrisberg C, Fisher L: Mental rehearsal during rehabilitation, *Athletic Therapy Today* 10(6):58, 2005.

67. Wrisberg C, Fisher L: Staying connected to teammates during rehabilitation, *Athletic Therapy Today* 10(2):62, 2005.

68. Yang, J: Social support patterns of collegiate athletes before and after injury, *J Athl Train,* 45(4):372–79, 2010.

## ANNOTATED BIBLIOGRAPHY

Afremow, J: *The champion's mind: How great athletes think, train, and thrive,* Emmaus, PA, 2014, Rodale Books.

*Provides tips and techniques based on high-performance psychology research, such as how to get in a "zone," thrive on a team, and stay humble.*

Arvinen-Barrow, M: *The psychology of sport injury and rehabilitation,* New York, NY, 2013, Routledge.

*Demonstrates the ways in which athletes and practitioners can transfer psychological skills to an injury and rehabilitation setting, to enhance recovery and the well-being of the athlete.*

Gould D, Weinberg R: *Foundations of sport and exercise psychology,* Champaign, IL, 2014, Human Kinetics.

*Discusses the techniques that a coach should use for contributing to the success of an athlete.*

Kreider RB et al.: *Overtraining in sport,* Champaign, IL, 1998, Human Kinetics.

*An excellent secondary reference covering the psychological, immunological, nutritional, and psychological considerations of overtraining in sport.*

Lane, A: *Sport and exercise psychology,* London, 2015, Routledge.

*This text takes an applied perspective that bridges the gap between sport and exercise by covering the key topics in the field, including confidence, anxiety, self-regulation, stress, and self-esteem.*

Pargman, D: *Psychological Bases of Sports Injuries,* Morgantown, WV, 2007, Fitness Information Technologies.

*Provides a thorough examination of the psychological aspects of prevention, treatment, and rehabilitation of sport injuries.*

Selye H: *Stress without distress,* New York, 1974, Lippincott.

*A practical guide to understanding the role of stress in life.*

Singer RN, Hausenblas HA, Janelle CM: *Handbook of sport psychology,* ed 2, New York, 2001, Wiley.

*A good resource for sport psychologists, coaches, and athletes searching for new and effective approaches to pain management, exercise psychology, and building self-confidence. It combines theoretical explanations and practical applications and emphasizes the value of basic and applied research to practice.*

Taylor J, Taylor S: *Psychological approaches to sports injury rehabilitation,* Gaithersburg, MD, 2004, Aspen.

*Provides practical techniques and strategies for sports rehabilitation.*

Tennenbaum, G, Eklund, R: *Handbook of sport psychology,* 3rd ed., New York, 2007, Wiley.

*A resource for sport psychologists, coaches, and athletes searching for new and effective approaches to pain management, exercise psychology, and building self-confidence. Combines theoretical explanation and practical applications and emphasizes the value of basic and applied research to practice.*

Van Raalte, JL, ed., *Exploring sport and exercise psychology,* 2nd ed. Washington, DC, 2013, American Psychological Association.

*Provides an overview of the field of sport and exercise psychology, connecting theory and practice, and discussing practical issues.*

Weinberg, RS, Gould, D: *Foundations of sport and exercise psychology,* Champaign, IL, 2010, Human Kinetics.

*Discusses the techniques that a coach should incorporate for contributing to the success of an athlete.*

Williams JM: *Applied sport psychology: personal growth to peak performance,* San Francisco, CA, 2014, McGraw-Hill.

*Leading sports psychologists presenting both the "whys" and "how tos" of the intervention techniques in sport psychology.*

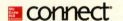

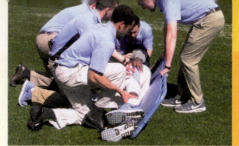
© William E. Prentice

# 12

# On-the-Field Acute Care and Emergency Procedures

## ■ Objectives

*When you finish this chapter you should be able to*

- Establish a plan for handling emergency situations.
- Explain the importance of knowing cardiopulmonary resuscitation and how to manage an obstructed airway.
- Describe the types of hemorrhage and their management.
- Assess the types of shock and their management.
- Describe the emergency management of musculoskeletal injuries.
- Describe techniques for moving and transporting the injured patient.

## ■ Key Terms

primary survey
secondary survey
systolic blood pressure
diastolic blood pressure
mm Hg

## ■ Connect Highlights    **connect**

*Visit connect.mcgraw-hill.com for further exercises to apply your knowledge:*

- Clinical application scenarios covering handling emergency situations, shock, and emergency management of musculoskeletal injuries
- Click-and-drag questions covering emergency action plans, emergency managements, and cardiopulmonary resuscitation
- Multiple-choice questions covering emergency management of musculoskeletal injuries, transporting an injured patient, emergency action plans, and management of hemorrhage
- Selection questions covering musculoskeletal injuries and vital signs

**A**n emergency is defined as "an unforeseen combination of circumstances and the resulting state that calls for immediate action." Certainly, most sports injuries do not result in life-or-death emergency situations, but when such situations do arise, prompt care is essential.[1] It has been suggested that the first hour following injury—the so-called Golden Hour—is most critical in treating injury. The Golden Hour refers to the time between injury and the initiation of the appropriate treatment. Although research evidence has shown that the Golden Hour is simply an arbitrary myth, it is certainly true that rapid intervention as soon as possible following traumatic injury improves the patients' chance of survival and thus a successful outcome.[62] Time is the critical factor, and assistance to the injured person must be based on knowledge of what to do and how to do it—on how to perform effective first aid immediately.[23] There is no room for uncertainty, indecision, or error. A mistake in the initial management of an injury can prolong the length of time required for recovery and can create a life-threatening situation for the athlete.[4]

> Time is critical in an emergency situation.

## THE EMERGENCY ACTION PLAN

The prime concern of emergency aid is to maintain cardiovascular function and, indirectly, central nervous system function.[42] Failure of either of these systems may lead to death. Regardless of the setting, whether on an athletic field or in a clinic, hospital, or fitness center, emergency action should be developed for every situation in which an athletic trainer works.[25] The key to emergency aid is the initial evaluation of the injured patient. Time is of the essence, so this evaluation must be done rapidly and accurately, so that proper first aid can be rendered without delay.[9] In some instances, these first steps not only will be lifesaving but also will determine the degree and extent of permanent disability.

As discussed in Chapters 1 and 3, any individual who provides emergency care—the athletic trainer, the team physician, the coach—must act reasonably and prudently at all times.[49] This behavior is especially important during emergencies.

All health care programs must have a prearranged emergency action plan (EAP) that can be implemented immediately when necessary.[4,28,67] The following issues must be addressed when developing the emergency action for athletic settings:

> All sports programs must have an emergency action plan.

1. Develop separate emergency action plans for each sport's field, courts, or gymnasiums[58] **SoR:C**

(see *Focus Box 12–1:* "Sample emergency action plan").
   a. Determine the personnel who will be on the field during practices and competitions (e.g., athletic trainers, athletic training students, physicians, emergency medical technicians, rescue squad). Each person should understand exactly what his or her role and responsibilities are if an emergency occurs. It is also recommended that the sports medicine team practice the use and operation of emergency equipment, such as stretchers and automated external defibrillators for each venue, and document that this has been done.[33,58]
   b. Decide what emergency equipment should be available for each sport. The emergency equipment needs for football will likely be different from those of the cross-country team.
2. Establish specific procedures and policies regarding the removal of protective equipment, particularly the helmet and shoulder pads.[41,61] These procedures are discussed later in this chapter.
3. Make sure phones are readily accessible. Wireless phones or satellite phones are easily available and accessible. However, a land line should also be easily accessible in case wireless phone service is not available. If wireless phones are not available, the athletic training students, coaches, all staff personnel, and athletes should know the location of the telephone; phones should be clearly marked. Use 911 if available, but realize that in some areas not all service is accessible by wireless phones and thus land lines should be used to access the emergency medical system.
4. All staff should be familiar with the community-based emergency health care delivery plan, including existing communication and transportation.[48] It is also critical for the athletic trainer to be familiar with emergency care facility admission and treatment policies, particularly when rendering emergency care to a minor. The athletic trainer should designate someone to make an emergency phone call. Most emergency medical systems can be accessed by dialing 911, which connects the caller to a dispatcher who has access to rescue squad, police, and fire personnel. The person making the emergency phone call must provide the following information:
   a. Type of emergency situation
   b. Type of suspected injury
   c. Present condition of the patient
   d. Current assistance being given (e.g., cardiopulmonary resuscitation)
   e. Location of telephone being used
   f. Exact location of emergency (give names of streets and cross-streets) and how to enter facility
   g. Any limitations in the building (such as no elevator to the third floor)

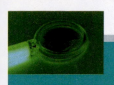

## FOCUS 12–1 Focus on Healthcare Administration and Professional Responsibilities

### Sample emergency action plan

*Emergency action plan for women's ice hockey*

**Emergency Personnel:**
Certified athletic trainer and athletic training students on-site for practice and competition; additional sports medicine staff accessible from main athletic training facility (across street from arena)

**Emergency Communication:**
Fixed telephone line in ice hockey satellite athletic training room (_____-_____)

**Emergency Equipment:**
Supplies (AED, trauma kit, splint kit, spine board) maintained in ice hockey satellite athletic training room; additional emergency equipment accessible from athletic training facility across street from arena (_____-_____)

**Roles of First Responders:**
Immediate care of the injured or ill student-athlete
Emergency equipment retrieval

**Activation of Emergency Medical System:**
911 call (provide name, title or position, address, telephone number, number of individuals injured, condition of injured, first, aid treatment, specific directions, other information as requested)
Direct EMS to scene
  Open appropriate doors
  Designate individual to "flag down" EMS and direct to scene
Scene control: Limit scene to first-aid providers and move bystanders away from area

**Venue Directions:**
Ice hockey arena is located on corner of _____ Street and _____ Street adjacent to _____. Two gates provide access to the arena:_____ Street: drive leads to arena as well as rear door of complex (locker room, athletic training room)

**Sports Medicine Staff and Phone Numbers:**
Athletic Trainer in Charge   929-0000 (cell)
Head Athletic Trainer       929-0001 (office)
Team Physician             929-0002 (office)

Source: From *NCAA Sports Medicine Handbook: 2011–2012.*

---

5. Make sure keys to gates or padlocks are easily accessible. The athletic trainer, staff members, and the coach should have the appropriate keys. Make sure an elevator in a building can accommodate a gurney or spine board.

6. Inform all coaches, athletic directors, school nurses, staff, and maintenance personnel of the emergency plan at a meeting held annually before the beginning of the school year and document that this has been done. Each individual must know his or her responsibilities, should an emergency occur. This plan should be reviewed, revised, and rehearsed at least once a year.

7. Assign someone to accompany the injured athlete to the hospital.

8. Carry contact information for all athletes, coaches, and other personnel at all times, particularly when traveling (see Figure 3–1). For minors, consent forms for medical treatment should also be available when traveling.

9. In certain situations in both secondary schools and colleges, the athletic trainer may be called upon to provide emergency services not only to athletes but also to coaches, referees, and in some cases parents and other spectators who develop an emergent condition during an athletic event. The emergency action plan should include plans for managing these situations that should be developed with the help and input of emergency medical services and other local health care providers.[26]

10. It has been recommended that a *time-out* be routinely included prior to the start of each athletic event.[40] This time-out should be used to have all of the individuals who will be involved with any aspect of athletic health care for that specific event meet to go over a checklist for that venue's emergency action plan to make certain that all parties involved are prepared to handle an emergency to ensure a decisive and coordinated response and outcome. In 2012, NATA released the Official Statement "Time Outs Before Athletic Events Recommended for Health Care Providers" (www.nata.org/sites/default/files/TimeOut.pdf).[40]

An athletic trainer working in a clinic, hospital, corporate, or industrial setting should also develop an emergency action plan to make certain that appropriate procedures will be followed, should an emergency occur. If the athletic trainer is working in a hospital, he or she should become familiar with the hospital's pre-established emergency action plan for dealing with in-house emergencies and should follow it. For emergent situations that occur in a clinic, corporate, or industrial setting, similar procedures and considerations should be followed as described for managing injuries in an athletic setting.

In 2002, the NATA released a position statement relative to an emergency action plan.[4] The objective was to provide guidelines for athletic trainers in the development of emergency plans and to advocate the documentation of emergency planning. A link to the NATA position statement "Emergency Planning in Athletics" can be found at www.nata.org/sites/default/files/EmergencyPlanning InAthletics.pdf.

In 2007, representatives from the NATA worked on an interassociation task force official statement *Recommendations on Emergency Preparedness and Management of Sudden Cardiac Arrest in High School and College Athletic Programs* (www.nata.org/sites/default/files/sudden -cardiac-arrest-consensus-statement.pdf).

## Cooperation between Emergency Care Providers

Individuals providing emergency care to injured athletes must cooperate and act professionally. The athletic trainer should make every effort to nurture the relationship with the emergency medical technicians (EMTs) and, if possible, incorporate them into the development and implementation of both the emergency action plan and also in time-outs held prior to the start of an athletic event. Occasionally, disagreements arise between rescue squad personnel, the physician, and the athletic trainer over exactly how the injured athlete should be handled and transported. The athletic trainer is usually the first to deal with the emergency situation. The athletic trainer has generally had more training and experience in moving and transporting an injured athlete than the physician has. If an athletic trainer or a physician is not available, the coach should not hesitate to call 911 to let the rescue squad handle an emergency situation. If the rescue squad is called and responds, the EMTs should have the final say on how that patient is to be transported in accordance with their established protocols while the athletic trainer assumes an assistive role.

To alleviate potential conflicts, the athletic trainer should establish procedures and guidelines and should arrange practice sessions at least once a year that include everyone responsible for handling an injured athlete.[19,58] **SoR:C** All individuals involved with providing athletic health care for a specific event should also routinely meet for a time-out prior to the start of every athletic event to go over the emergency action plan. Rescue squad personnel may not be experienced in dealing with someone who is wearing a football, lacrosse, or hockey helmet or other protective equipment; thus,

> Emergency practice sessions for athletic trainers and EMTs should be held at least once a year.

athletic trainer should make sure before an incident occurs that the EMTs understand the correct management of athletes wearing various types of athletic equipment.

## Parental Notification

If the injured patient is a minor, the athletic trainer should try to obtain consent from the parent before it becomes necessary to treat the patient during an emergency.[4] *Focus Box 12–2:* "Consent form for medical treatment of a minor" provides an example of a consent form that may be signed by the parents or guardians of a minor. Consent may be given in writing either before or during an emergency. This consent is notification that the parent has been informed about what the athletic trainer thinks is wrong and what the athletic trainer intends to do, and parental permission is granted to give treatment for a specific incident. If the patient's parents cannot be contacted, the predetermined wishes of the parent given at the beginning of a season or school year can be enacted. The athletic trainer should have these consent forms available when traveling in case the need for medical care arises. If no informed consent exists, the patient's implied consent to save his or her life takes precedence.

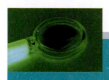

## FOCUS 12–2 Focus on Healthcare Administration and Professional Responsibilities

### Consent form for medical treatment of a minor

By this signature, I hereby consent to allow the physician(s) and other health care provider(s) selected by me or the school to perform a preparticipation examination on my child and to provide treatment for any injury or condition resulting from participating in athletics and activities for his or her school during the school year covered by this form. I further consent to allow said physician(s) or health care provider(s) to share appropriate information concerning my child that is relevant to participation in athletics and activities with coaches and other school personnel as deemed necessary.

_____
Parent or Guardian

_____
Date

# PRINCIPLES OF ON-THE-FIELD INJURY ASSESSMENT

The athletic trainer cannot deliver appropriate acute medical care to the injured patient until a systematic assessment of the situation has been made on the playing field or court where the injury occurs.[54] This *on-the-field assessment* helps determine the nature of the injury and provides direction in the decision-making process concerning the emergency care that must be rendered (Figure 12–1). The on-the-field assessment may be subdivided into a primary survey and a secondary survey.

The **primary survey**, which is done initially, determines the existence of potentially life-threatening situations, including problems with level of consciousness, airway, breathing, circulation, severe bleeding, and shock. The primary survey takes precedence over all other aspects of victim assessment and should be used to correct life-threatening situations.[42] Any patient who has a life-threatening situation should be transported to an emergency care facility as soon as possible.

Once the primary survey has ruled out the existence of a life-threatening injury or illness, the **secondary survey** takes a closer look at the injury. The secondary survey gathers specific information about the injury from the patient, systematically assesses vital signs and symptoms, and allows for a more detailed evaluation of the injury. The secondary survey is done to uncover problems that do not pose an immediate threat to life but that may do so if they remain uncorrected.[42]

An injured patient who is conscious and stable does not require a primary survey. However, an unconscious patient must be monitored for life-threatening problems throughout the assessment process.

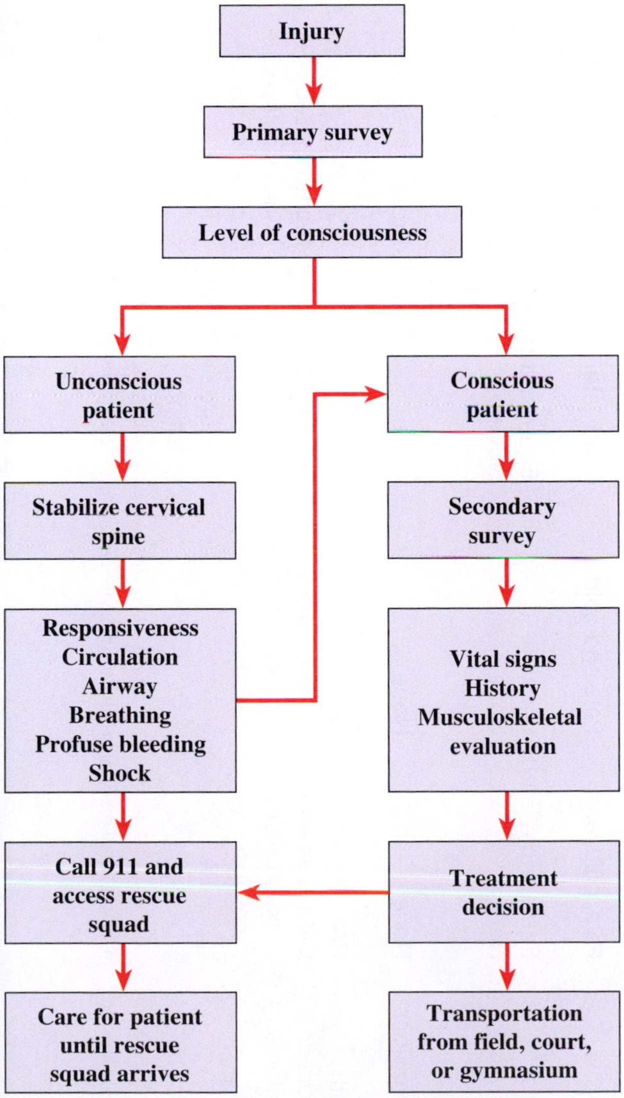

## THE PRIMARY SURVEY

### Treatment of Life-Threatening Injuries

Life-threatening injuries take precedence over all other injuries. Situations that are considered life-threatening include those that require cardiopulmonary resuscitation (i.e., obstruction of the airway, no breathing, no circulation), profuse bleeding, and shock. In the primary survey, it is first necessary to assess the level of consciousness.

> **Life-threatening conditions:**
> - Airway obstruction
> - No breathing
> - No circulation
> - Profuse bleeding
> - Shock

### Dealing with the Unconscious Patient

The state of unconsciousness provides one of the greatest dilemmas for the athletic trainer. Whether to move the injured athlete and allow the game to resume or to await the arrival of a physician is a decision that too often is resolved hastily and without much forethought. Unconsciousness is a state of insensibility in which the athlete exhibits a lack of conscious awareness. This condition can be brought about by a blow to either the head or the solar plexus; it may result from general shock, or it may result from fainting (syncope) due to inadequate blood flow to the brain. It is often difficult to determine the exact cause of unconsciousness (Table 12–1).

> With an unconscious victim, the athletic trainer should call 911 immediately.

The unconscious patient always must be considered to have a life-threatening injury, which requires that the athletic trainer call 911 immediately. The following

FIGURE 12–1 Flowchart showing the appropriate emergency procedures for the injured patient.

The flowchart shows:
- Injury → Primary survey → Level of consciousness
- Level of consciousness branches to: Unconscious patient and Conscious patient
- Unconscious patient → Stabilize cervical spine → Responsiveness, Circulation, Airway, Breathing, Profuse bleeding, Shock → Call 911 and access rescue squad → Care for patient until rescue squad arrives
- Conscious patient → Secondary survey → Vital signs, History, Musculoskeletal evaluation → Treatment decision → Transportation from field, court, or gymnasium
- Treatment decision → Call 911 and access rescue squad

**TABLE 12–1**    Evaluating the Unconscious Athlete

### Selected Conditions

| Functional Signs | Fainting | Concussion | Grand Mal Epilepsy | Brain Compression and Injury | Heatstroke | Diabetic Coma | Shock |
|---|---|---|---|---|---|---|---|
| Onset | Usually sudden | Usually sudden | Sudden | Usually gradual | Gradual or sudden | Gradual | Gradual |
| Level of consciousness | Complete unconsciousness | Confusion or unconsciousness | Unconsciousness | Unconsciousness, gradually deepening | Delirium or unconsciousness | Drowsiness, later unconsciousness | Listlessness, later unconsciousness |
| Pulse | Fast and weak | Weak and irregular | Fast | Gradually slower | Fast and weak | Fast and weak | Fast and weak |
| Respiration | Quick and shallow | Shallow and irregular | Noisy, later deep and slow | Slow and noisy | Difficult | Deep and sighing | Rapid and shallow, with occasional deep sighs |
| Skin | Pale, cold, and clammy | Pale and cold | Livid, later pale | Hot and flushed | Hot and limited sweating | Livid, later pale | Pale, cold, and clammy |
| Pupils | Equal and dilated | Equal | Equal and dilated | Unequal | Equal | Equal | Equal and dilated |
| Paralysis | None | None | None | May be present in leg, arm, or both | None | None | None |
| Convulsions | None | None | None | Present in some cases | Present in some cases | None | None |
| Breath | N/A | N/A | N/A | N/A | N/A | Acetone smell | N/A |
| Special features | Giddiness and sway before collapse | Signs of head injury, vomiting during recovery | Bites tongue, voids urine and feces, may injure self while falling | Signs of head injury, delayed onset of symptoms | Vomiting in some cases | In early stages, headache, restlessness, and nausea | May vomit; early stages shivering, thirst, defective vision, and ear noises |

Source: Modified from International medical guide, for ships, Geneva: World Health Organization.

guidelines should be used when working with an unconscious patient:

A football defensive back is making a tackle and drops his head on contact with the ball carrier. He hits the ground and does not move. When the athletic trainer gets to him, the patient is lying prone, is unconscious, but is breathing.

**?** How should the athletic trainer manage this situation?

1. The athletic trainer should immediately note the body position and determine the level of consciousness and responsiveness.
2. Circulation, airway, and breathing (CAB) should be established immediately if the patient is not breathing.
3. Injury to the neck and cervical spine should always be considered a possibility in the unconscious patient.[55]
4. Rescuers should immediately expose the airway by removing any protective equipment such as the face mask, helmet, and shoulder pads that could interfere with CPR.[57,58,61] **SoR:C**
5. If the patient is supine and breathing, monitor closely until he or she regains consciousness.
6. If the patient is prone and not breathing, he or she should be logrolled carefully to the supine position, and CPR should begin immediately.
7. If the patient is prone and breathing, monitor closely until he or she regains consciousness; then the patient should be carefully logrolled onto a spine board because CPR could be necessary at any time.
8. Life support supersedes spinal motion concerns and for the unconscious patient should be maintained and monitored until emergency medical personnel arrive.
9. Once the patient is stabilized (no longer exhibits a life-threatening condition), the athletic trainer should begin a secondary survey.

## Overview of Emergency Cardiopulmonary Resuscitation

A careful evaluation of the injured person must be made to determine whether CPR should be initiated. This overview of adult and child CPR is not intended to be used by persons who are not certified in CPR. Because of the serious nature of CPR, athletic trainers should routinely be recertified in *CPR/AED for the Professional Rescuer* through the American Red Cross, the American Heart Association, or the National Safety Council.[1,2,42]

The American Heart Association uses the acronym CAB—circulation, airway, breathing—to help individuals who are certified in CPR remember the order of the procedures to emphasize the importance of chest compressions in creating circulation.[43] *Focus Box 12–3: "CPR summary"* summarizes the basics of performing CPR for the adult, child, and infant.

**Establishing Unresponsiveness** Initially, the athletic trainer, who is a trained rescuer, should assess the situation to make sure there is no chance of additional injury and quickly check for any potentially life-threatening conditions (e.g., severe bleeding). The next step is to establish the responsiveness of the victim by asking "Are you okay?" and then tapping the shoulder or using a painful pinch of the distal extremity (Figure 12–2). Note that shaking should be avoided if there is a possible neck injury. Quickly check for signs of breathing and pulse taking no more than 10 seconds. If the victim does not respond to any stimuli, the emergency medical system (EMS) should be activated immediately by directing a specific person to dial 911. That person should also be directed to get an automated external defibrillator (AED) if available. A victim who is lying prone or on his or her side and is breathing should be placed on his or her left side in the recovery position (Figure 12–3). This position can be maintained for as long as 30 minutes. If the victim is not breathing or is gasping for air, he or she should be carefully placed in the supine position. If the victim is in a position other than supine, he or she must be carefully rolled over as a unit, minimizing movement of the spine, because

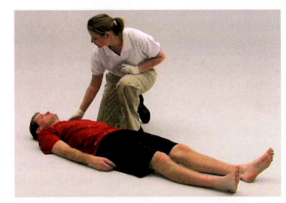

FIGURE 12–2 Establish responsiveness by gently tapping the victim's shoulder and asking "Are you okay?"
© William E. Prentice

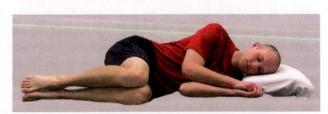

FIGURE 12–3 Victims who are breathing should be placed on their left side in the recovery position.
© William E. Prentice

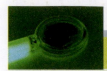

# FOCUS 12–3 Focus on Therapeutic Intervention

## CPR summary[1,2,43]

**Instructions for individuals certified in CPR**

### For an adult

- Establish unresponsiveness, then call 911.
- Look for no breathing and check pulse (<10 seconds).
- If an AED is available, deliver 1 shock if instructed by the device and begin CPR.
- Restore blood circulation, using chest compressions at a rate of 100–120 per minute.
- Perform 30 compressions.
- Use two hands for compression.
- Compress chest at least 2 inches (5 cm) and not greater than 2.4 inches (6 cm).
- Perform mouth-to-mouth breathing after opening the airway.
- Give two breaths (1 second per ventilation).
- Breathe until the chest rises.
- Resume chest compressions.
- After five cycles or 2 minutes with no response, use an automated external defibrillator (AED) (Figure 12-4).
- Administer one shock if instructed by the device, then continue CPR
- Continue CPR 30 compressions: 2 breaths until the person begins to breathe or EMS takes over.

### For a child (ages 1-12)

- Establish unresponsiveness, then call 911.
- Look for no breathing and check pulse (<10 seconds).
- Restore blood circulation, using chest compressions at a rate of 100 per minute.
- Perform 30 compressions.
- Use two hands for compressions.
- Compress chest about 2 inches (5 mm).

- Perform mouth-to-mouth breathing after opening the airway.
- Give two breaths (1 second per ventilation).
- Breathe until the chest rises.
- Resume chest compressions.
- After five cycles or 2 minutes with no response, use an automated external defibrillator (AED).
- Use pediatric pads if available.
- Administer 1 shock if instructed by the device, then continue CPR.
- Continue CPR 30 compressions: 2 breaths until the child begins to breathe or EMS takes over.

### For an infant (< 1 year)

- Establish unresponsiveness, then call 911.
- Restore blood circulation with chest compressions at a rate of 100 per minute.
- Perform 30 compressions.
- Use only two fingers on sternum just below nipple line for compressions.
- Perform mouth-to-mouth/nose breathing after opening the airway.
- Give two breaths.
- Breathe more gently than for an adult.
- Resume chest compressions.
- After five cycles or 2 minutes with no response, reassess.
- Continue CPR until the child begins to breathe or EMS takes over.

**Instructions for individuals who are not certified in CPR**

- Perform chest compressions only at a rate of 100 per minute continuously until EMS arrives.

---

CPR can be administered only with the victim lying flat on the back with knees straight or slightly flexed. In cases of suspected cervical spine injury, cervical movement must be minimized during logrolling by manually stabilizing the cervical spine while being careful not to apply cervical traction.[58] SoR:B Then CPR should be performed.[42] If an automated external defibrillator (AED) is available it should be used immediately after it has been determined that the victim is unresponsive. If not it should be used as soon as it becomes available.

**Using an Automated External Defibrillator** An AED is a device that evaluates the heart rhythm of a victim of sudden cardiac arrest.[51] It is capable of delivering an electrical charge to the heart and does not require the expertise of a medical professional.[53] To prevent

human error, all machines have computers that evaluate heart rhythm and decide if deployment is appropriate. AEDs have become an essential tool in the treatment of out-of-hospital cardiac arrest.[22] The American Heart Association estimates that 100,000 deaths could be prevented each year with rapid defibrillation. Over the years, the devices have become safer, more reliable, and more maintenance free. The new technologies used in these devices make them suitable for use by anyone who has had basic training.[53]

AEDs are extremely easy to use; anyone trained to use cardiopulmonary resuscitation (CPR) can be trained to use an AED. Most AEDs are designed to be used by people without medical backgrounds, such as police, firefighters, flight attendants, security guards, and lay rescuers, as long as the procedure is coordinated with existing

EMS systems and the person administering the procedure has received proper training. Public places where AEDs might be located include police cars, theaters, sports arenas, public buildings, business offices, and airports. An increasing number of commercial airplanes are now equipped with AEDs and enhanced medical kits. Formal training programs, such as those offered by the American Heart Association's Heartsaver AED course, can be taught in as little as 4 hours. However, operating an AED is so simple that it can be done successfully even without formal training. Training is recommended for as many people as possible. Local and state regulations determine the training requirements for public access defibrillator (PAD) programs.[53]

The legal requirements that allow the lay public to use AEDs are determined on a state-by-state basis. In some states, there is true public access defibrillation, meaning that anyone with knowledge of an AED can use one any time it is available. For example, a traveler in an airport may retrieve and use an AED mounted in a public location. In other states, use of AEDs is more restricted. Some states require a formal training program or the direct involvement of an authorizing doctor, or the AED rescuer must be part of a formal in-house response team. In most states, any individual using an AED in a good-faith attempt to save the life of a cardiac arrest victim will be covered by some form of a "good Samaritan" statute.[42]

Anyone can be certified to use an AED in most states and can learn to use an AED in about an hour.[64] AED users also need yearly training, not only on the use of the device but also in CPR. Athletic trainers must be certified in both CPR and AED use. Maintenance is minimal on AEDs. The devices are equipped with long-life batteries and have features that notify the users when the batteries need replacement. To date, most professional teams and college teams have AEDs readily available.

To use an AED, the rescuer simply applies the two electrodes to the right apex and the left base of the chest (Figure 12–4). To operate most devices, push the "on" button and listen for a voice on the machine to direct you whether to push the defibrillator button. If the pulse does not resume after one shock, perform CPR for two minutes; then deliver another shock from the AED. If the pulse resumes, place the victim into the recovery position on his or her left side (see Figure 12–3) until the rescue squad arrives. If the pulse does not resume, continue external compressions at a 30 (compressions) to two (breaths) ratio. The victim should not be on a metal stretcher, the ground should not be wet, and the chest should be dry (not sweaty). It is best to shave chest hair if quickly possible. NATA's official statement on using AEDs appears in *Focus Box 12–4:* "Official statement—automated external defibrillators."

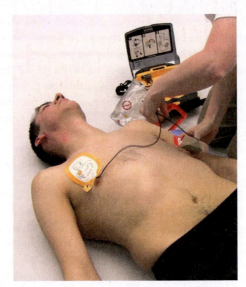

FIGURE 12–4  An automated external defibrillator (AED) can be used if the victim has no heartbeat.
© William E. Prentice

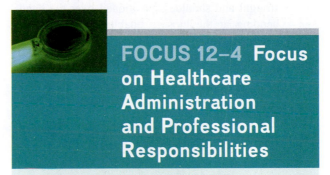

## FOCUS 12–4  Focus on Healthcare Administration and Professional Responsibilities

### Official statement—automated external defibrillators

The National Athletic Trainers' Association (NATA), as a leader in health care for the physically active, strongly believes that the treatment of sudden cardiac arrest is a priority. An AED program should be part of an athletic trainer's emergency action plan. NATA strongly encourages athletic trainers, in every work setting, to have access to an AED. Athletic trainers are encouraged to make an AED part of their standard emergency equipment. In addition, in conjunction and coordination with local EMS, athletic trainers should take a primary role in implementing a comprehensive AED program within their work setting.

From NATA official statement "Automated external defibrillators" www.nata.org/sites/default/files/AutomatedExternalDefibrillators.pdf "Reprinted with permission from the National Athletic Trainers' Association."

### Establishing Circulation by Performing Compressions

1. In the adult and child victim, a health care provider should take no more than 10 seconds to check for a

pulse at the carotid artery, performed simultaneously with the check for no breathing. To locate the carotid artery, place two fingers on the Adam's apple and slide them toward you into the groove on the side of the neck (Figure 12–5). Monitor for no more than 10 seconds.[43]

2. If an AED is available, use it as soon as possible (see the section on AED). Deliver one shock followed immediately by chest compressions.

3. If no AED is available and there are no evident signs of circulation (i.e., breathing, coughing, or movement), begin chest compressions immediately.

    a. Maintain an open airway. Position yourself close to the side of the victim's chest.

    b. Next, position the heel of the hand closest to the victim's head on the middle of the sternum. Place the other hand on top of the hand on the sternum, so that the heels of both hands are parallel and the fingers are directed straight away from you (Figure 12–6). Fingers can be extended or interlaced, but they must be kept off the chest wall.

    c. Keep elbows in a locked position, with arms straight and shoulders positioned over the hands, bending at the hips to enable the thrust to be straight down.

    d. In a normal-sized adult, apply enough force to depress the sternum at least 2 inches (5 cm) but no more than 2.4 inches (6 cm).[43] (In the child, the sternum

should be compressed up to 2 inches [5 cm].) After compression, completely release the sternum to allow the heart to refill. The time of release should equal the time of compression. For one rescuer, compression must be given at the rate of 100 to 120 compressions per minute, maintaining a ratio of 30 chest compressions to two full breaths (30:2) for all victims, from infants to adults.[43]

    e. Continue CPR for 2 minutes or five cycles of 30 compressions and two breaths (30:2), until prompted by the AED to allow a rhythm check.[43]

NOTE: The American Heart Association recommends Hands-Only CPR for untrained lay rescuers. This technique only requires a rescuer to call 911, then to perform uninterrupted chest compressions—100 to 120 a minute—until paramedics take over or an automated external defibrillator is available to restore a normal heart rhythm.[1] This action should be taken only for adults who unexpectedly collapse, stop breathing, and are unresponsive.

**Opening the Airway** There are several techniques that the athletic trainer can use to open the airway.[65] The most common method is to open the airway by using the head-tilt/chin-lift method (Figure 12–7A).[2] Lift under the chin with one hand while pushing down on the victim's forehead with the other, avoiding the use of excessive force. The tongue is the most common cause of airway obstruction; the forward lift of the jaw raises the tongue away from the back of the throat, thus clearing the airway.

In the modified jaw thrust technique, grasp each side of the mandible at the angles and pull upward to open the airway. Studies have shown that this technique (Figure 12–7B) does not consistently open the airway effectively, and even professional rescuers move the cervical spine when using it. Therefore, this technique is not recommended for the lay rescuer. The athletic trainer should use the head-tilt/chin-lift method to open the airway of a person with no suspected cervical injury. If there is a suspected cervical injury, rescuers should cause as little motion as possible, and thus the modified jaw

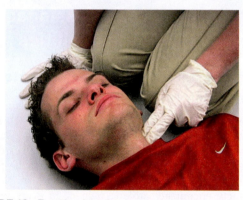

FIGURE 12–5  Checking for a pulse at the carotid artery.
© William E. Prentice

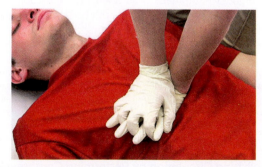

FIGURE 12–6  Chest compressions should be performed with pressure from both hands over the sternum and between the nipples.
© William E. Prentice

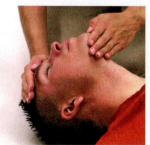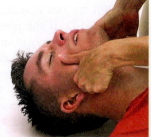

**A**                                         **B**

FIGURE 12–7  Opening the airway. **(A)** Head-tilt/chin-lift method. **(B)** Modified jaw thrust technique.
© William E. Prentice

thrust technique should be used.[58] **SoR:B** If the jaw thrust maneuver fails to open the airway, use the head-tilt/chin-lift method.

***Airway Adjunct Devices*** A suction device can be used if there is some substance (e.g., blood, fluids, vomitus) in the mouth or throat that appears to be obstructing the airway and that cannot be cleared by using a finger sweep.[2] Suction units can be portable manual units (hand-suctioning), portable mechanical units, or wall-mounted mechanical units (Figure 12–8). Each of these works by creating a negative pressure that suctions fluid and small particles into a collecting chamber. Suctioning helps to reduce the risk of aspiration into the lungs and should be done as quickly as possible so that normal ventilation procedures can be reimplemented. The suction tube should reach only to the base of the tongue, suctioning only what can be visualized. The length of the tube inserted into the throat can be estimated by measuring the distance from the corner of the mouth to the same side earlobe. Suctioning should move from back to front, using a small circular motion with the tip of the tube.

Oropharyngeal (OPA) airways, nasopharyngeal (NPA) airways, and supraglottic (SGA) airways are types of airway adjunct devices that are used to make it easier to maintain an open airway once it has been established. Their purpose is essentially to prevent the tongue from obstructing the airway. These devices may be used by certified first responders, EMTs, paramedics, and athletic trainers who have been properly trained in their use.[8]

An oropharyngeal airways is essentially a curved, J-shaped plastic tube, designed to fit the natural contour of the mouth and throat, that is inserted into the mouth and through the posterior pharynx (Figure 12–9). It should only be used in unconscious (unresponsive) patients with no gag reflex. If a victim gags, it should be removed immediately. OPAs come in different sizes from large adult to infant. It is critical to select the correct size to avoid displacing the tongue into the posterior pharynx, causing additional airway obstruction. The size of the OPA can be estimated by measuring the distance from the corner of the mouth to the same side earlobe. If there is difficulty ventilating the patient after the airway is inserted, it should be removed and reinserted. Once correctly inserted, the flange should lie on the patient's lips. The OPA can facilitate the delivery of adequate ventilation with a bag/valvemask by preventing the tongue from occluding the airway.[8]

A nasopharyngeal airway is a soft rubber tube that is passed through the right side of the nose into the posterior pharynx (Figure 12–10). It is used on a responsive, semiconscious patient and does not cause a gag reflex unless it is too long. Insertion of the NPA requires a water-soluble lubricating agent to avoid injuring the nasal mucosa. The tubes come in different sizes based on the diameter of the opening, which ranges from 6.5 to 8.5 mm. The length of the tube inserted into the nose can

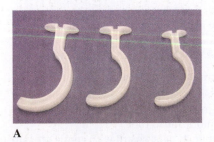
A

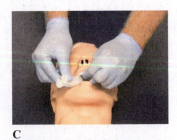
B

FIGURE 12–8   Using a suction device. **(A)** Rotate the head to the side or log roll the patient onto their side and perform a finger sweep. **(B)** Insert the suction tip into the throat and suction from the back of the throat outward using a circular movement. Always visualize the tip.
© William E. Prentice

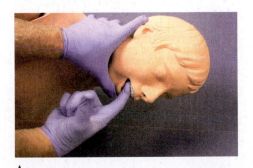
A

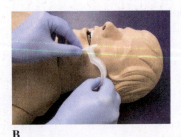
B

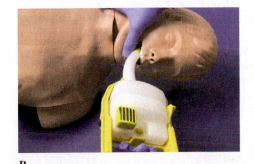
C

FIGURE 12–9   Establishing an oropharyngeal airway. **(A)** OPAs come in different sizes. **(B)** Measure from the corner of the mouth to the same side earlobe to select the correct size. **(C)** Insert the airway into the pharynx.
© William E. Prentice

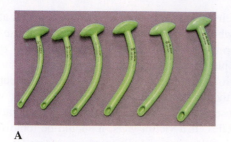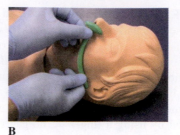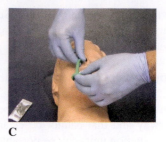

A                      B                      C

FIGURE 12–10    Establishing a nasopharyngeal airway. **(A)** NPAs come in different sizes. **(B)** Measure from the nostril to the same side earlobe to select the correct size. **(C)** Lubricate and insert the airway into the right nostril.

© William E. Prentice

be estimated by measuring the distance from the nostril to the same side earlobe. When correctly inserted, the flared end of the tube should rest just outside of the nasal passage and a bag/valve mask should fit easily over the airway. An NPA should not be used in any patient who has head trauma.[8]

A supraglottic airway is used with patients who are unresponsive with no gag reflex. The airway is inserted into the pharynx, without visualization, and is designed to create a seal in the posterior pharynx above the glottis (vocal chords), obstructing the esophagus and forcing air into the trachea. Currently, only EMTs and paramedics may use SGAs outside of a hospital.[8]

Using the airway adjunct devices has not traditionally been within the scope of practice for the athletic trainer. However, these skills are now considered a competency that athletic trainers should practice and master so they may be incorporated into clinical practice.[8]

See *Focus Box 12–5* "Procedures for using airway adjunct devices" for a more detailed description of specific techniques.

### Performing Breathing

1. When establishing unresponsiveness, the trained rescuer can quickly determine whether the victim is breathing, maintain the open airway; place your ear over the victim's mouth; observe the chest; and look, listen, and feel for breath sounds for 5 to no more than 10 seconds. If the victim is prone, look for the back to rise and fall with breathing (Figure 12–11).
2. To deliver rescue breaths:
   a. Using the hand on the victim's forehead, pinch the nose shut, keeping the heel of the hand in place to hold the head back (if there is no neck injury).
   b. In 1992, the Occupational Safety and Health Administration (OSHA) recommended the use of some barrier device, either a pocket mask or a bag/valve mask (and disposable gloves if available) protect the athletic trainer against disease transmission during CPR (see Figure 12–12 A through C).[44]

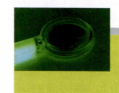

## FOCUS 12–5 Focus on Therapeutic Intervention

### Procedures for using airway adjunct devices

*Manual suction*

- If there is no cervical injury, logroll patient onto his or her side.
- Open patient's mouth and perform a finger sweep to remove large foreign bodies.
- Measure distance from corner of the mouth to the earlobe.
- Use this as a guide when inserting tube into the mouth. (Don't suction below base of tongue.)
- Suction from back to front in a circular pattern, moving quickly, for no more than 15 sec.
- If there is gag reflex, remove the suction tip.

*Oropharyngeal (OPA) airway*

- Choose the correct size by measuring from the corner of the mouth to the earlobe.
- Open the patient's mouth and lift the lower jaw and tongue up.
- Insert OPA with curved end up, then rotate tip down as it reaches the back of the throat.
- Slide it down the back of the throat behind the tongue.
- Flared end should rest on the patient's lips.

*Nasopharyngeal (NPA) airway*

- Choose the correct size by measuring from the nostril to the earlobe.
- Apply lubricant to tube.
- Insert tube in right nostril with gentle pressure (do not force), moving along the nasal floor.
- Flared end should rest on the patient's nostril.

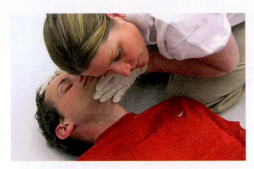

FIGURE 12–11   Once the airway is established, look, listen, and feel for breathing.
© William E. Prentice

These shields have a plastic or silicone sheet that spreads over the face and separates the athletic trainer from the victim. Some models have a tube-like mouthpiece, which may help in situations in which the athlete is wearing a face mask.

c. Take a normal breath, place your mouth over the barrier mask to provide an airtight seal, and give two slow, full breaths at a rate of one breath per second. Observe the chest rise and fall. Remove your mouth, and listen for the air to escape through passive exhalation. If the airway is obstructed, reposition the victim's head and try again to ventilate. If the airway is still obstructed, give thirty chest compressions; then look for an object in the mouth.

d. If the object is visible, clear visible objects from the mouth. Be careful not to push an object further into the throat. Continue to repeat this sequence until ventilation occurs.

e. If the victim is not breathing but has a pulse, give one ventilation every 5 to 6 seconds or 10 to 12 breaths per minute. Activate the EMS (if not already done) after 2 minutes in an adult. Recheck for breathing and pulse every 2 minutes.

3. If available, use a bag/valve mask for artificial respiration. Although the bag/valve mask is easy to use, some instruction and practice in its use is recommended (Figure 12–12B and D).

NOTE: Asthma is a chronic inflammatory condition that involves spontaneous spasm and narrowing of the bronchial airways and excessive production of mucus. The patient experiencing an asthma attack exhibits respiratory

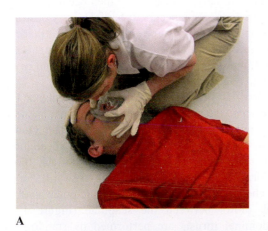

A

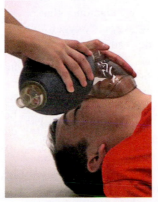

B

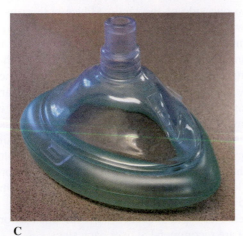

C

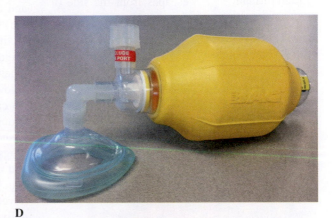

D

FIGURE 12–12   **(A&C)** A barrier pocket mask protects the athletic trainer from potential exposure to bloodborne pathogens. **(B&D)** A bag/valve mask can be used for respiration.
© William E. Prentice

distress in breathing and wheezing. However, this condition does not require basic life support intervention and is effectively managed using medication delivered via an inhaler. Asthma is discussed in detail in Chapter 29, and the use of an inhaler is discussed in Chapter 17.

***Administering Supplemental Oxygen*** Serious and life-threatening medical emergencies often cause oxygen to be depleted in the body, leaving the victim at risk for cardiac arrest or brain damage. Supplemental oxygen may prove to be a critical step in treating a severe or life-threatening illness or injury. An athletic trainer who has been specifically trained in supplemental oxygen administration should routinely give oxygen to a victim who is having trouble breathing. Administering supplemental oxygen requires using a bag/valve mask and a pressurized cylinder or canister containing oxygen (Figure 12–13).

The air that a person normally breathes contains about 21 percent oxygen. During rescue breathing, the victim receives only about 16 percent oxygen, but a bag/valve mask provides about 21 percent oxygen. Giving supplemental oxygen can provide the victim with a significantly higher oxygen concentration.[2]

All oxygen cylinders are easily identified because they are green with a yellow diamond that clearly says "oxygen." During administration, a face mask with an attached oxygen reservoir bag and a one-way valve between the mask and the bag are attached to the oxygen cylinder. As the patient breathes, the concentrated oxygen is inhaled from the bag, and exhaled air freely escapes from the side of the mask. As much as 90 percent oxygen can be delivered to the victim.[2] The oxygen should be delivered at a rate of 10 to 15 liters per minute as indicated by a flow rate meter.

In some states it is illegal to administer oxygen without a physician's prescription.

***Obstructed Airway Management*** Choking is a possibility in many sports activities; for example, an athlete may choke on a mouth guard, a broken piece of dental work, tongue rings, chewing gum, or even a chew of tobacco. When such emergencies arise, early recognition and prompt, knowledgeable action are necessary to avert a tragedy. An unconscious victim can have an obstructed airway

**All athletic trainers must have current CPR/AED.**

when the tongue falls back in the throat, thus blocking the upper airway.[46] Blood clots resulting from head, facial, or dental injuries may impede normal breathing, as may vomiting. When complete airway obstruction occurs, the individual is unable to speak, cough, or breathe.

***Conscious Victim*** If the victim is conscious, there is an effort made to breathe, the head is forced back, and the face initially is flushed and then becomes cyanotic as oxygen deprivation occurs. If partial airway obstruction is causing the choking, some air passage can be detected, but during a complete obstruction no air movement is discernible. If the victim is coughing, he or she should be encouraged to continue coughing.[2]

First, if the victim cannot cough, speak, or breathe, have someone call 911. Obtain consent from the victim before proceeding. In the conscious victim, back slaps, chest thrusts, and abdominal thrusts can all be effective in relieving airway obstructions. Back blows are performed by leaning the victim forward, supporting the chest with one hand and with the other hand deliver back blows between the scapulae (Figure 12–14A). Abdominal thrusts are performed by standing behind and to one side of the victim. Place both arms around the waist just above the belt line, and permit the victim's head, arms, and upper trunk to hang forward (Figure 12–14B). Grasp one of your fists with the other, placing the thumb side of the grasped fist immediately below the xiphoid process of the sternum, clear of the rib cage. Sharply and forcefully thrust the fists into the abdomen, inward, and upward, five times. This thrust pushes up on the diaphragm, compressing the air in the lungs, creating forceful pressure against the blockage, and thus usually causing the obstruction to be promptly expelled. Repeat the maneuver until the victim is relieved or becomes unconscious. Abdominal thrusts delivered in rapid sequence until the obstruction is relieved are recommended over back slaps.

***Unresponsive Victim*** If a conscious victim with an obstructed airway eventually becomes unresponsive, help

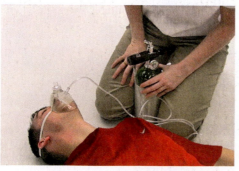

FIGURE 12–13  Administering supplemental oxygen to facilitate breathing.
© William E. Prentice

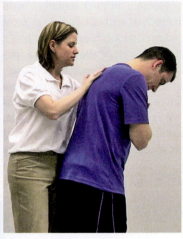
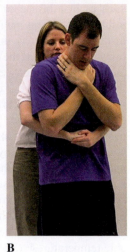

A                       B

FIGURE 12–14  In attempting to clear an obstructed airway for a conscious victim a rescuer may choose to deliver either **(A)** back blows or **(B)** abdominal thrusts.

© William E. Prentice

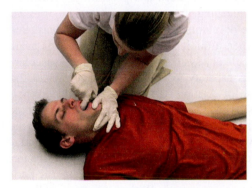

FIGURE 12–15  When the airway is opened look for a foreign object in the mouth and, if an object is found, remove it with your fingers.

© William E. Prentice

the victim get to the ground without falling. The victim must be on his or her back. Send someone to activate the EMS and begin CPR without a breath or pulse check. After performing 30 chest compressions, open the airway and look for an object in the mouth and, if found, remove it (Figure 12–15). Repeat this sequence as long as necessary. Victims who begin breathing on their own should be placed on their left side in the recovery position (see Figure 12–3).[1,2] Care must be taken to avoid applying extreme force over the rib cage because fractures of the ribs and damage to the organs can result.

*Finger Sweeping*  If a foreign object, such as a mouth guard, is lodged in the mouth or the throat and is visible, it may be possible to remove or release it with the fingers.[1] Care must be taken that the probing does not drive the object deeper into the throat. It is usually impossible to open the mouth of a conscious victim who is in distress, so the abdominal thrust technique should be used immediately. In the unconscious athlete, turn the head either to the side or face up, open the mouth by grasping the tongue

and the lower jaw, hold them firmly between the thumb and fingers, and lift—an action that pulls the tongue away from the back of the throat and from the impediment. If this action is difficult to do, the crossed finger method can usually be used effectively. The index finger of the free hand (or, if both hands are used, an assistant can probe) should be inserted into one side of the mouth along the cheek deeply into the throat; using a hooking maneuver, attempt to free the impediment, moving it into a position from which it can be removed (Figure 12–15). Once the object is removed, if the victim is not already breathing, attempt to ventilate.[1]

## Control of Hemorrhage

An abnormal discharge of blood is called a hemorrhage. The hemorrhage may be venous, capillary, or arterial and may be external or internal.

Venous blood is characteristically dark red with a continuous flow; capillary bleeding exudes from tissue and is a reddish color; and arterial bleeding flows in spurts and is bright red.

NOTE: The athletic trainer must be concerned with exposure to bloodborne pathogens and other diseases when coming into contact with blood or other body fluids. It is essential to take universal precautions to minimize this risk. The athletic trainer should use disposable latex gloves whenever he or she comes in contact with blood or other body fluids. This topic is discussed in detail in Chapter 14.

**External Bleeding**  External bleeding stems from open skin wounds, such as abrasions, incisions, lacerations, punctures, and avulsions (see Chapter 28 for further discussion). It can also occur from an open fracture. The control of external bleeding includes the use of direct pressure, elevation, and pressure points.[42]

*Direct Pressure*  Pressure is directly applied with the hand over a sterile gauze pad. The pressure is applied firmly against the resistance of a bone (Figure 12–16).

> External bleeding can usually be managed through direct pressure, elevation, or pressure points.

*Elevation*  Elevation in combination with direct pressure provides an additional means for reducing external hemorrhaging. Elevating a hemorrhaging part against gravity reduces hydrostatic blood pressure and facilitates venous and lymphatic drainage, which slows bleeding.

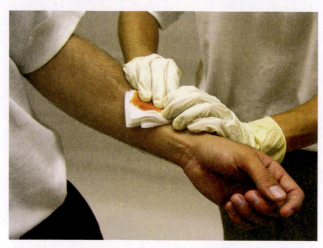

FIGURE 12–16 Direct pressure for the control of bleeding is applied with the hand over a sterile gauze pad.
© William E. Prentice

**Pressure Points** When direct pressure combined with elevation fails to slow hemorrhage, the use of pressure points may be the method of choice. Eleven points on each side of the body have been identified for controlling external bleeding, including the dosalis pedis, popliteal, femoral (anterior thigh), femoral (femoral triangle), radial and ulnar, brachial, axillary, subclavian, carotid, facial, and temporal pressure points. The two most commonly used are the brachial artery in the upper limb and the femoral artery in the lower limb. The brachial artery is compressed against the medial aspect of the humerus, and the femoral artery is compressed as it is detected within the femoral triangle (Figure 12–17).[7]

**Internal Hemorrhaging** Internal hemorrhage is invisible to the eye unless manifested through some body opening or identified through X-ray studies or other diagnostic techniques. Its danger lies in the difficulty of diagnosis. When internal hemorrhaging occurs—subcutaneously,

such as in a bruise or contusion; intramuscularly; or in joints—the patient may be moved without danger in most instances. However, the detection of bleeding within a body cavity, such as the skull, thorax, or abdomen, is a life-and-death situation. Because the symptoms are obscure, internal hemorrhage is difficult to diagnose properly. If an internal hemorrhage is suspected, blood pressure should be closely monitored.[33] As a result, patients with internal injuries require hospitalization under complete and constant observation by a medical staff to determine the nature and extent of the injuries. All severe hemorrhaging will eventually result in shock and should therefore be treated on this premise. Even if the patient shows no outward indication of shock, he or she should be kept quiet and body heat should be maintained at a constant and suitable temperature.[42] (See the following section for the preferred body position.)

## Shock

With any injury, shock is a possibility.[62] However, when severe bleeding, fractures, or internal injuries are present, the development of shock is more likely. Shock occurs when a diminished amount of blood is available to the circulatory system—that is, when the vascular system loses its capacity to hold the fluid portion of the blood because of dilation of the blood vessels.[62] When shock occurs, a quantity of plasma moves from the blood vessels into the tissue spaces of the body, leaving the blood cells within the vessels, causing stagnation and slowing the blood flow. As a result, not enough oxygen-carrying blood cells are available to the tissues, particularly those of the nervous system. With this general collapse of the vascular system comes widespread tissue death, which will eventually cause the death of the individual unless treatment is given.

Certain conditions, such as extreme fatigue, extreme exposure to heat or cold, extreme dehydration of fluids

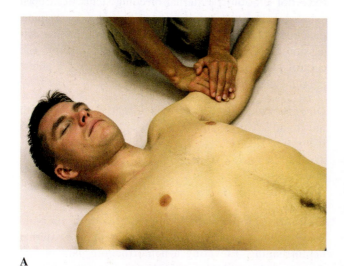

A

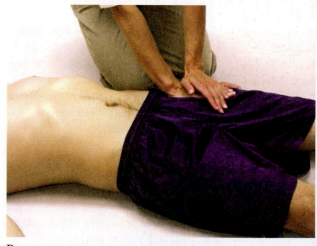

B

FIGURE 12–17 The two most common sites for compression of pressure points. **(A)** The brachial artery. **(B)** The femoral artery.
© William E. Prentice

and mineral loss, or illness, predispose a patient to shock. In a situation in which there is a potential shock condition, there are other signs by which the athletic trainer should assess the possibility of the patient's lapsing into a state of shock as an aftermath of the injury. The most important clue to potential shock is the recognition of a severe injury. It may happen that none of the usual signs of shock are present.[42]

The main types of shock are hypovolemic, respiratory, neurogenic, psychogenic, cardiogenic, septic, anaphylactic, and metabolic shock.[33]

*Hypovolemic shock* stems from trauma in which there is blood loss. Decreased blood volume causes a decrease in blood pressure. Without enough blood in the circulatory system, the organs are not properly supplied with oxygen.

*Respiratory shock* occurs when the lungs are unable to supply enough oxygen to the circulating blood. Trauma that produces a pneumothorax or an injury to the breathing control mechanism can produce respiratory shock.

*Neurogenic shock* is caused by the general dilation of blood vessels within the cardiovascular system. When it occurs, the typical 6 liters of blood can no longer fill the system. As a result, the cardiovascular system can no longer supply oxygen to the body.

*Psychogenic shock* is commonly known as fainting (syncope). It is caused by a temporary dilation of blood vessels that reduces the normal amount of blood in the brain.

*Cardiogenic shock* is the inability of the heart to pump enough blood to the body.

*Septic shock* occurs from a severe, usually bacterial, infection. Toxins liberated from the bacteria cause small blood vessels in the body to dilate.

*Anaphylactic shock* is the result of a severe allergic reaction caused by foods, insect stings, or drugs or by inhaling dusts, pollens, or other substances. Management of anaphylaxis, using an EpiPen (see Figure 17–2) is discussed in Chapter 17.

*Metabolic shock* happens when a severe illness, such as diabetes, goes untreated. Another cause is an extreme loss of body fluid (e.g., through urination, vomiting, or diarrhea).

**Symptoms and Signs** The major signs of shock are moist, pale, cool, clammy skin; weak and rapid pulse; increased and shallow respiratory rate; decreased blood pressure; and, in severe situations, urinary retention and fecal incontinence.[33,42] If conscious, the patient may display a disinterest in his or her surroundings, irritability, restlessness, or excitement. He or she may also exhibit extreme thirst.

> **A wrestler is thrown to the mat and suffers an open fracture of both the radius and the ulna in the forearm. There is significant bleeding from the wound. The patient begins to complain of light-headedness, his skin is pale and feels cool and clammy, and his pulse becomes rapid and weak.**
>
> **❓ What potential problem may be developing, and how should the athletic trainer manage this situation?**

> **Signs of shock:**
> - Blood pressure is low.
> - Systolic pressure is usually below 90 mm Hg.
> - Pulse is rapid and weak.
> - Patient may be drowsy and appear sluggish.
> - Respiration is shallow and extremely rapid.
> - Skin is pale, cool, and clammy.

**Management** Depending on the cause of the shock, the following emergency care should be given:

1. Maintain body temperature as close to normal as possible.
2. Elevate the feet and legs 8 to 12 inches (20 to 30 cm) for most situations. However, shock positioning varies according to the type of injury.[33] For a neck injury, for example, the athlete should be immobilized as found; for a head injury, the head and shoulders should be elevated; for a leg fracture, the legs should be kept level and should be raised after splinting.

Shock can also be compounded or even initially produced by the patient's psychological reaction to an injury situation. Fear or the sudden realization that a serious situation has occurred can result in shock. In the case of a psychological reaction to an injury, the patient should be instructed to lie down and avoid viewing the injury. The patient should be handled with patience and gentleness but also with firmness. Spectators should be kept away from the injured athlete. Reassurance is of vital concern to the injured individual. The person should be given immediate comfort through the loosening of clothing. Nothing should be given by mouth until a physician has determined that no surgical procedures are indicated.

# THE SECONDARY SURVEY

After the primary survey has determined that no life-threatening injuries or illnesses exist, and the patient appears to be in stable condition, the athletic trainer should conduct an on-the-field secondary survey to assess the existing injury more precisely.

## Recognizing Vital Signs

The ability to recognize physiological signs of injury is essential to the proper handling of potentially critical injuries. When evaluating the seriously ill or injured

> **Vital signs to observe:**
> - Level of consciousness
> - Pulse
> - Respiration
> - Blood pressure
> - Temperature
> - Skin color
> - Pupils
> - Movement
> - Abnormal nerve response

patient, the athletic trainer or physician must be aware of nine response areas: level of consciousness, pulse, respiration, blood pressure, temperature, skin color, pupils, movement, and abnormal nerve response. The three primary vital signs are pulse, respiration, and blood pressure.[33]

**Level of Consciousness** When recognizing vital signs, the examiner must always note the patient's level of consciousness. Normally, the individual is alert, is aware of the environment, and responds quickly to vocal stimulation. Head injury, heatstroke, and diabetic coma can alter the patient's level of conscious awareness.

The level of consciousness can be assessed by using several different scales: the AVPU scale, the ACDU scale, and the Glasgow Coma Scale. (See Chapter 27 for a discussion of the Glasgow Coma Scale.) The AVPU scale is widely used by EMTs for assessing the neurological status of trauma patients as originally taught in Advanced Trauma Life Support (ATLS). Both the AVPU and the ACDU scales are simpler to use than the Glasgow Coma Scale.

The AVPU scale is as follows:

- *A* for *alert* signifies that the patient is alert; awake; responsive to voice; and oriented to person, time, and place.
- *V* for *verbal* signifies that the patient responds to voice but is not fully oriented to person, time, or place.
- *P* for *pain* signifies that the patient does not respond to voice but does respond to a painful stimulus, such as a squeeze of the hand.
- *U* for *unresponsive* signifies that the patient does not respond to a painful stimulus.

The ACDU scale is as follows:

- Alert
- Confused
- Drowsy
- Unresponsive

**Pulse** The pulse is the direct extension of the functioning heart. In emergency situations, the pulse is usually determined at the carotid artery in the neck or the radial artery in the wrist (Figure 12–18). A normal pulse rate per minute for adults ranges between 60 and 100 beats, and in children, between 80 and 100 beats; however, well-conditioned athletes usually have slower pulses than the typical population.

**Respiratory patterns:**

- Apnea—temporary cessation of breathing
- Tachypnea—rapid breathing
- Bradypnea—slow breathing
- Dyspnea—difficult breathing
- Hyperventilation—labored breathing
- Obstructed—blocked airway caused by either partial or complete obstruction

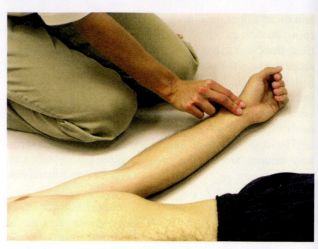

FIGURE 12–18    *Pulse rate taken at the radial artery.*
© William E. Prentice

An alteration of a pulse from normal may indicate the presence of a pathological condition. For example, a rapid but weak pulse could mean shock, bleeding, diabetic coma, or heat exhaustion. A rapid and strong pulse may mean heatstroke or severe fright; a strong but slow pulse could indicate a skull fracture or stroke; and no pulse means cardiac arrest or death.[33]

**Respiration** The normal breathing rate per minute is approximately 12 to 20 breaths in adults and 15 to 30 breaths in children. Breathing rate may be normal but breath may be shallow (indicating shock), labored, or noisy. Frothy blood being coughed up indicates a chest injury, such as a fractured rib, that has affected a lung. The athletic trainer should look, listen, and feel: look to ascertain whether the chest is rising or falling; listen for air passing into and out of the mouth, nose, or both; and feel where the chest is moving. If the victim is prone, look for the back to rise and fall with respiration.

**Blood Pressure** Blood pressure, as measured by the sphygmomanometer, indicates the amount of pressure exerted against the arterial walls. It is indicated at two pressure levels: systolic and diastolic. **Systolic blood pressure** occurs when the left ventricle contracts, thereby pumping blood, and **diastolic blood pressure** is the residual pressure present in the arteries when the heart is between beats. The resting blood pressure for 15 to 20-year-old males should be less than 120 **mm Hg** (systolic) and less than 80 mm Hg (diastolic). The normal blood pressure for females is usually 8 to 10 mm Hg lower than in males for both systolic and diastolic pressures. Between the ages of 15 and 20, a systolic pressure of greater than 120 mm Hg and a diastolic pressure of greater than 80 mm Hg may be excessive. Table 12–2 provides recommendations for blood pressure. A lowered blood pressure (hypotension) could indicate hemorrhage, shock, heart attack, or internal organ injury.[62]

| TABLE 12–2 | American Heart Association Recommended Blood Pressure Levels[1] | | |
|---|---|---|---|
| **Blood Pressure Category** | **Systolic (mm Hg)** | | **Diastolic (mm Hg)** |
| Normal | Less than 120 | and | Less than 80 |
| Prehypertension | 120–139 | or | 80–89 |
| High | | | |
|    Stage 1 | 140–159 | or | 90–99 |
|    Stage 2 | 160 or higher | or | 100 or higher |

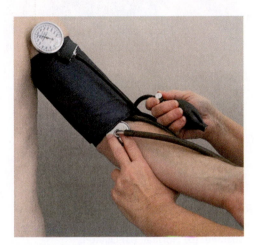

FIGURE 12–19   Blood pressure is measured using a sphygmomanometer and a stethoscope.

© William E. Prentice

Blood pressure is measured by applying the cuff circumferentially around the upper arm just proximal to the elbow (Figure 12–19). For individuals who have large or muscular upper arms, an extra-large sleeve should be used to get an accurate reading. The stethoscope should be placed on the anterior surface at the crease of the elbow joint directly over the brachial artery. The cuff should be inflated to 200 mm Hg, which occludes blood flow in the brachial artery distal to the cuff in the cubital fossa. The sounds, heard through the stethoscope are referred to as Korotkoff sounds. The cuff should be slowly deflated with the stethoscope in place; the first beating sound is recorded as systolic pressure. The cuff continues to be deflated until the beating sound disappears; diastolic pressure is then recorded.

**Korotkoffs sounds identify systolic and diastolic blood pressures**

**Temperature** Body temperature is maintained by water evaporation and heat radiation. It is normally 98.2°F (36.8°C) to 98.6°F (37°C). Temperature is measured with a thermometer, which is placed under the tongue, in the armpit, against the tympanic membrane in the ear, or, in case of unconsciousness, in the rectum. Core temperature is most accurately measured in the rectum (see *Focus Box 6–5:* "Measuring rectal temperature"). The technique using tympanic membrane temperature measurement in the ear (Figure 12–20) is easily done and is becoming a more accurate indication of core temperature. However, it is difficult to achieve the same temperature in consecutive trials due to difficulty replicating the depth and angle of insertion. A digital oral thermometer can also provide a reasonably accurate temperature measure (Figure 12–20C). Changes in body temperature can be reflected in the skin. For example, hot, relatively dry skin might indicate disease, infection, or overexposure to environmental heat. Cool, clammy skin could reflect trauma, shock, or heat exhaustion; cool, dry skin is possibly the result of overexposure to cold.

> **To convert Fahrenheit to centigrade (Celsius):**
> °C = (°F − 32) ÷ 1.8.
> **To convert centigrade to Fahrenheit:** °F = (1.8 × °C) + 32.

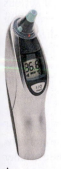
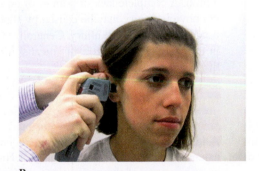
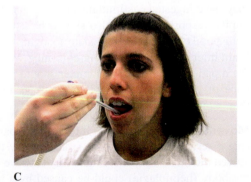

A              B                       C

FIGURE 12–20   Measuring temperature. **(A)** Digital tympanic membrane thermometer. **(B)** Measuring tympanic membrane thermometer. **(C)** Digital oral thermometer temperature measurement.

(a) Courtesy Welch Allyn; (b, c) © William E. Prentice

A rise or fall of internal temperature may be caused by a variety of circumstances, such as the onset of a communicable disease, cold exposure, pain, fear, or nervousness. Characteristically, a lowered body temperature is accompanied by chills with chattering teeth, blue lips, goose bumps, and pale skin.

**Skin Color** For individuals who are lightly pigmented, the skin can be a good indicator of the state of health. Normal skin tone is pink. A flushed or red skin color may indicate heatstroke, sunburn, allergic reaction, high blood pressure, or elevated temperature. A pale, ashen, or white skin can mean insufficient circulation, shock, fright, hemorrhage, heat exhaustion, or insulin shock. Skin that is bluish in color (cyanotic), primarily in the lips and fingernails, usually means an airway obstruction or a respiratory insufficiency. A yellowish or jaundice color may indicate liver disease or dysfunction.

Assessing skin color in a dark-skinned individual is more difficult. These individuals normally have pink coloration of the nail beds and inside the lips, mouth, and tongue. When a dark-skinned person goes into shock, the skin around the mouth and nose will often have a grayish cast, and the tongue, the inside of the mouth, the lips, and the nail beds will have a bluish cast. Shock resulting from hemorrhage will cause the tongue and inside of the mouth to become a pale, grayish color instead of blue. Fever in these individuals can be noted by a red flush at the tips of the ears.[33]

**Pupils** The pupils of the eyes are extremely sensitive to situations affecting the nervous system. Although most persons have pupils of regular outline and equal size, some individuals normally have pupils that are irregular and unequal. This disparity requires the athletic trainer to know which individuals deviate from the norm.

A constricted pupil may indicate the patient is using a central nervous system depressant drug. If one or both pupils are dilated, the patient may have sustained a head injury; may be experiencing shock, heatstroke, or hemorrhage; or may have ingested a stimulant drug (Figure 12–21). The pupils' response to light also should be noted. If one or both pupils fail to accommodate to light, there may be brain injury or alcohol or drug poisoning. When examining a patient's pupils, the examiner should note the presence of contact lenses. Pupil response is more critical than pupil size in an evaluation.

> Some athletes normally have irregular and unequal pupils.

**Movement** The inability to move a body part can indicate a serious central nervous system injury that has involved the motor system. An inability to move one side of the body (hemiplegia) could be caused by a head injury or cerebrovascular accident (stroke). Bilateral tingling and numbness or sensory or motor deficits of the upper extremity may indicate a cervical spine injury. Weakness or inability to move the lower extremities could mean an

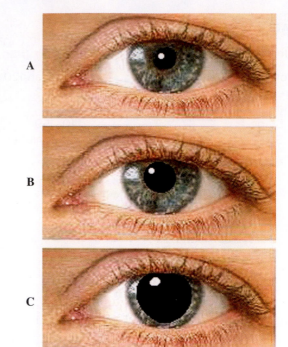

FIGURE 12–21 The pupils of the eyes are extremely sensitive to situations affecting the nervous system. **(A)** Constricted. **(B)** Normal. **(C)** Dilated.
© William E. Prentice

injury below the neck, and pressure on the spinal cord could lead to limited use of the limbs.[23]

**Abnormal Nerve Response** The injured patient's pain or other reactions to adverse stimuli can provide valuable clues to the athletic trainer. Numbness or tingling in a limb with or without movement can indicate nerve or cold damage. Blocking of a main artery can produce severe pain, loss of sensation, or lack of a pulse in a limb. A complete lack of pain or of awareness of serious but obvious injury may be caused by shock, hysteria, drug usage, or a spinal cord injury. Generalized or localized pain in the injured region probably means there is no injury to the spinal cord.

> **Decisions that can be made from the secondary survey:**
> - Seriousness of injury
> - Type of first aid required
> - Whether injury warrants physical referral
> - Type of transportation needed.

## Musculoskeletal Assessment and Management

A logical process must be used to evaluate accurately the extent of a musculoskeletal injury.[37] The athletic trainer must be aware of the major signs that reveal the site, nature, and, above all, severity of the injury. Detection of these signs can be facilitated by understanding the mechanism or traumatic sequence and by methodically inspecting the injury.[13] Knowledge of the mechanism of an injury is extremely important in determining which area of the body is most affected. When the injury mechanism has been determined, the examiner proceeds to the next phase: physical inspection of the affected region. At this point, information is gathered by what is seen, heard, and felt.[37]

In an attempt to understand the mechanism of injury, a detailed *history* of the complaint must be taken. The patient is asked, if possible, about the events leading up to the injury and how it occurred and what he or she heard or felt when the injury took place.[6] Sounds occurring at the time of injury or during manual inspection yield pertinent information about the type and extent of pathology present. Such uncommon sounds as grating or harsh rubbing may indicate fracture. Such sounds as a snap, crack, or pop at the moment of injury often indicate bone fracture or injury to ligaments or tendons. Joint sounds may be detected when either arthritis or internal derangement is present. Areas of the body that have abnormal amounts of fluid may produce crepitus when palpated or moved.

The athletic trainer should make a visual *observation* of the injured site, comparing it with the uninjured body part and looking for symmetry. The initial visual examination can disclose obvious deformity, swelling, and skin discoloration.

Finally, the region of the injury should be gently *palpated*. Feeling, or palpating, a part with trained fingers can, in conjunction with visual and audible signs, indicate the nature of the injury. Palpation is started away from the injury and gradually moved toward it. As the examiner gently feels the injury and surrounding structures with the fingertips, several factors can be revealed: the extent of point tenderness, the extent of irritation (whether it is confined to soft tissue alone or extends to the bony tissue), deformities that may not be detected by visual examination alone, and the presence of a pulse.[6]

### Assessment Decisions

After a quick on-site injury inspection and evaluation, the athletic trainer should make the following decisions:

1. The seriousness of the injury
2. The type of first aid and immobilization necessary
3. Whether the injury warrants immediate referral to a physician for further assessment

4. The manner of transportation from the injury site to the sidelines, athletic training room, or hospital

All information about the initial history, signs, and symptoms of the injury must be documented, if possible, so that they may be described in detail to the physician.

**Immediate Treatment** Musculoskeletal injuries are extremely common in sports. The athletic trainer must be prepared to provide appropriate first aid immediately.

For many years, the recommendation for managing acute musculoskeletal injuries has included the immediate application of ice, compression, and elevation in combination with some type of protection (e.g., elastic wrap, tape, crutches, walking boot, etc.) and/or rest or restricted activity. The acronyms **RICE** and **PRICE** have both been commonly used to refer to this combination of simultaneously applied treatment techniques that have been well accepted as a best practice recommendation by most health care providers. But despite this near-unanimous clinical consensus, there is limited evidence from high-quality randomized clinical trials that supports the use of these interventions.[31,66] Most recently, it has been recommended that a more appropriate acronym would be **POLICE,** which stands for protection, optimal loading, ice, compression, and elevation (Figure 12–22).[10]

The goals of treatment in acute care are to protect the injured tissue from further injury, to reduce the secondary hypoxic injury that results from the acute inflammatory response, and to control pain while limiting swelling. If swelling can be controlled initially, the amount of time required for injury rehabilitation will be significantly reduced.

*Protection* Protecting the damaged tissue from further injury is an extremely important component of any treatment program. Once a tissue is injured, it immediately begins the healing process. Subjecting the injured part to additional unnecessary external stresses and strains may cause additional bleeding and further damage that can interfere with the essential biological processes in the acute inflammatory stage of the healing process. Thus, short periods of protection (using crutches, braces, etc.), which include rest and

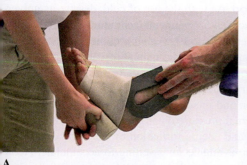 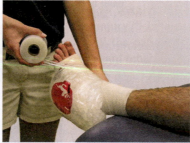 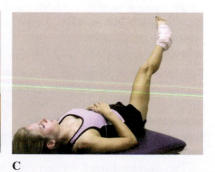

A                                   B                           C

FIGURE 12–22   POLICE technique. **(A)** A compression wrap should be applied over the horseshoe pad. **(B)** Ice bags should be secured in place by an elastic or plastic wrap. **(C)** The leg should be elevated as much as possible during the initial treatment period.

A field hockey player trips over an opponent's stick, plantar flexing and inverting her ankle, and she falls to the turf with a grade 2 ankle sprain. She has immediate effusion and significant pain. On examination, there appears to be some laxity in the ankle joint. The athletic trainer transports the patient to the training room so that the ankle sprain can be managed properly.

**?** What specifically should the athletic trainer do to most effectively control the initial swelling associated with this injury?

immobilization, are recommended immediately following acute soft tissue injury.[10] Although aggressive ambulation or exercise should be avoided immediately, rest should be of limited duration after trauma.

***Optimal Loading*** Longer periods of rest during which injured tissues are unloaded may produce adverse changes to joint biomechanics and tissue morphology. Progressive mechanical loading of injured tissues following the acute inflammatory stage of healing promotes cellular responses that improve the structural characteristics of collagen, and thus facilitating healing.[32] *Optimal loading* refers to determining and subsequently incorporating the appropriate progression from protecting the tissue to prevent exacerbation of the injury, to mechanically loading the tissue to facilitate healing. Early functional activity encourages early recovery.[30]

***Ice*** The use of ice application immediately following musculoskeletal injury has been accepted and routinely practiced by athletic trainers despite the fact that there is limited strong clinical evidence supporting its efficacy.[11,31] **SoR:C** Ice is most commonly used immediately after injury to decrease cell metabolism and pain in the injured area. Ice may also be beneficial in chronic inflammatory conditions, such as bursitis, and tendinopathies in which heat may cause additional pain and swelling. Cold is also used to reduce the muscle guarding that accompanies pain.

Cold applied to an acute injury will lower metabolism and tissue demands for oxygen and will reduce hypoxia.[39] This benefit extends to uninjured tissue, limiting secondary hypoxic tissue injury from occurring in adjacent normal cellular structures. Cellular metabolism is maximally decreased when the tissue temperature is between 50° to 59°F.[11]

The deceased need for oxygen likely causes reduced blood flow and there is vasoconstriction of the arterioles and reduced perfusion to the tissues. In fact, this decreased blood flow begins within 10 minutes and

> Protection, optimal loading, ice, compression, and elevation POLICE are essential in the emergency care of musculoskeletal injuries.

continues for approximately 13 minutes.[27] Thus, ice application limits edema formation and swelling as a result of decreased cell metabolism. Vasoconstriction reduces blood flow, which decreases intravascular pressure, thereby decreasing fluid movement out of the vessels and into the tissues.[20]

Evidence indicates that cold application is effective in decreasing pain.[11] The pain-reducing (analgesic) effect is likely to be one of the greatest benefits. One explanation of the analgesic effect is that cold slows the speed of nerve transmission, so the pain sensation is reduced. It is also possible that cold bombards pain receptors with so many cold impulses that pain impulses from peripheral skin receptors are blocked. With ice treatments, the patient usually reports an uncomfortable sensation of cold, followed by burning, then an aching sensation, and finally complete numbness.

Cold applied to the skin is capable of lowering the temperature of deeper tissues. The temperature to which the deeper tissues can be lowered depends on the type of cold that is applied to the skin, the duration of its application, the thickness of the subcutaneous (under the skin) fat, and the region of the body to which it is applied. Because the subcutaneous fat slowly conducts the cold, applications of cold for short periods of time will be ineffective in cooling deeper tissues. For this reason, treatments of at least 20 to 30 minutes have been traditionally recommended.[39] However, application of cold for prolonged periods can potentially cause tissue damage.

For best results, ice packs (crushed ice) or ice massage should be used because they produce the most rapid and significant temperature decreases. Frozen gel packs should not be used directly against the skin because they reach much lower temperatures than do ice packs and can damage the skin. Ice immersion in a tub or whirlpool should be avoided in acute treatment of an injured extremity since it requires the extremity to be in a dependent position.

High-quality studies focusing on developing modes, durations, and frequencies of ice application that will optimize outcomes after injury are necessary to create evidence-based guidelines on the use of ice.[11]

***Compression*** As with the use of cold, despite its universal acceptance as a treatment technique in acute injury, limited evidence from high-quality clinical trials supports the use of compression making treatment recommendations difficult.[31] **SoR:C** In most cases, immediate compression of an acute injury is considered to be at least as essential as cold and elevation and in some cases may be superior to them. Placing external pressure on an injury assists in decreasing hemorrhage and edema formation by mechanically reducing the space available for swelling to accumulate. Acute inflammation increases the permeability of capillary and arteriole walls allowing fluid leakage into interstitial spaces. This process is retarded by compression, and drainage into the lymphatic system is facilitated.

Many types of compression are available including elastic wraps, tape, and commercial pneumatic compression devices (i.e., Game-Ready). A compression wrap should be left in place for at least 72 hours after an acute injury. It has been demonstrated that using an elastic or plastic wrap to hold an ice bag in place significantly decreases subcutaneous tissue temperatures.[15] An elastic wrap that has been soaked in water and frozen in a freezer can provide both compression and cold when applied to a recent injury. Pads can be cut from felt or foam rubber to fit difficult-to-compress body areas. For example, a horseshoe-shaped pad placed bilaterally around the malleoli in combination with an elastic wrap and tape provides focal compression to reduce ankle edema.[72] Although cold is applied intermittently, compression should be maintained throughout the day and if possible throughout the night. Because of the pressure buildup in the tissues, the patient may find it painful to leave a compression wrap in place for a long time. In many chronic overuse problems, such as tendinopathies, and particularly bursitis, the compression wrap should be worn until the swelling is gone. CAUTION: Applying compression to an anterior compartment syndrome in the lower leg which swelling has significantly increased pressure in that area is contraindicated.

**Elevation** Along with cold and compression, elevation reduces capillary bleeding into the tissues. The injured part, particularly an extremity, should be elevated to eliminate the effects of gravity on blood pooling in the extremities. Elevation assists the lymphatic system, which drains blood and edema from the injured area, returning them to the central circulatory system. The greater the degree of elevation, the more effective the reduction in swelling. In an ankle sprain, for example, the leg should be placed so that the ankle is virtually straight up in the air to maximize the effects of gravity. The injured part should be elevated as much as possible during the first 72 hours.

**Emergency Splinting** Any suspected fracture should be splinted before the patient is moved.[38] Transporting a person with a fracture without proper immobilization can result in increased tissue damage, hemorrhage, and shock.[35] Conceivably, a mishandled fracture could cause death. Therefore, a thorough knowledge of splinting techniques is important. Applying splints should be a simple process using commercial emergency splints.[38,42] The athletic trainer usually does not have to improvise a splint because such devices are readily available in most sports settings. Whatever the type of splint used, the principles of good splinting remain the same. Two major concepts of splinting are to splint from one joint above the fracture to one joint below the fracture and to splint where the patient lies. If at all possible, do not move the patient until he or she has been splinted. *Focus Box 12–6:* "Guidelines for proper splinting" outlines the approach to be used.

> A suspected fracture must be splinted before the patient is moved.

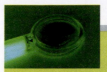

### Guidelines for proper splinting

- Put a dressing on any open wound before applying a splint.
- Splint the injury in the position in which it is found.
- Make sure the splint immobilizes the injury and doesn't permit movement.
- Immobilize the joints above and below the site of injury.
- Elevate the splinted extremity if possible.
- Apply a cold pack to the injury around the splint.
- Continuously check the color of the fingers and toes to make sure circulation is not impaired.

**Rapid form Vacuum Immobilizer** The rapid form vacuum immobilizer is widely used by both EMTs and athletic trainers.[50] It consists of styrofoam chips contained inside an airtight cloth sleeve that is pliable. This splint can be molded to the shape of any joint or angulated fracture through the use of Velcro straps. A handheld pump sucks the air out of the sleeve, giving it a cardboardlike rigidity. This splint is most useful for injuries that are angulated and must be splinted in the position in which they are found (Figure 12–23A).

**Air Splint** An air splint is a clear plastic splint that is inflated with air around the affected part and can be used for extremity splinting, but its use requires some special training. This splint provides support and moderate pressure to the body part and affords a clear view of the site for X-ray examination. The inflatable splint should not be used if it will alter a fracture deformity (Figure 12–23B).

**SAM® Splint** A SAM® Splint is made with a thin sheet of soft, pliable aluminum covered by padding. The material can be cut with a pair of taping scissors. However, when shaped into structural curves, the SAM® Splint's aluminum core becomes rigid. The material is reusable and can be folded and unfolded repeatedly, allowing the same sheet of splint material to be reused as many times as desired (Figure 12–23C).

**Half-Ring Splint** For fractures of the femur, the half-ring traction splint offers the best support and immobilization but takes considerable practice to master. An open fracture must be carefully dressed to avoid additional contamination (Figure 12–23D).

**Splinting of Lower-Limb Fractures** Fractures of the ankle or leg require immobilization of the foot and knee. Any fracture involving the knee, thigh, or hip

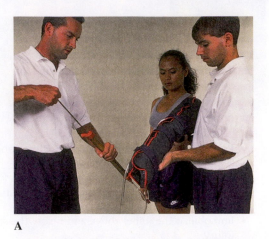

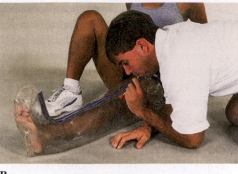

B

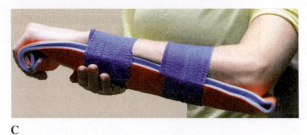

C

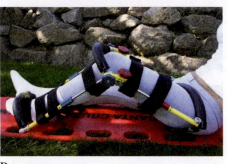

D

FIGURE 12–23 Examples of splints. **(A)** Rapid form vacuum immobilizer. **(B)** Air splint. **(C)** SAM® Splint (from SAM® Splint). **(D)** Half-ring splint (from Reel Research and Development).

(a, b) © William E. Prentice; (c) Courtesy SAM Medical Products; (d) Courtesy Reel Research and Development Corporation

needs splinting of all the lower-limb joints and one side of the trunk.

***Splinting of Upper-Limb Fractures*** Fractures around the shoulder complex are immobilized by a sling and swathe bandage, with the upper limb securely bound to the body. Upper-arm and elbow fractures must be splinted, with immobilization effected in a straight-arm position to lessen bone override. Lower-arm and wrist fractures should be splinted in a position of elbow flexion and should be supported by a sling. Hand and finger dislocations and fractures can be buddy-taped or may be splinted with tongue depressors, roller gauze, or aluminum splints.[52]

***Splinting of the Spine and Pelvis*** Injuries involving a possible spine or pelvic fracture are best splinted and the patient moved using a spine board. Recently, a full body mattress vacuum splint immobilizer has been developed for dealing with spinal injuries (Figure 12–24).[36] The effectiveness of this piece of equipment as an immobilization device has yet to be determined.[50]

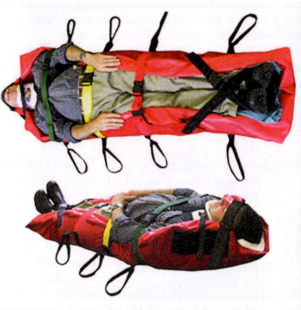

FIGURE 12–24 Full body mattress vacuum splint immobilizer. (From Neann, Victoria, Australia).

Courtesy RAPP Australia Pty Ltd.

# PROTECTIVE EQUIPMENT REMOVAL

For the athletic trainer who must decide how to manage a suspected cervical spine injury, the primary goal is to ensure that the cervical spine is immobilized and maintained in a neutral position while the vital life functions are accessible. It has been shown that football, ice hockey, or lacrosse helmets as well as the face mask and various types of shoulder pads will complicate lifesaving CPR procedures.[17,68] Exposure and access to the airway and chest should CPR, and the use of an AED, be necessary must be established or easily achieved in a reasonable and acceptable manner.[58] Over the years, significant debate has raged in the sports medicine community over removing the helmet and/or shoulder pads of an athlete with suspected cervical spine injury, and a number of differing opinions have been expressed.[45,55,58,69,70,71]

In the past, the recommendation has been that protective equipment (e.g., helmets and shoulder pads in football, hockey, and lacrosse) should be left in place for transport and removed after arrival in the hospital emergency department. Due primarily to recent changes in EMS protocols, the most current recommendation is that when appropriate, protective athletic equipment may be removed while maintaining cervical spine stabilization *prior* to transport to an emergency facility for a patient with suspected cervical spine instability.[41] Further, it is recommended that equipment removal be performed by at least three rescuers who have been trained and are experienced with equipment removal at the earliest possible time. If fewer than three people are present, the equipment should be removed as soon as possible after enough trained individuals arrive on the scene.[41]

The rationale for these recommendations is that athletic trainers have been exposed to more equipment removal training than the hospital emergency department staff, thus expediting access to the injured patient.[41]

After decades of controversy regarding the correct approach or sequence for removal of protective equipment in football, lacrosse, and ice hockey, it now appears that *both the helmet and shoulder pads may be removed prior to transport.* Removing one or the other independently may compromise the cervical spine.[58] **SoR:B**

## Face Mask Removal

It has been shown that removing the face mask and then the helmet creates significantly less motion (particularly less flexion-extension and axial rotation) and is thus safer for prehospital emergent access to the airway than direct removal of the helmet.[21,59] Although it has been suggested that newer helmet designs have made it significantly easier and faster to remove the helmet, research has shown that there is no difference between traditional and newer helmet designs even if the helmet's air bladder is deflated prior to removal.[59,60]

The face mask is attached to the football helmet, usually by four fasteners that must be removed. It is recommended that the two side fasteners be removed first, followed by the top fasteners.[58] Different types of fasteners are currently being used, including loop strap fasteners, shock-blocker fasteners, stabilizer fasteners, Revolution fasteners, and quick-release fasteners (Figure 12–25).[56] The most recent studies have shown

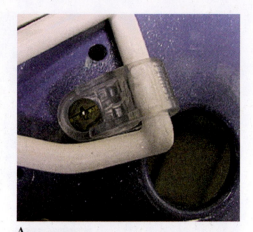

A

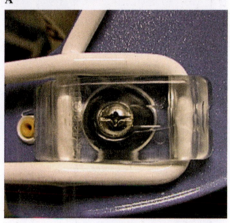

B

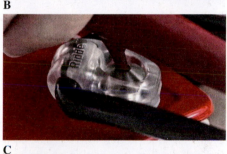

C

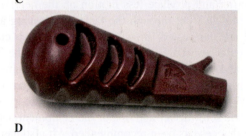

D

FIGURE 12–25 Helmet fasteners. **(A)** Loop strap. **(B)** Revolution. **(C)** Quick Release. **(D)** Quick Release tool.
© William E. Prentice

that helmet face masks with the quick-release fasteners allow for the fastest removal times with little additional motion.[57] Additionally, it has been recommended that helmet manufacturers consider incorporating quick-release face mask designs into all helmets that do not currently possess the technology and should design all future helmets with this feature.[57]

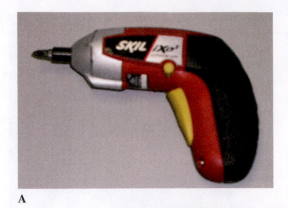

A

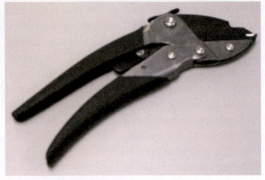

B

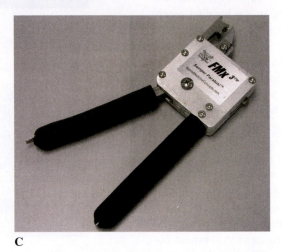

C

FIGURE 12–26   Tools for removing facemask. **(A)** Electric screwdriver. **(B)** Anvil Pruner. **(C)** FM Extractor.
© William E. Prentice

For those helmets that have fasteners other than quick release, it is recommended that the face mask be removed using the tool and technique that perform the task quickly and with minimal movement and difficulty.[58] **SoR:B** Using an electric screwdriver has been shown to be faster and produce less motion on the helmet than using tools that cut through the fasteners, as long as the screws are not rusted, in which case a backup cutting tool should be used.[16,29] Two cutting devices—the Anvil Pruner and the FM Extractor—have been recommended for their effectiveness in quickly cutting the plastic fasteners (Figure 12–26).[56] A combined-tool approach using an electric screwdriver and one of the equipment-specific cutting devices has been recommended.[24] It also has been suggested that the athletic trainer should be proficient in removing the face mask within 30 seconds.[58]

## Helmet and Shoulder Pad Removal[14] *

The following sequence should be followed when removing the helmet and shoulder pads:

1. One rescuer (Rescuer 1) maintains stabilization of the cervical spine. There are two techniques that are

*Based on Courson R; Personal communication, Athens, GA, 2016, University of Georgia

recommended for stabilizing the cervical spine; the head-squeeze technique (Figure 12–27A), where the rescuer holds the sides of the head with both hands and the trap-squeeze method (Figure 12–27B), where the rescuer grips the patient's trapezius muscles on either side of the neck and firmly squeezes the head between the forearms.

2. A second rescuer (Rescuer 2) cuts the front of the jersey from the waist to the neck and from sleeve to sleeve in a T pattern (Figure 12–28A).

3. Rescuer 2 cuts the right and left chest straps on the shoulder pads and opens the front of the shoulder pads either by cutting the front/center strings or straps (Figure 12–29A), or by pulling the tab on the Riddell RipKord system which provides a quick release for removal of the shoulder pads allowing for easy separation of both the chest and posterior parts of the shoulder pad[34] (Figure 12–29B). The quick release design allows for clinically acceptable removal times without inducing additional motion or difficulty.[57]

4. Before removing the helmet, the chinstrap is cut and removed (Figure 12–30A). Removing the jaw pads makes helmet removal easier (Figure 12–30B).

5. Rescuer 2 reaches under the shoulder pads from the front and takes over stabilization of the cervical spine

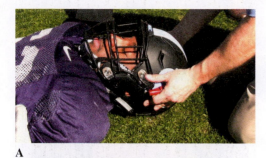

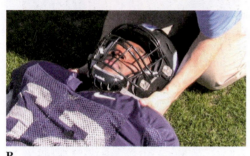

FIGURE 12–27   Cervical spine immobilization techniques.
**(A)** Head squeeze. **(B)** Trap squeeze.
© William E. Prentice

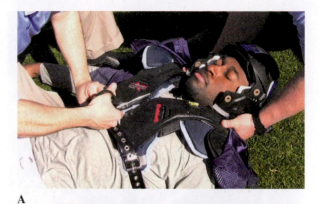

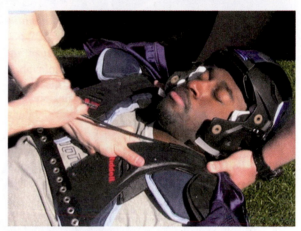

FIGURE 12–29   Expose the chest by opening the shoulder pads. **(A)** Cutting the straps or strings. **(B)** Pulling the Riddell RipKord tab.
© William E. Prentice

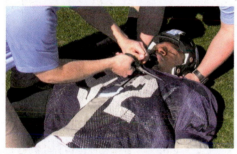

FIGURE 12–28   Cut the front of the jersey in a T pattern from waist to chest and sleeve to sleeve.
© William E. Prentice

saying "I have the c-spine" telling Rescuer 1 to release control (Figure 12–30C).

6. Rescuer 1 removes the helmet then resumes control of the cervical spine (Figure 12–30D).

7. The shoulder pads are removed using one of the following techniques depending on the number of available trained rescuers and the type of shoulder pads:

   a. **The elevated torso technique** is used when the shoulder pad straps have not been cut posteriorly. Rescuer 2 reaches inside shoulder pads and assumes control of the c-spine from Rescuer 1. Rescuers 3 and 4 tilt the athlete 30–45 degrees at the waist. Rescuer 1 removes the shoulder pads axially and then resumes control of the c-spine as the patient is lowered to the ground (Figure 12–31A). An alternative to this technique for smaller athletes would be for Rescuer 2 to straddle the athlete, reach under both shoulders, and lift the shoulder while Rescuer 3 slides the shoulder pads out axially.[28]

   b. **The flat torso technique** can only be used when the shoulder pads have been cut or separated (bivalved) both anteriorly and posteriorly. The c-spine must be stabilized by Rescuer 2 who takes over stabilization from Rescuer 1 from the front. Rescuers 1 and 3 may then slide the shoulder pads laterally  (Figure 12–31B).[28] Pulling the quick release tab on the **Riddell RipKord shoulder pads** automatically separates the pads in both the front and back. Thus, the flat torso technique can be used to remove the pads and the Rescuers can slide the pads laterally without having to elevate the torso (See Figure 12–29B).[34]

   c. In the **8-Person Lift** Rescuer 1 continues to stabilize the c-spine. On the command of Rescuer 1, Rescuers 2-7 (3 on each side) lift the athlete approximately 12" to allow for shoulder pad removal); Rescuer 8 slides the long spine board under the athlete from the feet (Figure 12–31C). A 9th Rescuer carefully slides the shoulder pads from under the athlete without interfering with Rescuer 1's c-spine control and says, "shoulder pads clear." The athlete is then lowered directly onto the long spine board.

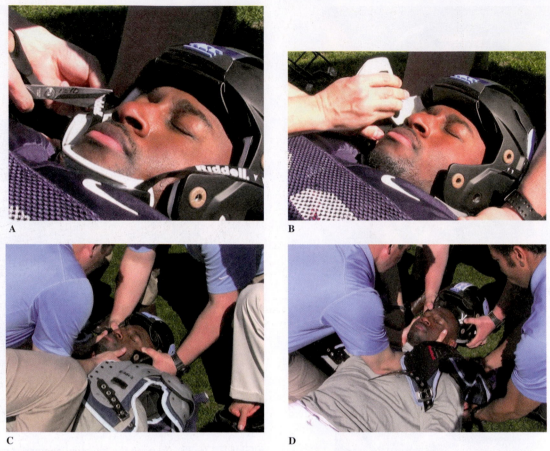

FIGURE 12–30    Removing the helmet. **(A)** Cutting and removing the chinstrap. **(B)** Removing the jaw pads. **(C)** Rescuer 2 stabilizes c-spine. **(D)** Rescuer 1 removing the helmet.
© William E. Prentice

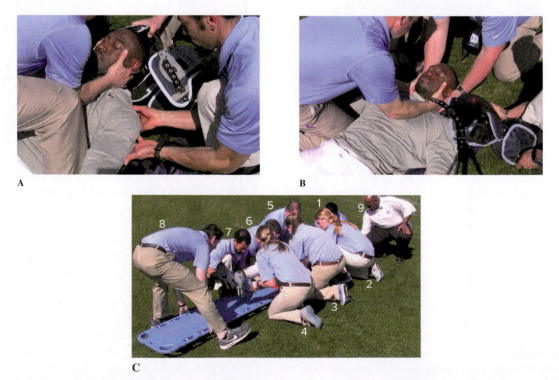

FIGURE 12–31    Removing the shoulder pads **(A)** Elevated torso technique. **(B)** Flat torso technique. **(C)** 8-Person lift technique.
© William E. Prentice

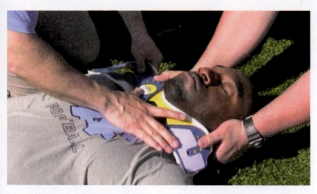

**FIGURE 12–32** Applying a rigid cervical collar.
© William E. Prentice

8. As soon as the helmet and shoulder pads are removed a rigid cervical collar should be applied while one rescuer continues to maintain in-line cervical spine stabilization (Figure 12–32).[41]

# MOVING AND TRANSPORTING THE INJURED PATIENT

Moving, lifting, and transporting the injured patient must be executed with the use of techniques that will prevent further injury. Moving or transporting the patient improperly causes more additional injuries than does any other emergency procedure.[33,42] There is no excuse for poor handling of the injured patient. Planning should take into consideration all the possible transportation methods and the necessary equipment to execute them.[42] Capable and well-trained personnel, spine boards, stretchers, and a rescue vehicle may be needed to transport the injured patient. Special consideration must be given to extracting an injured swimmer from a pool.

> Great caution must be taken when transporting the injured athlete.

In 2009, NATA developed a position statement "Acute management of the cervical spine injured athlete" (www.nata.org/sites/default/files/AcuteMgmtOfCervicalSpine-InjuredAthlete.pdf). More recently in 2015, an Inter-Association Task Force consensus statement entitled "Appropriate Prehospital Management of the Spine-Injured Athlete" provided significant changes to the previous recommendations.

## Placing the Patient on a Spine Board

Primary emergency care involves helping the patient maintain normal breathing, treating the patient for profuse bleeding or shock, and keeping the patient quiet and calm. In cases of suspected cervical spine injury, the athletic trainer should contact the EMS and then work closely with EMS personnel to move and transport the injured patient.

A suspected cervical spine injury requires extremely careful handling and is best left to properly trained paramedics, EMTs, or athletic trainers who are well prepared and have access to the proper equipment for transport.[63] Ideally, the patient with a suspected cervical spine injury should not be moved until a physician has examined the athlete and has given permission to move him or her. The most important principle in moving and transporting the injured patient is *spinal motion restriction (SMR)* to prevent further harm to the spinal cord by maintaining the head and neck in neutral alignment with the long axis of the body throughout the entire transport process.[5,35,41]

The following steps should be followed when managing a patient with a suspected cervical spine injury:

1. Have one person whose sole responsibility is to ensure and maintain proper stabilization of the head and neck immediately after injury, throughout transportation, first to the emergency vehicle, then to the hospital, and throughout the hospital procedure (see Figure 12–27).[18, 58] **SoR:B**

2. As soon as the equipment is removed a rigid cervical collar should be applied to immobilize cervical spinal motion (see Figure 12–32).[41,58] **SoR:B** Spinal motion restriction (SMR) is indicated when there is spinal pain and tenderness, sensory deficits or motor weakness, deformity of the spine, or altered level of consciousness due to blunt trauma.[41] It should be noted that rigid cervical collars do not completely control cervical spine motion but are more effective when combined with manual in-line cervical stabilization.[41]

3. Until recently the standard of care for cervical spine–injured patients has been to place the patient on a rigid, long spine board for transport. However, evidence now shows that prehospital spinal immobilization using a spine board may not be best for the patient. Concerns over the length of time the patient is in discomfort from lying on the rigid, unyielding board have led to recommendations that a scoop stretcher or a vacuum mattress may effectively provide the necessary stabilization while being more comfortable for the patient.[36,41] In the case of an injured athlete, the most current recommendation is to initially place the patient on a long spine board, scoop stretcher, or vacuum mattress for extraction from the field or court and then transfer him or her, as soon as possible, to a less-rigid stretcher for transport.[41]

4. If the patient is supine, an eight-person lift should be used to move the patient onto the long spine board using a lift and slide technique.[41] Eight rescuers are need for this technique; Rescuer 1 is responsible for stabilizing the patient's cervical spine; Rescuers 2 to 7 (three on each side) are responsible for lifting the patient's trunk, hips, and legs. On Rescuer 1's lift command, the patient is lifted about 12 inches while Rescuer 8 slides a spine board under the patient between Rescuers 2 to 7 (see Figure 12–31A). If the patient is wearing a jersey and shoulder pads both should be removed before being lowered onto the spine board. The eight-person lift has

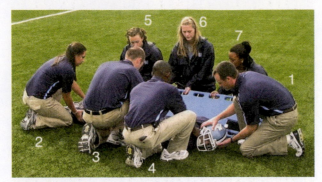

FIGURE 12–33   Logroll technique onto a spine board.
© William E. Prentice

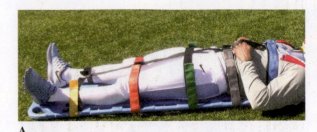

A

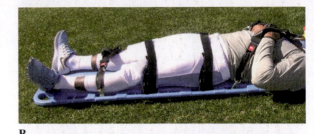

B

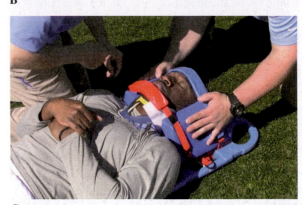

C

FIGURE 12–34   **(A)** Using spider straps to stabilize the patient on a long spine board. **(B)** Using seat belts to stabilize the patient on a long spine board. **(C)** Securing the head to the spine board.
© William E. Prentice

been shown to be more effective in restricting motion in the head, reducing both lateral flexion and axial rotation, compared with the logroll technique.[18]

5. If the patient is prone, he or she must be logrolled onto his or her back to be placed on either a long spine board, a scoop stretcher, or a vacuum mattress (Figure 12–33).[47] To logroll the patient requires Rescuer 1 to stabilize the cervical spine and carefully move the head into a neutral position as the patient is being rolled. Again, if the patient is wearing a jersey and shoulder pads, both should be cut down the back prior to logrolling. Rescuers 5-7 position the long spine board at an angle of 45 degrees on the side opposite to the direction that the patient's head is facing to facilitate moving the head and spine into neutral alignment. All extremities are placed in an axial alignment. Rescuers 2 to 4 are responsible for maintaining the axial alignment of the trunk, hips and thighs, and lower legs. With the spine board held close to the patient's side, Rescuer 1 gives the command for rescuers 2 to 4 to logroll and push the patient onto the spine board as one unit (Figure 12–33). Once the patient is supine on the long spine board the helmet and shoulder pads can be removed as described earlier, and a rigid cervical collar should be applied immediately.[41]

6. Once on the spine board the patient should be secured using spider straps applied across the chest, hips, thighs, and lower legs with the wrists secured across the chest by either tape or a Velcro strap (Figure 12–34A). Seat belt straps may also be used to secure the patient to the spine board (Figure 12–34B). Finally, the head should be secured with lateral restraint pads and then secured to the spine board with tape over the chin and forehead (Figure 12–34C).[14]

7. All rescuers place themselves in a position to stand, and then, on the command of Rescuer 1 stabilizing the cervical spine, they collectively lift and carry the patient on the spine board to a cart for removal from the field or to an emergency vehicle for transport to a hospital capable of delivering immediate, definitive care to a patient with a potential spinal cord injury (Figure 12–35).[41]

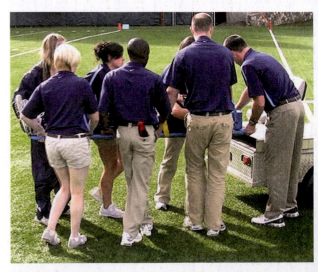

FIGURE 12–35   Carrying the spine board to the cart of rescue vehicle.
© William E. Prentice

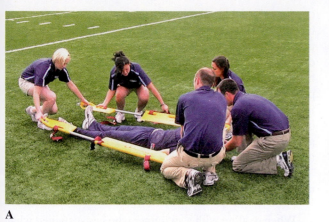
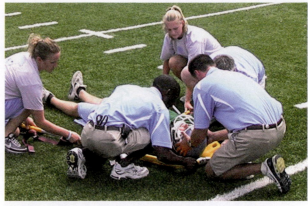

A           B

FIGURE 12–36   **(A)** Preparing a scoop stretcher. **(B)** Latching the top and bottom of a scoop stretcher.
© William E. Prentice

8. Once the patient arrives at the hospital emergency department, the patient should be transferred off of the spine board to the appropriate hospital bed to prevent potentially detrimental effects related to a prolonged length of time on the spine board or scoop stretcher.[41]

**Using a Scoop Stretcher** A scoop stretcher may also be used for transporting a patient with a potential injury to the spine. A scoop stretcher has detachable hinges at each end and thus can be split into two halves (Figure 12–36A). Each half of the stretcher is placed on either side of the supine athlete. The athletic trainer can easily slide each half of the stretcher under the patient until the hinges are locked together, in effect "scooping" the athlete onto the stretcher (Figure 12–36B). The advantage in using a scoop stretcher is that it is not necessary to lift or roll the injured patient onto his or her side to get the stretcher underneath.

## Ambulatory Aid

Ambulatory aid is support or assistance given to an injured patient who is able to walk (Figure 12–37). Before the patient is allowed to walk, he or she should be carefully scrutinized to make sure that the injuries are minor. Whenever serious injuries are suspected, walking should be prohibited. The patient should go from prone to supine or side lying to sitting and should sit for approximately 30 seconds before standing. Weight should be on the uninvolved extremity; the knee is bent; the athlete grasps the athletic trainer's hands and stands up. Two individuals who are approximately the same height should provide complete support on both sides of the patient. The patient's arms are draped over the assistants' shoulders, and their arms encircle his or her back.

## Manual Conveyance

Manual conveyance may be used to move a mildly injured individual a greater distance than the person could walk with ease (Figure 12–38). Any decision to carry the

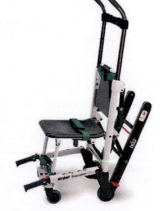

FIGURE 12–37   The ambulatory aid method of transporting a mildly injured athlete.
© William E. Prentice

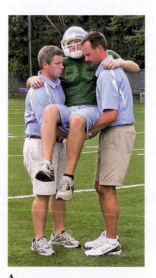

A           B

FIGURE 12–38   **(A)** Manual conveyance method for transporting a mildly injured athlete. **(B)** A stair chair can also be used if the athlete is too large for the athletic trainer to lift manually.
(a) © William E. Prentice; (b) Courtesy Stryker

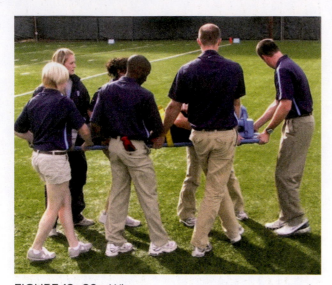

FIGURE 12–39 Whenever a serious injury is suspected, a stretcher is the safest method for transporting the patient. When loading the patient into a rescue vehicle, the head should go first.

© William E. Prentice

patient, such as a decision to use ambulatory aid, must be made only after a complete examination to determine the existence of potentially serious conditions. The most convenient carry is performed by two assistants.

## Stretcher Carrying

Whenever a serious injury is suspected, the best and safest mode of transportation for a short distance is by stretcher. With each segment of the body supported, the patient is gently lifted and placed on the stretcher, which is carried adequately by a minimum of four assistants, two supporting each side (Figure 12–39). The stretcher carriers should face the direction of travel and carry the patient feet first. However, they should carry a patient head first if going uphill or upstairs, or when loading the stretcher into a rescue vehicle. Any person with an injury serious enough to require the use of a stretcher must be carefully examined before being moved.

A suspected fracture must be splinted properly before the patient is transported. Patients with shoulder injuries are more comfortably moved in a semisitting position, unless other injuries preclude such positioning. If injury to the upper extremity is such that flexion of the elbow is not possible, the individual should be transported on a stretcher with the limb properly splinted and carried at the side, with adequate padding placed between the arm and the body.

## Pool Extraction

Removing an injured swimmer from a pool requires some special consideration on the part of the athletic trainer. Obviously, an athletic trainer who is providing

coverage for athletes training or competing in a pool must be able to swim and should have water safety or lifeguard training. The athletic trainer should routinely have immediate access to both a rescue tube and an aquatic spine board in case an athlete sustains an injury while in the pool. A rescue tube should always be used to extract an injured swimmer from the pool.[3] The rescue tube will not only serve as a flotation device but also can help prevent a swimmer who is distressed from grabbing the athletic trainer while in the water.

The following procedures are recommended for removing an injured swimmer from a pool:

1. When dealing with a swimmer who has sustained what appears to be a minor injury in the pool, if the swimmer is close to the edge of the pool, the athletic trainer can reach out to the swimmer with the rescue tube while standing on the pool deck and holding onto the shoulder strap with the other hand. The swimmer should grab the tube; then the athletic trainer can pull him or her to the edge of the pool (Figure 12–40A).[3]

2. If the swimmer is too far away from the pool deck, the athletic trainer should get into the water, approach the swimmer from the front, extend the rescue tube, have the swimmer grab the tube, and kick if possible, while the athletic trainer pulls the swimmer to the edge of the pool (Figure 12–40B).[3]

3. If a swimmer appears to be more severely injured, the athletic trainer should get into the water, approach the swimmer from behind, reach under the armpits, and grab the swimmer's shoulders while putting the rescue tube between the swimmer's back and the athletic trainer's chest. The athletic trainer should keep his or her head to either side to avoid being hit by the swimmer's head, should it fall backward. The athletic trainer should lean back, pulling the swimmer onto the rescue tube, which should support the swimmer, keeping the swimmer's mouth and face out of the water; the athletic trainer should pull the swimmer to the edge of the pool while attempting to keep him or her calm (Figure 12–41).[3]

4. Deciding to remove an injured swimmer from the water depends on several factors, including the

A diver, attempting a 2½ inward dive on a 3-meter board, hits her head on the end of the board. She lands on her face in the water, is briefly submerged, but floats quickly to the surface. She is conscious but disoriented; she has a bump on her forehead but is not bleeding. A teammate nearby jumps immediately in the water and, using a cross-chest technique, tows her about 10 feet to the side of the pool.

**?** The athletic trainer is concerned about both a head and a neck injury. What precautions should be taken when removing the injured athlete from the pool?

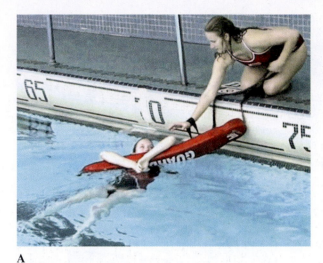 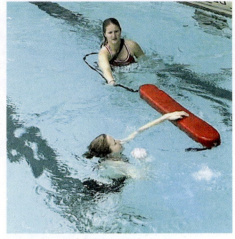

A                                                    B

FIGURE 12–40   Techniques for pool rescue. **(A)** The swimmer is close to the edge of the pool.
**(B)** The swimmer is in the middle of the pool, using a rescue tube.
© William E. Prentice

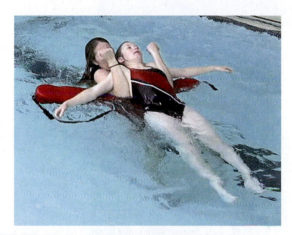

FIGURE 12–41   Technique for removing a severely
injured swimmer from the water.
© William E. Prentice

swimmer's condition and size and the availability of help or how long until help arrives. For example, an injured swimmer requiring CPR should be removed immediately from the water; rescue breathing should not be attempted in the water. A spine board should be used by two people to remove any swimmer from the water who is unable to get out on his or her own, even if a spinal injury is not suspected. The primary rescuer takes the injured swimmer to the side of the pool and turns him or her to face the pool deck. A second rescuer standing on the pool deck grabs the swimmer's opposite wrists and pulls the swimmer up, keeping the head above water and away from the edge of the pool (Figure 12–42A). The primary rescuer gets out of the water, grabs the spine board, then guides the spine board foot-end first down into the water between the swimmer and the edge of the pool (Figure 12–42B). The second rescuer then turns

the swimmer so that his or her back rests against the spine board (Figure 12–42C). Each rescuer then grasps a wrist with one hand and the spine board with the other. The rescuers pull the spine board upward and backward, leveraging the board onto the pool deck (Figure 12–42D).[3]

5. A swimmer with a suspected head or cervical neck injury or a swimmer who is unconscious requires special precaution. A swimmer's cervical spine can be immobilized in the water by a single primary rescuer placing the victim's arms overhead and compressing them against the head. Squeezing the arms together stabilizes the spine and head. The swimmer may be held face up in the water in this position until help arrives (Figure 12–43A). While the primary rescuer continues stabilizing the head and neck, a second rescuer submerges the spine board, positioning it appropriately under the swimmer. The primary rescuer maintains stabilization of the neck. Rescue tubes may be used to help float the spine board. The second rescuer moves to the swimmer's head and assumes responsibility for stabilizing the swimmer's head. The primary rescuer then securely straps the chest, hips, thighs, and head to the spine board (Figure 12–43B&C). Both rescuers then remove the spine board from the pool, head first, by initially lifting the board onto the edge of the pool while still in the water. Then one rescuer gets on the pool deck while the other remains in the water to complete the pool extraction (Figure 12–43D).[3]

## PROPER FIT AND USE OF THE CRUTCH OR CANE

Weight bearing may be contraindicated for a patient with a lower-limb injury, in which case a crutch or cane should be used for ambulation. The athletic

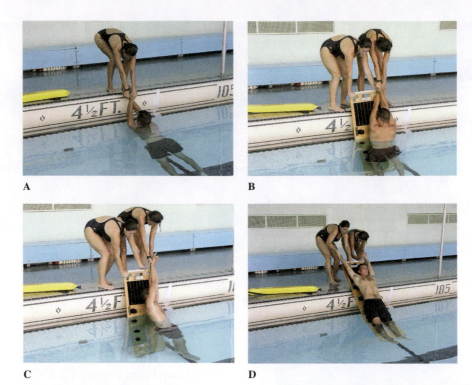

A

B

C

D

FIGURE 12–42   Technique for removing an athlete from the water who can't get out on his or her own.
© William E. Prentice

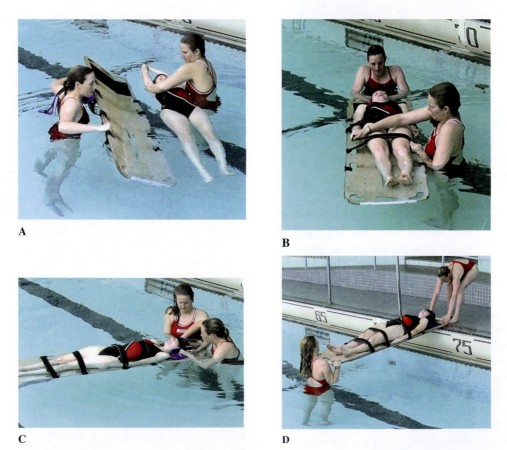

A

B

C

D

FIGURE 12–43   Technique for putting an athlete with a suspected spinal injury on a spine board and removing him or her from the pool.
© William E. Prentice

trainer must be responsible for properly fitting the crutch or cane to the injured patient and then for providing instruction in its use. If the crutch or cane is not properly fitted, the patient may experience discomfort in the axilla from excessive pressure as well as pain in the low back. Faulty mechanics in the use of the crutch or cane when ambulating and particularly when ascending or descending stairs can cause the patient to fall.

## Fitting the Patient

The adjustable aluminum or wooden crutch is well suited to the patient. Before fitting, the athletic trainer should inspect the crutch tops and the bolts and wing nut to make sure they are neither worn nor defective. For a correct fit, the patient should wear low-heeled shoes and stand with good posture and the feet close together. The crutch length is determined first by placing the tip 6 inches (15 cm) from the outer margin of the shoe and 2 inches (5 cm) in front of the shoe. The underarm crutch brace is positioned 1 inch (2.5 cm) below the anterior fold of the axilla. Next, the hand brace is adjusted so that it is even with the patient's hand when the elbow is flexed at approximately a 30-degree angle (Figure 12–44).

Fitting a cane to the patient is relatively easy. Measurement is taken from the crease of the wrist to the floor while the patient is wearing street shoes (Figure 12–45A). The patient holds the cane on the uninjured side and uses a 3-point gait to advance the cane 4 to 6 inches (10 to 15 cm) ahead of the uninjured foot while simultaneously bearing weight on the injured side on the cane (Figure 12–45B).

## Walking with the Crutch or Cane

Many elements of crutch walking correspond with normal walking. The technique commonly used is

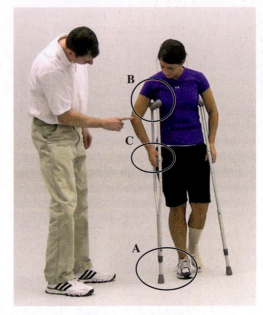

FIGURE 12–44   The crutch must be properly fitted to the patient. **(A)** The crutch tips are placed 6 inches (15 cm) from the outer margin of the shoe and 2 inches (5 cm) in front of the shoe. **(B)** The underarm crutch brace is positioned 1 inch (2.5 cm) below the anterior fold of the axilla. **(C)** The hand brace is placed even with the patient's hand, with the elbow flexed approximately 30 degrees.
© William E. Prentice

the tripod method. In this method, the patient swings through the crutches without

> **Properly fitting a crutch or cane is essential to avoid placing abnormal stresses on the body.**

making any surface contact with the injured limb or by partially bearing weight with the injured limb. The

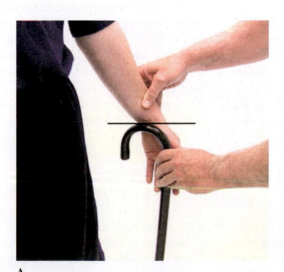
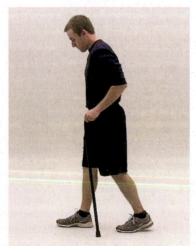

A                                                              B

FIGURE 12–45   Using a cane. **(A)** Top of cane should be at the crease of the wrist. **(B)** Patient should walk with cane on the uninjured side.
© William E. Prentice

12–7 Clinical Application Exercise

A fencer has a grade 2 ankle sprain. After spending an hour in the athletic training room applying ice, compression, and elevation, the athletic trainer decides that the patient should be sent home on crutches. The athlete indicates some reluctance to use the crutches because he has never used them before.

**?** What instructions should the athletic trainer give the patient, so that he can correctly and safely ambulate on crutches?

following sequence is performed:

1. The patient stands on the uninjured leg with no weight or partial weight on the injured leg.
2. Placing the crutch tips 12 to 15 inches (30 to 37.5 cm) ahead of the feet, the patient leans forward, straightens the elbows, pulls the upper crosspiece firmly against the side of the chest, and swings or steps with the uninjured leg between the stationary crutches (Figure 12–46A). The patient should avoid placing the major support in the axilla.
3. After moving through, the patient recovers the crutches and again places the tips forward repeating the sequence. The crutches and the injured or non–weight-bearing leg always move together.

An alternative method is the four-point gait. In this method, the patient stands on both feet, moves one crutch forward, and steps forward with the opposite foot. The patient moves the crutch on the same side as the foot that moved forward, to just ahead of the foot, steps forward, using the opposite foot, followed by the crutch on the same side, and so on (Figure 12–46B).

The tripod gait that is used for crutch walking on a level surface is also used on stairs. In going up stairs, the uninjured support leg moves up one step while the body weight is supported by the hands on the crutches. The full weight of the body is transferred to the uninjured leg, and the crutch tips and injured leg are moved to that step. In going down stairs, the crutch

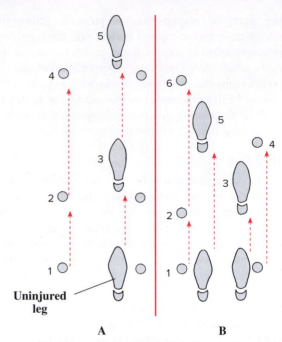

FIGURE 12–46  Crutch gait. **(A)** Tripod method. **(B)** Four-point gait.

tips and the injured leg move down one step, followed by the uninjured leg. If a handrail is available, the patient uses the tripod gait holding both crutches with the outside hand.

NOTE: The patient should exercise caution when ambulating on any wet surface.

Crutch walking will generally follow a progression from non–weight bearing (NWB) to touch-down weight bearing (TDWB), to partial weight bearing (PWB), to full weight bearing (FWB). The rate of progression will be dictated by the limitations of the injury as well as the capabilities of the patient.

When the injured patient needs to be partially weight bearing, a cane or a single crutch can be used to help with balance. In this case, the patient should hold the cane or crutch in the hand on the uninjured side and move the cane forward simultaneously with the uninjured leg. The patient should avoid leaning too heavily on the cane or crutch. If this is a problem, then the patient should use two crutches.

## SUMMARY

- An emergency is defined as "an unforeseen combination of circumstances and the resulting state that calls for immediate action." The primary concern of emergency aid is to maintain cardiovascular function and, indirectly, central nervous system function. An emergency action plan should be activated whenever a patient is seriously injured.

- The athletic trainer must make a systematic assessment of the injured patient to determine appropriate emergency care. A primary survey assesses and deals with life-threatening situations. Once the patient is stabilized, the secondary survey makes a more detailed assessment of the injury.

- In adult CPR, the ratio of compression to breaths is 30 to 2, with 100 compressions per minute. An obstructed airway is relieved by using backblows, abdominal thrusts, the finger sweep of the throat, or all of these.
- Hemorrhage can occur externally and internally. External bleeding can be controlled by direct pressure, by applying pressure at pressure points, and by elevation. Internal hemorrhage can occur subcutaneously, intramuscularly, or within a body cavity.
- Shock can occur from a variety of situations. Shock can be hypovolemic, respiratory, neurogenic, psychogenic, cardiogenic, septic, anaphylactic, or metabolic. Symptoms include pale skin, dilated eyes, weak and rapid pulse, and rapid, shallow breathing. Management includes maintaining normal body temperature and slightly elevating the feet.
- Protection, optimal loading, ice, compression, and elevation (POLICE) should be used for the immediate care of a musculoskeletal injury. Ice should be applied for at least 20 minutes every 1 to 1½ hours, and compression and elevation should be continuous for at least 72 hours after injury.
- Any suspected fracture should be splinted before the patient is moved. Commercial rapid form vacuum immobilizers and air splints are most often used as splints in an athletic training setting.
- Great care must be taken in moving the seriously injured patient. The unconscious patient must be handled as though he or she has a cervical spine injury. Moving a patient with a suspected serious neck injury must be performed only by persons specifically trained to do so. A spine board, scoop stretcher, or vacuum mattress should be used for transport to avoid any movement of the cervical region.
- After decades of controversy regarding the correct approach or sequence for removal of protective equipment in football, lacrosse, and ice hockey, it now appears that both the helmet and shoulder pads may be removed prior to transport.
- When removing an injured swimmer from a pool, the athletic trainer should make every effort to minimize movement of the head and cervical spine while placing the swimmer on a spine board in the water.
- The athletic trainer should be responsible for the proper fitting of and instruction in the use of crutches or a cane by a patient with an injury to the lower extremity.

## WEB SITES

**National Athletic Trainers Association Position, Official, Consensus, and Support Statements**

*Executive Summary: Appropriate Prehospital Management of the Spine Injured Athlete (June 2015):* www.nata.org/sites/default/files/Executive-Summary-Spine-Injury-updated.pdf

*"Time Outs" Before Athletic Events Recommended for Health Care Providers (August 2012):* www.nata.org/sites/default/files/TimeOut.pdf

*Preventing Sudden Death in Sports (2012):* www.nata.org/sites/default/files/Preventing-Sudden-Death-Position-Statement_2.pdf

*Acute Management of the Cervical Spine Injured Athlete (2009):* www.nata.org/sites/default/files/AcuteMgmtOfCervicalSpineInjuredAthlete.pdf

*Head Down Contact and Spearing in Tackle Football (2004):* www.nata.org/sites/default/files/HeadDownContactAndSpearingInTackleFB.pdf

*Emergency Planning in Athletics (2002);* www.nata.org/sites/default/files/EmergencyPlanningInAthletics.pdf

American Red Cross: www.redcross.org/en/aboutus
*The American Red Cross offers many emergency services and training. This site describes those services, introduces the information provided in various training opportunities, and explains how to obtain that training.*

American Heart Association: www.heart.org

Cervical Spine Stabilization: www.trauma.org/archive/spine/cspine-stab.html
*This brief article describes the considerations with cervical spine stabilization.*

First Aid with Parasol EMT: www.parasol.edu.au
*This site provides a comprehensive on-line first aid reference.*

First Aid: www.mayohealth.org
*This Web site on first-aid care is maintained by the Mayo Clinic.*

National Safety Council: www.nsc.org
*The National Safety Council is a membership organization with resources on safety, health, and environmental topics, training, products, publications, news, and more.*

## SOLUTIONS TO CLINICAL APPLICATION EXERCISES

12-1 Because of the mechanism of injury, the athletic trainer should suspect that the patient has a cervical neck injury, and the head should be stabilized throughout. Because the patient is prone and breathing, the athletic trainer should do nothing until the patient regains consciousness. An on-field exam should determine the athlete's neurological status. Then the player should be carefully logrolled onto a spine board because CPR could be necessary at any time. The face mask should be removed in case CPR is required. The helmet and shoulder pads should also be removed. The patient should then be transported to an emergency facility. In this situation, the worst mistake the athletic trainer can make is not exercising enough caution.

12-2 If the equipment is available, the athletic trainer should administer supplemental oxygen, using a bag/valve mask and a pressurized oxygen cylinder to facilitate recovery.

12-3 The athletic trainer should encourage her to continue to cough to attempt to dislodge the gum. If she cannot breathe at all, the athletic trainer should perform a series of abdominal thrusts to help dislodge the gum, continuing the abdominal thrusts until the obstruction is ejected.

12-4 The patient may be going into hypovolemic shock secondary to hemorrhage and trauma, which can be a life-threatening situation. The athletic trainer should first direct someone to dial 911 to access the emergency medical system. Next, the athletic trainer must control the bleeding by using direct pressure, elevation, and pressure points. If bleeding is controlled and the rescue squad has not arrived, the forearm should be immobilized in a rapid form vacuum immobilizer. The patient should be supine, and his feet should be elevated in the shock position. His body temperature should be maintained.

12-5 A rapid form vacuum immobilizer will work well for this injury because of its ability to mold the splint to the joint without causing unnecessary movement. Therefore, the ankle can be immobilized in the current position before transporting the patient.

12-6 The athletic trainer should place the swimmer on a spine board and secure her before extracting her from the pool. Several people may be required to get the swimmer appropriately positioned on the spine board while still in the water. The swimmer should be given a brief neurological exam to determine the extent of the injury. The swimmer should then be transported to an emergency facility in a rescue vehicle.

12-7 The athletic trainer should instruct the patient in the tripod gait, in which the patient swings through the crutches without making any surface contact with the injured limb. The tripod gait is also used on stairs. In negotiating stairs, the rule of thumb is go up with the good leg first, followed by crutches, and to go down with the crutches first, followed by the good leg. If the stairs have a handrail, the patient can hold both crutches with his outside hand. Crutch walking will generally follow a progression: NWB to TDWB, to PWB, to FWB.

## REVIEW QUESTIONS AND CLASS ACTIVITIES

1. What considerations are important in a well-planned system for handling emergency situations?
2. Discuss the rules for managing and moving an unconscious patient.
3. What are the life-threatening conditions that should be evaluated in the primary survey?
4. What are the ABCs of life support?
5. Identify the major steps in giving CPR and managing an obstructed airway. When might these procedures be used in a sports setting?
6. List the basic steps in assessing a musculoskeletal injury.
7. What techniques should be used to stop external hemorrhage?
8. Numerous types of shock can occur from a sports injury or illness; list them and their management.
9. What first-aid procedures are used to decrease hemorrhage, inflammation, muscle spasm, and pain from a musculoskeletal injury?
10. Describe the basic concepts of emergency splinting.
11. How should a patient with a suspected spinal injury be transported?
12. What techniques can be used to transport a patient with a suspected musculoskeletal injury?
13. Discuss the methods for extracting an injured swimmer from a pool.
14. Explain how to fit crutches properly.

## REFERENCES

1. American Heart Association: *Highlights of the 2015 American Heart Association guidelines update for cardiopulmonary resuscitation and emergency cardiovascular care*, Dallas, TX, 2015, American Heart Association.
2. American Red Cross: *CPR/AED for professional rescuers and health care providers handbook*, Boston, MA, 2011, StayWell Health and Safety Solutions.
3. American Red Cross: *American Red Cross lifeguarding manual*, Boston, MA, 2011, Krames-StayWell.
4. Andersen J: National Athletic Trainers' Association position statement: Emergency planning in athletics, *J Athl Train* 37(1):99, 2002.
5. Bailes J: Management of cervical spine injuries in athletes, *J Athl Train* 42(1):126–34, 2007.
6. Baxter R: *Pocket guide to musculoskeletal assessment*, St. Louis, MO, 2003, Saunders.
7. Berry D: Demonstrating external bleeding and shock, *Athletic Therapy Today* 11(4):22, 2006.
8. Berry D: Educating the educator: Teaching airway adjunct techniques in athletic training, *Athletic Training Education Journal,* 107–16, 2011.
9. Biddington C: Certified athletic trainers' management of emergencies, *J Sport Rehabil* 14(2):185, 2005.
10. Bleakley C: Price needs updating, should we call the POLICE? *British Journal of Sports Medicine* 46:220–21, 2012.
11. Bleakley C: The use of ice in the treatment of acute soft-tissue injury: A systematic review of randomized controlled trials, *Am J Sports Med* 32(1):251–61, 2004.
12. Brukner P: Sporting emergencies. In Brukner P: *Clinical sports medicine*, ed 2, Sydney, 2002, McGraw-Hill.
13. Courson R: Emergency assessment, *Athletic Therapy Today* 10(2):19, 2005.
14. Courson R: Personal communication, Athens, GA, 2016, University of Georgia.
15. Danielson R: Differences in skin surface temperature and pressure during the application of various cold and compression devices, *J Athl Train* 32:S34, 1997.
16. Decoster L: Football face mask removal with a cordless screwdriver on helmets used for at least one season of play, *J Athl Train* 40(3):169, 2005.
17. Delano T: Removal of a man's lacrosse helmet is faster and produces less cervical movement compared with removal of the face mask, *J Athl Train* 41(S):S-57, 2006.
18. Del Rossi G: A comparison of spine-board transfer techniques and the effect of training on performance, *J Athl Train* 38(3):204–8, 2003.
19. Dezner J: Interassociation task force recommendations on emergency preparedness and management of sudden cardiac arrest in high school and college athletic programs: A consensus statement, *J Athl Train* 42(1):143, 2007.
20. Dolan M: Effects of cold water immersion on edema formation after blunt injury to the hind limb in rats, *J Athl Train* 32:233, 1997.
21. DuBose D, et al.: Motion created in an unstable cervical spine during removal of a football helmet: Comparison of techniques, *Athletic Training and Sports Health Care* 7(6):242–47, 2015.
22. Farrell R: AEDs and cardiac resuscitation: Is prevention part of your plan? *Athletic Therapy Today* 6(3):46, 2001.
23. Fincher A: Managing medical emergencies, part 1, *Athletic Therapy Today* 6(3):44, 2001.
24. Gale S: The combined tool approach for face mask removal during on-field conditions, *J Athl Train* 43(1):14–20, 2008.
25. Herbert D: Emergency preparedness recommendations for high school and college athletic programs, *Exercise Standards and Malpractice Reporter* 21(4):58, 2007.
26. Herbert D: Plan to save lives: Create and rehearse an emergency response plan, *ACSM's Health and Fitness Journal* 1(5):34, 1997.
27. Ho S: The effects of ice on bloodflow and bone metabolism in the knee, *Am J Sports Med* 22:537, 1994.
28. Horodyski M: Comparison of the flat torso versus the elevated torso shoulder pad removal techniques in a cadaveric cervical spine instability model, *Spine* 34(7):687–91, 2009.
29. Jenkins H: Removal tools are faster and produce less force and torque on the helmet than cutting tools during face mask retraction, *J Athl Train* 37(3):246, 2002.
30. Jones M: Acute treatment of inversion ankle sprains: Immobilization versus functional

treatment, *Clin Orthop Relat Res* 455:169–72, 2007.

31. Kaminski T, et al.: National Athletic Trainer's Association position statement: Conservative management and prevention of ankle sprains in athletes, *J Athl Train* 48(4):528–45, 2013.

32. Khan K: Mechanotherapy: How physical therapists' prescription of exercise promotes tissue repair, *Br J Sports Med* 43:247–52, 2009.

33. Karren K: *First aid for colleges and universities,* Boston, MA, 2011, Benjamin Cummings.

34. Kordecki M: The Riddell RipKord System for shoulder pad removal in a cervical spine injured athlete: A paradigm shift, *International Journal of Sports Physical Therapy* 6(2):142–49, 2011.

35. LaPrade R: Cervical spine alignment in the immobilized ice hockey player: A computed tomographic analysis of the effects of helmet removal, *Am J Sports Med* 28(6):800, 2000.

36. Luscombe M: Comparison of a long spinal board and vacuum mattress for spinal immobilisation, *Emerg Med J* 20(5):476–78, 2003.

37. Magee DL: *Orthopedic physical assessment,* Philadelphia, 2013, Elsevier Health Science.

38. Meredith R: Field splinting of suspected fractures: Preparation, assessment, and application. *Physician Sportsmed* 25(10):29, 1997.

39. Merrick M: A preliminary examination of cryotherapy and secondary injury in skeletal muscle, *Med Sci Sport Exer* 31:1516, 1999.

40. National Athletic Trainers' Association: Official Statement on Athletic Healthcare Provider "Time Outs" Before Athletic Events, Dallas, TX, 2012, NATA.

41. National Athletic Trainers' Association: Appropriate prehospital management of the spine injured athlete, Dallas, TX, 2015, NATA.

42. National Safety Council: *Standard 2012. First aid and CPR and AED,* San Francisco, CA, 2012, McGraw-Hill

43. Neumar R, et al.: 2015 American Heart Association guidelines update for cardiopulmonary resuscitation and emergency cardiovascular care, *Circulation* 132:5315–67, 2015.

44. Occupational Safety and Health Administration (OSHA): *Personal protective equipment,* Washington, DC, 1992, U.S. Department of Labor.

45. Palumbo M: The effect of protective football equipment on alignment of the injured cervical spine: Radiographic analysis in a cadaveric model, *Am J Sports Med* 24(4):446, 1996.

46. Paluska A: Laryngeal trauma in sport, *Current Sports Medicine Reports* 7(1):16–21, 2008.

47. Petschauer M: Helmet fit and cervical spine motion in collegiate men's lacrosse athletes secured to a spine board, *J Athl Train ,* 45(3):215–21, 2010.

48. Potter B: Testing the emergency action plan in athletics, *Athletic Therapy Today* 14(6): 214, 2009.

49. Ransone J: Assessment of first-aid knowledge and decision making of high school athletic coaches, *J Athl Train* 34(3):267, 1999.

50. Ransone J: The efficacy of the rapid form cervical vacuum immobilizer in cervical spine immobilization of the equipped football player, *J Athl Train* 35(1):65, 2000.

51. Rothmier J: The role of the automated external defibrillators in sports, *Sports Health: A Multidisciplinary Approach* 1(1):16, 2009.

52. Sailer S: Rehabilitation and splinting of common upper-extremity injuries in athletes, *Clin Sports Med* 14(2):411, 1995.

53. Schnirring L: AEDs gain foothold in sports medicine, *Physician Sportsmed* 29(4):11–19, 2001.

54. Starkey C, Ryan J: *Examination of orthopedic and athletic injuries,* Philadelphia, 2015, F.A. Davis.

55. Swartz E: Cervical spine alignment during on-field management of potential catastrophic spine injuries, *Sports Health* 1(3):247–52, 2009.

56. Swartz E: Emergency face mask removal effectiveness: A comparison of traditional and nontraditional football helmet face mask attachment systems, *J Athl Train* 45(6):560–69, 2010.

57. Swartz E: Emergent access to the airway and chest in American football players, *J Athl Train* 50(7):681–87, 2015.

58. Swartz E, et al.: National Athletic Trainers' Association position statement: Acute management of the cervical spine-injured athlete, *J Athl Train* 44(3):306–31, 2009.

59. Swartz E: Face mask removal: Movement and time associated with cutting of the loop straps, *J Athl Train* 38(2):120, 2003.

60. Swartz E: Football equipment design affects face mask removal efficiency, *AMJ Sports Med* 3(8):1210, 2005.

61. Swartz E: Protective equipment removal in the prehospital setting: We got this, *Athletic Training and Sports Health Care* 7(6):219–21, 2015.

62. *Taber's cyclopedic medical dictionary,* Philadelphia, 2013, FA Davis.

63. Tator C: Recognition and management of spinal cord injuries in sports and recreation, *Physical Medicine and Rehabilitation Clinics of North America,* 20(1):69–76, 2009.

64. Terry G: Sudden cardiac arrest in athletic medicine, *J Athl Train* 36(2):205, 2001.

65. Toler J: Comparison of three airway access techniques during suspected spine injury management in American football, *Clinical Journal of Sports Medicine* 20(2):92–97, 2010.

66. Van den Bekerom M: What is the evidence for Rest, Ice, Compression, and Elevation therapy in the treatment of ankle sprains in adults? *J Athl Train* 47(4):435–43, 2012.

67. Walsh K: Thinking proactively: The emergency action plan, *Athletic Therapy Today* 6(5):57, 2001.

68. Waninger K: Adequate performance of cardiopulmonary resuscitation techniques during simulated cardiac arrest over and under protective equipment in football, *Clin J Sport Med* 24:280–83, 2014.

69. Waninger K: Cervical spine injury management in the helmeted athlete, *Current Sports Medicine Reports* 10(1):45–9, 2011.

70. Waninger K: Computed tomography is diagnostic in the cervical imaging of helmeted football players with shoulder pads, *J Athl Train* 39(3):2, 2004.

71. Waninger K: Management of the helmeted athlete with suspected cervical spine injury, *Am J Sports Med* 32(5):331, 2004.

72. Wilkerson, G: Treatment of the inversion ankle sprain through synchronous application of focal compression and cold, *J Athl Train* 26(3):220–37, 1991.

## ANNOTATED BIBLIOGRAPHY

American Red Cross: *CPR/AED For the Professional Rescuer and Health Care Providers manual,* Boston, MA, 2011, American Red Cross.

*This text provides CPR information at the level that athletic trainers need to know to be a professional rescuer.*

Karren KJ, Hafen BQ: *First aid for colleges and universities,* Boston, MA, 2011, Benjamin Cummings.

*A well-illustrated, simple approach to the treatment of emergency illness and injury.*

Leikin JB, Feldman BJ: *American Medical Association handbook of first aid and emergency care,* Philadelphia, PA, 2009, Random House.

*Covers urgent emergency situations as well as the common injuries and ailments that occur in every family, taking the reader step-by-step through basic first-aid techniques, the medical symptoms to recognize before an emergency occurs, and what to do when one does occur.*

Magee DJ: *Orthopedic physical assessment,* Philadelphia, PA, 2013, Elsevier Health Science.

*An extremely well-illustrated book with excellent coverage. Its strength lies in its coverage of injuries commonly found during athletic training.*

National Safety Council: *First aid CPR and AED,* San Francisco, CA, 2012, McGraw-Hill

*Well-written and extremely well-illustrated text that deals with first-aid and emergency procedures. Although most of the information is directed at the general population, the principles and techniques can certainly be applied to the injured athlete. An excellent resource for the athletic trainer.*

Swartz E, Boden B, Courson R, Decoster C: National Athletic Trainers' Association position statement: Acute management of the cervical spine injured athlete, *J Athl Train* 44(3):306, 2009.

*Provides athletic trainers, team physicians, emergency responders, and other health care professionals with recommendations on how to best manage a catastrophic cervical spine injury in the athlete.*

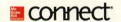

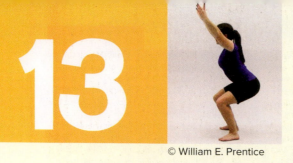

© William E. Prentice

# Off-the-Field Injury Evaluation

## ■ Objectives

*When you finish this chapter you should be able to*

- Discuss the athletic trainer's ability to make an accurate clinical diagnosis.
- Review the terminology used in injury evaluation.
- Apply the HOPS off-the-field evaluation scheme.
- Understand the value of using functional screening tests to identify characteristic movement impairments and minimize the risk for injury.
- Incorporate the best available evidence in the professional literature into the clinical decision making process.
- Organize the process for documenting the findings of an off-the-field secondary or progress evaluation.
- Recognize additional diagnostic techniques available to the athletic trainer through the team physician.
- Discuss how an ergonomic risk assessment can be performed to reduce workplace-related injuries.

## ■ Outline

## ■ Key Terms

biomechanics
pathomechanics
etiology
mechanism

pathology
symptom
sign
diagnosis

prognosis
sequela
syndrome
HOPS

active range of motion
passive range of motion
dermatome
myotomes

## ■ Connect Highlights ■ Mc Graw Hill Education **connect**

*Visit connect.mcgraw-hill.com for further exercises to apply your knowledge:*

- Clinical application scenarios covering ability to make an accurate clinical diagnosis, HOPS off-the-field evaluation scheme, process for documenting findings, and using additional diagnostic techniques
- Click-and-drag questions covering ability to make an accurate clinical diagnosis, terminology and anatomy, HOPS off-the-field evaluation scheme, process for documentation findings, and using additional diagnostic techniques
- Multiple-choice questions covering terminology, HOPS, documentation, diagnostic techniques, and ergonomic risk assessment to reduce workplace-related injuries
- Selection questions covering terminology and anatomy
- Video identification of joint ranges of motion
- Picture identification of additional diagnostic techniques and terminology

Injury evaluation is an essential skill for the athletic trainer.[8] In athletic training, four distinct evaluations are routinely conducted: (1) The *preparticipation examination*, which was discussed in Chapter 2, is done prior to the start of preseason practice; (2) the initial *on-the-field injury assessment*, which was discussed in great detail in Chapter 12, is done immediately after acute injury to rule out injuries that may be life-threatening, to determine the immediate course of acute care, necessary first aid, how the patient should be transported from the field, and the approach to handling emergency situations; (3) a more detailed *off-the-field injury evaluation* is performed routinely after the immediate on-the-field evaluation either on the sidelines or in the athletic training clinic, a hospital or an outpatient clinic, an emergency room, or a physician's office after appropriate first aid has been rendered; and (4) a *progress evaluation* is done periodically throughout the rehabilitative healing process to determine the progress and effectiveness of a specific treatment regimen. This chapter concentrates on the off-the-field evaluation and the progress evaluation.

> Athletic trainers use their evaluation skills to make an accurate clinical diagnosis.

The setting in which the athletic trainer is employed determines the type of evaluation that is appropriate. An athletic trainer working in a hospital or an industrial setting is likely doing mostly off-the-field injury evaluations and progress evaluations. Athletic trainers who are employed in an athletic setting can expect to be arranging preparticipation exams, performing both on- and off-the-field evaluations, and writing progress evaluations throughout the course of rehabilitation.

# BASIC KNOWLEDGE REQUIREMENTS

The athletic trainer who is examining a patient with an injury must have a general knowledge of normal human anatomy and biomechanics and an understanding of the potential hazards inherent in a particular activity. Without this information, accurate assessment is impossible.

> To examine sports injuries, the athletic trainer must have a thorough knowledge of human anatomy and its function and of the hazards inherent in a particular activity.

## Normal Human Anatomy

**Surface Anatomy** Understanding typical surface, or topographical, anatomy is essential when evaluating a possible injury.[36] Key surface landmarks provide the examiner with indications of the normal or injured anatomical structures lying underneath the skin.[20]

***Abdominopelvic Quadrants and Regions*** The abdominopelvic *quadrants* are the four corresponding regions of the abdomen that are divided for evaluative and diagnostic purposes (Figure 13–1A). A second division system divides the abdominopelvic area into nine *regions* (Figure 13–1B). Clinicians use the quadrants and regions as reference points for locating underlying organs or abdominopelvic pain or abnormality (Figure 13–1C&D). The regions tend to be more specific relative to organ location, whereas the quadrants are simpler and generally more commonly used.

**Musculoskeletal System Anatomy** Anyone examining the musculoskeletal system for injuries must have an in-depth knowledge of both structural and functional anatomy.[6] This knowledge encompasses the major joints and bony structures as well as skeletal musculature. A knowledge of neural anatomy is also of major importance, particularly that which is involved in movement control and sensation, along with the neural factors that influence superficial and deep pain.

***Standard Musculoskeletal Terminology for Bodily Positions and Deviations*** When assessing the musculoskeletal system, the athletic trainer must use a standard terminology to convey precise information to other health care providers who may become professionally involved with the athlete. These terms are found in Table 13–1.

***Body Planes and Anatomical Directions*** Associated with surface anatomy is the understanding of body planes and anatomical directions.[36] Body planes are used as points of reference from which positions of body parts are indicated. The three most commonly mentioned planes are the sagittal, transverse, and coronal (or frontal) planes (Figure 13–2). The sagittal plane runs vertically from front to back, or anterior/posterior, and divides the body into right and left sides.

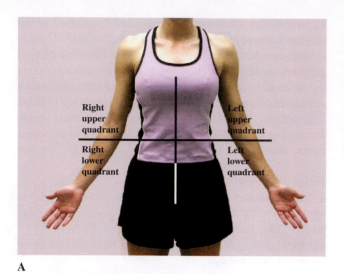

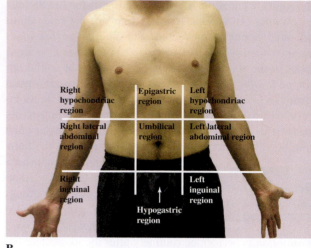

FIGURE 13–1   Division of the abdomen into quadrants and regions. **(A&C)** Four quadrants. **(B&D)** Nine regions.
(a, b) © William E. Prentice

The transverse plane runs horizontally and divides the body into upper and lower parts. The coronal, or frontal, plane runs vertically from right to left and divides the body into front (anterior) and back (posterior). Anatomical directions refer to the position of one part in relation to another (Figure 13–3).

## Biomechanics

The understanding of biomechanics is the foundation for the assessment of musculoskeletal injuries. **Biomechanics** is the application of mechanical forces, which may stem from within or outside the body, to living organisms. Of major concern is pathomechanics, which may precede an injury. **Pathomechanics** refers to mechanical forces that are applied to the body because of a structural body deviation, leading to

faulty alignment. Pathomechanics often cause overuse syndromes.

## Understanding the Activity

Understanding the activity that the injured patient is involved in is critical if the athletic trainer is to be effective in determining the mechanism of injury, making an accurate clinical diagnosis, and designing a rehabilitation program that will address the functional aspects of returning to that activity. To fully understand injuries that occur in a particular activity, the athletic trainer must possess detailed knowledge and be able to apply the correct kinesiological and biomechanical principles that can correct faulty movement patterns. For example, an athletic trainer working with a ballet dancer needs to understand the physical

TABLE 13–1

| Term | Definition |
|---|---|
| Abduction | To draw away or deviate from the midline of the body. |
| Adduction | To deviate toward or draw toward the midline of the body. |
| Eversion | Turning outward. |
| Extension | To straighten; when the part distal to a joint extends, it straightens; joint angle decreases toward 0 degrees. |
| External (lateral) rotation | Rotary motion in the transverse plane away from the midline. |
| Flexion | To bend; when a joint is flexed, the part distal to the joint bends; joint angle increases toward 180 degrees. |
| Internal (medial) rotation | Rotary motion in the transverse plane toward the midline. |
| Inversion | Turning inward. |
| Pronation | Applied to the foot and assuming the foot is in a prone position, it refers a combination of eversion and abduction movements, resulting in a lowering of the medial margin of the foot; applied to the hand, the palm is turned downward. |
| Supination | To assume a supine position; applied to the foot, raising the medial margin of the foot; applied to the hand, turning the palm upward. |
| Valgus | Deviation of a part or portion of the extremity distal to a joint away from the midline of the body. |
| Varus | Deviation of a part or portion of an extremity distal to a joint toward the midline of the body. |

Source: Adapted from Post, M: *Physical examination of the musculoskeletal system,* Chicago: Yearbook Medical Publishers, 1987.

demands of performing that artistic activity. Or, an athletic trainer overseeing a work hardening program must understand the ergonomics of a repetitive activity to correct the habits of a worker performing that job. The more the athletic trainer who evaluates a

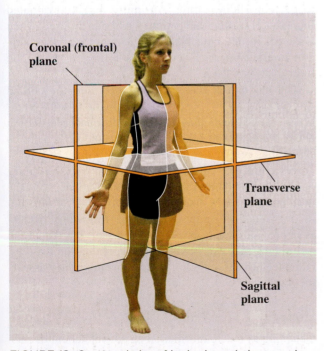

FIGURE 13–2  Knowledge of body planes helps provide points of reference.
© William E. Prentice

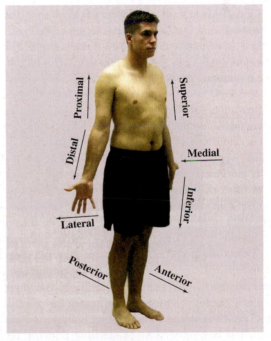

FIGURE 13–3  Anatomical directions refer to the position of one body part in relation to another.
anterior = in front of
posterior = in back of
superior = above
inferior = below
distal = farther away
proximal = closer to
medial = toward the middle
lateral = away from the middle
© William E. Prentice

sports-related injury knows about how a sport is performed, the physical requirements of different positions within that sport, and its potential for trauma, the better his or her injury assessment can be.[54]

## Descriptive Assessment Terms

When evaluating injuries, examiners use certain terms to describe and characterize what is being learned about the condition. The athletic training student should become familiar with these terms.

**Etiology** refers to the cause of an injury or disease (for example, a patient rolls the foot inward when landing after jumping). In sports medicine, the term *mechanism of injury (MOI)* is often used interchangeably with *etiology*. A **mechanism** is the mechanical description of the cause (for example, inversion and plantar flexion). **Pathology** refers to the structural and functional changes that result from the injury process.

After developing an understanding of an injury's etiology, the athletic trainer ascertains symptoms and signs. **Symptom** refers to a *perceptible* change in a patient's body or its functions that indicates an injury or a disease. Symptoms are subjective; the patient describes them to the athletic trainer or physician. In comparison, a **sign** is objective, a definitive and obvious indicator of a specific condition. Signs are often determined when the patient is examined.

After it is inspected, an injury may be assigned a *grade*. Grade 1, 2, or 3 corresponds to an injury that is mild, moderate, or severe, respectively. Sometimes the term *degree* is used in place of *grade*, depending on the athletic trainer's preference.

**Diagnosis** denotes the name of a specific condition. To establish the diagnosis of a patient's injury or illness, the athletic trainer must study all aspects of the condition. A *differential diagnosis* is a systematic method of diagnosing a disorder that lacks unique symptoms or signs. The differential diagnosis is a list of possible injuries that cannot be ruled out until more information is obtained, typically through diagnostic tests. Diagnosis involves a process of including, excluding, and prioritizing possibilities by expecting the most serious injury first.[16] Prioritizing means to list the possible injuries from the most likely to the least likely. Applying the differential diagnosis technique, the athletic trainer first develops a list of possible injuries. By obtaining a history, observing, palpating, and conducting tests, the clinician can include or exclude some of the possible causes. Occasionally, the terms *working diagnosis* and *hypothesis* are also used to refer to the differential diagnosis. These terms also suggest a process for determining the most likely diagnosis for that condition. Once all the possible information has been gathered about the patient's condition, a **prognosis** is made. A prognosis is a prediction of the course of the condition.

In other words, the patient is told what to expect as the injury heals. The amount of pain, swelling, or loss of function is discussed. *Prognosis* also refers to the projected outcome of an illness or injury and to the length of time predicted for complete recovery. For an athlete, prognosis translates into "the length of time before I can compete."

**Sequela** refers to a condition following and resulting from a disease or an injury. Sequela is an additional condition developed as a complication of an existing disease or injury. For example, pneumonia might result from a bout with the flu, or osteoarthritis might follow a severe joint sprain.

The term **syndrome** is refers to a group of symptoms and signs that, together, indicate a particular injury or disease.

## THE OFF-THE-FIELD INJURY EVALUATION PROCESS

The on-the-field primary and/or initial injury assessment discussed in detail in Chapter 12 is done on the field immediately after injury to rule out those injuries that may become life threatening, to assess musculoskeletal injuries, and to determine how the patient should be transported from the field. Once the patient has been transported from the site of initial injury, away from the excitement and confusion inherent in an athletic arena, a more detailed secondary off-the-field injury evaluation is performed. This detailed evaluation may be performed on the sideline, in the athletic training clinic, in an emergency room, or in a sports medicine clinic. An injury may be evaluated immediately after the patient has been injured when it is still in an acute phase, or it may take place several hours or perhaps even days following traumatic injury.

The evaluation scheme is divided into four broad categories: history, observation, palpation, and a number of special tests that provide additional information about the extent of injuries. This evaluation scheme is sometimes referred to as the **HOPS** format. HOPS involves collecting information about an existing injury or illness and then making a decision about what the problem might be (see *Focus Box 13–1:* "Off-the-field evaluation sequence"). The following discussion provides an overview of some of the steps and techniques that can be used in the evaluation process. (Chapters 18 through 27 provide specific injury assessment procedures.)

## History

Obtaining as much information as possible about the history of the injury is perhaps the single most important aspect of the injury evaluation.[20] Understanding how

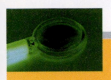

## Off-the-field evaluation sequence

### History

- Injuries to same body part
- Related injuries
- Present
- Mechanism of injury (MOI)
- Injury location
- Pain characteristics
- Joint responses
- Determining whether the injury is acute or chronic
- Past

### Observation

- Demeanor
- Movement
- Posture
- Asymmetrics
- Deformity
- Swelling, redness, warmth

### Palpation

- Bony palpation
- Soft-tissue palpation

### Special Tests

A. Movement assessment
- Active range of motion
  - Manual muscle testing
- Passive range of motion
  - Testing Joint Endpoints
    - Normal endpoints (end feels)
    - Abnormal endpoints (endpoints)
- Measuring Range of Motion
  - Goniometric measurement
  - Digital Inclinometer
- Testing accessory motions

B. Neurological examination
- Cerebral function
- Cerebellar function
- Cranial nerve function
- Sensory testing
- Reflex testing
- Determining projected/referred pain
- Motor testing

C. Testing Joint Stability

D. Postural examination

E. Anthropometric measurements

F. Volumetric measurements

G. Testing functional performance

H. Functional Screening Tests

---

the injury may have occurred (the mechanism of injury) and listening to the patient's complaints and answers to key questions can provide important clues to the exact nature of the injury. The athletic trainer becomes a detective in pursuit of as much accurate information as possible, which will lead to a determination of the true nature of the injury (see *Focus Box 13–2:* "History of musculoskeletal injuries"). From the history, the athletic trainer develops strategies for further examination and possible immediate and follow-up management.[6]

When obtaining a history, the athletic trainer should do the following:

- Be calm and reassuring.
- Ask open-ended questions that allow the patient to say anything that might be applicable rather than leading closed-end questions that require a yes or no response.

> **Taking a detailed history from the athlete is perhaps the most critical aspect of the off-the-field evaluation.**

- Listen carefully to the patient's complaints.
- Maintain eye contact to try to see what the patient is feeling (remove sunglasses to get eye contact).
- Record exactly what the patient says without interpretation.
- Try to obtain the history as soon after injury as possible.[5]

Questions might be stated under specific headings in an attempt to get as complete a historical picture as possible. In many cases, a history becomes clear-cut because the mechanism, trauma, and pathology are

---

**13–2 Clinical Application Exercise**

A fencer comes to a clinic complaining of pain in his shoulder, which he has had for about a week. He indicates that he first hurt the shoulder when lifting weights but did not think it was a bad injury. During the past week he has not been able to lift because of pain. He has continued to fence, but his shoulder seems to be getting worse instead of better.

**?** What is the standard evaluation scheme that the athletic trainer should use?

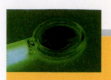

## History of musculoskeletal injuries

### Information to obtain

- The mechanism of injury or trauma that caused the problem
- Chief complaints and present problems
- If pain is present, its location, character, type, duration, variation, aggravation, distribution or radiation, intensity, and course
- If the pain is increased or decreased by specific activities or stresses
- The existing environmental conditions when the injury occurred
- The type of equipment being worn at the time of the injury
- If the problem has occurred before and, if so, when and how it was treated and if the treatment was successful

obvious; in other situations, symptoms and signs may be obscured.

It is alright to observe the patient when taking a history but there should be no palpation while the patient is explaining what happened and what he or she is feeling.[17]

**Present Injury** If the patient is conscious and coherent, the athletic trainer should encourage him or her to describe the injury in detail.

***Mechanism of Injury (MOI)*** If the athletic trainer did not see the injury happen, he or she should try to get the patient to describe in detail the mechanism of the injury by asking the following questions as an example:

- What is the problem?
- How did it occur?
- When did it occur?
- Did you fall? How did you land?
- Which direction did your joint move?
- Did you hear or feel anything when it occurred?

If the patient is unable to describe accurately how the injury occurred, perhaps someone who observed the event can do so.

***Injury Location*** The athletic trainer should ask the patient to locate the area of complaint by pointing to it

with one finger only. If the patient can point to a specific pain site, the injury is probably localized. If the exact pain site cannot be indicated, the injury may be generalized.

***Pain Characteristics*** The patient should describe as accurately as possible exactly what the pain feels like.

- What type of pain is it?
  - Nerve pain is sharp, bright, or burning.
  - Bone pain tends to be localized and piercing.
  - Pain in the vascular system tends to be poorly localized, aching, and referred from another area.
  - Muscle pain is often dull, aching, and referred to another area.[38]
- Where is the pain? Determining pain origin makes the evaluation of musculoskeletal injuries difficult. The deeper the injury site, the more difficult it is to match the pain with the site of trauma. This factor often causes treatment to be performed at the wrong site. Conversely, the closer the injury is to the body surface, the better the elicited pain corresponds with the site of pain stimulation.[5]
- Does the pain change at different times? Pain that subsides during activity usually indicates a chronic inflammation. Pain that increases in a joint throughout the day indicates a progressive increase in edema. Does pain increase at night?
- Does the patient feel sensations other than pain? Pressure on nerve roots can produce pain or a sensation of "pins and needles" (paresthesia). What movement, if any, causes pain or other sensations?
- Is there anything the patient does to relieve or alleviate pain?

### Joint Responses

- If the injury is related to a joint, is there instability laxity, or previous history?
- Does the joint feel as though it will give way?
- Does the joint lock and unlock?

Positive responses may indicate that the joint has a loose body that is catching or that is inhibiting the normal muscular support in the area. There may also be a structural injury or lesion that is causing instability.

***Determining Whether the Injury Is Acute or Chronic*** The examiner should ask the patient how long he or she has had the symptoms and how often they appear.

***History of Injury*** It is important to obtain information about the patient's previous or preexisting injuries.[21] The athletic trainer who is working with a patient or group of patients on a daily basis often has the advantage of being familiar with their medical history. Nevertheless, an off-the-field injury evaluation requires asking.

- Has this ever happened before? If so, when?

## Observation

The examiner gains knowledge and understanding of the patient's major complaint not only from a history but also through general observation, often done at the same time the history is taken. What is observed is commonly modified by the patient's complaints. The following are suggested as specific points to observe:

- Is there an obvious deformity?
- How does the patient move?
- Are there any obvious body asymmetries?
- Are there unnatural protrusions or lumps, such as occur with a dislocation or fracture?
- Is there a postural malalignment?
- Is there a limp?
- Are movements abnormally slow, jerky, and asynchronous?
- Is the patient unable to move a body part?
- Is the patient holding his or her body stiffly?
- Does the patient's facial expression indicate discomfort or lack of sleep?
- Does soft tissue appear swollen or wasted as a result of atrophy?
- Are there abnormal sounds, such as crepitus, when the athlete moves?
- Does a body area appear inflamed?
- Is there swelling, heat, or redness?
- Is there any type of discoloration (beyond redness)?

An athletic trainer is evaluating an assembly line worker who complains of pain in her elbow. During the evaluation, active and passive range of motion tests and manual muscle testing reveal pain when the elbow is moved into extension both actively and passively. However, there is no pain when the elbow is moved actively into flexion.

**?** Does the injury more likely involve the ligament or the musculotendinous unit?

## Palpation

Some examiners use palpation in the beginning of the examination procedure, whereas others use it only when they believe they have identified the specific injury site by other assessment means.[15,37] In some cases, palpation would be beneficial at both the beginning and the end of the examination. The two areas of palpation are bony and soft tissue. Like all examination procedures, palpation must be performed systematically.[41] The athletic trainer starts with very light pressure, followed by gradually deeper pressure, and usually begins away from the site of complaint and gradually moves distal to proximal.

**Bony Palpation** Both the injured and noninjured sites should be palpated and compared. The sense of touch might reveal an abnormal gap at a joint, swelling on a bone, joints that are misaligned, or abnormal protuberances associated with a joint or a bone.

**Soft-Tissue Palpation** Through palpation, with the patient as relaxed as possible, the athletic trainer can assess normal soft-tissue relationships.[57] Tissue deviations, such as swelling, lumps, gaps, abnormal muscle tension, and temperature variations, can be detected. The palpation of soft tissue can detect where ligaments or tendons have torn or where muscle/fascia tissue deformities may be present. The athletic trainer can determine variations in the shape of structures, differences in tissue tightness and textures, and differentiation of tissue that is pliable and soft from tissue that is more resilient. Involuntary muscle twitching or tremors may also be felt. Excessive skin dryness and moisture can also be noted. The athletic trainer can become aware of abnormal skin sensations, such as diminished sensation (dysesthesia), numbness (anesthesia), or increased sensation (hyperesthesia). Like bony palpation, soft-tissue palpation must be performed on both sides of the body for comparison.[57]

## Special Tests

Special tests have been designed for almost every body region to detect specific pathologies.[30] They are often used to substantiate what has been learned from the history, observation, and palpation portions of the evaluation process.[37] Special tests should be performed bilaterally beginning with the uninjured side to compare what is "normal" for that patient with what the injured side feels like. CAUTION: A joint should not be moved or stressed when a fracture is suspected.

**Movement Assessment** If a joint or soft-tissue lesion exists, the patient is likely to complain of pain on movement. Cyriax has developed a method for locating and identifying a lesion by applying tension selectively to each

> **Movement assessment:**
> - Active movement
> - Passive movement
> - Resistive movement

of the structures that might produce this pain.[15] Tissues are classified as *contractile* or *inert*. Contractile tissues are capable of lengthening and shortening and include muscles and their tendons. Inert tissues do not lengthen and shorten and include bones, ligaments, joint capsules, fascia, bursae, nerve roots, and dura mater.

If a lesion is present in contractile tissue, pain will occur on active motion in one direction and on passive motion in the opposite direction. Thus, a muscle strain would cause pain on both active contraction and passive stretch. Contractile tissues are tested through the midrange by an isometric contraction against maximum resistance. The specific location of the lesion within the musculotendinous unit cannot be identified by the isometric contraction.[11]

A lesion of inert tissue elicits pain on active and passive movement in the same direction. For example, a sprain of a ligament results in pain whenever that ligament is stretched, through either active contraction or passive stretching. It is not possible to identify a specific lesion of inert tissue by looking at movement patterns alone; other special tests must be done to identify injured structures.[5]

**Contractile tissue:**
- Muscles and their tendons

**Inert tissues:**
- Bones
- Ligaments
- Joint capsules
- Fascia
- Nerves
- Bursae
- Nerve roots
- Dura mater

***Active Range of Motion*** Movement assessment should begin with **active range of motion (AROM)**. The athletic trainer should evaluate quality of movement, range of movement, motion in other planes, movement at varying speeds, and strength throughout the range but in particular at the endpoint. If unable to perform the movement, make sure there are no contraindications before preceding. A complaint of pain on active motion will not distinguish contractile pain from inert pain, so the athletic trainer must proceed with an evaluation of both passive and resistive motion. A patient who seems to be pain free in each of these tests throughout a full range should be tested by applying passive pressure at the endpoint.

***Resistive Range of Motion through Manual Muscle Testing*** Manual muscle testing is an integral part of the physical examination process.[7,28] The ability of the injured patient to tolerate varying levels of resistance can indicate a great deal about the extent of the injury to the contractile units. For the patient, the limitation in muscular strength is generally caused by pain.[14] As pain diminishes and the healing process progresses, levels of muscular strength gradually return to normal. The development of isokinetic testing devices has enabled the athletic trainer to test levels of muscular strength objectively within the limitations of those devices.[29]

Manual muscle testing is usually performed with the patient positioned so that individual muscles or muscle groups can be isolated and tested through a full range of motion via the application of manual resistance. The ability of the patient to move through a full range of motion or to offer resistance to movement is subjectively graded by the athletic trainer according to various classification systems and grading criteria. Table 13–2 indicates a commonly used grading system for manual muscle testing. Examples of manual muscle testing techniques for most joint movements can be found in Appendix F.

***Passive Range of Motion*** When passive ROM is assessed, the patient should be positioned so that the contractile tissues are relaxed and do not influence the findings due to active muscle contraction. The athletic trainer then takes the limb through the desired passive movement pattern until the point of pain or end ROM. Upon reaching

| TABLE 13–2 | Manual Muscle Strength Grading | | |
|---|---|---|---|
| **Grade** | **Percentage (%)** | **Qualitative Value** | **Muscle Strength** |
| 5 | 100 | Normal | Complete range of motion (ROM) against gravity with full resistance |
| 4 | 75 | Good | Complete ROM against gravity with some resistance |
| 3 | 50 | Fair | Complete ROM against gravity with no resistance |
| 2 | 25 | Poor | Complete ROM with gravity omitted |
| 1 | 10 | Trace | Evidence of slight contractility with no joint motion |
| 0 | 0 | Zero | No evidence of muscle contractility |

the end ROM, gentle overpressure should be applied and particular attention should be directed toward the sensation of the endpoint feel.

***Testing Joint Endpoints*** Cyriax has described *normal endpoints* and *abnormal endpoints*.[47] Normal endpoints have also been referred to as *end feels* and are what the examiner is looking for in passive range of motion testing.[31] Abnormal endpoints, sometimes referred to simply as *endpoints* are what the examiner feels during ligamentous stress tests.[15] The athletic trainer should categorize the "feel" of the endpoints as described in the following sections.[15]

***Normal endpoints (end feels)*** Normal endpoints include the following:[33]

- Soft-tissue approximation—soft and spongy, a gradual, painless stop (e.g., knee flexion)
- Capsular feel—an abrupt, hard, firm endpoint with only a little give (e.g., endpoint of hip rotation)
- Bone to bone—a distinct and abrupt endpoint when two hard surfaces come in contact with one another (e.g., elbow in full extension)
- Muscular—a springy feel with some associated discomfort (e.g., end of shoulder abduction)

***Abnormal endpoints (endpoints)*** Abnormal endpoints include the following:

- Empty feel—movement is definitely beyond the anatomical limit, and pain occurs before the end of the range (e.g., a complete ligament rupture)
- Spasm—involuntary muscle contraction that prevents motion because of pain; also called guarding (e.g., back spasms)
- Loose—occurs in extreme hypermobility (e.g., previously sprained ankle)
- Springy block—a rebound at the endpoint (e.g., meniscus tear)

Throughout the passive range of movement, the athletic trainer is looking for limitation in movement and the presence of pain. A patient's report of pain before the end of the available range probably indicates acute inflammation, in which stretching and manipulation are both contraindicated as treatments. Pain occurring synchronous with the end of the range indicates that the condition is subacute and has progressed to some inert tissue fibrosis. If no pain occurs at the end of the range, the condition is chronic and contractures have replaced inflammation.[57]

### Measuring Range of Motion

***Goniometric Measurement*** Goniometry, which measures joint range of motion, is an essential procedure during the early, intermediate, and late stages of injury. Full range of motion of an affected body part is a major criterion for a patient to return to activity. Active and passive joint range of motion can be measured using goniometry (Figure 13–4A).[45]

Although a number of different types of goniometers are on the market, the most commonly used are ones that measure 0 to 180 degrees in each direction. The arms of the instrument are usually 12 to 16 inches (30 to 40 cm) long, with one arm stationary and the other fully movable.[11]

When measuring joint range of motion, the goniometer should generally be placed along the lateral surface of the extremity being measured. The 0, or starting, position for any movement is identical to the standard anatomical position. The patient should move the joint either actively or passively through the available range to the endpoint. The stationary arm of the goniometer should be placed parallel with the longitudinal axis of the fixed reference part. The movable arm should be placed along the longitudinal axis of the movable segment. (NOTE: The axis of rotation will change throughout the range as movement occurs. Thus, the axis of rotation is located at the intersection of the stationary and movable arms.) A reading in degrees of motion should be taken and recorded as either active or passive range of motion for that movement. Accuracy and consistency in goniometric measurement require practice

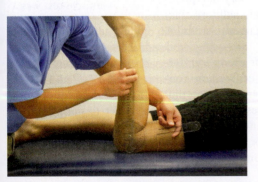
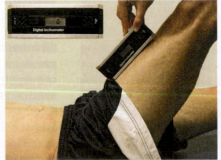
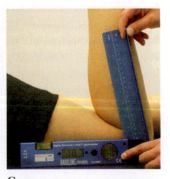

A                        B                       C

FIGURE 13–4  Measuring joint range of motion. (A) Goniometric measurement of knee joint flexion. (B) Inclinometer measurement of hip flexion. (C) Digital goniometer.

| TABLE 13–3 | Range of Joint Motion | |
|---|---|---|
| **Joint** | **Action** | **Degrees of Motion** |
| Shoulder | Flexion | 180 |
| | Extension | 50 |
| | Adduction | 40 |
| | Abduction | 180 |
| | Internal rotation | 90 |
| | External rotation | 90 |
| Elbow | Flexion | 145 |
| Forearm | Pronation | 80 |
| | Supination | 85 |
| Wrist | Flexion | 80 |
| | Extension | 70 |
| | Abduction | 20 |
| | Adduction | 45 |
| Hip | Flexion | 125 |
| | Extension | 10 |
| | Abduction | 45 |
| | Adduction | 40 |
| | Internal rotation | 45 |
| | External rotation | 45 |
| Knee | Flexion | 140 |
| Ankle | Plantar flexion | 45 |
| | Dorsiflexion | 20 |
| Foot | Inversion | 40 |
| | Eversion | 20 |

Source: Modified from Veterans Administration Standard Form;
A, Washington, DC: U.S. Government Printing Office.

and repetition. Digital inclinometers and goniometers are commonly used to provide a more accurate measure of joint range (Figures 13–4B and C).

The normal available range of motion for specific movements at individual joints is indicated in Table 13–3. Examples of goniometric measurement techniques for joint range of motion can be found in Appendix G.

***Digital Inclinometer*** Like a goniometer, an inclinometer is an instrument for measuring range of motion (Figure 13–4B). It measures the slope of elevation or the angle of movement relative to gravity. The inclinometer is placed on a body part and set to 0 degrees; it measures the total range of movement digitally. It provides accuracy, repeatability, and objective documentation of range of motion measurements. For this purpose, the digital inclinometer is considered to be a useful instrument because it is inexpensive and easy to use.

***Testing Accessory Motions*** *Accessory motions* refers to the manner in which one articulating joint surface moves relative to another.[3] Normal accessory component motions must occur for full-range movement to take place. Accessory motions are limited by tightness of the joint capsule and/or ligaments that surround a joint. It is critical for the athletic trainer to closely evaluate the injured joint to determine whether motion is limited by tightness of the musculotendinous units or by limitation in accessory motion involving the joint capsule and ligaments. If accessory motion is limited by some restriction of the joint capsule or the ligaments, joint mobilization techniques may be incorporated into the treatment program.[32] Joint mobilization is discussed in detail in Chapter 16.

**Neurological Examination** Performing a detailed and accurate neurological exam is difficult for everyone, including physicians. The exam consists of six major areas: cerebral function, cranial nerve function, cerebellar function, sensory testing, reflex testing, projected or referred pain, and motor testing. In cases of musculoskeletal injury that do not involve head injury, it is generally not necessary to assess cerebral function, cranial nerve function, and cerebellar function. The athletic trainer should concentrate instead on sensory testing, reflex testing, and motor testing to determine the involvement of the peripheral nervous system after injury.

> **Neurological examination:**
> - Cerebral function
> - Cranial nerve function
> - Cerebellar function
> - Sensory testing
> - Reflex testing
> - Projected or referred pain
> - Motor testing

***Cerebral Function*** Tests for general cerebral function include questions that assess general affect, level of consciousness, intellectual performance, emotional status, thought content, sensory interpretation (visual, auditory, tactile), and language skills.

***Cerebellar Function*** Because the cerebellum controls purposeful, coordinated movement and motor function, tests such as touching finger to nose, touching finger to finger of examiner, drawing alphabets in the air with the foot, and heel-toe walking may be used to determine dysfunction.

***Cranial Nerve Function*** The function of the 12 cranial nerves can be quickly determined by assessing the quality of the following: sense of smell, eye tracking, imitation of facial expressions, biting down, balance, swallowing, tongue

> A baseball player complains of pain in his right shoulder. A manual muscle test for shoulder external rotation was a grade 3.
>
> **?** What does this evaluation indicate about the tissue? If the result of the manual muscle test was a grade 3, what is a possible conclusion for this evaluation?

TABLE 13–4 ■ Cranial Nerves and Their Functions

| I. | Olfactory | Smell |
|---|---|---|
| II. | Optic | Vision |
| III. | Oculomotor | Eye movement, opening of eyelid, constriction of pupil, focusing |
| IV. | Trochlear | Inferior and lateral movement of eye |
| V. | Trigeminal | Sensation to the face, mastication |
| VI. | Abducens | Lateral movement of eye |
| VII. | Facial | Motor nerve of facial expression; taste; control of tear, nasal, sublingual salivary, and submaxillary glands |
| VIII. | Vestibulocochlear | Hearing and equilibrium |
| IX. | Glossopharyngeal | Swallowing, salivation, gag reflex, sensation from tongue and ear |
| X. | Vagus | Swallowing; speech; regulation of pulmonary, cardiovascular, and gastrointestinal functions |
| XI. | Accessory | Swallowing, innervation of sternocleidomastoid and trapezius muscle |
| XII. | Hypoglossal | Tongue movement, speech, swallowing |

protrusion, and strength of shoulder shrugs. Table 13–4 lists the cranial nerves and their functions.

***Sensory Testing*** A major component of musculoskeletal assessment is determining the distribution of peripheral nerves and dermatomes (Figure 13–5). A **dermatome** is an area of skin that is innervated by the sensory fibers of a single spinal nerve or cranial nerve. The term *dermatome* is sometimes confused with **myotomes**, which are found in developing embryos. Segmental myotomes eventually develop into a muscle or a group of muscles that are innervated by motor fibers from a specific spinal nerve. Table 13–5 shows myotome patterns at muscle weakness that can occur with lesions to specific spinal nerve roots.

Although peripheral nerve distribution varies with individuals, it is more predictable than dermatome distribution.[20] As the dermatome examination progresses, the examiner compares sensation from one side of the body to the other, using the following tests as examples:

- Superficial sensation—touch dermatomes with cotton
- Superficial pain—touch dermatomes with a pin
- Deep pressure pain—squeeze a muscle (e.g., gastrocnemius)
- Sensitivity of temperature—touch dermatomes with ice cube
- Sensitivity of vibration—touch dermatomes with a tuning fork
- Position sense—move fingers or toes passively and ask athlete to indicate direction

***Reflex Testing*** The term *reflex* refers to an involuntary response to a stimulus. In terms of the neurological examination, there are three types of reflexes: deep tendon (somatic) reflexes, superficial reflexes, and pathological reflexes.

***Deep Tendon Reflexes*** A deep tendon reflex is caused by stimulation of the stretch reflex (see Chapter 4) and results in an involuntary contraction of a muscle when its tendon is stretched. Deep tendon reflexes can be elicited at the tendons of the biceps (C5), brachioradialis (C6), extensor digitorum (C6), triceps (C7), adductor (L2), patella (L4), Achilles (S1), and hamstring (S2). Perhaps the best example of a deep tendon reflex is the "knee-jerk" response. Table 13–6 shows a grading system for deep tendon reflexes.[38]

***Superficial Reflexes*** Superficial reflexes are elicited by stimulation of the skin at specific sites, which produces a reflex muscle contraction. For example, stroking the abdomen at a specific area in a specific direction causes a predictable contraction of the abdominal muscles. Superficial reflexes include upper abdominal (T7, 8, 9), lower abdominal (T11, 12), cremasteric (T12, L1), plantar (S1, 2), and gluteal (L4, S3). An absence of a superficial reflex is indicative of some lesion in the spinal cord—specifically, the descending corticospinal tract in the spinal cord.

***Pathological Reflexes*** Most, but not all, pathological reflexes are also superficial reflexes. The presence of a pathological reflex indicates a lesion in the descending upper motor neuron, including the spinal cord; an absence indicates integrity. For example, Babinski's sign, in which stroking of the lateral plantar surface produces extension and splaying of the toes, is an example of a pathological reflex.[38] Chaddock's, Oppenheim's, and Gordon's are

**13–5 Clinical Application Exercise**

A receiver in football has his feet taken out from under him by a tackler and lands flat on his low back with his legs above him. An on-the-field evaluation reveals unilateral decreased muscle strength, decreased sensation, and a decreased patellar tendon reflex in the right lower extremity.

**?** Based on the findings of the evaluation, how should the athletic trainer manage this injury?

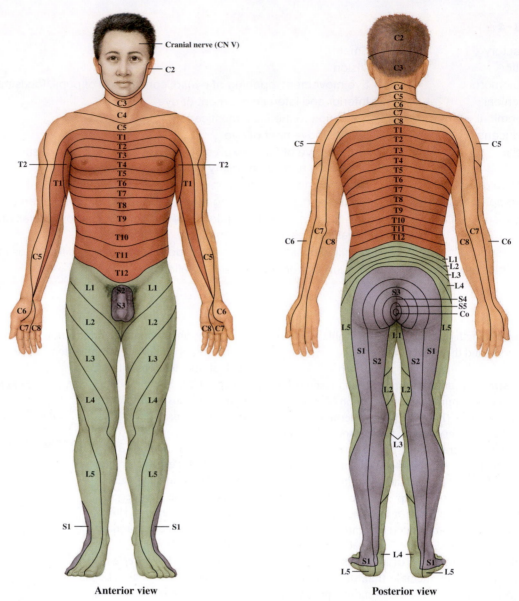

**FIGURE 13–5** Dermatomes. Numbness, referred pain, and other nerve involvements often follow the segmental distribution of spinal nerves on the skin's surface.

Anterior view        Posterior view

| TABLE 13–5 | Myotome Patterns of Weakness Resulting from Spinal Nerve Root Lesion | | |
|---|---|---|---|
| C1 | None | L1 | None |
| C2 | Neck flexion | L2 | Hip flexion |
| C3 | Neck lateral flexion and extension | L3 | Knee extension |
| C4 | Shoulder shrug | L4 | Ankle dorsiflexion |
| C5 | Shoulder abduction | L5 | Hallux extension |
| C6 | Elbow flexion/wrist extension | S1 | Plantar flexion/eversion/knee flexion/hip extension |
| C7 | Elbow extension/wrist flexion | S2 | Plantar flexion/knee flexion/hip extension |
| C8 | Ulnar deviation/thumb extension | S3 | None |
| T1 | None (finger abduction and adduction) | S4 | Bladder, rectum |

**TABLE 13–6** Deep Tendon Reflex Grading

| | Grade | Definition |
|---|---|---|
| Absence of a reflex | 0 | Areflexia |
| Diminished reflex | 1 | Hyporeflexia |
| Average reflex | 2 | |
| Exaggerated reflex | 3 | Hyperreflexia (increased but not pathological) |
| Markedly hyperactive | 4 | Often associated with clonus, but clonus is not required for grade 4 |

additional reflexes that are alternatives for eliciting a Babinski's response. For Chaddock's reflex, the lateral foot, from lateral malleolus to small toe, is stroked with a blunt instrument and there is extension of the great toe. For Oppenheim's reflex, the anterior tibia, from just below the patella to the foot, is firmly stroked with a knuckle and there is extension of the great toe. For Gordon's reflex, the calf muscles are squeezed and there is extension of the great toe or all of the toes.

In general, hyperactive reflexes, clonus (alternating contraction between antagonist muscle groups), Babinski's sign, and decreased superficial reflexes are all considered to be upper motor neuron signs and usually indicate a lesion somewhere in that tract as it courses through the brain, brain stem, and spinal cord.

*Projected or Referred Pain* As discussed in Chapter 10, a complaint of deep, burning pain, an ache that is diffused, or a painful area with no signs of disorder or malfunctioning is most likely referred pain. Cyriax considers that the common sites for pain referral are, in order of importance, joint capsule, tendon, muscle, ligament, and bursa.[15] Pressures from the dura mater or nerve sheath can also produce referred pain or other sensory responses. Palpation of what is thought to be the area at fault often is misleading. Detecting the selective tension of the tissue at fault is one of the best means for gathering correct data. Some musculoskeletal pain is caused by myofascial trigger points, which are not related to deep, referred pain. Palpation is used to determine the presence or absence of tense tissue bands and tender trigger points.

*Motor Testing* Motor tests are done by evaluating strength in muscles that are innervated by a specific nerve root level to test neurological function of that nerve root. The manual muscle tests discussed earlier in this chapter are used to test the function of the motor neurons in both the upper and lower extremities.

*Testing Joint Stability* A number of specific tests for determining the integrity of the ligaments surrounding a particular joint are described in Chapters 18 through 25.

Joint stability tests provide information about the grade of a sprain of a particular ligament and can determine the extent of the functional instability of the joint.

**Postural Examination** As is discussed in Chapter 25, many cases of injuries can be attributed to body malalignments. Musculoskeletal assessment might be one area of a postural examination. It is designed to test for malalignments and asymmetries by viewing the body compared with a grid or plumb line (see Figures 25–7 through 25–9).

**Anthropometric Measurements** Anthropometry is the science of measuring the human body. Anthropometric measurements include osteometry (measurement of the dimensions of the skeletal system), craniometry (measurement of the bones of the skull), skin-fold measurements to determine body composition (see Chapter 5), and height and weight measurements (see Chapter 2). Limb girth measurements taken during a rehabilitation program are also considered a type of anthropometric measurement. Anthropometric measurements are seldom used by athletic trainers in a sports medicine setting.

**Volumetric Measurements** Volumetric measurements can be taken to determine changes in limb volume caused by swelling, which can be attributed to hemorrhage, edema, or inflammation.[48] Limb volume may be measured in a volumetric tank that essentially measures the amount of water displaced by immersion of the limb in the tank. *Focus Box 13–3:* "Constructing and using a volumetric tank" describes the tank and the procedure for measuring limb volume.

**Testing Functional Performance** Functional performance testing may be done as part of an initial evaluation to determine whether an injury is severe enough to keep the patient from activity. It may also be used to evaluate progress during a rehabilitation program. Decisions about when a patient is ready to return to full activity following injury should be based to a large extent on performance on functional tests.[30] Functional testing should proceed

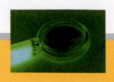
## Constructing and using a volumetric tank

A volumetric tank is constructed of five 0.6-centimeter sheets of acrylic plastic molded together to form a container, which is mounted on a platform. The internal dimensions of the tank are length = 35.6 centimeters (14 in.), width = 17.8 centimeters (7 in.), and depth = 20.3 centimeters (8 in.). All the walls form right angles with each other as well as with the floor of the tank. The bottom of the tank has three adjustable leveling screws. Two of these screws are at one end of the tank base, and the third is centrally located on the opposite end. The end with one screw is classified as the front of the tank. A piece of acrylic plastic that measures 1.3 centimeters (0.5 in.) wide by 6 centimeters (2.4 in.) long is attached to the side of the tank, 4 centimeters (1.6 in.) from the back of the tank, to ensure consistent limb positioning in the tank.

A glass tube, 7.3 millimeters (0.29 in.) in diameter by 7.6 centimeters (3 in.) passes through the front of the tank. The tube extends 3.2 centimeters (1.25 in.) outside the front wall of the tank. The tube is 5.1 centimeters (2 in.) from the top of the front wall and is perpendicular to the wall of the tank. A 10.2-centimeter (4 in.) piece of rubber tubing is attached to the end of the glass tube. This tubing combination allows for displaced water to be collected. A centimeter ruler, a skin thermometer, and a 500- and 1,000-milliliter (19.7 in. and 39.4 in.) graduated cylinder is used for all measurements. A water collection container is used to catch the runoff when the tubing is unclamped.

### Procedure for measuring water displacement

The volumetric tank is placed on the floor and leveled using the adjusting screws. The tank is then filled to the 17-centimeter (6.7 in.) mark on the ruler with 33.58C (92.3°F) water. The subject places the limb against the back wall of the tank. The tank is then shaken gently to eliminate any air bubbles in the tank or on the surface of the limb. When the water is completely motionless, the tubing is unclamped and the runoff is collected in the container. Any water remaining in the tubing should be shaken out into the collection container. The amount of water collected in the runoff container is measured in the graduated cylinders and the measurements are noted.

---

> Functional examination determines whether the athlete has full strength, joint stability, and coordination, and whether the part is pain free.

full activity. The major concern is whether the patient has regained full range of motion, strength, speed, endurance, and neuromuscular control and is pain free.

## FUNCTIONAL SCREENING TESTS

Functional screening tests may be performed as part of the preparticipation physical examination to identify individuals that may be at risk for injury. There is little scientific research on what the athletic trainer should focus on during injury risk screening. However, knowledge of basic biomechanics and anatomy can help the athletic trainer identify movement patterns that put stress and strain on tissue, hence increasing risk of injury.

Traditionally the clinician has used an assessment model based on anatomy that identifies a structure that generates anatomic pain that exhibits signs and symptoms that are consistent with a specific diagnosis. The trend is to shift toward a newer model that focuses more gradually from minimal stress to tests that mimic the actual stress that would normally come from

on a kinesiologic assessment rather than on an anatomic assessment. This new paradigm identifies characteristic movement impairments within the human movement system and suggests how to treat these movement-related impairments and not just the structural abnormalities.

When the athlete is at greater risk of injury, he or she can devise an injury prevention training program to address the cause of the inefficient movements. By incorporating training in injury prevention, the athletic trainer may be able to reduce the incidence of injury. This has been demonstrated in several research studies looking at the incidence of lower-extremity injury, specifically ACL injury.[9,26,56]

Several clinicians have developed functional evaluation screening protocols that give more attention to functional movement deficits, which may limit performance and predispose the individual to injury.[10,12,44,46] The overhead and single leg squat tests, the functional movement screen (FMS), the landing error scoring system (LESS), and the tuck jump test are four examples of functional screening tests that are evidence-based.[10,12,27,44,46] All of these functional screening tests have moderate to excellent intra- and inter-rater reliability.

In general, these protocols involve the individual performing a dynamic movement in a controlled manner. The athletic trainer then observes the individual's movement pattern at each of the involved joints. By noting inefficient movement patterns, the athletic trainer may be able to identify preexisting muscle imbalances that alter the normal force-couple relationships, postural alignment, joint kinematics, and neuromuscular control.

## Overhead and Single Leg Squat Tests

The overhead and single leg squat tests were developed by Clark to identify movement impairments, determine the underlying causes, and then use this information to direct treatment.[10] In the overhead squat, the patient performs a squat maneuver while extending the arms above his or her head (Figure 13–6). In the single leg squat, with the hands on the hips the patient squats on one leg to a comfortable level and returns to the standing position (Figure 13–7).

Essentially, the athletic trainer observes whether the subject can maintain a neutral alignment of limb segments while performing a dynamic movement. The athletic trainer looks for compensation patterns at the foot, knee, hip, lumbar spine, and shoulder.

If the patient's limb segment moves out of neutral alignment, it can be due to muscle tightness or weakness. Muscle tightness may be present in the muscles in the direction of limb motion. Excessively tight muscles are believed to pull the limb into the direction of tightness, away from neutral alignment. Muscle inhibition or weakness might also be present in the muscles acting in the opposite direction of limb motion. Weak and inhibited muscles are believed to be unable to generate the magnitude of force necessary to maintain neutral alignment.

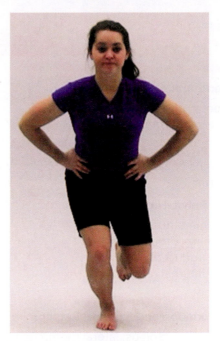

FIGURE 13–7    Single leg squat
© William E. Prentice

Both situations cause altered joint kinematics that can place greater stress on the surrounding tissues and push these tissues closer to their point of failure during repeated movements. Tables 13–7 and 13–8 identify the compensation patterns that the patient may exhibit when performing the overhead squat and the single leg squat and the recommendations relative to how the athletic trainer should interpret those findings.

## Landing Error Scoring System

LESS was developed by Padua to identify individuals at high risk for ACL injury.[46] The test involves a jump-landing task incorporating vertical and horizontal movements as the patient jumps from a 30-cm high box to a distance of 50 percent of his or her height away from the box, and immediately rebounds for a maximal vertical jump on landing (Figure 13–8).

The LESS score is simply a count of landing technique "errors" on a range of readily observable items of human movement. The landing technique is analyzed from both a side view and a frontal view by the athletic trainer. There are 17 scored items in the LESS (Table 13–9). A higher LESS score indicates poor technique in landing from a jump; a lower LESS score indicates better jump-landing technique.

## Tuck Jump Test

Like the LESS, the tuck jump test developed by Myer may be useful to the clinician for the identification of lower extremity landing technique flaws during a plyometric activity that may cause ACL injury.[44] In this test,

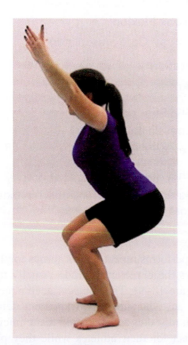

FIGURE 13–6    Overhead Squat
© William E. Prentice

| TABLE 13–7 | Overhead Squat Compensation Patterns |
|---|---|

**Compensations at**

**Foot and Ankle**

- Foot pronation:            Y / N
- Externally rotation:    Y / N

**Knees**

- Valgus collapse:        Y / N
- Varus:                 Y / N

**Lumbo-Pelvic-Hip Complex**

- Asymmetrical weight shift:   Y / N
- Lumbar lordosis:        Y / N
- Hip adduction:          Y / N
- Hip internal rotation:    Y / N

*What to Do with Findings*

**Foot Pronation and External Rotation**

- Tightness: Soleus, lateral gastrocnemius, biceps femoris, peroneals, piriformis

**Knee Valgus and Internal Rotation**

- Tightness: Gastrocnemius/soleus, adductors, IT band
- Weakness: Gluteus medius

**Lumbar Lordosis**

- Tightness: Erector spinae and psoas
- Weakness: Transverse abdominis, internal obliques

**Hip Adduction**

- Tightness: Hip adductors
- Weakness: Gluteus medius

**Hip Internal Rotation**

- Weakness: Gluteus maximus, hip external rotators

| TABLE 13–8 | Single Leg Squat Compensation Patterns |
|---|---|

**Compensations at**

**Foot and Ankle**

- Foot pronation:            Y / N
- Externally rotation:    Y / N

**Knees**

- Valgus collapse:        Y / N
- Varus:                 Y / N

**Lumbo-Pelvic-Hip Complex**

- Lumbar lordosis:        Y / N
- Lateral trunk flexion:    Y / N
- Trunk rotation:         Y / N
- Hip adduction:          Y / N
- Hip internal rotation:    Y / N

*What to Do with Findings*

**Foot Pronation and External Rotation**

- Tightness: Soleus, lateral gastrocnemius, biceps femoris, peroneals, piriformis

**Knee Valgus and Internal Rotation**

- Tightness: Gastrocnemius/soleus, adductors, IT band
- Weakness: Gluteus medius, adductors, IT band

**Lumbar Lordosis**

- Tightness: Erector spinae and psoas
- Weakness: Transverse abdominis, internal obliques

**Lateral Trunk Flexion**

- Weakness: Core musculature

**Trunk Rotation**

- Weakness: Core musculature

**Hip Adduction**

- Tightness: Hip adductors
- Weakness: Gluteus medius

**Hip Internal Rotation**

- Weakness: Gluteus maximus, hip external rotators

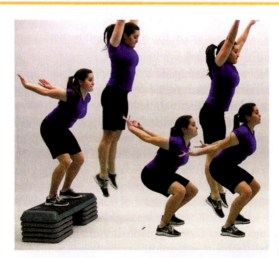

FIGURE 13–8   Landing Error Scoring System (LESS)

© William E. Prentice

the subject performs repeated tuck jumps for 10 seconds, which allows the clinician to grade visually the outlined criteria (Figure 13–9). The subjects' technique is subjectively rated as either having an apparent deficit or not. Six common mistakes are identified that clinicians should aim to correct for their athletes while they perform the tuck jump exercise (Table 13–10). The deficits are tallied for the final assessment score. Patients who demonstrate

| TABLE 13–9 | Landing Technique "Errors" |
|---|---|

**Sagittal (Side) View Score**

| | | |
|---|---|---|
| • | Hip flexion angle at contact—hips are flexed | Yes = 0, No = 1 |
| • | Trunk flexion angle at contact—trunk in front of hips | Yes = 0, No = 1 |
| • | Knee flexion angle at contact—greater than 30 degrees | Yes = 0, No = 1 |
| • | Ankle plantar flexion angle at contact—toe to heel | Yes = 0, No = 1 |
| • | Hip flexion at max knee flexion angle—greater than at contact | Yes = 0, No = 1 |
| • | Trunk flexion at max knee flexion—trunk in front of the hips | Yes = 0, No = 1 |
| • | Knee flexion displacement—greater than 30 degrees | Yes = 0, No = 1 |
| • | Sagittal plane joint displacement - Large motion (soft) = 0, Average = 1, Small motion (loud/stiff) = 2 | |

**Coronal (Frontal) View Score**

| | | |
|---|---|---|
| • | Lateral (side) trunk flexion at contact—trunk is flexed | Yes = 0, No = 1 |
| • | Knee valgus angle at contact—knees over the mid-foot | Yes = 0, No = 1 |
| • | Knee valgus displacement—knees inside of large toe | Yes = 1, No = 0 |
| • | Foot position at contact—toes pointing out greater than 30 degrees | Yes = 1, No = 0 |
| • | Foot position at contact—toes pointing out less than 30 degrees | Yes = 1, No = 0 |
| • | Stance width at contact—less than shoulder width | Yes = 1, No = 0 |
| • | Stance width at contact—greater than shoulder width | Yes = 1, No = 0 |
| • | Initial foot contact—symmetric | Yes = 0, No = 1 |
| • | Overall impression | Excellent = 0, Average = 1, Poor = 2 |

**Total Score_____**

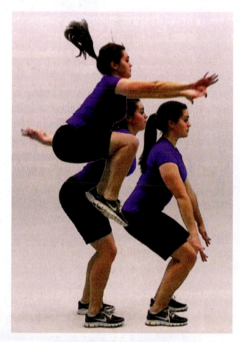

FIGURE 13–9   Tuck Jump Test
© William E. Prentice

six or more flawed techniques should be targeted for further technique training.

## Functional Movement Screen

FMS was developed by Cook to bridge the gap between preparticipation exams and performance testing by examining individuals performing fundamental movement patterns.[12,27] It is not intended to be a diagnostic tool that will direct patient treatment. FMS consists of seven fundamental movement patterns that require a balance of stability and mobility including the (1) deep squat, (2) hurdle step, (3) in-line lunge, (4) shoulder mobility test, (5) active straight-leg raise, (6) trunk stability push-up, and (7) rotary stability test (Figure 13–10). The FMS is scored on an ordinal scale, with four possible scores ranging from 0 to 3 (Table 13–11). The maximum score on the FMS is 21.

## Fusionetics

Fusionetics is a new screening tool that assesses global movement quality to identify injury risk and athletic performance ability. Fusionetics uses seven tasks including a two-leg squat, two-leg squat with a heel lift, one-leg squat, push-up, shoulder movement, trunk/lumbar spine movement, and cervical spine movements. The individual scores from each of the seven tasks are based on specific compensations and asymmetries observed while performing that task. Scores on the seven functional tasks are added to generate an overall composite score out of 100. The composite score is used to predict injury risk and athletic performance. Based on the compensations and asymmetries observed during the tasks, a list of corrective exercises is generated for the individual patient, consisting of suggested sets, repetitions, and times per week the individual should complete each exercise. To date there

TABLE 13–10    Tuck Jump Test Technique Flaws

| Tuck Jump Assessment: | Pre | Mid | Post |
|---|---|---|---|
| **Knee and Thigh Motion** | | | |
| Knee valgus at landing | | | |
| Thighs not parallel at peak | | | |
| Thighs not equal side-to-side during flight | | | |
| **Foot Position during Landing** | | | |
| Feet not shoulder width apart | | | |
| Feet not parallel on landing | | | |
| Foot contact timing not equal | | | |
| | ___ Total | ___ Total | ___ Total |

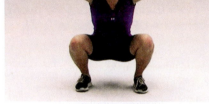
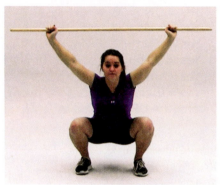
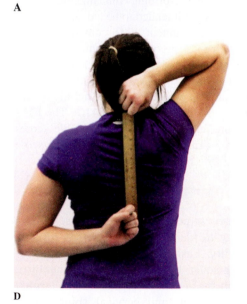

A

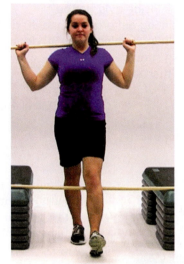

B

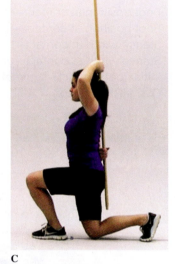

C

D

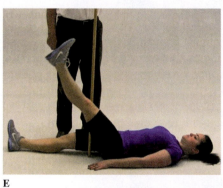

E

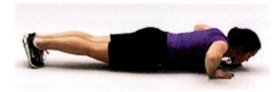

F

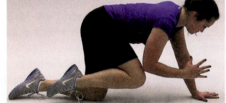

G

FIGURE 13–10   Functional movement screen (FMS). **(A)** deep squat. **(B)** hurdle step. **(C)** in-line lunge. **(D)** shoulder mobility test. **(E)** active straight-leg raise. **(F)** trunk stability push-up, and **(G)** rotary stability test.
© William E. Prentice

TABLE 13–11    Functional Movement Screen

| FMS Test | Right | Left | Score* |
|---|---|---|---|
| • Overhead deep squat | _____ | _____ | _____ |
| • Trunk stability push-up | _____ | _____ | _____ |
| • Hurdle step | _____ | _____ | _____ |
| • In-line lunge | _____ | _____ | _____ |
| • Shoulder mobility | _____ | _____ | _____ |
| • Active straight leg raise | _____ | _____ | _____ |
| • Rotary stability | _____ | _____ | _____ |
| | | Total Score /21 | _____ |

*Scoring
- Performs pattern correctly without compensation = 3
- Completes pattern with some compensation = 2
- Unable to complete pattern = 1
- Pain at any time when performing movement pattern = 0

is no evidence-based data to support the efficacy of the Fusionetics program.

# USING THE BEST AVAILABLE EVIDENCE IN CLINICAL DECISION MAKING

As a clinician, incorporating an evidence-based approach as a part of the clinical decision-making process is critical to successful practice. The clinician has two primary responsibilities: (1) to determine the correct diagnosis of an injury and (2) to choose the correct treatment. Decisions about the correct treatment are made on the basis of diagnostic test results.[58]

The athletic trainer has hundreds of special evaluative diagnostic tests to choose from, which have been described in the professional literature. Many of these are discussed in Chapters 18 to 25 of this text. For example, when evaluating an injured knee, there may be 25 different tests described in the literature that can be used to determine whether an injury actually exists. Certainly when performing an injury assessment it is not necessary to use all of those tests to determine the diagnoses of the injury. The athletic trainer should choose to incorporate specific tests that are the most appropriate based on (1) the history and symptoms of the patient's injury, and (2) the reliability and accuracy of that test in identifying an injury. To a large extent, clinicians rely on studies published in the professional literature to provide evidence-based data relative to the reliability and accuracy of specific diagnostic clinical tests in correctly diagnosing an injury. But there are still many tests being used by clinicians on a daily basis that have yet to be studied and are not very accurate. Some tests may eventually prove to be reliable and accurate, whereas others will not be reliable or accurate as a diagnostic tool.

## Determining the Reliability and Accuracy of a Diagnostic Test

**Reliability** The first step in determining a test's usefulness is to establish *intra-rater* and *inter-rater reliability*. **Intra-rater reliability** is determined by the extent to which the same examiner obtains the same result on the same patient. **Inter-rater reliability** is determined by the extent to which different examiners obtain the same result on the same patient.[58] Statisticians use both an intraclass correlation coefficient (ICC) and a Kappa coefficient (K) to calculate a reliability value that can range between 0.0 and 1.0. The closer to 1.0 the more reliable a diagnostic test is (Table 13–12).

**Diagnostic Accuracy** It is also important that the diagnostic tests the athletic trainer chooses be as accurate as possible in identifying whether an injury actually exists. If there is an injury, the diagnostic test is said to be positive, and if there is not an injury the test is said to be negative. Ideally, a perfect diagnostic test would be accurate in correctly identifying the presence or absence of an injury 100 percent of the time. However, it is not likely that any clinical test would be correct 100 percent of the time. Therefore, to calculate the accuracy of a clinical diagnostic test, it can be compared with some "gold standard" test that has been defined as the best available test and has been demonstrated to have the highest diagnostic accuracy (Figure 13–11A).

| TABLE 13–12 | Clinical Test Reliability |
|---|---|
| Coefficient | Reliability of a diagnostic test |
| 0.0–0.5 | Poor clinical reliability |
| 0.5–0.75 | Moderate clinical reliability |
| 0.75–1.0 | Good clinical reliability |

| | Gold Standard | | |
|---|---|---|---|
| | Condition positive | Condition negative | |
| Diagnostic Test Outcome positive | True positive (a) | False positive (b) | Positive predictive value = a / a+b |
| Outcome negative | False negative (c) | True negative (d) | Negative predictive value = d / d+c |
| | Sensitivity = a / a+c | Specificity = d / d+b | |

**(A)**

| | | Gold Standard (Radiographs) | |
|---|---|---|---|
| | | Condition positive | Condition negative |
| Tuning Fork Test | Outcome positive | 10 | 5 |
| | Outcome negative | 2 | 20 |

| Sens = | 0.83 | PPV = | 0.67 | LR(+)= | 4.17 |
|---|---|---|---|---|---|
| Spec = | 0.80 | NPV = | 0.91 | LR(−)= | 0.21 |

**(B)**

FIGURE 13–11  **(A)** The accuracy of a clinical diagnostic test is compared with some "gold standard" test to determine the number of patients that the clinician correctly classifies as true positives and true negatives, compared to the total number of patients examined. **(B)** An example of using a tuning fork compared to a radiograph for determining the diagnostic accuracy of using a tuning fork.

There will be instances where an injury truly exists and a clinician would correctly determine that a clinical test is positive (True positive "a"). But there may be other instances where the clinician incorrectly determines the test is positive, with no existing injury (False positive "b").

Conversely, there will be instances where an injury does not exist and a clinician would correctly determine that a clinical test is negative (True negative "d"). But there may be other instances where the clinician incorrectly determines the test is negative, and yet there is an existing injury (False negative "c"). Accuracy of a specific clinical test is determined by the number of patients that the clinician correctly classifies as true positives and true negatives, compared to the total number of patients examined. For example, radiographic imaging is considered the gold standard for determining a fracture while the tuning fork test is a diagnostic test commonly used by athletic trainers in the clinic (Figure 13–11B).[43]

**Sensitivity and Specificity** The properties of the diagnostic test that tell us about the *accuracy* of a test are called *sensitivity (Sn)* and *specificity (Sp)*. Sensitivity and specificity describe how well a test discriminates between patients with and without an injury. Sensitivity is the ability of a diagnostic test to rule out a condition or injury. The higher the sensitivity (Sn), the greater the chance that a negative test (N) correctly rules out an injury (indicated by the acronym SnNout).[49]

High sensitivity + negative test = rule condition out (SnNout)

Specificity is the ability of a test to rule in a condition. The higher the specificity (Sp), the greater the chance that a positive test (P) correctly rules in an injury (indicated by the acronym SpPin).[49]

High specificity + positive test = rule condition in (SpPin)

A perfect diagnostic test would be described as 100 percent sensitive and 100 percent specific in discriminating between patients with and without an injury. For example, the tuning fork test identifies the presence of a fracture 100 percent of the time and identifies the absence of a fracture 100 percent

In Chapters **18** to **25** the sensitivity, specificity, and likelihood ratios (identified in the literature) for most of the special tests discussed are included in bold red at the end of the paragraph to help the reader evaluate the diagnostic accuracy and clinical usefulness of that particular test.

of the time (Figure 13–11B). If sensitivity is low and specificity is high, a positive test means low false positives and the injury is likely. A negative test means high false negatives, meaning that the test is not very helpful because sensitivity is low. Conversely, if sensitivity is high and specificity is low, a negative test means low false negatives and the injury is not likely while a negative test means high false positives. In this case, the test is not very helpful because specificity is low. In the tuning fork example, the test is 83 percent sensitive and the test identified 10 out of the 12 condition positive fractures as outcome positive fractures. The test is 80 percent specific or the test identified 20 out of 25 condition negative fractures as outcome negative fractures.

**Predictive Values** In the literature, accuracy of a diagnostic technique may be reported as predictive values. Predictive values answer the question: given a certain test result, what is the probability of the injury? A positive predictive value (PPV) indicates the probability of actually having an existing injury in patients with a positive test. A negative predictive value (NPV) indicates the probability that there is no injury in patients with a negative test.[39] In the tuning fork example, PPV of 67 percent means 10 out of 15 patients with a positive tuning fork test for fracture actually had a fracture. An NPV of 91 percent means 20 out of 22 patients with a negative tuning fork test for fracture did not really have a fracture.

Predictive values tell us how many of the patients who have a positive test are true positives or how many of the patients who have a negative test are true negatives. The closer to 100 percent (1.0) the better the predictive value.

A small positive predictive value (e.g., PPV = 10 percent [0.1]) indicates that many of the positive results from the diagnostic test are false positives. Thus, a more reliable test will be necessary to obtain a more accurate assessment as to whether an injury is actually present.

Positive and negative predictive values are directly related to the prevalence of the injury in the population where prevalence is the number of injured divided by the size of the population. A PPV will increase with increasing prevalence while the NPV will decrease with increasing prevalence.[39]

**Likelihood Ratios** A clinical test is only accurate if it alters the pretest probability, which is the likelihood that a specific injury is present before the diagnostic test results are known.[18] Does a positive test confirm what a clinician suspects based on the mechanism of injury, symptoms, and the like? Does a negative test help a clinician rule out an injury?

Likelihood ratios are calculated from sensitivity and specificity. A positive likelihood ratio (+LR) indicates the likelihood that a positive test means the condition is present. A negative likelihood ratio (–LR) indicates the likelihood that a negative test means the condition is absent.[18]

| TABLE 13–13 | Interpreting Likelihood Ratios | |
|---|---|---|
| **+LR** | **–LR** | **Probability That the Condition Is Present** |
| If the +LR is > 10 or the –LR is <0.1 | | Often conclusive (large shift) |
| If the +LR is 5–10 or the –LR is 0.1–0.2 | | Usually important (moderate shift) |
| If the +LR is 2–5 or the –LR is 0.2–0.5 | | Sometimes important (small shift) |
| If the +LR is 1–2 or the –LR is 0.5–1.0 | | Usually unimportant (very small shift) |

Table 13–13 provides a summary of the values for interpreting the clinical interpretation of likelihood ratios. A +LR over 1 indicates at least a minimal shift in pretest probability, which suggests the injury is present. A –LR less than 0.5 indicates a minimal shift in pretest probability, which suggests the injury is not present. LRs equal or close to 1 indicate no change in pretest probability. In general, tests with +LR greater than (>) 5 are useful in ruling in an injury and a –LR less than (<) 0.2 are useful in ruling out an injury. +LRs >10 and –LRs <0.1 indicate a large shift in pretest probability and thus would be considered conclusive. In the tuning fork test example, the +LR of 4.17 indicates it would not be useful ruling in a fracture; however, –LR of 0.2 indicates the potential for ruling out a fracture.[18]

## Clinical Prediction Rules

Clinical prediction rules (CPRs) are medical algorithms that are used as evidence-based tools which may help to improve and standardize medical care.[52] They may help the athletic training clinician with clinical decision making when identifying subgroups of patients who are likely to respond favorably to certain interventions or in diagnosing specific pathologic musculoskeletal conditions. A CPR integrates a combination of relevant clinical findings with medical signs and symptoms that can collectively predict the probability of an existing medical condition or an outcome for a patient who has been provided with a specific treatment.[4]

Before clinical prediction rules can be integrated into patient care as accurate and reliable clinical tools, they must first be developed or derived statistically and subsequently validated by prospective, longitudinal, randomized controlled statistical trials that compare outcomes after selected interventions. At this point, many CPRs are in the derivation stage, but only a few of the exiting CPRs used by athletic trainers have been validated. Generally the existing CPRs used by athletic trainers are very specific and less sensitive; they are thus better at ruling in a target outcome but not as useful for ruling out a target outcome.[13] Currently, there is little evidence that CPRs are useful for predicting the effects of interventions used in treating various musculoskeletal conditions.[52]

CPRs can be classified as being either (1) prescriptive, (2) diagnostic, or (3) prognostic. Athletic trainers most often use prescriptive CPRs that determine the most effective treatment interventions for patients who meet a similar score on the CPR. Studies that focus on predictive factors related to a specific diagnosis are known as *diagnostic* CPRs. Clinical prediction rules that are designed to predict an outcome such as success or failure are considered *prognostic*.

Table 13–14 identifies clinical prediction rules that have either completed or are currently in the derivation stage of development and are at least accurate prescriptive studies for musculoskeletal interventions or diagnosis for specific conditions.

| TABLE 13–14 | Clinical Prediction Rules Currently Used in Diagnosis and Clinical Practice |
| --- | --- |

**Shoulder**

Rotator cuff pathology
Subacromial impingement
Anterior shoulder instability
Cervicothoracic manipulation for shoulder pain

**Hand**

Carpal tunnel syndrome

**Spine**

Cervical manipulation for neck pain
Canadian cervical spine rules
Cervical myelopathy
Cervical radiculopathy
Cervical closed fracture
Vertebral compression fracture
Lumbar spinal stenosis
Manipulation for low back pain
Mechanical traction for low back pain
Mechanical traction for neck pain
Stabilization for low back pain
Thoracic manipulation for neck pain
Sacroiliac joint pain

**Hip**

Hip osteoarthritis
Hip mobilization for knee osteoarthritis

**Knee**

Manipulation for patellofemoral pain syndrome
Orthotics for patellofemoral pain syndrome
Patellar taping for patellofemoral pain syndrome
Medial collateral ligament pathology
Meniscal pathology
Ottawa knee rules
Pittsburgh knee rules

**Ankle**

Ottawa ankle rules

## PROGRESS EVALUATIONS

The athletic trainer who is overseeing a rehabilitation program must constantly monitor the progress of the patient toward full recovery throughout the rehabilitative process. In many instances, the athletic trainer will be able to treat the injured patient on a daily basis. This close supervision affords the athletic trainer the luxury of being able to continuously adjust or adapt the treatment program based on the progress made by the patient on a day-to-day basis.

The progress evaluation should be based on the athletic trainer's knowledge of exactly what is occurring in the healing process at any given time. The timelines of injury healing provide the framework that dictates the progress of the rehabilitation program. The athletic trainer must understand that the aggressive approach taken in rehabilitation does little to speed up the healing process. Progression will be limited by the constraints of the healing process.

Progress evaluations will be more limited in scope than the detailed off-the-field evaluation sequence described in this chapter. The off-the-field evaluation should be thorough and comprehensive. The athletic trainer should take time to systematically rule out information that is not pertinent to the present injury. Once the extraneous information has been eliminated, the subsequent progress evaluation can focus specifically on how the injury appears today compared with yesterday. Is a positive patient outcome evident from the previous day's treatment? Is the patient better or worse as a result of the treatment program rendered on the previous day?

To ensure that the progress evaluation will be complete, the athletic trainer still needs to go through certain aspects of history, observation, palpation, and special tests.

A gymnast is 4 months post-anterior cruciate ligament (ACL) reconstruction. She was last seen in the clinic 3 months ago prior to leaving for summer vacation. She has returned for the beginning of classes and visits the athletic trainer to see what kind of activities she should be doing in her rehabilitation program.

**?** To generate a progress note, what type of information does the athletic trainer need to know?

## History

The athletic trainer should ask the patient the following questions:

- How is the pain today compared with yesterday?
- Are you able to move better and with less pain?
- Do you think that the treatment done yesterday helped or made you more sore?

## Observation

The athletic trainer should make the following observations:

- Is the swelling today more or less than it was yesterday?
- Is the patient able to move better today?
- Is the patient still guarding and protecting the injury?
- How is the patient's affect? Is he or she upbeat and optimistic or depressed and negative?

## Palpation

The athletic trainer should palpate the injured area to determine the following:

- Does the swelling have a different consistency today, and has the swelling pattern changed?
- Is the injured structure still as tender to the touch?
- Is there any deformity present today that was not obvious yesterday?

## Special Tests

The athletic trainer should use special tests to make the following determinations:

- Does ligamentous stress testing cause as much pain? Has the athletic trainer's assessment of the grade of instability changed?
- How does a manual muscle test compare with yesterday?
- Has either active or passive range of motion changed?
- Does accessory movement appear to be limited?
- Can the athlete perform a specific functional test better today than yesterday?

## CLINICAL EVALUATION AND DIAGNOSIS

Making a diagnosis is the use of scientific or clinical methods to establish the cause and nature of a patient's illness or injury and the subsequent functional impairment caused by the pathology. The diagnosis forms the basis for patient care and ultimately for patient outcomes.[53] Physicians are responsible for making a *medical* diagnosis, which is regarded as the ultimate determination of a patient's physical condition. Athletic trainers and other health care professionals use their evaluation and assessment skills to make a *clinical* diagnosis.[54] The clinical diagnosis accurately identifies the pathology of injury, the limitations and the possible disabilities associated with a condition.[53] A certified athletic trainer has an academically based credential and in most states has some form of regulation that both recognizes the ability and empowers the athletic trainer to make an accurate clinical diagnosis. The term *diagnosis* is truly representative of what an athletic trainer actually does when evaluating an injury or illness.[53]

> Athletic trainers make a clinical diagnosis.

## DOCUMENTING INJURY EVALUATION INFORMATION

Complete and accurate documentation of findings from an evaluation is essential. As stressed in Chapter 3, accurate documentation can be a strong ally, should the athletic trainer become involved in litigation. For the athletic trainer working in a clinical setting, clear, concise, accurate record keeping is necessary for third-party reimbursement. Although the process may seem at times cumbersome and time-consuming, the athletic trainer must develop proficiency not only in evaluation skills but also in generating an accurate report of the findings from that evaluation, which is based on patient outcome measures.

In documenting medical information, it is common practice for the clinician to use abbreviations for words that routinely appear in medical notes or evaluations.[25] Table 13–15 provides many terms and their corresponding abbreviations that an athletic trainer might use in documenting injury information during an evaluation.

### Soap Notes

Documentation of acute injury can be effectively accomplished through a system designed to record subjective and objective findings and to document the immediate and future treatment plan for the patient.[35] The SOAP note format (subjective, objective, assessment, and plan) provides a standard format for recording

> SOAP note format:
> - Subjective
> - Objective
> - Assessment
> - Plan

| | |
|---|---|
| ↑ | increase |
| ↓ | decrease |
| < | less than |
| > | greater than |
| Δ | change |
| c̄ | with |
| p̄ | after |
| s̄ or w/o | without |
| 1° | primary |
| 2° | secondary |
| +tive | positive |
| A&O | alert & oriented |
| abnor. | abnormal |
| AC | acromioclavicular or acute |
| ADL | activities of daily living |
| ant. | anterior |
| ante | before |
| AOAP | as often as possible |
| AP | anterior-posterior; assessment and plans |
| AAROM | active assistive range of motion |
| AROM | active range of motion |
| ASAP | as soon as possible |
| ASIS | anterior superior iliac spine |
| AT | athletic training |
| B | bilateral |
| BID or bid | twice a day |
| C/O | complained of; complaints; under care of |
| CC | chief complaint; chronic complainer |
| ck. | check |
| CP | cold pack; chronic pain |
| CPR | cardiopulmonary resuscitation |
| CWI | crutch walking instruction |
| D/C | discharge |
| DF | dorsiflexion |
| DOB | date of birth |
| DTR | deep tendon reflex |
| DVT | deep vein thrombosis |
| Dx | diagnosis |
| E | edema |
| EENT | eyes, ears, nose, throat |
| ELOP | estimated length of program |
| EMS | emergency medical services |
| EMT | emergency medical technician |
| EOA | examine, opinion, and advice |
| ES | electrical stimulation |
| EV | eversion |
| exam. | examination |
| FH | family history |
| FROM | full range of movement |

| | |
|---|---|
| FWB | full weight bearing |
| Fx | fracture |
| G1–4 | grades 1 to 4 |
| GA | general appearance |
| H&P | history and physical |
| H/O | history of |
| HA | headache |
| HP | hot pack |
| HPI | history of present illness |
| ht | height; heart |
| HTN | hypertension |
| Hx | history |
| IN | inversion |
| IPPA | inspection, percussion, palpation, and auscultation |
| L | left |
| LAT | lateral |
| LBP | low back pain |
| LE | lower extremity |
| MAEEW | moves all extremities equally well |
| MEDS | medications |
| mm | muscle; millimeter |
| MMT | manual muscle testing |
| MOD | moderate |
| N | normal, never, no, not |
| NC | neurological check; no complaints; not completed |
| NEG | negative |
| NKA | no known allergies |
| NP | no pain |
| NPT | normal pressure and temperature |
| NSA | no significant abnormality |
| NSAID | nonsteroidal antiinflammatory drug |
| NT | not tried |
| NWB | non–weight bearing |
| o | negative, without |
| O | objective finding |
| OH | occupational history |
| ORIF | open reduction/internal fixation |
| OT | occupational therapy |
| P&A | percussion and auscultation |
| p.o. | postoperatively |
| PA | posterior-anterior (X-ray); physician's assistant |
| PE | physical examination |
| PF | plantar flexion |
| PH | past history; poor health |
| PMH | past medical history |
| PNF | proprioceptive neuromuscular facilitation |
| PNS | peripheral nervous system |

*Continued*

**TABLE 13–15** continued

| | | | |
|---|---|---|---|
| PPPBL | peripheral pulses palpable both legs | S | subjective findings |
| PT | point tender | SLR | straight leg raises |
| PRE | progressive resistance exercise | SOAP | subjective, objective, assessment, plan |
| pre-op | preoperatively | stat | immediately |
| prog. | prognosis | STG | short-term goals |
| PROM | passive range of motion | Sx | signs; symptom |
| PT | physical therapy | T | temperature |
| Pt./pt. | patient | TENS | transcutaneous electrical nerve stimulation |
| PWB | partial weight bearing | tid | three times a day |
| Px | physical exam; pneumothorax | TTWB | toe touch weight bearing |
| qd | once daily | UE | upper extremity |
| qid | four times a day | UK | unknown |
| R | right | US | ultrasound |
| R/O | rule out | WBAT | weight bearing as tolerated |
| rehab | rehabilitation | Whp | whirlpool |
| ROM | range of motion | WNL | within normal limits |
| RROM | resistive range of motion | x | times |
| RTP | return to play | y.o. | year old |
| Rx | prescription, including therapy and treatment | Y/O | years old |

injury information obtained from on-site, sideline, or clinical evaluations.[23] This method combines information provided by the patient and observations of the examiner.[34] Figure 13–12 presents a recommended SOAP note injury report form that includes the components of documentation. This form also includes a provision to document findings arising from more definitive evaluation or from the examiner's subsequent evaluation.

**S (Subjective)** History taking is designed to elicit the subjective impressions of the patient relative to time, mechanism, and site of injury. The type and course of the pain and the degree of disability experienced by the patient are also noteworthy. The subjective evaluation is the foundation for the rest of the evaluation process. Perhaps the single most revealing component of the injury evaluation is the information gathered during the subjective evaluation. Essentially, during the subjective evaluation the athletic trainer engages in an orderly, sequential process of questions and dialogue with the patient. In addition to gathering information about the injury, the subjective evaluation serves to establish a level of comfort and trust between the patient and the athletic trainer. The injury history and the symptoms are the key elements of the subjective evaluation. A detailed injury history is the most important portion of the evaluation. The remainder of the evaluation will focus on confirming the information taken from the patient's history.

**O (Objective)** Objective findings result from the athletic trainer's visual inspection, palpation, and assessment of active, passive, and resistive motion. Findings of special testing should also be noted here. Thus, the objective report would include assessment of posture, presence of deformity or swelling, and location of point tenderness. Also, limitations of active motion and pain arising or disappearing during passive and resistive motion should be noted. Finally, the results of special tests relative to joint stability or apprehension are also included.

**A (Assessment)** Assessment of the injury is the athletic trainer's professional judgment with regard to impression and nature of injury. Although the exact nature of the injury will not always be known initially, information pertaining to the suspected site and anatomical structures involved is appropriate. A judgment of severity may be included but is not essential at the time of acute injury evaluation.

**P (Plan)** The plan should include the first-aid treatment rendered to the patient and the athletic trainer's intentions relative to disposition. Disposition may include referral

A professional bull rider is thrown from the bull and, on landing, twists his knee. There is immediate swelling and pain. After evaluation, the athletic trainer is not sure what the injury is and sends the patient directly to the physician for a medical diagnosis. The physician decides that additional diagnostic tests are necessary to determine the exact pathology.

**?** What diagnostic tests is the physician likely to order to determine the exact nature and extent of the knee injury?

13–7 Clinical Application Exercise

**SUBJECTIVE**: The patient is a _____ -year-old athlete with the above diagnosis. The patient notes a _____onset on _____ . Past history for this condition is remarkable for_____unremarkable. Diagnostic testing of_____ . Medications include_____ . The patient's goals are to_____ . General medical history is remarkable for/unremarkable. The patient will follow with MD on_____ .

**OBJECTIVE**: Measurable, Reproducible, Observable findings—Be Objective
*(The following Objective Measurements may not all be relevant depending on the injury)*
OBSERVATION: (e.g., movement quality, gait, affect etc.):
PALPATION
• Bones:
• Soft tissue:
MOVEMENT ASSESSMENT
• Active range of motion/Resistive range of motion
 – Manual muscle testing:
• Passive range of motion
 – Goniometric or digital inclinometer measurements of joint range:
 – Accessory motions:
NEUROLOGIC EXAM
• Cerebral function:
• Cerebellar function:
• Cranial nerve function:
• Sensory testing (compare sides):
• Reflex testing:
• Determining projected/referred pain:
• Motor testing (compare sides):
JOINT STABILITY TESTS:
POSTURAL EXAMINATION:
ANTHROPOMETRIC MEASUREMENTS:
VOLUMETRIC MEASUREMENTS:
FUNCTIONAL PERFORMANCE TEST AND SCORES:
FUNCTIONAL SCREENING TEST SCORES:

**ASSESSMENT**: Your professional opinion of the patient's problem
The patient presents with the following problems (1)_____ , (2)_____ ,
(3) _____ , (4)_____ .

**PLAN**: Describe how you will manage the patient's care regarding frequency of treatment, what the treatment will include (i.e., modalities, therapeutic exercise, home program, and follow up with you).
Plan for referral (if necessary) _____

Short-term goals include (1)_____ , (2)_____ , (3)_____ ,
(4) _____ .

Long-term goals include _____ .

Comments: _____

Signature _____ ATC

FIGURE 13–12    SOAP note form.

for more definitive evaluation or simply application of splint, wrap, or crutches and a request to report for reevaluation the next day. If the injury is chronic, the examiner's plan for treatment and therapeutic exercise would be appropriate. The treatment plan should establish specific short-term goals for the rehabilitation program and should provide criteria-based guidelines for accomplishing these goals (e.g., progress from touch-down gait on two crutches to weight bearing on one crutch). A specific long-term goal should also be clearly identified in the plan (e.g., normal gait without a limp).

## Progress Notes

Progress notes should be routinely documented after each progress evaluation done throughout the course of the rehabilitation program. Progress notes can follow the SOAP format, as indicated in the previous sections. They can be generated in the form of an expanded treatment note or done as a weekly summary. Information in the progress note should concentrate on the types of treatment received and the patient's response to that treatment, progress made toward the short-term goals established in the SOAP note, changes in the previous treatment plan and goals, and the course of treatment planned over the next several days.[2]

# ADDITIONAL DIAGNOSTIC TESTS USED BY A PHYSICIAN

The physician, like the athletic trainer, often performs a detailed musculoskeletal examination on the injured patient. Often, the physician and the athletic trainer will discuss and compare their individual findings. Because the physician is charged with determining a medical diagnosis and deciding on a course of treatment, he or she may have to acquire and compare additional information. This information can come from imaging techniques, including plain film radiographs (X-rays), arthrography, arthroscopy, myelography, computed tomography, positron emission tomography, bone scanning, DEXA scans, magnetic resonance imaging, ultrasonography, and echocardiography.[42,55] Other tests include electrocardiography, electroencephalography, electromyography, nerve conduction velocity, synovial fluid analysis, blood testing, and urinalysis.[19,22,40]

## Imaging Techniques

**Plain Film Radiography (X-rays)** An X-ray examination helps the physician identify fractures and dislocations or any bone abnormality that may be present. It may also be used to rule out serious disease, such as an infection or a neoplasm. A trained radiologist can detect some soft-tissue factors, such as joint swelling and ectopic bone development in ligaments and tendons (Figure 13–13A).[42]

**Arthroscopy** The fiber-optic arthroscope is widely used by orthopedists in surgery. It is considered more accurate than the arthrogram but is more invasive, requiring anesthesia and a small incision for the introduction of the arthroscope (endoscope) into the joint space. While the arthroscope is in the joint, the surgeon can perform surgical procedures, such as removing loose bodies and, in some cases, suturing torn tissues (Figure 13–13B).[42]

> Arthroscopy uses a fiber-optic arthroscope to view the inside of a joint.

**Myelography** During myelography, an opaque dye is introduced into the spinal canal (epidural space) through a lumbar puncture. While the patient is tilted, the dye is allowed to flow to different levels of the spinal cord. Using this contrast medium, physicians can detect conditions such as tumors, nerve root compression, and disk disease, as well as other diseases within the spinal cord (Figure 13–13C).

**Computed Tomography** Computed tomography (CT) penetrates the body with a thin, fan-shaped X-ray beam, producing a cross-sectional view of tissues. Unlike X-ray images, CT images allow the injured structure to be viewed from many angles. As the machine scans, a computer compares the many views; these electrical signals are then processed by a computer into a visual image (Figure 13–13D).

**Positron Emission Tomography (PET)** Positron emission tomography is a nuclear medicine imaging technique that uses an injection of a radioactive tracer chemical to produce a three-dimensional (3-D) image. A PET scan, unlike the other diagnostic imaging techniques that only confirm the presence of a mass, can help distinguish between living and dead tissue or between benign and malignant tissue. It can detect abnormal cellular activity in the very early stages, which is extremely valuable for oncology patients. A PET scan is often used in conjunction with an MRI and/or a CT to produce both anatomical and metabolic information (Figure 13–13E).

**Bone Scan** A bone scan involves the intravenous introduction of a radioactive tracer, such as technetium-99. By imaging the entire skeleton or part of a skeleton, bony lesions in which there is some inflammation, such as stress fractures, can be detected (Figure 13–13F).

**DEXA Scan** Dual-energy X-ray absorptiometry, or DEXA scanning, is currently the most widely used method to measure bone mineral density. For the test, a patient lies down on an examining table, and the scanner directs an X-ray toward the bone being examined. The greater the bone mineral density, the greater the signal picked up. DEXA scanning more precisely documents small changes in bone mass and is more flexible than a bone scan, because it can be used to examine both the spine and the extremities. DEXA scanning is less expensive, exposes the patient to less radiation, and is more sensitive and accurate at measuring subtle changes in bone density over time (Figure 13–13G).

**Magnetic Resonance Imaging** Magnetic resonance imaging (MRI) surrounds the body with powerful electromagnets, creating a field as much as 600,000 times as strong as that of the earth.[3] The magnetic current focuses on hydrogen atoms in water molecules and aligns them; when the current is shut off, the atoms continue to spin, emitting an energy that is detected by the computer. The hydrogen atoms in different tissues spin at different rates,

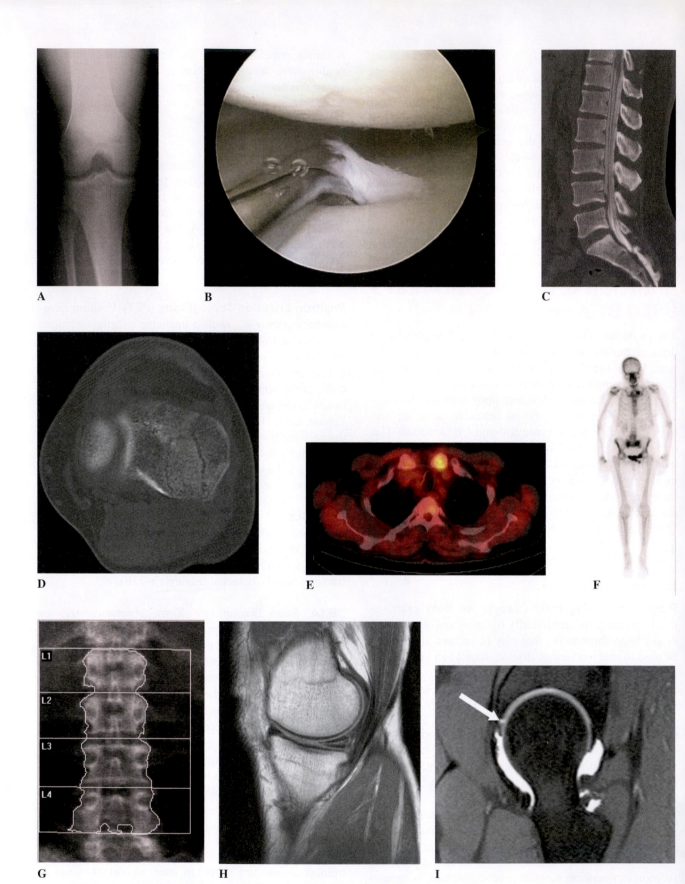

FIGURE 13–13  **(A)** X-ray of knee. **(B)** Arthroscope of knee. **(C)** Myelogram of spine. **(D)** Computed tomography (CT) of knee. **(E)** Positron emission tomography (PET) of chest. **(F)** Bone scan. **(G)** DEXA scan of spine. **(H)** MRI of knee. **(I)** MR arthrography of shoulder.

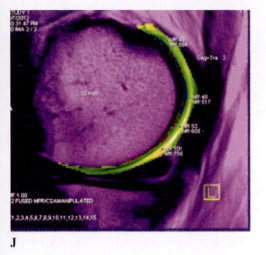

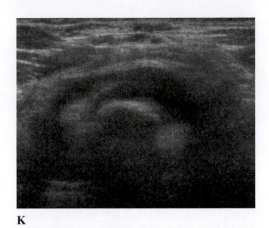

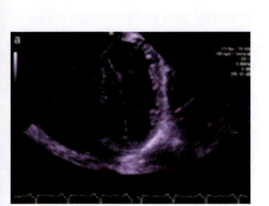

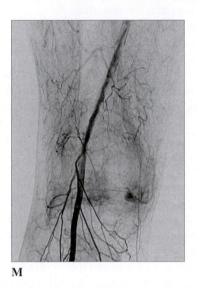

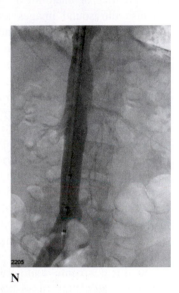

**J**

**K**

**L**

**M**

**N**

FIGURE 13–13    continued

**(J)** T1-Rho imaging of normal articular cartilage. **(K)** Musculoskeletal ultrasound of hip. **(L)** Echocardiogram of heart chambers. **(M)** Arteriogram of knee. **(N)** Venogram of femoral vein.

thus producing different images. In many ways, MRI provides clearer images than does CT scanning. Despite the expense of MRI, it is currently physicians' test of choice for detecting soft-tissue lesions (Figure 13–13H).

**MR Arthrography** MR arthrography is an imaging study involving injection of a contrast agent into a joint prior to MRI to obtain more detail of the interior of the joint than standard MRI. The contrast agent is used to highlight certain areas of the body during imaging exams (Figure 13–13I).

***T1-Rho*** T1-rho is another MRI-based imaging technique that is used to detect subtle early degeneration in articular cartilage resulting from osteoarthritis. This technique helps monitor the course of progression of osteoarthritis and allows clinicians to evaluate the success of patient treatments for those who exhibit early stages of osteoarthritis (Figure 13–13J).[61]

**Ultrasonography** Ultrasound imaging, also called *diagnostic ultrasound* or *sonography*, involves exposing part of the body to high-frequency sound waves to produce pictures of anatomical structures inside the body. Because ultrasound images are captured in real time, they can show the structure and movement of the body's musculoskeletal structures, internal organs, and blood flowing through blood vessels. Conventional ultrasound displays the images in thin, flat two-dimensional sections of the body. Advancements in ultrasound technology include 3-D ultrasound that formats the sound wave data into 3-D images.

***Musculoskeletal Ultrasound*** Musculoskeletal ultrasound, or diagnostic ultrasound, is used for imaging and evaluating soft-tissue musculoskeletal disorders. It offers an excellent complementary imaging technique to traditional magnetic resonance imaging (MRI) or computed tomography (CT) studies.[24] Imaging is accomplished by placing a transducer over the area to be visualized. Ultrasound is nonpainful and noninvasive, and it allows the patient to watch while his or her anatomical structures are being imaged on a video monitor. Compared with other cross-sectional modalities, diagnostic ultrasound is the most cost-effective imaging procedure available, other than plain X-ray (Figure 13–13K). Using a combination of physical and ultrasound data collected during the acute phase of sport-related muscle injury has been shown to be effective in helping to predict time until sport resumption.[24]

**Doppler Ultrasonography** This test uses ultrasound to examine the blood flow in the major arteries and veins in the arms and legs. It is done as an alternative to arteriography and venography and may help diagnose a blood clot, venous insufficiency, arterial occlusion (closing), or abnormalities in the blood flow caused by a narrowing of the vessels.

**Echocardiography** Echocardiography uses ultrasound to produce a graphic record of internal cardiac structures. An echocardiogram is most often used to visualize the cardiac valves and to determine the dimensions of the left atrium and both ventricles (Figure 13–13L).

**Arteriogram** Arteriography is a procedure in which a catheter is inserted into a specific blood vessel, contrast material is injected, and radiographs are taken, allowing the physician to see the vessel. An arteriogram can be used to examine almost any artery. In general, arteriograms give the best pictures of the body's blood vessels. Arteriograms are used to make specific diagnoses and to help determine the best treatment. Often, the treatment itself can be performed using the same type of catheters used in the arteriogram, instead of requiring a more extensive surgery in an additional procedure (e.g., angioplasty) (Figure 13–13M).

**Venogram** A venogram is a radiographic procedure used to image veins filled after injecting a contrast medium. This imaging technique is most often used to detect thrombophlebitis. It provides a visual tracing of a venous pulse (Figure 13–13N).

## Other Diagnostic Tests

**Electrocardiography** An electrocardiogram (ECG) records the electrical activity of the heart at various phases in the contraction cycle to determine whether impulse formation, conduction, and depolarization and repolarization of the atria and ventricles follows a normal pattern. It is of value in diagnosing causes of abnormal cardiac rhythm and myocardial damage. Several apps are available for smartphones that allow the phone to serve as an ECG and instantly provide the user with an ECG tracing of electrical activity in the heart. Figure 13–14 shows a visual representation of an ECG for a normal heart.

**Electroencephalography** The electroencephalogram (EEG) records electrical potentials produced in the brain on an instrument called an electroencephalograph. It is used to detect changes or abnormalities in brain wave patterns.

**Electromyography** Electromyography (EMG) involves the graphic recording of a muscle contraction and the

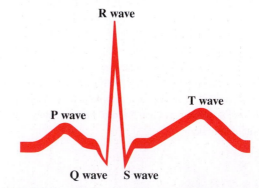

FIGURE 13–14 Electrocardiogram (ECG) tracing. This wave shows a graphic representation of the electrical activity in the heart at different points in the contraction cycle. P = atrial contraction, QRS = ventrical depolarization, T = ventrical repolarization.

amount of electrical activity generated in a muscle using either surface or needle electrodes. Motor unit potentials can be observed on an oscilloscope screen or from a graphic recording called an electromyogram. Various muscular conditions can be evaluated.

**Nerve Conduction Velocity** Determining the conduction velocity of a nerve may provide key information to the physician about a number of neuromuscular conditions. After a stimulus is applied to a peripheral nerve, the speed with which a muscle action occurs is measured. Delays in conduction might indicate nerve compression or other muscular or nerve disease.

**Pulse Oximetry** A pulse oximeter is a device used for assessing breathing by indirectly measuring the oxygen saturation of arterial blood. A pulse oximeter works by placing the device directly over a spot where there is a strong pulse, such as the tip of a finger (Figure 13–15). It emits two beams of light of different wavelengths, one red and one infrared, that pass through the finger to a photodetector.[60] The oximeter then calculates the ratio of red-to-infrared light that has passed through the finger.

Pulse oximeters are commonly used in hospitals to monitor oxygen saturation and pulse rate in patients who have some type of respiratory difficulty (i.c, asthma, emphysema). In athletes, a pulse oximeter can help them be aware of their breathing rates and technique, which together can help maintain oxygen saturation levels above 95 percent during high-intensity training periods.[51]

**Synovial Fluid Analysis** The primary purpose of synovial fluid analysis is to detect the presence of an infection in the joint. The test also confirms the diagnosis of gout and differentiates noninflammatory joint disease, such as degenerative

> Analysis of synovial fluid and blood can be used to detect musculoskeletal infections.

arthritis, from inflammatory conditions, such as rheumatoid arthritis.

**Blood Testing** The physician may decide to run a complete blood count (CBC) on a patient for many different reasons. The most common reasons are to screen for anemia (too few red cells) or infection (too many white cells).[59] Samples may be taken in a syringe from a vein in the arm or from a needle stick in the finger. A routine CBC addresses the following:

- The red blood cell count looks at the number of cells per unit volume to detect anemias, prolonged infections, iron deficiencies, internal bleeding, and certain types of cancers.
- Hemoglobin levels are closely associated with red blood cell count and tend to reflect overall blood volume.
- The hematocrit measures how much of the total blood volume is made up of red blood cells. A low hematocrit indicates certain types of anemias.
- The white blood cell count is used to determine the presence of bacteria. Differentiation of white cell types microscopically can identify specific types of infection.
- A deficiency in the platelet count can lead to dangerous internal bleeding.
- Blood testing can also measure levels of serum cholesterol. The recommended desirable range is <200 mg/dL.

Normal laboratory values for the CBC are summarized in Table 13–16. Normal laboratory values for blood electrolyte levels are summarized in Table 13–17.

**Glucometer** A glucometer is a small handheld device that is used to determine the approximate concentration of glucose in the blood (Figure 13–16). It is most commonly used by patients who have hypoglycemia or diabetes, to provide immediate feedback on levels of blood glucose. The skin must be pricked with a small lancet on the meter that draws a drop of blood, which is analyzed by the glucometer. In just a few seconds, the glucometer digitally displays the glucose level in mg/dl. A normal blood glucose level is less than 100 mg/dl when fasting and less than 140 mg/dl 2 hours after eating. Patients usually must repeat this test several times per day.

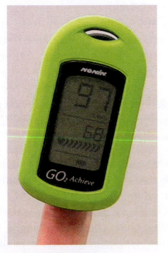

FIGURE 13–15  Pulse oximeter.
© William E. Prentice

| TABLE 13–16 | Normal Laboratory Values of a Complete Blood Count* |
|---|---|
| **Test** | **Normal Values** |
| Red blood cell count | Males: 4.7–6.1 million cells/mcL |
| | Females: 4.2–5.4 million cells/mcL |
| White blood cell count | 4,500–10,000 cells/mcL |
| Platelet count | 150–450 billion/L |
| Hematocrit | Males: 40.7%–50.3% |
| | Females: 36.1%–44.3% |
| Hemoglobin | Males: 13.8–17.2 grams/dL |
| | Females: 12.1–15.1 grams/dL |
| Cholesterol | <200 mg/dl |
| HDL | <40 mg/dl |
| LDL | <100 mg/dl |
| Triglycerides | <150 mg/dl |
| Glucose | 70–100 mg/dl |

*From https://www.nlm.nih.gov/medlineplus/ency/article/003642.htm

| TABLE 13–17 | Blood Electrolyte Levels (normal adult range) |
|---|---|
| Sodium | 135–145 mEq/L |
| Potassium | 3.7–5.2 mEq/L |
| Chloride | 96–106 mEq/L |
| Calcium | 8.5–10.2 mg/dl |
| Phosphorus | 2.4–4.1 mEq/dl |
| Carbon dioxide ($CO_2$) | 23–29 mEq/L |
| Bicarbonate | 24–30 mEq/dl |

From https://www.nlm.nih.gov/medlineplus/ency/article/003468.htm

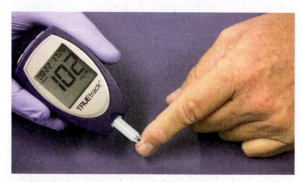

FIGURE 13–16   A glucometer is a device that measures blood glucose levels.
© William E. Prentice

**Urinalysis** Urinalysis is a common test that can yield a large quantity of information. In most cases, a sample of urine in a small, dry container is all that is needed. If the urine will not be analyzed within 1 hour, the sample

| TABLE 13–18 | Normal Laboratory Values of a Urinalysis |
|---|---|
| **Test** | **Normal Values** |
| Output | 1,000–1,500 ml |
| Color | Yellow to amber and clear |
| Specific gravity | 1.015–1.025 |
| Osmolality | 500–800 mosm/kg water |
| pH | 4.6–4.8 |
| Uric acid | 250–750 mg/day |
| Urea | 23–25 g/24 hr |
| Creatine | 1–2 g/24 hr |

should be refrigerated. A routine urinalysis addresses the following:[59]

- Specific gravity indicates the ability of the kidney to concentrate and dilute fluids.
- The pH refers to how acid or alkaline the urine is. It may be acidic in cases of diabetes or dehydration. Alkaline urine is present in urinary tract infections and kidney disease. The presence of glucose may indicate diabetes.
- The presence of ketones, a by-product of fat metabolism, may also indicate diabetes.
- Hemoglobin may appear in urine after intense exercise or from kidney disease.
- The presence of protein indicates kidney disease.
- The presence of nitrate indicates infection.
- A small amount of urine is examined under a microscope to find red blood cells, white blood cells, and bacteria.
- If bacteria are present, a urine culture may be necessary to determine the specific bacteria causing an infection.
- Many additional tests may also be done on urine, including electrolytes, hormones, and drug levels.

Normal laboratory values for a standard urinalysis are listed in Table 13–18.

Urinalysis using dip-and-read test strips (such as Chemstrips) can provide fast, accurate results for a wide range of test parameters, such as specific gravity, leukocytes, nitrate, pH, protein, glucose, ketones, urobilinogen, bilirubin, and blood. Large test areas on each strip are impregnated with reagents that provide clear, easy-to-read color changes when dipped in urine. Color comparison charts are often located on the box.

***Refractometer*** An accurate method of measuring hydration status uses a refractometer (Figure 13–17). A refractometer offers a precise reading of specific gravity of urine (USG). This measurement is less subjective than comparing urine color and is also simple to use. When measuring urine for specific gravity, urine that is collected midstream for analysis by the refractometer is best for consistency and accuracy. USG measurements should be

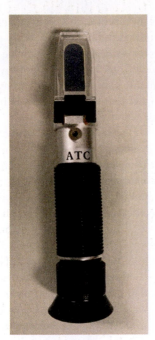

FIGURE 13–17 A refractometer measures the specific gravity of urine.
© William E. Prentice

taken before exercise. A urine-specific gravity of <1.010 indicates an individual is well hydrated (euhydrated), whereas a USG of 1.010 to 1.020 indicates that the individual is dehydrated (hyohydrated), and a USG >1.020 indicates significant dehydration.[1]

**Peak Flow Meter** A peak flow meter is a small handheld device that quickly assesses a patient's peak expiratory flow rate or the ability to quickly expire or breathe air out of the lungs (Figure 13–18). These meters are most often used in patients who have some type of disease or condition that obstructs airflow through the bronchii. Asthma patients are typically evaluated using a peak flow meter. Peak expiratory flow is measured in l/min. There is a high degree of variability in peak flow measurement, thus readings should be taken using the same peak flow meter, by the same clinician.

# ERGONOMIC RISK ASSESSMENT (ERA)

In addition to performing injury evaluations, an athletic trainer working in a clinic, corporate, or industrial setting may be required to perform an *ergonomic risk assessment (ERA)*. An ergonomic risk assessment is the evaluation of factors within a job that increase the risk of someone suffering a workplace-related ergonomic injury and what aspects of, or movements within, that job should be focused on to reduce this risk. These factors include awkward postures, repetitive movements without variation, forceful movements, and vibration. The ERA aims at finding a solution through ergonomic control measures to make it safer for everyone performing that task. By combining information from the ERA with injury statistics, the physical demands of the job can be evaluated to prioritize ergonomic interventions.

Incorporating ergonomics into the introduction or design stage of a specific job task will prove a more efficient use of time and resources than dealing with the results of costly injuries and decreases in production at some point in the future. Likewise, when a process is being modified significantly, it is important to consider how the changes could impact the physical requirements to perform the work. Investigating complaints or concerns raised by the workers performing the work is a proactive step toward reducing the costly aspects of work-related injuries, lost time injuries, absenteeism, and workers compensation premiums. Workers who are tired or sore cannot produce at the same level of quality and productivity as healthy workers. Workers will know which jobs contain ergonomic risks. The discomfort or pain that workers experience is enough of an indicator that there is likely a better, safer, more efficient way of doing their work.

When an employee suffers a work-related injury, his or her body is reacting to an ergonomic stress. If the ergonomic risk is not identified and controlled, the possibility remains for another worker performing similar movements, or the same worker upon returning to an unmodified job, to develop a similar problem.

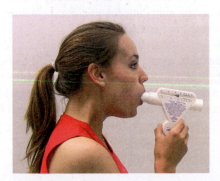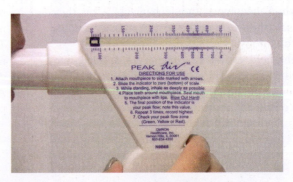

FIGURE 13–18 A peak flow meter assesses the ability to quickly and forcefully expire or breathe air out of the lungs.
© William E. Prentice

The first step in an ergonomic risk assessment is to identify the jobs most in need of attention. Prioritizing those jobs with the greatest potential for injury will assist in ensuring that the ergonomic interventions will have the greatest impact possible. Performing an ERA is an effective means of reducing the frequency and severity of workplace-related injuries. The workers need to be briefed on why the assessment is being completed and how they are involved in the solution process. This is done by reviewing injury statistics, worker concerns and complaints, and a physical demands analysis. An ergonomic risk assessment should include the following groups of employees:

- The *worker(s)* performing the job, so they understand what the ERA process is going to accomplish
- The worker's direct *supervisor*, who must understand why a job (or part of the job) needs to be modified and what the new expectations of work will be
- *Management*, so that they are aware of the costs associated with work-related musculoskeletal injuries and the benefits that the ERA can provide to the company
- Company support professionals, such as a nurse, an engineer, or safety personnel, because they will bring more resources to the group performing the ERA

Video can be an effective assessment tool; therefore, the athletic trainer should consider its use in the ERA. Video allows more people access to the assessment process than would be possible with everyone huddled around, watching the worker performing the job. Video can also be used for training purposes in addition to determining best work practices.

An ERA will result in a list of the ergonomic risk factors that exist in a specific job. The athletic trainer should identify risk factors to be controlled to minimize or eliminate the chance of a worker suffering from a workplace-related injury. These control measures should be decided in consultation with the workers affected, their supervisors, and management. The control measures can include making physical changes to the job (for example, providing a sit/stand option or tilting work surfaces) or making administrative changes (such as job rotation or a two-person lift policy). When either of these options is not reasonably practicable, personal protective equipment (such as antivibration gloves) may be beneficial. Proposed changes should also be subject to an ergonomic risk assessment to ensure that the original ergonomic risks are reduced and others are not being introduced.

## SUMMARY

- Once the patient has been transported from the site of initial injury, a detailed off-the-field injury evaluation may be performed on the sideline, in the athletic training clinic, in an emergency room, or in a sports medicine clinic.
- Athletic trainers evaluate injuries and decide on a clinical diagnosis, whereas physicians are responsible for providing a medical diagnosis.
- To accurately evaluate an injury, the athletic trainer must possess a thorough background in human anatomy, including surface anatomy, body planes, and anatomical directions. The athletic trainer also needs an in-depth understanding of the musculoskeletal system, with special focus on adverse biomechanical forces, which become pathomechanical. After they are assessed, injuries must be described using appropriate terminology.
- The off-the-field evaluation scheme is divided into four broad categories: history, observation, palpation, and special tests that provide additional information about the extent of injuries.

- Functional screening tests are used to identify characteristic movement impairments and suggest interventions for these impairments to reduce an athlete's individuals risk for injury.
- To be an effective clinician, the athletic trainer must consistently incorporate the best available evidence in the professional literature into the clinical decision making process.
- The progress evaluation focuses specifically on how the injury appears today compared with yesterday, and it is more limited in scope than the detailed off-the-field evaluation sequence.
- The SOAP note (subjective, objective, assessment, and plan) provides a standard format for documenting and recording injury information. Progress notes may also be recorded in the SOAP format.
- To make an accurate medical diagnosis, the physician may need to use a particular imaging technique or one of several additional specific diagnostic tests.
- An ergonomic risk assessment (ERA) can identify tasks performed in the workplace that can result in injury.

## WEB SITES

Cramer First Aider:
  www.cramersportsmed.com/first-aider.html

National Athletic Trainers' Association:
  www.nata.org

# SOLUTIONS TO CLINICAL APPLICATION EXERCISES

13–1 The athletic trainer must realize that the physician should have been consulted earlier in this case. Despite the fact that the athletic trainer correctly identified the MCL sprain, the meniscus tear was completely overlooked. Although the athletic trainer's actions were not inappropriate, it would have been better to refer the injured patient to the physician for medical diagnosis. In most cases, the athletic trainer's clinical diagnosis should reveal the same results as the physician's medical diagnosis.

13–2 The athletic trainer should first take a subjective history from the injured patient and follow that with an objective examination that includes observation, palpation, movement assessment (active, passive, resistive), neurological examination, testing joint stability, postural examination, anthropometric measurements, volumetric measurements, vascular screening, and testing functional performance.

13–3 In this case, a ligamentous injury is more likely. A lesion of inert tissue will elicit pain on active and passive movement in the same direction. If a lesion is present in contractile tissue, pain will occur on active motion in one direction and on passive motion in the opposite direction. A sprain of a ligament will result in pain whenever that ligament is stretched either through active contraction or passive stretching.

13–4 A grade 3 manual muscle test suggests there is a gross lesion of contractile tissue in the shoulder, such as the rotator cuff. A weak and painful contraction indicates there may be a complete rupture of the tissue or a potential nervous system disorder.

13–5 Generally, injury to the spinal cord would result in bilateral symptoms. Unilateral changes are more indicative of peripheral nerve injury. However, any change in the neurological status of the athlete is cause for great concern. The athletic trainer should remove the patient from the playing field using a stretcher or, preferably, a spine board.

13–6 To ensure that the progress evaluation will be complete, the athletic trainer needs to go through history, observation, palpation, and special testing. The patient should be asked pertinent questions, such as "What types of exercises have you done for the past 3 months?" and "What type of pain, if any, are you still experiencing?" Observation of the symmetry to the other knee and palpation of the injured structures should be done. Range of motion, muscle strength, joint stability, and neuromuscular control should also be assessed.

13–7 Initially, it is likely that standard knee X-rays would be used to determine the presence of a fracture. An MRI is widely used by sports medicine physicians to determine injury to ligamentous, meniscal, and other soft tissues. On occasion, a diagnostic arthroscopy might be done to directly observe the injured structures.

13–8 Both the hematocrit and the hemoglobin levels are low and it is likely that the office worker does have anemia. However, depending on other signs and symptoms, the physician may need to order additional diagnostic tests to determine what may be causing this problem.

# REVIEW QUESTIONS AND CLASS ACTIVITIES

1. Differentiate between a clinical diagnosis made by an athletic trainer and a medical diagnosis made by a physician.
2. What basic knowledge must the athletic trainer have before performing an injury assessment?
3. Explain the key terminology needed to communicate the results of an assessment.
4. Identify the various descriptive assessment terms.
5. How should an athletic trainer take a history? What questions should be asked?
6. Describe palpation and when and how it should be performed.
7. What can be ascertained from active, passive, and resisted isometric movement?
8. Explain how muscle testing, reflex testing, and sensory testing are performed.
9. What part do special tests play in injury assessment?
10. When should a functional evaluation be given?
11. What information should be included in a SOAP note?
12. What insights can a physician gain by having special laboratory tests performed? Describe each test in detail.
13. How can an ergonomic risk assessment be used to minimize the chances of workplace-related injuries?

# REFERENCES

1. Armstrong L: Hydration assessment techniques, *Nutrition Review* 63(6):S40–S54, 2005.
2. Arrigo C: Clinical documentation. In Konin J, ed: *Clinical athletic training,* Thorofare, NJ, 2011, Slack.
3. Barak T: Mobility: Passive orthopedic manual therapy. In Gould J, Davies G, eds: *Orthopedic and sports physical therapy,* St. Louis, MO, 1997, Mosby.
4. Beattie P: Clinical prediction rules: What are they and what do they tell us? *Aust J Physiother* 52(3):157–63, 2006.
5. Berry D: Athletic and Orthopedic Injury Assessment: A Case Study Approach, 2010, Holcomb Hathaway.
6. Bickley L: *Bates' guide to physical examination and history taking,* Philadelphia, PA, 2008, Lippincott, Williams and Wilkins.
7. Bohannon R: Manual muscle testing: Does it meet the standards of an adequate screening test? *Clinical Rehabilitation* 19(6):662, 2005.
8. Booher J: *Athletic injury assessment,* San Francisco, CA, 2001, McGraw-Hill.
9. Chaudhari A: ACL Research Retreat VI: An Update on ACL Risk and Prevention, *Journal of Athletic Training* 47(5):591–603, 2012.
10. Clark M: Movement assessments. In Clark M, Luckett S, eds: *NASM essentials of corrective exercise training,* Baltimore, MD, 2011, Lippincott, Williams and Wilkins.
11. Clarkson H: *Musculoskeletal assessment: Joint range of motion and manual muscle strength,* Philadelphia, PA, 2012, Lippincott, Williams and Wilkins.
12. Cook G: Pre-participation screening: the use of fundamental movements as an assessment of function—part 1. *N Am J Sports Phys Ther* 1:62–72, 2006.
13. Cook C: Potential pitfalls of clinical prediction rules, *J Man Manip Ther* 16(2):69–71, 2008.
14. Cutter N, Kevorkian G: *Handbook of manual muscle testing,* New York, 1999, McGraw-Hill.
15. Cyriax J: *Cyriax's illustrated manual of orthopaedic medicine,* London, 1996, Butterworth-Heinemann.
16. Delforge G: Sports injury assessment and problem identification. In Delforge G, ed: *Musculoskeletal trauma: Implications for sports injury management,* Champaign, IL, 2002, Human Kinetics.
17. DeMont R: The place for palpation, *Athletic Therapy Today* 8(2):42, 2003.
18. Denegar C: Application of statistics in establishing diagnostic certainty, *Journal of Athletic Training* 47(2):233–36, 2012.
19. Deyle G: Musculoskeletal imaging in physical therapist practice, *J Orthop Sports Phys Ther* 35(11):708, 2005.
20. Evans R: *Illustrated orthopedic physical assessment,* St. Louis, MO, 2008, Mosby.
21. Gabbe B: How valid is a self-reported 12 month sports injury history? *British Journal of Sports Medicine* 37(6):545, 2003.
22. Garber M: Diagnostic imaging and differential diagnosis in two case reports, *J Orthop Sports Phys Ther* 35(11):745, 2005.
23. Gottlieb J: *SOAP for orthopedics,* Philadelphia, 2013, Lippincott, Williams and Wilkins.
24. Guillodo Y: Value of sonography combined with clinical assessment to evaluate muscle injury severity in athletes, *J Athl Train* 46(5):500–04, 2011.

25. Gylys B: *Medical terminology simplified: A programmed learning approach by body systems,* ed 3, Philadelphia, PA, 2014, F.A. Davis.

26. Hewitt T: Current concepts for injury prevention in athletes after anterior cruciate ligament reconstruction, *American Journal of Sports Medicine* 41(1):216–24, 2013.

27. Hoogenboom B: Functional movement assessment. In Hoogenboom B, Voight M, Prentice W, eds: *Musculoskeletal interventions: Techniques for therapeutic exercise,* ed 3, New York, 2014, McGraw-Hill.

28. Hilsop H: *Daniels and Worthingham muscle testing,* San Diego, CA, 2013, Elsevier Science.

29. Hoppenfeld S: *Physical examination of the spine and extremities,* New York, 2013, Pearson.

30. Hubbard T: How accurate is that clinical assessment test? *Athletic Therapy Today* 9(6):63, 2004.

31. Hurley W: Agreement of clinical judgments of end-feel between two sample populations, *J Sport Rehabil* 11(3):209, 2002.

32. Kaltenborn F: *Manual mobilization of the joints: The extremities,* Minneapolis, MN, 2014, Orthopedic Physical Therapy Products.

33. Kendall F: *Muscles testing and function,* Philadelphia, PA, 2005, Lippincott, Williams and Wilkins.

34. Kettenbach G: *Writing SOAP notes with patient/client management formats,* Philadelphia, PA, 2004, F.A. Davis.

35. Konin J: *Documentation for athletic training,* Thorofare, NJ, 2011, Slack.

36. Lumley J: *Surface anatomy—the anatomical basis of clinical evaluation,* Philadelphia, PA, 2008, Churchill-Livingstone.

37. Mattacola C: Introduction to clinical evaluation and testing, *Athletic Therapy Today* 8(2):24, 2003.

38. Magee D: *Orthopedic physical assessment,* Philadelphia, PA, 2013, Elsevier Health Sciences.

39. McGee S: Understanding the evidence In McGee S, ed: *Evidence-based physical diagnosis,* Philadelphia, PA, 2012, Elsevier Saunders.

40. McKinnis L: *Fundamentals of musculoskeletal imaging,* Philadelphia, PA, 2014, F.A. Davis.

41. McRae R: *Clinical orthopaedic examination,* Philadelphia, PA, 2010, Elsevier Health Sciences.

42. Milbauer D: Principles of radiographic evaluation and imaging techniques. In Nicholas J, Hershman E, eds: *The lower extremity and spine in sports medicine,* St. Louis, MO, 1995, Mosby.

43. Moore M: The use of a tuning fork and stethoscope to identify fractures, *Journal of Athletic Training* 44(3):272–74, 2009.

44. Myer G: Tuck jump assessment for reducing ACL injury risk, *Athletic Therapy Today* 13(5):39–44, 2008.

45. Norkin C: *Measurement of joint motion: A guide to goniometry,* Philadelphia, PA, 2009, F.A. Davis.

46. Padua D, et al.: The landing error scoring system (LESS) prospectively identifies ACL injury, *J Athl Train* 45(5):539, 2010.

47. Petersen C: Construct validity of Cyriax's selective tension examination: Association of end-feels with pain at the knee and shoulder, *J Orthop Sports Phys Ther* 30(9):512, 2002.

48. Peterson E, et al.: Reliability of water volumetry and the figure eight method on subjects with ankle joint swelling, *J Orthop Sports Phys Ther* 29(10):609, 1999.

49. Pewsner D: Ruling a diagnosis in or out with "SpPIn" and "SnNOut": A note of caution, *British Medical Journal* 329:209–13, 2004.

50. Sackett D: *Clinical epidemiology: A basic science for clinical medicine,* ed 2, New York, 1991, Little Brown.

51. Sinex J: Pulse oximetry: Principles and limitations, *The American Journal of Emergency Medicine,* 17(1):59–66, 1999.

52. Stanton T: Critical appraisal of clinical prediction rules that aim to optimize treatment selection for musculoskeletal conditions, *Phys Ther* 90(6):843–54, 2010.

53. Starkey C: Diagnosis appropriate? Physicians agree, *NATA News* 5:48, 2006.

54. Starkey C: *Evaluation of orthopedic and athletic injuries,* Philadelphia, PA, 2015, F.A. Davis.

55. Suetens P: *Fundamentals of medical imaging,* Cambridge, 2009, Cambridge University Press.

56. Sugimoto D: Compliance with neuromuscular training and anterior cruciate ligament injury risk reduction in female athletes: A meta-analysis. *Journal of Athletic Training* 47(6):714–23, 2012.

57. Taxa S: *Atlas of palpatory anatomy of limbs and trunk,* Teteroboro, NJ, 2007, Icon Learning Systems.

58. VanLunen B: *Evidence guided practice: A framework for clinical decision making in athletic training,* Thorofare, NJ, 2015, Slack.

59. Wurman R: *Medical access,* Los Angeles, 1985, Access Press.

60. Yamaya Y: Validity of pulse oximetry during maximal exercise in normoxia, hypoxia and hyperoxia, *Journal of Applied Physiology,* 92(1):162–68, 2002.

61. X Li: In vivo T! Rho mapping of articular cartilage in osteoarthritis of the knee using 3T MRI, *Osteoarthritis and Cartilage* 15(7):789–97, 2007.

## ANNOTATED BIBLIOGRAPHY

Booher JM, Thibodeau GA: *Athletic injury assessment,* ed 4, St. Louis, MO, 2001, McGraw-Hill.

*Addressed the practitioner in sports medicine or athletic training. It considers all aspects of musculoskeletal and internal sports injuries.*

Cyriax J, Cyriax P: *Cyriax's Illustrated manual of orthopaedic medicine,* London, 1996, Butterworth-Heinemann.

*A color-illustrated text designed for diagnosing and providing Cyriax management to musculoskeletal conditions.*

Gross J, Fetto J, Rosen E: *Musculoskeletal examination,* Cambridge, MA, 2015, Blackwell.

*An evaluation text is written primarily for physicians.*

Hoppenfeld S: *Physical examination of the spine and extremities,* New York, 2013, Pearson.

*Presents an easy-to-follow, methodical, and in-depth procedure for examining musculoskeletal conditions.*

Konin J, Wiksten D, Isear J: *Special tests for orthopedic examination,* Stamford, CT, 2006, Thomson Learning.

*A well-illustrated text that details examination techniques used in evaluating musculoskeletal injuries.*

Magee DJ: *Orthopedic physical assessment,* Philadelphia, PA, 2013, Elsevier Health Sciences.

*An extremely well-illustrated book with excellent depth of coverage of injuries commonly found during athletic training.*

Starkey C: *Evaluation of orthopedic and athletic injuries,* Philadelphia, PA, 2015, F.A. Davis.

*A detailed, well-illustrated text addressing all aspects of injury assessment for the athletic trainer.*

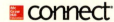

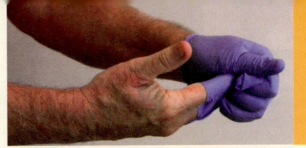

© William E. Prentice

# 14

# Infectious Diseases, Bloodborne Pathogens, and Universal Precautions

## ■ Objectives

*When you finish this chapter you should be able to*

- Discuss how infectious diseases are transmitted from person to person.
- Describe how the immune system neutralizes and eliminates an antigen that invades the body.
- Explain what bloodborne pathogens are and how they can infect patients and athletic trainers.
- Describe the transmission, symptoms, signs, and treatment of hepatitis B.
- Describe the transmission, symptoms, signs, and treatment of hepatitis C.

- Describe the transmission, symptoms, and signs of human immunodeficiency virus.
- Explain how human immunodeficiency virus is most often transmitted.
- List the pros and cons of athletes with hepatitis B virus, hepatitis C virus, or human immunodeficiency virus participating in sports.
- Evaluate universal precautions as mandated by the Occupational Safety and Health Administration and how they apply to the athletic trainer.

## ■ Key Terms

immune system                OSHA
retrovirus

## ■ Connect Highlights    connect

*Visit connect.mcgraw-hill.com for further exercises to apply your knowledge:*

- Clinical application scenarios covering universal precautions and signs, symptoms, and transmission of disease
- Click-and-drag questions covering disease transmission, bloodborne pathogens, and disease identification
- Multiple choice questions covering signs, symptoms, and transmission of disease, immune system and transmission of infectious diseases

Like other health care providers, athletic trainers must be aware of and take universal precautions against the spread of infectious diseases and bloodborne pathogens.[20,59] It has always been important for the athletic trainer as a health care provider to be concerned with maintaining an environment in the athletic training clinic that is as clean and sterile as possible.[20] In our society, it has become critical for everyone to take measures to prevent the spread of infectious diseases.[17] Failure to do so may predispose any individual to life-threatening situations. The athletic trainer must take every precaution to minimize the potential for exposure to blood or other infectious materials. The NATA official statement "Communicable and infectious diseases in secondary school sports" can be found at www.nata.org/sites /default/files/CommunicableInfectiousDiseasesSecondary SchoolSports.pdf.

# INFECTIOUS DISEASES

Infectious diseases are the invasion or infection of a *host* (person or animal) by microorganisms called *pathogens*.[17,26,40] A pathogen causes disease by either disrupting a vital body process or stimulating the immune system to mount a defensive reaction. An immune response against a pathogen, which can include a high fever, inflammation, and other damaging symptoms, can be more devastating than the direct damage caused by the pathogen itself.[53] The most common pathogens are various bacteria, viruses, parasites, and fungi (Table 14–1).[31] A microorganism can live harmlessly in a host (such as an animal) without causing infection. Over time, these hosts gradually become resistant to the microorganisms. However, when a microorganism is somehow transmitted from that animal host to a human, it may cease being harmless and become a pathogen in the new host.

## TABLE 14–1 — Common Infectious Diseases

### Viral infectious diseases

| | | | |
|---|---|---|---|
| AIDS | Hepatitis A,B,C,D,E | Marburg haemorrhagic fever | Viral encephalitis |
| AIDS-related complex | Herpes simplex | Infectious mononucleosis | Viral gastroenteritis |
| Chickenpox (varicella) | Herpes zoster | Mumps | Viral meningitis |
| Common cold | Human immuno-deficiency disease | Poliomyelitis | Viral pneumonia |
| Cytomegalovirus infection | Human papillomavirus | Rabies | West Nile disease |
| Ebola haemorrhagic fever | Influenza (flu) Type B | Rubella | Yellow fever |
| Hand, foot, and mouth disease | H1N1 | SARS | |
| | Measles | Smallpox | |

### Bacterial infectious diseases

| | | | |
|---|---|---|---|
| Anthrax | Lyme disease | Pneumococcal pneumonia | Syphilis |
| Bacterial meningitis | MRSA (methacillin-resistant staphylococcus aureus) infection | Rocky Mountain spotted fever (RMSF) | Tetanus |
| Cat scratch disease | | | Tuberculosis |
| Cholera | Pertussis (whooping cough) | Salmonellosis | Typhoid fever |
| Diphtheria | | Scarlet fever | Typhus |
| Gonorrhea | | Shigellosis | Urinary tract infections |
| Impetigo | | | |

### Parasitic infectious diseases

| | | |
|---|---|---|
| Giardiasis | Pinworm infection | Trichinosis |
| Malaria | Scabies | Tropical parasite diseases |
| Pediculosis | Toxoplasmosis | |

### Fungal infectious diseases

| | | |
|---|---|---|
| Candidiasis | Histoplasmosis | Tinea pedis |

Infectious disease requires an *agent* and a *mode of transmission*, as is the case when a mosquito is carrying malaria and injects that microorganism into the human. This microorganism becomes a pathogen and the person is now infected.[59]

An infectious disease is termed *contagious* if it is transmitted from one person to another. Transmission can be either direct or indirect. There are three types of direct transmission: contact between body surfaces (touching, sexual intercourse), droplet spread (inhalation of contaminated droplets from someone who sneezes in close proximity), and fecal-oral spread (feces on the host's hands are brought into contact with the new host's mouth).[47]

Transmission does not have to occur through direct human contact. Indirect transmission from an infected person to an uninfected person occurs when infectious agents travel by means of inanimate objects, such as water, food, towels, clothing, and eating utensils. Infectious agents can also be indirectly transmitted through *vectors*, which are living things, such as insects, birds, or animals, that carry diseases from human to human or animal to human.[38] Airborne transmission of infected particles that have been suspended in an air source for an extended time can occur by sharing air with infected people who were in the same room earlier (such as passengers on an airplane).[59]

Pathogens can enter the body through the skin, respiratory system, digestive system, or reproductive system. Whether the pathogen will actually infect the new host is determined by factors such as acquired immunity, overall health, and health-related behavior.

When a pathogen infects a new host, a sequence of five stages predictably occurs. The *incubation* stage lasts from the time a pathogen enters the body until it multiplies to the point where signs and symptoms of a disease begin to appear. This stage can last from a few hours to years in the case of herpes, HIV, or shingles.[52] depending on the concentration of organisms, the virulence of the organisms, the level of the immune response in the host, and the presence of additional health problems.

During this stage, a host may be infected but is not infectious. In the *prodromal* stage, a variety of signs and symptoms (watery eyes, runny nose, slight fever, malaise) may briefly develop. During this stage, the pathogenic agent continues to multiply and the host is capable of transferring pathogens to a new host. The person should be isolated to prevent transmission to others. In the *acute* stage, the disease reaches its greatest development, and the likelihood of transmitting the disease to others is highest. The body is resisting further damage from the pathogen. In the *decline* stage, the first signs of recovery appear, signaling

| Stages of pathogen infection: |
| :--- |
| • Incubation stage |
| • Prodromal stage |
| • Acute stage |
| • Decline stage |
| • Recovery stage |

that the infection is ending. However, patients can experience a relapse if they overextend themselves. The *recovery* stage is characterized by apparent recovery from the invading pathogen. However, because overall health has been compromised, the patient is susceptible to other pathogens. Following the recovery stage, subsequent exposure to that pathogen may not result in infection, because the body has built up immunity. It must be stressed that immunity is not necessarily permanent.[58]

## The Immune System

The **immune system** consists of several types of cells and molecules that protect the body from invading pathogens (Figure 14–1). Once a pathogen breaches mechanical defenses, such as skin and mucous membranes, the immune system mounts a cellular response to combat the invading pathogen. The immune system consists of two branches, the *innate immune response* and the *adaptive immune response*.[42]

Upon infection by a pathogen, the cells of the innate immune response, such as neutrophils, quickly recognize the invasion. These cells can remove the infectious agent through the release of antimicrobial molecules. This response directs more innate immune cell types to the site of infection. Innate immune cells, such as macrophages and dendritic cells (DCs), can also engulf the invading pathogen and digest it into small protein fragments, known as antigens. Antigens are recognizable by adaptive immune cells. The innate immune cells then display antigen on the cell surface. This process, termed *antigen presentation*, activates cells of the adaptive immune response.[42]

The major cell types involved in the adaptive immune response are B cells and T cells. T cells activate upon recognition of antigen presented by innate immune cells, and differentiate into specialized effector cell subsets.[37] These subsets direct many immune cell types to the site of infection and signal the cells to destroy the pathogen. These subsets are referred to as CD4+ T helper cells. Other T cells, CD8+ cytotoxic T cells, directly kill host cells that have been compromised by the infection, which stalls the progression of the infection. T cells can become memory T cells, which activate quickly after a second exposure to the same antigen.[42]

T helper cells assist B cells in recognition of foreign antigen. After antigen recognition, B cells differentiate into a more mature type of B cells, called plasma cells. Plasma cells secrete antibodies. Antibodies bind specific regions on pathogens, which decreases the pathogen's ability to propagate infection. Antibody-bound pathogens cannot enter host cells, as the antibody neutralizes the mechanisms necessary for entry. Additionally, a pathogen bound by antibody is a signal for other immune cells to engulf and destroy the pathogen. In a process similar to T cells, B cells can acquire immunological memory (memory B cells), which allows for a fast and efficient response upon secondary exposure to the same antigen.[42]

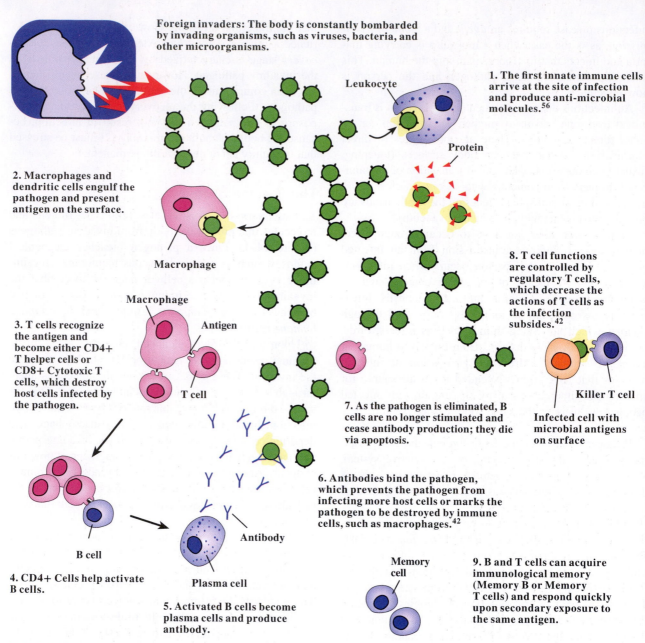

Foreign invaders: The body is constantly bombarded by invading organisms, such as viruses, bacteria, and other microorganisms.

Leukocyte

**1. The first innate immune cells arrive at the site of infection and produce anti-microbial molecules.**[56]

Protein

**2. Macrophages and dendritic cells engulf the pathogen and present antigen on the surface.**

Macrophage

Macrophage

**3. T cells recognize the antigen and become either CD4+ T helper cells or CD8+ Cytotoxic T cells, which destroy host cells infected by the pathogen.**

Antigen

T cell

**8. T cell functions are controlled by regulatory T cells, which decrease the actions of T cells as the infection subsides.**[42]

Killer T cell

Infected cell with microbial antigens on surface

**7. As the pathogen is eliminated, B cells are no longer stimulated and cease antibody production; they die via apoptosis.**

**6. Antibodies bind the pathogen, which prevents the pathogen from infecting more host cells or marks the pathogen to be destroyed by immune cells, such as macrophages.**[42]

B cell

Antibody

Plasma cell

**4. CD4+ Cells help activate B cells.**

**5. Activated B cells become plasma cells and produce antibody.**

Memory cell

**9. B and T cells can acquire immunological memory (Memory B or Memory T cells) and respond quickly upon secondary exposure to the same antigen.**

FIGURE 14–1    The immune system response.

**Immunity** When the immune system successfully eliminates the effects of an invading antigen, it is primed to respond quickly and effectively, should the same antigens appear again. Thus, the body has developed natural *acquired immunity*. Acquired immunity can also be developed either artificially, when the body is exposed to weakened pathogens through vaccination or immunization, or passively, when antibodies are injected to provide immediate protection until the body can develop natural immunity. Collectively, these forms of immunity can provide important protection against infectious disease.[14]

**Immunizations** Vaccinations against several potentially serious infectious conditions are available and should be

given to everyone.[55] These include the following: diphtheria, pertussis (whooping cough), hepatitis B, haemophilus influenza type B, tetanus, rubella (German measles), measles (red measles), polio, mumps, and chickenpox. This immunization process has markedly reduced the incidence of several childhood communicable diseases and minimized the infection rate of hepatitis B, influenza, and tetanus.[13]

Immunization has virtually eradicated many infectious diseases worldwide. Epidemiology is a tool used to study infectious disease in a population. For infectious diseases, it helps to determine whether a disease outbreak is *sporadic* (occasional occurrence), *endemic* (regular cases often occurring in a region), *epidemic* (an unusually high number of cases in a region), or *pandemic* (a global epidemic).

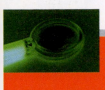

## Preventing Spread of Infectious Diseases

The athletic trainer, like other health care professionals, must be diligent in efforts to minimize the chances of transmitting infectious diseases.[36,39]

A number of administrative measures should be implemented by the athletic trainer to help to limit the spread of infectious diseases. The institution must provide the necessary fiscal and human resources to maintain infection control, and employees must be held accountable for adherence to recommended infection-control practices.[62] **SoR:B** The institution's policies and procedures manual should include infection-control policies.[62] **SoR:C** A detailed, documented cleaning schedule must be implemented for all areas and procedures should be reviewed regularly.[62] **SoR:C** Adequate hygiene materials must be provided to the athletes, and the custodial staff should be vigilant in providing antimicrobial liquid (not bar) soap in the shower and by all sinks.[62] **Sor:B**

Without question, the most effective practice to prevent spreading infectious diseases is for the athletic trainer to wash his or her hands frequently with an antimicrobial soap when treating patients.[62] **SoR:A** This is particularly important after caring for a sick person, after using the bathroom, and after

> **Handwashing is the single most important practice for preventing the spread of infectious diseases.**

blowing the nose, and/or using hands to cover sneezing or coughing. The athletic trainer should review medical histories of the patients being treated or cared for to make sure that all potential immunizations are up to date. The athletic trainer should also make sure that patients who are sick understand that taking antibiotics is not useful in treating infections caused by viruses and that antibiotics should be taken exactly as prescribed. Taking them unnecessarily will reduce their ability to combat subsequent bacterial infections. All patients should be routinely encouraged to develop healthy lifestyle habits, such as eating well, getting enough sleep, exercising, and avoiding tobacco and substance abuse (see *Focus Box 14–1*: "Suggestions for preventing the spread of infectious diseases").

## BLOODBORNE PATHOGENS

Despite the media attention given to bloodborne pathogens in recent years, many athletic trainers have only a moderate understanding of the magnitude of the problem (Figure 14–2).[28] The most common bloodborne pathogens are viruses, but there are several bacterial bloodborne pathogens as well.[52] A virus is a submicroscopic parasitic organism that is dependent on the nutrients within cells. A virus consists of a strand of either deoxyribonucleic acid (DNA) or ribonucleic acid (RNA). A virus contains one or the other, but not both.

> **Modes of transmission:**
> - Human blood
> - Semen
> - Vaginal secretions
> - Cerebrospinal fluid
> - Synovial fluid

A virus consists of a shell of proteins surrounding genetic material. It is a parasite that depends on a host cell for metabolic and reproductive requirements. In general, viruses make their cell hosts ill by redirecting cellular activity to create more viruses (Figure 14–3).

Bloodborne pathogens are pathogenic microorganisms that can cause disease and are present in human blood and other body fluids, including semen, vaginal secretions, cerebrospinal fluid, synovial fluid, and any other fluid contaminated with

> **Bloodborne pathogens:**
> - Hepatitis B virus (HBV)
> - Hepatitis C virus (HCV)
> - Human immunodeficiency virus (HIV)

blood (Table 14–2).[34] The three most significant bloodborne pathogens are the hepatitis B virus (HBV), the hepatitis C virus (HCV), and the human immunodeficiency virus (HIV).[1] Although HIV has been widely addressed in the media, HBV and HCV have a higher possibility for spread than does HIV, and thus athletic trainers should be more concerned about contracting HBV and HCV.[2,28,43] The hepatitis B virus is stronger and more durable than HIV and can be spread more easily via sharp objects, open wounds, and body fluids.[18]

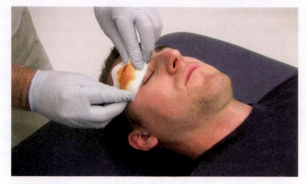

FIGURE 14–2 The athletic trainer must take precautions to prevent exposure to and transmission of bloodborne pathogens.

© William E. Prentice

## Hepatitis B Virus

The hepatitis B virus attacks the liver, resulting in life-long infection, cirrhosis (scarring) of the liver, liver cancer, liver failure, and death.[24] Hepatitis B is not spread through food or water or by casual contact. HBV is spread when blood from an infected person enters the body of a person who is not infected. For example, HBV is spread through having unprotected sex (no condom), intravenous drug use, or in health care providers through needlesticks or sharps exposures on the job. Health care personnel who have received the hepatitis B vaccine and developed immunity to the virus are at virtually no risk of infection. An estimated 350 to 400 million people worldwide have chronic HBV

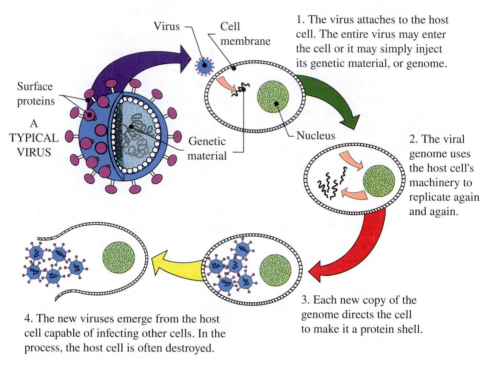

1. The virus attaches to the host cell. The entire virus may enter the cell or it may simply inject its genetic material, or genome.

2. The viral genome uses the host cell's machinery to replicate again and again.

3. Each new copy of the genome directs the cell to make it a protein shell.

4. The new viruses emerge from the host cell capable of infecting other cells. In the process, the host cell is often destroyed.

FIGURE 14–3 The reproducing virus.

| TABLE 14–2 | Body Fluids |
| --- | --- |
| Universal precautions should be practiced in any environment where individuals are exposed to bodily fluids, such as<br>• Blood<br>• Semen<br>• Vaginal secretions<br>• Synovial fluid<br>• Amniotic fluid<br>• Cerebrospinal fluid<br>• Pleural fluid<br>• Peritoneal fluid<br>• Pericardial fluid | Body fluids that do not require such precautions include<br>• Feces<br>• Nasal secretions<br>• Urine<br>• Vomitus<br>• Perspiration<br>• Sputum<br>• Saliva |

infection (compared, with 35 million living with HIV). In the United States, it is estimated that 1.4 million have chronic hepatitis B and about 5,000 die per year of sickness caused by HBV.[4] An estimated 8,700 health care workers contract HBV each year, and as many as 200 of these cases end in death.[4]

**Symptoms and Signs** The symptoms and signs in a person infected with HBV include flulike symptoms, such as fatigue, weakness, and nausea; abdominal pain; headache; fever; dark urine; and possibly jaundice (yellowing of the skin or eyes). It is possible that an individual infected with HBV will exhibit no signs or symptoms, and the virus may go undetected. In these individuals, the HBV antigen will always be present. Thus, the disease may be unknowingly transmitted to others through exposure to blood or other body fluids or through intimate contact. Cases of chronic active hepatitis may occur because of a problem with the immune system that prevents the complete destruction of virus-infected liver cells.

> The athletic trainer is responsible for taking every precaution to prevent infection by bloodborne pathogens.
>
> **?** How are bloodborne pathogen infections prevented from spreading from one person to another?

An infected person's blood may test positive for the HBV antigen within 2 to 6 weeks after the symptoms develop. Approximately 85 percent of those infected recover within 6 to 8 weeks.

**Prevention** Good personal hygiene and avoiding high-risk activities are the best ways to avoid HBV.[29] Hepatitis B virus can survive for at least 1 week in dried blood or on contaminated surfaces and may be transmitted through contact with these surfaces. Caution must be taken to avoid contact with any blood or other fluid that potentially contains a bloodborne pathogen.[29] Several vaccines have been developed for preventing HBV.[13] However vaccination does not help individuals already infected by HBV.

> A participant in a corporate wellness program has been diagnosed with hepatitis B virus.
>
> **?** What are the symptoms and signs of HBV infection?

***Management*** Vaccination against HBV must be made available by employers at no cost to any individual who may be exposed to blood or other body fluids and thus may be at risk of contracting HBV.[55] **All athletic trainers and any individual working in an allied health care profession should receive immunization**. The vaccine is given in three doses over a 6-month period. Approximately 87 percent of those receiving the vaccine are immune after the second dose, and 96 percent develop immunity after the third dose. Postexposure vaccination is available when individuals have come in direct contact with the body fluids of an infected person.[6]

## Hepatitis C Virus

Originally referred to as non-A, non-B hepatitis, hepatitis C is both an acute and a chronic form of liver disease caused by the hepatitis C virus (HCV). HCV is the most common chronic bloodborne infection in the United States. At least 85 percent of those infected acutely with HCV become chronically infected, and 67 percent develop chronic liver disease. It is the leading indication for liver transplant. Three percent of those with chronic liver disease die from cirrhosis or liver cancer. It is estimated that 170 million people worldwide and 4.5 million Americans have been infected with HCV, of whom 2.7 million are chronically infected.[45]

**Symptoms and Signs** Eighty percent of those infected with HCV have no signs or symptoms. Those who are symptomatic may be jaundiced and/or have mild abdominal pain, particularly in the upper right quadrant, loss of appetite, nausea, fatigue, muscle or joint pain, and/or dark urine.

**Prevention** HCV is not spread by sneezing, hugging, coughing, food or water, eating utensils or drinking glasses, or casual contact. It is rarely spread through sexual contact. It is spread by contact with the blood of an infected person.[45] It is most commonly transmitted by sharing needles or syringes. However, it can also be transmitted by sharing personal care items that might have blood on them (razors, toothbrushes). Consider the risks of getting a tattoo or body piercing. Athletic trainers should always follow routine barrier precautions and safely handle needles and other sharp objects.

**Management** Unlike for HBV, presently there is no vaccine for preventing HCV transmission.[13] Several blood tests can be done to determine whether a person has been infected with HCV. A physician may order just one or a combination of these tests. It is possible to find HCV within 1 to 2 weeks after being infected with the virus. A single positive test indicates infection with HCV. However, a single negative test does not prove that a person is not infected. When hepatitis C is suspected, even though an initial test is negative, the test should be repeated.[45]

HCV-positive persons should be evaluated by their doctor for liver disease. Interferon and ribavirin are two drugs used in combination that appear to be the most effective for the treatment of persons with chronic hepatitis C. Drinking alcohol can make liver disease worse.

# Human Immunodeficiency Virus

Human immunodeficiency virus is a **retrovirus** that combines with a host cell. HIV can enter only three types of immune cells: macrophages, dendritic cells, and CD4+ T cells. HIV replication occurs only in CD4+ T cells. These cells die once HIV replicates. HIV can be passed to CD4+ T cells via macrophages and dendritic cells, but it does not affect their function.[42]

When CD4+ T cells are infected and destroyed by HIV the immune system breaks down, which is why people with HIV usually die from secondary infections, or cancers that normally don't kill non-immunocompromised people.[42]

As of 2013, an estimated 35 million people worldwide were living with HIV/AIDS. Worldwide, an estimated 8 percent of adults ages 15 to 49 are infected with HIV. An estimated 2.1 million new HIV infections occurred worldwide during 2013. In 2013 alone, HIV/AIDS-associated illnesses caused approximately 1.5 million deaths worldwide.[61]

**Symptoms and Signs** As is the case with HBV, HIV is transmitted by exposure to infected blood or other body fluids and by intimate sexual contact.[9] In the acute phase of HIV, symptoms may include fatigue, weight loss, muscle or joint pain, painful or swollen glands, night sweats, and fever. Antibodies to HIV can be detected in a blood test within 1 year after exposure. Following the acute phase, people with HIV enter an asymptomatic phase during which they may be unaware that they have contracted the virus and may go for 8 to 10 years before developing any signs or symptoms. After these two phases, AIDS symptoms occur.[42] Unfortunately, most individuals who test positive for HIV will ultimately develop acquired immunodeficiency syndrome (AIDS). Table 14–3 summarizes information on HBV, HCV, and HIV.

*Acquired Immunodeficiency Syndrome* A syndrome is a collection of signs and symptoms that are recognized as the effects of an infection. An individual with AIDS has no protection against even the simplest infections and thus is extremely vulnerable to developing a variety of illnesses, opportunistic infections, and cancers (such as Kaposi's sarcoma and non-Hodgkin's lymphoma) that cannot be stopped.[16,33]

According to the Centers for Disease Control and Prevention (CDC), it is estimated that, as of 2013, 1.2 million U.S. residents are living with HIV infection and that approximately 50,000 new HIV infections occur each year. Overall, an estimated 1,194,039 people in the United States have been diagnosed with AIDS, and since 1981 an estimated 658,507 people with AIDS in the United States have died.[7]

A positive HIV test cannot predict when the individual will show the symptoms of AIDS.[10] About 50 percent of people develop AIDS within 10 years of becoming HIV infected. Those individuals who develop AIDS generally die within 2 years after the symptoms appear.

**Management** Unlike HBV, there is no vaccine for HIV. Even though some drug therapy may extend their lives, there is currently no available treatment to cure patients with AIDS. Much research is being done to find a preventive vaccine and an effective treatment. Presently, the most effective treatment seems to be a therapy consisting of a combination of three drugs. One drug blocks the action of an enzyme that the virus needs to make some of the components for new virus cells. A second drug blocks the copying of viral genes that can enter the host cell's nucleus (a process called reverse transcription) and thus disables the synthesis of new viruses. A third drug helps protect the T cells and thus slows the progression of HIV.[47]

| TABLE 14–3 | Transmission of Hepatitis B and C Viruses and Human Immunodeficiency Virus | | |
|---|---|---|---|
| **Disease** | **Symptoms and Signs** | **Mode of Transmission** | **Infectious Materials** |
| Hepatitis B virus | Flulike symptoms, jaundice | Direct and indirect contact | Blood, saliva, semen, feces, food, water, other products |
| Hepatitis C virus | Jaundice, upper right quadrant pain, loss of appetite, nausea, fatigue, dark urine | Direct and indirect contact with blood | Blood |
| Human immunodeficiency virus/ acquired immunodeficiency syndrome | Fever, night sweats, weight loss, diarrhea, severe fatigue, swollen lymph nodes, lesions | Direct and indirect contact | Blood, semen, vaginal fluid |

It has been recommended that HIV-infected patients engage in an exercise or training program for the purpose of improving muscle and aerobic fitness. It appears that a fitness program has no negative effect on the patient's immunologic function.[12]

Although new treatments have extended the healthy life span of many people with AIDS, HIV prevalence has continued to increase. As the number of AIDS cases declines because of these new treatments, the number of people with HIV will increase, which means there will be a greater need for both prevention and treatment services.

**Prevention  It is essential to understand that the greatest risk of contracting HIV is through intimate sexual contact with an infected partner.**[51] Practicing safe sex is of major importance. Anyone engaging in sexual activities must choose nonpromiscuous sex partners and use condoms for vaginal or anal intercourse. Latex condoms provide a barrier against both HBV and HIV. Male condoms should have reservoir tips

> **Human immunodeficiency virus is most often transmitted through intimate sexual contact.**

to reduce the chance of ejaculate being released from the sides of the condom. Condoms that are prelubricated are less likely to tear. Water-based, greaseless spermicides or lubricants should be

> **The use of latex condoms can reduce the chances of contracting HIV.**

avoided.[31] If the condom tears, a vaginal spermicide should be used immediately. The condom should carefully be removed and discarded.[47] Additional ways to reduce the risk of HIV infection can be found in *Focus Box 14–2*: "HIV risk reduction."

## Additional Hepatitis Viruses

Three additional viruses—hepatitis A, D, and E—exist, which, while related, are not generally considered to be bloodborne pathogens.

**Hepatitis A Virus** Hepatitis A (HAV) is a virus that causes inflammation of the liver but does not lead to chronic disease of the liver. HAV is transmitted by the fecal or oral routes, through close personal contact, or through ingestion of contaminated food or water. For example, it may be transmitted by an infected food preparer who doesn't wash his or her hands after going to the bathroom. In food, HAV is most commonly transmitted in milk, shellfish, salad, and sliced meat. HAV may show no outward symptoms or signs, but adults may have dark urine, light stools, fatigue, fever, and jaundice. HAV persists acutely for up to 21 days, but the effects last considerably longer. Death is rare with HAV infection.[4]

**Hepatitis D Virus** Hepatitis D (HDV), like HAV, causes inflammation of the liver and those infected are prone to

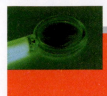

developing hepatitis and cirrhosis. HDV may be transmitted by sexual activity, injected drugs, or needlesticks in health care workers. It is most likely to infect those individuals who are already infected with HBV. Symptoms are more severe than with HBV and there is at least a 2 percent mortality rate.[17]

**Hepatitis E Virus** Like HAV and HDV, hepatitis E (HEV) causes inflammation of the liver. It is transmitted through the fecal and oral routes.[48] Hepatitis E is a waterborne disease, and contaminated water and food supplies have been implicated in major outbreaks in foreign countries with poor sanitation standards. Person-to-person transmission is uncommon. There is no evidence for sexual transmission or for transmission by transfusion. HEV is a self-limiting viral infection followed by recovery, with mortality rates between 0.5 percent and 4.0 percent.[17]

## Bloodborne Pathogens in Athletics

In general, the chances of transmitting HIV among athletes is low.[2,16,19,36,41] There is minimal risk of on-field transmission of HIV from one player to another in sports.[22] One study involving professional football estimated that the risk of transmission from player to player is less than 1 per 1 million games.[41] At this time there have been no validated reports of HIV transmission in sports.[43]

Some sports may have a higher risk of transmission because of close contact and the possibility of passing blood on to another person.[2] Sports such as the martial arts, wrestling, and boxing have more theoretical potential for transmission (see *Focus Box 14–3*: "Risk categories for HIV transmission in sports").[36]

**Policy Regulation** Athletes participating in organized sports are subject to procedures and policies about the

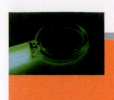

## FOCUS 14–3 Focus on Immediate and Emergency Care

### Risk categories for HIV transmission in sports

Although the risk of HIV transmission in athletics is minimal, the following classifications of sports indicate risks relative to one another:

- Highest risk: boxing, martial arts, wrestling, rugby
- Moderate risk: basketball, field hockey, football, ice hockey, judo, soccer, team handball
- Lowest risk: archery, badminton, baseball, bowling, canoeing/kayaking, cycling, diving, equestrianism, fencing, figure skating, gymnastics, modern pentathlon, racquetball, rhythmic gymnastics, roller skating, rowing, shooting, softball, speed skating, skiing, swimming, synchronized swimming, table tennis, volleyball, water polo, weight lifting, yachting

transmission of bloodborne pathogens.[43] The National Athletic Trainers' Association, U.S. Olympic Committee, National Collegiate Athletic Association, National Federation of State High School Athletic Associations, National Basketball Association, National Hockey League, National Football League, and Major League Baseball all have established policies to help prevent the transmission of bloodborne pathogens.[20,43] These organizations have also initiated programs to help educate athletes under their control. The Centers for Disease Control and Prevention is another useful resource for the athletic trainer seeking information and guidelines for medical assistance on disease control, epidemic prevention, and notification.[7]

All institutions should take responsibility for educating their student-athletes about how bloodborne pathogens are transmitted.[43] In the case of a secondary-school athlete, efforts should also be made to educate the parents.[2,20] Professional, collegiate, and secondary-school athletes should be made aware that the greatest risk of contracting HBV or HIV is through their off-the-field activities, which may include unsafe sexual practices and sharing of needles, particularly in the use of steroids.[33]

**14–3 Clinical Application Exercise**

A wrestler comes into the athletic training clinic very concerned that his wrestling partner got a bloody nose and that he came in contact with a few drops of that athlete's blood.

**?** What should the athletic trainer tell the athlete about the transmission of HIV from this type of contact?

Athletes, perhaps more than other individuals in the population, think that they are immune and that infection will always happen to someone else. The athletic trainer should also assume the responsibility of educating and informing athletic training students about exposure control policies.

Each institution should implement policies and procedures concerning bloodborne pathogens.[23] A recent survey of NCAA institutions found that a large number of athletic trainers and other health care providers at many colleges and universities demonstrated significant deficits in following the universal guidelines mandated by OSHA. Universal precautions in a sports medicine or other health care setting protect both the athlete and the health care provider.[46]

**Human Immunodeficiency Virus and Athletic Participation** There is no definitive answer to whether asymptomatic HIV carriers should participate in sports.[30] Body fluid contact should be avoided, and the participant should avoid engaging in exhaustive exercise that may lead to an increased susceptibility to infection.[30]

The Americans with Disabilities Act of 1991 says that athletes infected with HIV cannot be discriminated against and may be excluded from participation only on a medically sound basis.[30] Exclusion must be based on objective medical evidence and must take into consideration the extent of risk of infection to others, the potential harm to the athlete, and what means can be taken to reduce this risk.[30]

A female patient has had unprotected sex with a male she has dated only once previously. She knows that she should be tested for HIV but is so worried and embarrassed that she has avoided going to a medical facility to have a test. Finally, she goes to the athletic trainer and confides her concerns.

**?** What should the athletic trainer tell her about being tested for HIV?

**Testing for Human Immunodeficiency Virus** Testing for HIV should not be used as a screening tool to determine if an athlete can participate in sports.[30] Mandatory testing for HIV may not be allowed because of legal reasons related to the Americans with Disabilities Act and the Health Insurance Portability and Accountability Act (HIPAA).[44] In terms of importance, mandatory testing should be secondary to education to prevent the transmission of HIV.[54] Neither the NCAA nor the Centers for Disease Control and Prevention recommends mandatory HIV testing for athletes.[7,44]

Individuals who engage in high-risk activities should be encouraged to seek voluntary anonymous testing for HIV.[47] A blood test analyzes serum using an enzyme-linked immunosorbent assay (ELISA). This test detects antibodies to HIV proteins. Positive ELISA tests should be repeated to rule out false-positive results. A second positive test requires the Western blot examination, which is a more sensitive test.[49] Detectable antibodies may appear from 3 months to 1 year after exposure. Testing, therefore, should occur at 6 weeks, 3 months, and 1 year.[49]

Home testing kits are also available in which an individual can collect a sample for testing in the privacy of his or her home and then send it to a laboratory for analysis. There are more than a dozen different HIV home test kits being advertised on the market today. Only the Home Access test system is FDA approved and legally marketed in the United States. This approved system uses a simple finger prick process for home blood collection, which results in dried blood spots on special paper. The dried blood spots are mailed to a laboratory with a confidential and anonymous personal identification number (PIN). The sample is then analyzed by trained clinicians in a certified medical laboratory using the same procedures that are used for samples taken in a doctor's office. The purchaser obtains results by calling a toll-free telephone number and using the PIN; posttest counseling is provided by telephone when results are obtained.[44]

Many states have enacted laws that protect the confidentiality of the HIV-infected person. The athletic trainer should be familiar with state law and make every effort to guard the confidentiality and anonymity of HIV testing for athletes.

> For additional information on HIV and AIDS care, contact the CDC National AIDS Hotline: 1 (800) 342-2437.

# UNIVERSAL PRECAUTIONS IN AN ATHLETIC ENVIRONMENT

In 1991, the Occupational Safety and Health Administration (**OSHA**) established standards for an employer to follow that govern occupational exposure to bloodborne pathogens.[46]

The guidelines instituted by OSHA were developed to protect the health care provider and the patient against bloodborne pathogens.[46] OSHA has mandated that training programs for dealing with bloodborne pathogens be repeated each year to provide the most current information.[46] It is essential that every program develop and carry out a bloodborne pathogen exposure control plan.[60] NATA has established specific guidelines for athletic trainers.[43] This plan should

> Throughout the remainder of this text, whenever there is a discussion of an injury or a technique of care that requires universal precautions, the biohazard icon will appear in the margin.

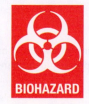

**BIOHAZARD**

include counseling, education, volunteer testing, and the management of body fluids.[43]

Universal precautions should be practiced by anyone coming into contact with blood or other body fluids (see Table 14–3).[3,25,60] Following are considerations specifically in the sports arena.

## Preparing the Athlete

Before an athlete participates in practice or competition, all open skin wounds and lesions must be covered with a dressing that is fixed in place and does not allow for transmission to or from another athlete.[59] An occlusive dressing lessens the chances of cross-contamination. One example is the hydrocolloid dressing, which is considered a superior barrier. This type of dressing also reduces the chances that the wound will reopen because it keeps the wound moist and pliable.[36]

## When Bleeding Occurs

As mandated by the NCAA and the USOC, open wounds and other skin lesions considered a risk for disease transmission should be given aggressive treatment.[44] Athletes with active bleeding must be removed from participation as soon as possible and can return only when it is deemed safe by the medical staff.[5] Uniforms containing blood must be evaluated for infectivity. A uniform that is saturated with blood must be removed and changed before the athlete can return to competition. All personnel managing potential infective wound exposure must follow universal precautions.[44,54]

> A hospital-based sports medicine program must initiate and carry out a bloodborne pathogen exposure control plan.
>
> **?** What are the universal precautions, as proposed by OSHA, that must be followed?

14–5 Clinical Application Exercise

## Personal Precautions

The health care personnel working directly with body fluids on the field or in the athletic training clinic must make use of the appropriate protective equipment in all situations in which there is potential contact with bloodborne pathogens. Protective equipment includes disposable nonlatex gloves, nonabsorbent gowns or aprons, masks and shields, eye protection, and disposable mouthpieces for resuscitation devices.[3] Equipment for dealing with bloodborne pathogens should be included in sideline emergency kits.[39] Disposable nonlatex gloves must be used when handling any potentially infectious material. Double gloving is suggested when there

> Nonlatex gloves should be worn whenever the athletic trainer handles blood or body fluids.

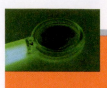

### Glove use and removal

1. Avoid touching personal items when wearing contaminated gloves.
2. Remove the first glove and turn it inside out.
3. Place the first glove in the second gloved hand and then turn the second glove inside out so as to contain the first glove.
4. Remove the second glove, making sure not to touch soiled surfaces with the ungloved hand.
5. Discard gloves that have been used, discolored, torn, or punctured.
6. Wash hands immediately after glove removal.

is heavy bleeding or sharp instruments are used. Gloves should always be removed carefully after use. In cases of emergency, heavy toweling may be used until gloves can be obtained[2] (see *Focus Box 14–4*: "Glove use and removal") (Figure 14–4).

**Hand Washing** Hands and all skin surfaces that come in contact with blood or other body fluids should be washed immediately with soap and water or other antigermicidal agents.[50] Hands should also be washed between each patient treatment.[35] If there is a possibility of body fluids becoming splashed, spurted, or sprayed, the mouth, nose, and eyes should be protected. Aprons or nonabsorbent gowns should be worn to avoid clothing contamination.

> Hands should be washed frequently to minimize the spread of diseases.

First-aid kits must contain protection for hands, face, eyes, and resuscitation mouthpieces. Kits should also contain towelettes for cleaning skin surfaces.[3]

**Latex Sensitivity and Using Nonlatex Gloves** It is recommended that athletic trainers use nonlatex, vinyl, or nitrile rubber gloves.[6] A number of manufacturers produce nonlatex gloves. Latex, a sap from the rubber tree, is composed of compounds that may cause an allergic reaction that can range from contact dermatitis to a systemic reaction.[11] Recognizing the signs and symptoms of these reactions may help prevent a more severe reaction from occurring. Some individuals are more at risk of latex allergies due to repetitive exposure to latex through their career paths, multiple surgeries, other allergies, or respiratory conditions.[11] Management of an acute reaction involves removing the irritant, cleansing the affected area, monitoring vital signs for changes, and seeking additional medical assistance as warranted.[6]

> During a basketball game, one of the players sustains a nosebleed. Blood is visible on the court and on the player's jersey and skin.
>
> ❓ What actions need to take place before the game can resume?

## Availability of Supplies and Equipment

In keeping with universal precautions, the sports program must have available chlorine bleach, antiseptics, proper receptacles for soiled equipment and uniforms, wound care bandages, and a designated container for disposal of sharp objects, such as needles, syringes, and scalpels.[44]

> Universal precautions minimize the risk of exposure and transmission.

Biohazard warning labels should be affixed to containers for regulated wastes, refrigerators containing blood, and other containers used to store or ship potentially infectious materials (Figure 14–5). The labels are fluorescent orange or red. Red bags or containers should be

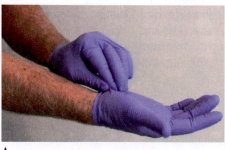
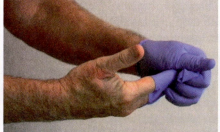
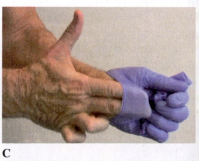

A                                   B                                   C

**FIGURE 14–4** Technique for removing nonlatex gloves. (A) Grasp one gloved hand at the wrist with the opposite hand and peel that glove off. (B) Ball up the removed glove and hold it in the opposite gloved hand. (C) Then peel off the second glove trapping the first glove inside.

(a–c) © William E. Prentice

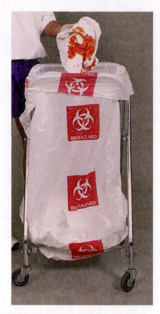

FIGURE 14–5  Soiled linens should be placed in a leakproof bag marked as a biohazard.
© William E. Prentice

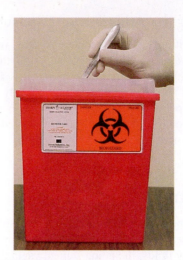

FIGURE 14–6  Sharps should be disposed of in a red or orange puncture-resistant plastic container marked as a biohazard.
© William E. Prentice

used for the disposal of potentially infected materials. If you're not sure whether a substance qualifies as biohazardous waste, the best practice is to use a biohazard bag to dispose of it.

**Disinfectants**  All contaminated surfaces, such as treatment tables, taping tables, work areas, and floors, should

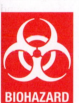

be cleaned immediately with a disinfectant approved by the Environmental Protection Agency.[8,15] The manufacturer's recommendations for amount, dilution, and contact time should be followed precisely.[67] SoR:B A solution consisting of 1 part bleach to 10 parts water (1:10) has been recommended for immediate cleaning following contamination.[54] Disinfectants should inactivate the HIV virus.

**Contaminated Laundry**  Towels and other linens that have been contaminated should be bagged and separated from other laundry. Soiled linen should be transported in red or orange containers or bags that prevent soaking or leaking and are labeled with biohazard warning labels (see Figure 14–4). Contaminated laundry should be washed in hot water (71°C/159.8°F for 25 minutes) using a detergent that deactivates the virus.[46] Laundry done outside the institution should be sent to a facility that follows OSHA standards. Gloves must be worn during bagging and cleaning of contaminated laundry.

**Sharps**  *Sharps* refers to sharp objects used in athletic training, such as needles, razor blades, and scalpels. Extreme care should be taken when handling and disposing of sharps to minimize the risk of puncturing or cutting the skin. Athletic trainers rarely use needles, but it is not unusual for them to use scalpels or razor blades. Whenever needles are used, they should not be recapped, bent, or removed from a syringe. Sharps should be disposed of in a leakproof and puncture-resistant container.[46] The container should be red or orange and should be labeled as a biohazard (Figure 14–6). Scissors and tweezers are not as likely to cause injury as sharps are, but they should be sterilized with a disinfecting agent and stored in a clean place after use.

| Sharps: |
| --- |
| • Scalpels |
| • Razor blades |
| • Needles |

## Protecting the Athletic Trainer

OSHA guidelines for bloodborne pathogens are intended to protect the coach, athletic trainer, and other employees.[46] Coaches do not usually come in contact with blood or other body fluids from an injured athlete, so their risk is considerably reduced. It is the responsibility of the secondary school, college, professional team, or clinic to ensure the safety of the athletic trainer as a health care provider by instituting and annually updating policies for education on the prevention of transmitting bloodborne pathogens through contact with athletes. The institution must provide the necessary supplies and equipment to carry out these recommendations.

The athletic trainer has the personal responsibility of adhering to these policies and guidelines and enforcing them in the athletic training clinic. Athletic trainers may further minimize the risk of exposure in the athletic training setting by not eating, drinking, applying cosmetics or lip balm, handling contact lenses, or touching the face before washing hands. Food products should never be placed in a refrigerator containing contaminated blood.[46]

## Protecting the Athlete from Exposure

Several additional recommendations may further help protect the athlete. The USOC supports the required use of mouthpieces in high-risk sports. It is also recommended that all athletes shower immediately after practice or competition. Athletes who may be exposed to HIV, HBV, or HCV should also be evaluated for immunization against HBV.

## Postexposure Procedures

After a report of an exposure incident, the athletic trainer should have a confidential medical evaluation that includes documentation of the exposure route, identification of the source individual, a blood test, counseling, and an evaluation of reported illness. Again, the laws that pertain to the reporting and confidentiality of test results notification vary from state to state.[46]

## SUMMARY

- Bloodborne pathogens are microorganisms that can cause disease and are present in human blood and other body fluids, including semen, vaginal secretions, cerebrospinal fluid, synovial fluid, and any other fluid contaminated with blood. Hepatitis B virus, hepatitis C virus, and HIV are bloodborne pathogens.
- A virus is a submicroscopic organism that contains either DNA or RNA, but not both. It is dependent on the host cell to function and reproduce.
- A vaccine is available to prevent HBV. Currently, no effective vaccine exists for HCV or HIV.
- An individual infected with HIV may develop AIDS, which is fatal.
- The risks of contracting HBV, HCV, or HIV may be minimized by avoiding exposure to blood and other body fluids and by practicing safe sex.

- The risk of an athlete being exposed to bloodborne pathogens on the field is minimal. Off-the-field activities involving risky sexual behaviors pose the greatest threat for transmission.
- Various national medical and sports organizations have established policies and procedures for dealing with bloodborne pathogens in the athletic population.
- The Occupational Safety and Health Administration has established rules and regulations that protect the health care employee.
- Universal precautions must be taken to avoid bloodborne pathogen exposure. All sports programs must carry out a plan for counseling, education, volunteer testing, and the management of exposure.

## WEB SITES

**National Athletic Trainers Association Official Statement**
*Communicable and Infectious Diseases in Secondary School Sports (2007) www.nata.org/sites/default/files/Communicable InfectiousDiseasesSecondarySchoolSports.pdf*
Centers for Disease Control and Prevention: www.cdc .gov

Department of Health and Human Services: www.hhs .gov
HIV/AIDS Prevention: cdc.gov/hiv
Occupational Safety and Health Administration (OSHA): www.osha.gov
National Institutes of Health: www.nih.gov

## SOLUTIONS TO CLINICAL APPLICATION EXERCISES

14–1 During competition or practice, the athlete should be most concerned about coming in contact with blood from another athlete. There should be little or no concern about exposure to sweat or saliva. The chances of contracting HIV during athletic participation are minimal. Certainly, the athlete is most likely to be exposed to HIV during unprotected intimate sexual contact.

14–2 The participant complained of flulike symptoms, such as headache, fever, fatigue, weakness, nausea, and some abdominal pain. A blood test revealed the presence of the HBV antigen.

14–3 The greatest risk of contracting HIV is through intimate sexual contact with an infected partner. The athletic trainer should explain to the athlete that there is little chance of HIV transmission among athletes. There is a theoretical potential risk of transmission among athletes in close contact who pass blood from one to the other.

14–4 The athletic trainer should inform her that it is best if she waits for 6 weeks before being tested. The athletic trainer should strongly encourage her to seek testing and should explain to her that if she is uncomfortable with being tested in a medical care facility, there

is a home test available that has been approved by the FDA and provides confidentiality. The athletic trainer should add that if the athlete were to test positive on the home test, it would become imperative that she seek additional testing at a medical care facility.

14–5 Universal precautions should be practiced by anyone coming in contact with blood or other body fluids. This plan must include counseling, education, volunteer testing, and management of body fluids.

14–6 To prevent possible transmission of bloodborne pathogens, several precautions need to be followed. The athlete must be removed from the game until active bleeding has ceased and he or she has been cleared by the medical staff. The jersey must be removed and changed if the uniform is saturated with blood. Any blood on the skin must be cleaned off before the athlete can return to play. In addition, the basketball court needs to be properly cleaned and disinfected. The solution used to clean the court should be 1 part bleach to 10 parts water or a solution approved by the Environmental Protection Agency. All contaminated products need to be properly disposed of according to OSHA standards.

# REVIEW QUESTIONS AND CLASS ACTIVITIES

1. What can the athletic trainer do to prevent the spread of infectious disease?
2. How are infectious diseases transmitted from person to person?
3. How does the immune system respond to an infectious antigen?
4. Define and identify the bloodborne pathogens.
5. Describe HBV and HCV transmission, symptoms, signs, prevention, and treatment.
6. Explain the pros and cons of allowing an athlete who is an HBV carrier to participate.
7. Describe HIV transmission, symptoms, signs, prevention, and treatment.
8. How is HIV transmitted, and why is it eventually fatal at this time?
9. Should an athlete who tests positive for HBV or HIV be allowed to participate in sports? Why or why not?
10. How can an athlete reduce the risk of HIV infection?
11. Define OSHA universal precautions for preventing bloodborne pathogen exposure.
12. What precautions would you, as an athletic trainer, take when caring for a bleeding wound on the field?

# REFERENCES

1. American Academy of Orthopedic Surgeons: *Bloodborne pathogens*, 2011, Jones and Bartlett.
2. American Academy of Pediatrics: Human immunodeficiency virus and other bloodborne viral pathogens in the athletic setting, *Pediatrics*, 104(6):1400–03, 2009.
3. American Red Cross: *Responding to emergency*, San Bruno, CA, 2012, Staywell.
4. Barreto M: Infectious diseases epidemiology, *Journal of Epidemiology and Community Health* 60(3):192, 2006.
5. Berry D: Teaching wound care management: A model for the budget conscious educator, *Athletic Training Education Journal* 7(3):140, 2012.
6. Binkley H: Latex allergies: A review of recognition, evaluation, management, prevention, education, and alternative product use, *J Athl Train* 38(2):133, 2003.
7. Centers for Disease Control and Prevention: HIV in the United States: At a glance, www.cdc.gov/hiv/statistics/basics/ataglance.html, 2013.
8. Clark G: Blood on the gym floor: Application of universal precautions, *Strategies* 21(3):15, 2008.
9. Clem K: HIV and the athlete. *Clinics in Sports Medicine* 26(3):413, 2007.
10. Dittman D: *Sports and HIV/AIDS prevention*, Saarbrücwken, Germany, 2008, VDM Verlag.
11. Epling C: Latex symptoms among health care workers: Results from a university health and safety surveillance system, *International Journal of Occupational and Environmental Health* 17(1):17–23, 2011.
12. Farinatti P: Effects of a supervised exercise program on the physical fitness and immunological function of HIV-infected patients, *Journal of Sports Medicine and Physical Fitness* 50(4):511–18, 2010.
13. Gartner B: Vaccination in elite athletes, *Sports Medicine* 44(10):1361, 2014.
14. Gleeson M: Exercise, nutrition and immune function, *Journal of Sports Sciences* 22(1):115, 2004.
15. Grindle M: Appropriate disinfection techniques for playing surfaces to prevent the transmission of bloodborne pathogens, *International Journal of Athletic Therapy and Training* 19(5):12–15, 2014.
16. Gutierrez R: Bloodborne infections and the athlete, *Dis Mon* 56(7):436–42, 2010.
17. Hamann B: *Disease: Identification, prevention, and control*, New York, 2006, McGraw-Hill.
18. Harrington D: Viral hepatitis and exercise, *Medicine & Science in Sports and Exercise*, 32(7):422–30, 2000.

19. Harris M: Infectious disease in athletes, *Current Sports Medicine Reports* 10(2):84–89, 2011.
20. Hart P: Complying with the bloodborne pathogen standard: Protecting health care workers and patients, *AORN Journal* 94(4):393–99, 2011.
21. Honshik K: Sideline skin and wound care for acute injuries, *Current Sports Medicine Reports* 6(3):147, 2007.
22. Hoogenboom B: Management of bleeding and open wounds in athletes, *International Journal of Sports Physical Therapy* 7(3):350–56, 2012.
23. Hosey R: Training room management of medical conditions: Infectious diseases, *Clinics in Sports Medicine* 24(3):477–506, 2005.
24. Howe W: The athlete with chronic illness. In Birrer RB, ed: *Sports medicine for the primary care physician*, ed 3, Boca Raton, FL, 2004, CRC Press.
25. Irion G: *Comprehensive wound management*, ed 2, Thorofare, NJ, 2009, Slack.
26. Jaworski C: Infectious disease, *Clinics in Sports Medicine* 30(3):575–90, 2011.
27. Kahanov L: Certified athletic trainers' knowledge of methicillin-resistant Staphylococcus aureus and common disinfectants, *Journal of Athletic Training* 46(4):415–23,2011.
28. Kordi R: Risk of hepatitis B and C infections in Tehranian wrestlers, *J Athl Train*, 46(4):445–50, 2011.
29. Kordi R: Blood borne infections in sport: Risks of transmission, methods of prevention, and recommendations for hepatitis B vaccination, *Br J Sports Med* 38:678–84, 2004.
30. Kukka C: Bloodborne infections: Should they be disclosed? Is differential treatment necessary? *The Journal of School Nursing* 20(6): 324–30, 2004.
31. Landry G, Bernhardt D: Common infectious diseases. In Landry G: *Essentials of primary care sports medicine*, Champaign, IL, 2003, Human Kinetics.
32. Landry G: Sexually transmitted diseases and blood-borne infections. In Landry G: *Essentials of primary care sports medicine*, Champaign, IL, 2003, Human Kinetics.
33. LaPeniere A: Acquired immune deficiency syndrome. In American College of Sports Medicine: *ACSM's exercise management for persons with chronic disease and disabilities*, Champaign, IL, 2009, Human Kinetics.
34. Lindsey J: *Bloodborne pathogens*, Boston, MA, 2008, Jones and Bartlett.
35. Lindsey J: *Preventing infectious diseases*, Boston, MA, 2007, Jones and Bartlett.

36. Luke A: Prevention of infectious disease in athletes, *Clinics in Sports Medicine* 26(3):321–44, 2007.
37. MacDonald T: Suppressor T cells, rebranded as regulatory T cells, emerge from the wilderness bearing surface markers, *Gut* 51(3): 311–12, 2002.
38. Madigan M: *Brock biology of microorganisms*, San Francisco, 2012, Benjamin Cummings.
39. Maloney G: Infectious disease update 2006: How to protect yourself and your patients, *Journal of Emergency Medical Services* 31(5):120, 2006.
40. Minoee A: Sports: The infectious hazards. In Schlossberg D: *Infections of leisure*, Philadelphia, PA, 2009, ASM Press.
41. Midgley A: Infection and the elite athlete: A review, *Research in Sports Medicine: An International Journal* 11(4):235–60, 2003.
42. Murphy K: *Janeway's immunobiology*, New York, 2012, Garland Science.
43. National Athletic Trainers' Association: Bloodborne pathogens guidelines for athletic trainers, *J Athl Train* 30(3):203, 1995.
44. National Collegiate Athletic Association: *NCAA 2014–2015 Sports Medicine Handbook*, Indianapolis, 2014, NCAA.
45. Negro F: *Handbook of hepatitis C management*, New Zealand, 2016, Adis.
46. Occupational Safety and Health Administration: OSHA's bloodborne pathogens standard, Washington, DC: OSHA, 2011.
47. Payne W: *Understanding your health*, San Francisco, CA, 2012, McGraw-Hill.
48. Pirozzolo J: Blood-borne infections, *Clinics in Sports Medicine* 26(3):425–31, 2007.
49. Porter R: *The Merck manual of diagnosis and therapy*, ed 19, Whitehouse Station, NJ, 2011, Merck.
50. Rani S: The in vitro antimicrobial activity of wound and skin cleansers at nontoxic concentrations, *Advances in Skin and Wound Care* 27(2):65–69, 2014.
51. Reel J: Reducing high-risk sexual behaviors among college athletes, *Journal of Sport Psychology in Action* 3(1):21–9, 2012.
52. Schaechter M: *Schaechter's mechanisms of microbial disease*, Philadelphia, 2013, Wolters Kluwer Health/Lippincott Williams and Wilkins.
53. Shetty N: *Infectious diseases: Pathogenesis, prevention and case studies*, New York, 2009, Wiley.
54. Schultz S: Preventing transmission of bloodborne pathogens. In Schultz SJ, ed: *Sports medicine handbook*, Indianapolis, IN, 2005, National Federation of State High School Associations.

55. Strikas R: Immunizations: Recommendations and resources for active patients, *Physician Sportsmed* 29(10):33, 2001.
56. Summers C, et al.: Neutrophil kinetics in health and disease, *Trends Immunol* 31(8):318–24, 2010.
57. Thygerson A: *First aid, CPR, and AED Advanced,* Boston, MA, 2011, Jones and Bartlett.
58. Tuberville S: Infectious disease outbreaks in competitive sports: A review of the literature, *Am J Sports Med* 34(11):1860, 2006.
59. Walsh K: Infection and disease transmission in the athletic training setting, *Athletic Therapy Today* 9(3):11, 2004.
60. U.S. Departments of Labor and Occupational Safety and Health Administration: *Model plans and programs for the OSHA bloodborne pathogens and hazards communication standards*, CreateSpace Independent Publishing Platform, 2012.
61. World Health Organization: Global Health Observatory data, www.who.int/gho/hiv/en/, 2013.
62. Zinder S: National Athletic Trainers' Association position statement: Skin diseases, *J Athl Train*, 45(4): 411–28, 2010.

## ANNOTATED BIBLIOGRAPHY

Porter R,: *The Merck manual of diagnosis and therapy*, ed 19, Whitehouse Station, NJ, 2011, John Wiley and Sons.

*This excellent guide discusses diagnosis, symptoms, signs, and treatment of bloodborne pathogens.*

Negro F: *Handbook of Hepatitis C Management,* New Zealand, 2016, Adis.

*This definitive guide outlines the course of the disease and associated symptoms. It discusses available treatment and lifestyle changes and contains an extensive section on herbs, vitamins, and nutritional supplements.*

Friend, M., & Kohn, J. 2010. *Fundamentals of occupational safety and health.* Lanham, MD: Government Institutes.

*Provides a thorough and up-to-date overview of the occupational safety and health field and the issues safety professionals face today, and does so in an accessible and engaging manner.*

Hamann B: Disease: *Identification, prevention, and control*, St. Louis, MO, 2006, McGraw-Hill.

*This text is designed for health educators and covers in detail both AIDS and hepatitis.*

NCAA: *National Collegiate Athletic Association* 2014–2015 *sports medicine handbook*, Indianapolis, IN, 2014, National Collegiate Athletic Association.

*This text offers a complete discussion of bloodborne pathogens and intercollegiate athletic policies and administration.*

National Safety Council: *Bloodborne pathogens*, Boston, MA, 2012, Jones and Bartlett.

*This manual is dedicated to presenting OSHA regulations specific to bloodborne pathogens.*

Occupational Safety and Health Administration:. OSHA's Bloodborne Pathogens Standard. Washington, DC: OSHA. 2011.

*Presents OSHA standards, with special emphasis on bloodborne pathogens and incident and injury reporting.*

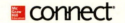

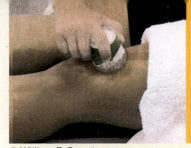

© William E. Prentice

# 15

# Using Therapeutic Modalities

## ■ Objectives

*When you finish this chapter you should be able to*

- Recognize the legal ramifications of treating a patient with therapeutic modalities.
- Explain how therapeutic modalities are classified according to the type of energy they produce.
- Describe the theoretical uses of the various types of modalities.
- Correctly demonstrate a variety of thermotherapy and cryotherapy techniques.

- Discuss the physiological basis and therapeutic uses of electrical stimulating currents.
- Examine the use of ultrasound in an athletic training setting.
- Describe how massage, traction, and intermittent compression can be used as therapeutic agents.

## ■ Outline

## ■ Key Terms

| | | | | |
|---|---|---|---|---|
| ischemia | hunting response | watts | effective radiating area | petrissage |
| conduction | cryokinetics | frequency | beam nonuniformity | friction |
| convection | amperes | tetany | ratio (BNR) | tapotement |
| radiation | ohms | attenuation | coupling medium | vibration |
| conversion | voltage | piezoelectric effect | effleurage | |

## ■ Connect Highlights   connect

*Visit connect.mcgraw-hill.com for further exercises to apply your knowledge:*

- Clinical application scenarios covering application of thermotherapy and cryotherapy techniques, use of ultrasound, use of electrical stimulating currents, and the use of massage, traction, and intermittent compression
- Click-and-drag questions covering thermotherapy and cryotherapy techniques, therapeutic modality nomenclature, and electrical stimulating currents
- Multiple-choice questions covering legal ramifications of the use of therapeutic modalities, theoretical use of modalities, and physiological uses of therapeutic modalities
- Picture identification of therapeutic modalities

Most athletic trainers routinely incorporate the use of therapeutic modalities into their rehabilitation programs.[12] When used appropriately, therapeutic modalities can be an effective adjunct to various techniques of therapeutic exercise. Rehabilitation protocols and progressions must be based primarily on the physiological responses of the tissues to injury and on an understanding of how various tissues heal. The decisions the athletic trainer makes on how and when therapeutic modalities may best be used should be based on his or her recognition of signs and symptoms as well as some awareness of the time frames associated with the various phases of the healing process. This chapter is an introduction to the therapeutic modalities that an athletic trainer may use: thermotherapy, cryotherapy, electrical stimulating currents, shortwave diathermy, low-level laser therapy, ultrasound, phonophoresis, traction, intermittent compression and massage.

## LEGAL CONCERNS

Therapeutic modalities must be used with the greatest care possible; they should not be used indiscriminately.

> **The athletic trainer must carefully follow laws that prohibit him or her from the use of certain therapeutic modalities.**

Specific laws governing the use of therapeutic modalities vary considerably from state to state. The athletic trainer must follow laws that specifically dictate how athletic trainers can use certain therapeutic modalities. An athletic trainer who uses any type of therapeutic modality must have a thorough understanding of the functions and the indications or contraindications for its use.[52]

The athletic trainer should avoid using a shotgun approach when deciding to incorporate therapeutic modalities into a treatment program. Selection of the appropriate modality should be based on an accurate clinical diagnosis of the injury and a decision about which modality can most effectively reach the desired target tissue to achieve specific results. The manufacturers of therapeutic modality equipment often provide recommended protocols for using their equipment in treating specific problems. The athletic trainer should certainly be familiar with these recommended treatment protocols. However, the athletic trainer does not necessarily have to follow the manufacturers' treatment protocols precisely. These are only recommendations. Decisions to alter recommended treatment protocols should be based on sound theory and previous experience. If used appropriately, modalities can be an integral part of a treatment and rehabilitation program.[52]

## CLASSIFICATION OF THERAPEUTIC MODALITIES

There is considerable confusion among even the most experienced clinicians regarding the different forms of energy involved with the various therapeutic modalities. The forms of energy that are relevant to the use of therapeutic modalities are thermal conductive energy, electrical energy, electromagnetic energy, sound energy, and mechanical energy.[51]

Thermotherapy and cryotherapy techniques transfer thermal energy. The electrical stimulating currents and iontophoresis use electrical energy. Shortwave and microwave diathermy, infrared lamps, ultraviolet light therapy, and low-power lasers use electromagnetic energy. Ultrasound and extracorporal shockwave therapy use sound energy. Intermittent compression, traction, and massage use mechanical energy.

> **Classifications of modalities:**
> - Thermal conductive energy
> - Electrical energy
> - Electromagnetic energy
> - Sound energy
> - Mechanical Energy

When these different forms of energy come in contact with human biological tissue, they can be reflected, refracted, absorbed, or transmitted. In human tissue, the energy must be absorbed before any physiological effects can take place.[51]

Each of these therapeutic agents transfers energy in one form or another into or out of biologic tissues. Different forms of energy can produce similar effects in biologic tissues. For example, tissue heating is a common effect of several treatments that use different types of energy. Electrical currents that pass through tissues will generate heat as a result of the resistance of the tissue to the passage of electricity. Electromagnetic energy such as light waves will heat any tissues that absorb it. Ultrasound treatments will also warm tissues through which the sound waves travel. Although the electrical, electromagnetic, and sound energy treatments all heat tissues, the physical mechanism of action for each is different.[51]

The mechanism of action of each therapeutic modality depends on which form of energy is used during its application.

## THERMAL CONDUCTIVE ENERGY MODALITIES

### Thermotherapy

The application of heat to treat disease and injuries has been used for centuries. Athletic trainers working in all settings use thermotherapy.

**Physiological Effects of Heat** The body's response to heat depends on the type of heat energy applied, the intensity of the heat energy, the duration of application, and the unique tissue response to heat. For a physiological response to occur, heat must be absorbed into the tissue and spread to adjacent tissue. To effect a therapeutic change that results in normal function of the absorbing tissue, the correct amount of heat must be applied. With too little, no change occurs; with too much, the tissue may be damaged.

The desirable therapeutic effects of heat include increasing the extensibility of collagen tissues; decreasing joint stiffness; reducing pain; relieving muscle spasm; reducing inflammation, edema, and exudates in the postacute phase of healing; and increasing blood flow.[53]

Heat increases the extensibility of collagen tissue, thus permitting an increase in extensibility through stretching. Muscle fibrosis, the joint capsule, contractures and scar tissue can all be effectively stretched after heating.[53] An increase in extensibility does not occur unless heat treatment is associated with stretching exercises.

> Heat has the capacity to increase the extensibility of collagen tissue.

Both heat and cold relieve pain via the gate control theory of pain modulation (see Chapter 10).[22] Muscle spasm caused by **ischemia** can be relieved by heat, which increases blood flow to the area of injury. Heat is also believed to assist the healing process by a number of mechanisms, such as raising temperature, increasing metabolism, reducing oxygen tension, lowering the pH level, increasing capillary permeability, and releasing histamine and bradykinin which cause vasodilation.

Thermal energy is transmitted through conduction, convection, radiation, and conversion. **Conduction** occurs when heat is transferred from a warmer object to a cooler one. The ratio of this heat exchange depends on the temperature and the exposure time. Skin temperatures are influenced by the type of heat or cold medium, the conductivity of the tissue, the quantity of blood flow in the area, and the speed at which heat is being dissipated.[45] To avoid tissue damage, the temperature should never exceed 116.6°F (47°C). An exposure that includes close contact with a hot medium that has a temperature of 113°F (45°C) should not exceed 30 minutes. Examples of conductive therapeutic modalities are hydrocollator packs, paraffin baths, electric heating pads, ice packs, and cold packs. **Convection** refers to the transference of heat through the movement of fluids or gases. Factors that influence convection heating are temperature, speed of movement, and the conductivity of the part.[53] The best example of modalities that use convection is hot and cold whirlpools. **Radiation** is the process whereby heat energy is transferred from one object through space to another object. Shortwave diathermy relies on the process of radiation for energy transfer. **Conversion** refers to the generation of heat from another energy form, such as sound, electricity, and chemical agents. The mechanical energy produced by high-frequency ultrasound sound waves changes to heat energy at tissue interfaces (ultrasound therapy).[53] The deep heat of shortwave diathermy can be produced by applying electrical currents of specific wavelengths to the skin. Chemical agents, such as liniments and balms, create a heating sensation through counterirritation of sensory nerve endings.[53]

Heat applied superficially to the skin directly increases the subcutaneous temperature and indirectly spreads to the deeper tissues. Muscle temperature increases through a reflexive effect on circulation and through conduction.[53] Comparatively, when heat is applied at the same temperature, moist heat causes a greater indirect increase in the deep-tissue temperature than does dry. Dry heat, in contrast to moist heat, can be tolerated at higher temperatures.

For the most part, moist heat aids the healing process in some local conditions by causing higher superficial tissue temperatures; however, joint and muscle circulation increase little in temperature. Superficial tissue is a poor thermal conductor, and temperature rises quickly on the skin surface as compared with the underlying tissues. The physiological responses to tissue heating are summarized in Table 15–1.

| TABLE 15–1 | Physiological Responses to Thermotherapy |
|---|---|
| **Variable** | **Response to Therapy** |
| Muscle spasm | Decreases |
| Pain perception | Decreases |
| Blood flow | Increases |
| Metabolic rate | Increases |
| Collagen elasticity | Increases |
| Joint stiffness | Decreases |
| Capillary permeability | Increases |
| Edema | Increases |

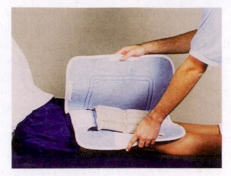

FIGURE 15–1   Protective layers of toweling or a commercially produced hydrocollator pack cover should be applied between the skin and a moist heat pack.
© William E. Prentice

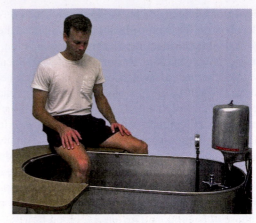

FIGURE 15–2   A whirlpool bath provides therapy through heat conduction and convection.
© William E. Prentice

## Hydrocollator Packs

**Equipment** Hydrocollator packs contain silicate gel in a cotton pad, which is immersed in thermostatically controlled hot water at a temperature of 160°F (71.1°C) to 170°F (76.7°C). Each pad retains water and a constant heat level for 20 to 30 minutes. Multiple layers of toweling or a commercially produced hydrocollator pack cover should be used between the packs and the skin (Figure 15–1).

**Indications** The major value of the hydrocollator pack is that its use results in general relaxation and reduction of the pain-spasm-ischemia-hypoxia-pain cycle. There are limitations of the hydrocollator pack in that the deeper tissues, including the musculature, are usually not significantly heated because the heat transfer from the skin surface into deeper tissues is inhibited by the subcutaneous fat, which acts as a thermal insulator, and by the increased blood flow to the skin, which cools and carries away the heat externally applied.[46]

**Application** Remove the pack from water and allow it to drain for a few seconds. Cover the pack dry toweling or commercial cover. Treat the area for 15 to 20 minutes. As the pack cools, remove layers of toweling to continue the heating.

**Special Considerations** The patient should not be lying on packs. Be sure the patient is comfortable at all times.[47]

## Whirlpool Baths

**Equipment** Whirlpool therapy is a combination of massage and water immersion. There are generally three types of whirlpools: the *extremity tank*, which is used for treating legs and arms; the *lowboy tank*, used for full-body immersion; and the *highboy tank*, which is designed for the hip or the leg.[7]

> The whirlpool bath combines heated water and massaging action.

The whirlpool is essentially a tank and a turbine motor, which regulates the movement of water and air. The amount of movement (agitation) is controlled by the amount of air that is emitted. The more air there is, the more water movement. The turbine motor can be moved up and down on a tubular column. It can also be rotated on the column and locked in place at a specific angle.

**Indications** The whirlpool provides both conduction and convection. Conduction is achieved by the skin's contact with the higher water temperature. As the water swirls around the skin surface, convection occurs (Figure 15–2).

This medium assists the body part by reducing swelling, muscle spasm, and pain. Because of the buoyancy of the water, active movement of the part is also assisted.

**Application** The water temperature should be set according to Table 15–2. As the volume of the body part submerged increases, the recommended water temperature

| TABLE 15–2 | Whirlpool Temperatures for Treatment of the Extremities |
|---|---|
| **Descriptive Terms** | **Temperature** |
| Very cold | >55°F (12.8°C) |
| Cold | 55°F–65°F (12.8°C–18.3°C) |
| Cool | 66°F–79°F (19°C–26°C) |
| Tepid | 80°F–90°F (27°C–33.5°C) |
| Neutral | 92°F–96°F (33.5°C–35.5°C) |
| Warm | 96°F–98°F (35.5°C–36.5°C) |
| Hot | 98°F–104°F (36.5°C–40°C) |
| Very hot | 104°F–110°F (40°C–43°C)* |

*Do not use water above 110°F.

should be decreased. A temperature that exceeds 104°F (40°C) should not be used for full body immersion. Some athletic trainers prefer to perform only cold-water treatments, whereas others prefer to increase the temperature according to the healing phase of an injury. Whirlpool use is contraindicated in acute injury because of the potential to increase swelling due to gravity-dependent positioning.[64] Chronic conditions normally require a higher water temperature.

Once the tank has been filled with water at the desired temperature, the patient is comfortably positioned so that the body part to be treated can be easily reached by the agitated water. In many cases, the water jet should not be placed directly on the body part but to the side of the tank. This placement is particularly relevant in the early stages of the acute injury.[64] In cases in which the stream is concentrated directly toward the injury site, the site should be at least 8 to 10 inches (20 to 25 cm) from the jet.

Treatment duration can be affected by many factors, including:

- whirlpool water temperature
- thickness of the subcutaneous fat in the area being treated
- the degree of tissue temperature increase necessary to accomplish the treatment goal

Therefore there is no universally recommended evidence-based treatment duration. In clinical practice treatment duration typically ranges between 20 and 30 minutes.

**Special Considerations** Caution should be taken anytime a patient is fully immersed in a whirlpool because of the possibility that the patient will experience lightheadedness.[46] Proper whirlpool maintenance is absolutely necessary to avoid infection—in particular, to prevent the spread of methicillin-resistant staphylococcus aureus (MRSA) (see Chapter 29). The whirlpool should be emptied and thoroughly disinfected after every patient. Both the inside and the outside of the tank as well as the turbine should be disinfected and dried.

Safety is of major importance in the use of the whirlpool. All electrical outlets should have a ground fault circuit interrupter. At no time should the patient turn the motor on or off. Ideally, the on/off switch should be a considerable distance from the machine.[46]

### Paraffin Bath

**Equipment** Paraffin is a popular method for applying heat to the distal extremities. The commercial paraffin bath is a thermostatically controlled unit that maintains a temperature of 126°F to 130°F (52°C to 54°C). The paraffin mixture consists of a ratio of 25 kilograms of paraffin wax to 1 liter of mineral oil. Slats at the bottom of the container protect the patient from burns

and collect the settling dirt. Also required for treatment are plastic bags, paper towels, and towels.

**Indications** The mineral oil acts to lower the melting point of the paraffin and thus the specific heat. Consequently, the ability to tolerate the heat from the paraffin is greater than it would be from water at the same temperature.[53]

This therapy is especially effective in treating chronic injuries occurring to the more angular areas of the body, such as the hands, wrists, elbows, ankles, and feet.

> Paraffin bath therapy is particularly effective for injuries to the more angular body areas.

**Application** Therapy by means of the paraffin bath can be delivered in several ways. The body part can be dipped and wrapped in a plastic bag, or it can be dipped and re-immersed to form eight to ten layers. The paraffin can be painted on in several layers, or the body part can be soaked in the paraffin.

Before therapy, the body part to be treated is thoroughly cleaned and dried. Then the patient dips the affected part into the paraffin bath and quickly pulls it out, allowing the accumulated wax to dry and form a solid covering. The process of dipping and withdrawing is repeated 6 to 12 times until the wax coating is ¼ to ½ inch (0.6 to 1.25 cm) thick.

If the dip and wrap technique is used, the accumulated wax is allowed to solidify on the last withdrawal; then the wax is completely wrapped in a plastic material, which in turn is wrapped with a towel. The packed body part is placed in a position of rest until heat is no longer generated. The covering is then removed and the paraffin is scraped back into the container.

If the soak technique is selected, the patient is instructed to soak the wax-coated part in the hot wax container for 15 to 20 minutes without moving it, after which the part is removed from the container and the paraffin on it is allowed to solidify. The part can be packed in towels following the soak, or the paraffin coating can be scraped back into the container immediately after it hardens. Once the paraffin has been removed from the part, an oily residue remains that provides an excellent surface for massage (Figure 15–3).

**Special Considerations** Avoid paraffin bath therapy on body areas that have open wounds or a decrease in normal circulation.

It is essential that the patient clean the body part thoroughly before therapy to avoid contaminating the mixture. In most cases, if this rule is closely adhered to, the mixture will only have to be replaced approximately every 6 months.[53]

**Fluidotherapy** Fluidotherapy creates a therapeutic environment with dry heat and forced convection through a suspended airstream.

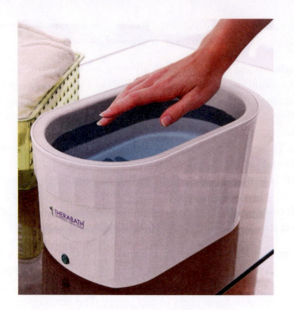

FIGURE 15–3 A paraffin bath is an excellent form of therapeutic heat for the distal extremities. After paraffin coating has been accomplished, the part is covered by a plastic material. When heat is no longer generated, the paraffin is scraped back into the container.
Courtesy WR Medical Electronics Company

**Equipment** Fluidotherapy units come in a variety of sizes, ranging from ones that treat distal extremities to ones that treat large body areas. The unit contains fine cellulose particles in which warm air is circulated. As the air is circulated, the cellulose particles become suspended, giving them properties that are similar to liquid.[53] Fluidotherapy allows the patient to tolerate much greater temperatures than would be possible using water or paraffin heat (Figure 15–4).

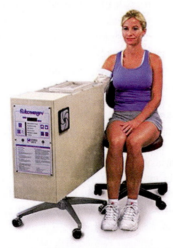

FIGURE 15–4 Fluidotherapy units contain fine cellulose particles in which warm air is circulated.
Courtesy DJO Global

**Indications** Fluidotherapy is effective in decreasing pain, increasing joint range of motion, decreasing muscle guarding.

**Application** Treatment temperature usually ranges from 100°F to 113°F (37.8°C to 45°C). Particle agitation should be controlled for comfort. Exercise can be performed while the patient is in the cabinet. The athlete should be positioned for comfort. Treatment duration is 15 to 20 minutes.

## Cryotherapy

The application of cold for the first aid of trauma to the musculoskeletal system is a widely used practice in sports medicine. When applied intermittently after injury, along with compression, elevation, and rest, it reduces many of the adverse conditions related to the inflammatory or reactive phase of an acute injury.[32,40,45] Depending on the severity of the injury, protection, optimal loading, ice, compression, and elevation (POLICE) may be used from the first day to as long as 2 weeks after injury.[40]

**Physiological Effects of Cold** In cryotherapy, the most common method for cold transfer to tissue is through conduction. The extent to which tissue is cooled depends on the cold medium that is being applied, the length of cold exposure, and the conductivity of the area being cooled.[45] In most cases, the longer the cold exposure, the deeper the cooling. At a temperature of 38.3°F (3.5°C), muscle temperatures can be reduced as deep as 1½ inches (4 cm). Cooling is dependent on the type of tissue. For example, tissue with a high water content, such as muscle, is an excellent cold conductor, whereas fat is a poor conductor. Because of fat's low cold conductivity, it acts as the body's insulator.[64] If no activity is involved, tissue that has previously been cooled takes longer to return to a normal temperature than does tissue that has been heated.

When cold is applied to skin for 20 minutes or less at a temperature of 50°F (10°C) or less, vasoconstriction of the arterioles and venules in the area occurs. This vasoconstriction is caused in part by the reflex action of the smooth muscles.[53]

It has been hypothesized that when local temperature is lowered considerably for a period of about 30 minutes, intermittent periods of vasodilation occur, lasting 4 to 6 minutes. This phenomenon has come to be known as the **hunting response** and is said to be necessary to prevent local tissue injury caused by cold. The hunting response has been accepted for a number of years as fact; in reality, however, it actually refers to measured temperature changes rather than circulatory changes. Some clinicians have taken the liberty of inferring that temperature changes produce circulatory changes, and this is simply not what the hunting response is. The hunting response is more likely a measurement artifact than an actual change in blood flow in response to cold.[53]

Trauma is a result of compromised circulation, which decreases the amount of oxygen being delivered to the cells in the area of injury. The immediate use of ice after injury decreases the extent of ischemic injury to those cells on the periphery of the primary injury by slowing their metabolic rate.[38] This slowdown results in less damage to the tissues and thus decreases rehabilitation time.[40]

Because cold lowers the metabolic rate and produces vasoconstriction, swelling will be reduced in an acute inflammatory response. Cold does not reduce swelling that is already present.[44]

Cooling tissues can directly decrease muscle guarding by slowing metabolism in the area, thus decreasing the waste products that may have accumulated—waste products that act as muscle irritants and cause spasm.

Because the local application of cold can decrease acute muscle guarding, the muscle becomes more amenable to stretch. A gentle stretch of a muscle after an acute injury may be indicated; however, the stretching of long-standing contractures is contraindicated. The use of either cold or heat does not appear to help increase muscle length when used in combination with proprioceptive neuromuscular facilitation (PNF) stretching.[53] Cold tends to cause collagen stiffness.[53]

Cold decreases free nerve ending excitability as well as the excitability of peripheral nerves.[10] Analgesia is caused by raising the nerve's threshold.[53]

> The extent of cooling depends on the thickness of the subcutaneous fat layer.

Nerve fiber response to cold depends mainly on the presence of myelination and the diameter of the fiber.[46] For example, most sensitive to cold are gamma efferent myelinated fibers to the muscle spindles.[53] The next most sensitive to cold are alpha motor nerves. The least sensitive to cold are the unmyelinated pain fibers and sympathetic nerves. During the application of cold, the patient experiences a progression of sensations from *cold*, to *burning*, to *aching*, and finally to *numbness* (CBAN). Table 15–3 indicates the usual outward sequential response to cold application.

Cold, in general, is more penetrating than heat. Once a muscle has been cooled through the subcutaneous fat layer, cold's effects last longer than heat effects do because fat acts as an insulator against rewarming.[53] The major problem is to penetrate the fat layer initially, so that muscle cooling occurs. In individuals with less than ½ inch (1.25 cm) of subcutaneous fat, significant muscle cooling can occur after 10 minutes of cold application. In persons with more than ⅘ inch (2 cm) of subcutaneous fat, muscle temperatures barely drop after 10 minutes (Table 15–4).[45,49]

## TABLE 15–3  Skin Response to Cold

| Stage | Response | Estimated Time after Initiation |
|---|---|---|
| 1 | Cold sensation | 0 to 3 minutes |
| 2 | Mild burning, aching | 2 to 7 minutes |
| 3 | Relative cutaneous numbness | 5 to 12 minutes |

## TABLE 15–4  Physiological Variables of Cryotherapy

| Variable | Response to Therapy |
|---|---|
| Muscle guarding | Decreases |
| Pain perception | Decreases |
| Blood flow | Decreases up to 10 minutes |
| Metabolic rate | Decreases |
| Collagen elasticity | Decreases |
| Joint stiffness | Increases |
| Capillary permeability | Increases |
| Edema | Controversial |

Another unique quality of cooling is its ability to decrease muscle fatigue and increase and maintain muscular contraction. This ability is attributed to the decrease of the local metabolic rate and the tissue temperature.[53] Although adverse reactions to therapeutic cold application are uncommon, they do happen and are described in *Focus Box 15–1*: "Adverse reactions to cold."

The two most common means of delivering cold as therapy to the body are ice or cold packs and immersion in cool or cold water. The most effective type of pack contains wet ice rather than ice in a plastic container or in a commercial chemical pack (e.g., Cryogen).[53] Wet ice is a more effective coolant because of (1) the extent of internal energy needed to melt the ice, and (2) the increased surface area contact which enhances conduction.[53] It has also been shown that ice that undergoes a phase change (i.e., ice melting to water) is more effective at lowering skin and intramuscular temperatures.[45]

### Ice Massage

***Equipment*** Water is frozen in a foam or waxed-paper cup, which forms a cylinder of ice. The foam is removed approximately an inch (2.5 cm) from the top of the cup. The remaining foam provides a handle for the athletic trainer to grasp while massaging. Another method is to fill a cup with water and insert a tongue depressor to act as a handle

> Cold therapy can begin immediately following injury.

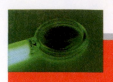

# FOCUS 15–1 Focus on Injury/Illness Prevention and Wellness Promotion

## Adverse reactions to cold

- Cooling for an hour at 30.2°F to 15.8°F (−1°C to −9°C) produces redness and edema that lasts for 20 hours after exposure. Frostbite has been known to occur in subfreezing temperatures of 26.6° to 24.8°F (−38 to −4°C).[40]
- Immersion at 41°F (5°C) increases limb fluid volume by 15 percent due to placing the limb in the dependent position.
- Exposure for 90 minutes at 57.2°F to 60.8°F (14°C to 16°C) can delay resolution of swelling up to 1 week.[40]
- Some individuals are allergic to cold and react with hives and joint pain and swelling.[53]
- Icing through a towel or an elastic bandage limits the reduction in temperature, which could influence the effectiveness of the treatment.[65]

- Raynaud's phenomenon is a condition that causes vasospasm of digital arteries lasting for minutes to hours, which could lead to tissue death. The early signs of Raynaud's phenomenon are attacks of intermittent skin blanching or cyanosis of the fingers or toes, skin pallor followed by redness, and finally a return to normal color. Pain is uncommon, but numbness, tingling, or burning may occur during and shortly after an attack.
- Although it is relatively uncommon, the application of ice can cause nerve palsy. Nerve palsy occurs when cold is applied to a part that has motor nerves close to the skin surface, such as the peroneal nerve at the fibular head. Usually, the condition resolves spontaneously with no significant problem. As a general rule, ice should not be applied longer than 45 minutes to an hour at any one time.

---

when the water is frozen. A towel should be present to absorb the water that is collected.

**Indications** Ice massage is commonly used over tendons, the belly of a muscle, bursae, or myofascial trigger points.

**Application** Ice massage is a cryotherapeutic method that is performed on a small body area. It can be applied by the athletic trainer or the patient. Grasping the ice cylinder, the athletic trainer rubs the ice over the patient's skin in overlapping circles in a 4- to 6-inch (10 to 15 cm) area for 5 to 10 minutes. The patient should experience the sensations of cold, burning, aching, and numbness. When analgesia has been reached, the patient can engage in stretching or exercise (Figure 15–5).

**Special Considerations** In a patient with normal circulation, tissue damage seldom occurs from cold application. The temperature of the tissue seldom goes below 59°F (15°C). However, when applying ice massage superficially, if an individual is going to have an adverse reaction to the cold, it tends to happen fairly early in the treatment.[34] The comfort of the patient must be considered at all times.

### Cold- or Ice-Water Immersion
**Equipment** Depending on the body part to be immersed, a variety of containers or basins can be used. In some cases, a small whirlpool can be used. Water and crushed ice are mixed together to reach a temperature of 50°F to 60°F (10°C to 15°C). Towels must be available for drying.

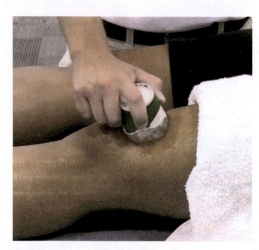

FIGURE 15–5 Ice massage can lead to analgesia, which can be followed by gentle muscle stretching.
© William E. Prentice

**Indications** Where circumferential cooling of a body part is desired, cold- or ice-water immersion is preferred.

**Application** The patient immerses the body part in the water and proceeds through the four stages of cold response. This process may take 10 to 15 minutes. Cold water

A dancer has Achilles tendinitis.

**?** What different methods of cryotherapy can be used to control pain and inflammation for this condition? Describe the benefits of each application.

immersion used in combination with electrical stimulation has been shown to minimize edema formation.[11]

**Special Considerations**  With immersion techniques, the extremities are in a gravity-dependent position thus increasing the likelihood of swelling. Overcooling can lead to frostbite. Any allergic response to cold should also be noted.

### Ice Packs (Bags)

**Equipment**  There are a number of types of ice packs. Wet ice packs provide the best cooling properties. Flaked or crushed ice can be encased in a wet towel and placed on the body part to be treated. An ice pack can be made by placing crushed or chipped ice in a self-sealing plastic bag. The packs easily fit the contour of the body part.

**Indications**  The patient experiences cold, burning aching and finally numbness (CBAN) and then proceeds with normal movement patterns (Figure 15–6).

**Application**  Two types of chemical cold packs are available. One is a gel pack that may be refrozen after use and is hypoallergenic. The gel pack is commonly used in many athletic training settings. The other type is a liquid bag within a bag of crystals. When the inner bag is ruptured, the chemicals mix, causing an endothermic reaction. If allowed contact with the skin, these chemicals can cause a chemical burn and a liability problem.[40] Plastic flexiwrap or an elastic wrap should be used to hold the pack firmly in place.

**Special Considerations**  Excessive cold exposure must be avoided. With chemical gel packs, it is recommended that a single layer of toweling be used. Crushed or flaked ice packs may be applied directly to the skin. With any indication of allergy to cold or of abnormal pain, the treatment should be discontinued.

### Vapocoolant Sprays

**Equipment**  The most popular vapocoolant is fluorimethane, a nonflammable, nontoxic substance. Under pressure in a bottle, it gives off a fine spray when it is inverted and an emitter is pressed.

**Indications**  The major value of a vapocoolant spray is its ability to reduce muscle guarding and increase range of motion. It is also a major treatment for myofascial pain and trigger points.

> Fluori-methane spray is used in the spray and stretch technique.

**Application**  When vapocoolant spray is used to increase the patient's range of motion in an area in which there is no trigger point, the following procedure is performed:

1. Hold the vapocoolant at a 30-degree angle, 12 to 18 inches (30 to 47 cm) from the skin.
2. Spray the entire length of the muscle from its proximal attachment to its distal attachment.
3. Cover the skin at a rate of approximately 4 inches (10 cm) per second; apply the spray two or three times as a gradual stretch is applied.

When dealing with a trigger point, the procedure is first to determine its presence, then to alleviate it. One method by which the athletic trainer can determine an active trigger point is to reproduce the injured patient's major pain complaint by pressing firmly on the site for 5 to 10 seconds. Another assessment technique is to elicit a jump response by placing the patient's muscle under moderate tension, applying firm pressure, and briskly pulling a finger across the tight band of muscle. This procedure causes the tight band of muscle to contract and the patient to wince.[53]

The spray and stretch method for treating trigger points and myofascial pain (Figure 15–7) using vapocoolant spray is performed as follows:[53]

1. Position the athlete in a relaxed but well-supported position. The muscle that contains the trigger point is stretched.
2. Alert the patient that the spray will feel cool.
3. Hold the fluori-methane bottle approximately 12 inches (30 cm) away from the skin to be sprayed.
4. Direct the spray at an acute angle in one direction toward the reference zone of pain.
5. Direct the spray to the full length of the muscle, including the reference zone of pain.
6. Begin firm stretching that is within the patient's pain tolerance.
7. Continue spraying in parallel sweeps that are approximately ¼ inch (0.6 cm) apart at a speed of approximately 4 inches (10 cm) every second.

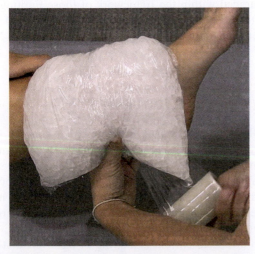

FIGURE 15–6  Ice packs are another way to apply cryotherapy. Use flexiwrap to hold the ice pack in place.
© William E. Prentice

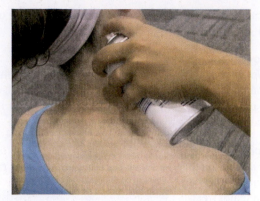

FIGURE 15–7 A vapocoolant spray, such as fluori-methane, can assist in reducing muscle spasm.

© William E. Prentice

8. Cover the skin area one or two times.
9. Continue passive stretching while spraying. Do not force the stretch; allow time for the muscle to let go.
10. After the first session of spraying and stretching, warm the muscle with a hot pack or by vigorous massage.
11. If necessary, perform a second session after step 10.
12. When a stretch has been completed, have the patient actively but gently move the part in a full range of motion.
13. Do not overload a muscle with strenuous exercise immediately after a stretch.
14. After an initial spraying and stretching session, instruct the patient about stretch exercises that should be performed at home on a daily basis.

### Cryokinetics

**Indications** **Cryokinetics** is a technique that combines cryotherapy, or the application of cold, with exercise.[40] The goal of cryokinetics is to numb the injured part to point of analgesia and then work toward achieving normal range of motion through progressive active exercise.

**Equipment** The technique uses ice immersion, cold packs, or ice massage.

**Application** The technique begins by numbing the body part. Patients report a feeling of numbness within 12 to 20 minutes. If numbness is not perceived within 20 minutes, the athletic trainer should proceed with exercise regardless. The numbness usually lasts for 3 to 5 minutes, at which point ice should be reapplied for an additional 3 to 5 minutes until numbness returns. This sequence should be repeated five times (see *Focus Box 15–2*: "Summary of cryokinetics"). Exercises are performed during the periods of numbness. The exercises selected should be pain free and progressive

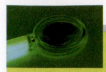

### Summary of cryokinetics[40]

1. Immerse ankle in ice water until numb (12 to 20 min).
2. Exercise within limits of pain (see progression in step 6) (3 to 5 min).
3. Renumb ankle by immersion (3 to 5 min).
4. Exercise within limits of pain (3 to 5 min).
5. Repeat steps 3 and 4 three more times.
6. Principles of exercising:
   a. All exercise should be active–that is, performed totally by the patient.
   b. All exercise must be pain free.
   c. All exercise must be performed smoothly, without limping, twitching, or any other abnormal motion.
   d. The exercise must be aggressively progressive– that is, it must progress to more complex and difficult levels as quickly as possible (remember–*no pain*).

Knight K: *Cryotherapy in sports injury management*, Champaign, Ill., 1995, Human Kinetics.

in intensity; the patient should concentrate on both flexibility and strength.[57]

***Special Considerations*** Changes in the intensity of the activity should be limited by both the nature of the healing process and individual patient differences in perception of pain. However, progression always should be encouraged within the framework of those limiting factors; the ultimate goal is to return the athlete to full sport activities.[40]

## ELECTRICAL ENERGY MODALITIES

**Physical Properties of Electricity** In general, electricity is a form of energy that displays magnetic, chemical, mechanical, and thermal effects on tissue.[25] It implies a flow of electrons between two points. Electrons are particles of matter that have a negative electrical charge and revolve around the core, or nucleus, of an atom.

An electrical current is a string of electrons that pass along a conductor, such as a nerve or wire. The volume or amount of the current is measured in **amperes** (A); 1 A equals the rate of flow of 1 coulomb (C) per second.

A coulomb is a unit of electrical charge and is defined as the quantity of an electrical charge that can be transferred by 1 A in 1 second.

Resistance to the passing of an electrical current along a conductor is measured in **ohms** ($\Omega$), and the force that moves the current along is called **voltage** (V). One volt is the amount of electrical force required to send a current of 1 A through a resistance of 1 $\Omega$. In terms of electrotherapy, currents of 0 to 150 V are considered low-voltage currents, and currents above 150 V are considered high-voltage. The intensity of a current varies directly with the voltage and inversely with the resistance. Electrical power is measured in **watts** (amps × volts).[60]

An electrical current applied to nerve tissue at a sufficient intensity and duration to reach that tissue's excitability threshold will result in a membrane depolarization, or firing, of that nerve. There are three major types of nerve fibers: sensory, motor, and pain. As current intensity or duration is increased, the threshold for depolarization will be reached first for sensory fibers, then for motor fibers, and then for pain fibers. Thus, it is possible to produce different physiological responses by adjusting the treatment parameters.[29]

**Equipment** Electrotherapeutic devices generate three types of current, which, when introduced into biological tissue, are capable of producing specific physiological changes. These three types of current are monophasic (DC), biphasic (AC), and pulsatile.[29]

> Electrical currents include monophasic (DC), biphasic (AC), and pulsatile.

A great deal of confusion has developed about the terminology used to describe electrotherapeutic currents. All therapeutic electrical generators, regardless of whether they deliver biphasic, monophasic, or pulsatile currents through electrodes attached to the skin, are *transcutaneous electrical stimulators.* The majority of these generators are used to stimulate peripheral nerves and are correctly called *transcutaneous electrical nerve stimulators (TENS)* (Figure 15–8). Occasionally, the terms *neuromuscular electrical stimulator (NMES)* and *electrical muscle stimulator (EMS)* are used; however, these terms are appropriate only when the electrical current is being used to stimulate muscle directly, as would be the case with denervated muscle in which peripheral nerves are not functioning. A type of transcutaneous electrical stimulator that uses current intensities too small to excite peripheral nerves has been called a *microcurrent electrical nerve stimulator (MENS)*, although this type is currently being referred to as a *low-intensity stimulator (LIS).*[29]

**Monophasic Current (DC)** Monophasic current, also called direct current, flows in one direction only from the

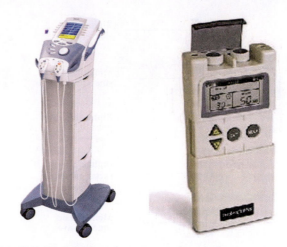

FIGURE 15–8   Many therapeutic electrical generators are transcutaneous electrical nerve stimulators (TENS).
Courtesy DJO Global

positive pole to the negative pole. DC may be used for pain modulation or muscle contraction or to produce ion movement. Specific physiological effects are determined by how the treatment parameters are set on the stimulating unit. Most electrical stimulators currently used in athletic training settings are monophasic units which deliver pulsed high-voltage currents.

**Biphasic Current (AC)** With biphasic current, also called alternating current, the direction of current flow reverses itself once during each cycle. Biphasic current may be used for pain modulation or muscle contraction.

**Pulsatile Current** Pulsatile currents usually contain three or more pulses grouped together. These groups of pulses are interrupted for short periods of time and repeat themselves at regular intervals. Pulsatile currents are used in interferential pre-modulated and so-called Russian currents.

**Current parameters**

*Waveform* A waveform is a graphic representation of the shape, direction, amplitude, and direction of a particular electrical current. Electrical stimulating units can take on various waveforms depending on the capability of the generator. Biphasic, monophasic,

> **Current parameters:**
> - Waveform
> - Modulation
> - Intensity
> - Duration
> - Frequency
> - Polarity
> - Electrode setup

and pulsatile units can produce currents with waveforms that are sine, rectangular, square, or spiked in shape (Figure 15–9).

*Modulation* Current modulation is the ability of the electrical stimulating unit to change the magnitude or

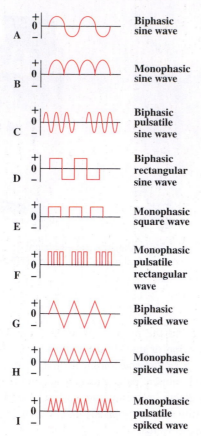

FIGURE 15–9    Waveforms of monophasic, biphasic, or pulsatile current may be either sine, rectangular, square, or spiked in shape.

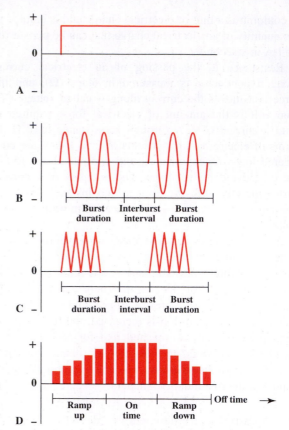

FIGURE 15–10    Current may be modulated using. **(A)** Continuous current. **(B)** Burst-modulated alternating current. **(C)** Burst-modulated pulsatile current. **(D)** Ramp-up and ramp-down modulation.

duration of a waveform. Modulation may be continuous, bursts, or surging for biphasic, monophasic, and pulsatile currents (Figure 15–10).

***Intensity*** Current intensity is the voltage output of the stimulating unit. Generators that produce voltage outputs of up to 150 V are low-voltage generators. Those that produce up to 500 V are high-voltage generators. Low-voltage generators are almost always monophasic; high-voltage generators may be either biphasic or monophasic. The majority of the electrical stimulators used in athletic training settings are high-voltage monophasic generators.

***Duration*** *Duration* refers to the length of time that current is flowing. It is also referred to as pulse width or pulse duration. Duration is preset on most of the high-voltage monophasic stimulators.

***Frequency*** **Frequency** refers to the number of waveforms being emitted by the electrical stimulating unit in 1 second. Frequency is identified in pulses per second (pps), cycles per second (cps), or hertz (Hz). Frequencies range from one pps to several thousand pps.

***Polarity*** Polarity is the direction of current flow toward either a positive or a negative pole.

***Electrode setup*** In electrotherapy, electrode pads are affixed directly to the skin. Electrodes are of different sizes. Using a large *(dispersive)* electrode remote from the treatment area while placing a smaller *(active)* electrode as close as possible to the nerve or muscle motor point will give the greatest effect at the small electrode. The large electrode disperses the current over a large area; the small electrode concentrates the current in the area of the motor point. The physiological effects can occur anywhere between the two pads, but they usually occur at the active electrode because current density (the amount of current in a given area) is greater at this point.[25] Many newer electrical stimulating units have pads that are of equal size; thus, both electrodes are considered active electrodes.

**Indications** Monophasic, biphasic, and pulsatile currents may all be used to achieve a specific therapeutic effect.[29] Clinically, athletic trainers use electrical currents for several purposes: to produce the depolarization of sensory nerves to modulate pain, to produce a depolarization of motor nerve fibers to elicit a muscle contraction, to create an electrical field to the biological tissues to stimulate or alter the healing process at the cellular level, and to create an electrical field on the skin surface to transport ions beneficial to the healing process into deeper target tissues.[29]

## Application

***Pain Modulation*** Electrical stimulating currents can reduce pain associated with injury.[29] The neurophysiological mechanisms associated with pain modulation—including gate control, descending pathway pain control, and opiate pain control—were discussed in Chapter 10.

***Gate control*** Electrical stimulation of sensory nerves will evoke the gate control mechanism and diminish awareness of painful stimuli. As long as the stimulation is causing the sensory nerves to fire, the gate to pain should be closed. If the stimulus stops, the gate is then open, and pain returns to perception. The following parameters can be used for gate control: Intensity should be adjusted to create a tingling sensation but should not cause a muscular contraction, and frequency should be set as high as possible to create as much sensory cutaneous stimulation as possible.[29]

***Descending pathway pain control*** Intense electrical stimulation of the smaller pain fibers at trigger and acupuncture points for short time periods causes stimulation of descending neurons, which then affect the transmission of pain information by closing the gate at the spinal cord level. Current intensity should be very high, approaching a noxious level; pulse duration should be 10 microseconds (msec); frequency should be 80 pulses per second.[29]

***Opiate pain control*** Electrical stimulation of sensory nerves stimulates the release of enkephalin from local sites throughout the central nervous system and the release of β-endorphins from the pituitary gland into the cerebrospinal fluid. Pain modulation is caused by applying an electrical current to areas close to the site of pain or to acupuncture or trigger points both local to and distant from the pain area. A point stimulator can be used, with current intensity set as high as tolerable; pulse duration should be set at the maximum possible on the machine; frequency should be set at 1 to 5 pps.[29]

**Muscle Contraction** The quality of a muscle contraction changes according to the changes in current parameters. As the frequency of stimulation increases, the muscle develops more tension because of progressive shortening of the muscle, until a tetanic contraction is achieved.[29] **Tetany** occurs for virtually all muscles at approximately 50 pps. Increases in intensity spread the current over a larger area and increase the number of motor units activated by the current. Increases in current duration also cause more motor units to be activated. A variety of therapeutic gains can be made by electrically stimulating a muscle contraction; these gains include muscle pumping contractions, muscle strengthening, retardation of atrophy, and muscle reeducation.

A muscle contraction can be used for

- Muscle pumping
- Muscle strengthening
- Retardation of atrophy
- Muscle reeducation

***Muscle pumping*** This type of contraction is used to help stimulate circulation by pumping fluid and blood through the venous and lymphatic channels back to the heart. High-voltage monophasic current is recommended. Intensity should be increased to elicit a muscle contraction at a frequency of 20 to 40 pps, using a surged mode with on/off times set at 5 seconds each. The injured body part should be elevated, and active contraction should be encouraged. Treatment time is twenty to thirty minutes.[25]

***Muscle strengthening*** Electrical stimulation can be used to facilitate strength gains. High-frequency biphasic current is recommended. Intensity should be increased at a frequency of 50 to 60 pps to elicit a tetanic muscle contraction using surging current set at 15 seconds on and 50 seconds off. Treatment should include 10 repetitions three times per week. For best results, the patient should combine this electrically induced tetanic contraction with maximal active contraction against some resistance.[29]

***Retardation of atrophy*** Electrically induced muscle contraction can be used to minimize the atrophy and loss of muscle function that typically occurs with immobilization after injury. High-frequency biphasic current is recommended. Intensity should be increased to 30 to 60 pps to elicit a tetanic contraction using interrupted current mode. The athlete should incorporate voluntary isometric contraction. Treatment time should be 15 to 20 minutes.[29]

**Muscle Reeducation** Muscular inhibition after surgery or injury can be reduced by electrically stimulating a muscle. Intensity should be increased to a level necessary for a comfortable contraction at 30 to 50 pps using either interrupted or surged current. The athlete should watch and feel the contraction and attempt to initiate a voluntary contraction. Treatment time is 15 to 20 minutes; treatment is repeated several times daily.[29]

## Iontophoresis

Iontophoresis is a therapeutic technique that involves the introduction of ions into the body tissues by means of a direct electrical current.[60]

Iontophoresis uses electrical current to drive ions.

**Equipment** The iontophoresis generator must output continuous monophasic current to ensure the unidirectional migration of ions, which cannot be accomplished using a biphasic current. Current intensity ranges between 1 and 5 milliamps.

**Indications** Clinically, iontophoresis is used in the treatment of inflammatory musculoskeletal conditions; for analgesic effects, scar modification, and wound healing; and in treating edema, calcium deposits, and hyperhydrosis.[6]

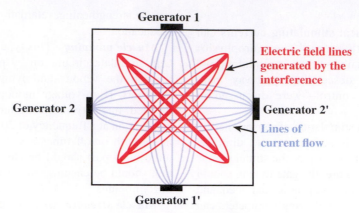

**Generator 1**

**Electric field lines generated by the interference**

**Generator 2**

**Generator 2'**

**Lines of current flow**

**Generator 1'**

FIGURE 15–11   Pattern created by interferential currents.

**Application** A self-adhering, prepared electrode, either reusable or commercially produced, must be securely attached to the skin. There are three techniques of application: An active pad is applied over gauze that is saturated with a solution containing the ions (this pad is positioned as close as possible to the involved tissue); the active electrode is suspended in a container of the ion solution, and then the body part to be treated is immersed in the container; or a special active electrode with a reservoir into which a treatment ion can be injected and stored is positioned as close to the involved tissue as possible. In all cases, a large dispersive pad is applied to the patient. The manner in which ions move in solution forms the basis for iontophoresis. Positively charged ions are transported into the tissue from the positive pole, and negatively charged ions are transported under the negative pole. Treatment time varies from 10 to 20 minutes, depending on the intensity of the current or the current density at the active electrode, the duration of the current flow, and the concentration of ions in solution.[60] Dexamethasone and hydrocortisone are two of the most commonly used ions in iontophoresis.[6]

**Special Considerations** The athletic trainer needs to be knowledgeable in the selection of the most appropriate ions for treating specific conditions. Perhaps the single most common problem associated with iontophoresis is a chemical burn, which usually occurs as a result of the direct current itself, not because of the ion being used in treatment.

## Interferential Currents

**Equipment** Interferential currents make use of two separate electrical generators that emit currents at two slightly different frequencies. Two pairs of electrodes are arranged in a square pattern such that the currents cross one another, creating an interference pattern at a central point of stimulation. The interference pattern creates a larger area of stimulation (Figure 15–11).[15]

**Indications** Interferential currents have been used for a variety of clinical conditions, including pain, joint pain with swelling, neuritis, retarded callus formation following fracture, and restricted mobility.

**Application** Positioning of the electrodes is critical to the success of the treatment. The athletic trainer must move the electrodes around until the patient indicates that the stimulation is centered over the area of pain. A frequency of stimulation should be selected with interferential currents that is similar to using other electrical stimulators: 20 to 25 pps for muscle contraction and 50 to 120 pps for pain management.

**Special Considerations** Although interferential currents are more complex from an engineering perspective than other electrical stimulating currents, the potential therapeutic effects are essentially the same.

## Low-Intensity Stimulators

**Equipment** Low-intensity stimulators (LIS) were originally referred to as microcurrent electrical nerve stimulators, or MENS. Low-intensity stimulators deliver current to the patient at very low frequencies (1 pps) and at low intensities (less than 1 milliamp) that are subsensory.

**Indications** This type of current is used to stimulate the healing process in both soft tissue and bone by altering the electrical activity to mimic a normal electrical field in normal individual cells. Specifically, it has been used to modulate pain and promote healing of wounds, nonunion fractures, and tendons and ligaments.

**Application** The electrical currents used by low-intensity stimulators are no different than those described previously. The athletic trainer need only turn the unit on and slightly increase the intensity. A large dispersive electrode keeps the current density low enough that threshold levels for depolarization of sensory nerves are not achieved.

**Special Considerations** The effectiveness of LIS therapy is currently based primarily on theory; there is little research information to support its use.[29]

# ELECTROMAGNETIC ENERGY MODALITIES

## Shortwave Diathermy

**Physiological Effects of Diathermy** Shortwave diathermy emits electromagnetic energy that is capable of producing temperature increases in the deeper tissues. Tissues with a higher water content (e.g., muscle) selectively absorb the heat delivered by shortwave diathermy.[55] The extent of muscle heating depends on the thickness of the subcutaneous fat layer.[55] Shortwave diathermy provides heat penetration similar to that of ultrasound. In contrast to shortwave diathermy, ultrasonic vibration is not absorbed by fat and is therefore not influenced by its thickness.[30]

Shortwave diathermy heats deeper tissues by introducing a high-frequency electrical current. Shortwave diathermy is in essence a radio transmitter; the Federal Communications Commission (FCC) has assigned a wavelength of 7.5 to 22 meters and a frequency of 13.56 or 27.12 megacycles per second for therapeutic purposes.[55]

Shortwave diathermy can be used in two ways: through capacitance that uses electrostatic field heating or through induction that uses electromagnetic field heating.[55] In electrostatic field heating, the patient is a part of the circuit. Heating is uneven because of different tissue resistance to energy flow, an application of Joule's law, which states that the greater the resistance, the more heat will develop. In electromagnetic field heating, the patient is not part of the circuit, but is heated by an electromagnetic field.[55]

Pulsed shortwave diathermy (PSWD), also referred to as pulsed electromagnetic energy (PEME) or pulsed electromagnetic fields (PEF) is a relatively new form of diathermy.[50] Pulsed diathermy is created by simply interrupting the output of continuous shortwave diathermy at consistent intervals. Pulsing reduces the likelihood of any significant tissue temperature increase and reduces the patient's perception of heat. Generators that deliver pulsed shortwave diathermy typically use a drum type of electrode. Pulsed diathermy is claimed to have therapeutic value and to produce nonthermal effects with minimal thermal

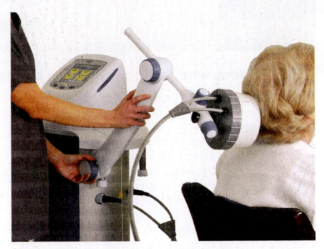

FIGURE 15–12 A shortwave diathermy unit: Courtesy DJO Global

physiological effects, depending on the intensity of the application. When pulsed diathermy is used in intensities that create an increase in tissue temperature, its effects are no different from those of continuous shortwave diathermy.[50]

### Shortwave Diathermy Treatments

*Equipment* In general, the shortwave diathermy unit consists of a power supply to a power amplifier and a frequency generator. It has an oscillator that produces high frequency (either 13.56 or 27.12 megacycles) and a power amplifier that converts biphasic current to monophasic current.[55] It also has a circuit that tunes in the patient automatically or manually as part of the circuitry (Figure 15–12).

The shortwave diathermy treatment applicators or electrodes are either capacitor or inductive types.[55] With the capacitor type electrodes the patient is a natural part of the circuit. The capacitor electrodes use a piece of flexible or rigid metal housed in either a pad or in plastic air space plates.

An inductive-type electrode is the drum unit that makes up of one or more coils that are rigidly fixed inside some kind of housing. If a small area is to be treated, particularly a small flat area, then a one-drum setup is fine. However, if the area is contoured, then two or more drums, which may be on a hinged apparatus or hinged arm, may be more suitable.[30]

*Indications* Shortwave diathermy is used to treat bursitis, capsulitis, osteoarthritis, and muscle strains. The depth of the inductive technique can be as much as 2 inches (5 cm). The capacitance technique penetrates from 1 to 2 inches (2.5 to 5 cm). Tissue temperature can reach 107°F (41.7°C).[55] Although shortwave diathermy has been used in connection with stretching, it is not clear whether using both diathermy and

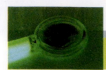

# FOCUS 15–3 Focus on Therapeutic Intervention

| TABLE 15–5 | Sample Shortwave Diathermy Dosage | |
|---|---|---|
| **Dosage** | **Effect** | **Application** |
| Lowest dose (I) | Just below the point of any sensation of heat (acute inflammatory process) | 20 to 30 minutes daily for 2 weeks |
| Low dose (II) | Mild heat sensation, barely felt (subacute, resolving inflammatory process) | 20 to 30 minutes daily for 2 weeks |
| Medium dose (III) | Moderate but pleasant heat sensation (subacute, resolving inflammatory process) | 20 to 30 minutes from 2 to 3 times weekly for 1 to 4 weeks |
| Heavy dose (IV) | Vigorous heating that causes a sensation that is well tolerated (chronic conditions): pain threshold should not be exceeded | 20 to 30 minutes from 2 to 3 times weekly for 1 to 4 weeks |

stretching increases flexibility more than stretching alone.[16,50]

**Application** If more superficial heating is desired, a capacitance electrode is used; when deeper therapy is desired, the induction electrode should be used. When the patient is as comfortable as possible, he or she is tuned in with the oscillating circuit of the unit. In most cases, the treatment times range from 20 to 30 minutes (Table 15–5).[55] *Focus Box 15–3*: "Precautions when using shortwave diathermy" offers important information about this technique.

**Special Considerations** Shortwave diathermy and ultrasound are both considered to be deep-heating modalities. Shortwave diathermy has been shown to be as effective as 1 Mhz ultrasound in increasing tissue temperature at a depth of 1⅛ inches (3 cm). Although ultrasound is much more widely used than shortwave diathermy, shortwave diathermy would be the modality of choice in certain treatment situations. If the treatment area is large, diathermy is more effective than ultrasound

in effectively heating it. If any condition exists in which pressure from an ultrasound transducer exacerbates pain, then shortwave diathermy is preferable. Unlike an ultrasound treatment, once a shortwave diathermy unit has been appropriately set up, it does not require constant monitoring by the athletic trainer.

## Low-Level Laser Therapy

*LASER* is an acronym that stands for **l**ight **a**mplification by **s**timulated **e**mission of **r**adiation (Figure 15–13).[59]

**Equipment** Helium neon (HeNe, a gas) and gallium arsenide (GaAs, a semiconductor) lasers are two low-level lasers currently used in the United States and other countries for wound and soft-tissue healing and pain relief.[42] HeNe lasers deliver a characteristic red beam with a direct penetration of 0.07 to 0.5 inch (2 to 13 mm) and an indirect penetration of 0.4 to 0.6 inch (10 to 15 mm). GaAs lasers are invisible and have a direct penetration of 0.4 to 0.8 inch (1 to 2 cm) and an indirect penetration to 2 inches (5 cm).

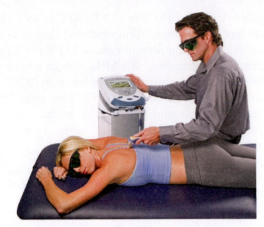

FIGURE 15–13 Low-level laser unit.
Courtesy DJO Global

**Indications** The proposed therapeutic applications of lasers in physical medicine include acceleration of collagen synthesis, decrease in microorganisms, increase in vascularization, and reduction of pain and inflammation.[41,59] Trigger or acupuncture points are also treated for painful conditions.

**Application** The technique of laser application ideally is done with gentle contact with the skin surface and should be perpendicular to the target surface.[35] Dosage appears to be the critical factor in eliciting the desired response, but exact dosimetry has not been determined. Dosage fluctuates by varying the pulse frequency and the treatment times. The laser is applied by developing an imaginary grid over the target area. The grid comprises 1 cm squares, and the laser is applied to each square for a predetermined time.

**Special Considerations** Although no deleterious effects have been reported, certain precautions and contraindications exist. Contraindications include lasing over cancerous tissue, directly into the eyes, and during the first trimester of pregnancy. Occasionally, pain may increase when laser treatments begin but does not indicate cessation of treatment. A low percentage of patients have experienced a syncope episode during laser treatment, but this is usually self-resolving.[31]

# SOUND ENERGY MODALITIES

## Therapeutic Ultrasound

Ultrasound is another widely used modality in athletic training. It is a valuable therapeutic tool in the rehabilitation of many different injuries because it stimulates the repair of soft-tissue injuries and relieves pain.[17] Ultrasound is a deep-heating modality and is used primarily for elevating tissue temperatures. It is a form of acoustic rather than electromagnetic energy. Ultrasound is defined as inaudible, acoustic vibrations of high frequency that may produce either thermal or nonthermal physiological effects.[17] The use of ultrasound as a therapeutic agent may be extremely effective if the athletic trainer has an adequate understanding of its effects on biological tissues and of the physical mechanisms by which these effects are produced.[17]

The number of movements, or oscillations, in 1 second is referred to as the frequency of a sound wave and is known as a hertz (Hz) unit. More commonly, 1 Hz equals 1 cycle per second, 1 kHz equals 1,000 cycles per second, and 1 MHz equals 1 million cycles per second.[17] The human ear cannot detect sound greater than 20,000 Hz; therefore, inaudible sound is considered ultrasound. When sound scatters and absorbs as it penetrates tissue, its energy is decreased (**attenuation**). Absorption of sound increases with an increase in frequency.

Tissue penetration depends on impedance or acoustical properties of the media that are proportional to tissue density.[20] Sound reflection occurs when adjacent tissues have different impedance. The greater the impedance, the greater the reflection, and the more heat produced. The greatest heat is developed between bone and the adjacent soft-tissue interface.

**Equipment** The main piece of equipment for delivering therapeutic ultrasound is a high-frequency generator, which provides an electrical current through a coaxial cable to a transducer contained within an applicator. In the applicator or transducer are synthetic crystals, such as barium titanate or lead zirconate titanate, that possess the property of piezoelectricity. These crystals are in disks 0.07 to 0.1 inch (2 to 3 mm) thick and 0.4 to 1.2 inches (1 to 3 cm) in diameter.[17] The **piezoelectric effect** causes expansion and contraction of the crystals, which produce oscillation voltage at the same frequency as the sound wave.[17]

**Frequency** Therapeutic ultrasound has a frequency range between 0.75 and 3.0 MHz. The majority of ultrasound generators are set at a frequency between 1 and 3 MHz. A generator that can be set between 1 and 3 MHz affords the athletic trainer the greatest treatment flexibility. Ultrasound energy generated at 1 MHz is transmitted through the more superficial tissues and absorbed primarily in the deeper tissues at depths of 1.2 to 2 inches (3 to 5 cm).[43] A 1 MHz frequency is most useful in individuals with high percent body fat cutaneously and whenever the desired effects are in the deeper structures.[17,43] At 3 MHz the energy is absorbed in the more superficial tissues with a depth of penetration between 0.4 and 0.8 inch (1 and 2 cm).[18]

> Ultrasound can be applied either to the skin or through a water medium.

***Ultrasound beam*** The portion of the surface of the ultrasound transducer that produces the sound wave is referred to as the **effective radiating area**. Energy is delivered to the tissues in a collimated cylindrical beam. The beam from ultrasound generated at 1 MHz is more divergent than at 3 MHz. Within this beam, the distribution of ultrasound energy is nonuniform. The amount of variability of intensity in the beam is indicated by the **beam nonuniformity ratio (BNR)**. The lower the BNR, the more uniform the energy output. Optimally, the BNR would be 1:1.

***Intensity*** The intensity of the ultrasound beam is determined by the amount of energy delivered to the sound head (applicator). It is expressed in the number of watts per square centimeter ($W/cm^2$). As a therapeutic modality used in sports medicine, the intensity ranges from 0.1 to 3 $W/cm^2$.

***Pulsed versus continuous ultrasound*** Virtually all therapeutic ultrasound generators can emit either continuous or pulsed ultrasound waves. If continuous ultrasound is used, the sound intensity remains constant throughout the treatment and the ultrasound energy is being produced 100 percent of the time. With pulsed ultrasound, the output is periodically interrupted and no ultrasound energy is produced during the off period. The percentage of time that ultrasound is being generated is referred to as the *duty cycle*. If the pulse duration is 1 millisecond and the total pulse period is 5 milliseconds, the duty cycle is 20 percent. Therefore, the total amount of energy being delivered to the tissues is only 20 percent of the energy that would be delivered if a continuous wave were being used.

> Ultrasound can be continuous or pulsed.

> The duty cycle is the percentage of time that ultrasound is being generated.

Continuous ultrasound is most commonly used to produce thermal effects. The use of pulsed ultrasound results in a reduced average heating of the tissues. Pulsed ultrasound or continuous ultrasound at a low intensity produces nonthermal or mechanical effects, which may be associated with soft-tissue healing.[57]

### Indications

***Thermal versus nonthermal effects*** Therapeutic ultrasound produces both *thermal* and *nonthermal effects*.[34] Traditionally, ultrasound has been used primarily to produce a tissue temperature increase. The clinical effects of using ultrasound to heat the tissues are similar to those of other forms of superficial heat, discussed in earlier sections. For the majority of these effects to occur, the tissue temperature must

> Ultrasound produces effects that are thermal or nonthermal.

be raised to a level of 104°F to 113°F (40°C to 45°C) for a minimum of five minutes.[26] Temperatures below this range are ineffective, and temperatures above 113°F (45°C) may be damaging.[17] Ultrasound at 1 MHz with an intensity of 1 $W/cm^2$ can raise soft-tissue temperature by 0.2°C per minute; at 3 MHz, by as much as 0.6°C per minute.[17,25]

Whenever ultrasound is used to produce thermal changes, nonthermal changes also occur. However, if appropriate treatment parameters are selected, nonthermal effects can occur with minimal thermal effects.[69] The nonthermal effects of therapeutic ultrasound include *cavitation* and acoustic *microstreaming*. Cavitation is the formation of gas-filled bubbles that expand and compress because of ultrasonically induced pressure changes in tissue fluids.[34] Cavitation results in an increased flow in the fluid around these vibrating bubbles. Microstreaming is the unidirectional movement of fluids along the boundaries of cell membranes, resulting from the mechanical pressure wave in an ultrasonic field.[17] Microstreaming can alter cell membrane structure and function because of changes in cell membrane permeability to sodium and calcium ions important in the healing process. As long as the cell membrane is not damaged, microstreaming can be of therapeutic value in accelerating the healing process.[17] These nonthermal effects have been reported to alter membrane properties, alter cellular proliferation, and produce increases in proteins associated with inflammation and injury repair, implying that ultrasound can modify the inflammatory response.[34] The proposed *frequency resonance hypothesis* relates to the absorption of the mechanical energy of ultrasound by proteins and protein complexes, resulting in alterations to signaling mechanisms within the cell and disturbance of the cellular membrane and the molecular structures within the cell. This may help explain the mechanisms responsible for changes in cell membrane permeability as well as an increase in protein production, which collectively may facilitate healing.

> Nonthermal effects include cavitation and microstreaming.

The nonthermal effects of therapeutic ultrasound in the treatment of injured tissues may be as important as the thermal effects and perhaps are even more important. The nonthermal effects—cavitation and microstreaming—can be maximized and the thermal effects minimized by using an intensity of 0.1 to 0.2 $W/cm^2$ with continuous ultrasound or 1.0 $W/cm^2$ at a duty cycle of 20 percent.

Acute conditions require frequent treatments over a short period of time, whereas chronic conditions require fewer treatments over a longer period of time.[17] Ultrasound treatments should begin as soon as possible after injury, ideally within hours but definitely within 48 hours, to maximize their effects on the healing process.[17] Acute conditions may be treated using low-intensity

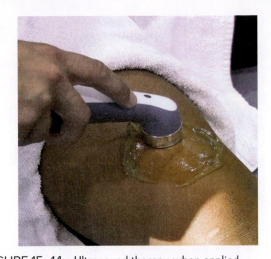

FIGURE 15–14   Ultrasound therapy, when applied directly to the skin, must be performed over a coupling medium because acoustic energy cannot travel through air.
© William E. Prentice

ultrasound once or twice daily for 6 to 8 days until acute symptoms, such as pain and swelling, subside. In chronic conditions, when acute symptoms have subsided, treatment may be done on alternating days for a total of 10 to 12 treatments.

**Application**   There are a number of options for using ultrasound in sports medicine.

*Direct skin application*   Because acoustic energy cannot travel through air and is reflected by the skin, there must be a **coupling medium** applied to the skin.[17] Coupling media include a variety of materials, such as mineral oil and water-soluble creams or gels. The purpose of a coupling medium is to provide an airtight contact with the skin and a slick, low-friction surface. When a water-soluble material is used, the skin should first be washed and dried to prevent air bubbles from hampering the flow of acoustic energy into the skin (Figure 15–14). The use of topical analgesics as a coupling medium has also been recommended, although their effectiveness has not been clearly demonstrated.[48]

*Underwater application*   Underwater ultrasound is suggested for such irregular body parts as the wrist, hand, elbow, knee, ankle, and foot. The part is fully submerged in water; then the ultrasound head is submerged and positioned approximately 1 inch (2.5 cm) from the body part to be treated. The water medium provides an airtight coupling and allows sound waves to travel at a constant velocity. To ensure uninterrupted therapy, air bubbles that form on the skin must be continually wiped away. The sound head is moved slowly in a circular or longitudinal pattern.[17]

Underwater application should be done in a plastic or rubber (nonmetal), container to avoid reflection of energy off metal walls.

*Gel pad technique*   If, for some reason, the treatment area cannot be immersed in water, a gel pad technique can be used. In this technique, a gel pad is applied to the treatment area, and the ultrasound energy is transmitted from the transducer to the treatment surface through this pad. Both sides of the pad should be coated with gel to ensure good contact.[5]

*Moving the transducer*   Moving the transducer during treatment leads to a more even distribution of energy within the treatment area and can reduce the likelihood of developing hot spots. The transducer should be moved slowly at approximately 1½ inches (4 cm) per second. The transducer should be kept in maximum contact with the skin via some coupling agent throughout the treatment.

Movement of the transducer can be in a circular pattern or a stroking pattern. In the circular pattern, the transducer is applied in small, overlapping circles. In the stroking pattern, the transducer is moved back and forth, overlapping the preceding stroke by half. Both techniques are performed slowly and deliberately. The field covered should not exceed 3 to 4 inches (7.5 to 10 cm). The pattern is determined mainly by the skin area to be treated. For example, the circular pattern is best for highly localized areas, such as the shoulder, whereas the stroking pattern is best used in larger, more diffuse areas. When a highly irregular surface area is to be given therapy, the underwater method should be used.[17]

*Dosage and treatment time*   Dosage of ultrasound varies according to the depth of the tissue treated and the state of injury, such as subacute or chronic.[17] Basically, 0.1 to 0.3 W/cm$^2$ is regarded as low intensity, 0.4 to 1.5 W/cm$^2$ is medium intensity, and 1.5 to 3 W/cm$^2$ is high intensity.[26] The duration of treatment ranges from 5 to 10 minutes.

**Special Considerations**   Although ultrasound is a relatively safe modality, certain precautions must be taken, and ultrasound should never be used in some situations. Great care must be taken when treating anesthetized areas because the sensation of pain is one of the best indicators of overdosage. Great precaution must be used in areas that have reduced circulation. In general, ultrasound must not be applied to highly fluid areas

> A field hockey player has a 3-week-old deep quadriceps contusion. She has returned to full practice. There is still a palpable swollen area present and some remaining purplish-yellow discoloration. The injury is no longer tender to the touch, but the athlete does not have full range of motion in flexion.
>
> **?** At this point in the process of healing, what modalities would be most appropriate?

15–3 Clinical Application Exercise

of the body, such as the eyes, ears, testes, brain, spinal cord, and heart. Reproductive organs and women who are pregnant must not receive ultrasound. Acute injuries should not be treated with thermal ultrasound, although nonthermal ultrasound is useful in managing acute injury. Epiphyseal areas in children should have only minimal ultrasound exposure.[17]

***Ultrasound in combination with other modalities*** In an athletic training environment, it is not uncommon to combine modalities to accomplish a treatment goal.[30] Ultrasound is frequently used with other modalities, including hot packs, cold packs, and electrical stimulating currents.

> Ultrasound is commonly used in conjunction with other modalities.

Hot packs and ultrasound are a useful combination because of the relaxing effects of hot packs in muscle spasm or muscle guarding. Hot packs produce more superficial heating, whereas ultrasound produces heating in the deeper tissues. The use of a hot pack and 1 MHz ultrasound treatments appears to have an additive effect on muscle temperature.[14]

Cold packs are frequently used before ultrasound application. However, if the treatment goal is an increase in deep-tissue temperature, the use of a cold pack before ultrasound interferes with heating and is not recommended.[17,19]

Ultrasound is often used with electrical stimulating currents and is thought to be particularly effective in treating trigger points and acupuncture points. Ultrasound increases the blood flow to the deep tissues, and the electrical currents produce a muscle contraction or modulate pain associated with an injury (Figure 15–15).[17]

## Phonophoresis

**Equipment** Phonophoresis is a method of transporting medications through the skin using the mechanical vibrations produced by an ultrasound generator.[1]

**Indications** Phonophoresis is predominantly used to introduce hydrocortisone and an anesthetic into the tissues. Many clinicians prefer to use a 10 percent hydrocortisone ointment.[1] Sometimes lidocaine is added to the cortisone to provide

> Phonophoresis is a method of transporting molecules through the skin with ultrasound.

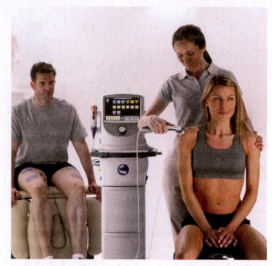

**FIGURE 15–15** Combination ultrasound and electrical stimulator units.
Courtesy DJO Global

a local anesthetic effect. This method has been proposed for treating painful trigger points, tendinitis, and bursitis.[17]

**Application** This medicine is massaged into the skin over an area of tendinitis, bursitis, or other chronic soft-tissue condition. A coupling gel is then spread over the medication, and the ultrasound is applied. Chempads are commercially produced pads that are impregnated with medication; they may be used instead of the traditional medicated ointment application. The effectiveness of phonophoresis as a treatment technique is questionable and needs further research.[1]

**Special Considerations** The techniques of phonophoresis and iontophoresis are often confused, and occasionally the two terms are erroneously interchanged. Both techniques are used to deliver chemicals to various biological tissues. Phonophoresis involves the use of acoustic energy in the form of ultrasound to transport whole molecules across the skin into the tissues, whereas iontophoresis uses an electrical current to transport ions into the tissues. Some athletic trainers prefer phonophoresis to iontophoresis, indicating that it is less hazardous to the skin and that there is greater penetration.[17]

# MECHANICAL ENERGY MODALITIES

## Traction

Traction is a drawing tension applied to a body segment. It is most commonly used in the cervical and lumbar regions of the spine.[28]

**Physiological Effects** Traction is used to produce separation of the vertebral bodies and in so doing can effect stretching of the ligaments and joint capsules of the spine, stretching of spinal and paraspinal muscles, increased separation of the articular facet joints, relief in pressure on nerves and nerve roots, decrease in the central pressure of the intervertebral disks. (allowing for the movement of herniated disk material back into the center of the disk), increases of and changes in joint proprioception, and relief of the compressive effects of normal posture.[28]

> Traction is commonly used in the cervical and lumbar spine.

**Indications** Traction is most commonly used for the treatment of spinal nerve root impingement, which has many causes, including vertebral disk herniation or prolapse and spondylolisthesis (see Chapter 25). It may also be used to decrease muscle guarding, treat muscle strain or sprain of the spinal ligaments, and relax discomfort resulting from normal spinal compression.

**Application** Traction may be applied to the spine through the use of manual techniques or mechanical traction, including table traction units, wall-mounted traction units, and inverted traction techniques.

**Manual traction** Manual traction is infinitely more adaptable and offers greater flexibility than mechanical traction. Changes in force, direction, duration, and patient position can be made instantaneously as the athletic trainer senses relaxation or resistance (Figure 15–16).

**Mechanical traction** For mechanical lumbar traction, a split table with a movable section to eliminate friction must be used to allow for smooth, nonrestricted traction. A nonslip traction harness applied directly to the skin is needed to transfer the traction force comfortably to the patient and to stabilize the trunk while the lumbar spine is placed under traction (Figure 15–17).

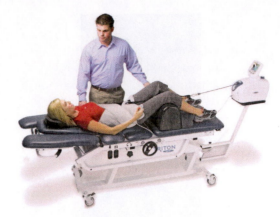

FIGURE 15–17   Lumbar traction using a split table and a traction machine.
Courtesy DJO Global

For cervical traction, the patient may be either in the supine or the sitting position. A nonslip cervical harness should be secured under the chin and back of the head.

**Positional traction** Positional traction is used on a trial-and-error basis to determine maximum position of comfort or to accomplish a specific treatment goal. For example, placing a patient with a lumbar disk problem in a back-lying position with the hips and knees flexed and supported at 90 degrees increases the opening of the foramen and takes pressure off the disk, thus minimizing pain and making the athlete more comfortable.[28]

**Wall-mounted traction** Cervical traction can be accomplished with a wall-mounted system. Plates, sand bags, or water bags can be used for weights. These units are relatively inexpensive and effective (Figure 15–18).

**Inverted traction** Specialized equipment or simply hanging upside down places the person in an inverted position. The spine is lengthened because of the stretch provided by the weight of the trunk (Figure 15–19).[13]

**Special Considerations** Good results have been achieved using both intermittent and sustained traction. In most cases of lumbar disk problems, sustained traction seems to be the treatment of choice. Intermittent traction is considered to be more comfortable.[28] Progressive traction increases the traction force gradually in a preselected number of steps, which allows the athlete to adapt slowly to the traction and helps him or her stay relaxed. Recommendations on length of treatment and on/off times vary depending on the specific problem to be treated. For the lumbar spine, a traction force equal to one-half the patient's body weight is a good guideline to use in selecting a force high enough to cause vertebral separation. Cervical traction forces can be adjusted from 20 to 50 pounds (9 to 23 kg), depending on patient comfort and response.

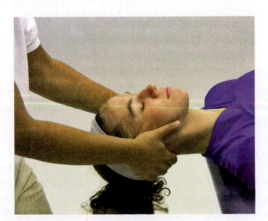

FIGURE 15–16   Manual cervical traction.
© William E. Prentice

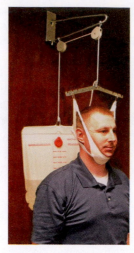

FIGURE 15–18   Cervical traction using a wall-mounted unit.
© William E. Prentice

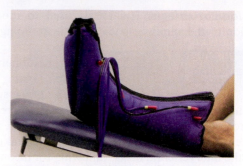

FIGURE 15–20   Intermittent compression devices are designed to reduce edema after injury.
© William E. Prentice

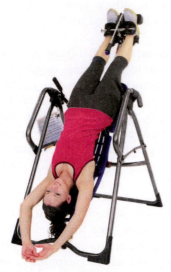

FIGURE 15–19   Inverted traction apparatus.
Teeter EP-970 Inversion Table, teeter.com

## Intermittent Compression

**Equipment**  Intermittent compression makes use of a nylon pneumatic inflatable sleeve applied around the injured extremity (Figure 15–20).[38] The sleeve can be inflated to a specific pressure that forces excessive fluid accumulated in the interstitial spaces into vascular and lymphatic channels, through which it is removed from the area of injury. Compression facilitates the movement of lymphatic fluid, which helps eliminate the byproducts of the injury process.[38]

**Indications**  Intermittent compression units are used for controlling or reducing swelling after one acute injury or for pitting edema, which tends to develop in the injured area several hours after injury.[27] The extremity should be elevated during treatment.[66] It is also common to use electrical stimulating currents to produce muscle pumping, thus facilitating lymphatic flow.

**Application**  Intermittent compression devices have three adjustable parameters: on/off time, inflation pressures, and treatment time. Recommended treatment protocols have been established through clinical trial and error, with little experimental data currently available to support any protocol.[27] On/off times are variable, including 1 minute on, 2 minutes off; 2 minutes on, 1 minute off; and 4 minutes on, 1 minute off. Again, these recommendations are not research based. Patient comfort should be the primary guide.

Recommended inflation pressures have been loosely correlated with blood pressures. The Jobst Institute recommends that pressure be set at 30 to 50 mm Hg for the upper extremity and at 30 to 60 mm Hg for the lower extremity. Because arterial capillary pressures are "approximately 30 mm Hg, any pressure that exceeds this level should encourage the absorption of edema and the flow of lymphatic fluid."[27] Clinical studies have demonstrated a significant reduction in limb volume after 30 minutes of compression.[3,27] Thus, a 30-minute treatment time seems to be efficient in reducing edema.

**Special Considerations**  Some intermittent compression units have the capability of combining cold along with compression, which is more effective in reducing edema.[3,27] The *Cryo-Cuff* is a device that uses both cold and compression simultaneously (Figure 15–21A). The Cryo-Cuff is used

A gymnast has been told by a physician that she has a sprain of a ligament between two lumbar vertebrae in her low back. He tells her that it is important to stretch her low back. Because she was extremely flexible before her injury, she does not feel that the stretching she has been doing is effectively stretching the injured ligament.

**?** The gymnast asks the athletic trainer whether any other therapeutic technique will help her stretch the injured ligament.

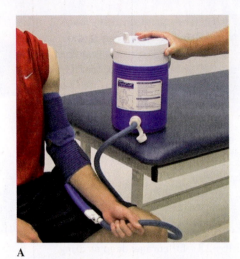

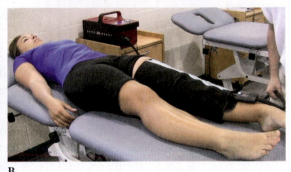

**B**

FIGURE 15–21 Portable compression and cold systems.
**(A)** Cryo-Cuff. **(B)** Game Ready Accelerated Recovery
System.
© William E. Prentice

A patient who stepped off a curb comes to the hospital with a 2-day-old postacute ankle sprain. The initial injury was not managed appropriately; as a result, the patient has a considerable amount of swelling. He has little range of motion and is capable of only touch down weight bearing.

❓ The patient will have a difficult time regaining function until the swelling is reduced. What therapeutic modalities can reduce this postacute lymphedema?

both acutely following injury and postsurgically. It is made of a nylon sleeve that connects via a tube to a 1-gallon (3.8 L) cooler/jug. Cold water flows into the sleeve from the cooler. As the cooler is raised, the pressure in the cuff is increased. During the treatment, the water warms and can be rechilled by lowering the cooler to drain the cuff, mixing the warmer water with the colder water, and then again raising the jug to increase pressure in the cuff. The only drawback to this simple yet effective piece of equipment is that the water in the cuff must be continually rechilled. However, the Cryo-Cuff is portable, easy to use, and inexpensive. Other cold and compression units include the *Game Ready Accelerated Recovery System*, *VitalWrap*, and the *Polar Cub*.

The *Game Ready Accelerated Recovery System* consists of various soft wraps and a control unit designed to simultaneously deliver cold therapy and intermittent compression (Figure 15–21B). The wraps are made from flexible fabric designed to fit various body parts. The wraps fit snugly to apply consistent cooling and intermittent pressure to an injury. To operate the system, the control unit reservoir is filled with ice water, which is circulated through the wraps over the course of a standard treatment program, which can be customized for various time, temperature, and compression settings.

## Massage

Massage is the systematic manipulation of the soft tissues of the body. The movements of gliding, compressing, stretching, percussing, and vibrating are regulated to produce specific responses in the patient.[23]

***Indications*** Massage seems to be regaining popularity among athletic trainers as a treatment modality. Manipulation of soft tissue by massage is a useful adjunct to other modalities.[4] Massage causes mechanical, physiological, and psychological responses.[54]

***Mechanical responses*** Mechanical responses to massage occur as a direct result of the graded pressures and movements of the hand on the body. Such actions encourage venous and lymphatic drainage and mildly stretch superficial and scar tissue.[70] Connective tissue can be stretched effectively by friction massage, which helps prevent rigidity in scar formation. When a patient is forced to remain inactive while an injury heals or when edema surrounds a joint, the stagnation of circulation may be prevented by using certain massage techniques.[24]

***Physiological responses*** Massage can increase circulation and, as a result, increase metabolism to the musculature and aid in the removal of metabolites.[23] It also helps overcome venostasis and edema by increasing circulation at and around the injury site, assisting in the normal venous blood return to the heart.[71]

The reflex effects of massage are processes that, in response to nerve impulses initiated through rubbing the body, are transmitted to one organ by afferent nerve fibers and then back to another organ by efferent fibers.

**Physiological responses to massage:**

- Reflex effects
- Relaxation
- Stimulation
- Increased circulation

Reflex responses elicit a variety of organ reactions, such as body relaxation, stimulation, and increased circulation.[54]

Relaxation can be induced by slow, superficial stroking of the skin. It is a type of massage that is beneficial for tense, anxious patients who may require gentle treatment.

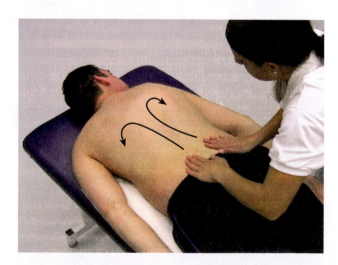

A javelin thrower has a muscle strain in his back. He comes into the sports medicine clinic on the sixth day after the initial injury, complaining of pain. He asks the athletic trainer whether anything can be done to help modulate his pain.

❓ What modalities can the athletic trainer use to modulate the pain?

Stimulation is attained by quick, brisk action that causes a contraction of superficial tissue. The benefits derived by the patient are predominantly psychological. He or she feels invigorated after intense manipulation of the tissue.

Increased circulation is accomplished by mechanical and reflex stimuli. Together they cause the capillaries to dilate and be drained of fluid as a result of firm outside pressure, thus stimulating cell metabolism, eliminating toxins, and increasing lymphatic and venous circulation. In this way the healing process is aided.[71]

***Psychological responses*** The tactile system is one of the most sensitive systems in the human organism. From earliest infancy, humans respond psychologically to being touched. Because massage is the act of laying on of hands, it can be an important means for creating a bond of confidence between the athletic trainer and the patient.[54]

**Application** Massage strokes can be separated into five basic categories: effleurage, petrissage, friction, tapotement, and vibration.

***Effleurage*** **Effleurage**, or stroking (Figure 15–22), is divided into light and deep methods. Light stroking is designed primarily to be sedative. It is also used in the early stages of injury treatment. Deep stroking is a therapeutic

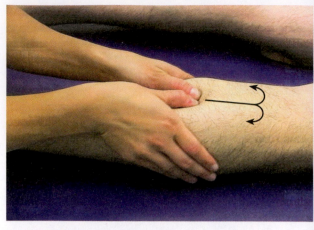

FIGURE 15–23   Effleurage: deep stroking.
© William E. Prentice

compression of soft tissue, which encourages venous and lymphatic drainage. A different application of effleurage may be used for a specific body part (Figure 15–23).

There are many variations in effleurage massage; some that are of particular value to sports injuries are pressure variations, the hand-over-hand method, and the cross-body method.[23] Pressure variations range from very light to deep and vigorous stroking. Light stroking, as discussed previously, can induce relaxation or may be used when an area is especially sensitive to touch; on the other hand, deep massage is designed to bring about definite physiological responses. Light and deep effleurage can be used alternately when both features are desired. The hand-over-hand stroking method is of special benefit to those surface areas that are particularly unyielding. It is performed by an alternate stroke in which one hand strokes, followed immediately by the other hand, somewhat like shingles on a roof. The cross-body effleurage technique is an excellent massage for the low back region. The athletic trainer places a hand on each side of the patient's spine. Both hands first stroke simultaneously away from the spine; then both hands at the same time stroke toward the spine (Figure 15–24).

***Petrissage*** Kneading, or **petrissage** (Figure 15–25), is a technique adaptable primarily to loose and heavy tissue areas (e.g., the trapezius, latissimus dorsi, or triceps muscles). The procedure consists of picking up the muscle and skin tissue between the thumb and forefinger of each hand and rolling and twisting them in opposite directions. As one hand is rolling and twisting, the other begins to pick up the adjacent tissue. The kneading action wrings out the muscle, thus loosening adhesions and squeezing congestive materials into the general circulation. Picking up skin may cause an irritating pinch. Whenever possible, deep muscle tissue should be gathered and lifted.

***Friction*** The **friction** massage (Figure 15–26) is used often around joints and other areas where tissue is thin and on tissues that are especially unyielding, such as scars, adhesions, muscle spasms, and fascia. The action is initiated

FIGURE 15–22   Effleurage: light stroking.
© William E. Prentice

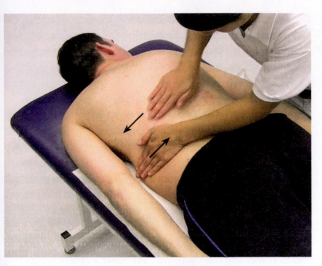

FIGURE 15–24   Cross-body effleurage.
© William E. Prentice

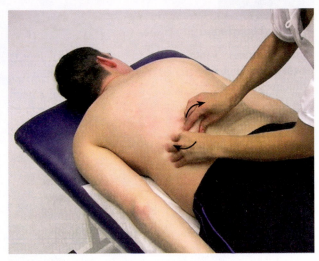

FIGURE 15–25   Petrissage (kneading).
© William E. Prentice

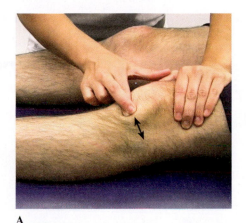

**A**

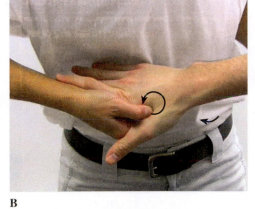

**B**

FIGURE 15–26   Friction massage. **(A)** Transverse friction technique—one finger crossed over another. **(B)** Circular friction technique using the thumb.
© William E. Prentice

by bracing with the heels of the hands, then either holding the thumbs steady and moving the fingers in a circular motion or holding the fingers steady and moving the thumbs in a circular motion. Each method is adaptable to the type of area or articulation that is being massaged. The motion is started at a central point, and then a circular movement is initiated, with the hands moving in opposite directions away from the center point. The purpose is to stretch the underlying tissue, develop friction in the area, and increase circulation around the joint.[54]

*Tapotement*   The most popular methods of **tapotement**, or percussion, are cupping, hacking, and pinching movements.

*Cupping*   The cupping action produces an invigorating and stimulating sensation. It is a series of percussion movements rapidly duplicated at a constant tempo. The hands are cupped to such an extent that the beat emits a dull and hollow sound, unlike the sound of the slap of the open hand. The hands move alternately, from the wrist, with the elbow flexed and the upper arm stabilized

(Figure 15–27A). The cupping action should be executed until the skin in the area develops a pinkish coloration.

*Hacking*   Hacking can be used in conjunction with cupping to bring about a varied stimulation of the sensory nerves (Figure 15–27B). Hacking is similar to cupping except that the hands are rotated externally and the ulnar, or little finger, border of the hand is the striking surface. Only the heavy muscle areas should be treated in this manner. (Avoid using vigorous hacking over the kidneys and behind the knees.)

*Pinching*   Although pinching is not in the strictest sense percussive, it is categorized under tapotement because of the vigor with which it is applied. Alternating hands lift small amounts of tissue between the first finger and thumb in quick, gentle pinching movements (Figure 15–27C).

*Vibration*   **Vibration** is rapid movement that produces a quivering or trembling effect. It is used in sports because of its ability to relax and soothe. Although vibration can be done manually, the machine vibrator is usually the preferred modality.

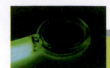
## Guidelines for an effective massage

Besides knowing the different kinds of massage, the athletic trainer should understand how to give the most effective massage. The following rules should be used whenever possible:

1. Make the patient comfortable.
   a. Place the body in the proper position on the table.
   b. Place a pad under the areas of the body that are to be massaged.
   c. Keep the room at a constant 72°F (22.2°C) temperature.
   d. Respect the patient's privacy by draping him or her with a blanket or towel, exposing only the body parts to be massaged.

2. Develop a confident, gentle approach when massaging.
   a. Assume a position that is easy both on you and on the patient.
   b. Avoid using too harsh a stroke, or further injury may result.
3. To ensure proper lymphatic and venous drainage, stroke toward the heart whenever possible.
4. Know when not to use massage.
   a. Never give a massage if the patient may have a local or general infection. To do so may encourage the infection's spread or may aggravate the condition.
   b. Never apply massage directly over a recent injury; limit stroking to the periphery. Massaging over recent injuries may dislodge the clot organization and start bleeding.

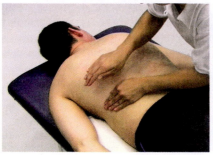
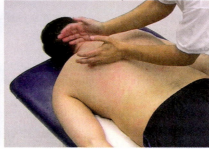
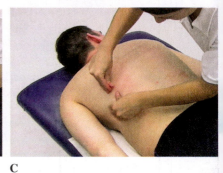

A  B  C

FIGURE 15–27  Tapotement. **(A)** Cupping. **(B)** Hacking. **(C)** Pinching.
© William E. Prentice

**Special Considerations**  Therapeutic massage performed by athletic trainers is usually confined to a specific area and is seldom given to the full body.[4] The time required for giving an adequate and complete body massage is excessive. It is not usually feasible to devote this much time to one patient; 5 minutes is usually all that is required for massaging a given area. *Focus Box 15–4*: "Guidelines for an effective massage" provides suggestions for giving an effective massage.

**Massage lubricants**  To enable the hands to slide easily over the body, a friction-reducing medium must be used. Rubbing the dry body can cause gross skin irritation by tearing and pulling on the hair. Many media (e.g., fine powders, oil liniments, or almost any substance having a petroleum base) can be used as a lubricant.

**Positioning the patient**  It is important to position a patient properly for a massage. The injured body part must be easily accessible, the patient must be comfortable, and the part to be massaged must be relaxed (Figure 15–28).

**Confidence**  Inexperienced hands can transmit a lack of confidence. Every effort should be made to think out the procedure to be used and to present a confident appearance to the patient.

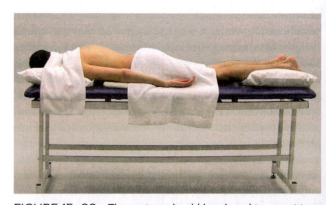

FIGURE 15–28  The patient should be placed in a position of comfort and appropriately draped with towels or sheets.
© William E. Prentice

*Ensuring patient privacy and athletic trainer Integrity*   As is the case with a number of other therapeutic techniques, massage involves direct physical contact between the athletic trainer and the patient. It is critical that the athletic trainer be aware of and, if necessary, take the required precautions to ensure that this physical contact can in no way be construed or misinterpreted as being inappropriate. This is particularly important when dealing with a patient of the opposite sex or with patients who are under legal age. The athletic trainer should always make certain that only the body part or body region being treated is exposed and that the rest of the body is appropriately covered or draped. It is also advisable to perform the massage with another patient or athletic trainer physically present in the same room or to do the massage in plain view of others in the athletic training clinic. There is no good reason not to take these precautions, and failure to do so may create situations that unnecessarily threaten the athletic trainer's professional and personal integrity.

## Deep Transverse Friction Massage

**Indications**   The transverse, or Cyriax, method of deep friction massage is a specific technique for treating muscles, tendons, ligaments, and joint capsules. The major purpose of transverse massage is to move transversely across a ligament or tendon to mobilize it as much as possible. This technique often precedes active exercise. Deep transverse friction massage restores mobility to a muscle in the same way that mobilization frees a joint.[23]

> Transverse massage is a method of deep transverse friction massage.

**Application**   The position of the athletic trainer's hands is important in gaining maximum strength and control. Four positions are suggested: index finger crossed over middle finger, middle finger crossed over index finger, two fingers side by side, and opposed finger and thumb.

The massage must be directly over the site of lesion and pain. The fingers move with the skin and do not slide over it. Massage must be across the grain of the affected tissue. The thicker the structure, the more friction is given.[23] The technique is to sweep back and forth over the full width of the tissue.

**Special Considerations**   Massage should not be given to acute injuries or over highly swollen tissues.

## Acupressure Massage

**Indications**   Acupressure is a type of massage based on the ancient Chinese art of acupuncture. Physiological explanations of the effectiveness of acupressure massage may likely be attributed to some interaction of the various mechanisms of pain modulation.

**Application**   The athletic trainer uses acupuncture/acupressure charts to select specific points that are described in the literature as having some relationship to the area of pain. The charts provide a general idea of where these points are located. Two techniques may be used to specifically locate acupressure points. Because it is known that electrical impedance is reduced at acupuncture points, an ohmmeter may be used to locate the points. Perhaps the easiest technique is for the athletic trainer simply to palpate the area until he or she feels either a small, fibrous nodule or a strip of tense muscle tissue that is tender to the touch.

Once the point is located, the athletic trainer begins massage with the index or middle finger, the thumb, or the elbow, using small, circular motions on the point. The amount of pressure applied to these acupressure points should be submaximal and determined by patient tolerance.

Effective treatment times range from one to five minutes at a single point per treatment. It may be necessary to massage several points during the treatment to obtain the greatest effects. If so, the athletic trainer should work distal points first and move proximally.

*Special Considerations*   During the massage, the patient will report a dulling or numbing effect and will frequently indicate that the pain has diminished or subsided totally during the massage. The lingering effects of acupressure massage vary tremendously from patient to patient. The effects may last for only a few minutes in some but may persist in others for several hours.

**Dry Needling**   *Dry needling* is a therapeutic treatment that involves inserting a thin, solid filament needle through the skin and usually directly into a myofascial trigger point located within a muscle (Figure 15–29).[67] With dry needling there is no injection of any type of medication. Dry needling and traditional Chinese acupuncture are similar in that they use the same kind of needles. But while dry needling focuses on treating pain associated with myofascial trigger points, acupuncture treats not only muscular

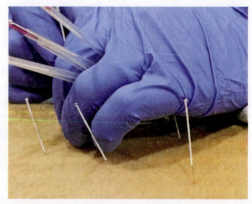

FIGURE 15–29   Dry needling focuses primarily on treating myofascial trigger points.
© William E. Prentice

conditions but also many nonmuscular medical conditions. When the needles are inserted into the skin, the patient feels minimal if any discomfort. But as the needle goes into the muscle, and particularly into an active trigger point, the sensation is similar to a muscle cramp typically with an associated "twitch response." Dry needling can be used in conjunction with stretching, joint mobilization, neuromuscular reeducation, strengthening, functional retraining, and other therapeutic interventions. A limited number of studies have shown evidence that dry needling works as an analgesic, but only moderate evidence for improving range of motion and disability.[8,39] The legality of athletic trainers and especially physical therapists using dry needling in clinical practice is currently a hotly debated topic and varies significantly with practice acts in each state.

# MODALITIES NOT COMMONLY USED BY ATHLETIC TRAINERS

Several therapeutic modalities marketed as therapeutic devices are seldom used by athletic trainers. Magnet therapy has little evidence-based support in the professional literature, although a search of the Internet reveals significant anecdotal information about magnet use. Extracorporal shock wave therapy has been used for many years for a variety of purposes. This modality has been approved by the FDA, and there is considerable experimental evidence in the professional literature to support its use. Nevertheless, athletic trainers rarely use these modalities, and they are included here for informational purposes only.

## Magnet Therapy

Magnet therapy has become popular among both competitive and recreational athletes. An increasing number of athletic trainers are using magnets as a treatment modality for a variety of musculoskeletal ailments. Although a wealth of anecdotal information on magnet therapy can be found in the popular literature, a careful review of the medical literature indicates few data-based research articles on the efficacy or potential therapeutic benefits of using magnets.

Magnet therapy is the application of a magnetic field to the human body. A magnet is a natural ferrous material with inseparable positively and negatively charged poles that characteristically attract particles of opposite charge and repel particles of similar charge. The strength of a magnetic field is measured in Gauss units. Most therapeutic magnets range between 300 and 1,000 Gauss. The explanations of the potential beneficial physiological effects of magnets include changes in polarity within a damaged cell, increased blood flow and thus increased oxygen saturation, increased muscle strength, increased hormone secretions, increased cell division rate, increased enzyme activity, increased lymphatic flow, and changes in blood

pH. It has been shown that magnets do not appear to cause a local increase in tissue temperature.[62]

Although magnet therapy appears to be a relatively safe treatment modality, athletic trainers should use it with caution until some definitive basis for use has been determined scientifically.

## Extracorporeal Shock Wave Therapy (ESWT)

Extracorporeal shock wave therapy (ESWT) is a pulsed, high-pressure, short-duration (<1 ms) acoustic sound wave that is produced by a generator and transmitted through a coupling medium over a large skin area to a specific target region with little attenuation.[61] This acoustic energy is concentrated in a focal area 0.08 to 0.3 inch (2 to 8 mm) in diameter. The treatment uses a sequence of 1,000 to 4,000 shock wave pulses at 1 to 4 pps. Focusing is checked every 200 to 400 shocks, and treatment lasts for 15 to 30 minutes. Shock wave therapy was first used for kidney stone fragmentation in the early 1980s.

Currently, because of its high cost, this modality is most likely to be found in a hospital, although there are a few athletic training facilities that have ESWT available. Imaging devices (e.g., ultrasound, X-ray) are sometimes used to target energy precisely but are not necessary in extremities.[63] Shock waves are applied to the point of maximal tenderness at the lowest energy setting. With direct patient feedback, the exact site of pain and pathology is identified. The intensity is slowly increased within the patient's level of tolerance. Anesthesia is sometimes used to minimize the pain associated with the treatment. However, anesthesia is not only unnecessary but also undesirable, because only the patient can verify that the correct site has been targeted. If the pain is not reproduced by the shock wave, the condition is unlikely to respond. Since the mid-1990s, ESWT has been approved for use in treating tennis elbow, plantar fasciitis, and nonunion fractures as well as for its analgesic effects. The mechanism of action is not well understood, but the healing that occurs with EWST has been attributed to enhanced metabolism, circulation, and revascularization.[68]

Because this is a relatively new modality, techniques for using ESWT have not yet been standardized. Precise dosages and optimal frequency of application have not been studied extensively. It has not been demonstrated whether shock waves should be directed to the target area by radiological or ultrasound imaging. Also, it is not yet clear whether local anesthetic injections should be used in the target area prior to treatment to reduce pain.[37]

## Cupping Therapy

Cupping therapy is an alternative therapeutic technique that has roots in several cultures dating back to

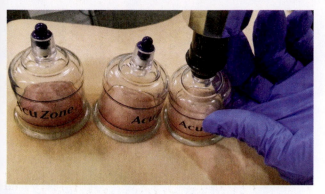

FIGURE 15–30   Therapeutic cupping technique creates suction of the skin.

© William E. Prentice

3,000 B.C. Two techniques of cupping are used therapeutically: dry cupping and wet cupping.

The dry cupping technique uses medical grade cups made of glass, silicone, or rubber to create suction of the skin. Suction may be created using either heat or a mechanical pump. The air inside the cup is heated with an open flame and then the cup is placed against the skin. When the air cools, it lowers the air pressure inside the cup and creates a vacuum, thus drawing the skin upward and causing reddening as the blood vessels expand inside the cup (Figure 15–30). Suction can also be created using a mechanical suction pump. A single cup can be used for treatment but most often, multiple cups are used. The length of the recommended treatment ranges from 5 to 15 minutes.

In wet cupping, suction is again created in the cup for 3 to 5 minutes. The clinician removes the cup and uses a scalpel to make small incisions superficially in the skin. Suction is then reapplied to draw out blood. After treatment, antiseptics or antibiotic ointment is used to prevent infection.

Both techniques create a residual circular area of discoloration or bruising that dissipates over a couple of days. Treatments are not usually painful.

Cupping has been used therapeutically to improve blood flow, reduce swelling, reduce pain, and to treat scar tissue in connective tissue. However, there is minimal evidence in the research literature to support the efficacy of cupping. A meta-analysis found that cupping therapy may be effective if combined with medications or other treatments in treating herpes zoster, acne, facial paralysis, and cervical spondylosis.[9]

# RECORDING THERAPEUTIC MODALITY TREATMENTS

Athletic trainers who use a therapeutic modality in treatment need to record the procedure. The specifics of the modality treatment should be recorded on the original SOAP note, the progress note, and a therapeutic modalities treatment log like the one shown in Figure 15–31. Changes in the treatment parameters should be noted on the treatment log, so that anyone administering a treatment modality can consult the log to determine the appropriate parameters.

Patient's Name _____

Diagnosis _____ Date of Injury _____

Athletic Trainer _____

Therapeutic Modality _____

Treatment Parameters

    Intensity/Output _____

    Frequency _____

    Duty Cycle _____

    Temperature _____

    Duration of Treatment _____

    Electrode Placement _____

Special Instructions:

Month/Year _____

Date Administered:

1 2 3 4 5 6 7 8 9 10 11 12 13 14 15 16 17 18 19 20 21 22 23 24 25 26 27 28 29 30 31

FIGURE 15–31   Therapeutic modalities treatment log.

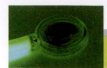

### Safe use of therapeutic modalities[27]

The following safety practices should be considered when using any type of electrical therapeutic modality:

- The entire electrical system of the building or athletic training room should be designed or evaluated by a qualified electrician. Problems with the electrical system may exist in older buildings or in rooms that have been modified to accommodate therapeutic devices (e.g., putting a whirlpool in a locker room where the concrete floor is always wet or damp).
- It should not be assumed that all three-pronged wall outlets are grounded. The ground must be checked.
- Ground fault interrupters (GFIs) should be used with all modalities that plug into a wall outlet. GFIs detect decreases in voltage output and can shut down electrical current automatically, should a problem occur.
- The athletic trainer should become very familiar with the equipment being used and with any potential or existing problems. Any defective equipment should be immediately removed from the clinic.
- The plug should not be jerked out of the wall by pulling on the cable.
- Extension cords or multiple adapters should never be used.
- Equipment should be calibrated yearly and should conform to *National Electrical Code* guidelines. If a clinic or an athletic training facility is not in compliance with this Code, then there is no legal protection in a lawsuit.
- Common sense should always be exercised when using electrotherapeutic devices. A situation that appears to be dangerous may, in fact, result in injury or death.

Hooker D, Prentice, W: Basic principles of electricity and electrical stimulating currents. In Prentice W, editor: *Therapeutic Modalities in Rehabilitation*, ed 4, New York, 2011, McGraw-Hill.

## SAFETY IN USING THERAPEUTIC MODALITIES

When using any type of therapeutic modality, the athletic trainer must ensure that the equipment is used and maintained in an appropriate manner.[3,27] Manufacturers of therapeutic modality equipment usually provide written guidelines and recommendations for appropriate care and maintenance in the manuals that accompany new equipment. There is usually a regular maintenance schedule for each piece of equipment, designed to discover any defects or breakdowns that occur due to normal wear and tear. The athletic trainer should be familiar with and closely follow the manufacturer's recommendations for equipment maintenance. Failure to do so may make the athletic trainer legally negligent, should an incident occur that results in an unnecessary injury to a patient. The athletic trainer should arrange to have the maintenance done either by the manufacturer or by some other qualified agency. *Focus Box 15–5*: "Safe Use of Therapeutic Modalities" lists recommended safety practices for using and maintaining therapeutic equipment.

## EVIDENCE-BASED DATA REGARDING THERAPEUTIC MODALITY USE

Despite the fact that therapeutic modalities are widely used by athletic trainers, as well as physical therapists, occupational therapists, and chiropractors, in general, their clinical effectiveness in treating a variety of conditions has yet to be established. For many years, health care professionals have tended to rely on information from therapeutic modality manufacturers, rather than on scientific evidence-based data generated by competent researchers from within the health care professions. A review of the evidence-based studies, which include randomized controlled trials, systematic reviews, and meta-analysis in the scientific literature should lead the athletic trainer to seriously question how therapeutic modalities should be most appropriately incorporated into clinical treatment regimens. Some of the conclusions in these systematic reviews support the efficacy of treatments using different therapeutic modalities while others do not. But most, if not all, conclude that the evidence base to support the common practice of using a therapeutic modality is limited, and there is a need for future higher-quality randomized controlled trials.[2,10,21,36,56] As health care professionals, athletic trainers have a responsibility to put the best available evidence to use when selecting clinical techniques for treating their patients.[33] An analysis of patient outcomes following the use of specific therapeutic modalities should guide clinical decision making relative to the effectiveness of incorporating a modality into the treatment regimen. Knowing that the evidence for the therapeutic effects of a particular modality is inadequate and applying it anyway presents a problematic level of accountability that the athletic trainer must consider.[33] Athletic trainers should work with equipment manufacturers to produce solid scientific data that determine the clinical efficacy of using a particular therapeutic modality as a treatment tool.

# SUMMARY

- To avoid legal problems, athletic trainers must use therapeutic modalities with extreme care. Athletic trainers must be familiar with the laws of their state regarding therapeutic modality use. Before using any modality, the athletic trainer must have a thorough understanding of its function and when it should and should not be used.

- The forms of energy that are relevant to the use of therapeutic modalities are thermal conductive energy, electrical energy, electromagnetic energy, sound energy, and mechanical energy.

- Thermotherapy increases blood flow, increases collagen viscosity, decreases joint stiffness, and reduces pain and muscle spasm. When the body's temperature is raised, tissue metabolism is increased, vascular permeability is increased, and chemicals (such as histamine, bradykinin, and serotonin) are released.

- Heat energy is transmitted through conduction, convection, radiation, and conversion. Conduction occurs when heat is transferred from a warmer object to a cooler one. Convection heating occurs by means of fluid or gas movement. Radiation is heat energy that is transmitted through empty space. Conversion is heat that is generated when one type of energy is changed to another.

- Superficial therapeutic heat should not be applied when there is a loss of sensation, immediately after an acute injury, and when there is decreased arterial bleeding. Superficial therapeutic heat should not be used over the eyes or genitals or over the abdomen of a pregnant woman. Types of superficial heat are moist heat packs, whirlpool baths, paraffin baths, and fluidotherapy.

- The use of cold for therapeutic purposes and as part of an emergency procedure is extremely popular in sports medicine. Cold penetrates more deeply than superficial heat. Therapy is usually performed when the tissue has reached a state of relative anesthesia. Cryotherapy decreases muscle spasm, pain perception, and blood flow. It increases the inelasticity of collagen fibers, joint stiffness, and capillary permeability. Common cryotherapy procedures and tools are ice massage, cold-water immersion, ice packs, vapocoolant sprays, and cryokinetics.

- The use of electrical stimulating currents is popular in sports medicine. Electrical stimulating units produce monophasic current (DC), biphasic current (AC), or pulsatile current. Both monophasic and biphasic current can be used for pain modulation and muscle contraction. Direct current can also be used for iontophoresis. The physiological effects of electrical current are determined by the treatment parameters and equipment selected. Current parameters include waveform, modulation, intensity, duration, frequency, polarity, and electrode setup. Interferential currents and low-intensity stimulators are two of the newest electrical stimulating currents available to the athletic trainer.

- Shortwave diathermy units produce heat through electromagnetic energy, whereas ultrasound produces heat through acoustic energy. The contraindications for the use of shortwave diathermy are the same as for superficial heating, with the additional restrictions of no implants, jewelry, or intrauterine devices.

- The low-level laser may be used to stimulate the healing process or to modulate pain.

- Ultrasound is a form of sound energy. It creates a mechanical vibration that is converted to heat energy within the body. Heating occurs in the denser tissues, such as bone and connective tissue. More heat is built up at tissue interfaces. Ultrasound has both thermal and nonthermal physiological effects. It can be combined with electrical stimulation or used to transport molecules through the skin with the method known as phonophoresis.

- Traction is used to produce separation of the vertebrae, most commonly for the treatment of spinal nerve root impingement and associated abnormalities. It is typically used in the cervical and lumbar spine and may involve either manual or mechanical traction.

- Intermittent compression devices are used to control swelling after acute injury and to reduce pitting edema.

- Massage is a useful modality for many sports-related injuries. Techniques include effleurage, petrissage, friction, tapotement, and vibration. Deep transverse massage is used on connective tissue.

# SOLUTIONS TO CLINICAL APPLICATION EXERCISES

15–1 The decision is subjective to some extent. The athletic trainer must understand what is going on with the healing process. On the fifth day, the inflammatory process is ending and the fibroblastic stage is establishing itself. At this point it is still advisable to avoid any treatment that may increase swelling, which can interfere with healing. Heat would increase circulation, which might increase swelling. The athletic trainer would not likely exacerbate the injury by using heat, but it is recommended that cold be used during this time. A rule of thumb is that, when the tenderness is gone, it is safe to change to some form of heat.

15–2 Ice massage may be used for Achilles tendinitis and is beneficial, since this area of the body is small. Cold-water immersion is an alternative for cryotherapy. Ice-water immersion is indicated because the injury is in a distal area and the entire area can be iced easily. The athlete is also able to perform cryokinetics simultaneously with the cryotherapy. Another alternative for cryotherapy is the use of ice packs, which can be formed around the ankle.

15–3 At this point, some form of heat to increase blood and lymphatic flow to the injured area is warranted. Increased blood flow will help facilitate the process of healing, and an increased lymphatic flow will help remove the byproducts of the inflammatory process. Hot packs provide superficial heat and would not be effective in this case. Both diathermy and ultrasound would be recommended because they have a depth of penetration great enough to affect the injured area; ultrasound would be somewhat more effective. For best results, stretching and strengthening exercises should always be used along with modalities.

15–4 In this case, the best treatment is to not use ultrasound at all. A better decision would be to use either hydrocollator packs or diathermy, both of which are more useful in treating larger areas. If depth of penetration is a concern, then shortwave diathermy would be the treatment modality of choice.

15–5 The athletic trainer should try using manual lumbar traction techniques, which, if done properly, can be effective in isolating a specific ligament between two lumbar vertebrae. If the athletic trainer cannot manually generate enough traction force to stretch the ligament, a table traction unit or an inverted traction technique may prove to be more useful.

15–6 Proper initial management of the injury could have prevented a great deal of the swelling that has occurred. At this point, the athletic trainer should make use of ice to modulate pain; intermittent compression and electrical stimulating currents to induce a muscle pumping contraction (both of which can help the lymphatic system remove the swelling); and low-intensity ultrasound ($>0.2$ W/cm²), which can help facilitate the healing process. In addition, the patient should continually wear a compressive elastic wrap. He must also progress to full weight bearing, concentrating on regaining a normal gait as soon as it can be tolerated.

15–7 Effleurage massage strokes are ideal during the initial stages of injury to help encourage venous and lymphatic drainage, especially if swelling is present. This method also is sedative for the athlete. Friction massage is beneficial for patellar tendinitis to increase circulation in the area and to develop friction.

15–8 The athletic trainer can use cryotherapy, heat, or electrical stimulating currents to help reduce pain. Electrical stimulating currents may be the most useful if the athletic trainer also wants to elicit a muscle contraction to help decrease muscle guarding. Massage also is useful for modulating pain and for relaxing muscles. Regardless of the modality chosen, the athlete should engage in some stretching and strengthening exercises after the treatment.

## REVIEW QUESTIONS AND CLASS ACTIVITIES

1. Explain the legal factors that an athletic trainer should consider before using a therapeutic modality.
2. Give examples of modalities that heat through conduction, convection, radiation, and conversion.
3. What physiological changes occur when heat is applied to the body?
4. Discuss the physiological effects of using cryotherapy.
5. Demonstrate the proper technique for a variety of cryotherapeutic approaches.
6. Compare therapy delivered through heat to that delivered through cold. When would you use each?
7. What is a TENS unit?
8. Identify the potential treatment goals of an electrically stimulated muscle contraction.
9. What is shortwave diathermy used for?
10. Discuss how ultrasound can be used during a rehabilitation program.
11. Compare phonophoresis with iontophoresis.
12. List the mechanical effects of cervical and lumbar traction.
13. How is massage best used in a sports medicine setting?
14. Explain when and how intermittent compression can best be used as a treatment modality.

## REFERENCES

1. Abrahams S: Phonophoresis of non-steroidal drugs: A review of the clinical evidence, *International Journal of Musculoskeletal Medicine* 30(1):37–41, 2008.
2. Alves A: Effects of low-level laser therapy on skeletal muscle repair: A systematic review, *American Journal of Physical Medicine and Rehabilitation* 93(12):1073–85, 2014.
3. Angus J: A comparison of two external intermittent compression devices and their effect on post acute ankle edema, *J Athl Train* 29(2):178, 1994.
4. Archer P: Three clinical sports massage approaches for treating injured athletes, *Athletic Therapy Today* 6(3):14, 2001.
5. Bishop S: Human tissue—temperature rise during ultrasound treatments with the Aquaflex gel pad, *J Athl Train* 39(2):126, 2004.
6. Brown C: Evidence-based guidelines for utilization of dexamethasone Iontophoresis, *Athletic Therapy and Training*, 16(4):33–36, 2011.
7. Burke D: The effect of hot or cold water immersion and proprioceptive neuromuscular facilitation on hip joint range of motion, *J Athl Train* 36(1):16, 2001.
8. Cagnie B: Evidence for the use of ischemic compression and dry needling in the management of trigger points of the upper trapezius in patients with neck pain: A systematic review, *Am J Phys Med Rehabil* 94(7):573–83, 2015.
9. Cao, H: An updated review of the efficacy of cupping therapy, *PLoS One* 7(2):e31793, 2012. doi:10.1371/journal.pone.0031793.
10. Costello J: Cryotherapy and joint position sense in healthy participants: A systematic review, *J Athl Train*, 45(3):306–16, 2010.
11. Danielle A: Ultrasound therapy for musculoskeletal disorders: A systematic review, *Pain* 81(3):257–71, 1999.
12. Dolan M: Cool water immersion and high-voltage electric stimulation curb edema formation in rats, *J Athl Train* 38(3):225–30, 2003.
13. Draper D: Are certified athletic trainers qualified to use therapeutic modalities? *J Athl Train* 37(1):11, 2002.
14. Draper D: Inversion table traction as a therapeutic modality, Part 1: Oh my aching back, *Athletic Therapy Today* 10(3):42, 2005.
15. Draper D, et al.: Hot-pack and 1-MHz ultrasound treatments have an additive effect on muscle temperature, *J Athl Train* 33(1):21, 1998.
16. Draper D: Interferential current therapy: Often used but misunderstood, *Athletic Therapy Today* 11(4):29, 2006.
17. Draper D: The carryover effects of diathermy and stretching in developing hamstring flexibility, *J Athl Train* 37(1):37, 2002.
18. Draper D: Therapeutic ultrasound. In Prentice W, ed.: *Therapeutic modalities in rehabilitation*, ed 4, New York, 2011, McGraw-Hill.
19. Draper D: Rate of temperature decay in human muscle following 3-Mhz ultrasound: The stretching window revealed, *J Athl Train* 30(4):304, 1995.
20. Draper D: The effect of cooling the tissue prior to ultrasound treatment, *J Athl Train* 29(2):154, 1994.
21. Draper D: Examination of the law of Grotthus Draper: Does ultrasound penetrate subcutaneous fat? *J Athl Train* 28(3):246, 1993.
22. French S: A Cochrane review of superficial heat or cold for low back pain, *Spine* 31(9):998–1006, 2006.
23. French D: The effects of contrast bathing and compression therapy on muscular performance, *Med Sci Sport Exer* 40(7):1297–1306, 2008.
24. Fritz S: *Mosby's fundamentals of therapeutic massage,* St. Louis, MO, 2012, Elsevier Health Sciences.
25. Gazzillo L: Therapeutic massage techniques for three common injuries, *Athletic Therapy Today* 6(3):5, 2001.
26. Holcomb W: A practical guide to electrical therapy, *J Sport Rehabil* 6(3):272, 1997.
27. Holcomb WA: Comparison of temperature increases produced by two commonly used ultrasound units, *J Athl Train* 38(1):24, 2003.
28. Hooker D: Intermittent compression devices. In Prentice W, ed: *Therapeutic modalities in rehabilitation*, ed 4, New York, 2011, McGraw-Hill.
29. Hooker D: Traction as a specialized modality. In Prentice W, ed: *Therapeutic modalities in rehabilitation*, ed 4, New York, 2011, McGraw-Hill.
30. Hooker D, Prentice W: Basic principles of electricity and electrical stimulating currents. In Prentice W, ed: *Therapeutic Modalities in Rehabilitation*, ed 4, New York, 2011, McGraw-Hill.
31. Hopkins J: Cryotherapy and transcutaneous electric neuromuscular stimulation decrease arthrogenic muscle inhibition of the vastus

medialis after knee joint effusion, *J Athl Train* 37(1):25, 2002.

32. Hopkins J: Low-level laser therapy facilitates superficial wound healing in humans: A tripleblind, sham-controlled study, *J Athl Train* 39(3):223, 2004.

33. Hubbard T: Does cryotherapy hasten return to participation? A systematic review, *J Athl Train* 39(1):88, 2004.

34. Ingersoll C: It's time for evidence, *J Athl Train* 41(1):7, 2006.

35. Johns L: Nonthermal effects of therapeutic ultrasound, *J Athl Train* 37(3):293, 299, 2002.

36. Johnson D: Low-level laser therapy in the treatment of carpal tunnel syndrome, *Athletic Therapy Today* 8(2):30, 2003.

37. Johnson M: Efficacy of electrical nerve stimulation for chronic musculoskeletal pain: A meta-analysis of randomized controlled trials, *Pain* 130(1)157–65, 2007.

38. Kaltenborn J: The efficacy of extracorporeal shock-wave treatment: A new perspective, *Athletic Therapy Today* 10(6):50, 2005.

39. Khanna A: Intermittent pneumatic compression in fracture and soft-tissue injuries healing, *British Medical Bulletin*, 88(1):147–56, 2008.

40. Kietrys D: Effectiveness of dry needling for upper-quarter myofascial pain: A systematic review and meta-analysis, *J Orthop Sports Phys Ther* 43(9):620–34, 2013.

41. Knight K: *Cryotherapy in sports injury management*, Champaign, IL, 1995, Human Kinetics.

42. McBrier N: Low-level laser therapy for stimulating muscle regeneration following injury, *Athletic Therapy Today* 14(3):104, 2009.

43. McLeod I: Low-level laser therapy in athletic training, *Athletic Therapy Today* 9(5):17, 2005.

44. Merrick M: Does 1-MHz ultrasound really work? *Athletic Therapy Today* 6(6):48, 2001.

45. Merrick M: Secondary injury after musculoskeletal trauma: A review and update, *J Athl Train* 37(2):209, 2002.

46. Merrick M: Cold modalities with different thermodynamic properties produce different surface and intramuscular temperatures, *J Athl Train* 38(1):28, 2003.

47. Michlovitz S, ed: *Modalities for therapeutic intervention*, Philadelphia, 2012, F.A. Davis.

48. Myrer J, et al.: Cold- and hot-pack contrast therapy: Subcutaneous and intramuscular temperature change, *J Athl Train* 32(3):238, 1997.

49. Myrer J: Intramuscular temperature rises with topical analgesics used as coupling agents during therapeutic ultrasound, *J Athl Train* 36(1):20, 2001.

50. Otte J: Subcutaneous adipose tissue thickness changes cooling time during cryotherapy, *Journal of Athletic Training* 36(2S):S-91, 2001.

51. Peres S: Pulsed shortwave diathermy and long-duration stretching increase dorsiflexion range of motion more than identical stretching without diathermy, *J Athl Train* 37(1):43, 2002.

52. Prentice W: The basic science of therapeutic modalities. In Prentice W, ed: *Therapeutic modalities in rehabilitation*, ed 4, New York, 2011, McGraw-Hill.

53. Prentice W: Preface. In Prentice W, ed: *Therapeutic modalities in rehabilitation*, ed 4, New York, 2011, McGraw-Hill.

54. Prentice W: Thermotherapy and cryotherapy. In Prentice W, ed: *Therapeutic modalities in Rehabilitation*, ed 4, New York, 2011, McGraw-Hill.

55. Prentice W: Therapeutic massage. In Prentice W, ed: *Therapeutic modalities in rehabilitation*, ed 4, New York, 2011, McGraw-Hill.

56. Prentice W, Draper D: Shortwave and microwave diathermy. In Prentice W, ed: *Therapeutic modalities in rehabilitation*, ed 4, New York, 2011, McGraw-Hill.

57. Robertson V: A review of therapeutic ultrasound: Effectiveness studies, *Physical Therapy* 81(7):1339–50, 2001.

58. Rubley M: Thermal ultrasound: It's more than power and time, *Athletic Therapy Today* 14(1):62, 2009.

59. Rubley M: Cryotherapy, sensation, and isometric-force variability, *J Athl Train* 38(2):113, 2003.

60. Saliba E: Low-power laser. In Prentice W, ed: *Therapeutic modalities in rehabilitation*, ed 4, New York, 2011, McGraw-Hill.

61. Snyder-Mackler L: *Clinical electrophysiology: Electrotherapy and electrophysiology*, Baltimore, MD, 2007, Lippincott, Williams and Wilkins.

62. Stemmans C: Low-energy extracorporeal shock-wave therapy, *Athletic Therapy Today* 8(2): 44, 2003.

63. Sweeney K: Therapeutic magnets do not affect tissue temperature, *J Athl Train* 36(1):27, 2001.

64. Thigpen C: Extracorporal shockwave therapy. In Prentice W, ed: *Therapeutic modalities in rehabilitation*, ed 4, New York, 2011, McGraw-Hill.

65. Tomchuk D: The magnitude of tissue cooling during cryotherapy with varied types of compression, I 45(3):230–37, 2010.

66. Tsang K, et al.: The effects of cryotherapy applied through various barriers, *J Sport Rehabil* 6(4):343, 1997.

67. Tsang K: Volume decreases after elevation and intermittent compression are negated by gravity dependent positioning, *J Athl Train* 38(4): 320, 2003.

68. Unverzagt C: Dry needling for myofascial trigger point pain: A clinical commentary, *Int J Sports Phys Ther* 10(3):402–18, 2015.

69. Wang C: Shock wave therapy for patients with lateral epicondylitis of the elbow: A one- to two-year follow-up study, *Am J Sports Med* 30(3):422, 2002.

70. Watson T: Ultrasound in contemporary physiotherapy practice, *Ultrasonics*, 48(4):321–29, 2008.

71. Whitehill W: Massage and skin conditions: Indications and contraindications, *Athletic Therapy Today* 7(3):24, 2002.

72. Zainuddin Z: Effects of massage on delayed-onset muscle soreness, swelling, and recovery of muscle function, *J Athl Train* 40(3): 174, 2005.

## ANNOTATED BIBLIOGRAPHY

Cameron M: *Physical agents in rehabilitation: From research to practice*, Philadelphia, PA, 2012, WB Saunders.

*A guide for the physical therapist using therapeutic modalities.*

Denegar C: *Therapeutic modalities for athletic injuries*, Champaign, IL, 2015, Human Kinetics.

*Focuses on the neurophysiological mechanisms of pain control as mediated by a variety of therapeutic modalities.*

Knight KL: *Cryotherapy in sports injury management*, Champaign, IL, 1995, Human Kinetics.

*Excellent coverage, both theoretical and practical, of one of the most widely used therapeutic approaches in sports medicine and athletic training—cryotherapy; clearly written and easily applied.*

Knight KL, Draper DO: *Therapeutic modalities: The art and science*, 2012, Philadelphia, PA: Lippincott Williams & Wilkins.

*Addresses all facets of therapeutic modality use.*

Michlovitz SL, editor: Modalities for therapeutic intervention. Philadelphia, PA, 2011, F.A. Davis.

*An excellent text about understanding the foundations and use of thermal agents in sports medicine and athletic training. Provides detailed discussions of inflammation, pain, superficial heat and cold, and the therapeutic use of ultrasound and shortwave diathermy.*

Prentice W: *Therapeutic modalities in rehabilitation*, New York, 2011, McGraw-Hill.

*A comprehensive guide to using therapeutic modalities in treating a variety of patient populations. Contains pertinent case studies and laboratory activities.*

Prentice W, editor: *Therapeutic modalities for sports medicine and athletic training*, ed 5, St. Louis, MO, 2010, McGraw-Hill.

*A comprehensive guide to the use of therapeutic modalities in the sports medicine setting. Addresses all aspects of modality use, including massage, traction, and intermittent compression. An excellent blend of theory and practical application.*

Starkey C: *Therapeutic modalities for athletic trainers*, Philadelphia, PA, 2013, F.A. Davis.

*Discusses many of the modalities used by athletic trainers in a clinical setting.*

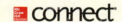

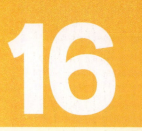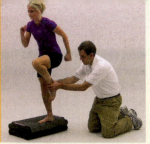

# 16

© William E. Prentice

# Using Therapeutic Exercise in Rehabilitation

## ■ Objectives

*When you finish this chapter you should be able to*

- Explain how the athletic trainer approaches rehabilitation.
- Contrast therapeutic exercise and conditioning exercise.
- Describe the consequences of sudden inactivity and injury immobilization.
- Recognize the primary components of a rehabilitation program.
- Discuss the concept of open versus closed kinetic chain exercises.
- Explain the importance of incorporating core stabilization training into a rehabilitation program.

- Evaluate the value of aquatic exercise in rehabilitation.
- Identify the techniques and principles of proprioceptive neuromuscular facilitation.
- Demonstrate the use of mobilization, traction, and Mulligan techniques for improving accessory joint motions.
- Discuss how muscle energy, myofascial release, strain/counterstrain, positional release, active release, and biofeedback techniques can be incorporated into a rehabilitation program.

## ■ Outline

## ■ Key Terms

proprioception                kinesthesia                buoyancy

## ■ Connect Highlights   ![McGraw Hill Education] connect

*Visit connect.mcgraw-hill.com for further exercises to apply your knowledge:*

- Clinical application scenarios covering primary components of rehabilitation, core stabilization, aquatic exercises, and mobilization techniques
- Click-and-drag questions covering components of a rehabilitation program, rehabilitation exercises, and joint mobilization
- Multiple-choice questions covering core stabilization, aquatic rehabilitation, joint mobilization, traction, therapeutic exercises, conditioning, and consequences of inactivity

# THE ATHLETIC TRAINER'S APPROACH TO REHABILITATION

The process of rehabilitation begins immediately after injury. Initial first-aid and management techniques can have a substantial impact on the course and ultimate outcome of the rehabilitative process. Thus, in addition to possessing a sound understanding of how injuries can be prevented, the athletic trainer must also be competent in providing correct and appropriate initial care when injury occurs. In a sports medicine setting, the athletic trainer most often assumes the primary responsibility for design, implementation, and supervision of the rehabilitation program for the injured patient.

> The athletic trainer is responsible for design, implementation, and supervision of the rehablitation program.

Designing programs for rehabilitation is relatively simple and involves several basic components: minimizing swelling, controlling pain, reestablishing neuromuscular control, establishing or enhancing core stability, restoring or increasing muscular strength and endurance, regaining or improving range of motion, regaining balance and postural control, and maintaining levels of cardiorespiratory endurance. Addressing each of these components is the easy part of supervising a rehabilitation program. The difficult part comes in knowing exactly when and how to change the rehabilitation protocols to most effectively accomplish both long- and short-term goals. Progression during the rehabilitation program should be based on specific criteria, and return to play decisions must be based on level of function and patient outcomes. Certainly, the athletic trainer plays a key role in return to play decisions.

The approach to rehabilitation in an athletic environment is considerably different than in most other rehabilitation settings. The competitive nature of athletics necessitates an aggressive approach to rehabilitation. Because the competitive season in most sports is relatively short, the long-term goal is for the patient to return to activity as soon as safely possible. Thus, the athletic trainer who is supervising the rehabilitation program must perform a balancing act between not pushing the patient hard enough and being overly aggressive. In either case, a mistake in judgment on the part of the athletic trainer may hinder the patient's return to activity.

> A soccer player has been diagnosed as having a grade 2 sprain of the medial collateral ligament in her knee. The team physician has referred the athlete to the athletic trainer, who is responsible for overseeing the rehabilitation program.
>
> **?** What are the components that need to be addressed in a rehabilitation program, and how can the athletic trainer best incorporate these components?

Decisions as to when and how to alter and progress a rehabilitation program should be based within the framework of the healing process. The athletic trainer must possess a sound understanding of both the sequence and the time frames for the various phases of healing and must realize that certain physiological events must occur during each of the phases.[62] Any actions taken during a rehabilitation program that interfere with this healing process will likely increase the length of time required for rehabilitation and slow the patient's return to full activity. The healing process must have an opportunity to accomplish what it is supposed to. At best, the athletic trainer can only try to create an environment that is conducive to the healing process. Little can be done to speed up the process physiologically, but many things can be done during rehabilitation to impede healing.[62]

Athletic trainers have many tools at their disposal that can facilitate the rehabilitative process. How the athletic trainer chooses to use those tools is often a matter of individual preference and experience. Additionally, each patient is different, and the responses to various treatment protocols vary. Thus, a cookbook approach to rehabilitation, with specific protocols that can be followed like a recipe, is impossible. In fact, the use of rehabilitation recipes is strongly discouraged. Instead, the athletic trainer must develop a broad theoretical knowledge base from which he or she can select and apply specific rehabilitation techniques to each athlete.

# THERAPEUTIC EXERCISE VERSUS CONDITIONING EXERCISE

Exercise is an essential factor in fitness conditioning, injury prevention, and injury rehabilitation. To compete successfully at a high level, the athlete must be fit. An athlete who is not fit is more likely to sustain an injury. Improper conditioning is one of the major causes of sports injuries. It is essential that the athlete engage in training and conditioning exercises that minimize the possibility of injury while maximizing performance.

The basic principles of conditioning that were discussed in Chapter 4 also apply to therapeutic, rehabilitative, and reconditioning exercises for restoring normal body function following injury. The term *therapeutic exercise* is perhaps most widely used to indicate exercises that are used in a rehabilitation program.[46]

> Therapeutic exercises are concerned with restoring normal body function after injury.

# SUDDEN PHYSICAL INACTIVITY AND INJURY IMMOBILIZATION

The human body is a dynamic, moving entity that requires physical activity to maintain proper physical function. When an injury occurs, two problems immediately arise that must be addressed. First is the generalized loss of physical fitness that occurs when activity is stopped, and second is the specific inactivity of the injured part, resulting from protective splinting of the soft tissue and, in some cases, immobilization by some external means.

## Effects of General Inactivity

An individual who is highly conditioned will experience a rapid, generalized loss of fitness when exercise is suddenly stopped.[1] This sudden lack of activity causes a loss of muscle strength, endurance,

> A sudden loss of physical activity leads to a generalized loss of physical fitness.

and coordination. Whenever possible, the patient must continue to exercise the entire body without aggravating the injury.

## Effects of Immobilization

An injured body part that is immobilized for a period of time causes a number of disuse problems that adversely affect muscle, joints, ligaments and bones, and the cardiorespiratory system.

**Muscle and Immobilization** When a body part is immobilized for even as short a period as 24 hours, definite adverse muscular changes occur.

*Atrophy and Fiber-Type Conversion* Disuse of a body part quickly leads to a loss of muscle mass. The greatest atrophy occurs in the type I (slow-twitch) fibers. Over time, the slow-twitch

> Immobilization of a part causes atrophy of slow-twitch muscle fibers.

fibers develop fast-twitch characteristics. Slow-twitch fibers also diminish in number without type II (fast-twitch) fibers lessening in number.[1] A muscle that is immobilized in a lengthened or neutral position tends to atrophy less. In contrast, immobilizing a muscle in a shortened position encourages atrophy and greater loss of contractile function.[1] Atrophy can also be prevented through isometric contraction and electrical stimulation of the muscles. As the unused muscle decreases in size because of atrophy, protein is also lost. When activity is resumed, normal protein synthesis is reestablished.

*Decreased Neuromuscular Efficiency* Immobilization causes motor nerves to become less efficient in recruiting and stimulating individual muscle fibers within a given motor unit.[4] Once immobilization ends, the original motor neuron discharge returns within about 1 week.

**Joints and Immobilization** The immobilization of joints causes a loss of normal compression, which in turn leads to a decrease in lubrication within the joint, caus-

> Joint immobilization decreases normal lubrication.

ing degeneration. This degeneration occurs because the articular cartilage is deprived of its normal nutrition. The use of continuous passive motion, electrical muscle stimulation, or rehabilitative hinged braces (see Figure 7–30C) has in some cases retarded the loss of articular cartilage.[53]

**Ligament and Bone and Immobilization** Both ligaments and bones adapt to normal stress by maintaining or increasing their strength. However, when stress is eliminated or decreased, ligament and bone become weaker.[58] Once immobilization has been removed, high-frequency, short-duration endurance exercise positively enhances the mechanical properties of ligaments. Endurance activities tend to increase both the production and the hypertrophy of the collagen fibers. Full remodeling of ligaments after immobilization may take 12 months or more.

**Cardiorespiratory System and Immobilization** Like other structures, the cardiorespiratory system is adversely affected by immobilization. The resting heart rate increases approximately one-half beat per minute each day of immobilization. The stroke volume, maximum oxygen uptake, and vital capacity decrease concurrently with the increase in heart rate.

## The Mental Aspects of Sudden Inactivity

The mental aspects of how an individual deals with an injury are a critical yet often neglected factor in the rehabilitation process. Injury and illness produce a wide range of emotional reactions; therefore, the athletic trainer needs to develop an understanding of the psyche of each patient.[9] Individuals vary in terms of pain threshold, cooperation, and compliance, competitiveness, denial of disability, depression, intrinsic and extrinsic motivation, anger, fear, guilt, and the ability to adjust to injury. These factors, both individually and collectively, can dictate the ultimate course of the rehabilitative process (see Chapter 11).

# MAJOR COMPONENTS OF A REHABILITATION PROGRAM

**Components of a rehabilitation program:**

- Minimizing swelling
- Controlling pain
- Reestablishing neuromuscular control
- Establishing or enhancing core stability
- Regaining or improving range of motion
- Restoring or increasing muscular strength and endurance
- Regaining balance and postural control
- Maintaining cardiorespiratory endurance
- Incorporating functional progressions

A well-designed, functional rehabilitation program should routinely address several key components before an injured athlete can return to preinjury competitive levels. Those components include minimizing swelling through appropriate first aid and management of initial injury, controlling pain, reestablishing neuromuscular control, establishing or enhancing core stability, regaining or improving range of motion, restoring or increasing muscular strength and endurance, regaining balance and postural control, maintaining levels of cardiorespiratory endurance, and incorporating functional progressions.[58]

## Minimizing Initial Swelling

The process of rehabilitation begins immediately after acute injury. The manner in which the injury is first managed unquestionably has a significant impact on the course of the rehabilitative process. The one problem all acute injuries, regardless of type, have in common is swelling. Swelling during the inflammatory stage of healing is caused by any number of factors, including bleeding, the production of synovial fluid, an accumulation of inflammatory byproducts, edema, or a combination of several factors. Once swelling has occurred, the healing process is significantly retarded. The injured area cannot return to normal until all the swelling is gone. Therefore, all first-aid management of these conditions should be directed toward controlling the swelling.[58] If the swelling can be controlled initially in the acute stage of injury, the time required for rehabilitation is likely to be significantly reduced. To control and significantly limit the amount of swelling, the POLICE principle—protection, optimal loading, ice, compression, and elevation—should be applied (see Chapter 12).

## Controlling Pain

When an injury occurs, the athletic trainer must realize that the patient will experience some degree of pain (see Chapter 10). The extent of the pain is determined by the severity of the injury, the patient's individual response to and perception of pain, and the circumstances under which the injury occurred. The athletic trainer can modulate acute pain by using the POLICE technique immediately after injury.[61] A physician may also make use of various medications to help ease pain.

Persistent pain can make strengthening or flexibility exercises more difficult and thus interfere with the rehabilitation process. The athletic trainer should routinely address pain during each treatment session. Making use of appropriate manual therapy techniques and therapeutic modalities, including various techniques of cryotherapy, thermotherapy, and electrical stimulating currents, will help modulate pain throughout the rehabilitation process (see Chapter 15).[61,72]

## Reestablishing Neuromuscular Control

After injury and subsequent rest and immobilization, the central nervous system "forgets" how to put together information coming from muscle and joint mechanoreceptors and from cutaneous, visual, and vestibular input.[26] *Neuromuscular control* is the mind's attempt to teach the body conscious control of a specific movement.[40] Successful repetition of a patterned movement using correct form makes its performance progressively less difficult and thus requires less concentration; eventually, the movement becomes automatic. Reestablishing neuromuscular control requires many repetitions of the same movement through a step-by-step progression from simple to more complex movements.[76] Strengthening exercises, particularly those that tend to be more functional, are essential for reestablishing neuromuscular control (Figure 16–1).[83]

Regaining neuromuscular control means regaining the ability to follow a previously established sensory pattern.[40] The central nervous system compares the intent and production of a specific movement with stored information, continually adjusting until any discrepancy in movement is corrected.[17] Four elements are critical for reestablishing neuromuscular control: (1) proprioception and kinesthesia, (2) dynamic stability, (3) preparatory and reactive muscle characteristics, and (4) conscious and unconscious functional motor patterns.[83]

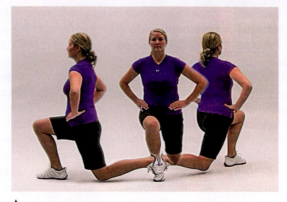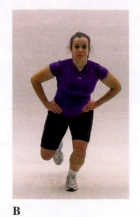

**A**                                                                **B**

FIGURE 16–1   Reestablishing neuromuscular control involves performing multiple repetitions of the same functional strengthening movements while concentrating on using correct form. **(A)** Multiplanar lunges. **(B)** Single-leg squat.

© William E. Prentice

Relearning correct functional movement and timing after injury to a joint may require several months. Addressing neuromuscular control is critical throughout the recovery process but may be most critical during the early stages of rehabilitation to avoid reinjury.[83]

Reestablishing proprioception and kinesthesia should also be of primary concern to the athletic trainer in all rehabilitation programs.[40] **Proprioception** is the ability to determine the position of a joint in space; **kinesthesia** is the ability to detect movement.[68] The ability to sense the position of a joint in space is mediated by mechanoreceptors found in both muscles and joints and by cutaneous, visual, and vestibular input. Neuromuscular control relies on the central nervous system to interpret and integrate proprioceptive and kinesthetic information and then to control individual muscles and joints to produce coordinated movement.[68,73]

> Neuromuscular control produces coordinated movement.

**Joint Mechanoreceptors**   Joint mechanoreceptors are found in ligaments, capsules, menisci, labria, and skin:

- Ruffini's corpuscles in the joint capsules, ligaments, and skin are sensitive to touch, tension, and possibly heat; these receptors are sensitive to changes in the position of the joint and to the rate and direction of movement of the joint. They are most active in the end ranges of motion.[61]

> Joint mechanoreceptors include Ruffini's corpuscles, Pacinian corpuscles, Merkel's corpuscles, Meissner's corpuscles, and free nerve endings.

- Pacinian corpuscles in the skin respond to deep pressure.
- Merkel's corpuscles in the skin respond to deep pressure, but more slowly than Pacinian corpuscles.

- Meissner's corpuscles in the skin are activated by light touch.
- Free nerve endings are sensitive to extreme mechanical, thermal, or chemical energy. They respond to noxious stimuli—in other words, to impending or actual tissue damage (for example, sprains, cuts, and burns).

Before the 1970s, these receptors in the joint capsules and ligaments were thought to be primarily responsible for joint proprioception. Since then, there has been considerable debate concerning the role of the joint mechanoreceptors in proprioception and whether joint mechanoreceptors and muscle mechanoreceptors do, in fact, interact with one another. At this point, it has become apparent that the joint mechanoreceptors are not solely responsible for determining joint position. The contemporary viewpoint is that, although joint and muscle mechanoreceptors work in a complementary manner, muscle mechanoreceptors play a more important role in signaling joint position.[76] Any single receptor working in isolation from the others is generally ineffective in signaling information about the movements of the body.[40]

**Muscle Mechanoreceptors**   The function and role of muscle spindles and Golgi tendon organs were discussed in detail in Chapter 4. Muscle spindles, located in the muscle, are sensitive to changes in the length of that muscle, whereas Golgi tendon organs, found at the musculotendinous juncture, are sensitive to changes in muscle tension.[60]

> Muscle mechanoreceptors include muscle spindles and Golgi tendon organs.

### Establishing or Enhancing Core Stability

Muscular-based stability of the trunk is referred to as *core stability,* which ensures a near static posture of the trunk even under the influence of destabilizing external forces.[2] A dynamic core stabilization training program should be an important component of all comprehensive strengthening and injury rehabilitation programs.[35] The *core* is defined as the lumbo-pelvic-hip complex. The core is where the center of gravity is located and where all movement begins. Twenty-nine muscles have their attachment to the lumbo-pelvic-hip complex. The key lumbar spine muscles are the transversospinalis group, erector spinae, quadratus lumborum, and latissimus dorsi. The key abdominal muscles are the rectus abdominus, external oblique, and internal oblique. The key hip muscles are the gluteus maximus, gluteus medius, and psoas.[10] The inner core or *deep core* muscles include the transversus abdominis and the multifidus, which work with the pelvic floor muscles, and the diaphragm to play perhaps the most critical role in the stability of the trunk and pelvis.

A core stabilization program improves dynamic postural control, ensures appropriate muscular balance and joint movement around the lumbo-pelvic-hip complex, allows for the expression of dynamic functional strength, and improves neuromuscular efficiency throughout the body.[10] This permits optimal acceleration, deceleration, and dynamic stabilization of all of functioning interconnected segments of the entire body, referred to as the kinetic chain, during functional movements. It also provides proximal stability for efficient lower-extremity movements.[12]

> **Kinetic Chain** Series of functioning interconnected segments throughout the entire body.

Many individuals have developed the functional strength, power, neuromuscular control, and muscular endurance in specific muscles that enable them to perform functional activities. However, relatively few have developed the muscles required for stabilization of the spine (see Chapters 4 and 25). The body's stabilization system has to be functioning optimally to effectively use the strength, power, neuromuscular control, and muscular endurance that individuals have developed in their prime movers. If the extremity muscles are strong and the core is weak, then there will not be enough force created to produce efficient movements.[12] A weak core is a fundamental problem of inefficient movements that leads to injury.

A core stabilization training program is designed to help an individual gain strength, neuromuscular control, power, and muscle endurance in the lumbo-pelvic-hip complex.[35] This approach facilitates a balanced muscular functioning of the entire kinetic chain. Greater neuromuscular control and stabilization strength offer a more biomechanically efficient position for the entire kinetic chain, therefore allowing optimal neuromuscular efficiency throughout the kinetic chain.[77]

A comprehensive core stabilization training program should be systematic, progressive, and functional.[10] When designing a functional core stabilization training program, the athletic trainer should select the appropriate exercises to elicit a maximal training response. The exercises must be safe yet challenging, stress multiple planes, incorporate a variety of resistance equipment (physioball, medicine ball, bodyblade, weight vest, dumbbells, tubing, etc.), derive from fundamental movement skills, and be activity specific (Figure 16–2). The athletic trainer should follow a progressive functional continuum to allow optimal adaptations. The patient starts with the exercises at the highest level at which he or she can maintain stability and optimal neuromuscular control. Patients then progress through the program as they achieve mastery of the exercises at each level.[10]

## Regaining or Improving Range of Motion

Injury to a joint will always be associated with some loss of motion. That loss of movement may be attributed to contracture of connective tissue (i.e., ligaments, joint capsules), resistance to stretch of the musculotendinous unit (i.e., muscle, tendon, and fascia), or a combination of the two.

**Physiological versus Accessory Movements** Two types of movement govern range of motion about a joint. *Physiological movements* result from an active muscle contraction that moves an extremity through flexion, extension, abduction, adduction, and rotation. *Accessory motions* refers to the manner in which one articulating joint surface moves relative to another; such motions are *spin, roll,* and *glide.*[31] Physiological movements are voluntary, and accessory movements normally accompany physiological movements. The two occur simultaneously. Normal accessory motions must occur for full-range physiological movements to take place. If any of the accessory component motions are restricted, normal physiological cardinal plane movements will not occur.[59]

> **Physiological movements:**
> - Flexion
> - Extension
> - Abduction
> - Adduction
> - Rotation

> **Accessory motions:**
> - Spin
> - Roll
> - Glide

Traditionally, rehabilitation programs tended to concentrate more on passive physiological movements and not pay much attention to accessory motions. It is critical for the athletic trainer to closely evaluate the injured joint to determine whether motion is limited because of

> **Restricted physiological** movement requires stretching.

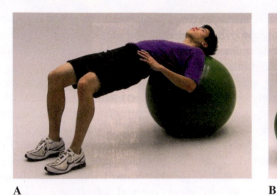
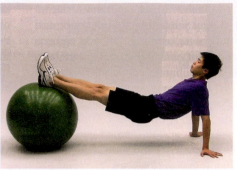

A                           B

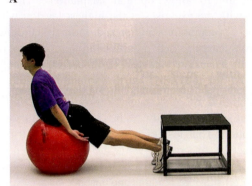
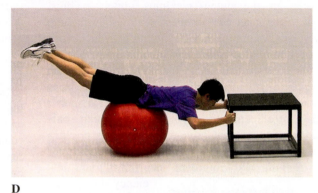

C                           D

FIGURE 16–2   Core stabilization training exercises using a stability ball to increase strength and control in the lumbo-pelvic-hip complex.
© William E. Prentice

**Restricted accessory motion requires joint mobilization.** physiological movement constraints involving musculotendinous units or because of limitation in accessory motion involving the joint capsule and ligaments. If physiological movement is restricted, the patient should engage in stretching activities designed to improve flexibility.[3] Stretching exercises should be used whenever there is musculotendinous resistance to stretch.[14] If accessory motion is limited because of some restriction of the joint capsule or the ligaments, the athletic trainer should incorporate mobilization techniques into the treatment program. Mobilization techniques should be used whenever there are tight articular structures.[59]

## Restoring or Increasing Muscular Strength and Endurance

Muscular strength is one of the most essential factors in restoring the function of a body part to preinjury status. Isometric, progressive resistance, and isokinetic exercises can benefit rehabilitation. A major goal in performing strengthening exercises is for the patient to work through a full, pain-free range of motion.

**Isometric Exercises** Isometric exercises are commonly performed in the early phase of rehabilitation when a joint is immobilized for a period of time. They are useful when resistance training though a full range of motion may make the injury worse. Isometrics increase static strength and assist in decreasing the amount of atrophy. Isometrics can also lessen swelling by causing a muscle-pumping action to remove fluid and edema. Isometric exercise can be used to increase strength at whatever angle weakness exists.

Strength gains are limited primarily to the angle at which the joint is exercised. No functional force or eccentric work is developed. Other difficulties are motivation and measurement of the force that is being applied.

**Progressive Resistance Exercises** Progressive resistance exercises are the most commonly used strengthening technique in a reconditioning program. These exercises may be done using free weights, exercise machines, rubber tubing, or manual resistance (Figure 16–3).[75] Progressive resistance exercises use isotonic contractions, in which force is generated while the muscle is changing in length.

*Concentric and Eccentric Muscle Contractions* Isotonic contractions may be either concentric or eccentric. Traditionally, patients engaging in progressive resistance exercises have concentrated primarily on the concentric component, without paying much attention to

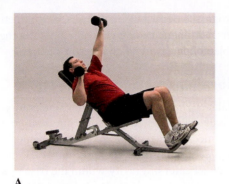

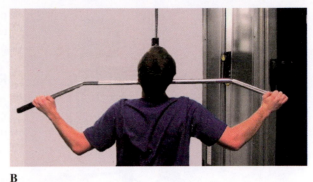

A                B

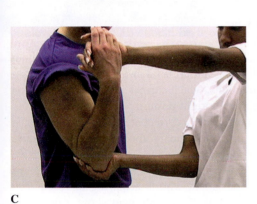

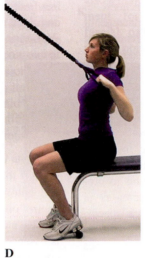

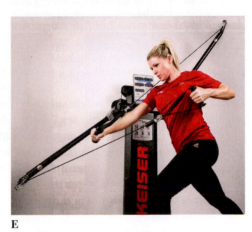

C              D             E

FIGURE 16–3  Progressive resistance exercise techniques. **(A)** Free weights. **(B)** Exercise machines. **(C)** Manual resistance. **(D)** Elastic bands or tubing. **(E)** Position-adjustable cable system.

(a-d) © William E. Prentice; (e) Courtesy Keiser

the importance of the eccentric component. The use of eccentric contractions, particularly in the rehabilitation of various injuries related to sport, has received considerable emphasis in recent years.[57] Eccentric contractions are critical for deceleration of limb motion, especially during high-velocity dynamic activities. For example, a baseball pitcher relies on an eccentric contraction of the external rotators at the glenohumeral joint to decelerate the humerus, which may be internally rotating at speeds as high as 8,000 degrees per second. Strength deficits or the inability of a muscle to tolerate these eccentric forces can predispose an athlete to injury. Eccentric contractions are used to facilitate concentric contractions in plyometric exercises and may be incorporated into functional proprioceptive neuromuscular facilitation strengthening exercises. Thus, the athletic trainer should include both eccentric and concentric strengthening exercises in a rehabilitation program.

Both concentric and eccentric contractions are possible with free weights, most isotonic exercise machines, and rubber tubing or an elastic band (Figure 16–3A–D). A disadvantage of most exercise machines is that they do not allow exercises to be performed in diagonal

or functional planes. It is also difficult to exercise at functional velocities without producing additional injuries. Several newer exercise machines have been developed that use position-adjustable cable systems that allow for more functional multiplanar resistance at higher velocities (e.g., Keiser Functional Trainer) (Figure 16–3E). Resistive exercise using rubber tubing allows both concentric and eccentric resistance and is not encumbered by the design of an exercise machine. It offers a wide range of usefulness at an extremely low cost.

**Isokinetic Exercises** If isokinetic exercises are used in the rehabilitation process, they are most often incorporated during the later phases.[54] Isokinetics uses a fixed speed with accommodating resistance to provide maximal resistance throughout the range of motion (Figure 16–4). Isokinetic devices are generally capable of calculating measures of torque, average power, and total work, and ratios of torque to body weight, each of which may be used diagnostically by the athletic trainer. Isokinetic measures are commonly used as a criterion for return of the athlete to functional activity after injury.

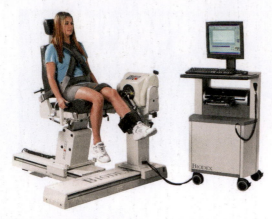

FIGURE 16−4   Isokinetics are primarily used as a diagnostic tool to determine levels of strength.
Courtesy Biodex Medical Systems, Inc.

The speed of movement can be altered in isokinetic exercise. Gains in strength from training at slower speeds (60 to 120 degrees per second) are fairly specific to the angular velocity used in training. Isokinetic machines allow the athlete to exercise at speeds that are somewhat more functional. Training at faster speeds seems to produce more general improvement because increases in torque values can be seen at both fast and slow speeds. Isokinetic exercises performed at high speeds tend to decrease the joint's compressive forces. Fast exercises produce fewer negative effects on joints than do slow exercises. Short-arc submaximal isokinetic exercise spreads out synovial fluid, helping nourish the articular cartilage and preventing deterioration.[54] It also develops neuromuscular patterning for the functional speed and movements demanded by specific sports.

**Testing Strength, Endurance, and Power** Testing for improvement in muscular strength, endurance, or power can be accomplished through manual muscle tests, progressive resistance exercises, or isokinetic dynamometers. Isokinetic testing generally provides the most reliable objective measure of changes in strength.

## Regaining Balance and Postural Control

Balance involves the complex integration of muscular forces, neurological sensory information received from the mechanoreceptors, and biomechanical information.[16] Achieving postural control involves positioning the body's center of gravity within the base of support. When the center of gravity extends beyond the base of support, the limits of stability are exceeded, even though the base of support has not changed, and a corrective step or stumble is necessary to prevent a fall. Even when an individual appears to be motionless, the body is undergoing constant postural sway caused by reflexive muscle contractions, which correct and maintain dynamic equilibrium in an upright posture.[16] When balance is disrupted, the response to correct it is primarily reflexive and automatic.[3] The primary mechanisms for postural control occur in the joints of the lower extremity.[82]

> Postural control involves the integration of muscular, neurological, and biomechanical information.

The ability to balance and maintain postural control is essential to a patient who is acquiring or reacquiring complex motor skills.[16] Patients who show a decreased sense of balance or lack of postural control after injury may lack sufficient proprioceptive and kinesthetic information or muscular strength, either of which may limit the patient's ability to generate an effective correction response to disequilibrium.[3] A rehabilitation program must include functional exercises that incorporate balance and proprioceptive training to prepare the patient for return to activity. Failure to address balance problems may predispose the patient to reinjury (Figure 16–5).

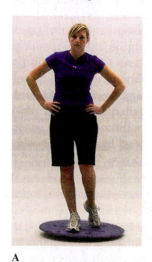
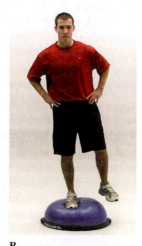
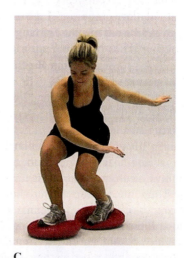

A                          B                          C

FIGURE 16−5   Balance training is essential in the rehabilitation program. Many balance training products are available. **(A)** BAPS Board. **(B)** Bosu Balance Trainer. **(C)** Dynadisc.
© William E. Prentice

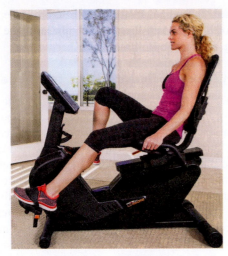

**FIGURE 16-6** Stationary cycling provides a means of maintaining cardiorespiratory fitness during rehabilitation.
Courtesy LifeCORE Fitness, Inc.

## Maintaining Cardiorespiratory Endurance

Although strength and flexibility are commonly regarded as essential components in any injury rehabilitation program, relatively little consideration is given to maintaining levels of cardiorespiratory endurance. An athlete spends a considerable amount of time preparing the cardiorespiratory system to be able to handle the increased demands made on it during a competitive season. When injury occurs and the athlete is forced to miss training time, levels of cardiorespiratory endurance may decrease rapidly. Thus, the athletic trainer must design or substitute alternative activities that allow the individual to maintain existing levels of cardiorespiratory endurance during the rehabilitation period.

Depending on the nature of the injury, a number of possible activities are open to the athlete. For a lower-extremity injury, non–weight bearing activities should be incorporated. Pool activities provide an excellent means for injury rehabilitation. Cycling can also positively stress the cardiorespiratory system (Figure 16–6).

## Incorporating Functional Progressions

The purpose of any rehabilitation program is to restore normal function after injury. Functional progressions involve a series of gradually progressive activities designed to prepare the individual for return to a specific sport.[17] Functional progressions should be incorporated into the treatment program as early as possible. Well-designed functional progressions will gradually assist the injured patient in achieving normal, pain-free range of motion, restoring adequate strength levels, and regaining neuromuscular control throughout the rehabilitation process.[59] Ultimately, the focus becomes a safe return to activity. Those skills necessary for successful participation in a given activity are broken down into component parts, and the patient gradually reacquires those skills within the limitations of his or her progress.[17] The athletic trainer should transfer those skills observed in the performance of a specific activity into a progression of rehabilitative exercises.

Functional activities follow a consistent progression from simple to complex skills, slow to fast speeds, short to longer distances, or light to heavy activities.[81] The athletic trainer must monitor every new activity introduced to determine the athlete's ability to perform as well as his or her physical tolerance. If an activity does not produce additional pain or swelling, the level should be advanced; new activities should be introduced as quickly as possible. Thus, the injured patient would be gradually introduced to the stresses imposed by a particular demand until function is adequate for the patient to return to *sport-specific activity*.[17]

In the case of an athlete, the optimal functional progression program would be designed such that the athlete would have an opportunity to practice every possible skill that is required in a sport before he or she returns to competition. This

> Functional progressions incorporate sport-specific skills into the rehabilitation program.

program would minimize the normal anxiety and apprehension the athlete would experience on return to a competitive environment.[47] Supervised functional progression activities can be done during team practice sessions. This arrangement allows athletes to be around teammates and coaches, which should help them feel more accepted as team members.[47]

**Functional Testing** Functional testing involves having the patient perform certain tasks appropriate to his or her stage in the rehabilitation process in order to isolate and address specific deficits.[63] As a result, the athletic trainer is able to determine the patient's current functional level and set functional goals. Functional testing can be used to determine risk of injury due to limb asymmetry, provide objective measure of progress during a treatment or rehabilitation program, and measure the ability of the individual to tolerate forces.[47]

**16-3 Clinical Application Exercise**

A runner complains of anterior knee pain. She has greatly cut back on the distance of her training runs and indicates that she has been taking antiinflammatory medication to help her continue to train. However, she is frustrated because her knee seems to be getting worse instead of better.

**?** What can the athletic trainer recommend to most effectively help the patient deal with her knee pain?

Functional testing can provide the athletic trainer with objective data for review. Traditional rehabilitation programs and improvements in strength and range of motion do not always correlate with functional ability. Functional testing should have a better correlation with functional ability.

When contemplating the use of a functional test or battery of tests, the athletic trainer must evaluate the test(s) chosen. Validity and reliability must be considered. A test should measure what it intends to measure (validity) and should consistently provide similar results (reliability) regardless of the evaluator. Other factors must be considered before releasing a patient to full activity. These include a subjective evaluation of the injury, performance on functional tests, presence or absence of signs and symptoms, other recognized clinical tests (isokinetic testing, special tests, etc.), and the physician's approval. Functional testing should attempt to look at unilateral function and bilateral function in an attempt to determine whether the patient is compensating with the uninjured limb. Other considerations should include the stage of healing for the patient, appropriate rest time, and self-evaluation.[63]

Obviously, a patient who cannot complete the test(s) is not ready for a return to play. If the athletic trainer has normative values or has collected preinjury baseline values, comparison with postinjury testing values makes a return to activity decision easier. Usually, the athletic trainer has to make a subjective decision based on the test result. But if the normative data or preinjury data are available, the athletic trainer can make an objective decision. If a soccer player is able to complete a sprint test with a mean of 20 seconds but her preinjury time was 17 seconds, then she is only 85 percent functional. Without the preinjury data, the athletic trainer might be unable to determine the patient's functional level.[47]

For years, athletic trainers have used a variety of functional tests to assess a patient's progress, including sprinting tests, agility runs, figure eights, shuttle runs, carioca tests, side stepping, vertical jumps, hopping for time or distance, and balance tests. Functional testing should be an easy task for athletic trainers and should be equally simple for patients to understand. Cost efficiency, time demands, and space demands are important concepts when considering the tests to use.[17,47]

# DEVELOPING A REHABILITATION PLAN

No rehabilitation program can be effective without a carefully designed plan. Athletic trainers overseeing a rehabilitation program must have a complete understanding of the injury, including knowledge of how the injury was

> All exercise rehabilitation must be conducted as part of a carefully designed plan.

sustained, the major anatomical structures affected, the grade of trauma, and the stage or phase of the injury's healing.

## Setting Long-term and Short-term Goals

Setting goals is the best way to achieve a successful rehabilitation outcome. The athletic trainer should work with patients to develop long-term and short-term measurable goals and insure that the goals agreed upon are realistic and attainable.[21] When beginning a rehabilitation program, the patient must have at least some idea of what he or she ultimately wants to accomplish at the end of the program. For an athlete, the long-term goal is almost always to return to practice and competition as soon as safely possible. For the office worker or the soccer mom who has been injured, the long-term goal may simply be to return to performing normal daily activities.

Short-term goals should be a means to help the patient achieve the long-term goal. For example, if a runner has sprained an ankle and the long-term goal for completing rehabilitation is to run a 5K road race, the early phases of rehabilitation should include two short-term goals: (1) walking once around a running track (400 yards) without a limp and then (2) jogging 1 mile in under 8 minutes without increased pain or swelling.

The short-term goals need to be linked to the problem that the patient is seeking help for, or the majority of patients will not stick with the program. When patients understand that their care has been customized for them and has been designed to restore the function that is important to them, two important things happen. First, they accept some ownership of the rehabilitation program because they were involved in the development of the plan. Patients are more likely to follow a procedure that they can see direct relevance in, and less likely to follow programs that they see as meaningless. Second, short-term goals provide the patient with a road map to follow. Because the goals are measurable, the patient is able to self-assess, and the plan provides the patient with a means of recognizing when he or she is on the expected path to full recovery.[21]

Generally, when designing an exercise program, it is better to have two or three simple exercises that are executed faithfully and correctly than to have an elaborate program that will not be done due to lack of time, understanding, or some other perceived barrier. Thus, another key element that goes hand-in-hand with the development of short-term goals is to keep the instruction simple.[47]

## Exercise Phases

Rehabilitation progressions can be subdivided into three phases based primarily on the three stages of the healing process: phase 1, the acute inflammatory response phase;

phase 2, the fibroblastic repair phase; and phase 3, the maturation-remodeling phase (see Chapter 10). If surgery is necessary, a fourth phase, the preoperative phase, must also be considered. Depending on the type and extent of injury and the individual response to healing, phases will usually overlap. Each phase must include carefully considered goals and criteria for advancing from one phase to another.

**Preoperative Exercise Phase** The preoperative exercise phase applies only to those patients who sustain injuries that require surgery. If surgery can be postponed, exercise may be used as a means to improve its outcome. By allowing the initial inflammatory response phase to resolve and by maintaining or increasing muscle strength and flexibility, cardiorespiratory fitness, and neuromuscular control, the patient may be better prepared to continue the rehabilitation program after surgery.

**Phase 1: Acute Inflammatory Response Phase** Phase 1 begins immediately when injury occurs and may last as long as 4 days. This phase of the healing process is attempting to control and clean up the injured tissues, thus creating an environment that is conducive to the fibroblastic repair stage. The primary focus of rehabilitation during this phase is to control swelling and to modulate pain by using protection, optimal loading, ice, compression, and elevation (POLICE) immediately after injury. Throughout this phase, ice, compression, and elevation should be used as much as possible.[58]

Rest of the injured part is critical during this phase. It is widely accepted that early mobility during rehabilitation is essential. However, if the athletic trainer becomes overly aggressive during the first 48 hours after injury and does not allow the injured part to rest during the inflammatory stage of healing, the inflammatory process never gets a chance to accomplish its purpose. Consequently, the length of time required for inflammation may be extended. Immobility during the first 2 days after injury is necessary to control inflammation.

Rest does not mean that the patient does nothing. The term *rest* applies only to the injured body part. During this period, the patient should work on cardiorespiratory endurance and should do strengthening and flexibility exercises for the parts of the body not affected by the injury. When immobilized, muscle tensing or isometrics may be used to maintain muscle strength.

By day 3 or 4, swelling begins to subside and eventually stops altogether. The injured area may feel warm to the touch, and some discoloration may be apparent. The injury is still painful to the touch, and some pain is elicited when the injured part is moved. At this point, the patient may begin active mobility exercises, working through a pain-free range of motion. If the injury involves the lower extremity, the patient should be encouraged to bear progressively more weight.

A physician may choose to have the patient take nonsteroidal antiinflammatory drugs (NSAIDs) to help control swelling and inflammation. It is usually helpful to continue this medication throughout the rehabilitative process.

**Phase 2: Fibroblastic Repair Phase** Once the inflammatory response has subsided, the fibroblastic repair phase begins. During this stage of the healing process, fibroblastic cells are laying down a matrix of collagen fibers and forming scar tissue. This stage may begin as early as 4 days after the injury and may last for several weeks. At this point, swelling has stopped completely. The injury is still tender to the touch but is not as painful as during phase 1. Pain is also less with active and passive motion.[58]

As soon as inflammation is controlled, the athletic trainer should immediately begin to incorporate into the rehabilitation program activities that can help the patient maintain levels of cardiorespiratory endurance, restore full range of motion, restore or increase strength, and reestablish neuromuscular control.

Modalities in this phase, as in phase 1, should be used to control pain and swelling. Cryotherapy should be used during the early portion of this phase to reduce the likelihood of swelling. Electrical stimulating currents can help control pain and improve strength and range of motion.[61]

**Phase 3: Maturation-Remodeling Phase** The maturation-remodeling phase is the longest of the three phases and may last for several years, depending on the severity of the injury. The ultimate goal during this phase of the healing process is return to activity. The injury is no longer painful to the touch, although some progressively decreasing pain may still be felt on motion. The collagen fibers must be realigned according to tensile stresses and strains placed on them during functional sport-specific exercises.[48]

The focus during this phase should be on regaining activity-specific skills. Dynamic functional activities related to performance should be incorporated into the rehabilitation program. Functional training involves the repeated performance of a particular skill for the purpose of perfecting that skill. Strengthening exercises should progressively place stresses and strains on the injured structures that would normally be encountered during that activity. Plyometric strengthening exercises can be used to improve muscle power and explosiveness.[17] Functional testing should be done to determine specific skill weaknesses that need to be addressed before full return to activity.

At this point, some type of heating modality is beneficial to the healing process. The deep-heating modalities, ultrasound, or diathermy should be used to increase circulation to the deeper tissues. Massage and gentle mobilization may also be used to reduce spasm, increase circulation, reduce pain, and for tissue remodeling. Increased blood flow delivers the essential nutrients to the injured area to promote healing, and increased lymphatic flow assists in the breakdown and removal of waste products.[61] As the maturation-remodeling phase begins, aggressive, active range of motion and strengthening exercises should be incorporated to facilitate tissue remodeling and realignment.

Engaging in exercise that is too intense or too prolonged can be detrimental to the progress of rehabilitation. Any increase in the amount of swelling, an increase in pain, a loss or plateau in strength, a loss or plateau in range of motion, an increase in the laxity of a healing ligament, or exacerbation of other clinical symptoms during or after a particular exercise or activity indicates that the load is too great for the level of tissue repair or remodeling.[17]

## Adherence to a Rehabilitation Program

For a rehabilitation program to be successful, the injured patient must comply with and adhere to the plan of rehabilitation.[7,42] In the field of athletic injury, compliance is the biggest deterrent to successful rehabilitation.[24] The athletic trainer can take several steps to enhance adherence:

- The athletic trainer can provide the encouragement and positive reinforcement necessary for the patient to make a commitment. Patients who are committed to the rehabilitation

program work harder and thus return to activity more quickly with better results than those who are not committed.[22,24,64]

- The athletic trainer can be creative in designing and varying the exercise routine to keep the patient interested and motivated.[41]
- Support from peers, family, and rehabilitation staff is important in influencing compliance. Those patients with support show a greater effort to fit the rehabilitation effort into their schedules.[20]
- The athletic trainer's attitude is another important consideration when dealing with injured patients. An athletic trainer who feels that a patient is not going to adhere to the treatment program is less likely to motivate the patient to comply with the program.[56]
- The patient is more likely to follow treatment plan instructions that are clearly explained verbally and then written down.[55]
- Encourage the coach to support the rehabilitation concept and to discipline the athlete if he or she does not participate in the rehabilitation process.
- Almost all rehabilitation should be pain free. Painful exercise not only is harmful but also reduces compliance, especially in the nonadherent patient. The athletic trainer should examine rehabilitation programs to determine the aspects that may be painful.[20]

## Criteria for Full Return to Activity

All exercise rehabilitation plans must determine what is meant by complete recovery from an injury. Often, it means that the patient is fully reconditioned and has achieved full range of motion, strength, neuromuscular control, cardiovascular endurance, and activity-specific functional skills. Besides physical well-being, the patient must also have regained full confidence to return to his or her activity.

The decision to release a patient recovering from injury to a full return to activity is the final stage of the rehabilitation and recovery process. The decision should be carefully considered by each member of the sports medicine team involved in the rehabilitation process. The physician should be ultimately responsible for deciding that the patient is ready to return to practice or competition. The decision to return a patient to activity should address the following concerns:

- *Physiological healing constraints*—Has rehabilitation progressed to the later phases of the healing process?
- *Pain status*—Has pain disappeared, or is the patient able to function within his or her own levels of pain tolerance?
- *Swelling*—Is there still a chance that swelling will be exacerbated by a return to activity?

- *Range of motion*—Is the patient's range of motion adequate to allow him or her to perform both effectively and with minimized risk of reinjury?
- *Strength*—Is strength, endurance, or power great enough to protect the injured structure from reinjury?
- *Neuromuscular control/proprioception/kinesthesia*—Has the patient relearned how to use the injured body part?
- *Cardiorespiratory endurance*—Has the patient been able to maintain cardiorespiratory endurance at or near the level necessary for competition?
- *Sport-specific demands*—Are the demands of the activity or a specific position such that the patient will not be at risk of reinjury?
- *Functional testing*—Does the patient's performance on appropriate functional tests indicate that his or her extent of recovery is sufficient to allow successful performance?
- *Prophylactic strapping, bracing, padding*—Are any additional supports necessary for the injured patient to return to activity?
- *Responsibility of the patient*—Is the patient capable of listening to his or her body and recognizing a potential reinjury situation?
- *Predisposition to injury*—Is this patient prone to reinjury or to a new injury when he or she is not fully recovered?
- *Psychological factors*—Is the patient capable of returning to activity and competing at a high level without fear of reinjury?
- *Athlete education and preventive maintenance program*—Does the patient understand the importance of continuing to engage in conditioning exercises that can greatly reduce the chances of reinjury?

# ADDITIONAL APPROACHES TO THERAPEUTIC EXERCISE IN REHABILITATION

## Open versus Closed Kinetic Chain Exercises

The concept of the kinetic chain deals with the functional anatomical relationships that exist in the upper and lower extremities. In a weight-bearing position, the lower-extremity kinetic chain involves the transmission of forces among the foot, ankle, lower leg, knee, thigh, and hip. In the upper extremity, the hand as a weight-bearing surface transmits forces to the wrist, forearm, elbow, upper arm, and shoulder girdle.[57]

An open kinetic chain exists when the foot or hand is not in contact with the ground or some other surface.[27] In a closed kinetic chain, the foot or hand is weight bearing. Movements of the more proximal anatomical segments are affected by open and closed kinetic chain positions.[43] For example, the rotational components of the ankle, knee, and hip reverse direction when changing from an open to a closed kinetic chain activity. In a closed kinetic chain, the forces begin at the ground and work their way up through each joint. In a closed kinetic chain, forces must be absorbed by various tissues and anatomical structures rather than simply dissipating, as would occur in an open chain.[19]

> An open kinetic chain occurs when the foot or hand is off the ground.

> A closed kinetic chain occurs when the foot or hand is on the ground.

The use of closed chain strengthening techniques has become the rehabilitation treatment of choice for many athletic trainers.[57] Because most activities involve some aspect of weight bearing with the foot in contact with the ground or with the hand in a weight-bearing position, closed kinetic chain strengthening activities are more functional than are open chain activities. Closed kinetic chain exercises are more sport- or activity-specific, involving exercise that more closely approximates the desired activity. Specificity of training must be emphasized to athletes for them to maximize carryover to functional activities on the playing field.[57] Therefore, the treatment program should incorporate rehabilitative exercises that emphasize strengthening the entire kinetic chain rather than an isolated body segment.[66]

Closed kinetic chain exercises use varying combinations of isometric, concentric, and eccentric contractions, which must occur simultaneously in different muscle groups within the chain. Isolation exercises typically make use of one type of muscular contraction to produce or control movement.[32] Consequently, there must be some neuromuscular adaptation to this type of strengthening exercise.

In the athletic training setting, several different closed kinetic chain exercises have gained popularity and have been incorporated into rehabilitation protocols.[29] Exercises commonly used for the lower extremity are minisquats, leg presses, forward and lateral step-ups, terminal knee extensions using tubing, and exercises that use equipment such as stair climbing or stepping machines, slide boards, and stationary bicycles.[57] Push-ups and weight-shifting exercises on a medicine ball are two of the more typically used upper-extremity exercises (Figure 16–7).[48,77]

## Aquatic Exercise

Aquatic exercise is a popular rehabilitative tool. An athletic trainer who has access to a swimming pool is fortunate. Water submersion offers an excellent environment for

> Aquatic exercise provides an excellent means for rehabilitation.

beginning a program of exercise therapy, and it can complement all phases of rehabilitation.[27,72]

Because of **buoyancy** and water resistance, submersion in a pool presents a versatile exercise environment that can be varied easily according to individual needs.[2] With the proper technique, the patient can reduce muscle guarding; relax tense muscles; increase the range of joint motion; reestablish correct movement patterns; and, above all, increase strength, power, and muscular endurance.[27]

Aquatic exercise uses the water's buoyancy and pressure; it can be described as assistive, supportive, and resistive.[74] As an assistive medium, the water's buoyancy can increase range of motion, strength, and control. The patient starts by placing the body part below the water level and allows the part to be carried passively upward, keeping within pain-free limits. As the patient gains strength, he or she actively engages in movement, again

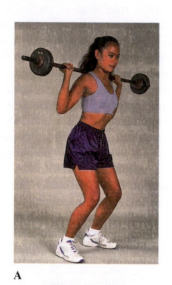

A

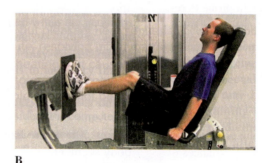

B

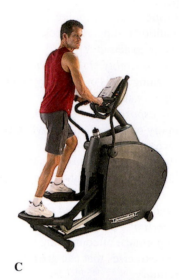

C

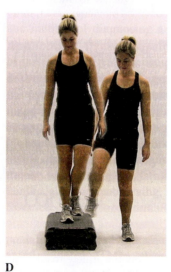

D

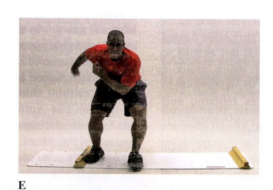

E

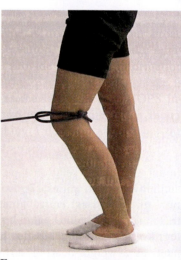

F

FIGURE 16–7    Closed kinetic chain exercises. **(A)** Minisquats. **(B)** Leg press. **(C)** Stepping machines. **(D)** Lateral step-ups. **(E)** Slide boards. **(F)** Terminal knee extensions using tubing.

(a, b, d-f, i, j) © William E. Prentice; (c, g) Courtesy Sports Authority; (h) Courtesy Contemporary Design, Glacier, WA.; (k) Courtesy Fitter International, Inc.

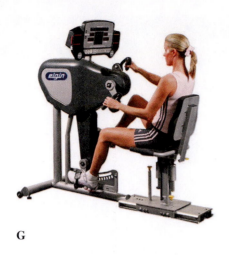

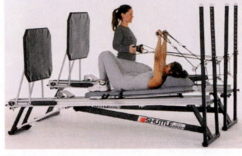

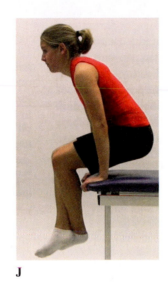

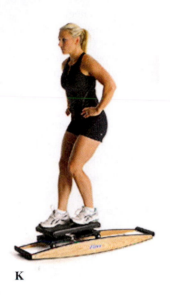

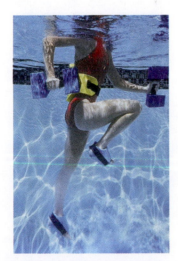

G

H

I

J

K

FIGURE 16–7 continued
**(G)** Stationary bicycling. **(H)** Shuttle 2000. **(I)** Weight shifting. **(J)** Seated push-ups. **(K)** Fitter.

assisted by the buoyancy of the water. Progression of the movement can be initiated by increasing speed and by using the water above the body part as a resistive medium (Figure 16–8).[52]

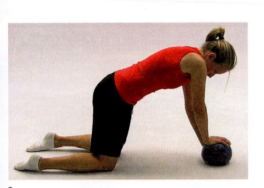

FIGURE 16–8 Using water's buoyancy and pressure for progressive exercise.
© William E. Prentice

A second use of water buoyancy is for support.[34] The limb normally will float just below the water's surface. In this position, the limb is parallel to the surface of the water. An increase in speed will make movement more difficult. Progression also can be accomplished if the part is less streamlined. In exercising the arm, for example, the athlete can increase the difficulty by moving across the water with the flat of the hand or by using a hand paddle or webbed glove. Flippers can increase resistance to the leg.

Resistance is the third use of water buoyancy.[34] The injured body part is moved downward against the upward thrust of the water. Maximum resistance is attained by keeping the limb at a right angle to the water's surface. Like the supportive technique, the resistive technique can be made progressively more difficult by the use of different devices. Extra resistance is added by pushing or dragging flotation devices down into the water.[5]

Besides engaging in specific exercises, the patient can practice sports skills, using the water's buoyancy and resistance to his or her advantage. For example, locomotor or throwing skills can be practiced to regain normal movement patterns.[49] The swimming pool can

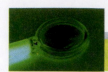

## Suggested aquatic workouts

*Swim workout**

| Activity | Time |
|---|---|
| Warm-up (jog in place) | 5 minutes |
| Scissors (abduction/adduction) | 1 minute |
| Kicking (standing position with toes dorsiflexed–increase difficulty by plantar flexing toes) | 1 minute |
| High knees | 1 minute |
| Heels to butt | 1 minute |
| Rest (passive) | 45 seconds |
| Repeat sequence three times | |
| Running in place (sprinting) | 10 times–30 seconds on, 15 seconds off |
| Active cool-down | 3:30 minutes |
| | Total time: 30 minutes |

*Kick workout with a kickboard*

Use flutter kick for this workout (prone to work hip flexors/knee extensors or supine to work hip extensors/knee flexors, using a kickboard).

| Activity | Time |
|---|---|
| Warm-up | 5 minutes |
| Prone | 20 seconds hard, 10 seconds easy for 5 minutes |
| Rest (passive) | 1 minute |
| Supine | 20 seconds hard, 10 seconds easy for 5 minutes |
| Rest (passive) | 1 minute |
| Sprint the middle 15 yards[†] | 5 minutes |
| Active cool-down | 5 minutes |
| | Total time: 27 minutes |

*Increase difficulty by adding arm and leg buoys. Scissors and kicking should focus on both speed and a medium range of motion. Patient needs to be suspended in the water by a waist belt or tethered to the side of the pool. Patient should not worry about treading during the workout.

[†]Each lane is 25 yards. Have patient kick easy for the first 5 yards of the lap, kick hard for the middle 15 yards, and kick easy for the final 5 yards. Repeat for 5 minutes.

also be an excellent medium for retaining or restoring functional capacities as well as restoring cardiovascular endurance. Wearing a flotation device around the waist, the patient can perform a variety of upper- and lower-limb movement patterns (Figure 16–9). Movements of straight-ahead running, backward running, side stepping, figure eights, and carioca can be performed by a patient bearing full weight while in 3 to 5 feet (0.9 to 1.5 m) of water.

*Focus Box 16-1:* "Suggested aquatic workouts" suggests aquatic workouts using a swim program and a kickboard program.

## Proprioceptive Neuromuscular Facilitation Techniques

Proprioceptive neuromuscular facilitation (PNF) is an approach to therapeutic exercise that uses propriocep-tive, cutaneous, and auditory input to produce func-tional improvement in motor output and can be a vital

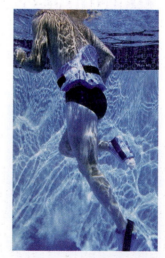

FIGURE 16–9   A wet vest can facilitate exercise programs in the water by making the patient more buoyant.
© William E. Prentice

element in the rehabilitation process of many injuries.[37] These techniques have been recommended and are widely used in sports medicine for increasing strength, flexibility, and coordination, as well as decreasing deficits in kinesthetic sense in response to demands placed on the neuromuscular system.[36,79] The principles and techniques of PNF are based primarily on the neurophysiological mechanisms involving the stretch reflex, which was discussed in detail in Chapter 4.[60] The PNF techniques are generally used in rehabilitation for facilitating strength and increasing range of motion. Flexibility is increased by the techniques of contract-relax, hold-relax, and slow-reversal-hold-relax. In contrast, strength can be facilitated by repeated contraction and the slow-reversal, rhythmic initiation, and rhythmic stabilization techniques.[60]

**Strengthening Techniques** To assist the patient in developing muscle strength, muscle endurance, and coordination, use the following techniques.[60]

> **PNF strengthening techniques:**
> - Rhythmic initiation
> - Repeated contraction
> - Slow reversal
> - Slow-reversal-hold
> - Rhythmic stabilization

*Rhythmic Initiation* Rhythmic initiation consists of a progressive series, first of passive movement, then of active assistive movement, followed by an active movement through an agonist pattern. This technique can be initiated within the first day following injury and is progressed over the next few days or weeks as the patient can tolerate. This approach helps patients with limited movement progressively regain strength through the range of motion.

*Repeated Contraction* Repeated contraction of a muscle or a muscle group is used for general weakness or weakness at one specific point. The patient moves isotonically against the maximum resistance of the athletic trainer until he or she experiences fatigue. At the time fatigue is felt, stretch is applied to the muscle at that point in the range to facilitate greater strength production. All resistance must be carefully accommodated to the strength of the patient. Because the patient is resisting as much as possible, this technique may be contraindicated for some injuries.

*Slow Reversal* The patient moves through a complete range of motion against maximum resistance. Resistance is applied to facilitate antagonist and agonist muscle groups and to ensure smooth and rhythmic movement. It is important that reversals of the movement pattern be instituted before the previous pattern has been fully completed. The major benefit of this PNF technique is that it promotes normal reciprocal coordination of agonist and antagonist muscles.

*Slow-Reversal-Hold* In this technique, the patient moves a body part isotonically, using agonist muscles, and immediately follows that movement with an isometric contraction. The patient is instructed to hold at the end of each isotonic movement. The primary purpose of this technique is to develop strength at a specific point in the range of motion.

> **PNF stretching techniques:**
> - Contract-relax
> - Hold-relax
> - Slow-reversal-hold-relax

*Rhythmic Stabilization* Rhythmic stabilization uses an isometric contraction of the agonists, followed by an isometric contraction of the antagonists. With repeated contraction of these muscles, strength is maximum at this point.

**Stretching Techniques** To produce muscle relaxation through an inhibitory response for increasing range of motion, the following PNF techniques may be used.

*Contract-Relax* The affected body part is passively moved until resistance is felt. The patient is then told to contract the antagonistic muscle isotonically. The athletic trainer resists the movement for 10 seconds or until the patient feels fatigued. The patient is instructed to relax for 10 seconds. The athletic trainer passively moves the limb to a new stretch position, and the exercise is repeated three times.

*Hold-Relax* The hold-relax technique is similar to contract-relax except that an isometric contraction is used. The patient moves the body part to the point of resistance and is told to hold that position. The athletic trainer isometrically resists the muscles for 10 seconds. The patient is then told to relax for 10 seconds, and the body part is moved to a new range, either actively by the patient or passively by the athletic trainer. This exercise is repeated three times.

*Slow-Reversal-Hold-Relax* The patient moves the body part to the point of resistance and is told to hold that position. The athletic trainer isometrically resists the muscles for 10 seconds. The patient is then told to relax for 10 seconds, thus relaxing the antagonist while the

> A patient was injured in karate and was immobilized in a cast for 6 weeks after a fracture of the olecranon process of the ulna. The cast was removed 3 weeks ago, and the patient has been working hard on stretching exercises to regain elbow extension. At this point, he is still lacking 16 degrees of extension and does not seem to be gaining any additional motion.
>
> **?** Because the stretching seems to be ineffective at this point, what can the athletic trainer do to help the patient regain range of motion?
>
> 16–7 Clinical Application Exercise

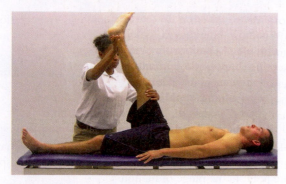

FIGURE 16–10    The slow-reversal-hold-relax stretching technique for the hamstring muscle.
© William E. Prentice

agonist is contracted, moving the part to a new limited range (Figure 16–10).

**Basic Principles of Using PNF Techniques**  These principles are the basis of PNF and must be used with any specific techniques. Application of the following principles may assist in promoting a desired response in the individual being treated.[37]

1. The patient must be taught, through brief, simple descriptions, the PNF patterns for sequential movements from starting position to terminal positions.
2. When learning the patterns, the patient should look at the moving limb for feedback on directional and positional control.
3. Verbal commands should be firm and simple—push, pull, or hold.
4. Manual contact with the hands can facilitate a movement response.
5. The athletic trainer must use correct body mechanics when providing resistance.
6. The amount of resistance given should facilitate a maximal response that allows smooth, coordinated motion.
7. Rotational movement is a critical component in all the PNF patterns.
8. The distal movements of the patterns should occur first and should be completed by no later than halfway through the pattern.
9. The stronger components are emphasized to facilitate the weaker components of a movement pattern.
10. Pressing the joint together causes increased stability, whereas traction pulls the joint apart and facilitates movement.
11. Giving a quick stretch causes a reflex contraction of that muscle.

**PNF Patterns**  The PNF exercise patterns involve three component movements: flexion-extension, abduction-adduction, and internal-external rotation. Human movement is patterned and rarely involves straight motion because all muscles are spiral in nature and lie in diagonal directions.[37]

The PNF patterns involve distinct diagonal and rotational movements of upper extremity, lower extremity, upper trunk, lower trunk, and neck. The exercise pattern is initiated with the muscle groups in the lengthened or stretched position. The muscle group is then contracted, moving the body part through the range of motion to a shortened position.

The upper and lower extremities each have two separate patterns of diagonal movement for each part of the body, which are referred to as the diagonal 1 (D1) and diagonal 2 (D2) patterns. These two diagonal patterns are subdivided into D1 moving into flexion, D1 moving into extension, D2 moving into flexion, and D2 moving into extension. The patterns are named according to the movement occurring at either the shoulder or the hip.

Manually resisted PNF patterns  are most often used with the patient supine on a treatment table as shown in Figures 16–11 for the upper extremity and 16–12 for the lower extremity. Figure 16–13 shows examples of how PNF patterns can also be used in both standing and kneeling. PNF techniques for specific joints are discussed in Chapters 18 through 24.

## Muscle Energy Techniques

Muscle energy techniques have been established to treat complex kinetic chain dysfunction.[18] *Muscle energy techniques (MET)* are manually applied stretching techniques that use principles of neurophysiology to relax overactive muscles and/or stretch chronically shortened muscles.[8] Muscle energy is a manual therapy technique that is a variation of the PNF contract-relax and hold-relax techniques. Like the PNF techniques, the muscle energy techniques are based on the same neurophysiological mechanisms involving the stretch reflex discussed in Chapter 4. Muscle energy techniques involve the voluntary contraction of a muscle in a specifically controlled direction at varied levels of intensity against a distinctly executed counterforce applied by the athletic trainer.[69] The patient provides the corrective *intrinsic* forces and controls the intensity of the muscular contractions, while the athletic trainer controls the precision and localization of the procedure. The amount of effort by the patient can vary from a minimal muscle twitch to a maximal muscle contraction.

Five components are needed to make muscle energy techniques effective:

1. Active muscle contraction by the patient
2. A muscle contraction oriented in a specific direction
3. Some control of contraction intensity by the patient

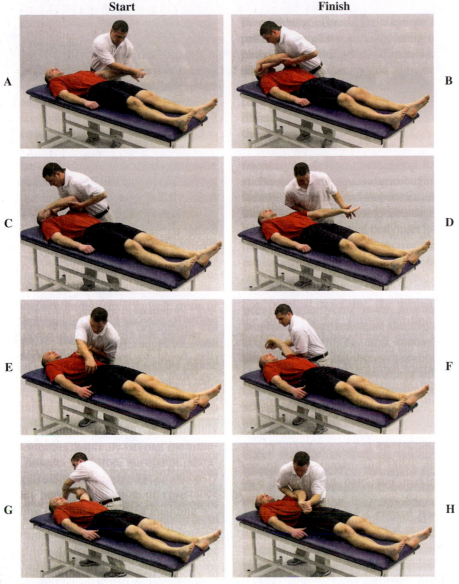

**Start**      **Finish**

A    B

C    D

E    F

G    H

FIGURE 16–11   Upper-extremity PNF patterns. **(A&B)** D1 moving into flexion. **(C&D)** D1 moving into extension. **(E&F)** D2 moving into flexion. **(G&H)** D2 moving into extension.

© William E. Prentice

4. Control of the joint position by the athletic trainer
5. Appropriate counterforce applied by the athletic trainer

The specific muscle energy technique begins by locating a point of resistance to stretch that is referred to as a *resistance barrier*. This is not necessarily a pathological barrier, but does represent the point in the range of motion at which movement will not occur without some degree of passive assistance.[23] Beginning at the resistance barrier, the patient is asked to contract the antagonist (muscle to be stretched) isometrically for 10 seconds. At this point, the patient is asked to relax completely and to inhale and exhale maximally. As the patient exhales, the athletic trainer moves the body part to the new resistance barrier. This process should be repeated three to five times or until there is no further gain in range of motion.[8]

## Joint Mobilization and Traction

The techniques of joint mobilization are used to improve joint mobility and to decrease joint pain by restoring accessory movements to the joint, thus allowing for full, nonrestricted, pain-free range of motion.[59] Mobilization techniques may be used to attain a variety of treatment goals, such as the following: reducing pain; decreasing muscle guarding; stretching or lengthening tissue surrounding a joint, especially capsular and ligamentous tissue; either inhibiting or facilitating muscle tone or the

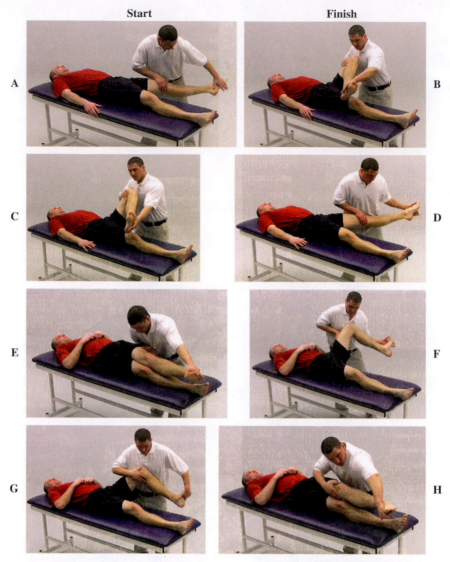

FIGURE 16–12   Lower-extremity PNF patterns. **(A&B)** D1 moving into flexion. **(C&D)** D1 moving into extension. **(E&F)** D2 moving into flexion. **(G&H)** D2 moving into extension.

© William E. Prentice

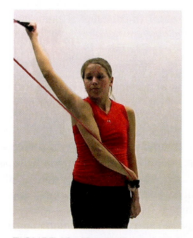
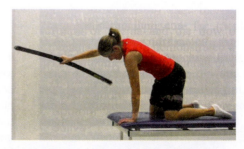

FIGURE 16–13   PNF patterns may also be done in either standing or kneeling positions, in this case using a BodyBlade.

© William E. Prentice

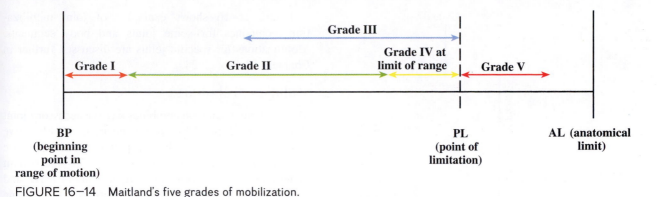

FIGURE 16–14   Maitland's five grades of mobilization.

stretch reflex; and proprioceptive effects that improve postural and kinesthetic awareness.

**Mobilization Techniques** Mobilization techniques are used to increase the accessory motions about a joint.[59] Treatment techniques designed to improve accessory motion involve small-amplitude oscillating movements called

*glides*, within a specific part of the range.[25,59] Mobilization should be done with both the patient and the athletic trainer in comfortable and relaxed positions. The athletic trainer should mobilize one joint at a time. The joint should be stabilized as near one articulating surface as possible; the other surface should be held with a firm, confident grasp.[59]

Maitland has categorized mobilization techniques into five grades as follows:[25]

- Grade I—a small-amplitude glide at the beginning of the range of motion. It is used when pain and spasm limit movement early in the range of motion.
- Grade II—a large-amplitude glide within the midrange of movement. It is used when spasm limits movement sooner with a quick oscillation than with a slow one, or when slowly increasing pain restricts movement halfway into the range.
- Grade III—a large-amplitude glide up to the pathological limit in the range of motion. It is used when pain and resistance from spasm, inert tissue tension, or tissue compression limit movement near the end of the range.
- Grade IV—a small-amplitude glide at the end of the range of motion. It is used when resistance limits movement in the absence of pain and spasm.
- Grade V—a small-amplitude, quick thrust delivered at the end of the range of motion, usually accompanied by a popping sound called a manipulation. It is used when minimal resistance limits the end of the range. Manipulation is most effectively accomplished

by the velocity of the thrust rather than by the force of the thrust. Most authorities agree that manipulation should be used only by individuals trained specifically in these techniques because a great deal of skill and judgment is necessary for safe and effective treatment.

In Maitland's system, grades I and II are used primarily to treat pain, and grades III and IV are used to treat stiffness. It is necessary to treat pain first and stiffness second.[25] Figure 16–14 shows the various grades of oscillation that are used in a joint with some limitation of motion.

The shape of the articulating surfaces usually dictates the direction of the mobilization being performed.[59] Generally, one articulating surface may be considered to be concave and the other to be convex. When the concave surface is stationary and the convex surface is moving, the glide should be done in the opposite direction of the bone movement. If the convex surface is stationary and the concave surface is moving, the glide should be done in the same direction as the bone movement. If mobilization in the appropriate direction exacerbates complaints of pain or stiffness, the athletic trainer should apply the technique in the opposite direction until the patient can tolerate the application of the technique in the appropriate direction.

In many cases, traction can be combined with mobilization.[31] *Traction* is a technique in which one articulating segment is pulled to produce some separation of the two joint surfaces. Both mobilization and traction techniques use a translational movement of one joint surface relative to the other. This translation may be in one of two directions: either perpendicular or parallel to the *treatment plane*. The treatment plane falls perpendicular to, or at a right angle to, a line running from the axis of rotation in the convex surface to the center of the concave articular surface (Figure 16–15). Mobilization techniques use glides that translate one articulating surface along a line parallel with the treatment plane. Traction techniques translate one of the articulating surfaces perpendicular

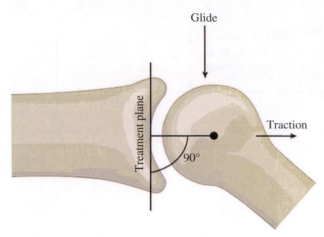

Glide

Treatment plane

90°

Traction

FIGURE 16–15   The treatment plane is perpendicular to a line drawn from the axis of rotation to the center of the articulating surface of the concave segment.

to the treatment plane. Mobilization glides are done parallel to the treatment plane; traction is performed perpendicular to the treatment plane. Like mobilization techniques, traction may be used either to decrease pain or to reduce joint hypomobility.[31,38]

Figure 16–16 shows examples of joint mobilization techniques for some joints and body segments. Mobilizations for specific joints are discussed further in Chapters 18 through 24.

## Mulligan Technique

The Mulligan technique combines passive accessory joint mobilization, applied by an athletic trainer, with active physiological movement by the patient for the purpose of correcting positional faults and returning the patient to normal pain-free function.[50] It is a noninvasive and comfortable intervention with applications for the spine and the extremities. Mulligan's concept uses what are referred to as either *mobilizations with movement (MWMs)* for treating the extremities or *sustained natural apophyseal glides (SNAGs)* for treating problems in the spine. Instead of the athletic trainer using oscillations or thrusting techniques, the patient moves in a specific direction as the athletic trainer guides the restricted body part. MWMs and SNAGs have the potential to quickly restore functional movements in joints, even after many years of restriction.[50]

**Principles of Treatment**   The basic premise of the Mulligan technique for an athletic trainer choosing to

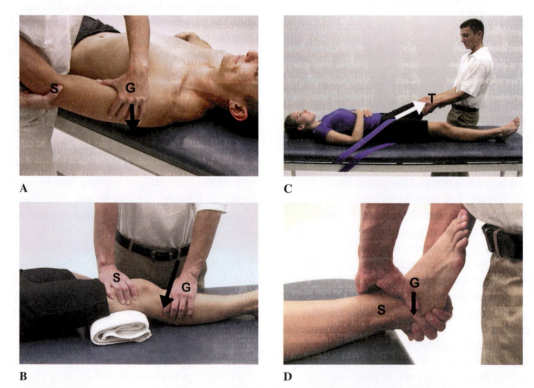

FIGURE 16–16   Joint mobilization and traction. **(A)** Posterior humeral glide (for increasing flexion and medial rotation). **(B)** Posterior tibial glide (for increasing flexion). **(C)** Inferior femoral traction (increases flexion and abduction). **(D)** Posterior talar glides (for increasing dorsiflexion). (S = stabilize, G = glide, T = traction)
© William E. Prentice

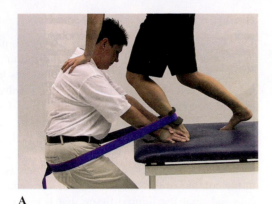
A

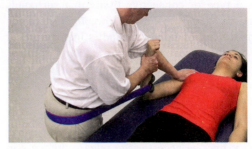
B

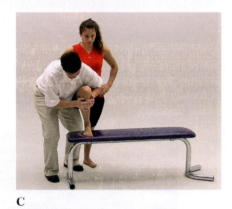
C

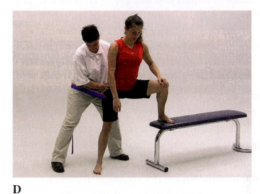
D

FIGURE 16–17 Mulligan technique. **(A)** Mobilization with manipulation (MWM) for restricted ankle dorsiflexion. **(B)** MWM for movement loss in the elbow. **(C)** MWM for restricted knee flexion. **(D)** MWM for restricted hip abduction.

© William E. Prentice

make use of MWMs in the extremities or SNAGS in the spine is to never cause pain in the patient.[50] During assessment, the athletic trainer should look for specific signs, including a loss of joint movement, pain associated with movement, or pain associated with specific functional activities. A passive accessory joint mobilization is applied either parallel or perpendicular to the joint plane.[11] The athletic trainer must continuously monitor the patient's reaction to ensure that no pain is re-created during this mobilization. The athletic trainer experiments with various combinations of parallel or perpendicular glides until he or she discovers the appropriate treatment plane and grade of movement that together significantly improve range of motion and/or significantly decrease or, better yet, eliminate altogether the original pain. Failure to improve range of motion or decrease pain indicates that the athletic trainer has not found the correct contact point, treatment plane, grade, or direction of mobilization. The patient then actively repeats the restricted and/or painful motion or activity while the athletic trainer continues to maintain the appropriate accessory glide. Further increases in range of motion or decreases in pain may be expected during a treatment session that typically involves three sets of 10 repetitions. Additional gains may be realized through the application of pain-free, passive overpressure at the end of available range.

An example of MWM might refer to a patient with restricted ankle dorsiflexion.[11] The patient stands on a treatment table with the athletic trainer manually stabilizing the foot (Figure 16–17). A nonelastic belt passes around both the distal leg of the patient and the waist of the athletic trainer, who applies a sustained anterior glide of the tibia by leaning backward away from the patient. The patient then performs a slow dorsiflexion movement until the first onset of pain or end of range. Once this end point is reached, the position is sustained for 10 seconds. The patient then relaxes and returns to the standing position, followed by release of the anteroposterior glide, followed by a 20 second rest period.

## Myofascial Release

*Myofascial release* refers to a group of techniques used to relieve soft tissue from the abnormal grip of tight fascia.[33] It is essentially a form of stretching that has been reported to have significant impact in treating a variety of conditions.[45] Some specialized training is necessary for the athletic trainer to understand specific techniques of myofascial release.[65] It is also essential to have an in-depth understanding of the fascial system.

Fascia is a type of connective tissue that surrounds muscles, tendons, nerves, bones, and organs. It is essentially continuous from head to toe and is interconnected in various sheaths or planes. Fascia is composed primarily of collagen along with some elastic fibers. During movement, the fascia must stretch and move freely. If there is damage to the fascia from injury, disease, or inflammation, it will affect not only local, adjacent structures but also areas far removed from the site of the injury. Thus, it may be necessary to release tightness in both the area of injury and distant areas. Tightness in these areas tends to soften and release in response to gentle pressure over a relatively long period of time.[44]

Myofascial release has also been referred to as *soft-tissue mobilization*, although technically all forms of massage involve the mobilization of soft tissue. Soft-tissue mobilization should not be confused with joint mobilization, although the two are closely related. Joint mobilization is used to restore normal joint arthrokinematics, and specific rules exist regarding direction of movement and joint position based on the shape of the articulating surfaces. Myofascial restrictions are considerably more unpredictable and may occur in many different planes and directions. Myofascial treatment is based on localizing the restriction and moving into the direction of the restriction, regardless of whether that follows the arthrokinematics of a nearby joint.[70] Thus, myofascial manipulation is considerably more subjective and relies heavily on the experience of the clinician.

Myofascial manipulation focuses on large treatment areas, whereas joint mobilization focuses on a specific joint. Releasing myofascial restrictions over a large treatment area can have a significant impact on joint mobility.[44] Once a myofascial restriction is located, the massage should be directly through the restriction. The progression of the technique is from superficial to deep. Once more superficial restrictions are released, the deep restrictions can be located and released without causing any damage to superficial tissues. Joint mobilization should follow myofascial release and will likely be more effective once soft-tissue restrictions are eliminated.

As the extensibility is improved in the myofascia, elongation and stretching of the musculotendinous unit should be incorporated.[45] In addition, strengthening exercises are recommended to enhance neuromuscular reeducation, which helps promote new, more efficient movement patterns.[70] As freedom of movement improves, postural reeducation may help to ensure the maintenance of the less restricted movement patterns.

Generally, acute cases tend to resolve in just a few treatments. The longer a condition has been present, the longer it will take to resolve. Occasionally, dramatic results occur immediately after treatment. It is usually recommended that treatment be done at least three times per week.

## Graston Technique®

The Graston technique® is an advanced method of instrument-assisted soft tissue mobilization (GISTM) that is combined with rehabilitation exercises to improve musculoskeletal function. The technique involves a warm up, the treatment, and therapeutic exercise. Graston enables clinicians to break down scar tissue and fascial restrictions. It can also be used to stretch both connective tissue and muscle fibers (Figure 16–18).[15,29] The technique utilizes six handheld stainless steel instruments, shaped to fit the contour of the body, to scan an area and then to locate and treat the injured tissue that is causing pain and restricting motion.[29] A clinician normally palpates a painful area, looking for unusual nodules, restrictive barriers, or tissue tensions. The instruments help magnify existing restrictions, and the clinician can feel these through the instruments.[39] Then the clinician can use the instruments to supply precise pressure to break up scar tissue, which relieves the discomfort and helps restore normal function.

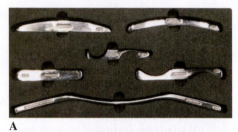

A

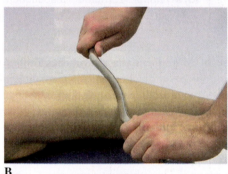

B

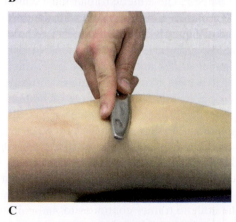

C

FIGURE 16–18 The Graston technique® **(A)** uses a variety of curved instruments to **(B)** supply precise pressure and **(C)** break down scar tissue and fascial restrictions.
© William E. Prentice

The instruments, with a narrow surface area at their edge, have the ability to separate fibers.

A specially designed lubricant is applied to the skin prior to using an instrument, allowing the instrument to glide over the skin without causing irritation. Using a cross-friction massage in multiple directions, which involves using the instruments to stroke or rub against the grain of the scar tissue, the clinician creates small amounts of trauma to the affected area.[15] This temporarily causes inflammation, which increases the rate and amount of blood flow in and around the area. The theory is that this process helps initiate and promote the healing process of the affected soft tissues. It is common for the patient to experience some discomfort during the procedure and possibly some bruising. Ice application following the treatment may ease the discomfort. It is recommended that an exercise, stretching, and strengthening program be used in conjunction with the technique to help the injured tissues heal.[39]

## Strain/Counterstrain

*Strain/counterstrain* is an approach to decreasing muscle tension and guarding that may be used to normalize muscle function. It is a passive technique that places the body in a position of greatest comfort, thereby relieving pain.[80]

In this technique, the athletic trainer locates "tender points" on the patient's body that correspond to areas of dysfunction in specific joints or muscles that are in need of treatment. These tender points are not located in or just beneath the skin, as are many acupuncture points, but deeper in muscle, tendon, ligament, or fascia. They are characterized by tense, tender, edematous spots on the body; they are ⅜ inch (1 cm) or less in diameter, with the most acute point ¹⁄₁₀ of an inch (3 mm) in diameter, although they may be a few centimeters long within a muscle; there may be multiple points for one specific joint dysfunction; they may be arranged in a chain; and points are often found in a painless area opposite the site of pain and/or weakness.[80]

With the patient completely relaxed, the athletic trainer monitors the tension and level of pain elicited by the tender point as he or she moves the patient into a position of ease or comfort. This is accomplished by markedly shortening the muscle.[71] When this position of ease is found, the tender point is no longer tense or tender. When this position is maintained for a minimum of 90 seconds, the tension in the tender point and in the corresponding joint or muscle is reduced or cleared. By slowly returning to a neutral position, the tender point and the corresponding joint or muscle remain pain free with normal tension. For example, with neck pain and/or tension headaches, the tender points may be found on either the front or back of the patient's neck and shoulders. The athletic trainer has the patient lie on his or her back and gently and slowly bends the patient's neck until that tender point is no longer tender. After the patient has held that position for

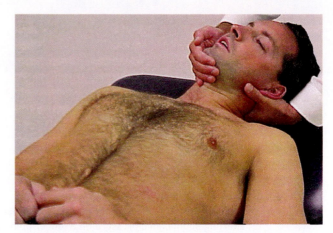

**FIGURE 16–19** Strain/counterstrain technique. The body part is placed in a position of ease for 90 seconds and then slowly moved back to neutral position.
© William E. Prentice

90 seconds, the athletic trainer gently and slowly returns the patient's neck to its resting position. Upon pressing that tender point again, the patient should notice a significant decrease in pain (Figure 16–19).[71]

The physiological rationale for the effectiveness of the strain/counterstrain technique can be explained by the stretch reflex. The stretch reflex was discussed in detail in Chapter 4. When a muscle is placed in a stretched position, impulses from the muscle spindles create a reflex contraction of the muscle in response to stretch. With strain/counterstrain, the joint or muscle is not placed in a position of stretch but rather a slack position. Thus, muscle spindle input is reduced and the muscle is relaxed, allowing for a decrease in tension and pain.[80]

## Positional Release Therapy

Positional release therapy (PRT) is based on the strain/counterstrain technique. The primary difference between the two is the use of a facilitating force (compression) to enhance the effect of the positioning.[9]

Like strain/counterstrain, PRT is an osteopathic mobilization technique in which the body is brought into a position of greatest relaxation.[13] The athletic trainer finds the position of greatest comfort and muscle relaxation for a particular joint with the help of movement tests and diagnostic tender points. Once located, the tender point

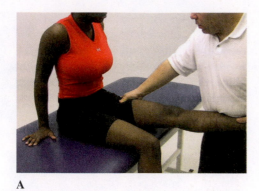
A

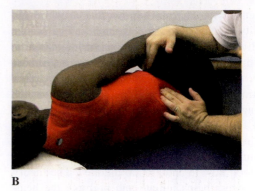
B

FIGURE 16–20   Positional release therapy uses a position of comfort, with the finger or thumb exerting submaximal pressure on a tender point. **(A)** Quadriceps. **(B)** Quadratus lumborum.
© William E. Prentice

is maintained with the palpating finger at a subthreshold pressure.[67] The patient is then passively placed in a position that reduces the tension under the palpating finger and causes a subjective reduction in tenderness as reported by the patient. This specific position is adjusted throughout the 90-second treatment period. It has been suggested that maintaining contact with the tender point during the treatment period exerts a therapeutic effect.[9] This technique is one of the most effective and most gentle methods for the treatment of acute and chronic musculoskeletal dysfunction (Figure 16–20).[67]

## Soft-Tissue Mobilization

Soft-tissue mobilization (active release technique, or ART®) is a manual therapy technique that has been developed to correct soft-tissue problems in muscle, tendon, and fascia caused by the formation of fibrotic adhesions as a result of acute injury, repetitive or overuse injuries, and constant pressure or tension injuries.[6] When a muscle, tendon, fascia, or ligament is torn (strained or sprained) or a nerve is damaged, the tissues heal with adhesions or scar tissue formation rather than the formation of brand new tissue. Scar tissue is weaker, less elastic, less pliable, and more pain sensitive than healthy

tissue. These fibrotic adhesions disrupt the normal muscle function, which in turn affects the biomechanics of the joint complex and can lead to pain and dysfunction. Soft-tissue mobilization provides a way to diagnose and treat the underlying causes of cumulative trauma disorders that, left uncorrected, can lead to inflammation, adhesions/fibrosis, muscle imbalances that result in weak and tense tissues, decreased circulation, hypoxia, and symptoms of peripheral nerve entrapment, including numbness, tingling, burning, and aching.[6]

Soft-tissue mobilization is a deep-tissue technique used for breaking down scar tissue/adhesions and restoring function and movement. In soft-tissue mobilization, the athletic trainer should first locate through palpation those adhesions in the muscle, tendon, or fascia that are causing the problem. Once these are located, the athletic trainer traps the affected muscle by applying pressure or tension with the thumb or finger over these lesions in the direction of the fibers. Then the patient is asked to actively move the body part so that the musculature is elongated from a shortened position while the athletic trainer continues to apply tension to the lesion (Figure 16–21). This should be repeated three to five times per treatment session. By breaking up the adhesions, the technique improves the patient's condition by softening and

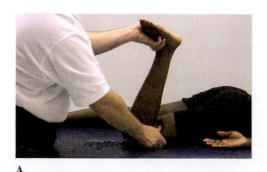
A

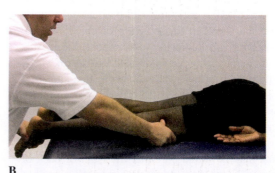
B

FIGURE 16–21   Soft-tissue mobilization. **(A)** Starting position. **(B)** Muscle is elongated from a shortened position while static pressure is applied to the lesion.
© William E. Prentice

stretching the scar tissue, resulting in increased range of motion, increased strength, and improved circulation, which optimizes healing. Treatments tend to be uncomfortable during the movement phases as the scar tissue or adhesions tear apart. This is temporary and subsides almost immediately after the treatment. An important part of soft-tissue mobilization is for the patient to heed the athletic trainer's recommendations regarding activity modification, stretching, and exercise.

## Structural Integration

Structural integration is a system that uses manual therapy and sensorimotor movement education, which is based on a type of massage called Rolfing that was developed more than 50 years ago. Unlike massage, which focuses primarily on muscle, structural integration focuses instead on connective tissue or fascia, which surrounds muscles, groups of muscles, bones, nerves, blood vessels, and organs. Ideally, fascia is elastic and functions to bind different tissues together providing shape and structure while permitting free movement. However, factors such as repetitive movements, the stresses of normal daily activities, injury, or even the normal aging process can cause the fascia to become more dense, less elastic, and thus tighter and shorter. These factors eventually cause postural malalignment of musculoskeletal structures, which affects normal biomechanical function.[30]

Structural integration attempts to lengthen, stretch, soften, and release fascial adhesions to reduce mechanical stress and nociceptive irritation, restore postural balance, and thus efficiency of movement.[30] The technique involves an organized series of 10 hour-long sessions designed to progressively restore postural balance of the body in segments using fascial mobilization to achieve optimal vertical alignment. During the sessions practitioners identify habitual patterns of movement and existing imbalances in the body and help educate the patient about making corrective changes in these patterns in his or her daily life.[51]

Structural integration practitioners receive extensive training at schools and institutions in accordance with the standards established by the International Association of Structural Integrators (IASI).

## Postural Restoration

Postural restoration (PRI) is a treatment technique that is used to identify and correct asymmetrical postural patterns that negatively influence normal sitting, standing, walking, and breathing.[28] These asymmetries create adaptive and compensatory changes in soft tissue and bone structures that eventually result in movement patterns that restrict functional range and negatively influence structural alignment and thus postural control. Several muscles such as the diaphragm and transversus abdominis are important for both postural control/stabilization and for respiration. Maintaining a balance between

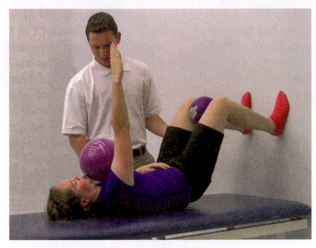

FIGURE 16–22 The 90/90 Bridge with Ball and Balloon technique is a postural restoration technique.
© William E. Prentice

the two is challenging.[7] A goal of postural restoration is to maintain what is referred to as a *zone of apposition* (ZOA), which is an area of the diaphragm that directly opposes the rib cage.

PRI has been used in treating low back and SI joint pain, acetabular labral tear, anterior knee pain, thoracic outlet syndrome, sciatica, asthma, and chronic obstructive pulmonary disease.[7] Treatment focuses on asymmetrical patterns and multiple joint muscles in combination with diaphragmatic breathing. PRI recommends the use of an exercise called the 90/90 Bridge with Ball and Balloon technique designed to help restore the ZOA and spine to an optimal position, thus allowing the diaphragm to optimally perform both its respiratory and postural roles (Figure 16–22).[7] The patient lies supine with the feet flat on the wall and the knees flexed at 90 degrees. The hamstrings are contracted pressing the heels into the wall. Lift the pelvis up by rotating it posteriorly. A 4- to 6-inch ball is squeezed between the knees. The right arm is placed above the head while the left hand holds a balloon. The patient slowly inhales through the nose (4 seconds), then slowly exhales through the mouth to inflate the balloon, then pause (4 seconds) and repeat 3 times.

It must be added that there is little published evidence regarding the efficacy of this exercise.

## Biofeedback

In rehabilitation, athletic trainers use biofeedback to help a patient develop greater voluntary control for the purpose of enhancing either neuromuscular relaxation or muscle reeducation following injury.[78] A biofeedback unit is an electronic or electromechanical instrument that accurately measures, processes, and feeds back reinforcing information to the patient via auditory or visual signals (Figure 16–23). Perhaps the biggest advantage of biofeedback is that it provides the patient with immediate feedback on how effectively he or she is able to either

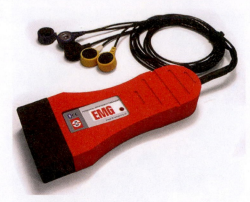

**FIGURE 16-23** The biofeedback unit is connected via a series of electrodes to the skin over the contracting muscle and measures electrical activity in that muscle.

Courtesy Kamran Fallahpour, PhD, Brainquiry (www.brainquiry .com), Brain Resource Center (brainresourcecenter.com)

contract or relax a muscle. Effective contraction or relaxation is immediately noted and rewarded so that eventually larger changes or improvements in these capabilities can be accomplished.[61]

Several types of biofeedback units are available for use in rehabilitation; EMG biofeedback is the most widely used in a clinical setting.[61] An EMG biofeedback unit measures the electrical activity produced by depolarization of a muscle fiber as an indicator of the quality of a muscle contraction. The EMG biofeedback unit detects small amounts of electrical energy generated during muscle contraction through active electrodes. The biofeedback unit processes and interprets this electrical activity and subsequently quantifies this information into either visual or auditory feedback that the patient can easily understand. Biofeedback

**16-9 Clinical Application Exercise**

A patient is having difficulty contracting her quadriceps muscle on the second day after a surgical reconstruction of her knee. She has some swelling in the vastus medialis, and she is still experiencing some pain.

❓ What modality can the athletic trainer use to help her achieve a quadriceps contraction?

information is displayed either visually using lights or meters or auditorily using tones, beeps, buzzes, or clicks.[78]

## PURCHASING AND MAINTAINING THERAPEUTIC EXERCISE EQUIPMENT

The extent and variety of therapeutic exercise equipment available to use in injury rehabilitation can at times be overwhelming. Prices of rehabilitation equipment can range from $2 for a piece of resistance tubing to $4,000 for an electrical stimulating unit to $80,000 for certain computer-driven isokinetic or balance devices. It is certainly not necessary to purchase expensive exercise equipment to see good results. It is likely that an injured patient can achieve many of the same physiological benefits from using a $2 piece of surgical tubing as from exercising on an $80,000 isokinetic device. Many athletic trainers would argue that the most useful pieces of rehabilitation equipment available are the hands and the creativity of a well-trained and experienced clinician. Others maintain that the greater the extent and variety of rehabilitation equipment available, the more flexibility the athletic trainer has in devising rehabilitation programs.

For almost everyone, budgetary constraints, at least to some extent, will limit the pieces of rehabilitation equipment that can be purchased. Decisions to purchase pieces of rehabilitation equipment should be based on a realistic assessment of the usefulness and functionality of that piece of equipment, the extent to which it will be used, and its durability. Perhaps the most important question that should be asked when purchasing a new piece of equipment is whether this piece of equipment will help the patient reach the goals of the rehabilitation program.

Once rehabilitation equipment has been purchased, the athletic trainer should assume the responsibility of making sure that it is being used correctly and for the intended purpose as stated in the manufacturer's instructions for use. It is also essential that the athletic trainer apply the manufacturer's guidelines for the periodic inspection and maintenance of the equipment to ensure that it is operating safely.

## SUMMARY

- When injuries occur, the athletic trainer usually assumes the primary responsibility for the design, implementation, and supervision of the rehabilitation program for the injured patient. Two major goals of rehabilitation are to prevent deconditioning and to restore the injured part to a preinjury state. Besides the

physical aspect, the mental and emotional aspects of rehabilitation must always be considered.
- When an injured body part is immobilized for a period of time, a number of disuse problems adversely affect muscle, joints, ligaments, bones, cartilage, neuromuscular efficiency, and the cardiorespiratory system.

- Designing rehabilitation programs is relatively simple and involves several basic components: minimizing swelling, controlling pain, reestablishing neuromuscular control, establishing or enhancing core stability, regaining or improving range of motion, restoring or increasing muscular strength and endurance, regaining balance and postural control, maintaining cardiorespiratory endurance, and incorporating functional progressions. The long-term goal is to return the injured athlete to practice or competition as quickly and safely as possible.
- Rehabilitation programs can be subdivided into three phases, based primarily on the three stages of the healing process: phase 1, the acute inflammatory response phase; phase 2, the fibroblastic repair phase; and phase 3, the maturation-remodeling phase. If surgery is necessary, a fourth phase, the preoperative phase, must also be considered.
- The decision to release a patient recovering from injury to full activity is the final stage of the rehabilitation and recovery process. The decision should be carefully considered by each member of the sports medicine team involved in the rehabilitation process.
- An open kinetic chain exists when the foot or hand is not in contact with the ground or some other surface. In a closed kinetic chain, the foot or hand is weight bearing. The use of closed chain strengthening techniques is the rehabilitation treatment of choice for many athletic trainers. Closed kinetic chain strengthening activities are more functional than are open kinetic chain activities.
- Aquatic exercises can be an important rehabilitative tool for the athletic trainer, particularly with injuries involving the lower extremity. Aquatic exercises allow for resistance with motion without weight bearing.
- Proprioceptive neuromuscular facilitation is a manual therapy technique that can be used for strengthening muscle or increasing range of motion. The PNF movement patterns involve a sequential series of specific movements for the lower extremity, lower trunk, upper trunk, and upper extremity.
- Mobilization, traction, and Mulligan techniques are manual therapy techniques used to improve joint mobility or to decrease joint pain by restoring accessory movements to the injured joint, which allows full, pain-free range of motion.
- A variety of manual therapy techniques, including muscle energy, myofascial release, the Graston technique®, strain/counterstrain, positional release, soft-tissue mobilization, and biofeedback can be incorporated into a rehabilitation program.

## WEB SITES

Archives of Physical Medicine and Rehabilitation: www.archives-pmr.org

Cramer First Aider: www.cramersportsmed.com/first-aider.html

International Association of Structural Integrators (IASI): www.theiasi.net
*IASI is the professional membership organization for structural integration.*

Journal of Sport Rehabilitation: http://journals.humankinetics.com/JSR

National Athletic Trainers' Association: www.nata.org
*Accesses rehabilitation in the athletic training journals.*

Postural Restoration Institute: www.posturalrestoration.com
*Explains kinetic and kinematic movement dysfunction, and provides details of courses offered in Lincoln, Nebraska.*

The Physician and Sportsmedicine: www.physsportsmed.com
*Search back issues and access the ones specifically geared toward weight training and rehabilitation.*

## SOLUTIONS TO CLINICAL APPLICATION EXERCISES

16–1 The components that should be addressed in any rehabilitation program are minimizing swelling, controlling pain, reestablishing neuromuscular control, establishing or enhancing core stability, regaining or improving range of motion, restoring or increasing muscular strength and endurance, regaining balance and postural control, maintaining cardiorespiratory endurance, and incorporating functional progressions. The approach to rehabilitation should be aggressive, and decisions as to when and how to alter and progress specific components within a rehabilitation program should be based on and are limited by the healing process.

16–2 After injury and subsequent rest and immobilization, it is not unusual for the patient to "forget" how to walk. The athletic trainer must help the patient relearn neuromuscular control, which means regaining the ability to follow some previously established motor and sensory pattern by regaining conscious control of a specific movement until that movement becomes automatic. Strengthening exercises, particularly those that tend to be more functional, such as closed kinetic chain exercises, are essential for reestablishing neuromuscular control. Addressing neuromuscular control is critical throughout the recovery process but may be most critical during the early stages of rehabilitation to avoid reinjury or overuse injuries to additional structures.

16–3 Anterior knee pain can result from many different causes. Strengthening the quadriceps can be helpful. If full-range-of-motion strengthening exercises increase pain, the patient should begin with positional isometric exercises done at different points in the range, progressing to full-range concentric and eccentric exercise as tolerated. Closed kinetic chain exercises, such as minisquats, stepping exercises, and leg presses, are excellent quadriceps-strengthening exercises and tend to be more functional than traditional open kinetic chain exercises.

16–4 The patient should have minimal signs of inflammation, such as pain and swelling. The appropriate healing time frame should also be reached before the patient progresses.

16–5 The athletic trainer can provide the encouragement and positive reinforcement necessary for the patient to make a commitment. Support from peers, coaches, and rehabilitation staff is important. The athletic trainer should clearly explain the instructions verbally to the athlete and then write them down. The rehabilitation program should fit into the patient's schedule. The athletic trainer must be creative in designing and varying the exercise routine. The rehabilitation program should be as pain free as possible. The coach needs to support the rehabilitation process.

16–6 Perhaps the best recommendation is to have the patient engage in an aquatic exercise program. In the water, the patient would not be weight bearing and could exercise the injured knee through a pain-free range of motion while working on maintaining levels of fitness by engaging in water-resisted conditioning exercises.

16–7 To achieve a full physiological range of motion, the joint must have normal accessory motions. Stretching techniques address motion restriction caused by tightness of the musculotendinous unit. The athletic trainer should incorporate joint mobilization techniques that address restriction of motion caused by some tightness of capsular and ligamentous structures that surround the affected joint.

16–8 To some extent, the answer depends on exactly what is causing her pain. In general, the athletic trainer may choose to use one of several or a combination of manual therapy techniques, including myofascial release, strain/counterstrain, positional release, and soft-tissue mobilization.

16–9 A biofeedback unit can help the patient relearn how to fire the quadriceps muscle. The biofeedback unit can provide both visual and auditory feedback to indicate the strength of a contraction as well as the timing of a contraction. Biofeedback can be used almost immediately following surgery.

## REVIEW QUESTIONS AND CLASS ACTIVITIES

1. What occurs physiologically when an athlete is suddenly forced to stop physical activity?
2. Discuss the physiological effects of immobilization on muscles, ligaments, joints, bones, neuromuscular efficiency, and the cardiovascular system.
3. Discuss the similarities and differences between training and conditioning exercises and therapeutic exercise.
4. Why must an athlete condition the entire body while an injury heals?
5. Why is it important to modulate pain during a rehabilitation program?
6. Discuss the difference between proprioception and kinesthesia, and explain how they are related to neuromuscular control.
7. What is the significance of having the patient engage in core stabilization training during a rehabilitation program?
8. Critically compare the use of isometric, isotonic, and isokinetic exercises in rehabilitation.
9. How is range of motion restored after an injury?
10. How and when should functional progressions be incorporated into the rehabilitation program?
11. Describe how to determine whether a patient is ready to return to activity after injury.
12. What is the importance of developing a rehabilitation plan? Include the criteria for moving to various phases.
13. What are the important considerations during each of the three phases of rehabilitation?
14. Why are closed kinetic chain exercises more useful than open kinetic chain exercises in the rehabilitation of injuries?
15. How may aquatic exercise be incorporated into a rehabilitation program?
16. Proprioceptive neuromuscular facilitation includes stretching, strengthening, and movement-patterning techniques. How can these techniques apply to sports injuries?
17. How can a muscle energy technique be used to increase range of motion?
18. Explain why it is necessary to use stretching techniques to increase physiological movement and to use mobilization techniques to improve accessory motions.
19. How does a Mulligan technique help in treating pain and restricted motion?
20. How are the strain/counterstrain technique and positional release therapy related to one another?

## REFERENCES

1. Anderson J: Effects of strength training on muscle fiber types and size; consequences for athletes training for high-intensity sport, *Scandinavian Journal of Medicine and Science in Sports* 20(Supplement): 32–38, 2010.
2. Barr K, et al.: Lumbar stabilization: Core concepts and current literature, *American Journal of Physical Medicine and Rehabilitation* 84:473–480, 2005.
3. Becker B: Aquatic Therapy: Scientific foundations and clinical rehabilitation applications, *Physical Medicine and Rehabilitation* 1(9): 859–72, 2009.
4. Bialosky J: The mechanisms of manual therapy in the treatment of musculoskeletal pain, *Manual Therapy* 14(5):531–38, 2009.
5. Binkley H: Aquatic therapy in the treatment of upper extremity injuries, *Athletic Therapy Today* 7(1):49, 2002.
6. Blanchette M: Augmented soft tissue mobilization vs. natural history in the treatment of lateral epicondylitis, *Journal of manipulative and physiological therapeutics* 34(2):123–30, 2011.
7. Boyle K: The value of blowing up a balloon, *North American Journal of Sports Physical Therapy* 5(3):179–88, 2010.
8. Chaitlow L: *Muscle energy techniques,* Philadelphia, PA, 2013, Churchill Livingstone.
9. Chaitlow L: *Positional release techniques,* Philadelphia, 2015, Elsevier Science.
10. Clark M, Hoogenboom, B: Establishing core stability in rehabilitation. In Prentice W, ed: *Rehabilitation techniques in sports medicine and athletic training.* Thorofare, NJ: 2015, Slack.
11. Collins N: The initial effects of a Mulligan's mobilization with movement technique on dorsiflexion and pain in subacute ankle sprains, *Manual Therapy* 2(May 9):77, 2004.
12. Colston M: Abdominal muscle training and core stabilization: The past, present, and future, *Athletic Therapy Today* 10(4): 6, 2005.
13. D'Ambrogio K, Roth G: *Positional release therapy: Assessment and treatment of musculoskeletal dysfunction,* Philadelphia, PA, 1997, Elsevier Science.
14. DeDeyne P: Application of passive stretch and its implications for muscle fibers, *Phys Ther* 81:819, 2001.
15. DeLuccio J: Instrument assisted soft tissue mobilization utilizing Graston Technique: A physical therapist's perspective, *Orthopedic Physical Therapy Practice* 18(3): 32–34, 2006.
16. DiStefano L: Evidence supporting balance training in healthy individuals: A systematic review, *Journal of Strength and Conditioning Research* 23(9):2718–31, 2009.

17. Ellenbecker T: *Effective functional progressions in sport rehabilitation,* Champaign, 2009, Human Kinetics.

18. Giammetto T: *Integrative manual therapy: For biomechanics application of muscle energy and beyond technique,* vol. 3, Berkeley, CA, 2003, North Atlantic Books.

19. Glass R: The effects of open versus closed kinetic chain exercises on patients with ACL deficient or reconstructed knees: A systematic review, *N Am J Sports Phys Ther.* 5(2):74–84, 2010.

20. Granquist M: Development of a measure of rehabilitation adherence for athletic training, *Journal of Sport Rehabilitation* 19:249–67, 2010.

21. Halle J: Designing home exercise programs. In Hoogenboom B, Voight M, Prentice W, eds: *Musculoskeletal interventions techniques of therapeutic exercise,* New York, 2013, McGraw-Hill.

22. Hamson-Utley, J: Athletic trainers' and physical therapists' perceptions of the effectiveness of psychological skills within sport injury rehabilitation programs, *J Athl Train.* 43(3):258–64, 2008.

23. Harris A: Immediate effects of static stretching and muscle energy technique on hamstring flexibility, *J Athl Train* 39 (2 Suppl): S-99, 2004.

24. Hedgepath E, Gieck J: Psychological considerations for rehabilitating the injured athlete. In Prentice W, ed: *Rehabilitation techniques in sports medicine and athletic training,* Thorofare, NJ, 2015, Slack.

25. Hengeveld E: *Maitland's peripheral manipulation,* Waltham, MA, 2013, Butterworth-Heinemann.

26. Hertel J: A rehabilitation paradigm for restoring neuromuscular control following athletic injury, *Athletic Therapy Today* 3(5):12, 1998.

27. Hoogenboom B: Aquatic therapy in rehabilitation. In Prentice W, ed: *Rehabilitation techniques in sports medicine and athletic training,* Thorofare, NJ, 2015, Slack Inc.

28. Hruska, R: Influences of dysfunctional respiratory mechanics on orofacial pain, *Dental Clinics of North America* 41(2):211–27, 1997.

29. Hyde T: Graston technique: A soft tissue treatment for athletic injuries. *D.C. Tracts,* 15(3): 2–4, 2003.

30. Jacobson E: Structural integration, an alternative method of manual therapy and sensorimotor education, *Journal of Alternative and Complementary Education* 17(10): 89–199, 2011.

31. Kaltenborn F: *Manual mobilization of the joints: The Kaltenborn method of joint examination and treatment: The extremities,* vol. 1, and *The spine,* vol. 2, Minneapolis, 2003, Orthopedic Physical Therapy Products.

32. Karandikar N: Kinetic chains: A review of the concept and its clinical applications, *Physical Medicine and Rehabilitation,* 3(8): 739–45, 2011.

33. Keirns M: *Myofascial release in sports medicine,* Champaign, IL, 2000, Human Kinetics.

34. Kersey R: Aquatic therapy, *Athletic Therapy Today* 10(5):48, 2005.

35. King M: Core stability: Creating a foundation for functional rehabilitation, *Athletic Therapy Today* 5(2):6, 2000.

36. Kitani I: The effectiveness of proprioceptive neuromuscular facilitation (PNF) exercises on shoulder joint position sense in baseball players, *J Athl Train* 39(2 Suppl):S-62, 2004.

37. Knott M: *Proprioceptive neuromuscular facilitation: Patterns and techniques,* ed 2, Philadelphia, PA, 1985, Lippincott, Williams and Wilkins.

38. Konin J: Joint mobilization to decrease glenohumeral-joint impingement, *Athletic Therapy Today* 11(3):50, 2006.

39. Larkins P: Graston Technique, *Podiatry Management* 27(1):37–38, 2008.

40. Lephart S, Swanik C: Reestablishing neuromuscular control. In Prentice W, ed: *Rehabilitation techniques in sports medicine and athletic training,* Thorofare, NJ, 2015, Slack.

41. Levy A: Sport injury rehabilitation adherence: Perspectives of recreational athletes, *International Journal of Sport and Exercise Psychology* 7(2):212–29, 2011.

42. Levy A: Mental toughness as a determinant of beliefs, pain, and adherence in sport injury rehabilitation, *J Sport Rehabil* 15(3): 246, 2006.

43. Lim G: The effects of closed kinetic chain exercise and open kinetic chain exercise on knee position sense in normal adults, *Journal of International Academy of Physical Therapy Research* 1(2):126, 2010.

44. Manheim C: *Myofascial release manual,* Thorofare, NJ, 2008, Slack.

45. McClellan E, Prentice W: Effects of myofascial release and static stretching on active range of motion and muscle activity, *J Athl Train* 39(2 Suppl):S-98, 2004.

46. McGee D: *Athletic and sport issues in musculoskeletal rehabilitation,* Philadelphia, PA, 2010, Saunders.

47. McGee M: Functional progressions and functional testing in rehabilitation. In Prentice W, ed: *Rehabilitation techniques in sports medicine and athletic training,* Thorofare, NJ, 2015, Slack.

48. McMullen J: A kinetic chain approach for shoulder rehabilitation, *J Athl Train* 35(3):329, 2000.

49. Miller M: Comparisons of land-based and aquatic-based plyometric programs during an 8-week training period, *J Sport Rehabil* 11(4):268, 2002.

50. Mulligan B: Manual therapy: NAGS, SNAGS, MWMS, etc., *Journal of Orthopedic and Sports Physical Therapy* 35(10)674–78, 2004.

51. Myers, T: Structural integration- developments in Ida Rolf's recipe-Part 1, *Journal of Bodywork and Movement Therapies* 8(2):131–42, 2004.

52. O'Neill D: Return to function through aquatic therapy, *Athletic Therapy Today* 5(2): 14, 2000.

53. O'Sullivan, S: 2013,. *Physical rehabilitation,* Philadelphia, PA, F.A. Davis.

54. Perrin D: *Isokinetic exercise and assessment,* Champaign, IL, 1993, Human Kinetics.

55. Piccininni J: Athlete-patient education in rehabilitation: developing a self-directed program, *Athletic Therapy Today* 4(6):51, 1999.

56. Pizzari T: Adherence to rehabilitation after anterior cruciate ligament reconstructive surgery: Implications for outcome, *J Sport Rehabil* 14(3):201, 2005.

57. Prentice W: Closed kinetic chain exercise. In Prentice W, ed: *Rehabilitation techniques in sports medicine and athletic training,* St. Louis, MO, 2010, McGraw-Hill.

58. Prentice W: The healing process and pathophysiology of musculoskeletal injury. In Prentice W, ed: *Rehabilitation techniques in sports medicine and athletic training,* Thorofare, NJ, 2015, Slack.

59. Prentice W: Mobilization and traction techniques in rehabilitation. In Prentice W, ed: *Rehabilitation techniques in sports medicine and athletic training,* Thorofare, NJ, 2015, Slack.

60. Prentice W: Proprioceptive neuromuscular facilitation techniques. In Prentice W, ed: *Rehabilitation techniques in sports medicine and athletic training,* Thorofare, NJ, 2015, Slack.

61. Prentice W: *Therapeutic modalities in rehabilitation,* ed 4, New York, 2011, McGraw-Hill.

62. Prentice W: Understanding and managing the healing process through rehabilitation. In Prentice W, ed: *Rehabilitation techniques in sports medicine and athletic training,* Thorofare, NJ, 2015, Slack.

63. Reiman M: 2009. *Functional testing in human performance,* Champaign, Human Kinetics.

64. Scherzer C: Psychological skills and adherence to rehabilitation after reconstruction of the anterior cruciate ligament, *J Sport Rehabil* 10(3):165, 2001.

65. Sefton J: Myofascial release for athletic trainers, Part I, *Athletic Therapy Today* 9(1):40, 2004.

66. Smith D: Incorporating kinetic-chain integration, Part 2: Functional shoulder rehabilitation, *Athletic Therapy Today* 1(5):63, 2006.

67. Speicher T: Top 10 positional release therapy techniques to break the chain of pain, Part 1, *Athletic Therapy Today* 1(5):60, 2006.

68. Stillman B: Making sense of proprioception: The meaning of proprioception, kinesthesia and related terms, *Physiotherapy* 88(11): 667–76, 2002.

69. Stone J: Muscle energy technique, *Athletic Therapy Today* 5(5):25, 2000.

70. Stone J: Myofascial release, *Athletic Therapy Today* 5(4):34, 2000.

71. Stone J: Strain-counterstrain, *Athletic Therapy Today* 5(6):30, 2000.

72. Swann E: Uses of manual-therapy techniques in pain management, *Athletic Therapy Today* 7(4):14, 2002.

73. Swanson K: Improving proprioception and neuromuscular control following shoulder injury, *Athletic Therapy Today* 3(5):30, 1998.

74. Thien-Brody L: *Aquatic exercise for rehabilitation and training,* Champaign, IL, 2009, Human Kinetics.

75. Thomas M: Comparison of tension in theraband and cando tubing, *J Orthop Sports Phys Ther* 32(11):576, 2002.

76. Tripp B: Integrating sensorimotor control into rehabilitation, *Athletic Therapy Today* 1(5):24, 2006.

77. Ubinger M: Effect of closed kinetic chain training on neuromuscular control in the upper extremity, *J Sport Rehabil* 8(3):184, 1999.

78. Wasielewski N: Evaluation of electromyographic biofeedback for the quadriceps femoris: A systematic review, *J Athl Train* 46(5):543–54, 2011.

79. Westwater-Wood S: The use of proprioceptive neuromuscular facilitation in physiotherapy practice, *Physical Therapy Reviews* 15(1):23–28, 2010.

80. Wong C: Strain counterstrain: Current concepts and clinical evidence, *Manual Therapy* 17(1):2–8, 2012.

81. Yoke M: *Functional exercise progressions,* Monterey, CA, 2003, Healthy Learning.

82. Zech A: Balance training for neuromuscular control and performance enhancement: A systematic review, *J Athl Train* 45(4):392–403, 2010.

83. Zech A: Neuromuscular training for rehabilitation of sports injuries: A systematic review, *Medicine and Science in Sports and Exercise* 41(10):1831–41, 2009.

# ANNOTATED BIBLIOGRAPHY

Brotzman S: *Clinical orthopedic rehabilitation*, Philadelphia, PA, 2011, Elsevier Health Sciences.

*Discusses the rehabilitation of injuries that occur in specific sports.*

Chaitlow L: *Muscle energy techniques*, Philadelphia, PA, 2013, Elsevier Health Sciences.

*Discusses muscle energy techniques (manipulative treatments in which a patient engages a muscle against a counterforce) for osteopaths, chiropractors, athletic trainers, physical therapists, and massage therapists.*

Chaitlow L: *Positional release techniques*, 2015, Churchill-Livingston.

*Organizes the concept of strain/counterstrain and positional release into a systemic approach that is easy to use and document. Contains examples demonstrating each release position with an awareness of the clinician's body mechanics.*

Edmond S: *Manipulation and mobilization: Extremity and spinal techniques*, New York, 2006, Mosby.

*Provides the entry-level student and the practicing clinician with a comprehensive text on mobilization and manipulation techniques.*

Ellenbecker T: *Effective functional progressions in sport rehabilitation*, Champaign, IL, 2009, Human Kinetics.

*Presents scientific principles and practical applications for using functional exercise to rehabilitate athletic injuries.*

Kisner C, Colby A: *Therapeutic exercise: Foundations and techniques*, Philadelphia, PA, 2012, F.A. Davis.

*A clear, concise presentation of the field of therapeutic exercise well suited to sports medicine. Covers exercise for increasing range of motion and for treating soft tissue, bone, and postsurgical problems.*

McGee D: *Athletic and sport issues in musculoskeletal rehabilitation*, Philadelphia, PA, 2010, Saunders.

*An extremely detailed, scientifically based, advanced text dealing with athletic injury rehabilitation.*

Prentice W: *Mobilization and traction: Principles and techniques* (video, 33 minutes), St. Louis, MO, 1993, Mosby/McGraw-Hill.

*A thorough overview of mobilization and traction and includes detailed demonstrations of various techniques.*

Prentice W: *Proprioceptive neuromuscular facilitation: Principles and techniques* (video, 26 minutes), St. Louis, MO, 1993, Mosby/McGraw-Hill.

*An introduction to PNF stretching and strengthening exercises, complete with a detailed, hands-on demonstration of specific techniques.*

Prentice W: *Rehabilitation techniques in sports medicine and athletic training*, ed 6, Thorofare, NJ, 2015, Slack.

*A comprehensive text dealing with all aspects of rehabilitation used in a sports medicine setting.*

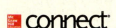

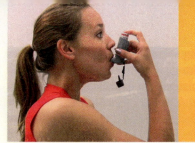
© William E. Prentice

# Pharmacology, Drugs, and Sports

## ■ Objectives

*When you finish this chapter you should be able to*

- Define the term *drug*.
- Identify the various methods by which drugs can be administered.
- Analyze pharmacokinetics relative to absorption, distribution, metabolism, and excretion.
- Explain the difference between administering and dispensing medications.
- Express legal concerns for administering medications to the athletic population.
- Apply the various protocols that the athletic trainer should follow for administering over-the-counter medications to patients.

- Categorize the various drugs that can be used to treat infection, reduce pain and inflammation, relax muscles, treat gastrointestinal disorders, treat symptoms of colds and congestion, and control bleeding.
- Recognize the problem of substance abuse in the athletic population.
- Describe the ergogenic aids used by athletes to improve performance.
- Discuss the abuse of alcohol, drugs, and tobacco by athletes.
- Evaluate drug-testing policies and procedures, and list the types of banned drugs.

## ■ Outline

## ■ Key Terms

pharmacology
drug
pharmacokinetics

drug vehicle
bioavailability

volume of
  distribution
efficacy

potency
biotransformation
metabolism

half-life
steady-state
bioequivalent drugs

## ■ Connect Highlights  connect

*Visit connect.mcgraw-hill.com for further exercises to apply your knowledge:*

- Clinical application scenarios covering administering and dispensing medications, drug classifications and therapeutic uses, and the use of alcohol, drugs, and tobacco by athletes and banned substances for athletes
- Click-and-drag questions covering various methods by which drugs can be administered, regulating governing agencies for drugs, drug classifications and therapeutic uses, dispensing and application of medications, and banned drugs for athletes
- Multiple-choice questions covering various methods to administer/dispense drugs, legal concerns, drug classifications and therapeutic uses, substance abuse, ergogenic aids, and drug-testing policies and procedures
- Picture identification of various drug classifications and therapeutic uses

**P**harmacology is the branch of science that studies the actions of drugs on biological systems, especially drugs that are used in medicine for diagnostic and therapeutic purposes.[30] Pharmaceutical care is the direct provision of medication-related care for the purpose of achieving definite outcomes that improve quality of life.[23] Medications of all types, both prescription and over-the-counter, are as commonly used by athletes as they are by others in the population.[1]

Unfortunately, the abuse of various drugs and other substances for performance enhancement or for recreational mood alteration is also widespread among athletes. Thus, the athletic trainer must be knowledgeable about drug use and substance abuse within the population with which he or she works.[30]

# WHAT IS A DRUG?

A **drug** is a chemical agent used in the prevention, treatment, or diagnosis of disease.[42] The use of substances for the express purpose of treating some infirmity or disease dates back to early history. The ancient Egyptians were highly skilled in making and using medications, treating a wide range of external and internal conditions.

Many of our common drugs, such as aspirin and penicillin, are derived from natural sources. Historically, medications were composed of roots, herbs, leaves, or other natural materials that were identified as having, or were believed to have, medicinal properties. Today many medications that originally came from nature are produced synthetically.

# PHARMACOKINETICS

**Pharmacokinetics** is the method by which drugs are absorbed, distributed, metabolized, and eliminated or excreted by the body. The term *pharmacodynamics* is often confused with *pharmacokinetics. Pharmacodynamics* refers to the actions or the effects of a drug on the body and will be discussed in more detail throughout this chapter.[9,42]

## Administration of Drugs

To be effective therapeutically, a drug must first enter the system and then reach a receptor in a target tissue. The administration of medications can be either internal or external and is based on the type of local or general response desired.

> Drugs can be administered internally or externally.

**Internal Administration** Drugs can be taken internally through inhalation, or they can be administered intradermally or subcutaneously, intramuscularly, intranasally, intraspinally, intravaginally, intravenously, orally, rectally, or sublingually and buccally.

*Inhalation* is a means of bringing medication or substances to the respiratory tract. This method is most often used in sports to relieve the athlete of the symptoms of respiratory illnesses, such as asthma. The vehicle for inhalation is normally water vapor, oxygen, or highly aromatic medications.

*Intradermal* (into the skin) or *subcutaneous* (under the cutaneous tissues) administration is usually accomplished through a hypodermic needle injection. Such introduction of medication is initiated when a rapid response is needed, but this method does not produce as rapid a response as intravenous injection offers.

*Intramuscular* injection means that the medication is given directly into the muscle tissue. The site for such an injection is usually the gluteal area or the deltoid muscle of the upper arm.

*Intranasal* application varies according to the condition that is to be treated. The introduction of a decongestant intranasal solution by using a dropper or an atomizer may relieve the discomfort of head colds and allergies.

*Intraspinal* injection may be indicated for any of the following purposes: introduction of drugs to combat specific organisms that have entered the spinal cord; injection of a substance, such as procaine, to anesthetize the lower limbs; or withdrawal of spinal fluid to be studied.

*Intravaginal* administration involves placement of a drug or drug-containing device inside the vagina. Drugs are readily absorbed through the vaginal mucosa.

*Intravenous* injection (into a vein) is given when an immediate reaction to the medication is desired. The drug enters the venous circulation and is spread rapidly throughout the body.

*Oral* administration of medicines is the most common method of all. Forms such as tablets, capsules, powders, and liquids are easily administered orally.

*Rectal* administration of drugs is limited. In the past, some medications have been introduced through the rectum to be absorbed by its mucous lining. Such methods have difficulties in regulating dosage.

*Sublingual* and *buccal* introductions of medicines usually consist of placing easily dissolved agents, such as troches (lozenges) or tablets, under the tongue. They dissolve slowly and are absorbed by the mucous lining.

**External Administration** Medications administered externally include inunctions, ointments, pastes, plasters, transdermal patches, and solutions.

*Inunctions* are oily or medicated substances that are rubbed into the skin and result in a local or systemic reaction. Oil-based liniments and petroleum analgesic balms used as massage lubricants are examples of inunctions.

*Ointments* consisting of oil, petroleum jelly, or lanolin combined with drugs are applied for long-lasting topical medication.

TABLE 17–1    Drug Vehicles

**Liquid preparations**

| | |
|---|---|
| Aqueous solution | Sterile water containing a drug substance. |
| Elixir | Alcohol, sugar, and flavoring with a drug dissolved in solution, designed for internal consumption. |
| Liniment | Alcohol or oil containing a dissolved drug, designed for external massage. |
| Spirit | A drug dissolved in water and alcohol or in alcohol alone. |
| Suspension | Undissolved powder in a fluid medium; must be mixed well by shaking before use. |
| Syrup | A mixture of sugar and water containing a drug. |

**Solid preparations**

| | |
|---|---|
| Ampule | A closed glass receptacle containing a drug. |
| Capsule | A gelatin receptacle containing a drug. |
| Ointment (emollient) | A semisolid preparation for external application of such consistency that it may be applied to the skin by inunction. |
| Paste | An inert powder combined with water. |
| Tablet | A solid pharmaceutical dosage compressed into a small oval, circle, square, or other form. |
| Plaster | A substance intended for external application, made of such materials and of such consistency as to adhere to the skin and thereby attach a dressing. |
| Powder | Finely ground drug plus vehicle or effervescent granules. |
| Suppository | A medicated gelatin molded into a cone for placement in a body orifice (e.g., the anal canal). |

*Pastes* are ointments with a nonfat base. They are spread on cloth and usually produce a cooling effect on the skin.

*Plasters* are thicker than ointments and are spread either on cloth or paper or directly on the skin. They usually contain an irritant, are applied as a counterirritant, and are used for relieving pain, increasing circulation, and decreasing inflammation.

*Transdermal patches* are patches resembling adhesive bandages that contain various types of slow-release medications that are absorbed gradually through the skin. Some patches may be left in place for only several hours, whereas others may be left on for several days.

*Solutions* can be administered externally and are extremely varied, consisting principally of bacteriostatics. Antiseptics, disinfectants, vasoconstrictors, and liquid rubefacients (alcohol, turpentine) are examples.

**Drug Vehicles** A **drug vehicle** is a therapeutically inactive substance that transports a drug. A drug is housed in a vehicle that may be either a solid or a liquid. Some of the more common drug vehicles are listed in Table 17–1.

**Absorption of Drugs** Once a drug is in the system, it must be dissolved before it can be absorbed. The rate and extent of absorption are determined by the chemical characteristics of the drug, the dosage form (e.g., tablet or solution), and the gastric-emptying time. Solutions in which the drug is already dissolved have the fastest absorption rate, and time-release medications have the slowest rate.[9]

**Bioavailability** Refers to how completely a particular drug is absorbed by the system and available to produce a response.[9] Bioavailability is most dependent on the characteristics of the drug and not on the dosage form, whereas absorption rate is largely determined by dosage form.

**Distribution** Once absorbed, the drug is transported through the blood to a specific target tissue. The drug will be distributed to other parts of the body as well. The **volume of distribution** is the volume of plasma, or fluid, in which the drug is dissolved and indicates the extent of distribution of that drug. The **efficacy** of a drug is its capability of producing a specific therapeutic effect once it reaches a particular receptor site in a target tissue. **Potency** is the dose of the drug that is required to produce a desired therapeutic effect.[42]

**Metabolism** The **biotransformation** of drugs into water-soluble compounds that can be excreted is referred to as **metabolism**. Most of the metabolism takes place in the liver, with some occurring in the kidneys and blood. Metabolism of drugs in the liver transforms most active drugs into inactive compounds. Occasionally, when an active drug is metabolized, the metabolites (byproducts of this process) are toxic.[9]

**Excretion** The excretion of a drug or its metabolites is controlled primarily by the kidneys. Drugs are filtered through the kidneys and are usually excreted in the urine, although some are reabsorbed. Some drugs are excreted in saliva, sweat, and feces.[9]

## Drug Half-Life

The rate at which a drug disappears from the body—through metabolism, excretion, or a combination of the two—is called the drug's **half-life**. This rate is the amount of time required for the plasma drug level to be reduced by one-half. For most drugs, the half-life is measured in hours, but for some it is measured in minutes or days. Knowing the half-life of a drug is critical in determining how often and in what dosage a drug must be administered to achieve and maintain therapeutic levels of concentration. The dosage interval, or time between the administration of individual doses, may be equal to the half-life of that drug.[9]

How often a drug will be administered is determined in part by the drug's **steady state**, which is reached when the amount that is taken is equal to the amount that is excreted. A steady state is usually reached after five half-lives of the drug have occurred. Drugs with long half-lives may take several days to weeks to reach a steady state.[9]

## Effects of Physical Activity on Pharmacokinetics

In general, exercise decreases a drug's absorption after oral administration, whereas exercise increases absorption after intramuscular or subcutaneous administration because of an increased blood flow in the muscle.[9] Thus, exercise has an influence on the amount of a drug that reaches a receptor site, which significantly affects the pharmacodynamic activity of that drug.[9]

# LEGAL CONCERNS IN ADMINISTERING VERSUS DISPENSING DRUGS

Administering a drug is defined as providing a single dose of medication for immediate use by the patient. Dispensing is providing the patient with a drug in a quantity sufficient for multiple doses.[24]

NOTE: The degree of variation between state laws and regulations is too vast to cover in this text. The athletic trainer should become familiar with the laws and regulations of the state in which he or she practices.

## Dispensing Prescription Drugs

*At no time can anyone other than a person licensed by law legally prescribe or dispense prescription drugs for a patient.* An athletic trainer, unless specifically allowed by state licensure, is not permitted to dispense a prescription drug.[25] Failure to heed this fact can be a violation of federal laws and state statutes. Table 17–2 lists information about how medication dispensing is controlled. A violation of these laws could mean legal problems for the physician, athletic trainer, clinic, school, school district, or league.[24]

A link to the NATA consensus statement "Managing prescription and nonprescription medication in the athletic training facility" can be found at www.nata.org /sites/default/files/ManagingMedication.pdf.

> At no time can anyone other than a person licensed by law legally prescribe or dispense prescription drugs for a patient.

## Administering Over-the-Counter Drugs

The situation is not as clear-cut for nonprescription drugs. Basically, the athletic trainer may be allowed to administer a single dose of a nonprescription medication. For example, most secondary schools do not allow the athletic trainer to administer nonprescription (over-the-counter [OTC]) drugs that the patient is to take internally, including aspirin and OTC cold remedies. Some secondary schools allow application of nonprescription wound medications under the category of first aid. On the other hand, some secondary-school athletic trainers in the United States are not allowed to apply even a wound medication in the name of first aid but can only clean the wound with soap and water. The patient must then be sent to the school nurse for medication. The dispensing of vitamins and even dextrose may be specifically disallowed by some school districts. At the college or professional level, minors are not usually involved, and the administration of nonprescription medications may be less restrictive. It is assumed that patients who are of legal age have the right to use whatever nonprescription drugs they choose. However, this right does not preclude the fact that the athletic trainer must be reasonable and prudent about the types of nonprescription drugs offered to the patient.[31]

A 2003 study indicated, that 9 years after a National Collegiate Athletic Association (NCAA) drug-distribution study of university athletic programs, many problem areas persisted, including unqualified personnel dispensing medications, inappropriately packaged and labeled medications, and a lack of record keeping.[25] In most athletic training clinics, athletic trainers (55.9 percent) and students (13.3 percent) still dispensed prescription drugs. In addition, in most athletic training clinics, athletic trainers (53.8 percent) administered any amount of over-the-counter medication necessary, and many did not record the transaction (46.2 percent). In virtually every state, this practice is against the law. Athletic trainers should

| TABLE 17–2 | Agencies and Regulations That Govern the Provision of Pharmaceutical Care | |
|---|---|---|
| **Regulation** | **Enforced/Administered by** | **Purpose** |
| Federal Food, Drug, and Cosmetic Act (FDCA) of 1938 | Food and Drug Administration | Regulates the quality, strength, bioequivalence, and labeling of prescription and nonprescription drugs |
| Durham–Humphrey Amendment of 1951 | Food and Drug Administration | Separates prescription from nonprescription drugs |
| Current Good Manufacturing Practice Regulations of 1962 | Food and Drug Administration | Mandates standards for repackaging of medications |
| Federal Controlled Substances Act of 1970 | Food and Drug Administration | Regulates controlled substances (drugs that have potential for abuse) |
| Poison Prevention Packaging Act (PPPA) of 1970 | Food and Drug Administration | Regulates packaging of prescription and nonprescription drugs in child-resistant safety containers |
| Medical Device Act of 1976 | Food and Drug Administration | Regulates classification and performance standards of medical devices |
| Federal Anti-Tampering Act of 1983 | Food and Drug Administration | Mandates tamper-resistant packaging on all nonprescription drugs |
| Fair Packaging and Labeling Act | Food and Drug Administration | Mandates labeling of the contents of nonprescription drugs to assist consumers in identifying similar products |
| Prescription Drug Marketing Act of 1987 | Food and Drug Administration | Mandates accountability of sample drugs from receiving through administering or dispensing |
| Anti–Drug Abuse Act of 1988 | Drug Enforcement Authority | Regulates anabolic steroids as controlled substances |
| Omnibus Reconciliation Act of 1990 (OBRA '90) | Food and Drug Administration | Mandates drug review, patient medication records, and verbal patient education as part of dispensing of prescription medications |
| State pharmacy practice acts | Individual state boards of pharmacy | Regulates the provision of pharmaceutical care within each state; laws and regulations may vary considerably among states |
| State medical acts | Individual state boards of medicine | Regulates the practice within each state |
| Health Insurance Portability-Accountability Act of 1996 (HIPAA) | Department of Health and Human Services | Provides national standards to protect the privacy of personal health information |
| Anabolic Steroid Control Act of 2004 | Drug Enforcement Administration | Added anabolic steroids and prohormones to the list of controlled substances regulated by the DEA |
| Combat Methamphetamine Act 2005 | Drug Enforcement Administration | Established retail sales and purchase transaction limits of pseudoephedrine products |
| Dietary Supplement and Nonprescription | Food and Drug Administration | Mandates reporting of serious adverse events for dietary supplements and Drug Consumer Protection Act 2006 nonprescription drugs |
| Affordable Care Act 2010 | Department of Health and Human Services | Increases access to health coverage and introduce new protections for people with health insurance |
| Drug Quality and Security Act 2013 | Food and Drug Administration | Amends the Federal Food, Drug, and Cosmetic Act with respect to drug compounding and drug supply chain security |

work in conjunction with members of the sports medicine team to review federal and state laws and revise institutional drug policies and procedures to comply with regulations to provide the best health care in a legal and safe manner.[25]

Generally, the administration of single doses of non-prescription medicines by a member of the athletic staff to any athlete depends on the philosophy of the school district and must be under the direction of the team physician.[43] In this area, as in all other areas of sports medicine and athletic training, the athletic trainer is obligated to act reasonably and prudently.

## Record Keeping

Those involved in any health care profession are acutely aware of the necessity of maintaining complete, up-to-date medical records, whether paper or electronic. The athletic training setting is no exception. The athletic trainer who administers medications must realize that maintaining accurate records of the types of medications administered is just as important as recording progress notes, treatments given, and rehabilitation plans.[37] The athletic trainer may be dealing with a number of different patients simultaneously while trying to get a team ready for practice or competition. Situations may become hectic, and stopping to record each time a medication is administered is difficult. Nevertheless, the athletic trainer should include the following information on the medication administration log:[24]

1. Name of the patient
2. Complaint or symptoms
3. Current medications
4. Any known drug allergies
5. Name of medication given
6. Lot number if available (identifies manufacturer, date, and place of production)
7. Expiration date
8. Quantity and dosage of medication given
9. Method of administration
10. Date and time of administration

Each athletic trainer should be aware of state regulations and laws that pertain to ordering, prescribing, distributing, storing, and dispensing or administering medications. Obtaining legal counsel, working with the state board of pharmacy or a student health clinic, working in cooperation with a physician, and establishing strict written policies are all actions that can minimize the chances of violating state laws that regulate the use of medications.[24,60]

**Labeling Requirements** OTC drugs are required to have directions for use and precautions that are adequate and readable. In 2011, the FDA finalized a regulation requiring OTC drugs to have clear and simple labeling. Standardized headings and subheadings make it easier for consumers to understand information about products, benefits, and risks, and how the drugs should be used most effectively.

The following "Drug Facts" must be included on the labels of prescription drugs:[51]

1. Name of the product
2. Active ingredient(s)
3. Purpose
4. Use(s)
5. Warnings, such as contraindications to using the product and side effects that could occur
6. Directions for use including dosage and when, how, or how often to take
7. Other information
8. Inactive ingredients
9. Questions? (optional) followed by a telephone number

Additionally, the Food and Drug Administration Amendments Act of 2007 made it mandatory for human drug products to include a toll-free number for reporting adverse events. Nonprescription drugs may not be repackaged without meeting labeling criteria. All drugs dispensed from the athletic training room must be properly labeled. Legal violations may occur if a portion of a nonprescription drug is removed from an original, properly labeled package and dispensed to an athlete. This practice carries the same liability as does dispensing prescription drugs, because the athlete is not given the opportunity to review the label for name, contents, precautions, directions, and other information considered essential for the safe use of the product. Liability for any adverse patient outcome is therefore transferred to the dispenser of the improperly labeled OTC drug.[24]

An athletic trainer is covering a youth league soccer practice, and one of the soccer moms complains of a sore throat and stuffy head and asks the athletic trainer to give her some "drugs" to get rid of her problem.

**?** Is the athletic trainer legally allowed to give her any type of medication, and, if so, how should the athletic trainer give it to this individual?

## Safety in the Use of Pharmaceuticals

No drug can be considered completely safe and harmless. If a drug is potent enough to effect some physiological action, it is also strong enough, under some conditions, to be dangerous. All persons react individually to any drug.[27] A given amount of a specific medication may produce no adverse reaction in one person and a pronounced adverse response in another. Both the patient and the athletic trainer should be fully aware of any untoward effect a drug may have. It is essential that the patient be instructed clearly about when specifically to take medications, with meals or not, and what not to combine with the drug, such as other drugs or specific foods.[27] Some drugs can nullify the effect of another drug or can cause a serious antagonistic reaction. For example, calcium, which is found in a variety of foods and in some vitamins and medications, can nullify the effects of the antibiotic doxycycline.

**Drug Responses** Individuals react differently to the same medication, and different conditions may alter the effect of a drug on the athlete. Drugs themselves can be changed through age or improper preservation, as well as through the manner in which they are administered. Response variations also result from differences in each individual's size and age.

Alcohol should not be ingested with a wide variety of drugs, both prescription and nonprescription. Alcohol is a central nervous system depressant and can increase or decrease the effects of other drugs. Alcohol may intensify drowsiness if used in combination with another depressant. It is also important to realize that alcohol is used in many liquid preparations that are being used as medications. Warnings concerning the use of alcohol should be listed on the drug label.

Medications can affect certain physiological functions that are related to dehydration, such as sweating, urination, and the ability to control and regulate body temperature. Some medications cause fluid depletion that results in dehydration, which can increase the risk of heat illness. Other medications can make an individual more sensitive to sunlight, increasing the risk of sunburn or allergic reactions to sunlight. A fatty diet may decrease a drug's effectiveness by interfering with its absorption. Excessively acidic foods, such as fruits, carbonated drinks, and vegetable juice, may cause adverse drug reactions. Athletic trainers must thoroughly know the individuals with whom they work. The possibility of an adverse drug reaction is ever present and requires continual education and vigilance.

Table 17–3 is a list of general body responses sometimes produced by drugs and medications.

| TABLE 17–3 | General Body Responses Produced by Drugs |
|---|---|
| Addiction | Body response to certain types of drugs that produces both a physiological need and a psychological craving for the substance. |
| Antagonistic action | Result observed when medications, used together, have adverse effects or counteract one another. |
| Cumulative effect | Exaggerated drug effects, which occur when the body is unable to metabolize a drug as rapidly as it is administered; the accumulated, unmetabolized drug may cause unfavorable reactions. |
| Depressive action | Effect from drugs that slow down cell function. |
| Habituation | Individual's development of a psychological need for a specific medication. |
| Hypersensitivity | Allergic response to a specific drug; such allergies may be demonstrated by a mild skin irritation, itching, a rash, or a severe anaphylactic reaction, which could be fatal. |
| Idiosyncrasy | Unusual reaction to a drug; a distinctive response. |
| Irritation | Process, as well as effect, caused by substances that result in a cellular change; mild irritation may stimulate cell activity, whereas moderate or severe irritation by a drug may decrease cell activity. |
| Paradoxical reaction | A drug-induced effect that is the exact opposite of that which is therapeutically intended. |
| Potentiating agent | A pharmaceutical that increases the effect of another; for example, codeine is potentiated by aspirin, and therefore less of it is required to relieve pain. |
| Specific effect | Action usually produced by a drug in a select tissue or organ system. |
| Side effect | The result of a medication that is given for a particular condition but affects other body areas or has effects other than those sought. |
| Stimulation | Effect caused by drugs that speed up cell activity. |
| Synergistic effect | Result that occurs when drugs given together produce a greater reaction than when given alone. |
| Tolerance | Condition existing when a certain drug dosage is no longer able to give a therapeutic action and must therefore be increased. |

## Buying Medications

One of the athletic trainer's best friends is the local pharmacist. The pharmacist can assist in the selection and purchase of nonprescription drugs, can save money by suggesting the lower-priced generic drugs, and can act as a general advisor on the effectiveness of drugs, the dose of a medicine, and even the dangers inherent in a specific drug.

All pharmaceuticals must be properly labeled, indicating clearly the content, the expiration date, and any dangers or contraindications for use. Pharmaceutical manufacturers place the expiration date on drugs, and athletic trainers should locate this date on the package. When storing medications;

1. Always keep both prescription and over-the-counter medications in a locked cabinet or secured place.
2. Keep them in the original container.
3. Store them away from heat, direct light, damp places, and extreme cold.
4. Keep over-the-counter medications in single-dose packs.[25]

## Traveling with Medications

When traveling with a team or individually, the individual should be advised to do the following with regard to medications:

1. Medication should not be stored in a bag or luggage but carried by the athlete taking it.
2. A sufficient supply of medication should be packaged in case of emergency.
3. Make sure there is a source of medication while traveling.
4. Take copies of written prescriptions.
5. Keep medications in their original containers and in a secure place.
6. When traveling internationally, understand the restrictions of individual jurisdictions.

# SELECTED THERAPEUTIC DRUGS

The use of medicines is widespread in the athletic population, as it is in society in general. Thousands of drugs, both prescription and nonprescription, are available for physicians and consumers to choose from, and new drugs are being constantly developed. Pharmaceutical laboratories develop compounds *in vitro* and then test, retest, and refine the drug *in vivo* before submitting it for Food and Drug Administration (FDA) approval.

> *In vitro* means in a laboratory; *in vivo* means in the body.

A number of texts and databases (e.g., *Physician's Desk Reference* and *Drug Facts and Comparisons*) are widely used as references for comparison of **bioequivalent drugs** (drugs that produce similar biological effects) relative to their appropriateness and effectiveness in treating a specific condition or illness.[38] Table 17–4 summarizes the classification of drugs most commonly used in athletes.

The following sections discuss the most common pharmaceutical practices in athletic training to date and the specific drugs that are in use (Table 17–5). The discussions include both prescription and nonprescription drugs, with emphases on what should most concern the athletic trainer and what the medications or materials are designed to accomplish.

## Drugs to Combat Infection

Combating infection, especially skin infection, is of major importance in sports. Serious infection can cause countless hours of lost time and has even been the indirect cause of death.

> Drugs used to combat infection include local antiseptics and disinfectants, antifungal agents, and antibiotics.

**Local Antiseptics and Disinfectants** Antiseptics are substances that can be placed on living tissue for the express purpose of either killing bacteria or inhibiting their growth. Disinfectants are substances that combat microorganisms but should be applied only to nonliving objects. Types of antiseptics and disinfectants are germicides, which are designed to destroy bacteria; fungicides, which kill fungi; sporicides, which destroy spores; and sanitizers, which minimize contamination by microorganisms.

Many agents are used to combat infection. It is critical that agents have a broad spectrum of activity against infective organisms, including the human immunodeficiency virus (HIV).

***Alcohol*** Alcohol is one of the most widely used skin disinfectants. Ethyl alcohol (70 percent by weight) and isopropyl alcohol (70 percent) are equally effective. They are inexpensive and nonirritating; they kill bacteria immediately, with the exception of spores. However, they have no long-lasting germicidal action. Besides being directly combined with other agents to form tinctures, alcohol acts independently on the skin as an antiseptic and astringent. In a 70 percent solution, alcohol can be used for disinfecting instruments. Because of alcohol's rapid rate of evaporation, it produces a mild anesthetic action. Combined with 20 percent benzoin, it is used as a topical skin dressing to provide a protective skin coating and astringent action.

> Antiseptics and disinfectants include alcohol, phenol, halogens, and oxidizing agents.

***Phenol*** Phenol was one of the earliest antiseptics and disinfectants used by the medical profession. From its inception to the present, phenol has been used to control disease

## TABLE 17–4    List of Drug Classifications and Definitions

| | |
|---|---|
| Analgesics | Pain-relieving drugs. |
| Anesthetics | Agents that produce local or general numbness to touch, pain, or stimulation. |
| Antacids | Substances that neutralize acidity; commonly used in the digestive tract. |
| Antibiotics | Drugs that kill bacteria or inhibit their growth. |
| Anticholinergics | Drugs that block the action of the neurotransmitter acetylcholine in the brain. |
| Anticoagulants | Agents that prevent the coagulation of blood. |
| Anticonvulsants | Drugs used in the treatment of seizures. |
| Antidepressants | Drugs used for treatment of depression. |
| Antidotes | Substances that prevent or counteract the action of a poison. |
| Antifungals | Drugs that kill fungi or inhibit their growth. |
| Antihistamines | Class of drugs used to treat allergic reactions in the nose. |
| Antihypertensives | Drugs used to treat hypertension (high blood pressure). |
| Anti-inflammatories | Drugs that reduce and/or control inflammation. |
| Antipruritics | Agents that relieve itching. |
| Antipsychotics | Drugs used to manage psychosis (delusions, hallucinations, disordered thought) |
| Antipyretics | Drugs that reduce body temperature. |
| Antiseptics | Agents that kill bacteria or inhibit their growth and can be applied to living tissue. |
| Antispasmodics | Agents that relieve muscle spasm. |
| Antitussives | Agents that inhibit or prevent coughing. |
| Astringents | Agents that cause contraction or puckering action. |
| Anxiolytics | Drugs that inhibit anxiety. |
| Bacteriostatics and fungistatics | Agents that retard or inhibit the growth of bacteria and fungi, respectively. |
| Bronchodilators | Drugs used to relax and dilate the airways in the lungs. |
| Carminatives | Agents that relieve flatulence (caused by gases) in the intestinal tract. |
| Cathartics | Agents used to evacuate substances from the bowels; active purgatives. |
| Caustics | Burning agents, capable of destroying living tissue. |
| Chemotherapeutics | Drugs used in the treatment of cancer. |
| Counterirritants | Agents applied locally to produce an inflammatory reaction for the relief of a deeper inflammation. |
| Decongestants | Drugs used to relieve nasal congestion in the upper respiratory tract. |
| Depressants | Agents that diminish body functions or nerve activity. |
| Disinfectants | Agents that kill or inhibit the growth of microorganisms; should be applied only to nonliving materials. |
| Diuretics | Agents that increase the excretion of urine. |
| Emetics | Agents that cause vomiting. |
| Expectorants | Agents that suppress coughing. |
| Hemostatics | Substances that either slow down or stop bleeding. |
| Hormonal contraceptives | Birth control drugs that act on the endocrine system. |
| Irritants | Agents that cause irritation. |
| Narcotics | Drugs that produce analgesic and hypnotic effects. |
| Sedatives | Agents that relieve anxiety. |
| Skeletal muscle relaxants | Drugs that depress neural activity within skeletal muscles. |
| Stimulants | Agents that excite the central nervous system. |
| Suppressants | Agents that reduce or control appetite. |
| Vasoconstrictors and vasodilators | Drugs that constrict and dilate blood vessels, respectively. |

organisms, both as an antiseptic and as a disinfectant. It is available in liquids of varying concentrations and in emollients. Substances that are derived from phenol and that cause less irritation are now used more extensively. Some of these derivatives are resorcinol, thymol, and the common household disinfectant Lysol.

***Halogens*** Halogens are chemical substances (chlorine, fluoride, and bromine) that are used for their antiseptic and disinfectant qualities. Iodophors, or halogenated compounds, a combination of iodine and a carrier, create a much less irritating preparation than tincture of iodine is. A popular iodophor is povidone-iodine complex (Betadine),

| Generic Name | Trade Name | Primary Use of Drug/Precautions | Additional Considerations |
|---|---|---|---|
| **Analgesics, antipyretics, and anti-inflammatories (NSAIDs)** | | | |
| Aspirin | Many trade names | Analgesic, antipyretic, anti-inflammatory | Gastric irritation, nausea, tinnitus, prolonged bleeding if injured. |
| Acetaminophen | Tylenol, others | Analgesic, antipyretic | Do not combine with alcohol. Hepatotoxicity with acute overdose; chronic daily dosing can result in liver damage. |
| Flurbiprofen | Ansaid* | All are analgesic, antipyretic, anti-inflammatory (NSAIDs). | Gastric irritation less common than with aspirin except for indomethacin. These medications should be used for reducing pain and inflammation; they should not be substituted for acetaminophen in cases of mild headache or low fever. Adequate hydration reduces the risk of adverse effects in the renal system. |
| Ketoprofen | Orudis* | Notify doctor immediately for skin rash, itching, visual disturbances, weight gain, edema, black stools, dark urine, or persistent headache. | |
| Indomethacin | Indocin* | | |
| Ibuprofen | Advil, Motrin | | *NSAID hypersensitivity:* Because of cross-sensitivity, to aspirin and all other NSAIDs, do not give these agents to athletes in whom aspirin, iodides, or other NSAIDs have caused symptoms of asthma, rhinitis, rash, nasal polyps, bronchospasm, or other symptoms of allergic reactions. |
| Naproxen | Naprosyn,* Anaprox,* Aleve | | |
| Diflunisal | Dolobid* | | |
| Piroxicam | Feldene* | *Drug interactions:* salicylates, other NSAIDs, probenecid, cimetidine, diuretics, lithium, phenytoin, beta blockers, ACE inhibitors, anticoagulants, digoxin | |
| Tolmetin | Tolectin* | | |
| Fenoprofen | Nalfon* | | |
| Meclofenamate | Meclomen* | | |
| Diclofenac | Voltaren,* Cataflam* | | |
| Ketorolac | Toradol* | NSAIDs carry a Black Box warning regarding possibilities of increased risk of cardiovascular events, especially in those with existing CV disease or risk factors for CV disease, and increased risk of gastrointestinal adverse events, especially in the elderly. | |
| Etodolac | Lodine* | | |
| Mefenamic acid | Ponstel* | | |
| Nabumetone | Relafen* | | |
| Meloxicam | Mobic* | | |
| Oxaprozin | Daypro* | | |
| Sulindac | Clinoril* | | |
| Celecoxib | Celebrex* | | |
| **Antifungal agents** | | | |
| Ketoconazole | Nizoral* | Systemic (oral) antifungal. Drug has been associated with hepatic toxicity including fatalities. Ketoconazole has a Black Box warning due to the risk of serious hepatotoxicity as well as drug interactions that can result in life-threatening dysrhythmias. Should only be used when other antifungal therapies are unavailable or not tolerated. Notify doctor immediately for unusual fatigue, anorexia, nausea, jaundice, dark urine, pale stools, abdominal pain, fever, or diarrhea. | Should not be taken within 2 hours of antacids. May cause dizziness or drowsiness. |
| Griseofulvin | Fulvicin P/G,* Gris-Peg* | Oral antifungal. Notify doctor immediately for fever, sore throat, or skin rash. Reduces the effectiveness of oral contraceptives. | *Hypersensitivity:* Anaphylaxis has been reported. |
| Fluconazole | Diflucan* | Oral antifungal. Warnings: Hepatic injury, anaphylaxis, | Photosensitivity may occur: Patient should avoid prolonged exposure to sunlight or sunlamps. |

| Generic | Trade | Action/Use | Notes |
|---|---|---|---|
| Terbinafine | Lamisil* | Oral antifungal for treatment of toenails or fingernails, scalp, body, groin, or feet

Notify doctor immediately for skin rash, itching, aching joints, dark urine, difficulty swallowing, fever, chills, pale skin, pale stool, redness, blistering, peeling or loosening of skin, unusual tiredness, and yellowing of skin or eyes

*Drug interactions:* cimetidine, rifampin, caffeine | Weeks to months may be required to resolve infection. Alcohol consumption during treatment increases risk of liver toxicity. Liver enzymes should be checked at baseline and periodically during therapy |

**Antibiotics**

| Generic | Trade | Action/Use | Notes |
|---|---|---|---|
| Penicillins | V-Cillin-K,* Pen Vee K,* Trimox* | *Drug interactions:* beta blockers, erythromycin, tetracycline | If diarrhea occurs, do not give Imodium AD. |
| Cephalosporins | Keflex,* Ceftin* | *Drug interactions:* alcohol, probenecid | Patients allergic to penicillin may have cross-sensitivity to cephalosporins. |
| Macrolides | Ery-Tab,* Zithromax,* Biaxin* | *Drug interactions:* fluconazole, zidovudine, theophylline, nonsedating antihistamines, carbamazepine, ergot alkaloids, penicillins | |
| Fluoroquinolones | Cipro,* Noroxin,* Floxin,* Levaquin* | Notify doctor immediately for agitation, confusion, tremors, fever, and skin rash.

*Drug interactions:* antacids, sucralfate, Pepto-Bismol, cimetidine, caffeine, probenecid, phenytoin, theophylline

Avoid administration with milk products and calcium-fortified juices | Photosensitivity; avoid overexposure to sunlight or sunlamps. May cause dizziness. Rarely associated with pain, inflammation, or rupture of a tendon. Fluoroquinolones carry a Black Box warning regarding the risk of tendinitis and tendon rupture at all ages, increased risk with concomitant steroid therapy. Risk of peripheral neuropathy—notify doctor immediately if symptoms occur. |
| Tetracyclines | Sumycin,* Vibramycin* | *Drug interactions:* antacids, anticoagulants, cimetidine, insulin, lithium, penicillins, sodium bicarbonate | Should not be taken with milk, antacids, or minerals because of reduced absorption. Photosensitivity may occur. |

**Drugs that affect the respiratory tract**

| Generic | Trade | Action/Use | Notes |
|---|---|---|---|
| Chlorpheniramine | Chlor-Trimeton | Antihistamine for allergies Used primarily for treatment of allergic rhinitis; causes drowsiness and decreased coordination | |
| Cromolyn | Nasalcrom | Nasal allergy symptom controller; prevents and relieves nasal allergy symptoms such as Allergic rhinitis, seasonal allergies | |
| Oxymetazoline | Afrin, Dristan Long Lasting, Neosynephrine 12 Hour, Allerest | Adrenergic decongestant applied topically as spray or nose drops | Do not exceed recommended duration of treatment because of rebound congestion; may cause sneezing, dryness of nasal mucosa, and headache. |
| Pseudoephedrine | Sudafed, others | Adrenergic decongestant used orally | Produces stimulation of the central nervous system; topically applied decongestants work faster, but oral decongestants are preferred for long-term use. Federal and state laws require record keeping and accountability. |
| Diphenhydramine | Benadryl, Benylin cough syrup | Antihistamine used primarily for allergic reaction; also used for sleep | Produces drowsiness and dry mouth; found in over-the-counter sleeping medications. |

*Continued*

*Requires a prescription.

| TABLE 17–5 | Athletic Trainers' Guide to Frequently Used Medications—continued | | |
|---|---|---|---|
| **Generic Name** | **Trade Name** | **Primary Use of Drug/Precautions** | **Additional Considerations** |
| Dextromethorphan | Robitussin DM, Benylin DMO, Sucrets lozenges | Nonnarcotic antitussive used for cough suppression *Drug interaction:* newer antidepressants | Very effective in cases of unproductive cough; rarely produces drowsiness and other side effects, can be abused for its dissociative effects. |
| Cetirizine | Zyrtec | Antihistamine; effective for some allergic reactions | May cause some sedation but less than traditional antihistamines. |
| Fexofenadine, loratidine | Allegra, Claritin | Antihistamines | Nonsedating. |
| Benzonatate | Tessalon* | Peripherally acting antitussive that acts as an anesthetic | May cause dizziness; should not be chewed. |
| Codeine | Robitussin AC* | Narcotic antitussive that depresses the central cough mechanism | Used in combination with expectorant; can produce sedation, dizziness, constipation, or nausea. The FDA says that in those < 18 years old, there is a potential for serious side effects with codeine, including slowed or difficult breathing, especially in children with preexisting breathing difficulties. |
| Guaifenesin | Mucinex, Robitussin | Expectorant used for symptomatic relief of unproductive cough | Used for treating dry or sore throat; good hydration maximizes effects. |
| *Drugs that affect the gastrointestinal tract* | | | |
| Sodium bicarbonate | Soda Mint | Antacid used for quick relief of upset stomach | Produces gas and belching; overuse may cause systemic alkalinity. |
| Aluminum hydroxide | Amphojel, Dialume | Antacid used for upset stomach | May produce constipation. |
| Calcium carbonate | Titralac, Mallamint, Tums | Antacid used for upset stomach and for calcium supplementation | May produce constipation and acid rebound; high acid neutralizing capacity. |
| Magnesium hydroxide | Milk of Magnesia | Laxative used for constipation | May cause diarrhea. |
| Histamine-2 antagonists Cimetidine, nizatidine, ranitidine, famotidine | Tagamet HB, Axid AR Zantac 75 Pepcid AC | Histamine-2 antagonists used for relief of upset stomach, heartburn, and acid indigestion Histamine-2 antagonists used for relief of upset stomach, heartburn, acid indigestion | Numerous drug interactions. |
| Combination antacids | Alka-Seltzer, Digel, Gaviscon, Gelusil, Maalox, Mylanta, others | Combination drugs for controlling gastric upset | May produce either diarrhea or constipation. |
| Promethazine | Phenergan* | Antiemetic used for preventing motion sickness, nausea, and vomiting | Produces sedation and drowsiness. |
| Diphenoxylate HCL Loperamide Combination antidiarrheals | Lomotil* Imodium AD Donnagel, Kaopectate, Pepto-Bismol | Narcotic antidiarrheals Nonnarcotic systemic antidiarrheal Relief of diarrhea | Cause dry mouth, nausea, and drowsiness. Abdominal discomfort and drowsiness with large doses. Relatively safe with few side effects; effective for traveler's diarrhea. |
| Proton pump inhibitor | Prilosec, Prevacid, Protonix, Nexium, others | Relief of heartburn; prevention of NSAID-induced ulcers | Do not use Pepto-Bismol in a patient with an aspirin allergy. |

which is an excellent germicide commonly used as a surgical scrub. Betadine as an antiseptic and germicide in athletic training has proved extremely effective on skin lesions, such as lacerations, abrasions, and floor burns.

**Oxidizing Agents** Oxidizing agents, as represented by hydrogen peroxide (3 percent), are commonly used in athletic training. Hydrogen peroxide is an antiseptic that, because of its oxidation, affects bacteria but readily decomposes in the presence of organic substances, such as blood and pus. For this reason, it has little effect as an antiseptic. Contact with organic material produces an effervescence, during which no great destruction of bacteria takes place. The chief value of hydrogen peroxide in the care of wounds is its ability to cleanse the infected cutaneous and mucous membranes. Application of hydrogen peroxide to wounds results in the formation of an active, effervescent gas that dislodges particles of wound material and debris and, by removing degenerated tissue, eliminates the wound as a likely environment for bacterial breeding. Hydrogen peroxide also possesses compounds that are widely used as antiseptics. Because it is nontoxic, hydrogen peroxide may be used for cleansing mucous membranes. A diluted solution (50 percent water and 50 percent hydrogen peroxide) can be used for treating inflammatory conditions of the mouth and throat.

**Antifungal Agents** Many medicinal agents on the market are designed to treat fungi, which are commonly found in and around athletic facilities. The three most common fungi are *Epidermophyton*, *Trichophyton*, and *Candida albicans*.

In recent years, antifungal agents such as terbinafine (Lamisil), ketoconazole (Nizoral), amphotericin B (Fungizone), and griseofulvin have been developed and used. Both ketoconazole and amphotericin B seem to be effective against deep-seated fungus infections, such as those caused by *Candida albicans*. Ketoconazole, fluconazole, terbinafine, and griseofulvin, all of which can be administered orally, produce an effective fungistatic action against the specific fungus species of *Microsporum, Trichophyton,* and *Epidermophyton*, all of which are associated with common athlete's foot. Given over a long period of time, griseofulvin becomes a functioning part of the cutaneous tissues, especially the skin, hair, and nails, producing a prolonged and continuous fungistatic action. Any patient taking an oral antifungal agent must be carefully monitored by a clinician. Terbinafine (Lamisil), miconazole (Micatin), clotrimazole (Lotrimin), and tolnaftate (Tinactin, which does not treat *Candida* infections) are topical medications for a superficial fungus infection caused by *Trichophyton* and other fungi.

**Ketoconazole now has a Black Box warning:** Ketoconazole tablets should only be used when other antifungal therapies are unavailable or not tolerated, and the potential benefits of treatment outweigh its risks. Serious hepatotoxicity, including cases with a fatal outcome or requiring liver transplant, have occurred with the use of oral ketoconazole even in patients with no obvious risk factors for liver disease. Additionally, ketoconazole has significant drug interactions.

**Antibiotics** Antibiotics are bacteriostatic (inhibiting bacterial growth) or bacteriocidal (destroying bacteria). Their useful action is primarily a result of their interference with the necessary metabolic processes of pathogenic microorganisms. The physician can use antibiotics as either topical dressings or systemic medications. The indiscriminate use of antibiotics can produce extreme hypersensitivity or idiosyncrasies and can prevent the development of natural immunity to subsequent infections. The use of any antibiotic must be carefully controlled by the physician, who selects the drug on the basis of the suspected bacterial organism, most desirable type of administration, and the least amount of toxicity to the patient.

The antibiotics mentioned here are just a few of the many available. New types continue to be developed, mainly because, over a period of time, many microorganisms become resistant to a particular antibiotic, especially if it is indiscriminately used. Some of the more common antibiotics are penicillins and cephalosporins, bacitracin, tetracycline, erythromycin, and sulfonamides, and quinolones.[36]

> Antibiotics include penicillins and cephalosporins, bacitracin, tetracyclines, macrolides, sulfonamides, and quinolones.

**Penicillins and Cephalosporins** Penicillins and cephalosporins as prescription medications are probably the most important of the antibiotics; they are useful in a variety of skin and systemic infections. In general, penicillins and cephalosporins interfere with bacterial cell-wall synthesis.

**Bacitracin** Bacitracin has a broad spectrum of effectiveness as an antibacterial agent. Bacitracin plus polymixin (Polysporin) also has a broad spectrum of effectiveness as an antibacterial agent. Adding neomycin to the product (Neosporin) does not increase effectiveness, and some individuals are allergic to neomycin.

**Tetracyclines** Tetracyclines consist of a wide group of antibiotics that have a broad antibacterial spectrum. Their application, which is usually oral, modifies the infection rather than eradicating it completely. Tetracyclines cause sensitivity to sun exposure.

**Macrolides** Macrolides, such as erythromycin and azithromycin, are most often used for streptococcal infection and mycoplasma pneumoniae. Macrolides have the same general spectrum as penicillin and are a useful alternative in the penicillin-allergic patient.

**Sulfonamides** Sulfonamides are a group of synthetic antibiotics. In general, sulfonamides make pathogens vulnerable to phagocytes by inhibiting certain enzymatic actions. They are often used to treat urinary tract infections and skin infections.

**Quinolones** Quinolones have a broad spectrum of activity. Patients taking these antibiotics must be carefully monitored for adverse effects.

## Drugs for Asthma

Asthma is a chronic inflammatory lung disorder characterized by obstruction of the airways as a result of complex inflammatory processes, smooth muscle spasm, and hyperresponsiveness to a variety of stimuli.[18] Asthma triggers include exercise, viral infection, animal exposure, dust mites, mold, air pollutants, weather, and NSAIDs as well as other drugs. The National Asthma Education and Prevention Program (NAEPP) has established international guidelines for the diagnosis and management of asthma.[32,33] The goals of asthma therapy are to prevent chronic and troublesome symptoms, maintain normal lung function and activity levels, prevent asthma exacerbations, provide optimal pharmacotherapy with minimal adverse effects,

and meet athletes' expectation of and satisfaction with asthma care.[22]

Exercise-induced bronchospasm (EIB), also referred to as exercise-induced asthma (EIA), is a limiting and disruptive experience. Any asthma patient is subject to EIB. A bronchospastic event caused by loss of heat, water, or both from the lungs during exercise or exertion, EIB results from hyperventilation of air that is cooler and dryer than that in the respiratory tract.[56] EIB occurs during or minutes after physical activity, reaches its peak in 5 to 10 minutes after stopping the activity, and usually resolves in 20 to 30 minutes. In some asthma patients, exercise is the only precipitating factor.

The individual who has asthma must be monitored carefully. The NAEPP recommends measurements of the following: asthma signs and symptoms, pulmonary function (peak flow or spirometry), quality of life/functional status, history of asthma exacerbations, patient satisfaction, and pharmacotherapy.[33] Table 17–6 identifies

> An aerobics instructor has a recurrent breathing problem, especially during high-intensity fitness training. Since the weather has gotten warmer, her symptoms have gotten worse.
>
> **?** What should the athletic trainer expect is wrong with this patient and how should her condition be managed?

| TABLE 17–6 | Medications Recommended for the Management of Asthma |
|---|---|
| **Long-Term Control** | **Quick Relief** |
| **Inhaled corticosteroids (anti-inflammatories)** | **Short-acting beta₂ agonists** |
| • Beclomethasone (Beclovent, Vanceril)<br>• Budesonide (Pulmicort)<br>• Fluticasone propionate (Flovent)<br>• Triamcinolone acetonide (Azmacort)<br>• Mast cell stabilizers (anti-inflammatories)<br>• Cromolyn nebulized solution | • Albuterol (Proventil), Ventolin, Pro-Air<br>• Pirbuterol (Maxair)<br>• Levalbuterol (Xopenex)<br>• Metaproterenol (Alupent)<br>• Terbutaline oral tablets only in the United States |
| **Long-acting beta₂ agonists (bronchodilators)** | **Anticholinergics**<br>• Ipratropium bromide (Atrovent) |
| • Salmeterol (Serevent)<br>• Albuterol sustained release (VoSpire ER)<br>• Formoterol (Foradil Aerolizer) | **Oral Corticosteroids** |
| **Leukotriene modifiers** | • Methylprednisolone (Medrol)<br>• Prednisolone (various generics)<br>• Prednisone (various generics) |
| • Zafirlukast (Accolate)<br>• Zileuton (Zyflo).<br>• Montelukast (Singulair) | |
| **Monoclonal antibody** | |
| • Omalizumab (Xolair) | |
| **Combinations (anti-inflammatory and bronchodilator)** | |
| • Fluticasone plus salmeterol (Advair)<br>• Budesonide plus formoterol (Symbicort)<br>• Mometasone plus formoterol (Dulera) | |
| **Theophylline (bronchodilator)** | |

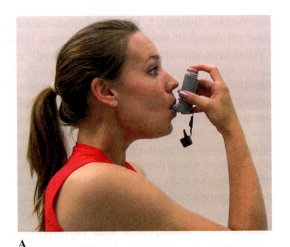
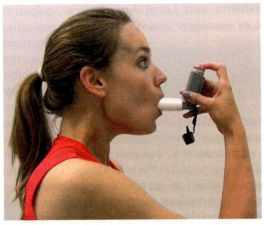

**A**                        **B**

FIGURE 17–1 **(A)** Metered-dose inhalers are commonly used by patients who have asthma. **(B)** A spacer helps keep medication from dissipating into the air.
© William E. Prentice

medications recommended in asthma management. A link to the NATA position statement "Management of asthma in athletes" can be found at www.nata.org/sites/default/files/MgmtOfAsthmaInAthletes.pdf.

**Using an Inhaler** The use of inhalers by individuals who have asthma and/or exercise-induced bronchospasm is common. Portable, handheld inhalers are convenient in that they deliver medicine directly to the lungs very rapidly. A variety of inhalers have been developed to relieve or control asthma symptoms. The two most common devices are *metered-dose inhalers (MDIs)* and *dry powder inhalers (DPIs)*. A metered-dose inhaler includes a pressurized canister with measured doses of medication inside.[57] The patient squeezes the top of the canister. The pressure within the canister converts the medication into a fine powder. To use an MDI, the individual places the mouthpiece of the inhaler between the teeth and closes the mouth around the mouthpiece. The person then breathes in slowly and presses down on the top of the inhaler. Using a metered-dose inhaler calls for coordinating two actions: squeezing the canister and inhaling the medication (Figure 17–1). Many individuals who use the metered-dose inhaler use it improperly; however, with careful and repeated instruction, more than 90 percent of people can use it correctly.[57] Metered-dose inhalers can use a spacer, which is a tube, 4 to 8 inches (10 to 20 cm) long, that attaches to the inhaler that allows time to inhale more slowly. The spacer acts as a holding chamber that keeps medication from escaping into the air.

Dry powder inhalers are not pressurized but rather release medication when the patient rapidly inhales. This type of inhaler requires the individual to place the lips on the mouthpiece and inhale more rapidly than with a traditional metered-dose inhaler. Generally, dry powder inhalers are easier to use than the conventional pressurized metered-dose inhalers because hand-lung coordination is not required. Spacers can't be used with dry powder inhalers.

People with asthma can rely too much on inhaled bronchodilators. Because these fast-acting medications can relieve symptoms quickly, there is a tendency, particularly among physically active individuals, to use them too often, leading to an overdose.[32] Signs of an overdose include irregular heartbeat, tremor, seizure, headache, nausea, and vomiting.

A device called a *nebulizer*, a compressor-driven pump that converts medication into a mist, is used by individuals who are not able to use an inhaler.

Using an inhaler is just one part of an asthma treatment plan. The treatment plan may also include checking lung function with a peak flow meter, eliminating asthma triggers, and exercising.

## Drugs That Inhibit Pain and Inflammation

**Pain Relievers** Controlling pain can involve innumerable drugs and procedures, depending on the beliefs of the athletic trainer or physician. As discussed in Chapter 9, the reason pain is positively affected by certain methods is not clearly understood; however, some of the possible reasons are as follows:

> Drugs used to inhibit pain or inflammation include counterirritants and local anesthetics, narcotic analgesics, and nonnarcotic analgesics and antipyretics.

- The excitatory effect of an individual impulse is depressed.
- An individual impulse is inhibited.
- The perceived impulse is decreased.
- Anxiety created by pain or impending pain is decreased.

## TABLE 17-7 Frequently Used NSAIDs

| Generic Name | Drug/Trade Name | Dosage Range (mg) and Frequency | Maximum Daily Dose (mg) |
|---|---|---|---|
| Celecoxib | Celebrex | 100–200 mg twice a day | 400 |
| Aspirin | Aspirin | 325–650 mg every 4 hours | 4,000 |
| Diclofenac | Voltaren | 50–75 mg twice a day | 200 |
| Diclofenac | Cataflam | 50–75 mg twice a day | 200 |
| Diflunasil | Dolobid | 500–1,000 mg followed by 250–500 mg 2 or 3 times a day | 1,500 |
| Fenoprofen | Nalfon | 300–600 mg 3 or 4 times a day | 3,200 |
| Ibuprofen | Motrin | 400–800 mg 3 or 4 times a day | 3,200 |
| Indomethacin | Indocin | 25–150 mg a day in 3 or 4 divided doses | 200 |
| Ketoprofen | Orudis | 75 mg 3 times a day or 50 mg 4 times a day | 300 |
| Mefenamic acid | Ponstel | 500 mg followed by 250 mg every 6 hours | 1,000 |
| Naproxen | Naprosyn | 250–500 mg twice a day | 1,250 |
| Naproxen | Anaprox | 550 mg followed by 275 mg every 6 to 8 hours | 1,375 |
| Piroxicam | Feldene | 20 mg a day | 20 |
| Sulindac | Clinoril | 200 mg twice a day | 400 |
| Tolmetin | Tolectin | 400 mg 3 or 4 times a day | 1,800 |
| Nabumatone | Relafen | 1,000 mg once or twice a day | 2,000 |
| Flurbiprofen | Ansaid | 50–100 mg 2 or 3 times a day | 300 |
| Keterolac | Toradol | 10 mg every 4 to 6 hours for pain; *not to be used for more than 5 days* | 40 |
| Etodolac | Lodine | 200–400 mg every 6 to 8 hours | 1,200 |
| Meloxicam | Mobic | 7.5 mg once a day | 15 |
| Oxaprosin | Daypro | 1,200 mg once a day | 1,800 |

- Neurological impairments (e.g., vertigo, headache, convulsions)
- Endocrine dysfunctions (e.g., menstrual irregularities)
- Ophthalmic conditions (e.g., glaucoma)
- Metabolic impairments (e.g., negative nitrogen balance, muscle wasting)

Cortisone is primarily administered by injection. Other methods of administration are iontophoresis and phonophoresis (see Chapter 15). Studies have indicated that cortisone injected directly into tendons, ligaments, and joint spaces can lead to weakness and degeneration. Strenuous activity may predispose the treated part to rupturing. Tennis elbow and plantar fasciitis have benefited from corticosteroid treatment.

## Drugs That Produce Skeletal Muscle Relaxation

Drugs that produce skeletal muscle relaxation include methocarbamol (Robaxin), cyclobenzaprine (Flexeril), and carisoprodol (Soma), which is classified as a Schedule IV controlled substance. There is growing speculation among physicians that because centrally acting muscle relaxants also act as sedatives or tranquilizers on the higher brain centers, these drugs are less specific to muscle relaxation than was once believed. Another major side effect is that they cause drowsiness.

Muscle spasm and guarding accompany many musculoskeletal injuries. Elimination of spasm and guarding should facilitate programs of rehabilitation. In many situations, centrally acting oral muscle relaxants are used to reduce spasm and guarding. However, to date the efficacy of using muscle relaxants has not been substantiated, and they do not appear to be superior to analgesics or sedatives in either acute or chronic conditions.

## Drugs Used to Treat Gastrointestinal Disorders

Disorders of the gastrointestinal tract include upset stomach or formation of gas because of food incompatibilities and acute or chronic hyperacidity, which leads to inflammation of the mucous membrane of the intestinal tract. Poor eating habits may lead to digestive tract problems, such as diarrhea or constipation. Drugs that elicit responses within the gastrointestinal tract include antacids, antiemetics, carminatives, cathartics

> Drugs used to treat gastrointestinal disorders include antacids, antiemetics, carminatives, cathartics (laxatives), antidiarrheals, histamine-2 blockers, and proton pump inhibitors.

(laxatives), antidiarrheals, histamine-2 blockers, and proton pump inhibitors.

**Antacids** The primary function of an antacid is to neutralize acidity in the upper gastrointestinal tract by raising the pH and inhibiting the activity of the digestive enzyme pepsin, thus reducing its action on the gastric mucosal nerve endings. Antacids are effective not only for the relief of acid indigestion and heartburn but also in the treatment of peptic ulcer. Antacids available on the market possess a wide range of acid-neutralizing capabilities and side effects.

One of the most commonly used antacid preparations is sodium bicarbonate, or baking soda. Other antacids include alkaline salts, which neutralize hyperacidity but are not easily absorbed in the blood. The ingestion of antacids containing magnesium tends to have a laxative effect. Those containing aluminum or calcium seem to cause constipation. Consequently, many antacid liquids and tablets are combinations of magnesium and either aluminum or calcium hydroxides. Overuse can cause electrolyte imbalance and other adverse effects.

**Antiemetics** Antiemetics are used to treat nausea and vomiting. Antiemetics act either locally or centrally. The locally acting drugs, such as most OTC medications (e.g., Pepto-Bismol), reportedly work by affecting the mucosal lining of the stomach. However, their effects of soothing an upset stomach may be more of a placebo effect. The centrally acting drugs affect the brain by making it less sensitive to irritating nerve impulses from the inner ear or stomach. A variety of prescription antiemetics can be used for controlling nausea and vomiting, including phenothiazines (Phenergan), antihistamines, anticholinergic drugs for preventing motion sickness, and sedative drugs. The primary side effect of these medications is drowsiness. Ondansetron (Zofran) is a very effective, nonsedating antiemetic that acts both centrally and peripherally by affecting select serotonin receptors. It is generally well tolerated with few side effects.

**Carminatives** Carminatives are drugs that give relief from flatulence (gas). Their action on the digestive canal is to inhibit gas formation and aid in its expulsion. Simethicone is the most commonly used carminative.

**Cathartics (Laxatives)** The use of laxatives in sports should always be under the direction of a physician. Constipation may be symptomatic of a serious disease condition. Indiscriminant use of laxatives may render an individual unable to have normal bowel movements. It may also lead to electrolyte imbalance. There is little need for healthy, active individuals to rely on artificial means for stool evacuation.

**Antidiarrheals** Diarrhea may result from many causes, but it is generally considered to be a symptom rather than a disease. It can occur as a result of emotional stress, allergies to food or drugs, adverse drug reactions, or many different types of intestinal problems. Diarrhea may be acute or chronic. Acute diarrhea, the most common, comes on suddenly and may be accompanied by nausea, vomiting, chills, and intense abdominal pain. It typically runs its course rapidly, and symptoms subside once the irritating agent is removed from the system. Chronic diarrhea, which may last for weeks, may result from more serious disease states.

Medications used for control of diarrhea are either locally acting or systemic. The locally acting medications most typically contain kaolin, which absorbs other chemicals, and pectin, which soothes irritated bowel. Some contain substances that add bulk to the stool. The systemic agents, which are generally antiperistaltic or antispasmodic medications, are considered to be much more effective in relieving symptoms of diarrhea, but most, except loperamide (Imodium AD), are prescription drugs. The systemic medications are either opiate derivatives or anticholinergic agents, both of which reduce peristalsis. Common side effects of the systemic antidiarrheals include drowsiness, nausea, dry mouth, and constipation. It is not advisable to treat antibiotic-induced diarrhea because diarrhea may be a protective symptom in antibiotic-induced pseudomembranous colitis.

**Histamine-2 Blockers** Histamine-2 blockers (H2 blockers) reduce stomach acid output by blocking the action of histamine on certain cells in the stomach. They are used to treat peptic and gastric ulcers and other gastrointestinal hypersecretory conditions. Cimetidine (Tagamet) and ranitidine (Zantac) are examples.

**Proton Pump Inhibitors** The mechanism of action of proton pump inhibitors (PPIs) is to suppress the gastric acid secretion by inhibition of the H+/K+-ATPase in the gastric parietal cell.

PPIs are used for treatment of erosive esophagitis, for maintaining symptom resolution and healing of erosive esophagitis, for treatment of symptomatic gastroesophageal reflux disease (GERD), as part of a multidrug regimen for *Helicobacter pylori* eradication in patients with duodenal ulcer disease, for prevention of gastric ulcers in patients at risk associated with continuous NSAID therapy, and for long-term treatment of pathological hypersecretory conditions. Omeprazole (Prilosec) is an over-the-counter example.

## Drugs Used to Treat Colds and Allergies

Drugs on the market designed to affect colds and allergies are almost too numerous to count. In general, they fall into four categories, all of which deal with the symptoms of the condition and not the cause.

> Drugs used to treat colds and allergies include nasal decongestants, antihistamines, cough suppressants, and sympathomimetics.

Those categories are drugs that deal with nasal congestion, with histamine reactions, with cough, and with exercise-induced bronchospasm.

**Nasal Decongestants** Topical nasal decongestants that contain mild vasoconstricting agents, such as oxymetazoline (Afrin), xylometazoline (Otrivin), and phenylephrine (neosynephrine) are on the market. These agents are relatively safe. However, prolonged use can cause rebound congestion and dependency.

An effective oral decongestant is pseudoephedrine hydrochloride (Sudafed). Repeated dosing does not lead to rebound congestion. The Combat Methamphetamine Epidemic Act bans over-the-counter retail sales of cold medicines that contain the ingredient pseudoephedrine, which is commonly used to make methamphetamine in illegal "meth labs." The sale of cold medicine containing pseudoephedrine is limited to behind the counter. In a few states, pseudoephedrine is available only by prescription. The amount of pseudoephedrine that an individual can purchase each month is limited, and individuals are required to present photo identification to purchase products containing pseudoephedrine. In addition, stores are required to keep personal information about purchasers for at least 2 years. This law became effective September 30, 2006.

In addition to these requirements, in order to comply with federal law, regulated sellers are mandated to complete a self-certification process that includes training their employees on the regulations and procedures. The final stage in the self-certification process is for regulated sellers to complete an online application on the Drug Enforcement Administration (DEA) Diversion Web site. Once this application is submitted, DEA sends a confirmation e-mail, which generates a self-certification certificate. Because the athletic training environment is not a "retail sales" operation, it is difficult to apply the federal law. Individuals must become familiar with individual state laws related to the provision of pseudoephedrine and develop procedures in compliance with state and federal regulations. Many states have enacted laws to limit the amount of pseudoephedrine that can be acquired, but the regulations vary from state to state.

**Antihistamines** Histamine is a protein substance contained in animal tissues that, when released into the general circulation, causes the reactions of an allergy. Histamine causes dilation of arteries and capillaries, skin flushing, and a rise in temperature. An antihistamine is a substance that opposes histamine action. Antihistamines offer little benefit in treating the common cold. They are beneficial in treating allergies, and antihistamines are often added to nasal decongestants. Examples are diphenhydramine hydrochloride (Benadryl), chlorpheniramine (Chlor-Trimeton), and loratidine (Claritin).

Antihistamines, as well as decongestants and diuretics, can decrease the peripheral mechanisms of sweating that impair the body's ability to dissipate heat and thus predispose the athlete to heat-related illness. The nonsedating antihistamines, such as loratidine (Claritin), may pose less risk of heat-related illnesses.

**Cough Medicines** Cough medicines either suppress the cough (antitussives) or increase the production of fluid in the respiratory system (expectorants). Antitussives are available in liquid, capsule, troche, and spray forms. Narcotic antitussives contain codeine (Robitussin AC); nonnarcotic antitussives contain diphenhydramine (Benylin cough syrup), dextromethorphan (Benylin DM, Sucrets), or benzonatate (Tessalon). The advantage of nonnarcotic antitussives is that they have few side effects and are not addictive. There is little evidence that expectorants (guaifenesin) are any more effective in the control of coughing than is simply drinking water.

**Sympathomimetics** Exercise-induced bronchospasm (EIB) is a spasm of smooth muscle in the bronchioles and shortness of breath. Drugs used to treat EIB are called sympathomimetics. An example is albuterol (Proventil, Ventolin). Bronchodilators generally reverse the symptoms. Sympathomimetics may cause heat-related problems if used in a hot environment.

***Epinephrine*** In some states, the athletic trainer may receive instructions and certification for the administration of epinephrine via an injective device (EpiPen) to treat anaphylaxis resulting from insect stings. Once it is clear that an individual is having an anaphylactic reaction, the EpiPen can be used to safely and easily inject medication into the thigh (Figure 17–2).

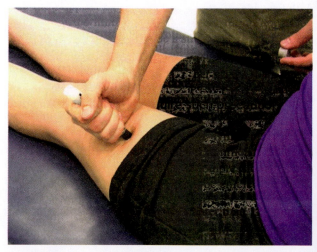

FIGURE 17–2   An EpiPen can be used to treat severe allergic reactions.
© William E. Prentice

## Drugs Used to Control Bleeding

Various drugs and medicines, including vasoconstrictors, hemostatic agents, and anticoagulants, cause selective actions on the circulatory system.

> Drugs used to control bleeding include vasoconstrictors, hemostatic agents, and anticoagulants.

**Vasoconstrictors** Vasoconstrictors are most often administered externally to sites of profuse bleeding. The drug most commonly used for this purpose is epinephrine (adrenaline), which is applied directly to a hemorrhaging area. It acts immediately to constrict damaged blood vessels and is extremely valuable in cases of epistaxis (nosebleed) in which normal procedures are inadequate.

**Hemostatic Agents** Drugs that immediately inhibit bleeding are currently being investigated. There are products such as zeolite granules (QuikClot) and chitosan (HemCon) that can be used as specialized dressings to temporize hemorrhage outside of the operating room, such as in a rescue or battlefield situations. These may be used by a physician in an athletic setting.

**Anticoagulants** The most common anticoagulants used by physicians are heparin and coumarin derivatives. Heparin prolongs the clotting time of blood but will not dissolve a clot once it has developed. Heparin is used primarily to control extension of a thrombus (clot) that is already present. Warfarin (Coumadin) acts by suppressing the formation of prothrombin in the liver. Given orally, it is used to slow clotting time in certain vascular disorders. Newer anticoagulants that directly target thrombin and factor Xa are increasingly being used. These newer agents have fewer drug interactions and require less frequent laboratory monitoring.

## DRUGS THAT CAN INCREASE THE RATE OF HEAT ILLNESS

Thermoregulation involves the central and peripheral nervous system and circulatory mechanisms.[7] Drugs that affect neurotransmitters in these systems could affect temperature regulation. Table 17–8 lists drugs that can predispose peoples to heat-related problems. Anticholinergics and antihistamines can decrease the peripheral mechanism of sweating and therefore eliminate the body's ability to lose heat from this mechanism. Sympathomimetic amines, including decongestants, are vasoconstrictors that can predispose an athlete to heat illness. Phenothiazines affect both hot and cold temperature regulation. Tricyclic antidepressants have been shown to affect hypothalamic heat control and to have anticholinergic activity. Diuretics can prevent volume expansion and limit cutaneous vasodilation.

Lithium carbonate can increase the risk of heatstroke by its effects on potassium levels. It is important that the athletic trainer recognize medications that can increase the risk of heat-related problems, especially when individuals are taking any of these medications and exercising in a warm climate.

## PROTOCOLS FOR USING OVER-THE-COUNTER MEDICATIONS

There is a major difference between prescription and nonprescription drugs. Drugs that require a prescription may pose a greater risk to the patient and therefore require the clinical skills and judgment of individuals trained and licensed to prescribe drugs. In most cases, the athletic trainer will be concerned only with nonprescription medications.

*Focus Box 17–1*: "Protocols for the use of over-the-counter drugs for athletic trainers" presents guidelines for

| TABLE 17–8 | Drugs Reported to Predispose to Heat Illness |
|---|---|
| **Sympathomimetics** | **Phenothiazines** |
| • Amphetamines | • Prochlorperazine |
| • Epinephrine | • Chlorpromazine hydrochloride |
| • Ephedrine | • Promethazine hydrochloride |
| • Cocaine | **Butyrophenones** |
| • Norepinephrine | • Haloperidol |
| • Pseudoephedrine | **Cyclic antidepressants** |
| **Anticholinergics** | • Amitriptyline hydrochloride |
| • Atropine sulfate | • Imipramine hydrochloride |
| • Scopolamine HBr | • Nortriptyline hydrochloride |
| • Benztropine mesylate | • Protriptyline hydrochloride |
| • Belladonna and synthetic alkaloids | **Monoamine oxidase inhibitors** |
| • Antihistamines | • Phenelzine |
| **Diuretics** | • Tranylcypromine sulfate |
| • Furosemide | **Alcohol** |
| • Hydrochlorothiazide | **Lysergic acid diethylamide (LSD)** |
| • Bumetanide | **Lithium** |

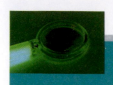

## FOCUS 17–1 Focus on Healthcare Administration and Professional Responsibilities

### Protocols for the use of over-the-counter drugs for athletic trainers

The athletic trainer is often responsible for the initial screening of individuals who have various illnesses or injuries. Frequently, the athletic trainer must make decisions regarding the appropriate use of over-the-counter medications. Subjective findings, such as onset, duration, medication taken, and known allergies, must be included in the screening evaluation.

The following protocols should be viewed as guidelines. The protocols are aimed at clarifying the use of over-the-counter drugs in the treatment of common problems encountered by the athletic trainer while covering an event or traveling with a team. These guidelines do not cover every situation the athletic trainer encounters in assessing and managing the patient's physical problems. Therefore, physician consultation is recommended whenever there is uncertainty in making a decision regarding the appropriate care of the athlete.

| Existing illness or injury | Appropriate treatment protocol |
|---|---|
| **Temperature** | |
| Greater than or equal to 102°F orally | Consult physician ASAP. |
| Less than 102°F but more than 99.5°F orally | Patient may be given acetaminophen. *See acetaminophen administration protocol.* |
| | Limit exercise of athlete. Do not allow participation in practice. |
| | If fever decreases to less than 99.5°F, the athlete may participate in practice. |
| | If patient is to be involved in an intercollegiate event, consult with a physician concerning participation. |
| Less than or equal to 99.5°F orally | Follow management guidelines for fever lower than 102°F, but allow patient to practice and/or compete. |
| **Throat** | |
| History | Advise saline gargles (½ tsp. salt in a glass of warm water). |
|   Sore throat | Patient may also be given Cepastat®/Chloraseptic® throat lozenges. |
|   No fever |   Before administering, determine: Is the patient allergic to Cepastat®/ |
|   No chills |   Chloraseptic® lozenges (which contain phenol)? If yes, do not administer. |
| Sore throat | Determine temperature. If fever, manage as outlined in temperature |
|   Fever |   protocol, and consult physician ASAP. |
| Sore throat and/or fever and/or swollen glands | Consult physician ASAP. |
| **Nose** | |
| Watery discharge | Patient may be given pseudoephedrine (Sudafed®) tablets. See *pseudoephedrine administration protocol.* |
| Nasal congestion | Patient may be given oxymetazoline HCl (Afrin®) nasal spray. See *oxymetazoline administration protocol.* |
| **Chest** | |
| Cough | You may administer Robitussin DM® (generic guaifenesin with |
|   Dry, hacking or clear, mucoid |   dextromethorphan). Before administering, determine: |
|   sputum |   Is the patient going to be involved in practice or a game within 4 hours of administration of medication? |
| |   If yes, do not give Robitussin DM®. |
| |   If indicated, you may administer one dose, 10 ml (2 tsp.). Inform the patient that drowsiness may occur. Repeat doses may be administered every 6 hours. Push fluids; encourage patient to drink as much as possible. |
| Green or rusty sputum | Consult physician ASAP. |
| Severe, persistent cough | Consult physician ASAP. |
| **Ears** | |
| Discomfort due to ears popping | Patient may be given pseudoephedrine (Sudafed®) tablets and/or oxymetazoline HCl (Afrin®) nasal spray. *See pseudoephedrine administration protocol and/or oxymetazoline protocol.* |
| Earache (external otitis) | Patient may be given acetaminophen. Consult physician ASAP. *See acetaminophen administration protocol.* |
| Recurrent earache | Consult physician ASAP. |

*Continued*

# Protocols for the use of over-the-counter drugs for athletic trainers—Cont'd

## *Prevention of Motion Sickness*

Complaint: history of nausea, dizziness, and/or vomiting associated with travel

Patient may be given dimenhydrinate (Dramamine®) or diphenhydramine (Benadryl®). Before administering, determine:

Is the patient sensitive or allergic to Dramamine®, Benadryl®, or any other antihistamine? If yes, do not administer.

Has the patient taken any other antihistamines (e.g., Actifed®, Chlor-Trimeton®, various cold medications) or other medications that cause sedation within the last 6 hours? If yes, do not administer.

Does the patient have asthma, glaucoma, or enlargement of the prostate gland? If yes, do not administer.

Is the patient going to be involved in practice or game within 4 hours from administration of medication? If yes, do not administer.

Administer Dramamine® or Benadryl® dose based on body weight, 30 to 60 minutes before departure time: Under 125 lbs: one Dramamine® 50 mg tablet. Over 125 lbs: two Dramamine 50 mg tablets.

Benadryl® dose: Under 125 lbs: one 25 mg capsule. Over 125 lbs: two 25 mg capsules.

Inform the patient that drowsiness may occur for 4 to 6 hours after taking this medication. Avoid alcoholic beverages. Avoid driving for 6 hours after taking. If travelling time is extended, another dose may be administered 6 hours after the first dose.

## *Nausea, Vomiting*

Prolonged and severe

Consult physician ASAP.

## *Nausea, Gastric Upset, Heartburn, Butterflies in the Stomach, Acid Indigestion*

Associated with dietary indiscretion or tension

You may administer an antacid as a single dose, as defined by label of particular antacid (e.g. Riopan®, Gelusil®, Maalox®, Pepto-Bismol®, Titralac®), or a histamine (H2) antagonist (Pepcid AC®, Tagamet HB®, Axid A®, Zantac 75®). *See histamine-2 blocker protocol. Pepto-Bismol® warning: Contains salicylates. Do not give to children or teenagers who have or are recovering from chickenpox or flu because of the risk of Reye's syndrome. Do not use this product with aspirin.*

Associated with abdominal or chest pain

Consult physician ASAP.

Vomiting, nausea–no severe distress

Monitor symptoms. Patient may be given dimenhydrinate (Dramamine®) or diphenhydramine (Benadryl®) orally. Same as instructions and precautions for motion sickness.

Vomiting: projectile, coffee ground, febrile

Consult physician ASAP.

## *Diarrhea*

Associated with abdominal pain or tenderness and/or dehydration, bloody stools, febrile, recurrent diarrhea

Consult physician ASAP.

Frequent, loose stools not associated with any of the above signs or symptoms

Encourage clear liquid diet. Encourage avoidance of dairy products and high-fat foods for 24 hours (BART diet–bananas, apples, rice, toast). If it persists, consult physician ASAP.

Patient may be given loperamide (Imodium AD®). Before administering, determine: How long has patient had diarrhea? If longer than 24 hours, see physician.

You may administer one dose (two caplets) of loperamide (Imodium AD®, 2 mg per caplet). One caplet may be administered after each loose stool not to exceed 8 mg (four caplets) per 24 hours. Inform the patient that dizziness or drowsiness may occur within 12 hours after taking this medication. Avoid alcoholic beverages. Use caution while driving or performing tasks requiring alertness.

## *Constipation*

Prolonged or severe abdominal pain or tenderness, nausea or vomiting

Consult physician ASAP.

*Continued*

## Protocols for the use of over-the-counter drugs for athletic trainers—Cont'd

### Constipation—Continued

| | |
|---|---|
| Discomfort associated with dietary change or decreased fluid intake | You may administer milk of magnesia, 30 ml as a single dose. Before administering, determine: Does the patient have chronic renal disease? If yes, do not administer.<br>Recommend increased fluid intake, increased intake of fruits, bulk vegetables, or cereals. |

### Headache

| | |
|---|---|
| Pain associated with elevated BP, temperature elevation, blurred vision, nausea, vomiting, or history of migraine | Consult physician ASAP. |
| Pain across forehead (mild headache) | Patient may be given acetaminophen or NSAID. *See acetaminophen administration or NSAID administration protocol.* |
| Tension headache, occipital pain | Patient may be given acetaminophen. *See acetaminophen administration protocol.* |
| Pain in antrum or forehead associated with sinus or nasal congestion | Patient may be given pseudoephedrine (Sudafed®) tablets and acetaminophen. *See protocols for pseudoephedrine and acetaminophen administration.* |

### Musculoskeletal Injuries

| | |
|---|---|
| Deformity | Consult physician ASAP. |
| Localized pain and tenderness, impaired range of motion | First aid to start as soon as possible:<br>  Ice<br>  Compression–Ace bandage<br>  Elevation<br>  Protection–crutches or sling and/or splint |
| Pain with swelling discoloration, no impaired movement or localized tenderness | If this injury interferes with the patient's normal activities, consult a physician within 24 hours.<br>Patient may be given acetaminophen or NSAID.<br>*See acetaminophen administration or NSAID administration protocol.* |

### Skin

| | |
|---|---|
| Localized or generalized rash accompanied by elevated temperature, enlarged lymph nodes, sore throat, stiff neck, infected skin lesion, dyspnea, wheezing | Consult physician ASAP. |
| Mild, localized, nonvesicular skin eruptions accompanied by pruritis | Hydrocortisone 1.0% cream may be applied.<br>Before administering, determine:<br>  Is the patient taking any medication? If yes, do not administer. Refer to physician.<br>  Are eyes or any large area of the body involved? If yes, do not administer. Refer to physician.<br>  Is there any evidence of lice infestation?<br>  The cream may be repeated every 6 hours if needed.<br>  Do not use more than three times daily. |
| Abrasions | Control bleeding. Clean with antibacterial soap and water. Apply appropriate dressing and antibiotic ointment. Monitor for signs of infection. Dressing may be changed 2 or 3 times a day if needed. |
| Localized erythema due to ultraviolet rays | Advise application of compresses soaked in a solution of cold water. |
| Jock itch or athlete's foot | Advise 10- to 15-minute application of compresses soaked in cool water to relieve intense itching.<br>Patient may be given terbinafine (Lamisil) or miconazole (Micatin®) cream topically. Before administering, determine:<br>  Is the patient sensitive or allergic to miconazole or terbinafine? If yes, do not administer. Consult physician ASAP.<br>  Is the patient receiving other types of treatment for rash in same area? If yes, do not administer. Consult physician ASAP.<br>  Instruct patient to wash and dry area of rash, and then apply ¼- to ½-inch ribbon of cream. Give patient the cream on a clean gauze pad and rub gently on the infected area. Spread evenly and thinly over rash. The dose may be repeated in 8 to 12 hours (twice a day). Consult physician within 24 hours. |

*Continued*

# Protocols for the use of over-the-counter drugs for athletic trainers—Cont'd

## Skin Wounds

| | |
|---|---|
| Lacerations | Control bleeding. Cleanse area with antibacterial soap and water. Apply steristrips. Consult physician immediately if there is any question about the necessity for suturing. |
| Extensive lacerations or other severe skin wounds | Control bleeding. Protect area with dressing. Refer to physician immediately. |

## Wound Infection

| | |
|---|---|
| Febrile, marked cellulitis, red streaks, tender or enlarged nodes | Consult physician ASAP. |
| Localized inflammation, afebrile, absence of nodes and streaks | Warm soaks to affected area. Consult physician ASAP. |

## Burns

| | |
|---|---|
| First-degree erythema of skin, limited area | Apply cold compresses to affected area. Dressing is not necessary on first-degree burns. If less than 45 minutes have elapsed since burn injury, clean gently with soap and water. Patient may be given acetaminophen. *See acetaminophen administration protocol.* |
| First-degree with extensive involvement over body | Consult physician ASAP. |
| Second-degree erythema with blistering | Consult physician ASAP. |
| Third-degree pearly white appearance of affected area, no pain | Consult physician ASAP. |

## Allergies

| | |
|---|---|
| Patient with known seasonal allergies who forgot to bring own medication | Patient may be given 10 mg tablet of loratidine (Claritin®). Before administering, determine: |

Is the patient sensitive to loratidine? If yes, do not administer. Consult physician ASAP.

Does the patient have liver or kidney disease? If yes, do not administer. Consult physician ASAP.

Has the patient taken any other antihistamines (e.g., Chlorpheniramine, Dramamine®, various cold medications) or other medications that cause drowsiness within the last 6 hours? If yes, do not administer. Consult physician ASAP.

You may administer one dose of loratidine (10 mg) every 24 hours. Avoid alcoholic beverages. Contact physician if symptoms do not abate.

## Contact Lens Care

Note: There are three types of contact lenses: hard, gas permeable, soft.

Solutions are labeled for use with a particular type of lens and should not be used for any other type of lens.

Do not use solutions preserved with thimersol or chlorhexidine because of possible allergy or irritation.

| | |
|---|---|
| Lens needs rinsing/wetting before insertion | Hard lens: use all-purpose wetting/soaking solution (e.g., Optimum®).<br>Gas permeable lens: use all-purpose wetting/soaking solution (e.g., Optimum®).<br>Soft lens: use rinsing/soaking solution (e.g., Opti-Free). |
| Lens needs soaking/storage | Hard lens: use all-purpose wetting/soaking solution (e.g., Optimum®).<br>Gas permeable lens: use all-purpose wetting/soaking solution (e.g., Boston Advance®).<br>Soft lens: use rinsing/soaking solution (e.g., Opti-Free®). |
| Lens needs cleaning | Hard lens: use cleaning solution (e.g., EasyClean®).<br>Gas permeable lens: use cleaning solution (e.g., Easy Clean®).<br>Soft lens: use cleaning solution (e.g., Opti-Free®). |

## Eye Care

| | |
|---|---|
| Foreign body–minor: sand, eyelash, etc. | Use eye wash irrigation solution (Dacriose®). |
| Irritation–minor | Use artificial tears. Do not use with contact lens in eye. |
| Severe irritation, foreign body not easily removed, trauma | Consult physician ASAP. |

*Continued*

## Protocols for the use of over-the-counter drugs for athletic trainers—Cont'd

*Red Eye*

| | |
|---|---|
| Only one eye affected | Consult physician ASAP. |
| Change in vision | Consult physician ASAP. |
| Pain in eye | Consult physician ASAP. |
| Sensitivity to light | Consult physician ASAP. |
| Thick discharge from eye, especially with lids sealed shut in morning | Consult physician ASAP. |
| Patient wears contacts | Consult physician ASAP. |
| Redness, tearing, both eyes itch | 1. Apply cold compresses.<br>2. Instill one or two drops of antihistamine/decongestant eye drop (e.g., Vasocon-A®) into each eye four times a day. (Do not use one bottle for more than one patient.)<br>3. If condition does not improve or worsens, consult physician ASAP.<br>4. If condition has not improved in 24 hours or persists for more than 48 hours, consult physician ASAP. |
| Redness, tearing, both eyes itch in patient with known allergies who forgot to bring own medication | 1. Apply cold compresses<br>2. Instill one or two drops of antihistamine/decongestant eye drop (e.g., Vasocon-A®) into each eye four times a day. (Do not use one bottle for more than one patient.)<br>3. *See also allergies treatment protocol.*<br>4. See No. 4 above. |

---

*Administration protocols for common over-the-counter drugs used in sports medicine Acetaminophen protocol (Tylenol®)*

Before *administering*, determine:

Is the patient allergic to acetaminophen? If yes, do not give acetaminophen.

You may *administer* acetaminophen 325 mg, two tablets. Repeat doses may be *administered* every 4 hours if needed. If *dispensing* occurs, use labeled 2/pack only. Patient instructions must accompany *dispensing*. The maximum dose must not exceed 4 g (4,000 mg) in 24 hours.

---

*Pseudoephedrine protocol (Sudafed®)*

Before *administering*, determine:

Is the patient allergic or sensitive to pseudoephedrine? If yes, do not give pseudoephedrine.

Does the patient have high blood pressure, heart disease, diabetes, urinary retention, glaucoma, or thyroid disease? If yes, do not give pseudoephedrine.

Does the patient have problems with sweating? If yes, do not give pseudoephedrine.

Do not administer 4 hours before practice or game.

Do not administer if patient is involved in postseason play.

You may *administer* pseudoephedrine (Sudafed®) 30 mg, two tablets. Repeat doses may be *administered* every 6 hours up to four times a day. If *dispensing* occurs, use labeled 2/pack only. Patient instructions must accompany *dispensing*.

---

*Oxymetazoline protocol (Afrin®)*

Before *administering*, determine:

Is the patient allergic or sensitive to Afrin® or Otrivin®? If yes, do not administer.

Does the patient react unusually to nose sprays or drops? If yes, do not administer.

You may *administer* two or three sprays of oxymetazoline (Afrin®) 0.05% nasal spray into each nostril. Repeat doses may be administered every 12 hours. (The container can be marked with the patient's name and maintained by the athletic trainer for repeat administration or dispensed to the patient. Patient instructions must accompany *dispensing*.) Do not use the same container for different patients.

Do not use for more than 3 days without MD supervision.

Use small package sizes to reduce risk of overuse/rebound congestion.

---

*NSAID Protocol (ibuprofen: Advil®, naproxen sodium: Aleve®, ketoprofen: Orudis KT®)*

Before *administering*, determine:

Is the patient allergic to aspirin, (e.g., asthma, swelling, shock, or hives associated with aspirin use)? If yes, do not give ibuprofen because, even though ibuprofen contains no aspirin or salicylates, cross-reactions may occur in patients allergic to aspirin.

Does the patient have renal disease or gastrointestinal ulcerations? If yes, do not administer ibuprofen.

You may *administer* ibuprofen 200 mg (Advil®), one or two tablets. Repeat doses may be *administered* every 6 hours if needed. Do not exceed six tablets in a 24-hour period without consulting an MD. Do not administer if patient is less than 12 years of age.

*Continued*

or

You may *administer* naproxen sodium 220 mg (Aleve®), one tablet every 8 to 12 hours or two tablets to start followed by one tablet 12 hours later. Do not exceed three tablets in a 24-hour period without consulting a physician. Do not administer if patient is less than 12 years of age.

or

You may *administer* ketoprofen 12.5 mg (Orudis KT®), one tablet or caplet every 4 to 6 hours if needed. If pain or fever persists after 1 hour, one more 12.5 mg tablet or caplet may be given. Do not exceed six tablets or caplets in a 24-hour period without consulting a physician. Do not administer if the patient is less than 16 years of age.

The patient should take the NSAID with a full glass of water and food if occasional and mild heartburn, upset stomach, or mild stomach pain occurs. Consult MD if these symptoms are more than mild or persist. Discontinue drug if patient experiences skin rash; itching; dark, tarry stools; visual disturbances; dark urine; or persistent headache. Instruct patient to avoid concurrent aspirin or alcoholic beverages.

*Histamine-2 Blocker Protocol (ranitidine: Zantac 75®, nizatidine: Axid AR®, famotidine: Pepsid AC®, cimetidine: Tagamet-HB®)*

Before *administering*, determine:

Is the patient less than 12 years of age? If yes, do not give histamine-2 blocker. Does the patient have difficulty swallowing or persistent abdominal pain? If yes, do not give histamine-2 blocker.

You may *administer* ranitidine (Zantac 75®), one 75 mg tablet with water up to two times a day. Do not administer more than two tablets in a 24-hour period.

or

You may *administer* nizatidine (Axid AR®), one 75 mg tablet with water up to two times a day. Do not administer more that two tablets in a 24-hour period.

or

You may *administer* famotidine (Pepcid AC®), one 10 mg tablet with water up to two times a day. Do not administer more than two tablets in a 24-hour period.

or

You may *administer* cimetidine (Tagamet-HB®), one 200 mg tablet with water up to two times a day. Do not administer more than two tablets in a 24-hour period. Do not administer cimetidine if the patient is taking phenytoin (Dilantin®) or theophylline (Theodur®).

Data from Lombardo, JA: Drugs in sports. In Krakurer, LJ: *The yearbook of sports medicine,* Chicago: Yearbook Medical Publishers, 1986.

---

treating a number of minor illnesses or conditions seen frequently in the athletic population. The authors and publisher have exerted every effort to ensure that the drug selection and dosage set forth in this text are in accord with current recommendations and practice at the time of publication. However, in view of ongoing research, changes in government regulations, and the constant flow of information relating to drug therapy and drug reactions, the reader is urged to check the package insert for each drug for any change in indications and dosage and for added warnings and precautions. Reading the package insert is especially important when the recommended agent is a new or infrequently used drug.

# SUBSTANCE ABUSE AMONG ATHLETES

Perhaps no other topic related to pharmacology has received more attention from the media during recent years than the use and abuse of drugs, especially by athletes. Much has been written regarding the use of performance-enhancing drugs among Olympic athletes and the widespread use of street drugs by collegiate and professional athletes. Clearly, substance abuse has no place in the athletic population.[44]

Although much of the information being disseminated to the public by the media may be based on hearsay and innuendo, the use and abuse of many different types of drugs can have a profound impact on athletic performance. To say that many experts in the field of sports medicine regard drug abuse among athletes with growing concern is a gross understatement. The athletic trainer must be knowledgeable about substance abuse in the athletic population and should be able to recognize signs that indicate when an individual is engaging in substance abuse[2] (see *Focus Box 17–2*: "Identifying the substance abuser").

## Performance-Enhancing Substances (Ergogenic Aids)

*Ergogenic aid* is a term used to describe any method, legal or illegal, used to enhance athletic performance.[48]

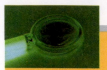

## FOCUS 17–2
### Focus on Examination, Assessment, and Diagnosis

### Identifying the substance abuser

The following are signs of drug abuse:

- Sudden personality changes
- Severe mood swings
- Changing peer groups
- Decreased interest in extracurricular and leisure activities
- Worsening grades
- Disregard for household chores and curfews
- Feelings of depression most of the time
- Breakdown in personal hygiene habits
- Increased sleep and decreased eating
- Smell of alcohol or marijuana on clothes and skin
- Sudden weight loss
- Lying, cheating, stealing
- Arrests for drunk driving or for possessing illegal substances
- Truancies from school
- Frequent loss or change of jobs
- Defensiveness at the mention of drugs or alcohol
- Increased isolation (spends time in room)
- Deteriorating family relationship
- Drug paraphernalia (needles, empty bottles, etc.)
- Observations by others about negative behavior
- Signs of intoxication
- Missed appointments
- Falling asleep in class or at work
- Financial problems
- Missed assignments or deadlines
- Diminished productivity

Athletic trainers should have a primary concern about the use of various pharmacological agents for enhancing performance. The NATA has prepared an official statement on this topic, "Steroids and performance-enhancing substances."

**Stimulants** People may ingest a stimulant to increase alertness, reduce fatigue, or increase competitiveness and even hostility. Some individuals respond to stimulants with a loss of judgment that may lead to personal injury or injury to others.

Two major categories of stimulants are psychomotor-stimulant drugs and adrenergic (sympathomimetic) drugs. Psychomotor stimulants are of two general types: amphetamines (e.g., methamphetamine) and nonamphetamines (e.g., methylphenidate and cocaine). The major actions of psychomotor stimulants result from the rapid turnover of catecholamines, which have a strong effect on the nervous and cardiovascular systems, metabolic rates, temperature, and smooth muscle.

Sympathomimetic drugs act directly on adrenergic receptors, or those that release catecholamines (i.e., epinephrine and norepinephrine) from nerve endings, and thus act indirectly on catecholamines. Ephedrine is an example of this type of drug and can, in high doses, cause mental stimulation and increased blood flow. As a result, it may also cause elevated blood pressure and headache, increased and irregular heartbeat, anxiety, and tremors.

Amphetamines and cocaine are the psychomotor drugs most commonly used. Cocaine is discussed in the section on recreational drug abuse in this chapter. Sympathomimetic drugs present an extremely difficult problem in sports medicine because they are commonly found in cold remedies.[55] The U.S. Olympic Committee (USOC) has approved some substances to be used by asthmatics who develop exercise-induced bronchospasms. These substances are selective $B_2$ agonists, consisting of albuterol (Proventil), salmeterol (Serevent), and formoterol (Foradil). Before an athlete engages in Olympic competition, his or her physician must notify the USOC Medical Subcommission in writing about the patient's use of these drugs.[59]

> Common ergogenic aids include stimulants, beta blockers, narcotic analgesics, diuretics, anabolic steroids, human growth hormone, and blood doping.

***Amphetamines*** Amphetamines are synthetic alkaloids that are extremely powerful and dangerous drugs. They may be injected, inhaled, or taken as tablets. Amphetamines are among the most abused of those drugs used to enhance performance. In ordinary doses, amphetamines can produce euphoria, with an increased sense of well-being and heightened mental activity, until fatigue sets in (from lack of sleep), accompanied by nervousness, insomnia, and anorexia. In high doses, amphetamines reduce mental activity and impair the performance of complicated motor skills. The patient's behavior may become irrational. The chronic user may be "hung up"—that is, stuck in a repetitive behavioral sequence. This perseveration may last for hours and become increasingly more irrational. The long-term or even short-term use of amphetamines can lead to amphetamine psychosis, manifested by auditory and visual hallucinations and paranoid delusions. Physiologically, high doses of amphetamines can cause mydriasis (abnormal pupillary dilation), increased blood pressure, hyperreflexia (increased reflex action), and hyperthermia.

Many athletes believe that amphetamines improve performance by promoting quickness and endurance, delaying fatigue, and increasing confidence, thereby causing increased aggressiveness. Studies indicate that there is no improvement in performance, but there is an increased risk of injury, exhaustion, and circulatory collapse.[16]

**Caffeine** Caffeine is found in coffee, tea, cocoa, and cola and is readily absorbed into the body (Table 17–9).[5] Caffeine is a central nervous system stimulant and diuretic, and it stimulates gastric secretion. One cup of coffee can contain from 100 to 150 milligrams of caffeine. In moderation, caffeine causes stimulation of the cerebral cortex and medullar centers, resulting in wakefulness and mental alertness. In larger amounts and in individuals who ingest caffeine daily, it raises blood pressure, decreases and then increases the heart rate, and increases plasma levels of epinephrine, norepinephrine, and renin. It affects coordination, sleep, mood, behavior, and thinking processes.[5]

In terms of exercise and sports performance, caffeine is controversial. Like amphetamines, caffeine can affect some athletes by acting as an ergogenic aid during prolonged exercise. The USOC considers caffeine a stimulant if the concentration in the athlete's urine exceeds 12 micrograms per milliliter. Some adverse effects of caffeine ingestion are tremors, nervousness, headaches, diuresis, arrhythmias, restlessness, hyperactivity, irritability, dry mouth, tinnitus, ocular dyskinesia (involuntary eye movement), scotomata (blind spots), insomnia, and depression.[5] A habitual user of caffeine who suddenly stops may experience withdrawal, including headache, drowsiness, lethargy, rhinorrhea, irritability, nervousness, depression, and loss of interest in work. Caffeine also acts as a diuretic when hydration may be important.[5]

**Narcotic Analgesic Drugs** Narcotic analgesic drugs are derived directly from opium or are synthetic opiates. Morphine and codeine (methylmorphine) are examples of substances made from the alkaloid of opium. Narcotic analgesics are used for the management of moderate to severe pain. Users risk physical and psychological dependency as well as many other problems stemming from the use of narcotics. It is believed that slight to moderate pain can be controlled effectively by drugs other than narcotics.

**Beta Blockers** The *beta* in beta blockers refers to the type of sympathetic nerve ending receptor that is blocked.[40] Medically, beta blockers are used primarily for hypertension and heart disease. Beta blockers have been used in sports that require steadiness, such as marksmanship, sailing, archery, fencing, ski jumping, and luge.[40] Beta blockers are one class of adrenergic agents that inhibit the action of catecholamines released from sympathetic nerve endings. Beta blockers produce relaxation of blood vessels. This relaxation in turn slows heart rate and decreases the contractility of heart muscle, thus decreasing cardiac output.

**Diuretics** Diuretic drugs increase kidney excretion by decreasing the kidney's resorption of sodium. The excretion of potassium and bicarbonate may also be increased. Therapeutically, diuretics are used for a variety of cardiovascular and respiratory conditions (e.g., hypertension) in which the elimination of fluids from tissues is necessary. Sports participants have misused diuretics mainly in two ways: to reduce body weight quickly and to decrease a drug's concentration in the urine (increasing its excretion to avoid the detection of drug misuse). In both cases, there are ethical and health grounds for banning certain classes of diuretics from use during competition.

**Anabolic Steroids** Anabolic steroids are synthetically created chemical compounds whose structure closely resembles naturally occurring sex hormones—in particular, the male hormone testosterone.[19,20] Anabolic

> A lacrosse player comes into the athletic trainer's office very concerned over the fact that she has been chosen for a random drug test later that afternoon. She met her boyfriend for lunch and drank a large cup of espresso. Now she is concerned that she will test positive for a performance-enhancing drug.
>
> **?** What should the athletic trainer tell the athlete to reduce her anxiety about the drug test?

| TABLE 17–9 | Examples of Caffeine-Containing Products |
|---|---|
| **Product** | **Dose** |
| Coffee (1 cup) | 100.0 mg |
| Diet Coke (12 oz) | 45.6 mg |
| Diet Pepsi (12 oz) | 36.0 mg |
| No-Doz (1) | 100.0 mg |
| Anacin (1) | 32.0 mg |
| Excedrin (1) | 65.0 mg |
| Midol (1) | 32.4 mg |
| Jolt (12 oz) | 200.0 mg |
| Mountain Dew (12 oz) | 54.0 mg |

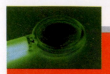

young male and female athletes are taking or have taken them, with most being purchased through the black market.[3] Approximately 6.5 percent of male athletes and 1.9 percent of female athletes are taking anabolic steroids.[39] An estimated 2.5 percent of intercollegiate athletes take anabolic steroids.[39] The more commonly used anabolic steroids are Anavar, Dianabol, Anadrol, and Finajet.[38]

Usage of anabolic steroids is a major problem in sports that involve strength. Powerlifting, the throwing events in track and field, and American football are some sports in which the use of anabolic steroids is a serious problem.

A football linebacker returns to school for preseason practice, and, to the shock of both his teammates and the coaches, he has gained 30 pounds and greatly increased his muscle bulk since leaving in June. Even though this athlete is known to be religious about his weight training, the coaches are fairly certain that he has engaged in steroid abuse. The athlete vehemently denies taking steroids and is willing to take a drug test to prove it.

**?** One of the coaches approaches the athletic trainer and asks if the athlete is using steroids. Without subjecting the athlete to a definitive drug test, what physical signs are indicative of steroid abuse?

steroids have both androgenic and anabolic effects. Androgenic effects include growth development and maintenance of reproductive tissues and masculinization in males.[20] Anabolic effects promote nitrogen retention, which leads to protein synthesis in skeletal muscles and other tissues, resulting in increased muscle mass and weight, general growth, and bone maturation.[8,19]

Individuals who choose to take anabolic steroids are seeking to maximize the anabolic effects while minimizing the androgenic side effects. The problem is that no steroids exist that have only anabolic effects; they all also have androgenic effects.[41]

In 1984 the American College of Sports Medicine (ACSM) reported that anabolic steroids taken with an adequate diet could contribute to an increase in body weight and, with a heavy resistance program, to a possible significant gain in strength.[61] However, when used in mass quantities, as individual athletes typically use them, anabolic steroids can have many deleterious and irreversible side effects that constitute a major threat to the health of the user (*Focus Box 17–3*: "Examples of deleterious effects of anabolic steroids").[3]

Anabolic steroids present an ethical dilemma for the sports world.[39] It is estimated that more than a million

**Tetrahydrogestrinone (THG)** Recently, a substance called tetrahydrogestrinone (THG) has reportedly been used by athletes to improve their performance. THG is currently thought to be undetectable on drug tests. Purveyors of THG may represent it as a dietary supplement, but it does not meet the dietary supplement definition. Rather, it is a purely synthetic "designer" steroid that is structurally related to two other synthetic anabolic steroids, gestrinone and trenbolone. It is derived by simple chemical modification from another anabolic steroid that is explicitly banned by the U.S. Anti-Doping Agency. It cannot be legally marketed without FDA approval under the agency's rigorous approval standards, and according to the FDA its use may pose considerable health risks.

**Androstenedione** Androstenedione is a relatively weak androgen that is produced primarily in the testes and in lower amounts by the adrenal cortex and ovaries.[47] It has been used in humans to produce transient increases in testosterone in males and particularly in females primarily for the purpose of enhancing athletic performance. To date there is no scientific evidence or research to support the efficacy or safety of using this ergogenic aid.[26] The Anabolic Steroid Control Act of

2004 added anabolic steroids and prohormones, including androstenedione, to the list of controlled substances regulated by the Drug Enforcement Administration. This makes possession of these substances without a prescription a crime. The use of androstenedione supplements is banned by the International Olympic Committee, the National Football League, the National Collegiate Athletic Association, and Minor League Baseball.

**Human Growth Hormone** Human growth hormone (HGH) is produced by the somatotropic cells of the anterior region of the pituitary gland, from which it is released into the circulatory system. The amount released varies with age and the developmental periods of a person's life. A lack of HGH can result in dwarfism. In the past, HGH was in limited supply because it was extracted from cadavers. Now, however, it can be made synthetically and is more readily available.[21]

Experiments indicate that HGH can increase muscle mass, skin thickness, connective tissues in muscle, and organ weight and can produce lax muscles and ligaments during rapid growth phases. It also increases body length and weight and decreases body fat percentage.[21]

The use of HGH by athletes throughout the world is on the increase because it is more difficult to detect in urine than are anabolic steroids.[49] There is currently a lack of concrete information about the effects of HGH on the athlete who does not have a growth problem. It is known that an overabundance of HGH in the body can lead to premature closure of long-bone growth sites or, conversely, can cause acromegaly, a condition that produces elongation and enlargement of bones of the extremities and thickening of bones and soft tissues of the face. Also associated with acromegaly is diabetes mellitus, cardiovascular disease, goiter, menstrual disorders, decreased sexual desire, and impotence. Acromegaly decreases the life span by up to 20 years. Like anabolic steroids, HGH presents a serious problem for the sports world. At this time there is no proof that an increase of HGH combined with weight training contributes to strength and muscle hypertrophy.[49]

**Blood Reinjection (Blood Doping, Blood Packing, and Blood Boosting)** Endurance, acclimatization, and altitude make increased metabolic demands on the body, which responds by increasing blood volume and the number of red blood cells to meet the increased aerobic demands.

Recently, researchers have replicated these physiological responses by removing 900 milliliters of blood, storing it, and reinfusing it after 6 weeks. The reason for waiting at least 6 weeks before reinfusion is that it takes that long for the athlete's body to reestablish a normal hemoglobin and red blood cell concentration. Athletes using this method have significantly improved their endurance performance. From the standpoint of scientific research, such experimentation has merit and is of interest. However, not only is the use of such methods in competition unethical, but use by nonmedical personnel could prove to be dangerous, especially when a matched donor is used.[48]

There are serious risks with transfusing blood and related blood products. The risks include allergic reactions, kidney damage (if the wrong type of blood is used), fever, jaundice, the possibility of transmitting infectious diseases (hepatitis B or HIV), and blood overload, which can result in circulatory and metabolic shock.[48]

## Recreational Substance Abuse

Just as it is of the world in general, recreational substance abuse is a part of the world of sports.[17] Reasons that individuals use these substances may include the desire to experiment, to temporarily escape from problems, and to just be part of a group (peer pressure). For some people, recreational drug use leads to abuse and dependence. Drug abuse may be defined as the use of drugs for nonmedical reasons—that is, with the intent of getting high or altering mood or behavior.[17]

> Recreational drugs include tobacco, alcohol, cocaine, and marijuana.

**Psychological versus Physical Dependence** There are two general aspects of dependence: psychological and physical. Psychological dependence is the drive to repeat the ingestion of a drug to produce pleasure or to avoid discomfort. Physical dependence is the state of drug adaptation that manifests itself as the development of tolerance and, when the drug is removed, causes a withdrawal syndrome. Tolerance of a drug is the need to increase the dosage to create the effect that was obtained previously by smaller amounts. The withdrawal syndrome consists of an unpleasant physiological reaction when the drug is abruptly stopped.

Some drugs that are abused overlap with those thought to enhance performance. Examples include amphetamines and cocaine. Tobacco (nicotine), alcohol, cocaine, and marijuana are the most abused recreational drugs. The athletic trainer might also come in contact with abuse of barbiturates, nonbarbiturate sedatives, psychotomimetic drugs, or different inhalants.

**Tobacco Use** Although cigarettes, cigars, and pipes are becoming increasingly rare in the athletic population, the use of smokeless tobacco and the passive exposure to others who are smoking are ongoing problems.

## Cigarette Smoking

On the basis of various investigations into the relationship between smoking and performance, the following conclusions can be drawn:

1. There is individual sensitivity to tobacco that may seriously affect performance in instances of relatively high sensitivity. Because more than one-third of the men studied indicated tobacco sensitivity, it may be wise to prohibit smoking by athletes.
2. Tobacco smoke has been associated with as many as 4,700 different chemicals, many of which are toxic.
3. As few as 10 inhalations of cigarette smoke cause an average maximum decrease in airway conductance of 50 percent. This decrease also occurs in nonsmokers who inhale secondhand smoke.
4. Smoking reduces the oxygen-carrying capacity of the blood. A smoker's blood carries 5 to 10 times more carbon monoxide than normal. Carbon monoxide inhibits the capability of oxygen molecules to bind to the hemoglobin molecule. Thus, the red blood cells are prevented from picking up enough oxygen to meet the demands of the body's tissues. The carbon monoxide also tends to make arterial walls more permeable to fatty substances, a factor in atherosclerosis.
5. Smoking aggravates and accelerates the heart muscle cells through overstimulation of the sympathetic nervous system.
6. Total lung capacity and maximum breathing capacity are significantly decreased in heavy smokers; this fact is important to the athlete because both changes would impair the capacity to take in oxygen and make it readily available for body use.
7. Smoking decreases pulmonary diffusing capacity.
8. After smoking, an accelerated thrombolic tendency is evidenced.
9. Smoking is a carcinogenic factor in lung cancer and is a contributing factor to heart disease.

The addictive chemical of tobacco is nicotine, which is one of the most toxic drugs. When inhaled, it causes blood pressure elevation, increased bowel activity, and an antidiuretic action. Moderate tolerance and strong physical dependence occur.

**Use of Smokeless Tobacco** It is estimated that more than 7 million individuals use smokeless tobacco, which comes in three forms: loose-leaf, moist or dry powder (snuff), and compressed. The tobacco is placed between the cheek and the gum. Then it is sucked and chewed. Aesthetically, this habit is an unsavory one, during which an athlete is continually spitting into a container. Besides the unpleasant appearance, the use of smokeless tobacco poses an extremely serious health risk.[45] Smokeless tobacco causes bad breath, stained teeth, tooth sensitivity to heat and cold, cavities, gum recession, tooth bone loss, leukoplakia (white patches in the mouth), and oral and throat cancer. Aggressive oral and throat cancer and periodontal destruction (with tooth loss) have been associated with this habit.[10]

The major substance ingested is nitrosonornicotine, which is the drug responsible for this habit's addictiveness. It is absorbed through the mucous membranes, and within a short period of time the level of nicotine in the blood is equivalent to that of a cigarette smoker. This chemical makes smokeless tobacco a more addictive habit than smoking. The user of chewing tobacco experiences the nicotine effects without exposure to the tar and carbon monoxide associated with a burning cigarette. Smokeless tobacco increases heart rate but does not affect reaction time, movement time, or total response time among athletes and nonathletes.[10]

In sports, the biggest problem with smokeless tobacco has historically been in baseball athletes.[11] Almost one-third of rookie baseball players entering professional baseball in 1999 used smokeless tobacco. Interventions targeting young baseball players are needed to prevent and stop the use of smokeless tobacco.[15]

**Passive Smoke** There are dangers associated with the passive inhalation of smoke (secondhand smoke) by nonsmokers. Both smokers and nonsmokers are exposed to smoke containing carbon monoxide, nicotine, ammonia, and cyanide. Obviously, smokers inhale the greater quantity of contaminated air. However, it has been estimated that, for each pack of cigarettes smoked, the nonsmoker who shares a common air supply will inhale the equivalent of three to five cigarettes. Significant numbers of individuals exposed to passive smoke develop nasal symptoms, eye irritation, headaches, cough, and allergies to smoke. For these reasons and others, many state, local, and private sector policies have been established that restrict or ban smoking in public areas. There is little doubt that passive smoking poses a significant health threat to the nonsmoker.

**Alcohol Use** Alcohol is the most widely used and abused substance.[34] Alcohol is a drug that depresses the central nervous system. It is absorbed from the digestive system into the bloodstream very rapidly. Factors that affect how rapidly absorption takes place include the number of drinks consumed, the rate of consumption, the alcohol concentration of the beverage, and the amount of food in the stomach.[54] Some alcohol is absorbed into the blood through the stomach, but the greater part is absorbed through the small intestine. Alcohol is transported through the blood to the liver, where it can be oxidized at a rate of 2/3 ounce per hour. An excess causes an increase in the level of alcohol circulating in the blood. As blood alcohol levels continue to increase, predictable signs of intoxication appear. At 0.1 percent, the person loses motor coordination; from 0.2 percent to 0.5 percent, the symptoms become progressively more profound and perhaps even life threatening.[55] Intoxication persists until the liver can metabolize the remainder of the alcohol. There is no way to accelerate the liver's metabolism of alcohol (the act of sobering up); it just takes time. Alcohol has no place in sports participation.

Approximately 20 percent of cases of alcoholism are associated with genetic reasons and 80 percent with overindulgence.[54] The individual who is suffering from alcohol abuse may display the following characteristics: mood changes, missed practices, isolation, attitude changes, fighting or inappropriate outbursts of violence, changes in appearance, hostility toward authority figures, complaints from family, and changes in peer group.[34]

## Abused Illegal Drugs

**Cocaine** Cocaine, also known as coke, snow, toot, happy dust, and white girl, is a powerful central nervous system stimulant with effects of very short duration. Cocaine use produces immediate feelings of euphoria and excitement, decreased sense of fatigue, and heightened sexual drive. Cocaine may be snorted, taken intravenously, or smoked (freebased). The initial effects are extremely intense, and, because they are pleasurable, strong psychological dependence is developed rapidly by users who can or cannot afford to support this expensive habit.

Habitual use of cocaine will not lead to physical tolerance or dependence but will cause psychological dependence and addiction. Long-term effects include nasal congestion and damage to the membranes and cartilage of the nose if snorted, bronchitis, loss of appetite leading to nutritional deficiencies, convulsions, impotence, cocaine psychosis with paranoia, depression, hallucinations, and disorganized mental function. An overdose can lead to overstimulation of the sympathetic nervous system and can cause tachycardia, hypertension, extra heartbeats, coronary vasoconstriction, strokes, pulmonary edema, aortic rupture, and sudden death.[17]

**Crack** Crack is a rocklike crystalline form of cocaine that is heated in a small pipe and then inhaled, producing an immediate rush. The effects last for only a matter of minutes and are frequently followed by a state of depression. This sudden, intense stimulation of the nervous system predisposes the user to cardiac failure or respiratory failure and makes this commonly available drug extremely dangerous.

**Marijuana** Marijuana is one of the most abused drugs in Western society. It is more commonly called grass, weed, pot, or dope. The marijuana cigarette is called a joint, jay, number, reefer, or root.

Marijuana is not a harmless drug. The components of marijuana smoke are similar to those of tobacco smoke, and the same cellular changes are observed in the user. Continued use leads to respiratory diseases, such as asthma and bronchitis, and a decrease in vital capacity of 15 percent to 40 percent (certainly detrimental to physical performance). Among other deleterious effects are lowered sperm counts and testosterone levels. Evidence of interference with the functioning of the immune system and cellular metabolism has also been found. The most consistent sign is the increase in pulse rate, which averages close to 20 percent higher during exercise and is a definite factor in limiting performance. Some decrease in leg, hand, and finger strength has been found at higher dosages. Like tobacco, marijuana must be considered carcinogenic.[43]

Psychological effects, such as a diminution of self-awareness and judgment, a slowdown of thinking, and a shorter attention span, appear early in the use of the drug. Postmortem examinations of habitual users reveal not only cerebral atrophy but also alterations of anatomical structures, which suggest irreversible brain damage. Marijuana also contains unique substances (cannabinoids) that are stored, in much the same manner as are fat cells, throughout the body and in the brain tissues for weeks and even months. These stored quantities result in a cumulative deleterious effect on the habitual user.

A drug such as marijuana has no place in sports. Claims for its use are unsubstantiated, and the harmful effects, both immediate and long-term, are too significant to permit indulgence at any time.

**Crystal Methamphetamine.** This drug is used by individuals of all ages and is increasingly gaining in popularity as a club drug. It is a colorless, odorless, and highly addictive synthetic stimulant. Crystal methamphetamine resembles small fragments of glass or shiny blue-white "rocks" of various sizes. Like powdered methamphetamine, it is abused because of the long-lasting euphoric effects it produces. But it has a higher purity level and may produce even longer-lasting and more intense physiological effects than the powdered form smoked in glass pipes similar to pipes used to smoke crack cocaine; or it may be injected. A user who smokes or injects the drug immediately experiences an intense sensation followed by a high that may last 12 hours or more.

Crystal methamphetamine use is associated with numerous serious physical problems, which may include rapid heart rate, increased blood pressure, and damage to the small blood vessels in the brain that can lead to stroke. Overdoses can cause increased temperature, convulsions, and death. People who use crystal methamphetamine may have episodes of paranoia, anxiety, violent behavior, confusion, and insomnia. The drug can produce psychotic symptoms that persist for months or years after an individual has stopped using the drug.

**Ecstasy.** Considered the most commonly used designer drug, Ecstasy is a close derivative of methamphetamine and can be described as a hallucinogenic stimulant. Designer drugs are illicit variations of other drugs. Ecstasy is most often found in tablet, capsule, or powder form and is usually consumed orally, although it can also be injected. Ecstasy can cause euphoria and feelings of well-being, enhanced mental or emotional clarity, anxiety, and paranoia. Heavier doses can cause hallucinations, sensations of lightness and floating, depression, paranoid thinking, and violent, irrational behavior. Physical reactions can include loss of appetite, nausea, vomiting, blurred vision, increased heart rate and blood pressure, muscle tension, faintness, chills, sweating, tremors, insomnia, convulsions, and loss of control over voluntary body movements. Some reactions have been reported to persist up to 14 days after taking Ecstasy.

**Abused Prescription Drugs** The misuse of drugs prescribed by a physician has become a huge problem in the athletic population.[60] Two prescription medications in particular, ADHD medication and OxyContin, are being widely misused.

**ADHD Medications.** The abuse of medications commonly used for treating attention deficit and hyperactivity disorder (ADHD) is a relatively new phenomenon, but one that has become a major cause for concern, especially in the college population. These medications usually are amphetamines such as Ritalin, Adderall, and Dexedrine. They are stimulants, but they also decrease an individual's distractibility and facilitate concentration and focus. Reasons for abusing or misusing stimulant medication include improving attention, partying, reducing hyperactivity, and improving grades. Some individuals are illegally or illicitly obtaining the medications for their own use or for sale. Common signs and symptoms include shakiness, rapid speech or movements, difficulty sitting still, difficulty concentrating, lack of appetite, sleep disturbance, and irritability.

**OxyContin (Oxycodone)** OxyContin is a prescription drug used to treat moderate to severe pain. Oxycodone is in a class of medications called opiate (narcotic) analgesics. It works by altering the way the brain and nervous system respond to pain. Although this is an extremely effective medication, it has become perhaps the most widely abused prescription drug. The drug is relatively inexpensive but may be sold on the street at 20 times the value. Tablets may be crushed, then snorted, chewed, or injected to obtain a heroin-like high. It is rare to become addicted to OxyContin when the drug is used as recommended. However, due to pharmacy break-ins, growing levels of illegal use, and increased media reports of OxyContin abuse, prescriptions are heavily regulated.

## Managing a Drug Overdose

Athletes, like others in society, are not immune to extreme instances of substance abuse. On occasion, an athlete can either accidentally or intentionally take too much of a particular drug or consume an excessive amount of alcohol. Sometimes the athletic trainer will get a phone call late at night from that athlete's friend or perhaps from a teammate who reports that the athlete is unconscious or not responding. They are scared that the athlete has "overdosed," and they are seeking advice as to how they should handle this emergency situation.

The athletic trainer should immediately insist that the rescue squad be called by dialing 911. In cases of suspected drug overdose, the athletic trainer should also insist that the poison control center be contacted. *Focus Box 17–4*: "Contacting the poison control center" tells how the poison control center can be contacted. It is imperative that the athletic trainer follow up to make certain that the right steps have been taken, either by telephone or by actually going to deal with the athlete in person.

## DRUG TESTING IN ATHLETES

Drug testing began with the 1968 Olympic Games. In 1985, the United States Olympic Committee (USOC) began drug testing athletes involved in both national and international competitions. In 2000, the USOC was aware that its drug testing program lacked credibility internationally. A decision was made to turn over the drug-testing program to an independent group called the U.S. Anti-Doping Agency (USADA). Today, both the USADA and the NCAA routinely conduct drug testing.[35,52]

> Both the NCAA and the USOC conduct drug-testing programs.

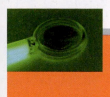

## FOCUS 17–4 Focus on Immediate and Emergency Care

### Contacting the poison control center

Each state has at least one and usually several poison control centers located in different regions of the state. The phone number of the poison control center is usually clearly accessible in the front of the phone book. The rescue squad can also contact the poison control center directly. The following information is necessary when communicating with the poison control center:

- Name and location of the person making the call
- Name and age of the person who has taken the medication
- Name and amount of the drug taken (if known)
- Time the drug was taken
- Signs and symptoms associated with the overdose, including vital signs

The experts at the poison control center will provide instructions for immediate care of the individual until the rescue squad arrives.

A Web site at Fast Health, www.fasthealth.com/poison/nc.php, provides a list of phone numbers for all the poison control centers in each state.

---

A university has recently implemented a drug-testing program for athletes in all sports. The athletic director has decided that the athletic trainer is the best individual to supervise the program.

? Should the athletic trainer be willing to take on the additional responsibilities of overseeing the drug-testing program for the athletes?

The legality and ethics of testing only those individuals involved with sports are still open to debate.[29] The pattern of drug usage among athletes may simply reflect that of our society in general. Great care must be taken that an athlete's personal rights are not violated.[46] USADA was given full authority to execute a comprehensive national anti-doping program encompassing testing, adjudication, education, and research and to develop programs, policies, and procedures for Olympic, Pan American, and Paralympic sports in the United States. In January 1986, the member institutions of the NCAA voted overwhelmingly to expand the NCAA drug-education program to include mandatory random drug testing in specific sports throughout the year and during and after NCAA championship events.[35] The major goals of both organizations are to protect the health of athletes and to help ensure that competition is fair and equitable.[29]

Most professional teams, individual colleges and universities, and many sport clubs and individual sport governing bodies, have initiated drug-testing programs for their athletes.[29] Unfortunately, drug testing is rarely done at the secondary school level because of cost constraints.

### The Drug Test

There are some slight differences between NCAA and USADA drug-testing procedures and protocols. Most of these differences have to do with how the athletes are selected for random tests. The NCAA requires all athletes to sign a consent form agreeing to participate in the drug-testing program throughout the year. The USADA tests athletes on a random basis throughout the year and tests all athletes before a USOC-sanctioned competition.[29]

During the drug test, the athlete must first provide positive identification. Then, under direct observation, the athlete must urinate into two separate specimen bottles (labeled A and B), which are sealed and submitted to an official NCAA or USOC testing laboratory for analysis. In the laboratory, specimen A is used for both screening and confirmation tests. A confirmation test uses analysis techniques that are more sensitive and accurate, should a positive test result occur during the screening test. Specimen B is used only when a reconfirmation is needed for a positive test of specimen A. The athlete is then notified of a positive test result and becomes subject to sanctions from either the NCAA or the USADA.[58]

**Sanctions for Positive Tests** For a first-time positive test, the NCAA will declare the athlete ineligible for all regular and postseason competitions for a minimum of 1 year. During that year, the athlete may be retested at any time. The athlete must be retested with a negative result and have eligibility restored before he or she may return to competition. Additional positive tests can result in a lifetime disqualification from NCAA competition.[35]

The USADA sanctions range from 3 to 24 months of disqualification, depending on the drug, for a first-time violation, and a minimum of 2 years to a lifetime ban for subsequent positive tests.[52]

### Banned Substances

Both the NCAA and the United States Olympic Committee have established lists of substances that

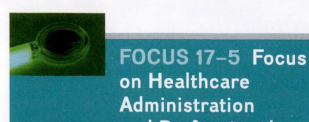

## FOCUS 17–5 Focus on Healthcare Administration and Professional Responsibilities

### Banned drugs—common ground

*Drugs banned by both NCAA and USOC*

Alcohol*
Anti-estrogens (promote the development and maintenance of female sex characteristics)
Anabolic steroids
Diuretics
Beta blockers (used to lower blood pressure, decrease heart rate, decrease cardiac arrythmias)
Hormones (human growth hormone, corticotropin, erythropoietin, human chorionic gonadotropin, etc.)
Stimulants
Blood doping
Marijuana

*Drugs banned by USADA only*

Narcotics (specific drugs prohibited)
Corticosteroids** (intramuscular, intravenous, rectal, and oral use is banned; most topical and inhaled use is permitted with written permission)

*Drugs banned by NCAA only*

Local anesthetics

*Dietary supplements*

Not banned, but both groups recommend using at your own risk

---

*Banned only for certain sports.
**Permits with prior written Therapeutic Use Exemption (TUE).

---

are banned from use by athletes. The lists include performance-enhancing drugs and street, or recreational, drugs, as well as many OTC and prescription drugs.

The list of drugs banned by either the NCAA or the USOC or by both is extensive and includes approximately 4,600 medications.[52] The list of drugs banned by the USOC is considerably more extensive than the NCAA list because the USOC is subject to internationally used drugs banned by the International Olympic Committee (IOC). *Focus Box 17–5*: "Banned drugs—common ground" summarizes the various categories of drugs that appear on the banned lists for the NCAA and the USOC.[29]

The athletic trainer working with athletes who may be tested for drug use by the NCAA or with world-class or Olympic athletes governed by the USOC should be thoroughly familiar with the list of banned drugs.[52] Having an athlete disqualified because of the indiscriminate use of some prescription or OTC medication would be very unfortunate. As is the case with others in the population, some athletes have conditions or illnesses that require them to take a particular medication. If that medication appears on the prohibited list, the athlete can apply for a Therapeutic Use Exemption (TUE) by completing a form that is available from the USADA, which may give that athlete permission to continue taking the needed medication.[52] Table 17–10 lists the drugs currently banned by the NCAA.

The National Federation of State High School Associations (NFHS) does not currently have a list of banned substances or specific policies on drug testing. They have left the choice of whether to drug test athletes up to individual states. To date only a few states have implemented mandatory drug-testing programs for athletes. However, they have provided guidelines for those schools wishing to institute a drug-testing program. Testing high school athletes for drugs has been occurring since the mid-1970s, when efforts to reduce drug use increased. Drug testing among high school athletes has been done infrequently and with varying degrees of success. However, court decisions in 1995 removed some hurdles for drug testing of high school athletes. Drug testing can be done for a variety of different drugs. It appears that high school drug-testing programs most commonly screen athletes for amphetamines, marijuana, cocaine, opiates, and phencyclidine (PCP). These standard drug-testing packages leave out several commonly used substances such as alcohol, tobacco, and steroids.

**Dietary Supplements** Many nutritional/dietary supplements contain NCAA-banned substances.[4,50] In addition, the U.S. Food and Drug Administration (FDA) does not strictly regulate the supplement industry; therefore, purity and safety of nutritional/dietary supplements cannot be guaranteed.[12] Impure supplements may lead to a positive NCAA drug test. The student-athlete is at his or her own risk when using supplements. Student-athletes should contact their institution's team physician or athletic trainer for further information.

TABLE 17–10    NCAA Banned Drug Classes

The following is a list of banned drug classes, with examples of substances under each class.

## A. Stimulants

amiphenazole
amphetamine
bemigride
benzphetamine
bromantan
caffeine* (guarana)
chlorphentermine
cocaine
cropropamide
crothetamide
dextroamphetamine
diethylpropion
dimethylamphetamine
doxapram
ephedrine (ephedra, ma huang)
ethamivan
ethylamphetamine
fencamfamine
lisdexamfetamine
meclofenoxate
methamphetamine

methylenedioxy-methamphetamine (MDMA) (ecstasy)
methylphenidate
nikethamide
pemoline
pentetrazol
phendimetrazine
phenmetrazine
phentermine
phenylephrine
phenylpropanolamine (ppa)
picrotoxine
pipradol
prolintane
strychnine
synephrine (citrus aurantium, zhi shi, bitter orange)
and related compounds

**The following stimulants are not banned:**
phenylephrine
pseudoephedrine

## B. Anabolic Agents

Anabolic steroids
androstenediol
androstenedione
boldenone
clostebol
dehydrochlormethyei-testosterone
dehydroepiandrosterone (DHEA)
dihydrotestosterone (DHT)
dromostanolone
epitrenbolone
fluoxymesterone
gestrinone
mesterolone
methandienone

methenolone
methyltestosterone
nandrolone
norandrostenediol
norandrostenedione
norethandrolone
oxandrolone
oxymesterone
oxymetholone
stanozolol
testosterone[†]
tetrahydrogestrinone (THG)
trenbolone
and related compounds

**Other Anabolic Agents**
clenbuterol

## C. Substances Banned for Specific Sports

Rifle

| | |
|---|---|
| alcohol | pindolol |
| atenolol | propranolol |
| metoprolol | timolol |
| nadolol | and related compounds |

## D. Diuretics

| | |
|---|---|
| acetazolamide | hydroflumethiazide |
| bendroflumethiazide | methyclothiazide |
| benzthiazide | metolazone |
| bumetanide | polythiazide |
| chlorothiazide | quinethazone |
| chlorthalidone | spironolactone |
| ethacrynic acid | triamterene |
| flumethiazide | trichlormethiazide |
| furosemide | and related compounds |
| hydrochlorothiazide | |

## E. Street Drugs

| | |
|---|---|
| heroin | THC (tetrahydrocannabinol) |
| marijuana[‡] | |

## F. Peptide Hormones and Analogues

corticotropin (ACTH)
growth hormone (hGH, somatotropin)
human chorionic gonadotropin (hCG)
insulin-like growth hormone (IGF-1)
leutenizing hormone (LH)

**All the respective releasing factors of the above-mentioned substances also are banned.**

erythropoietin (EPO)
sermorelin
darbepoetin

## G. Anti-Estrogens

anastrozole
clomiphene
tamoxifen
and related compounds

**Definitions of positive depend on the following:**

*For caffeine—if the concentration in the urine exceeds 15 micrograms/ml.

†For testosterone—if the administration of testosterone or the use of any other manipulation has the result of increasing the ratio of the total concentration of testosterone to that of epitestosterone in the urine to greater than 6:1, unless there is evidence that this ratio is due to a physiological or pathological condition.

‡For marijuana and THC—if the concentration in the urine of THC metabolite exceeds 15 nanograms/ml.

Source: Data from the NCAA.

## SUMMARY

- A drug is a chemical agent used in the prevention, treatment, or diagnosis of disease; a drug may be administered either internally or externally. It is transported in an inactive substance called a vehicle.
- Pharmacokinetics is the method by which drugs are absorbed, distributed, metabolized, and eliminated or excreted by the body.
- Administering a drug is providing a single dose of medication for immediate use. Dispensing is providing the patient with a drug in a quantity sufficient to be used for multiple doses. At no time can anyone other than a person licensed by law legally prescribe or dispense drugs. In certain situations, the athletic trainer may be allowed to administer a single dose of a non-prescription medication.
- Drugs used to combat infection include local antiseptics and disinfectants, antifungal agents, and antibiotics.
- Drugs used to inhibit pain or inflammation include counterirritants and local anesthetics, narcotic analgesics, nonnarcotic analgesics and antipyretics, acetylsalicylic acid (aspirin), nonsteroidal anti-inflammatory drugs, and corticosteroids.
- Drugs used to treat gastrointestinal disorders include antacids, antiemetics, carminatives, cathartics or laxatives, and antidiarrheals.
- Drugs used to treat colds and allergies include nasal decongestants, antihistamines, cough suppressants, and asthma drugs.
- Drugs used to control bleeding include vasoconstrictors, hemostatic agents, and anticoagulants.
- The athletic trainer is often responsible for the initial screening of patients who have various illnesses or injuries. Frequently, the athletic trainer must make decisions regarding the appropriate use of over-the-counter medications. Specific protocols have been established that can serve as a guide for the use of these medications by the athletic trainer.
- Substance abuse involves the use of performance-enhancing drugs and the widespread use of recreational drugs, or street drugs. The athletic trainer must be knowledgeable about substance abuse and should be able to recognize signs that an individual is engaging in substance abuse. Substance abuse has no place in the athletic population.
- The use of performance-enhancing drugs (ergogenic aids) must be discouraged because of potential health risks and to ensure equal competition. Among the more common ergogenic aids are stimulants, beta blockers, narcotic analgesics, diuretics, anabolic steroids, human growth hormone, and blood doping.
- Recreational drug abuse is of major concern. It can lead to serious psychological and physical health problems. The most prevalent substances that are abused are tobacco, alcohol, cocaine, and marijuana.
- Drug testing of athletes for the purpose of identifying individuals who may have some problems with drug abuse is done routinely by the NCAA and the USOC. The major goals of drug testing are to protect the health of athletes and to help ensure that competition is fair and equitable. Most professional teams and many individual colleges and universities have initiated drug-testing programs for their athletes. Unfortunately, drug testing is rarely done at the secondary school level because of cost constraints.
- Both the NCAA and the USOC have established lists of drugs that are banned for use by athletes competing in either NCAA- or USOC-sanctioned events.

## WEB SITES

NCAA Drug Testing Program: www.ncaa.org/health-and-safety/policy/drug-testing
*This site provides an updated list of banned drugs and drug-testing information.*

Wheeless' Textbook of Orthopaedics: www.wheelessonline.com
*Clicking on "medications" at this Web site allows the reader to search for information on dosages, indications, contraindications, and so on.*

National Center for Drug Free Sport, Inc. www.drugfreesport.com
*This agency is a provider of drug-testing services, drug-screening policies, and drug-testing education programs in sport.*

United States Anti-Doping Agency: www.usada.org
*This organization is dedicated to eliminating the practice of doping in sport.*

United States Olympic Committee: www.teamusa.org/Footer/Legal/Anti-Doping
*This site contains information about drug testing from the USOC.*

World Anti-Doping Agency: www.wada-ama.org
*This site offers a comprehensive list of all medicines (over 5,000), showing which are prohibited or permitted in international sport.*

# SOLUTIONS TO CLINICAL APPLICATION EXERCISES

17-1 At no time can anyone other than a person licensed by law legally prescribe or dispense drugs. An athletic trainer is not permitted to administer or dispense a prescription drug. However, the athletic trainer may be allowed to administer a single dose of a nonprescription medication. The athletic trainer must be reasonable and prudent about the types of nonprescription drugs offered to the patient. If medications are administered by an athletic trainer, he or she must maintain accurate records of the types of medications administered. Each athletic trainer should be aware of state regulations and laws that pertain to the use of medications.

17-2 It is possible that this patient has exercise-induced bronchospasm (EIB). EIB may be caused by loss of heat, water, or both from the lungs during exercise or exertion, resulting from hyperventilation of air that is cooler and dryer than that in the respiratory tract. The goals of asthma therapy are to prevent chronic and troublesome symptoms, maintain normal lung function and activity levels, prevent asthma exacerbations, provide optimal pharmacotherapy with minimal adverse effects, and meet patients' expectations of and satisfaction with asthma care.

17-3 The patient should use a nonsteroidal anti-inflammatory drug, such as ibuprofen or naproxen. Although acetaminophen is a drug with analgesic qualities, a nonsteroidal anti-inflammatory drug (NSAID) is advantageous because of its analgesic and anti-inflammatory capabilities. Aspirin is also an analgesic and anti-inflammatory drug; however, aspirin is associated with more frequent side effects and adverse reactions compared with an NSAID.

17-4 Ibuprofen is an NSAID. The NSAIDs are most effective for reducing pain, stiffness, swelling, redness, and fever associated with localized inflammation. Even though NSAIDs have analgesic and antipyretic capabilities, they should not be used in cases of mild headache or increased body temperature in place of aspirin or acetaminophen. However, they can be used to relieve many other mild to moderately painful somatic conditions, such as menstrual cramps and soft-tissue injury.

17-5 The athletic trainer should let the athlete know that her drug test is designed to screen for recreational drugs rather than for performance-enhancing drugs, so this should not be a problem. Additionally, even if the test were screening for performance-enhancing drugs, it is highly unlikely that one cup of espresso would contain enough caffeine for her to test positive.

17-6 The visible signs of steroid abuse include male pattern baldness, acne, voice deepening, mood swings, aggressive behavior, gynecomastia, reduction in testicle size, and changes in libido. Because the athlete denies steroid abuse, the athletic trainer might suspect that human growth hormone has been used to achieve these results.

17-7 The athletic trainer should first point out the potential long-term effects of using smokeless tobacco, which include bad breath, stained teeth, tooth sensitivity to heat and cold, cavities (with tooth loss), gum recession, periodontal destruction, and oral and throat cancer. The trainer may also try to give the players a substitute for the tobacco, such as gum or sunflower seeds, so that their habitual need to chew on something and spit while playing baseball is satisfied.

17-8 In this case, the issue of added responsibility is irrelevant. The athletic trainer should be more concerned with how this responsibility would affect his or her ability to perform normal job functions. Athletic trainers work hard to develop a sense of trust in the athletes for whom they must provide health care. Being forced to assume a role as a police officer or enforcer can only undermine that trust. Thus, this athletic trainer should be adamant in recommending to the athletic director that some other individual assume the responsibility of overseeing the drug-testing program.

# REVIEW QUESTIONS AND CLASS ACTIVITIES

1. What is the branch of science known as pharmacology, and what is the difference between a prescription and a nonprescription drug?
2. What is a drug vehicle? Give some examples of drug vehicles.
3. By what methods can drugs be administered to an individual?
4. Describe the pharmacokinetics of how a drug is handled by the body.
5. List procedures that should be followed in the selection, purchase, storage, record keeping, and safety precautions of over-the-counter drugs.
6. What are the legal implications if an athletic trainer administers prescription and nonprescription drugs?
7. List the responses that a patient may experience to a drug.
8. List examples of common drugs used to combat infection, to reduce pain and inflammation, to treat colds and allergies, to treat gastrointestinal disorders, to treat muscle dysfunctions, and to control bleeding.
9. Describe the specific protocols for administering over-the-counter medications.
10. Discuss the use of performance-enhancing drugs.
11. How do stimulants enhance performance?
12. What are the purposes of narcotic analgesic drugs? How do they affect performance?
13. What type of patient would use beta blockers? Why are they used?
14. Describe why individuals use anabolic steroids, diuretics, and growth hormone. What are their physiological effects?
15. Describe blood doping in sports. Why is it used? What are its dangers?
16. Contrast psychological and physical dependence, tolerance, and withdrawal symptoms.
17. List the dangers of smokeless tobacco. List the effects of nicotine on the body.
18. Why is cocaine use a danger to users?
19. Select a recreational drug to research. What are the physiological responses to it, and what dangers does it pose?
20. How can an individual who is abusing drugs be identified? Describe behavioral identification as well as drug testing.
21. Debate the issue of drug testing in athletics.

# REFERENCES

1. Alaranta A: Use of prescription drugs in sports, *Sports Medicine* 38(6):449–63, 2008.
2. Backhouse S: Doping in sport: A review of medical practioners' knowledge, attitudes and beliefs, *International Journal of Drug Policy* 22(11):198–202, 2011.
3. Bahrke M, Yesalis C, Kopstein A: Risk factors associated with anabolic-androgenic steroid use among adolescents, *Sports Med* 29(6): 397, 2000.
4. Baume N, Mahler N, Kamber M: Research of stimulants and anabolic steroids in dietary supplements, *Scandinavian Journal of Medicine and Science in Sports* 16(1):41, 2006.
5. Beck T, Housh T, Schmidt R: The acute effects of a caffeine-containing supplement on strength, muscular endurance and anaerobic capabilities, *J Strength Cond Res* 20(3):506, 2006.
6. Boissonnault W, Meek P: Risk factors for anti–inflammatory-drug- or aspirin-induced gastrointestinal complications in individuals receiving outpatient physical therapy services, *J Orthop Sports Phys Ther* 32(10): 510–17, 2002.
7. Bouchard M: Medications and exercise, *ACSM's Health and Fitness Journal* 16(2):34–36, 2010.
8. Brower K: Anabolic steroid abuse and dependence in clinical practice, *Physician and Sportsmedicine* 37(4):131–40, 2009.

9. Buxton I: Pharmacokinetics: The dynamics of drug absorption, distribution, metabolism, and elimination. In Brunton L: *Goodman and Gilman's the pharmacological basis of therapeutics,* New York, 2011, McGraw-Hill.

10. Cassisi NJ: Smokeless tobacco: Is it worth the risk? *NCAA Sports Sciences Education Newsletter,* Spring 2000.

11. Cooper J, Ellison J, Walsh M: Spit (smokeless)-tobacco use by baseball players entering the professional ranks, *J Athl Train* 38(2):126, 2003.

12. Earnest CP: Dietary androgen 'supplements': Separating substance from hype, *Physician Sportsmed* 29(5):63, 2001.

13. Elliott P: Nonsteroidal anti-inflammatory drugs. In Mottram D: *Drugs in sports,* New York, 2015, Taylor & Francis.

14. Feucht C: Analgesics and anti-inflammatory medications in sports: Use and abuse, *Pediatric Clinics of North America,* 57(3): 751–74, 2010.

15. Gansky S, Ellison J, Rudy D: Cluster randomized controlled trial of an athletic trainer-directed spit (smokeless) tobacco intervention for collegiate baseball athletes: Results after 1 year, *J Athl Train* 40(2):76, 2005.

16. Green G: Doping control for the team physician: A review of drug testing procedures in sport, *Am J Sports Med* 34(10):1690, 2006.

17. Green GA, Uryasz FD, Petr TA, Bray CD: NCAA study of substance use and abuse habits of college student-athletes, *Clin J Sports Med* 11(1):51, 2001.

18. Hackel J: Asthma overview, *Athletic Therapy Today* 9(2):28, 2004.

19. Hartgens F, Kuipers H: Effects of androgenicanabolic steroids in athletes, *Sports Med* 34(8):513, 2004.

20. Hartgens F, Van Marken Lichtenbelt WD, Ebbing S: Androgenic-anabolic steroid-induced body changes in strength athletes, *Physician Sportsmed* 29(1):49, 2001.

21. Holt R: Detecting growth hormone abuse in athletes, *Drug Testing and Analysis* 1(9): 426–433, 2009.

22. Houglum JE: Asthma medications: Basic pharmacology, *J Athl Train* 35(2):179, 2000.

23. Houglum J: *Principles of pharmacology for athletic trainers,* Thorofare, NJ, 2015, Slack.

24. Huff P: Drug distribution in the training room, *Clin Sports Med* 17(2):214, 1998.

25. Kahanov L: Adherence to drug-dispensation and drug administration laws and guidelines in collegiate athletic training rooms: A 5-year review, *J Athl Train* 45(3):299–305, 2010.

26. Kersey RD: What athletic trainers and therapists should know about androstenedione, *Athletic Therapy Today* 6(1):59, 2001.

27. Koda-Kimble MA, Young LL: *Applied therapeutics: The clinical use of drugs,* Philadelphia, PA, 2012, Lippincott, Williams and Wilkins.

28. Kraemer W, Gomez A, Ratamess H: Effects of vicoprofen and ibuprofen on anaerobic performance after muscle damage, *J Sport Rehabil* 11(2):104, 2002.

29. Landry G, Bernhardt D: Drug testing in the athletic setting. In Landry G, editor: *Essentials of primary care sports medicine,* Champaign, IL, 2003, Human Kinetics.

30. Loudon J: Principles of pharmacology for athletic trainers, *Physical Therapy,* 86(3):459, 2006.

31. Miller M: Questionable dispensing of medications in the athletic training room, *Athletic Therapy Today* 8(4):26, 2003.

32. Miller M, Weiler J, Baker R: National Athletic Trainers' Association position statement: Management of asthma in athletes, *J Athl Train* 40(3):224, 2005.

33. National Asthma Education and Prevention Program (NAEPP) Expert panel report 3: *Guidelines for the diagnosis and management of Asthma.* October 2007, NIH Publication 08–5846.

34. National Collegiate Athletic Association: Ergogenic drug use down: Binge-drinking on the rise according to a national study, *NCAA Sport Sciences Education Newsletter,* Winter 4:1, 1993.

35. National Collegiate Athletic Association: *NCAA drug testing program 2014–2015,* Indianapolis, IN, 2011, NCAA.

36. Neal M: *Medical Pharmacology at a Glance,* New York, 2015, Wiley-Blackwell.

37. Nickell R: Eight principles for managing prescription medications in the athletic training room, *Athletic Therapy Today* 10(1):6, 2005.

38. Orr E: Sources of drug information for the athletic therapist, *Athletic Therapy Today* 3(2): 18, 1998.

39. Parkinson A, Evans N: Anabolic androgenic steroids: A survey of 500 users, *Med Sci Sports Exerc* 38(4):644, 2006.

40. Pearson R: Beta-blockers in sports, *Sport and Medicine Today* 4(5):15, 2001.

41. Powers M: The safety and efficacy of anabolic steroid precursors: What is the scientific evidence? *J Athl Train* 37(3):300, 2002.

42. Reents S: *Sport and exercise pharmacology,* Champaign, IL, 2000, Human Kinetics.

43. Rich B: Drugs: A common link between physicians and athletic therapists, *Athletic Therapy Today* 3(2):13, 1998.

44. Schneider AJ, Butcher RB: An ethical analysis of drug testing. In Wilson W, Derse E, editors: *Doping in elite sport: The politics of drugs in the Olympic movement,* Champaign, IL, 2001, Human Kinetics.

45. Sinusas K, Coroso J: A 10-yr study of smokeless tobacco use in a professional baseball organization, *Med Sci Sports Exerc* 38(7): 1204, 2006.

46. Starkey C, Abdenour T, Finnane D: Athletic trainers' attitudes toward drug screening of intercollegiate athletes, *J Athl Train* 29(2):120, 1994.

47. Stilger V: Androstenedione and anabolicandrogenic steroids: What you need to know, *Athletic Therapy Today* 5(1):56, 2000.

48. Tokish J, Kocher M, Hawkins R: Ergogenic aids: A review of basic science, performance, side effects, and status in sports, *Am J Sports Med* 32(6):1543, 2004.

49. Trulock SC: Drug use in athletics: Abuse of the human growth hormone in amateur athletes, *Sports Med Update,* 14(4):18, 2000.

50. Tscholl P: The use of drugs and nutritional supplement in top level track and field athletes, *American Journal of Sports Medicine* 38(1):133–40, 2010.

51. U.S. Anti-doping Agency: *Athlete guide to the 2012 prohibited list,* Colorado Springs, CO, 2012, USADA.

52. U.S. Food and Drug Administration: Code of Federal Regulations Title 21 Volume 4 21CFR201.66, 2010.

53. VanHeest J, Stoppani J, Scheett T: Effects of ibuprofen and vicoprofen on physical performance after exercise-induced muscle damage, *J Sport Rehabil* 11(3):224, 2004.

54. Vella L: Alcohol, athletic performance and recovery, *Nutrients* 2(8):781–89, 2010.

55. Volpe S: Alcohol and athletic performance, *ACSM's Health and Fitness Journal* 14(3): 28–30, 2010.

56. Warrington R: Immunotherapy in asthma, *Immunotherapy,* 2(5):711–25, 2010.

57. Wennerberg D: Metered dose inhaler use and misuse by athletes, *Athletic Therapy Today* 15(5):30–33, 2010.

58. Whitehill W: The drug testing process, *Strength and Conditioning Journal* 31(6): 28–37, 2009.

59. Wilson W: Doping in elite sport: The politics of drugs in the Olympic movement, Champaign, IL, 2001, Human Kinetics.

60. Wolf D: National Collegiate Athletic Association Division I athletes' use of non-prescription medication, *Sports Health* 3(1): 25–28, 2011.

61. Yesalis CE, editor: *Anabolic steroids in sport and exercise,* ed 2, Champaign, IL, 2000, Human Kinetics.

62. Ziltener J: Non-steroidal anti-inflammatory drugs for athletes: An update, *Annals of Physical Medicine and Rehabilitation,* 53(4): 278–88, 2010.

## ANNOTATED BIBLIOGRAPHY

Bahrke M, Yesalis C: *Performance enhancing substances in sport and exercise,* Champaign, IL, 2002, Human Kinetics.

*A high-quality, evidence-based text on performance enhancing substances.*

Beamish R: *Steroids: A New Look at Performance Enhancing Drugs,* Westport, CT, 2011, Praeger.

*This book addresses a pressing issue in professional and high-performance sport—the use of steroids—by placing it within the historical context of the ongoing desire to achieve the pinnacle of human sport.*

Brenner G, Stevens C: *Pharmacology,* St. Louis, MO, 2012, Elsevier Health Sciences.

*Applies the most important basic science concepts to everyday clinical problem solving and decision making in pharmacology.*

Gauwitz D, Bayt P: *Administering medications,* New York, 2014, McGraw-Hill.

*Provides the fundamentals of drug administration, drug laws, principles of pharmacology, drug-handling procedures, physician's orders, routes of administration, dosage calculation, and drug actions related to specific body systems and disorders.*

Griffith HW: *Complete guide to prescription and nonprescription drugs*, New York, 2015, Perigee.

*User-friendly reference text listing dosage and usage information, actions in the body, generic equivalents, potential adverse interactions (including those with foods and other drugs), overdose symptoms, precautions, side effects from prolonged use, and guidelines for usage.*

Houglum J, Harrelson G,: *Principles of pharmacology for athletic trainers*, Thorofare, NJ, 2015, Slack.

*Designed to help athletic training students understand the basic principles of pharmacology, as well as the broad classification of drugs.*

Koester M: *Therapeutic Medications in Athletic Training*, Champaign, 2007, Human Kinetics.

*Provides the latest information on over-the-counter and prescription medications commonly used in athletics*

Magnus B, Miller M: *Pharmacology application in sports and Athletics*, Philadelphia, PA, 2005, F.A. Davis.

*Discusses pharmacological aspects of common medical conditions that certified athletic trainers may encounter in their careers. Describes the action of drugs for treating inflammation and pain, diabetes, cardiovascular arrhythmias, respiratory and gastrointestinal disorders, covers and infections. Also cover the adverse effects of performance enhancement and social drugs.*

Mamrack, M: *Exercise and Sport Pharmacology* Scottsdale, AZ: 2015, Holcomb Hathaway Publishers.

*This text will be useful for teaching upper-level undergraduates or entry-level graduate students about how drugs can affect exercise and as well as how exercise can affect the action of drugs.*

National Athletic Trainers' Association: *Consensus statement: managing prescription and nonprescription medication in the athletic training facility*, Dallas, TX, 2009, NATA.

*Discusses how athletic trainers should control the use of various medications in the clinical setting.*

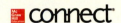

# 18

## The Foot

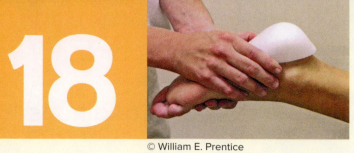

© William E. Prentice

### ■ Connect Highlights ■ connect

*Visit connect.mcgraw-hill.com for further exercises to apply your knowledge:*

- Clinical application scenarios covering evaluation of foot injuries, prevention of foot injuries, and management of foot injuries
- Click-and-drag questions covering anatomical features of the foot
- Multiple-choice questions covering injury evaluation, prevention of injury, and rehabilitation techniques for the foot
- Selection questions covering activities of the foot

Many activities involve some elements of walking, running, jumping, and changing direction. The foot is in direct contact with the ground, and the forces created by these athletic movements place a great deal of stress on the structures of the foot. Consequently, the foot has a high incidence of injury.[19,31,81]

The function of the foot is critical in walking, running, jumping, and changing direction. In one instant, the foot must act as a shock absorber to dissipate the ground reaction forces. In the next instant, it must become a rigid lever that propels the body forward, backward, or to the side.[22]

The foot forms the base for the entire kinetic chain, and different structural foot types can affect movement, stability, and the biomechanics throughout the kinetic chain.[32] Because of the stress that these movements place on the foot and because of the complex nature of the anatomical structures of this body part, recognition and management of injuries to the foot present a major challenge to the athletic trainer.

## FOOT ANATOMY

It has been proposed that a *core system* exists in the foot that is similar to the core system in the lumbo-pelvic-hip complex.[52] When the core is not functioning properly, the foundation becomes unstable and malaligned and abnormal movement of the foot ensues eventually resulting in injury. The foot core system consists of passive, active, and neural subsystems interacting collectively to provide stability and flexibility to cope with changing foot demands.

All of the ligaments of the foot in combination with the bony congruency of the joints and the plantar fascia form the *passive subsystem* of the foot core system. Muscles are the *active subsystem* of the foot in which both extrinsic muscles originating in the lower leg and intrinsic muscles on the plantar surface of the foot combine to produce foot stability and adaptability. The *neural subsystem* consists of the sensory receptors on the plantar surface of the foot and in the plantar fascia, ligaments, joint capsules, muscles, and tendons involved in the active and passive subsystems.[52]

### Bones

The foot consists of 26 bones: 14 phalangeal, 5 metatarsal, and 7 tarsal (Figure 18–1). Additionally, there are two sesamoid bones beneath the first metatarsal.

**Toes** The toes are somewhat similar to the fingers in appearance but are much shorter and serve a different function. The toes are designed to give a wider base both for balance and for propelling the body forward. The first toe, or hallux, has two phalanges, and the other toes each have three phalanges.

Two sesamoid bones are located beneath the first metatarsophalangeal joint. Their functions are to assist in reducing pressure in weight bearing, increase the mechanical advantage of the flexor tendons of the great toe, and act as sliding pulleys for tendons.

**Metatarsal Bones** The metatarsals are the five bones that lie between and articulate with the tarsals and the phalanges, thus forming the semimovable tarsometatarsal and metatarsophalangeal joints. Although little movement is permitted, the ligamentous arrangement gives elasticity to the foot in weight bearing. The metatarsophalangeal joints permit hinge action of the phalanges, which is similar to the action between the hand and fingers. The first metatarsal is the largest and strongest and functions as the main weight-bearing support during walking and running.

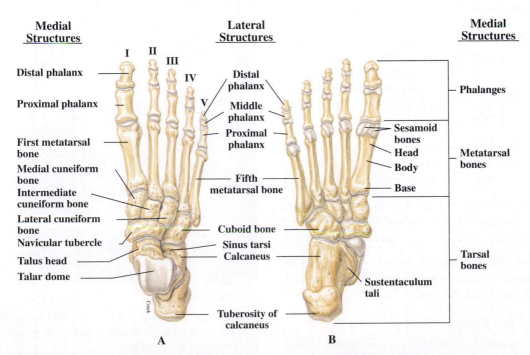

FIGURE 18–1   Bony structure of the foot. **(A)** Dorsal aspect. **(B)** Plantar aspect.

The medial and lateral sesamoid bones are located on the plantar aspect of the metatarsophalangeal joint of the great toe within the flexor hallucis brevis medial and lateral heads within each of the two tendons that attach to the first digit of the phalanx.[18] Their purposes are (1) to increase the mechanical efficiency of the tendon and (2) to decrease frictional stress as the tendon passes over bony prominances.

**Tarsal Bones**  The foot has seven tarsal bones, which are located between the bones of the lower leg and the metatarsals. These bones are important for body support and locomotion. They consist of the calcaneus, talus, navicular, cuboid, and first, second, and third cuneiform bones.

***Calcaneus***  The calcaneus is the largest tarsal bone. It supports the talus and shapes the heel; its main functions are to convey the body weight to the ground and to serve as an attachment for both the Achilles tendon and several structures on the plantar surface of the foot.

The wider portion on the posterior calcaneus is called the tuberosity of the calcaneus. The medial and lateral tubercles are located on the inferior lateral and medial aspects and are the only parts of this bone that normally touch the ground.

***Talus***  The irregularly shaped talus is the most superior of the tarsal bones. It is situated above the calcaneus over a bony projection called the sustentaculum tali. The talus consists of a body, neck, and head. The uppermost part of the talus is the trochlea, which articulates with the medial and lateral malleoli to form the ankle joint. The talus is broader anteriorly than posteriorly, thus preventing forward slipping of the tibia during locomotion.

Because the talus fits principally into the space formed by the malleoli, lateral movement is restricted by the stabilizing ligaments of the ankle. Since the talus is wider anteriorly, full dorsiflexion is the most stable position of the talocrural joint, primarily due to the bony congruency between the talus and the mortise. In contrast, plantar flexion relies most heavily on the ligaments for stability because the narrower posterior portion of the talus does not provide adequate surface area and contour for bony congruency. The average range of motion is 10 degrees in dorsiflexion and 23 degrees in plantar flexion.[88]

***Navicular***  The navicular bone is positioned anterior to the talus on the medial aspect of the foot. Anteriorly, the navicular bone articulates with the three cuneiform bones.

***Cuboid***  The cuboid is positioned on the lateral aspect of the foot. It articulates posteriorly with the calcaneus and anteriorly with the fourth and fifth metatarsals.

***Cuneiforms***  The three cuneiform bones are located between the navicular and the base of the three metatarsals on the medial aspect of the foot.

## Arches of the Foot

The foot is structured, by means of ligamentous and bony arrangements, to form several arches. The arches assist the foot in supporting the body weight; in absorbing the shock of weight bearing; and in providing a space on the plantar aspect of the foot for the blood vessels, nerves, and muscles.[62] There are four arches: the metatarsal, the transverse, the medial longitudinal, and the lateral longitudinal (Figure 18–2). These four arches actually work together to form a functional half dome of the foot.

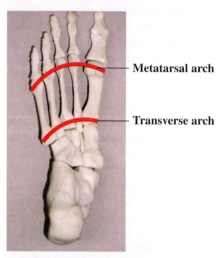

— **Metatarsal arch**

— **Transverse arch**

**A  Plantar view**

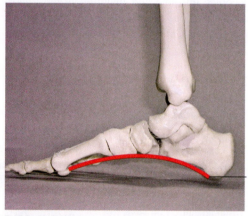

**Medial longitudinal arch**

**B  Medial view**

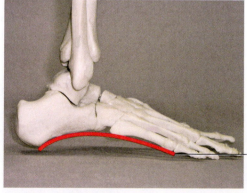

**Lateral longitudinal arch**

**C  Lateral view**

FIGURE 18–2   Arches of the foot. **(A)** Metatarsal and transverse arches. **(B)** Medial longitudinal arch. **(C)** Lateral longitudinal arch.
© William E. Prentice

**Metatarsal Arch** The metatarsal arch is shaped by the distal heads of the metatarsals. The arch has a half dome appearance, stretching from the first to the fifth metatarsal.

**Transverse Arch** The transverse arch extends across the transverse tarsal bones, primarily the cuboid and the internal cuneiform, and forms a half-dome. It gives protection to soft tissue and increases the foot's mobility.

**Medial Longitudinal Arch** The medial longitudinal arch originates along the distal medial border of the calcaneus and extends forward to the distal head of the first metatarsal. Bony support is provided by the calcaneus, talus, navicular, first cuneiform, and first metatarsal. The medial arch is governed by the position of the talus, which controls calcaneal and navicular motion. The main supporting ligament of the longitudinal arch is the plantar calcaneonavicular ligament, which acts as a spring by returning the arch to its normal position after it has been stretched. The arch is also supported by the plantar intrinsic muscles and the tendons of the extrinsic muscles that originate in the lower leg.[52] The tendon of the posterior tibialis muscle helps reinforce the plantar calcaneonavicular ligament.

**Lateral Longitudinal Arch** The lateral longitudinal arch is on the outer aspect of the foot and follows the same pattern as that of the medial longitudinal arch. It is formed by the calcaneus, cuboid, and fifth metatarsal bones. It is much lower and less flexible than the inner longitudinal arch and represents the lowest portion of the half dome.

## Plantar Fascia (Plantar Aponeurosis)

The plantar fascia is a thick, white band of fibrous tissue originating from the medial tuberosity of the calcaneus and ending at the proximal heads of the metatarsals. Along with ligaments, the plantar fascia supports the foot against downward forces (Figure 18–3). The plantar fascia is a distal continuation of fascia that runs posteriorly from the muscles of the thigh to the muscles of the calf

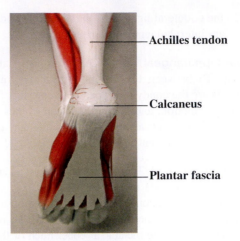

FIGURE 18–3 The Achilles tendon is continuous with the plantar fascia on the plantar surface of the foot.
© William E. Prentice

and continues under the calcaneus, where it thickens to become the plantar fascia. It is the most superficial layer on the plantar surface of the foot, lying just between the skin and the first layer of muscles.

## Articulations

The articulations (joints) of the foot are categorized into three regions: the forefoot (interphalangeal, metatarsophalangeal, intermetatarsal joints), the midfoot (tarsometatarsal and midtarsal joints), and the rearfoot (subtalar joint) (Figure 18–4).

**Interphalangeal Joint** The interphalangeal joints are articulations between the distal, middle, and proximal phalanges. The articulation between the distal and middle phalanges is called the distal interphalangeal joint (DIP) and the articulation between the middle and proximal phalanges is called the proximal interphalangeal joint (PIP). These joints are designed only for flexion and extension. All interphalangeal joints have reinforcing collateral ligaments on their medial and lateral sides. Also located

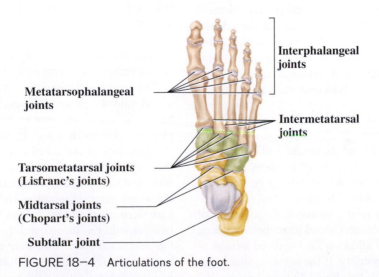

FIGURE 18–4 Articulations of the foot.

between the collateral ligaments on the plantar and dorsal surfaces are interphalangeal ligaments.

**Metatarsophalangeal Joint** The metatarsophalangeal joints (MTP) between the proximal phalanges and the metatarsals are the condyloid type, which permits flexion, extension, adduction, and abduction. Each of these joints has collateral ligaments as well as plantar and dorsal metatarsophalangeal ligaments.

**Intermetatarsal Joint** The intermetatarsal joints are sliding joints. They include two sets of articulations. One set consists of an articulation on each side of the base of the metatarsal bones, and the second articulations are on each side of the heads of the metatarsal bone. Each of these articulations permits only slight gliding movements. Shafts of the metatarsals are connected by interosseous ligaments. The bases are connected by plantar and dorsal ligaments, and the heads are attached by transverse metatarsal ligaments.

**Tarsometatarsal Joint (Lisfranc's Joint)** The tarsometatarsal joint is formed by the junction of the bases of the metatarsal bones with the cuboid and all three cuneiforms. The slight saddle shape of this joint allows for some gliding and thus for a restricted amount of flexion, extension, adduction, and abduction. Metatarsal bones are attached to the tarsal bones by the dorsal and plantar tarsometatarsal ligaments. Interosseous ligaments connect the three cuneiforms to the metatarsals. The tarsometatarsal joint is also known as Lisfranc's joint.

**Subtalar Joint** The subtalar joint is the articulation between the talus and the calcaneus. *Inversion, eversion, pronation,* and *supination* are normal movements that occur at the subtalar joint. Inversion is a movement of the calcaneus such that the sole of the foot turns inward, or medially. Eversion is a movement of the calcaneus such that the sole of the foot turns outward, or laterally.

In weight bearing, foot pronation is the combined movements of talar plantar flexion and adduction and calcaneal eversion. In contrast, foot supination is the combined movements of talar dorsiflexion and abduction and calcaneal inversion.[76] These movements, which occur at the subtalar joint, are triplanar movements—that is, movements that occur in all three planes simultaneously.[37] The movements of the talus during pronation and supination have profound effects on the lower extremity, both proximally and distally.

**Midtarsal Joint (Chopart's Joint)** The midtarsal joint, also referred to as Chopart's joint, consists of two distinct joints: the calcaneocuboid and the talonavicular joint. The midtarsal joint depends mainly on ligamentous and muscular tension to maintain position and integrity. Midtarsal joint stability is directly related to the position of the subtalar joint. If the subtalar joint is pronated, the joint axes of the talonavicular and calcaneocuboid joints become more parallel, thus effectively allowing for increased motion of the forefoot and hypermobility. If the subtalar joint is supinated, the axes of these two joints become less parallel

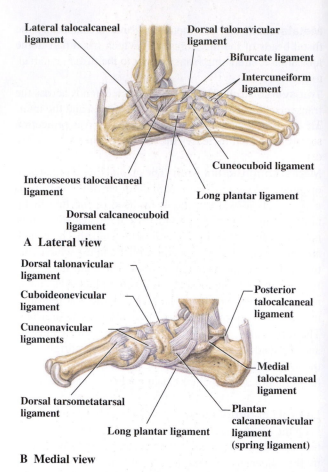

**FIGURE 18–5** Ligaments of the foot. **(A)** Lateral. **(B)** Medial.

creating hypomobility, thus locking the foot creating a rigid lever.[8] As the midtarsal joint becomes more or less mobile, it affects the distal portion of the foot because of the articulations at the tarsometatarsal joint.[76]

## Stabilizing Ligaments

The subtalar ligaments are the interosseus talocalcaneal and the anterior, posterior, lateral, and medial talocalcaneal (Figure 18–5). A major ligament is the plantar calcaneonavicular, which passes from the medial longitudinal arch. Because of its relatively large number of elastic fibers and its primary purpose of providing shock absorption, the plantar calcaneonavicular is commonly called the spring ligament.

The primary ligaments of the midtarsal joint are the dorsal talonavicular, bifurcate, and dorsal calcaneocuboid. The midtarsal joint is given added strength in its plantar aspect by the long plantar ligaments.

Ligaments of the anterior tarsal joints are divided into those of the cuneonavicular, cuboideonavicular, intercuneiform, and cuneocuboid joints. Each of these joints has both dorsal and plantar ligaments. The intercuneiform ligaments have three transverse bands; one band connects the first cuneiform with the second and the second with the third. A ligament also connects the third cuneiform with the cuboid bone. It should be added that all of the ligaments of the foot in combination with the bony congruency of the joints and the plantar fascia form the passive subsystem of the foot core system. Muscles are the active subsystem of the foot in which global movers and local stabilizers combine to produce foot stability and adaptability.

## Muscles and Movement

The movements of the foot are produced by both extrinsic and intrinsic muscles of the foot. Extrinsic muscles originate in the lower leg and intrinsic muscles originate in the foot (Figures 18–6 and 18–7). Dorsiflexion, plantarflexion, inversion, eversion, abduction, adduction, pronation, and supination are produced by the extrinsic muscles. Movements of the phalanges are produced by the intrinsic muscles. Table 18–1 summarizes the intrinsic muscles of the foot and their actions.

**Dorsiflexion and Plantar Flexion** Dorsiflexion and plantar flexion of the foot take place at the ankle joint and

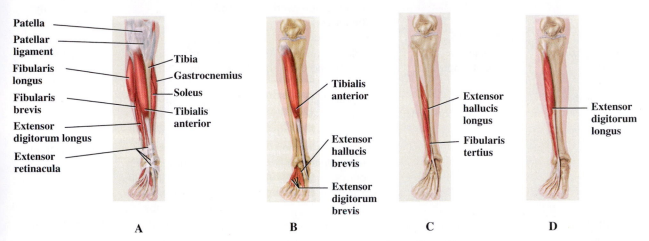

FIGURE 18–6   Extrinsic muscles and tendons of the anterior aspect of the ankle and foot.

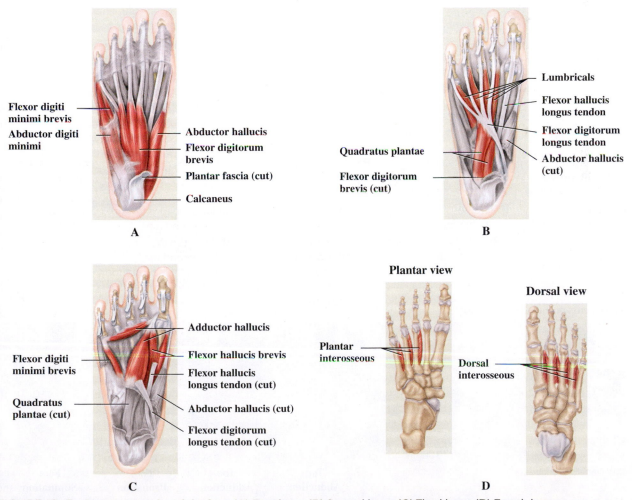

FIGURE 18–7   Intrinsic muscles of the foot. **(A)** First layer. **(B)** Second layer. **(C)** Third layer. **(D)** Fourth layer.

## TABLE 18–1 Intrinsic Muscles of the Foot

| Muscle | Origin | Insertion | Action | Nerve/Nerve Root |
|---|---|---|---|---|
| *Dorsal Muscle* | | | | |
| **Extensor digitorum brevis** | Lateral surface of the calcaneus | Tendon of the extensor digitorum longus | Extends the second through fifth toes | Deep peroneal (L5, S1) |
| *Plantar Muscles* | | | | |
| *First Layer* | | | | |
| **Abductor hallucis** | Calcaneus | Proximal phalanx of the great toe (with the tendon of the flexor hallucis brevis) | Abducts the great toe | Medial plantar (L4, L5, S1) |
| **Flexor digitorum brevis** | Calcaneus and plantar aponeurosis | Middle phalanx of the second through fifth toes | Flexes the second through fifth toes | Medial plantar (L4, L5, S1) |
| **Abductor digiti minimi** | Calcaneus and plantar aponeurosis | Proximal phalanx of the small toe | Abducts the small toe | Lateral plantar (S1, S2) |
| *Second Layer* | | | | |
| **Quadratus plantae** | Calcaneus | Into tendons of the flexor digitorum longus | Aids in flexing the second through fifth toes by straightening the pull of the flexor digitorum longus | Lateral plantar (S1, S2) |
| **Lumbricales** | From tendons of the flexor digitorum longus | Into tendons of the extensor digitorum longus | Flexes the second through fifth toes | Medial and lateral plantar (L4, L5, S1, S2) |
| *Third Layer* | | | | |
| **Flexor hallucis brevis** | Cuboid and lateral cuneiform | Proximal phalanx of the great toe | Flexes the great toe | Medial plantar (L4, L5, S1) |
| **Adductor hallucis** | *Oblique head:* second, third, and fourth metatarsals *Transverse head:* ligaments of the metatarsophalangeal joints | Proximal phalanx of the small toe | Adducts the great toe | Lateral plantar (S1, S2) |
| **Flexor digiti minimi brevis** | Fifth metatarsal | Proximal phalanx of the small toe | Flexes the small toe | Lateral plantar (S1, S2) |
| *Fourth Layer* | | | | |
| **Plantar interossei** | Third, fourth, and fifth metatarsals | Proximal phalanx of the same toe | Adducts the toes toward the second toe | Lateral plantar (S1, S2) |
| **Dorsal interossei** | Bases of the adjacent metatarsals | Proximal phalanges; both sides of the second toe; lateral side of the third and fourth toes | Abducts the toes from the second toe; moves the second toe medially and laterally | Lateral plantar (S1, S2) |

**Movements of the Foot and Toes***

Toe Flexion    Toe Extension    Toe Abduction    Toe Adduction    Foot Pronation    Foot Supination

© William E. Prentice

*Manual muscle tests and goniometric measurements of range of motion for the foot can be found in Appendix F and Appendix G of this text.

are discussed in greater detail in Chapter 19. These motions are regulated by the extrinsic foot muscles that originate in the lower leg. The gastrocnemius, soleus, plantaris, peroneus longus, peroneus brevis, tibialis posterior, flexor hallucis longus, and flexor digitorum longus muscles are the plantar flexors. Dorsiflexion is accomplished by the tibialis anterior, extensor digitorum longus, extensor hallucis longus, and peroneus tertius muscles (see Figure 18–6).

**Inversion, Adduction, and Supination** The medial movements of the foot are produced by the same muscles as inversion, adduction (medial movement of the forefoot), and supination (a combination of inversion and adduction). Muscles that produce these movements pass behind and in front of the medial malleolus. Muscles passing behind are the tibialis posterior (see Figure 19–5B), flexor digitorum longus, and flexor hallucis longus (see Figure 19–5D). Muscles passing in front of the medial malleolus are the tibialis anterior (see Figure 19–5A) and the extensor hallucis longus (see Figure 18–6C). The extensor retinaculum and flexor retinaculum provide pulleys for these tendons that maximize their lines of pull.

**Eversion, Abduction, and Pronation** The lateral movements of the foot are caused by the same muscles that produce eversion, abduction (lateral movement of the forefoot), and pronation (a combination of eversion and abduction). Muscles passing behind the lateral malleolus are the fibularis longus (peroneus longus) and the fibularis brevis (peroneus brevis). Muscles passing in front of the lateral malleolus are the fibularis tertius and extensor digitorum longus (see Figure 18–6C&D). The peroneal retinaculum and the extensor retinaculum provide pulleys for these tendons that maximize their lines of pull.

**Movement of the Phalanges** The movements of the phalanges are flexion, extension, abduction, and adduction. Flexion of the second, third, fourth, and fifth distal phalanges is executed by the flexor digitorum longus and the quadratus plantar muscles. Flexion of the middle phalanges is performed by the flexor digitorum brevis, and flexion of the proximal phalanges is performed by the lumbricales and the interossei. The great toe is flexed by the flexor hallucis longus. The extension of all the middle phalanges is done by the abductor hallucis and abductor digiti minimi the lumbricales, and the interossei. Extension of all distal phalanges is effected by the lumbricales, extensor digitorum longus, extensor hallucis longus, and extensor digitorum brevis. The adduction of the foot is performed by the interossei plantares and adductor hallucis; abduction is performed by the interossei dorsalis, abductor hallucis, and abductor digiti minimi.

## Nerve Supply and Blood Supply

**Nerve Supply** The medial and lateral plantar nerves, which are branches of the tibial nerve, supply all of the intrinsic muscles on the plantar surface of the foot. The deep peroneal nerve supplies the extensor digitorum brevis on the dorsal surface of the foot (Figure 18–8). Sensory receptors located on the plantar surface of the foot and in the plantar fascia, ligaments, joint capsules, muscles, and tendons involved in the active and passive subsystems are critical to gait and balance.[52]

**Blood Supply** The primary blood supply for the foot comes from the anterior and posterior tibial arteries. The dorsum of the foot is supplied by the dorsal pedal artery and the dorsal metatarsal arteries, which branch from the anterior tibial artery. The plantar aspect of the foot is supplied by the lateral plantar artery, the medial plantar artery, and the plantar arterial arch, which all branch from the posterior tibial artery (Figure 18–9A&B).

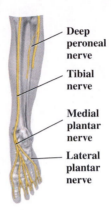

**Posterior view**

FIGURE 18–8    Nerves of the foot.

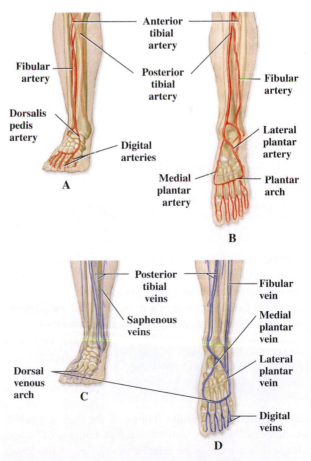

FIGURE 18–9    Blood supply of the foot. **(A)** Dorsal arteries. **(B)** Plantar arteries. **(C)** Dorsal veins. **(D)** Plantar veins.

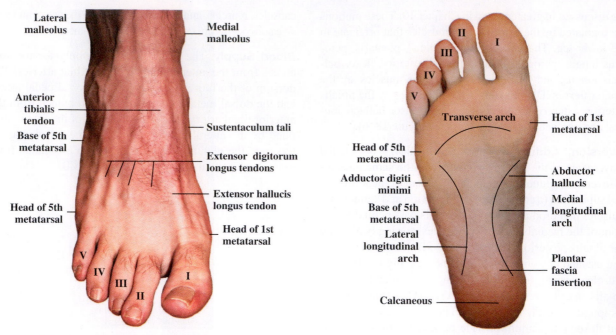

**FIGURE 18-10**   Surface anatomy showing pertinent landmarks of the foot from **(A)** dorsal view and **(B)** plantar view.
© William E. Prentice

The primary venous structure in the foot is the dorsal venous arch. On the plantar surface the digital veins drain into the dorsal venous arch which drain into the medial and lateral plantar veins. They combine to form the posterior tibial vein and the fibular vein.

On the dorsum of the foot the dorsal venous arch drains into the lesser and greater saphenous veins. (Figure 18–9C&D).

### Surface Anatomy

Figure 18–10A shows the pertinent surface anatomy for the dorsal surface of the foot, and Figure 18–10B shows the plantar surface of the foot.

# FUNCTIONAL ANATOMY AND FOOT BIOMECHANICS

Athletic trainers must realize, when considering foot, ankle, and leg injuries, that these segments are joined together to form a functional kinetic chain. Each movement of a body segment has a direct effect on proximal and distal body segments.[44] A study of lower-extremity chronic and overuse injuries related to sports participation must include some understanding of the biomechanics of the foot, especially in the act of walking and running. A number of biomechanical factors may be related to injuries of the lower-leg region.

> Most people will develop foot problems at some time in their lives.

### Normal Gait

The action of the lower extremity during a complete gait cycle in walking can be divided into two primary phases (Figure 18–11). The **stance phase** starts with initial contact of the heel on the ground and ends when the toe breaks contact with the ground (toe-off). This phase accounts for about 60 percent of the total gait cycle. The stance phase involves weight bearing in a closed kinetic chain. The stance phase has two functional demands: absorption and propulsion. This has been broken down into five phases: *initial contact, loading response,* and *midstance* are all associated with the absorption phase, whereas *terminal stance* and *preswing* are associated with propulsion. Consequently, within the absorption phase, muscles of the foot and ankle and up the lower extremity chain function eccentrically whereas during propulsion they function concentrically. At midstance and terminal stance, the body is supported by a single limb, whereas at initial contact and in the early portion of the loading response period, there is double support with both feet on the ground.[71,90]

The time between toe-off and the subsequent initial contact is termed the **swing phase**, which is a period of non–weight bearing. The swing phase can be subdivided into three periods: *initial swing, midswing,* and *terminal swing.* In normal gait, while one leg is in the stance phase, the other is in the swing phase.

As in the walking gait, a running gait has both stance and swing phases. However, there are several differences. In running, the loading response and midstance periods occur more rapidly. There is also a period after toe-off in which neither foot is in contact with the ground and there

| Stance Phase (60% of total) | | | | | Swing Phase | | |
|---|---|---|---|---|---|---|---|
| Initial Contact (heel contact) | Loading Response | Midstance | Terminal Stance | Preswing (toe-off) | Initial Swing | Midswing | Terminal Swing |
| External Rotation of Tibia | | Internal Rotation of Tibia | | External Rotation of Tibia | | | |
| Supination | | Pronation | | Supination | | | |

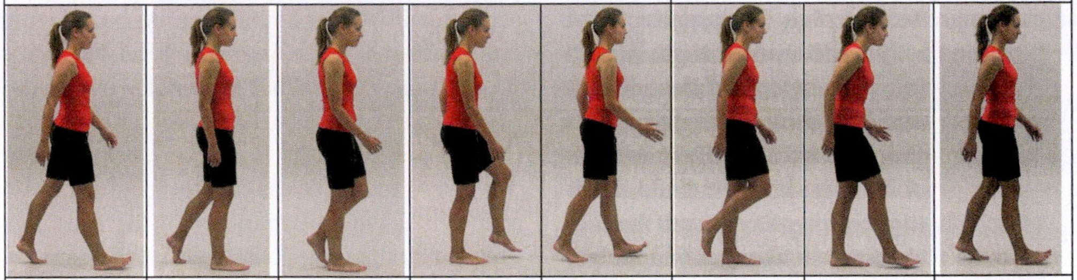

FIGURE 18–11   The stance and swing phases of a normal gait cycle.

is no time when both feet contact the ground simultaneously. In running, the stance phase accounts for only one-third of the gait cycle.

The foot's function during the stance phase of running is twofold as with a walking gait. At heel strike, the foot acts as a shock absorber to the impact forces and then adapts to the uneven surfaces. At toe-off, the foot functions as a rigid lever to transmit the propulsive force from the lower extremity to the running surface. In a heel-strike running gait, initial contact of the foot is on the lateral aspect of the calcaneus, with the subtalar joint in supination. It is estimated that 80 percent of distance runners use this heel-strike pattern, and the remainder are either midfoot or forefoot strikers.[88] Sprinters tend to be forefoot strikers, whereas a number of joggers are midfoot strikers.

At initial contact, the subtalar joint is supinated (Figure 18–12). Associated with this supination of the subtalar joint is an obligatory external rotation of the tibia.[71] As the foot is loaded, the subtalar joint moves into a pronated position until the forefoot is in contact with the running surface. The change in subtalar motion occurs between initial heel strike and 20 percent into the support phase of running.[71] As pronation occurs at the subtalar joint, there is obligatory internal rotation of the tibia. Transverse plane rotation occurs at the knee joint because of this tibial rotation. Pronation of the foot unlocks the midtarsal joint and allows the foot to assist in shock absorption and to adapt to uneven surfaces. It is important during initial impact to reduce the ground reaction forces and to distribute the load evenly on many different anatomical structures throughout the foot and leg. Pronation is normal and allows for this distribution

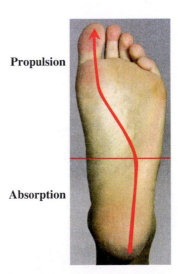

FIGURE 18–12   Foot bearing weight in walking as it moves from heel strike to toe-off.

of forces on as many structures as possible to avoid excessive loading on just a few structures. The subtalar joint remains in a pronated position through 55 to 85 percent of the stance phase, with maximum pronation being concurrent with the body's center of gravity passing over the base of support.[90]

The foot begins to resupinate and will approach the neutral subtalar position at 70 percent to 90 percent of the stance phase.[90] In supination, the midtarsal joints are locked, and the foot becomes stable and rigid to prepare for toe-off. This rigid position allows the foot to exert a great amount of force from the lower extremity to the running surface.

**Subtalar Joint Pronation and Supination** Pronation and supination of the foot and subtalar joint are normal during the stance phase of running. In pronation the foot functions to absorb ground reaction forces, and in supination the foot becomes rigid to allow propulsion of the body. However, excessive or prolonged pronation or supination often cause or contribute to overuse injuries. When structural or functional variations exist in the foot or leg, compensation is likely to occur at the subtalar joint. The subtalar joint compensates in a manner that allows the foot to make stable contact with the ground and get into a weight-bearing position (Figure 18–13). This excessive motion compensates for an existing structural deformity.[76]

18–1 Clinical Application Exercise

An athletic trainer working in a sports medicine clinic observes a forefoot valgus deformity in a soccer player during a preseason screening.

**?** Why might this deformity be a problem? What can be done to manage this condition?

**Structural Variations** The most typical structural variations of the foot that produce excessive pronation or supination include forefoot varus, forefoot valgus, and rearfoot varus (Figure 18–13).[71] These structural variations exist in a non–weight-bearing position. Structural forefoot varus and structural rearfoot varus variations are usually associated with excessive pronation.[67] A structural forefoot valgus causes excessive supination. The variations usually exist in one plane, but the subtalar joint will interfere with the normal functions of the foot and make it more difficult for the joint to act as a shock absorber, to adapt to uneven surfaces, and to act as a rigid lever for toe-off. The compensation, which occurs when the foot goes into weight bearing, rather than the deformity itself, usually causes overuse injuries.[76]

**Over-Pronation** Over-pronation, meaning that there is excessive or prolonged pronation during running, is one of the major causes of stress injuries. Overload of specific structures results when over-pronation is produced in the stance or absorptive phase or when pronation is prolonged into the propulsive phase of running.[15] Excessive pronation during the stance phase causes compensatory subtalar joint motion such that the midtarsal joint remains unlocked, resulting in an excessively loose foot.[30] As more motion occurs at the midtarsal joint, the first metatarsal and first cuneiform become more mobile. These bones constitute a functional unit known as the *first ray*. With pronation of the midtarsal joint, the first ray is more mobile because of its articulations with that joint. The first ray is also stabilized by the attachment of the fibularis longus tendon, which attaches to the base of the first metatarsal.[26]

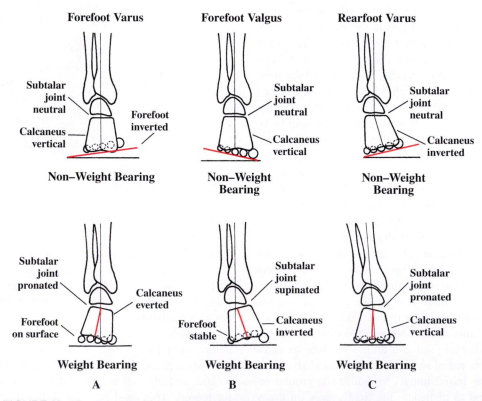

FIGURE 18–13   Structural foot deformities in non–weight bearing and compensations in weight bearing. **(A)** Forefoot varus. **(B)** Forefoot valgus. **(C)** Rearfoot varus.

The fibularis longus tendon passes posteriorly around the base of the lateral malleolus and then through a notch in the cuboid to cross the foot to the first metatarsal. The cuboid functions as a pulley to increase the mechanical advantage of the fibularis longus tendon. Stability of the cuboid is essential in this process. In the pronated position, the cuboid loses much of its mechanical advantage as a pulley; therefore, the fibularis longus tendon no longer stabilizes the first ray effectively. This condition creates hypermobility of the first ray and increased pressure on the other metatarsals. There is also an increase in tibial rotation, which forces the knee joint to absorb more transverse rotation motion.[76]

Prolonged pronation of the subtalar joint does not allow the foot to resupinate in time to provide a rigid lever for toe-off, resulting in a less powerful and efficient propulsive force. Thus, various foot and leg problems occur with excessive or prolonged pronation during the stance phase; these problems include stress fractures of the second metatarsal, plantar fasciitis, posterior tibial tendinitis, Achilles tendinitis, and medial knee pain.[37] There is strong evidence that over-pronation does not cause medial tibial stress syndrome or patellofemoral pain.[60]

**Over-Supination** At heel strike in prolonged or excessive supination, compensatory movement at the subtalar joint does not allow the midtarsal joint to unlock, which causes the foot to remain excessively rigid.[17] Because less movement occurs at the calcaneocuboid joint, the cuboid becomes hypomobile. The fibularis longus tendon has a greater amount of tension because the cuboid has less mobility and thus will not allow mobility of the first ray. In this case, the majority of the weight is borne by the first and fifth metatarsals. Thus, over-supination reduces the foot's ability to absorb ground reaction forces dynamically and effectively.[25] Therefore, other structures such as the second through fifth metatarsals begin to absorb the forces inappropriately.

Excessive supination limits tibial internal rotation. Injuries typically associated with excessive supination include inversion ankle sprains, medial tibial stress syndrome, fibularis tendinitis, iliotibial band friction syndrome, and trochanteric bursitis.[37]

# PREVENTION OF FOOT INJURIES

Certainly, the foot is highly vulnerable to a variety of injuries. The repetitive stresses and strains incurred by the foot during athletic activities are unquestionably sufficient to cause both acute traumatic and overuse injuries. Identifying the variations in foot posture and control that a person has can lend insight into how to best go about preventing injuries. Foot injuries can best be prevented by selecting appropriate footwear, using a shoe orthotic, and paying attention to appropriate foot hygiene and care.[72,87]

## Appropriate Footwear

The athletic and fitness shoe manufacturing industry has become extremely sophisticated and offers a number of options when it comes to purchasing shoes for different athletic activities. Shoe selection, parts of a shoe, and fitting were discussed in Chapter 7. Selecting an appropriate shoe can be helpful in preventing a foot problem. Before a shoe is selected, the athletic trainer should evaluate the patient's foot to determine the existence of a structural variation, such as a forefoot valgus or varus or a rearfoot varus.

As noted earlier, pronation is a problem of hypermobility. Individuals who excessively pronate need stability and firmness to reduce this excess movement. Research indicates that shoe compression, compared with a barefoot condition, may actually increase pronation.[40] The ideal shoe for a pronated foot is one that is less flexible and has good rearfoot control. Conversely, supinated feet are usually very rigid. Increased cushioning and flexibility benefit this type of foot.

Recently it has been suggested that a "good" running shoe would be a shoe that allows the bones, articulations, and supporting soft tissue structures of the skeleton to move in a "preferred movement path."[63] A good running shoe would, therefore, demand less muscle activity than a bad running shoe to ensure that the skeleton moves in the correct path. Furthermore, footwear that is more comfortable is associated with a lower movement-related injury frequency than shoes that are less comfortable. An athlete will likely choose the most comfortable shoe and avoid uncomfortable and potentially harmful footwear.[64,65]

Several construction factors may influence the firmness and stability of a shoe. The basic form upon which a shoe is built is called the last. The upper is fitted onto a last in several ways. Each method has its own flexibility and control characteristics (Figure 18–14). A slip-lasted shoe is sewn together like a moccasin and is very flexible. A board-lasted shoe contains a piece of fiberboard to which the upper is attached, which provides a very firm, inflexible base for the shoe. A combination-lasted shoe is boarded in the back half of the shoe and slip-lasted in the front, which provides rearfoot stability with forefoot mobility.

The shape of the last may also determine shoe selection (Figure 18–15). Most individuals with excessive pronation perform better in a straight-lasted shoe—that is, a shoe in which the forefoot does not curve inward in relation to the rearfoot.[24] Midsole design also affects the stability of a shoe. The midsole separates the upper from the outsole. More dense, less yielding material is often used under the medial aspect of the foot to control pronation.

In an effort to control rearfoot movement, many shoe manufacturers have reinforced the heel counter both internally and externally, often in the form

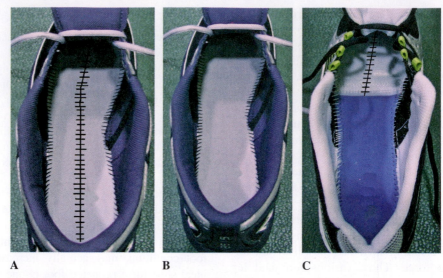

**FIGURE 18–14** Shoe lasts. **(A)** Slip-lasted. **(B)** Board-lasted. **(C)** Combination lasted.
© William E. Prentice

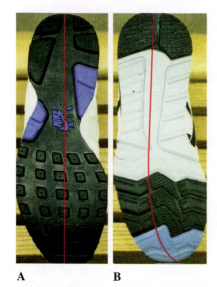

**FIGURE 18–15** Shape of the last. **(A)** Straight. **(B)** Curved.
© William E. Prentice

of extra plastic along the outside of the heel counter. Other factors that may affect the performance of a shoe are the outsole contour and composition, lacing systems, and forefoot wedges.[76]

Table 18–2 provides guidelines for choosing the correct shoe components based on the type of foot problem.

## Shoe Orthotics

Shoe inserts and orthotics for sport have been advocated and successfully used for many years. While there is some evidence that inserts or orthotics reduce or prevent movement-related injuries, knowledge about the specific function an orthotic or insert provides is limited.[64] They have been used to reduce the frequency of movement-related injuries, to align the bones, articulations, and supporting soft tissues of the skeleton properly to correct existing faulty biomechanics; to provide improved cushioning; to improve the sensory feedback; and/or to improve comfort.[63] Most recently it has been suggested that comfort of the orthotic as determined by proper fit, the degree of dynamic stability, and fatigue reduction are reasons to use an orthotic. However, comfort may be the single most important factor for determining the effectiveness of an orthotic in reducing lower extremity injuries.[63] The orthotic is a plastic, rubber, or leather support that is placed in the

| TABLE 18–2 | Suggested Shoe Components Based on Foot Type | | | | |
|---|---|---|---|---|---|
| **Type of Problem** | | | **Shoe Components** | | |
| Over-pronation | Stiff shoe | Dense midsole, medial wedge | Good rearfoot control | Board or combination last | Straight last | Rigid or semirigid orthotic |
| Over-supination | Flexible shoe | Soft midsole, lateral wedge | Rearfoot control not necessary | Slip last | Curved last | Soft or semirigid orthotic |

shoe as a replacement for the existing insert. Ready-made orthotics can be purchased in sporting goods and shoe stores. Some patients need to have orthotics that are custom-fitted or made by the athletic trainer or podiatrist.[66]

The use of orthotics for correcting specific problems are discussed in the section on rehabilitation at the end of this chapter.

## Barefoot Running

Running barefoot or in minimalist shoes has recently increased in popularity because of many claims that there is less chance of injury, greater running efficiency, and enhanced performance when compared with running in shoes. What is relatively clear is that biomechanical differences do exist when running barefoot, when running in minimalist shoes, and when running in shoes. But the current state of evidence strongly suggests that the potential risks and benefits of running barefoot as opposed to running in minimalist shoes or regular running shoes have yet to be clearly determined.[2,70]

## Foot Hygiene

Individuals who perform simple tasks—such as keeping their toenails trimmed correctly; shaving down excessive calluses; keeping their feet clean; wearing clean, correctly fitted socks; and keeping their feet as dry as possible to prevent the development of athlete's foot (see Chapter 28)—can individually and collectively reduce a number of problems that can cause them to miss days of practice or competition.

# FOOT ASSESSMENT

When assessing foot injuries, athletic trainers must clearly understand that the foot is part of a kinetic chain that includes both the ankle and the lower leg.[41] Acute injuries must be differentiated from injuries with a relatively slow onset.

## History

An athletic trainer making a decision about how to manage a foot injury must perform a quick assessment to determine the type of injury and its history. He or she should ask the following questions:

- Is this the first time this condition has occurred? If it has happened before, when, how often, and under what circumstances did it occur?
- How did the injury occur?
- Did it occur suddenly or come on slowly?
- Was the mechanism a sudden strain, twist, or blow to the foot?
- Where is the pain (ankle, heel, arches, toes)?
- What type of pain is the athlete experiencing?

- Is there muscle weakness?
- Is there any snapping, popping, or crepitus during movement?
- Is there any alteration in sensation?
- Can the patient point to the exact site of the pain?
- When is the pain or other symptoms more or less severe?
- On what type of surface has the patient been training?
- What type of footwear is being worn during training? Is it appropriate for the type of training? Is discomfort increased when footwear is worn?

## Observation

The athletic trainer should observe the patient to determine the following:

- Is the patient favoring the foot, walking with a limp, or unable to bear weight?
- Is the injured part deformed, swollen, or discolored?
- Does the foot change color when weight bearing and not weight bearing (changing rapidly from a darker to lighter pink when not weight bearing)?
- Is there pes planus (a flatfoot) or pes cavus (a high arch)?
- Is the foot well aligned? Does it maintain its shape on weight bearing?
- Do any abnormalities exist in the toes (e.g., hammertoes, mallet toes, claw toes, Morton's toe, hallux valgus, corns, bunions, plantar warts)?

**Looking for Structural Variations** The first step in looking for structural variations is to establish a position of subtalar neutral. The patient should be prone with the distal third of the leg hanging off the end of the table (Figure 18–16). A line should be drawn bisecting the leg from the start of the musculotendinous junction of the gastrocnemius to the distal portion of the calcaneus. With the patient still prone, the athletic trainer should palpate the talus while the forefoot is inverted and everted. One finger should palpate the talus at the anterior aspect of the fibula and another finger at the anterior portion of the medial malleolus. The position at which the talus is equally prominent on both sides is considered a neutral subtalar position in which the subtalar joint is neither pronated nor supinated.[76]

Once the subtalar joint is placed in a neutral position, the athletic trainer should apply mild dorsiflexion to lock the subtalar joint in place while observing the metatarsal heads in relation to the plantar surface of the calcaneus.[76] Forefoot varus is a rigid osseous deformity in which the medial metatarsal heads are inverted in relation to the plane of the calcaneus. Forefoot varus is the most common cause of over-pronation (see Figure 18–13A).[17] Forefoot varus can also be caused by soft-tissue tightness of the anterior tibialis muscle along with malposition of the calcaneocuboid joint. This has been referred to as

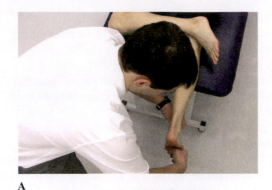

**A**

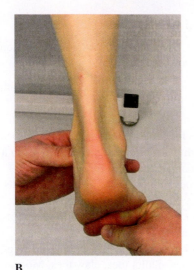

**B**

**FIGURE 18–16** **(A)** Position for assessing existing structural deformities. **(B)** Viewing the structural variation in subtalar neutral.

© William E. Prentice

forefoot supinatus and attributed to chronic subtalar joint pronation. Forefoot valgus is a rigid osseous variation in which the lateral metatarsals are everted in relation to the rearfoot (see Figure 18–13B).

These rigid forefoot variations are benign in a non–weight-bearing position; however, during weight bearing, the metatarsal heads must somehow make contact with the surface to bear weight. To accomplish this movement for a forefoot varus, the talus plantar flexes and adducts and the calcaneus everts. For the forefoot valgus, the calcaneus inverts and the talus abducts and dorsiflexes. A forefoot varus is the most common forefoot deformity.[17]

In a rearfoot varus variation, when the foot is in a subtalar neutral position and non–weight bearing, the medial metatarsal heads are elevated, as in a forefoot varus, and the calcaneus is also in an inverted position (see Figure 18–13C).[79] For the foot to bear weight, the subtalar joint must pronate.

An equinus foot, and particularly a rigid equinus foot, is another structural variation that is thought to be associated with poor shock absorption during running. In an equinus foot, the forefoot is plantar flexed relative to the rearfoot when the ankle is at 90 degrees of flexion. A similar condition, in which only the first metatarsal is plantar flexed relative to the rearfoot, is referred to as a plantar flexed first ray.[76]

**Shoe Wear Patterns** Individuals with over-pronation often wear out the front of the running shoe under the second metatarsal. Shoe wear patterns are commonly misinterpreted by athletes who think they must be pronators because they wear out the back outside edges of their heels. However, most people wear out the back outside edges of their shoes. Just before heel strike, the anterior tibialis fires to prevent the foot from slapping forward. The anterior tibialis not only dorsiflexes the foot but also slightly inverts it, hence the wear pattern on the lateral back edge of the shoe. An individual who over-supinates tends to show a wear pattern on the lateral border of the shoe. The key to inspection of wear patterns on shoes is observation of the heel counter and the forefoot.[37]

## Palpation

Besides determining pain sites, swelling, and deformities, palpation is used to determine and evaluate circulation.

**Bony Palpation** The following bony landmarks should be palpated:

**Medial aspect**
- Medial calcaneus
- Calcaneal dome
- Medial malleolus
- Sustentaculum tali (plantar aspect of medial calcaneus)
- Talar head
- Navicular tubercle
- First cuneiform
- First metatarsal
- First metatarsophalangeal joint
- First phalanx

**Lateral aspect**
- Lateral calcaneus
- Lateral malleolus
- Sinus tarsi
- Peroneal tubercle
- Cuboid bone
- Styloid process (proximal head of fifth metatarsal)
- Fifth metatarsal
- Fifth metatarsophalangeal joint
- Fifth phalanx

**Dorsal aspect**
- Second, third, fourth metatarsals
- Second, third, fourth metatarsophalangeal joints
- Second, third, fourth phalanges
- First, second, and third cuneiform bones

**Plantar aspect**
- Metatarsal heads
- Medial calcaneal tubercle
- Sesamoid bones

**Soft-Tissue Palpation** The following soft-tissue structures should be palpated:

**Medial and plantar aspect**
- Tibialis posterior tendon
- Flexor hallucis longus tendon
- Flexor digitorum longus tendon
- Deltoid ligament
- Calcaneonavicular ligament (spring ligament)
- Medial longitudinal arch
- Plantar fascia
- Transverse arch

**Lateral and dorsal aspect**
- Anterior talofibular ligament
- Calcaneofibular ligament
- Posterior talofibular ligament
- Peroneus longus tendon
- Peroneus brevis tendon
- Extensor hallucis longus tendon
- Extensor digitorum longus tendon
- Extensor digitorum brevis tendon
- Tibialis anterior tendon

**Pulses** To ensure that there is proper blood circulation to the foot, the pulse is measured at the posterior tibial and dorsalis pedis arteries (see Figure 18–9). Pulse in the dorsalis pedis artery is normally felt between the tendons of the extensor hallucis longus and extensor digitorum longus, on a line from the midpoint between the medial and lateral malleoli to the proximal end of the first intermetatarsal space.

Pulse in the posterior tibial artery is normally palpable behind the medial malleolus, 1 inch (2.5 cm) in front of the medial border of the Achilles tendon.[38]

## Special Tests

**Movement Assessment** Both the extrinsic and the intrinsic foot muscles should be assessed for pain and range of motion during active, passive, and resistive isometric movement.

**Morton's Test** With the foot in a neutral position, transverse compression is applied to the heads of the metatarsals, which may cause sharp pain in the forefoot. A positive test may indicate the presence of **metatarsalgia** or a **neuroma** (Figure 18–17A).

**Mulder's Sign**[58] With the patient in a sitting position the examiner squeezes the metatarsal heads together with one hand while the thumb and index finger of the other hand apply pressure to the interspace between the heads of the third and fourth metatarsal heads (Figure 18–17B). A click or pain radiating to the toes is a positive test.
Sn. 0.76 | Sp. 0.53 | +LR 0.90 | -LR 0.05

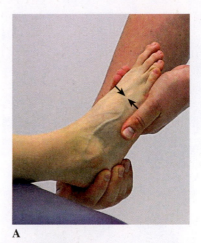

**A**

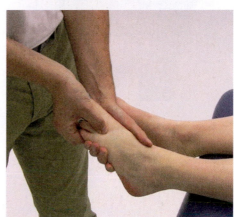

**B**

FIGURE 18–17   Tests for intermetatarsal neuroma.
**(A)** Morton's test. **(B)** Mulder's sign.
© William E. Prentice

**Neurological Assessment** Reflexes and cutaneous distribution should be tested. Skin sensation should be noted for any alteration.

Tendon reflexes, such as in the Achilles tendon (S1 nerve root), should elicit a response when gently tapped. Sensation is tested by running the hands over the anterior, lateral, medial, and posterior surfaces of the foot and toes.

**Tinel's Sign Test**[68] Tapping over the posterior tibial nerve produces tingling distal to that area. Numbness, tingling, and paresthesia may indicate the presence of tarsal tunnel syndrome (Figure 18–18A). Sn. 0.58 | Sp. NA | +LR NA | -LR NA

**Dorsiflexion-Eversion Test**[43] The dorsiflexion-eversion test is another test for tarsal tunnel syndrome. The ankle is passively, maximally everted and dorsiflexed while all of the metatarsophalangeal joints are maximally dorsiflexed and held in this position for 5 to 10 seconds.[43] Pain or numbness primarily in the tarsal tunnel or occasionally on the plantar surface of the foot indicates entrapment of the tibial nerve as it passes through a tunnel on the medial side of the ankle (Figure 18–18B). Sn. 0.57 | Sp. 1.0 | +LR Infinity | -LR 0.43

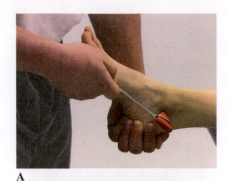

**FIGURE 18–18**   Tarsal tunnel syndrome tests. **(A)** Tinel's sign. **(B)** Dorsiflexion-eversion test.

© William E. Prentice

# RECOGNITION AND MANAGEMENT OF SPECIFIC INJURIES

Most people will at some time develop foot problems that can be attributed to the use of improper footwear, poor foot hygiene, or anatomical structural deviations that result from faulty postural alignments or abnormal stresses. Many activities place exceptional demands on the feet— far beyond what is considered normal. The athletic trainer should be well aware of potential foot problems and should be capable of identifying, ameliorating, and preventing them whenever possible.

## Injuries to the Tarsal Region

### Fractures of the Talus

***Etiology***   Fractures of the dome of the talus usually occur either laterally from a severe inversion and dorsiflexion force, or medially from an inversion and plantar flexion force, with external rotation of the tibia on the talus.[28]

The severity of the fracture may range from a nondisplaced compression fracture to a displaced osteochondral fracture. The presence of osteochondral fragments is referred to as *osteochondritis dissecans*.

***Symptoms and signs***   The patient often has a history of repeated trauma to the ankle. He or she feels pain on weight bearing and complains of catching and snapping along with intermittent swelling. The talar dome is tender on palpation over the anteromedial or anterolateral joint line.[4]

***Management***   For accurate diagnosis, a radiograph or MRI is essential. Nonsurgical management is appropriate for nondisplaced subchondral compression fractures. Treatment should include protective immobilization with non–weight bearing, progressing to full weight bearing, depending on symptoms. Rehabilitation should concentrate on strengthening and regaining full range of motion in the ankle joint. If conservative treatment fails and symptoms continue or if there is a displaced osteochondral fracture, surgical removal of the loose bodies arthroscopically may be necessary. Following surgery, the patient can expect to resume activity in 6 to 8 months.[4]

### Fracture of the Calcaneus

***Etiology***   A fracture of the calcaneus most often occurs from landing after a jump or fall from a height.[49] Avulsion fractures can also occur anteriorly at the attachment of the calcaneonavicular ligament to the sustentaculum tali or posteriorly at the attachment of the talocalcaneal ligament. Anterior avulsion fractures can be misdiagnosed as tendinitis of the posterior tibialis.[34]

***Symptoms and signs***   There is usually immediate swelling and pain and an inability to bear weight. Deformity is not normally present unless there is a displaced comminuted fracture.[54]

***Management***   POLICE must be used immediately to minimize pain and swelling before referring the athlete to X-ray for diagnosis. With nondisplaced fractures, immobilization and early range of motion exercises are recommended as soon as acute swelling and pain subside and motion is tolerated.[34]

### Calcaneal Stress Fracture

***Etiology***   Calcaneal stress fractures, along with stress fractures of the tibia and of the second metatarsal, are among the most common stress fractures in the lower extremity. A calcaneal stress fracture occurs with repetitive impact during heel strike and is most prevalent among distance runners. It is characterized by a sudden or gradual onset, which initially hurts in the plantar-calcaneal area with activity and eventually hurts even during rest.[49]

***Symptoms and signs***   Weight bearing, particularly on heel strike in running, increases pain. Complaints of pain tend to continue after exercise stops. The fracture may fail to appear during X-ray examination; a bone scan may be a better diagnostic tool.[54]

***Management***   Management is usually conservative for the first 2 or 3 weeks and includes rest and active range of motion exercises of the foot and ankle. Non–weight-bearing cardiovascular exercise, such as pool running, may continue during this period. After 2 weeks and when pain subsides, activity within pain limits can be resumed gradually, using proper running mechanics with the athlete wearing a cushioned shoe.

## Apophysitis of the Calcaneus (Sever's Disease)

*Etiology* Calcaneal **apophysitis**, or Sever's disease, occurs in young, physically active patients. Sever's disease is comparable to Osgood-Schlatter disease at the tibial tubercle of the knee (see Chapter 20).[74] Sever's disease is a traction injury at the **apophysis** of the calcaneus (bone protrusion) where the Achilles tendon attaches.[75]

*Symptoms and signs* Pain occurs at the posterior heel below the attachment of the Achilles tendon insertion of the child or adolescent athlete. Pain occurs during vigorous activity and does not continue at rest.

*Management* Apophysitis, like other overuse syndromes, is best treated with rest, ice, and anti-inflammatory medications. A heel lift can take some stress off the apophysis.

## Retrocalcaneal Bursitis

*Etiology* Retrocalcaneal bursitis is caused by inflammation of the bursa that lies between the Achilles tendon and the calcaneus. Retrocalcaneal bursitis often occurs from the pressure and rubbing of the heel counter of a shoe. This condition is chronic, developing gradually over a long period of time, and may take many days—sometimes weeks or months—to resolve.[17]

An **exostosis** is a benign bony outgrowth or callus that protrudes from the surface of a bone and is usually capped by cartilage. An exostosis that develops on the posterior aspect of the calcaneus, called a Haglund's deformity, causes ongoing inflammation of the retrocalcaneal bursa, sometimes referred to as a "pump bump" (Figure 18–19A).[22]

*Symptoms and signs* Pain may be elicited by palpating the bursa just above and anterior to the insertion of the Achilles tendon. There will likely be some swelling on both sides of the heel cord. If the source of irritation persists, a bony callus may also begin to form.

*Management* Initially, POLICE plus NSAIDs and analgesics are used as needed. Often, the use of ultrasound can reduce the inflammation. Stretching of the Achilles tendon should be routine. A heel lift should be used to take stress off the Achilles tendon. A doughnut heel pad can be used to take pressure off the bursa and an existing exostosis (Figure 18–19B). If necessary, larger shoes with wider heel contours should be worn.[22]

## Heel Contusion

*Etiology* Activities that demand a sudden stop-and-go response or a sudden change from a horizontal to a vertical movement (e.g., basketball, jumping, or the landing in long jumping) are particularly likely to cause heel contusions.[74] The calcaneus is protected by a thick, cornified skin layer and a heavy fat pad covering, but even this thick padding cannot always protect against the impact of jumping or running.[83]

The major function of the tissue heel pad is to sustain hydraulic pressure through fat columns. Tissue compression is monitored by pressure nerve endings from the skin and plantar aponeurosis. Often, the irritation is on the lateral aspect of the heel because of the heel strike in walking or running.[47]

*Symptoms and signs* When injury occurs, the patient complains of severe pain in the heel and is unable to withstand the stress of weight bearing. Often, there is warmth and redness over the tender area.[54]

*Management* A contusion of the heel may develop into chronic inflammation of the periosteum. The patient should not bear weight on the heel for at least 24 hours. POLICE is applied and NSAIDs should be administered. If pain when walking has subsided by the third day, the patient may resume moderate activity with the protection of a heel cup or protective doughnut (Figure 18–20). The patient should wear shock-absorbent footwear.

## Cuboid Subluxation Syndrome

*Etiology* Pronation and trauma have been reported to be prominent causes of cuboid subluxation.[77] This condition is sometimes incorrectly confused with plantar fasciitis. However, the patient usually complains of a midfoot sprain with pain on the dorsum of the foot and/or over the

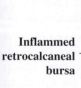
Inflammed retrocalcaneal bursa

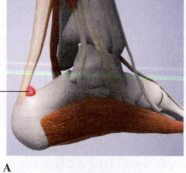
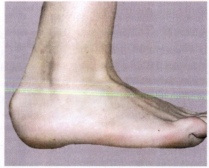
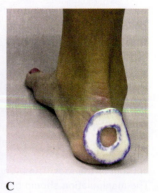

A         B         C

FIGURE 18–19 **(A)** Retrocalcaneal bursitis at the attachment of the Achilles tendon to the calcaneous. **(B)** A pump bump that develops. **(C)** Can be protected using a doughnut-type pad.

(b, c) © William E. Prentice

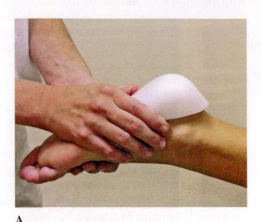 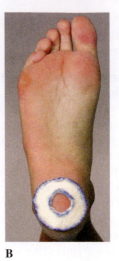

**FIGURE 18–20**   Heel protection. **(A)** Heel cup. **(B)** Protective heel doughnut.
© William E. Prentice

anterior/lateral ankle frequently after an inversion mechanism often accompanied by a lateral ankle sprain. The primary reason for pain is the stress placed on the fibularis longus muscle when the foot is in pronation. In this position, the fibularis longus muscle allows the cuboid bone to move downward medially.

*Symptoms and signs*   This displacement of the cuboid causes pain along the fourth and fifth metatarsals as well as over the cuboid. This problem often refers pain to the heel area and is often associated with plantar fasciitis. Many times this pain is increased when the patient stands after a prolonged non–weight-bearing period.

*Management*   Dramatic treatment results may be obtained by manipulating to restore the cuboid to its natural position (Figure 18–21). Once the cuboid is manipulated,

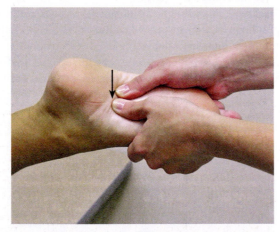

**FIGURE 18–21**   A cuboid manipulation is done with the patient prone. The lateral plantar aspect of the forefoot is grasped by the thumbs, with the fingers supporting the dorsum of the foot. The thumbs should be over the cuboid. The manipulation should be a thrust downward to move the cuboid into its more dorsal position. Often, a pop is felt as the cuboid moves back into place.
© William E. Prentice

an orthotic often helps support it in its proper position. If manipulation is successful, quite often the patient can return to play immediately with little or no pain. The patient should wear an appropriately constructed orthotic when practicing or competing to reduce the chances of recurrence.

**Tarsal Tunnel Syndrome**

*Etiology*   The tarsal tunnel is a loosely defined area behind the medial malleolus that forms a tunnel with an osseous floor and the roof composed of the flexor retinaculum. Through this tunnel pass the tibialis posterior, flexor hallucis longus, and flexor digitorum muscles with their surrounding synovial sheaths and the tibial nerve artery and vein.[23] Any condition that compromises the structures within this tunnel can cause tarsal tunnel syndrome, including tenosynovitis, previous fractures, excessive pronation, or any acute trauma.[85] It should be mentioned that this syndrome is similar to carpal tunnel syndrome which will be discussed in Chapter 24.

*Symptoms and signs*   Complaints of pain and paresthesia are typical, particularly along the medial and plantar aspects of the foot. Complaints of increased pain at night are also common. Tinel's sign will be positive in cases of tarsal tunnel syndrome (see Figure 18–18). If the condition persists, motor weakness and atrophy may gradually appear, following the course of the tibial nerve.

*Management*   Initial conservative management includes the use of antiinflammatory medication and other antiinflammatory modalities. The use of an appropriate orthotic to correct excessive pronation may effectively reduce the symptoms. Surgery may be necessary if the symptoms become recurrent.[73]

**Tarsometatarsal Fracture/Dislocation (Lisfranc Injury)**

*Etiology*   Named after a French surgeon who described amputations at the tarsometatarsal joint, this is

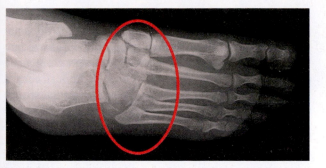

FIGURE 18–22  A Lisfranc injury is the dorsal displacement of the proximal end of the metatarsals.

Courtesy Jordan B. Renner, MD, Departments of Radiology and Allied Health Sciences, University of North Carolina

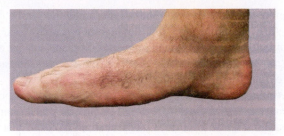

**A**

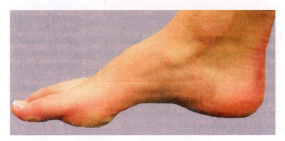

**B**

FIGURE 18–23  **(A)** Pes planus foot. **(B)** Pes cavus foot.

© William E. Prentice

an uncommon injury that can cause long-term disability. The ankle is plantar flexed with the rearfoot locked, and there is a sudden, forceful hyper–plantar flexion of the forefoot that results in dorsal displacement of the proximal end of the metatarsals. The dorsum of the foot rolls forward, with the body weight providing the force to displace the base of the metatarsals dorsally (Figure 18–22).[89]

***Symptoms and signs***  Symptoms may be relatively subtle. The patient complains of pain and an inability to bear weight. Swelling and tenderness are localized over the dorsum of the foot. There may be a fracture of the metatarsals. Sprain of the fourth and fifth proximal metatarsals causes ongoing pain. It is not uncommon to overlook the serious disruption of the supporting ligaments because attention is often focused on a metatarsal fracture.

***Management***  If the athletic trainer suspects this injury, the patient should be referred to the physician for evaluation. The key to treatment is first recognizing the injury, then restoring alignment, and finally maintaining stability.[89] Closed reduction often fails, and most likely it will be necessary to do an open reduction with internal fixation to stabilize the dislocation. Potential complications include metatarsalgia, limited motion of the metatarsophalangeal joints, and long-term disability.[89]

A patient comes to an outpatient clinic in a hospital, complaining of her flatfeet and that she has pain in her knees and a big callus under her second metatarsal.

**?** What is likely causing this problem, and how can it usually be corrected?

### Pes Planus Foot (Flatfoot)

***Etiology***  The term *pes planus* refers to a type of foot in which the medial longitudinal arch appears to be flat and is sometimes said to be fallen (Figure 18–23A). In general, pes planus is associated with excessive foot pronation and may be caused by a number of factors, including a structural forefoot varus variation shoes that are too tight,

trauma that weakens supportive structures (such as muscles and ligaments), overweight, and excessive exercise that repeatedly subjects the arch to severe pounding on an unyielding surface.

***Symptoms and signs***  The patient may complain of pain and a feeling of weakness or fatigue in the medial longitudinal arch. There may be calcaneal eversion, a bulging of the navicular bone, a flattening of the medial longitudinal arch, and dorsiflexing with lateral splaying of the first metatarsal.

***Management***  Regardless of how flattened the medial longitudinal arch appears to be, if it is not causing the individual any pain or related symptoms, then absolutely nothing should be done to try to correct the apparent problem. Attempts to do so may, in fact, create an unnecessary problem. However, if the patient is experiencing pain, an appropriately constructed orthotic designed to correct excessive pronation by using a medial wedge will most likely alleviate symptoms. In certain cases, incorporating an arch support into the orthotic or taping the arch for support may be helpful. Strengthening of the intrinsic muscles of the foot should also be incorporated.

### Pes Cavus Foot (High Arch Foot)

***Etiology***  The term *pes cavus* refers to a type of foot that has an arch that is higher than normal (Figure 18–23B). Sometimes called *clawfoot or hollow foot*, pes cavus is not as common as pes planus. A pes cavus is generally associated with excessive supination. The accentuated high medial longitudinal arch may be congenital or may indicate a neurological disorder.[15]

***Symptoms and signs***  In cases of pes cavus, shock absorption is poor, and thus problems such as general foot pain, metatarsalgia, and clawed or hammertoes are seen. Commonly associated with this condition are a structural forefoot valgus deformity and an abnormal shortening of the Achilles tendon. The Achilles tendon is directly linked with the plantar fascia (see Figure 18–3). Also, because of the abnormal distribution of body weight, heavy calluses develop on the ball and heel of the foot.[83]

***Management*** As is the case with pes planus, pes cavus may be asymptomatic, in which case no attempt should be made to correct the problem. If there are associated problems, then an orthotic should be constructed using a lateral wedge to correct a structural forefoot valgus deformity. Stretching of the Achilles tendon and the plantar fascia may also be helpful. Strengthening exercises for the intrinsic muscles in the foot should also be integrated into a rehabilitation program.

## Injuries to the Metatarsal Region

### Morton's Toe

***Etiology*** Normally, the first metatarsal is longer than the second. Morton's toe is a condition in which there is an abnormally short first metatarsal, and thus the second toe appears to be longer than the great toe (Figure 18–24). Much of the weight bearing is ordinarily on the first metatarsal. Because the first metatarsal is short, however, more weight must be borne by the second metatarsal instead. This uneven weight distribution becomes even more of a problem in a running gait, during which weight bearing tends to shift more to the second metatarsal.[58]

A Morton's toe is not an injury and can be a benign condition that causes no problems. However, if the second metatarsal is subjected to more stress, particularly during running, a stress fracture could develop.[58]

***Symptoms and signs*** Symptoms are those of stress fractures in general. The patient complains of pain both during and after activity, and there may be an area of point tenderness. A bone scan would be positive for a stress fracture. A callus is likely to form under the second metatarsal head.[58]

***Management*** If a Morton's toe is not causing any symptoms, nothing should be done to try to correct the problem. If a Morton's toe is associated with a structural forefoot varus variation an orthotic with a medial wedge would likely be helpful.

### Longitudinal Arch Strain

***Etiology*** Longitudinal arch strain is usually caused by subjecting the musculature of the foot to increased stress produced by repetitive contact with hard surfaces. In this condition, there is a flattening or depression of the longitudinal arch while the foot is in the midsupport phase, resulting in a strain to the arch.[39] Such a strain may appear suddenly, or it may develop slowly over a considerable length of time.

***Symptoms and signs*** As a rule, pain is experienced only during running or jumping. The pain usually appears just below the posterior tibialis tendon and is accompanied by swelling and tenderness along the medial aspects of the foot. This injury may also be associated with a sprain of the calcaneonavicular ligament as well as a strain of the flexor hallucis longus tendon.

***Management*** The management of a longitudinal arch strain involves immediate care, consisting of POLICE, followed by appropriate therapy and reduction of weight bearing.[51] Weight bearing must be performed

> A distance runner is experiencing pain in the left arch. There is palpable tenderness in the left foot's aponeurosis, primarily in the epicondyle region of the calcaneus.
>
> **?** What condition does this scenario describe, and how should it be managed?

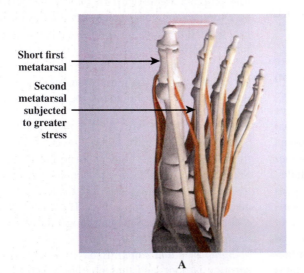

Short first metatarsal

Second metatarsal subjected to greater stress

A

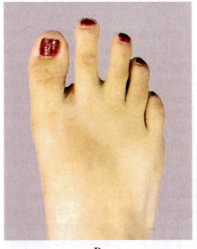

B

**FIGURE 18–24** In a Morton's toe, the first metatarsal is abnormally short.

(b) © William E. Prentice

pain free. Arch taping technique no. 1 or 2 might be used to allow earlier pain-free weight bearing (see Figure 8–20 through 8–23).

**Plantar Fasciitis** Heel pain is a very common problem in the athletic and nonathletic population. This phenomenon has been attributed to several etiologies, including heel spurs, plantar fascia irritation, and bursitis.[22] *Plantar fasciitis* is a catchall term that is commonly used to describe pain in the proximal arch and heel. The plantar fascia (plantar aponeurosis) runs the length of the sole of the foot (see Figure 18–3). It is a broad band of dense connective tissue that is attached proximally to the medial surface of the calcaneus. It fans out distally, with fibers and their various small branches attaching to the metatarsophalangeal articulations and merging into the capsular ligaments. The function of the plantar fascia is to assist in maintaining the stability of the foot and in securing or bracing the longitudinal arch.[42]

*Etiology* Tension develops in the plantar fascia both during extension of the toes and during depression of the longitudinal arch as a result of weight bearing.[1] When the weight is principally on the heel, as in ordinary standing, the tension exerted on the fascia is negligible. However, when the weight is shifted to the ball of the foot (on the heads of the metatarsals), fascial tension is increased. Also, as the gastrocnemius and soleus contract, tension is placed on the fascia. Combining eccentric contractions of the gastrocnemius and soleus with moving toward full dorsiflexion increases tension. In running, because the toe-off phase involves both a forceful extension of the toes and a powerful thrust by the ball of the foot (on the heads of the metatarsals), fascial tension is increased to approximately twice the body weight.[16] Tightening of the plantar fascia during dorsiflexion, thus shortening the longitudinal arch, has been described as the "windlass" mechanism.[9]

Plantar fasciitis can occur in individuals with pes cavus, in which case the foot has too little motion, or in those with a pes planus, in which case there is too much motion.[9]

Street shoes, by nature of their design, take on the characteristics of splints and tend to restrict foot action to such an extent that the arch may become somewhat rigid. This rigidity occurs because of shortening of the ligaments and other mild abnormalities. The athlete, changing from such footwear into a flexible gymnastic slipper or soft track shoe, often experiences trauma when the foot is subjected to stress. Trauma may also result from poor running technique.

A number of anatomical and biomechanical conditions have been studied as possible causes of plantar fasciitis. Those conditions include leg length discrepancy, excessive pronation of the subtalar joint, inflexibility of the longitudinal arch, and tightness of the gastrocnemius-soleus unit.[69] Wearing shoes without sufficient arch support, running with a lengthened stride, and running on soft surfaces are also potential causes of plantar fasciitis.[61]

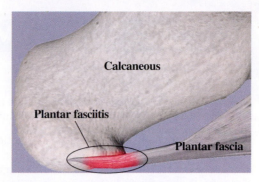

FIGURE 18–25   In plantar fasciitis, pain usually develops at the attachment to the medial portion of the calcaneous.

*Symptoms and signs* The patient complains of pain in the anterior medial heel, usually at the attachment of the plantar fascia to the calcaneus (Figure 18–25). The pain eventually moves into the central portion of the plantar fascia. This pain is increased when the patient rises in the morning or bears weight after sitting for a long period. However, the pain lessens after a few steps. Pain also will be intensified when the toes and forefoot are forcibly dorsiflexed. If irritation persists, a painful heel spur will probably develop at the attachment of the plantar fascia to the medial aspect of the calcaneus; the heel spur will be visible on an X-ray (Figure 18–26).

*Management* Management of plantar fasciitis generally requires an extended period of treatment.[81] It is not uncommon for symptoms to persist for as long as 8 to 12 weeks. Orthotic therapy is very useful in the treatment of this problem.[13,45,53] A soft orthotic works better than a hard orthotic. An extra-deep heel cup should be built into the orthotic. The orthotic should be worn at all times, especially when the athlete rises from bed in the morning.[76] Use of a heel cup compresses the fat pad under the calcaneus,

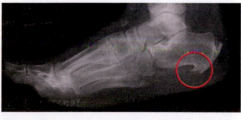

FIGURE 18–26   X-ray of a large plantar calcaneal exostotic spur.
Courtesy Jordan B. Renner, MD, Departments of Radiology and Allied Health Sciences, University of North Carolina

# MANAGEMENT PLAN

## Plantar Fasciitis

**Injury Situation** A marathon runner injured the proximal arch and heel when he stepped into a hole during a meet. The patient continued to run and work out for a week before reporting his injury to the athletic trainer.

**Symptoms and Signs** The patient complained of early pain in the medial arch and medial distal heel that tended to move centrally as the week progressed. He complained of severe pain when rising in the morning and after sitting for a long period. The area appeared slightly swollen with a severe, sharp pain on palpation at the plantar fascia insertion and medial aspect of the calcaneus. Pain increased with passive dorsiflexion of the great toe. An X-ray showed the beginning of a heel spur. The patient was found to have a cavus foot.

**Management Plan** The patient was diagnosed as having plantar fasciitis (heel spur syndrome), and a conservative plan was chosen.

### Phase 1 Acute Injury
**GOALS:** Minimize inflammation and pain.
**ESTIMATED LENGTH OF TIME (ELT):** 1 week.

- **Therapy** POLICE plus NSAID as needed to reduce pain and inflammation. Injection therapy consisting of a steroid and anesthetic for trigger points.
- **Exercise rehabilitation** Toe touch crutch walking. Begin heel cord stretching and rolling pin exercise to increase fascia flexibility. Integrate strengthening of the intrinsic and extrinsic muscles of the foot core.

### Phase 2 Repair
**GOALS:** Gain full weight bearing and walking pattern.
**ELT:** 1 to 3 weeks.

- **Therapy** Ultrasound to increase blood flow. Cross-friction massage over injury site. Apply shock absorption shoe insert with cutout 1 to 2 inches (3 to 5 cm) in the tender area. Apply arch taping.
- **Exercise rehabilitation** Continue heel cord stretching and rolling pin exercise to stretch the plantar fascia. Begin a program of gradual pain-free weight bearing. Continue foot core strengthening.

### Phase 3 Remodeling
**GOALS:** Focus on full pain-free weight bearing while engaged in running.
**ELT:** 2 weeks.

- **Therapy** Ultrasound as warranted. Continue cross-friction massage. Use a heel cup and arch taping when athlete is supporting weight.
- **Exercise rehabilitation** Continue heel cord and plantar fascia stretching. Use shoes with a reinforced heel counter for heel control. Continue foot core strengthening. Perform general exercise to the lower leg. Begin a running program that is pain free.

#### Criteria for Return to Competitive Cross-Country Running

1. Proximal arch and heel are pain free.
2. Heel cord and plantar fascia are stretched.
3. Lower leg has maximum strength.
4. Patient is able to run competitively without pain.
5. Patient is psychologically ready for competition.

---

providing a cushion under the area of irritation. When soft orthotics are not feasible, taping may reduce the symptoms. A simple arch taping or alternative taping often allows pain-free ambulation.[76] The use of a night splint to maintain a position of static stretch has also been recommended[53] (Figure 18–27). In some cases, the athlete may need to use a short leg walking cast for 4 to 6 weeks.

The patient should engage in vigorous Achilles tendon stretching and in exercises that stretch the plantar fascia in the arch, such as rolling the plantar surface of the foot back and forth over a tennis ball, a baseball, or some other rigid, round surface.[82] Exercises that increase dorsiflexion of the great toe also may be of benefit for this problem. Stretching should be done at least three times a day. Antiinflammatory medications are recommended. Steroidal injection may be warranted at some point if symptoms fail to resolve.

## Jones Fracture

**Etiology** Fractures may occur to any of the metatarsals and can be caused by inversion and plantar flexion of the foot; by direct force, such as being stepped on;

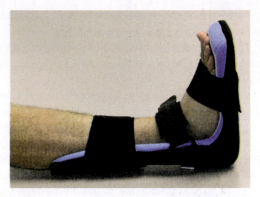

FIGURE 18–27   A night splint can be used to stretch the plantar fascia.

© William E. Prentice

would normally be bone tissue with cartilage between the fractured bone ends.

***Management***   Treatment for a Jones fracture is controversial, but it appears that the use of crutches with no immobilization, gradually progressing to full weight bearing as pain subsides, may allow the patient to return to activity in about 6 weeks. Early activity encourages early recovery, and the loading strategy should reflect the mechanical stresses placed on the fracture during functional activities.[35] However, nonunion may cause a refracture to occur. It has been recommended that patients be treated more aggressively using early internal fixation.[56] It has also been suggested that an electric or ultrasonic bone-growth stimulator will promote healing in a Jones fracture.[14]

### Metatarsal Stress Fractures

or by repetitive stress. By far the most common acute fracture is to the diaphysis at the base of the fifth metatarsal, which is referred to specifically as a Jones fracture (Figure 18–28).[57]

***Symptoms and signs***   A Jones fracture is characterized by immediate swelling and pain over the fifth metatarsal. Healing of a Jones fracture is slow and frustrating for the patient. This injury has a high nonunion rate, and the course of healing is unpredictable.[35] Nonunion fractures can occur as a result of several factors, including insufficient fracture immobilization (fixation), inadequate blood supply, chronic disease states (diabetes, renal failure, metabolic bone disease), fractures associated with tumors (pathological fractures), or infection. In a nonunion fracture, osteocytes and osteoblasts are replaced by chondroblasts. Thus, the fracture repairs itself by replacing what

***Etiology***   The most common metatarsal stress fracture in the foot involves the shaft of the second metatarsal and is often referred to as a *march fracture*. It occurs in the runner who has suddenly changed patterns of training, such as increasing mileage, running hills, or running on a harder surface. An individual who has an atypical condition, such as a structural forefoot

A triathlete changes her running patterns by increasing distance and performing more hill work. She complains to the athletic trainer of a gradually worsening pain in her forefoot. Inspection reveals point tenderness in the region of the fourth metatarsal bone. X-ray reveals a stress fracture.

**?** How should this condition be managed?

**18–6 Clinical Application Exercise**

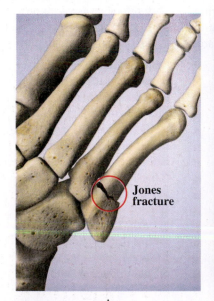
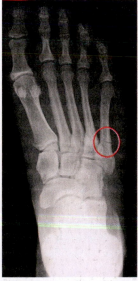

A                                    B

FIGURE 18–28   **(A)** A Jones fracture occurs at the neck of the fifth metatarsal. **(B)** Jones fracture X-ray.

(b) Courtesy Jordan B. Renner, MD, Departments of Radiology and Allied Health Sciences, University of North Carolina

varus, hallux valgus, flatfoot, or short first metatarsal (Morton's toe), is more predisposed to a second metatarsal stress fracture.[26]

A patient can also experience a stress fracture of the fifth metatarsal at the insertion of the peroneus brevis tendon, but this injury should not be confused with a Jones fracture.[5]

***Symptoms and signs*** Over a 2 to 3-week period, dull pain begins to occur during exercise, then progresses to pain at rest. Pain is initially diffuse, then localizes to the site of the fracture. Patients usually report having increased the intensity or duration of their exercise program.

***Management*** A bone scan is the best way to detect the presence of a stress fracture. Management of a metatarsal stress fracture usually consists of 2 to 4 days of partial weight bearing followed by 2 weeks of rest. Return to running should be very gradual. An orthotic that corrects excessive pronation can help take stress off the second metatarsal.[12]

## Bunions (Hallux Valgus Deformities) and Bunionettes (Tailor's Bunions)

***Etiology*** A bunion, one of the most frequent painful deformities, occurs at the head of the first metatarsal (Figure 18–29). The term *bunion* is often used to refer to an exostosis. Commonly, a bunion is associated with a structural forefoot varus in which there is poor foot control and over-pronation causing the first ray to splay outward, putting pressure on the first metatarsal head.[48] Bunions are often caused by shoes that are pointed, too narrow, or too short. It is generally believed that women's shoes play a predominant role in the development of a hallux valgus deformity.[3]

The bursa over the first metatarsophalangeal joint becomes inflamed and eventually thickens. Tendinitis may develop in the flexor tendons of the great toe.[59] The joint becomes enlarged and the great toe becomes malaligned, moving laterally toward the second toe, sometimes to such an extent that it eventually overlaps the second toe. This type of bunion is also associated with a depressed or flattened transverse arch and a pronated foot.

The bunionette, or tailor's bunion, is much less common than hallux valgus deformity, affecting the fifth metatarsophalangeal joint. In this case, the little toe angulates toward the fourth toe, causing an enlarged metatarsal head.[10]

In all bunions, both the flexor and extensor tendons are malaligned, creating more angular stress on the joint. NOTE: Sesamoid fractures and sesamoiditis can be secondary to hallux valgus.

***Symptoms and signs*** In the beginning of bunion formation, there is tenderness, swelling, and enlargement of the joint. Poorly fitting shoes increase the irritation and pain. As the inflammation continues, angulation of the toe progresses, eventually leading to painful ambulation.

***Management*** Each bunion has unique characteristics. Early recognition and care can often prevent increased irritation and deformity. Following are some management procedures:

1. Wear correctly fitting shoes with a wide toe box.
2. Wear an appropriate orthotic to correct a structural forefoot varus variation.
3. Place a felt or sponge rubber doughnut pad over the first and/or fifth metatarsophalangeal joint.

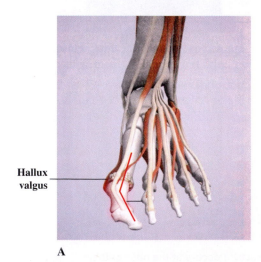
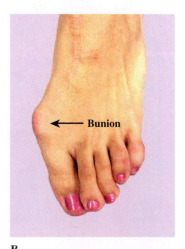

Hallux valgus

Bunion

A

B

**FIGURE 18–29** **(A)** A Hallux valgus deformity often causes the development of a **(B)** bunion.

(b) © William E. Prentice

4. Wear a tape splint along with a resilient wedge placed between the great toe and the second toe (see Figure 18–28).

5. Engage in daily foot exercises to strengthen the intrinsic and extrinsic muscles of the foot (core muscles). muscles. Ultimately, a surgical procedure called a bunionectomy may be necessary to correct the problem.

## Sesamoiditis

***Etiology*** Two sesamoid bones lie within the flexor hallucis brevis and adductor tendons of the great toe. These sesamoids transmit forces from the ground to the head of the first metatarsal. Sesamoiditis is caused by repetitive hyperextension of the great toe, which eventually results in inflammation. Sesamoiditis is most common in dancing and basketball. It is estimated that 30 percent of sesamoid injuries are sesamoiditis.[73] Fractures of the sesamoids are also common.

***Symptoms and signs*** The patient complains of pain under the great toe, especially during a push-off. There is palpable tenderness under the first metatarsal head.

***Management*** Sesamoiditis is treated with a variety of orthotic devices, including metatarsal pads, arch supports, and, most often, a metatarsal bar (Figure 18–30). Activity should be decreased to allow inflammation to subside.

## Metatarsalgia

***Etiology*** Although *metatarsalgia* is a general term used to describe pain in the ball of the foot, it is more commonly associated with pain under the second and sometimes the third metatarsal head. A heavy callus often forms in the area of pain (Figure 18–31).[20]

One of the causes of metatarsalgia is restricted extensibility of the gastrocnemius-soleus complex. Because of this restriction, the patient shortens the midstance phase of the gait and emphasizes the toe-off phase,

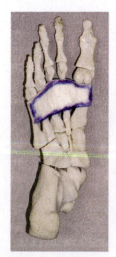

**FIGURE 18–30** Metatarsal bar to treat both sesamoiditis and metatarsalgia.
© William E. Prentice

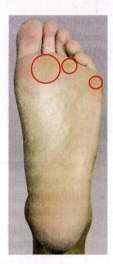

**FIGURE 18–31** A heavy callus often forms under the metatarsal heads in metatarsalgia.
© William E. Prentice

causing excessive pressure under the forefoot. This excess pressure over time causes a heavy callus to form in this region. As the forefoot bears weight, normal skin becomes pinched against the inelastic callus and produces pain.[20]

Another cause of metatarsalgia is a fallen metatarsal arch.

***Symptoms and signs*** As the transverse arch becomes flattened and the heads of the second, third, and fourth metatarsal bones become depressed, pain can result. A cavus deformity can also cause metatarsalgia.

***Management*** Management of metatarsalgia usually consists of applying a pad to elevate the depressed metatarsal heads. See *Focus Box 18–1:* "Metatarsal Pad Support." NOTE: The bar is placed behind and not under the metatarsal heads (Figure 18–30). Abnormal callus buildup should be removed by paring or filing. A patient for whom the etiology of metatarsalgia is primarily a gastrocnemius-soleus contracture should perform a regimen of static stretching several times per day. A patient whose metatarsal arch is depressed as a result of weakness should practice a daily regimen of exercise, concentrating on strengthening flexor and intrinsic muscles and stretching the Achilles tendon. A Thomas heel (Figure 18–32), which elevates the medial aspect of the heel from ⅛ to 3/16 inch (0.3 to 0.47 cm) also could prove beneficial.

## Metatarsal Arch Strain

***Etiology*** The patient who has a fallen metatarsal arch or who has a pes cavus is susceptible to strain.[22] Normally, the heads of the first and fifth metatarsal bones bear slightly more weight than the heads of the second, third, and fourth metatarsal bones. The first metatarsal head bears one-third of the body weight, the fifth bears slightly more than one-sixth, and the second, third, and fourth each bear approximately one-sixth. If the foot tends to pronate excessively or if the intermetatarsal

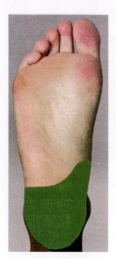

FIGURE 18–32 The Thomas heel extends anteriorly and elevates the medial aspect of the calcaneus ⅛ to ³⁄₁₆ inch (0.3 to 0.47 cm), which can help provide support to the medial longitudinal arch and relieve pronation and metatarsalgia.

© William E. Prentice

ligaments are weak, allowing the foot to spread abnormally (splayed foot), a fallen metatarsal arch may result (Figure 18–33).

***Symptoms and signs*** The patient has pain or cramping in the metatarsal region. There is **point tenderness** and weakness in the area. Morton's test may produce pain in the metatarsals (see Figure 18–17).

***Management*** Treatment of a metatarsal arch strain usually consists of applying a pad to elevate the depressed metatarsal heads. The pad is placed in the center and just behind the ball of the foot (metatarsal heads) (Figure 18–34). A teardrop-shaped pad will also work well with metatarsal arch sprains (Figure 18–35B). Exercises to increase foot strength and control have also been recommended.[51]

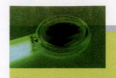

## Morton's Neuroma

***Etiology*** In the foot, a Morton's neuroma is a mass that occurs about the nerve sheath of the common plantar nerve at the point at which it divides into

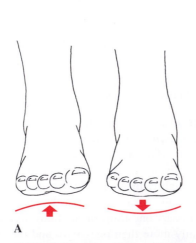

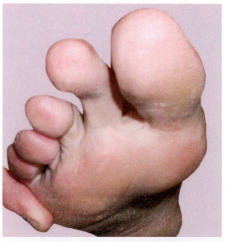

FIGURE 18–33 **(A)** Normal and fallen metatarsal arch. **(B)** Fallen metatarsal arch.

(b) © William E. Prentice

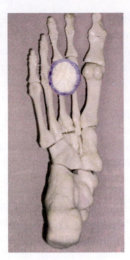

FIGURE 18–34   Metatarsal pad.

© William E. Prentice

the two digital branches to adjacent toes. A neuroma usually occurs between the metatarsal heads and is the most common nerve problem of the lower extremity.[66] A Morton's neuroma is located between the third and fourth metatarsal heads where the nerve is the thickest because it receives branches from both the medial and the lateral plantar nerves (Figure 18–35A).[29] It should be added that a neuroma can occur between any of the metatarsal heads.

Irritation increases with the collapse of the transverse arch of the foot, which puts the transverse metatarsal ligaments under stretch and thus compresses the common digital nerve and vessels. Excessive foot pronation or intrinsic muscle weakness can also be predisposing factors,

because more metatarsal shearing forces occur with the prolonged forefoot abduction.

*Symptoms and signs*   The patient complains of a burning paresthesia and severe intermittent pain in the forefoot that is often localized to the third web space and radiating to the toes. The pain is often relieved with non–weight bearing.[76] Hyperextension of the toes on weight bearing, as in squatting, stair climbing, or running, can increase the symptoms. Wearing shoes with a narrow toe box or high heels can increase the symptoms. If there is prolonged nerve irritation, the pain can become constant.[29]

*Management*   A bone scan is often necessary to rule out a metatarsal stress fracture. A teardrop-shaped pad is placed between the heads of the third and fourth metatarsals in an attempt to splay the metatarsals apart during weight bearing, which decreases pressure on the neuroma (Figure 18–35B). Often, this teardrop pad markedly reduces pain, and the patient can continue to play despite this condition. Shoe selection also plays an important role in the treatment of neuromas. Narrow shoes, particularly women's shoes that are pointed in the toe area and certain men's boots, may squeeze the metatarsal heads together and exacerbate the problem. A shoe that is wide in the toe box area should be selected. A straight-laced shoe often provides increased space in the toe box.[86] On rare occasions, surgical excision may be required.

## Injuries to the Toes

### Sprained Toes (Interphylangeal Joints)

*Etiology*   Sprains of the interphylangeal joints of the toes are caused most often by kicking some nonyielding

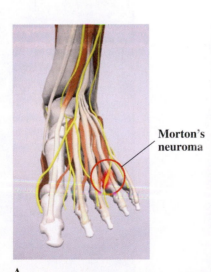

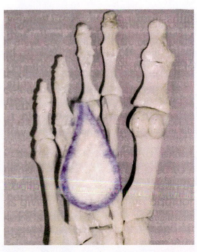

**Morton's neuroma**

A                                          B

FIGURE 18–35   **(A)** A Morton's neuroma between the third and fourth metatarsal heads can be treated using **(B)** a teardrop placed on the plantar surface of the foot as shown.

(b) © William E. Prentice

A football player who commonly plays on artificial turf complains of pain in his right great toe.

**?** What type of injury frequently occurs to the great toe of an athlete who plays on artificial turf?

object. Sprains result from a considerable force applied in such a manner as to extend the joint beyond its normal range of motion (jamming it) or to impart a twisting motion to the toe, thereby twisting and tearing the ligaments and joint capsule.

***Symptoms and signs*** Pain is immediate and intense but is generally short lived. There is immediate swelling with discoloration appearing during the first or second day. Stiffness and residual pain may last for several weeks.

***Management*** Casting or splinting of the small toes is difficult. Thus, buddy taping the injured toe to the adjacent toes is an effective technique of immobilization. The patient may begin weight bearing as soon as tolerated and may not need to be on crutches at all.

> Fractures and dislocations of the foot phalanges can be caused by kicking an object, stubbing a toe, or being stepped on.

### Great Toe Hyperextension (Turf Toe)

***Etiology*** A hyperextension of the great toe results in a sprain of the first metatarsophalangeal joint, either from a single trauma or from repetitive overuse (Figure 18–36).[6] Typically, this injury occurs on unyielding synthetic turf, although it can occur on grass also. Many of these injuries occur because sports shoes made for use on artificial turf often are more flexible and allow more dorsiflexion of the great toe.

***Symptoms and signs*** There is significant pain and swelling in and around the metatarsophalangeal joint of the great toe. Pain is exacerbated when the patient tries to push off the foot in walking and certainly in running and jumping.[21]

***Management*** Some shoe companies have addressed this problem by adding steel or other materials to the

forefoot of their turf shoes to stiffen them.[48] Flat insoles that have thin sheets of steel under the forefoot are also available. When commercially made products are not available, a thin, flat piece of thermoplastic (e.g., Orthoplast) may be placed under the shoe insole or may be molded to the foot. Taping the toe to prevent dorsiflexion may be done separately or with one of the shoe-stiffening suggestions (see Figure 8–27). Modalities of choice include ice and ultrasound. The patient should be discouraged from returning to activity until the toe is pain free.

### Fractures and Dislocations of the Phalanges

***Etiology*** Fractures of the phalanges (Figure 18–37) usually occur by kicking an object, stubbing a toe, or being stepped on. Dislocations of the phalanges are less common than fractures. If one occurs, it is most likely to be a dorsal dislocation of the middle phalanx proximal joint. The mechanism of injury is the same as for fractures. Frequently, fractures and dislocations accompany one another.[3]

***Symptoms and signs*** There is immediate, intense pain, which is increased when the toes are moved. In the case of a dislocation, deformity will be obvious. Swelling of the joint occurs rapidly, and there is subsequent discoloration in the area of injury.

***Management*** Toe dislocations should be reduced by a physician. Casting of toe fractures and dislocations is unnecessary unless multiple toes are involved or unless

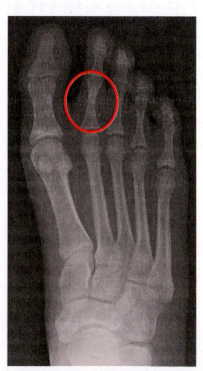

FIGURE 18–37 Fracture of the proximal phalanx of the second toe.

Courtesy Jordan B. Renner, MD, Departments of Radiology and Allied Health Sciences, University of North Carolina

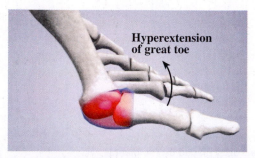

**Hyperextension of great toe**

FIGURE 18–36 A turf toe is a sprain of the metatarsophylangeal joint resulting from hyperextension of the great toe.

the injury is a great toe fracture, in which case a cast may be applied for as long as 3 weeks. Otherwise, buddy taping of the injured toe to adjacent toes usually provides sufficient support.

### Hallux Rigidus

***Etiology*** Hallux rigidus is a painful condition caused by the proliferation of bony spurs on the dorsal aspect of the first metatarsophalangeal joint, resulting in impingement and a loss of both active and passive dorsiflexion.[48] Hallux rigidus is a degenerative arthritic process, resulting in changes to the articular cartilage of the metatarsal head and in synovitis. In running and jumping activities, dorsiflexion of the metatarsophalangeal joint in the great toe is essential and, if restricted, causes the foot to roll onto the lateral border to compensate.

***Symptoms and signs*** The great toe is unable to dorsiflex, causing the patient to toe-off on the second, third, fourth, and fifth toes. Forced dorsiflexion increases pain. Walking becomes awkward because weight bearing is on the lateral aspect of the foot.

***Management*** Management usually includes a stiffer shoe with a larger toe box. An orthosis similar to that worn for a turf toe may also be helpful. Antiinflammatory medication may help reduce the inflammatory response. An osteotomy (surgically removing a piece of bone) to remove the mechanical obstruction to dorsiflexion may allow the patient to return to a normal level of function.[48]

### Hammertoe, Mallet Toe, and Claw Toe

***Etiology*** Deformities of the smaller toes can be either fixed or flexible. A hammertoe is a flexible deformity that becomes fixed. It is caused by a flexion contracture at the proximal interphalangeal (PIP) joint (Figure 18–38A). A mallet toe is caused by a flexion contracture at the distal interphalangeal (DIP) joint involving the flexor digitorum longus tendon (Figure 18–38B). It also eventually becomes a fixed deformity in which a callus develops dorsally over the DIP joint or on the tip of the toe. In a claw toe, a flexion contracture develops at the DIP joint, but there is also a hyperextension at the metatarsophalangeal (MP) joint (Figure 18–38C). A callus develops over the PIP joint and under the metatarsal head. Deformities of the lesser toes may be congenital, but more often the conditions are caused by wearing shoes that are too short over a long period of time, thus cramping the toes.[76]

***Symptoms and signs*** In all three conditions the MP, PIP, and/or DIP joints can become fixed. There may be blistering, swelling, pain, callus formation, and occasionally infection.

***Management*** Conservative treatment involves relieving pressure over the toes by wearing footwear with more room for the toes. The use of padding and protective taping (see Figure 8–28) can help prevent irritation. Shaving the calluses may also help reduce skin irritation. Once the deformities become fixed, it is likely that surgical procedures that involve straightening the toes and then maintaining positioning by using K-wire (Kirshner wire) inserted longitudinally through the phalanges into the metatarsals will be necessary.

### Overlapping Toes

***Etiology*** Overlapping of the toes (Figure 18–39) may be congenital or may be brought about by improperly fitting footwear, particularly shoes that are too narrow.

***Symptoms and signs*** At times, the condition indicates an outward projection of the great toe articulation or a drop in the longitudinal or metatarsal arch.

***Management*** As in the case of hammertoes, surgery is the only cure, but some therapeutic modalities, such as a whirlpool bath, can assist in alleviating inflammation. Taping may prevent some of the contractural tension within the sport shoe.

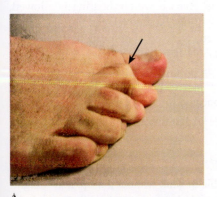
A

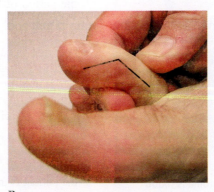
B

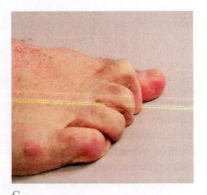
C

FIGURE 18–38 **(A)** Hammertoe. **(B)** Mallet toe. **(C)** Claw toes (all four toes).
© William E. Prentice

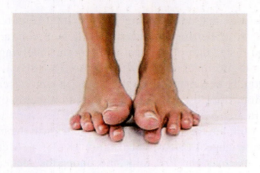

**FIGURE 18–39** Overlapping toes.
© William E. Prentice

### Blood under the Toenail (Subungual Hematoma)

*Etiology* Blood can accumulate under a toenail as a result of a direct blow to the nail bed, such as the toe being stepped on, dropping an object on the toe, or kicking another object. Repetitive shearing forces on toenails, as may occur in the shoe of a long-distance runner, may also cause bleeding into the nail bed. In any case, blood that accumulates in a confined space underneath the nail is likely to produce extreme pain and can ultimately cause loss of the nail (Figure 18–40).

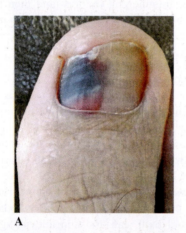

A

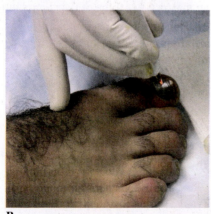

B

**FIGURE 18–40** **(A)** A subungual hematoma is blood accumulating under the nail **(B)** Draining a subungual hematoma using a electocautery tool.
© William E. Prentice

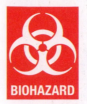

BIOHAZARD

*Symptoms and signs* Bleeding into the nail bed may be either immediate or slow, producing considerable pain. The area under the toenail assumes a bluish-purple color and gentle pressure on the nail greatly exacerbates pain.

*Management* An ice pack should be applied immediately, and the foot should be elevated to decrease bleeding. Within the next 12 to 24 hours, the pressure of the blood under the nail should be released by drilling a small hole through the nail into the nail bed. This drilling must be done under sterile conditions and is best done by either a physician or an athletic trainer. It is not uncommon to have to drill the nail a second time because more blood is likely to accumulate. An electrocautery tool that burns a hole through the nail can also be used to drain the hematoma and release the pressure (Figure 18–40A).

> A professional male soccer player is complaining about pain in the toes. Upon inspection, the athletic trainer observes that the second and third toes are heavily callused on the dorsal surface and on palpation realizes that the toes are stuck in a flexed, or clawlike, position.
>
> **?** What is this condition, and what steps can be taken to correct this problem?

## FOOT REHABILITATION

It is critical that the athletic trainer incorporate appropriate rehabilitation techniques in to the management of foot injuries. The foot is the base of support for the entire kinetic chain. Thus, injuries to the foot can affect the biomechanics of not only the foot but also the ankle, knee, hip, and spine.

### General Body Conditioning

Rehabilitation techniques for managing injuries to the lower extremity in general and to the foot in particular often require that the patient be non–weight bearing for some period of time. Even if weight bearing is allowed, the injured athlete will not be able to maintain his or her level of fitness by engaging in running activities. Thus, it becomes necessary to substitute alternative conditioning activities, such as running in a pool or working on an upper-extremity ergometer (Figure 18–41).[76] The patient should certainly continue to engage in strengthening and flexibility exercises as allowed by the constraints of the injury.

### Weight Bearing

If the patient is unable to walk without a limp, non–weight-bearing or limited weight-bearing crutch walking might be employed. Using incorrect gait mechanics certainly affects other joints within the kinetic chain, causing unnecessary

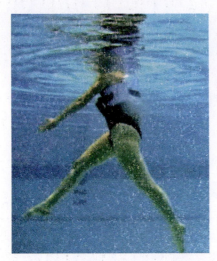

FIGURE 18–41 Pool exercises are useful in maintaining fitness while non–weight bearing.

© William E. Prentice

pain, and tends to do more harm than good. Progressing to full weight bearing as soon as it is tolerated is generally recommended.

## Joint Mobilization

Manual joint mobilization techniques are useful in maintaining or normalizing joint motions (Figure 18–42). The following joint mobilization techniques can be used in the foot:

- Anterior/posterior calcaneocuboid glides are used for increasing adduction and abduction. The calcaneus should be stabilized while the cuboid is mobilized (Figure 18–42A).
- Anterior/posterior cuboidmetatarsal glides are done with one hand stabilizing the cuboid and the other gliding the base of the fifth metatarsal. These glides are used for increasing mobility of the fifth metatarsal (Figure 18–42B).
- Anterior/posterior tarsometatarsal glides decrease hypomobility of the metatarsals (Figure 18–42C).
- Anterior/posterior talonavicular glides also increase adduction and abduction. One hand stabilizes the talus while the other mobilizes the navicular bone (Figure 18–42D).
- With anterior/posterior metatarsophalangeal glides, the anterior glides increase extension and the posterior glides increase flexion. Mobilizations are accomplished by isolating individual segments (Figure 18–42E).

## Flexibility

Maintaining normal flexibility is critical in the foot. Restoring full range of motion following various injuries to the phalanges is particularly important. It is also critical to engage in stretching activities in the case of plantar fasciitis (Figure 18–43). Stretching the gastrocnemius-soleus complex is also important for a number of injuries (see Figure 19–39).

## Muscular Strength

The concept of the foot "core" was discussed earlier in this chapter. Traditional exercises used primarily to strengthen the plantar intrinsic foot muscles include toe flexion exercises such as towel curls and marble pick-ups. While these exercises do activate some of the plantar intrinsic muscles, they also activate the extrinsic foot muscles that originate in the lower leg. These strengthening exercises for the toe flexors can be done using a variety of resistance methods, including rubber tubing, towel exercises, and manual resistance.

The following are traditional exercises commonly used in strengthening the muscles involved in foot motion:

- Writing the alphabet. With the toes pointed, the athlete writes the complete alphabet in the air three times.
- Picking up objects. The patient picks up small objects, such as marbles, with the toes and places them in a container.
- Gripping and spreading the toes. Gripping and spreading is repeated for up to 10 repetitions (Figure 18–44).
- Towel gathering. A towel is extended in front of the feet. The heels are firmly planted on the floor, with the forefoot on the end of the towel. The patient then attempts to pull the towel, with the feet, without lifting the heels from the floor. As execution becomes easier, a weight can be placed at the other end of the towel for added resistance. Each exercise should be performed 10 times (Figure 18–45A). This exercise can also be used for exercising the foot in abduction and adduction.
- Towel scoop. A towel is folded in half and placed sideways on the floor. The patient places the heel

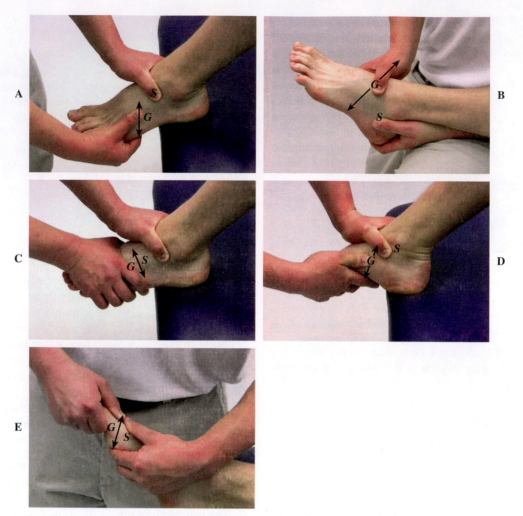

FIGURE 18–42 **(A)** Anterior/posterior calcaneocuboid glides. **(B)** Anterior/posterior cuboidmetatarsal glides. **(C)** Anterior/posterior tarsometatarsal glides. **(D)** Anterior/posterior talonavicular glides. **(E)** Anterior/posterior metatarsophalangeal glides. (S = stabilize, G = glide).
© William E. Prentice

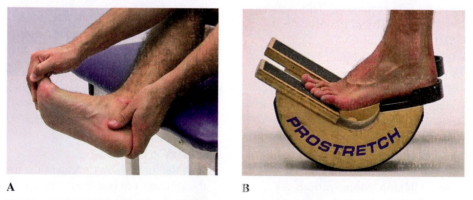

FIGURE 18–43 Plantar fascia stretches. **(A)** Manual. **(B)** Prostretch.
© William E. Prentice

firmly on the floor and the forefoot on the end of the towel. To ensure the greatest stability of the exercising foot, it is backed up with the other foot. Without lifting the heel from the floor, the athlete scoops the towel forward with the forefoot. Again, a weight resistance can be added to the end of the towel. The exercise should be repeated up to 10 times (Figure 18–45B).

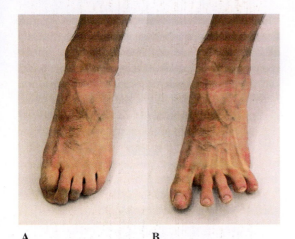

A                    B

FIGURE 18–44   **(A)** Gripping and **(B)** spreading of the toes can be an excellent rehabilitation exercise for the injured foot.
© William E. Prentice

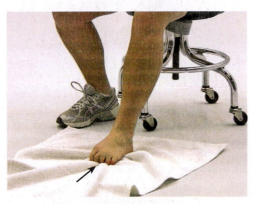

A

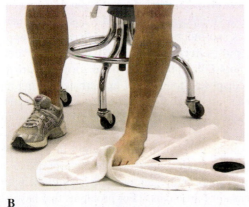

B

FIGURE 18–45   **(A)** Towel gathering exercise. **(B)** Towel scoop exercise.
© William E. Prentice

- Ankle circumduction. The ankle is circumducted in as extreme a range of motion as possible (10 circles in one direction and 10 circles in the other).

**Short Foot Exercise**   More recently, a *short foot exercise* has been recommended as a means to isolate contraction

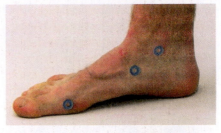

A

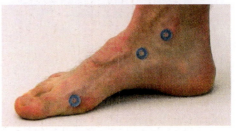

B

FIGURE 18–46   Short-foot exercise. **(A)** Foot relaxed. **(B)** Intrinsic muscles contracted, shortening and elevating the arch.
© William E. Prentice

of the plantar intrinsic muscles. This involves shortening of the foot in an anterior/posterior direction, pulling the first metatarsophalangeal joint toward the calcaneus while the long toe flexors are relaxed, thus activating the short toe flexors and foot intrinsics, causing the arch to rise (Figure 18–46).[80] Clinically, the short foot appears to enhance the longitudinal and transverse arches of the foot. The short foot exercise can be viewed as a foundational exercise for rehabilitative foot exercises that strengthen the intrinsic muscles similar to how the abdominal drawing-in maneuver is foundational to lumbo-pelvic core stability exercise programs. There is evidence to suggest that training the foot core via short foot exercise progressions can improve foot function.[51]

## Neuromuscular Control

Reestablishing neuromuscular control following foot injury is a critical component of the rehabilitative process and should not be overlooked. Although maintaining neuromuscular control while weight bearing may appear to be a rather simple motor skill for uninjured patients, neuromuscular control is compromised when injuries occur. Muscular weakness, proprioceptive deficits, and range of motion deficits may challenge a patient's ability to maintain a center of gravity within the body's base of support, causing the patient to lose balance. Neuromuscular control in the foot is the single most important element dictating movement strategies within the closed kinetic chain. The capability of adjusting and adapting to changing surfaces while creating a stable base of support is perhaps the most important function of the foot in weight bearing.[76]

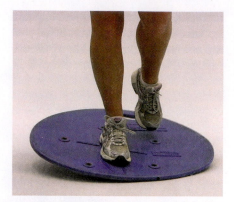

FIGURE 18–47    BAPS board exercises.
© William E. Prentice

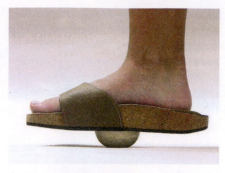

A

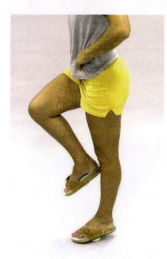

B

FIGURE 18–48    Exercise sandals are used to increase muscle activation and neuromuscular control in the foot.
© William E. Prentice

Neuromuscular control is a highly integrative, dynamic process involving multiple neurological pathways. Neuromuscular control relative to joint position sense, proprioception, and kinesthesia is essential to all performance but is particularly important to those activities that require weight bearing. Current rehabilitation protocols are therefore focusing more on closed kinetic chain exercises and neuromuscular control.

Exercises for reestablishing neuromuscular control in the foot should expose the injured patient to a variety of walking, running, and hopping exercises involving directional changes performed on varying surfaces. Balance board or wobble exercises can be useful to establish a dynamic base of support (Figure 18–47).

Exercise sandals can be incorporated into rehabilitation as a closed kinetic chain functional exercise that places increased proprioceptive demands on the patient.[7] The exercise sandals are wooden sandals with a rubber hemisphere located centrally on the plantar surface (Figure 18–48A). The patient can progress into the exercise sandals once he or she demonstrates proficiency in a barefoot single-leg stance. Prior to using the exercise sandals, the patient is instructed in the short-foot exercise. Once the patient can perform the short-foot exercise in the sandals, he or she progresses to walking in place and forward walking with short steps (see Figure 18–48B). The exercise sandals are excellent for increasing muscle activation in the foot and lower leg.[7]

## Foot Orthotics and Taping

There is strong evidence that foot orthotics, motion control footwear, and therapeutic adhesive taping are effective in controlling foot pronation compared with no intervention.[11] Taping techniques are thoroughly discussed in Chapter 8, and the use of orthotics was discussed earlier in this chapter. This section expands on the discussion of orthotic use relative to the various injuries described in this chapter.

The use of orthotics to correct foot deformities is a common practice by athletic trainers.[46] Orthotics, like any brace, provide external support but do not necessarily correct the biomechanical issues. Thus, a combination of orthotics and foot core strengthening exercises appears to be the most effective approach.[51] The normal foot functions most efficiently when no deformities are present that predispose it to injury or exacerbate existing injuries. Orthotics are used to control abnormal compensatory movements of the foot by "bringing the floor up to meet the foot."[37]

The foot functions most efficiently in a neutral position. By providing support so that the foot does not have to move abnormally, an orthotic should help prevent compensatory problems.[24] For problems that have already occurred, the orthotic provides a platform of support so that soft tissues can heal properly without undue stress (see Figure 7–26).[78]

Basically, there are three types of orthotics:[76]

1. Pads and flexible felt supports, referred to as *soft orthotics*. These soft inserts are readily fabricated and are advocated for mild overuse syndromes. Pads are particularly useful in shoes, such as track and field spikes and ski boots, that are too narrow to hold orthotics.

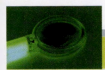

# FOCUS 18–2  Focus on Therapeutic Intervention

## Functional progression for the foot

- Non–weight bearing
- Partial weight bearing
- Full weight bearing
- Walking
  - Normal
  - Heel
  - Toe
  - Side step/shuffle slides
- Jogging
  - Straightaways on track

- Walk turns
- Jog complete oval of track
- Short sprints
- Acceleration/deceleration sprints
- Carioca
- Hopping
  - Two feet
  - One foot
  - Alternate
- Cutting, jumping, hopping on command

**A. Forefoot Varus**   **B. Forefoot Valgus**   **C. Rearfoot Varus**

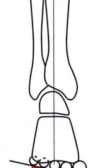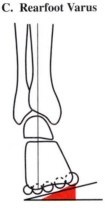

FIGURE 18–49   **(A)** Medial wedge for forefoot varus. **(B)** Lateral wedge for forefoot valgus. **(C)** Medial wedge for rearfoot varus.

2. *Semirigid orthotics* made of flexible thermoplastics, rubber, or leather.[55] These orthotics are prescribed for athletes who have increased symptoms. These orthotics are molded from a neutral cast. They are well tolerated by patients whose sports require speed or jumping.[27]
3. Functional, or *rigid, orthotics* are made from hard plastic and require neutral casting.[31] These orthotics allow control for most overuse symptoms.

Many athletic trainers make a neutral mold, put it in a box, mail it to an orthotic laboratory, and several weeks later receive an orthotic in the mail. Others like to construct the entire orthotic from start to finish, which requires a more skilled technician than does the mail-in method.[31]

**Orthotics for Correcting Over-Pronation and Supination**  For patients who are symptomatic, to correct a structural forefoot varus variation in which the foot over-pronates, the orthotic should be the rigid type and should have a medial wedge under the head of the first

metatarsal (Figure 18–49A).[33] It is also advisable to add a small wedge under the medial calcaneus to make the orthotic more comfortable.

Conversely, to correct a structural forefoot valgus variation in which the foot excessively supinates, the orthotic should be semirigid and have a lateral wedge under the head of the fifth metatarsal (Figure 18–49B). Again, adding a small wedge under the lateral calcaneus will make the orthotic more comfortable.

To correct a structural rearfoot varus variation the orthotic should be semirigid and have a wedge under the medial calcaneus and a small wedge under the head of the first metatarsal (Figure 18–49C).[37]

## Functional Progressions

Patients engage in functional progressions following injury to the foot in order to gradually regain the ability to walk, jog, run, change directions, and hop.[50] *Focus Box 18–2:* "Functional progression for the foot" details an appropriate functional progression for an injury to the foot.

Chapter Eighteen ■ The Foot     **541**

## SUMMARY

- The function of the foot is critical in running, jumping, and changing direction, and the complex nature of the anatomical structures of this body part makes recognition and management of foot injuries a major challenge to the athletic trainer.

- Many chronic and overuse injuries to the lower extremity can be related to faulty biomechanics of the foot because the foot is the part of the kinetic chain that is in direct contact with the ground.

- Essential movements that occur in the foot include pronation and supination, dorsiflexion and plantar flexion, adduction and abduction, and inversion and eversion.

- Foot injuries can best be prevented by selecting appropriate footwear, by correcting biomechanical structural deformities through the use of appropriate orthotics, and by paying attention to appropriate foot hygiene and care.

- Assessment of an injury to the foot includes a history and a palpation of soft-tissue and bony structures. In addition, observation should include a check for existing structural deformities, including forefoot varus, which might cause excessive pronation; forefoot valgus, which causes excessive supination; and rearfoot varus, which contributes to excessive pronation.

- Injuries to the foot can be classified into three categories: injuries to the tarsal region; injuries to the metatarsal region, including the arches; and injuries to the toes.

- A patient engaging in rehabilitation of an injury to the foot should maintain general body conditioning and should engage in exercises designed to regain essential joint mobility, strength, flexibility, and neuromuscular control through a series of functional progressions that gradually increase stress to the injured structures.

- The use of orthotics and taping techniques can be essential in treating many foot injuries.

## WEB SITES

American College of Foot and Ankle Surgeons: www.acfas.org
*Podiatric physicians and surgeons provide information on topics related to foot health.*

Dr. Pribut's Running Injuries Page: www.drpribut.com/sports/spsport.html
*This page lists common running injuries of the foot, ankle, knee, and hip.*

Medline Plus: Foot & Ankle Disorders: www.nlm.nih.gov/medlineplus/footinjuriesanddisorders.html

*This site can be a resource for many athletes related to foot injuries.*

Premiere Medical Search Engine: www.medscape.com
*This site allows the reader to enter any medical condition and will search the Internet to find relevant articles.*

Wheeless' Textbook of Orthopaedics: www.wheelessonline.com
*This Web page is great for injuries, anatomy, and X-rays.*

## SOLUTIONS TO CLINICAL APPLICATION EXERCISES

18-1 A forefoot valgus variation can cause excessive or prolonged supination. This condition may limit the ability of the foot and lower extremity to absorb ground reaction forces, resulting in injury. These injuries include inversion ankle sprains, tibial stress syndrome, peroneal tendinitis, iliotibial band friction syndrome, and trochanteric bursitis. The athlete can use an orthotic to correct this biomechanical problem or wear proper footwear with extra cushioning and flexibility.

18-2 Sever's disease is a traction injury to the apophysis of the calcaneal tubercle where the Achilles tendon attaches. The circulation becomes disrupted, resulting in a degeneration of the epiphyseal region.

18-3 It is likely that this athlete has a forefoot varus. To correct a structural forefoot varus variation where the foot excessively pronates, the orthotic should be the rigid type and should have a medial wedge under the head of the first metatarsal. It is also advisable to add a small wedge under the medial calcaneus to make the orthotic more comfortable. The athletic trainer should also recommend that this patient purchase a board-lasted shoe with a medial heel wedge and a firm heel counter.

18-4 This condition is characteristic of a plantar fascial strain. It should be managed symptomatically. A doughnut placed over the epicondyle region, a heel lift, and a shoe with a stiff shank may relieve some pain. The patient should stretch the plantar muscles and

gastrocnemius and perform arch exercises. Application of Low-Dye taping for pronation can also relieve pain.

18-5 A lateral sprain can produce an avulsion fracture of the proximal head of the fifth metatarsal bone.

18-6 Management of this stress fracture usually consists of 3 or 4 days' partial weight bearing followed by 2 weeks of rest. Return to running should be very gradual. An orthotic that corrects excessive pronation can help take stress off the second metatarsal.

18-7 This condition is a bunion, or hallux valgus deformity. It is associated with wearing dance shoes that are too pointed, narrow, or short. It may begin with an inflamed bursa over the metatarsophalangeal joint. It can be associated with a depressed transverse arch or a pronated foot.

18-8 A sprain of the first metatarsophalangeal joint (turf toe) stems from hyperextension, usually because of the unyielding surface of artificial turf. This injury is a tear of the joint capsule from the metatarsal head.

18-9 Kicking the locker with the great toe could cause a fracture of the proximal or distal phalanx. This injury may develop swelling, discoloration, and point tenderness.

18-10 This condition could be either hammertoes, mallet toes, or claw toes. It is likely that this condition developed from years of wearing shoes that were too tight or small. The athletic trainer could try padding the toes and recommend that the player wear a pair of shoes that has a larger toe box for the rest of the season. It is likely that, to permanently correct this problem, the soccer player will have to have surgery after the season.

18-11 Metatarsalgia can be caused by a restricted gastrocnemius-soleus complex that produces a pes cavus. It can also be caused by a fallen metatarsal arch that abnormally depresses the second or third metatarsal head and causes a heavy callus to develop.

18-12 The police officer has a Morton's neuroma. Conservatively, it is treated by having the patient wear a broad-toed shoe, a transverse arch support, and a metatarsal bar or teardrop pad.

## REVIEW QUESTIONS AND CLASS ACTIVITIES

1. Describe the anatomy of the foot.
2. How does the foot function during the gait cycle?
3. How can an injury on the plantar surface of the foot cause soreness and pain in the knee?
4. Demonstrate an appropriate procedure for assessing injuries of the foot.
5. How does a structural forefoot varus variation cause an individual to pronate excessively?
6. Identify the types of acute strains that occur in the region of the foot. How can they be prevented? How can they be managed?
7. What are the common fractures that occur in the foot, and how can they be managed?
8. How does plantar fasciitis occur, and what measures should be taken to treat it?
9. Where are the two most likely places for an exostosis to occur in the foot?
10. What is the difference between a pes cavus and a pes planus foot?
11. What is the difference between a Morton's toe and a Morton's neuroma?
12. How is a hallux valgus deformity related to excessive pronation?
13. Why does a Jones fracture often take such a long time to heal?
14. How would you construct the most appropriate orthotic for a patient who supinates excessively? Why?

## REFERENCES

1. Allen R: Toe flexors strength and passive extension range of motion of the first metatarsophalangeal joint in individuals with plantar fasciitis, *J Orthop Sports Phys Ther* 33(8):468, 2003.
2. Altman A: Barefoot running: Biomechanics and implications for running injuries, *Current Sports Medicine Reports* 11(5):244–50, 2011.
3. Anderson R: Management of common sports-related injuries about foot and ankle, *Journal of the American Academy of Orthopedic Surgeons* 18(10):546–56, 2010.
4. Baker C: Diagnostic and operative ankle arthroscopy. In Porter DM, ed: *Baxter's the foot and ankle in sports*, St. Louis, MO, 2007, Mosby.
5. Bender J: Fifth metatarsal fractures: Diagnosis and management, *Sports Medicine Alert* 6(3):18, 2000.
6. Bender J: Turf toe injuries: Correctly diagnosing an uncommon injury, *Sports Medicine Alert* 6(4):28, 2000.
7. Blackburn T: Exercise sandals increase lower extremity electromyographic activity during functional activities, *J Athl Train* 38(3):198, 2003.
8. Blackwood B, et al.: The midtarsal joint locking mechanism, *Foot and Ankle Int* 26(12):1074–80, 2005.
9. Bolgla L, Malone T: Plantar fasciitis and the windlass mechanism: A biomechanical link to clinical practice, *J Athl Train* 39(1):77, 2004.
10. Bruckner P: Foot pain. In Bruckner P, ed: *Bruckner and Kahn's clinical sports medicine*, Sydney, 2011, McGraw-Hill.
11. Cheng R: Efficacies of different external controls for excessive pronation: A meta-analysis, *British Journal of Sports Medicine* 45(9):743–51, 2011.
12. Cobb S: Custom-molded foot orthosis intervention and multisegment medial foot kinematics during walking, *J Athl Train* 46(4):358–65, 2011.
13. Cole C: Plantar fasciitis: Evidence-based review of diagnosis and therapy, *Am Fam Physician* 72:2237–48, 2005.
14. Conner C: Use of an ultrasonic bone growth stimulator to promote healing of a Jones fracture, *Athletic Therapy Today* 8(1):37, 2003.
15. Cornwall M: Common pathomechanics of the foot, *Athletic Therapy Today* 5(1):10, 2000.

16. Cornwall M: Plantar fasciitis: Etiology and treatment, *J Orthop Sports Phys Ther* 2 9(12):756, 2000.
17. Cote K: Effects of pronated and supinated foot postures on static and dynamic postural stability, *J Athl Train* 40(1):41, 2005.
18. Dedmond B: The Hallucal sesamoid complex, *J Am Acad Orthop Surg* 14:745–53, 2006.
19. Dolan MG: Preventing lower extremity injury with foot orthoses, *Athletic Therapy and Training* 17(1):17–19, 2012.
20. Espinosa N: Metatarsalgia, *Journal of the American Academy of Orthopedic Surgeons* 18(8):474–85, 2010.
21. Fair J: Turf toe injuries: Continuing to increase despite decline in artificial surfaces, *Sports Med Update* 15(1):8, 2000.
22. Ferber R: Suspected mechanisms in the cause of overuse running injuries: A clinical review, *Sports Health* 1(3):242–46, 2009.
23. Ferkel E: Entrapment neuropathies of the foot and ankle, *Clinics in Sports Medicine* 34(4):791–801, 2015.
24. Genova J: Effect of foot orthotics on calcaneal eversion during standing and treadmill walking for subjects with abnormal pronation, *J Orthop Sports Phys Ther* 30(11):664, 2000.
25. Glasoe W: Dorsal first ray mobility in women athletes with a history of stress fracture of the second or third metatarsal, *J Orthop Sports Phys Ther* 32(11):560, 2002.
26. Glasoe W: Comparison of first ray dorsal mobility among different forefoot alignments, *J Orthop Sports Phys Ther* 30(10):612, 2000.
27. Gross M: The impact of custom semirigid foot orthotics on pain and disability for individuals with plantar fasciitis, *J Orthop Sports Phys Ther* 32(4):149, 2002.
28. Grossman J: A review of osteochondral lesions of the talus, *Clinical Podiatric Medicine Surgery* 26:205–26, 2009.
29. 29. Gulick D: Differential diagnosis of Morton's neuroma, *Athletic Therapy Today* 7(1):38, 2002.
30. Hargrave M: Subtalar pronation does not influence impact forces or rate of loading during a single-leg landing, *J Athl Train* 38(1):18, 2003.
31. Henry T: Fabricating foot orthotics, *Athletic Therapy Today* 5(1):22, 2000.

32. Hertel J: Differences in postural control during single-leg stance among healthy individuals with different foot types, *J Athl Train* 37(2):129, 2002.
33. Houghlum P: Prefabricated foot orthotics decrease internal tibial rotation during hopping in females (abstract), *J Athl Train* 39(2 Suppl):S-29, 2004.
34. Hopton B: Fractures of the foot and ankle, *Surgery (Oxford)* 28(10):502–07, 2010.
35. Hunt K: Treatment of Jones fracture nonunions and refractures in the elite athlete, *American Journal of Sports Medicine* 39(9):1948–54, 2011.
36. Hunter S: Subtalar joint neutral and orthotic fitting, *Athletic Therapy Today* 5(1):6, 2000.
37. Hunter S: *Foot orthotics in therapy and sport*, Champaign, IL, 1996, Human Kinetics.
38. Hurwitz S: *Musculoskeletal examination of the foot and ankle: Making the complex simple*, Thorofare, NJ, 2011, Slack.
39. Jones M: Navicular stress fractures, *Clin Sports Med* 25(1):151, 2006.
40. Jungers W: Biomechanics: Barefoot running strikes back, *Nature* 463:433–34, 2010.
41. Kangas J: New approach to the diagnosis and classification of chronic foot and ankle disorders: Identifying motor control and movement impairments, *Manual Therapy* 6(6):522–30, 2011.
42. Karagounis P: Treatment of plantar fasciitis in recreational athletes: Two different therapeutic protocols, *Foot and Ankle Specialists* 4(4):226–34, 2011.
43. Kinoshita M et al.: The dorsiflexion-eversion test for diagnosis of tarsal tunnel syndrome, *J Bone Joint Surg Am* 83(12):1835–39, 2001.
44. Kindred J: Foot injuries in runners, *Current Sports Medicine Reports*, 10(5):249–54, 2011.
45. Lee S: Does the use of orthoses improve self-reported pain and function measures in patients with plantar fasciitis? A meta-analysis. *Phys Ther Sport* 10(1):12–18, 2009.
46. MacLean C: Short and long-term effects of a custom foot orthotic intervention on lower extremity dynamics, *Clinical Journal of Sport Medicine* 18(4):338–43, 2008.
47. Mancuso J: Posterior foot pain in a collegiate field hockey player, *J Sport Rehabil* 11(1):67, 2002.

48. Mann RA: Great toe disorders. In Porter DM, ed: *Baxter's the foot and ankle in sports* , St. Louis, MO, 2007, Mosby.

49. McCarvey W: Calcaneal fractures: Indirect reduction and external fixation, *Foot and Ankle International* 27(7):494, 2006.

50. McGee M: Functional progressions and functional testing in rehabilitation. In Prentice W, ed: *Rehabilitation techniques in sports medicine and athletic training*, Thorofare, NJ, 2015, Slack.

51. McKeon P: Freeing the foot: Integrating the foot core system into rehabilitation for lower extremity injuries, *Clinical Sports Medicine* 34(2):347–61, 2015.

52. McKeon P: The foot core system: A new paradigm for understanding intrinsic foot muscle function, *Br J Sports Med* 49:290–99, 2015.

53. McPoil T, et al.: Heel pain—plantar fasciitis: Clinical practice guidelines linked to the international classification of function, disability, and health from the orthopaedic section of the American Physical Therapy Association, *Journal of Orthopedic and Sports Physical Therapy* 4(38):A1–A18, 2008.

54. Meyer J: Differential diagnosis and treatment of subcalcaneal heel pain: A case report, *J Orthop Sports Phys Ther* 32(3):114, 2002.

55. Minert D: Foot orthoses: Materials and manufacturers, *Athletic Therapy Today* 5(1): 27, 2000.

56. Mologne T: Acute Jones fractures: Operative versus non-operative treatment, *Orthopedic Trauma Directions* 7(2):1–8, 2009.

57. Mologne T: Early screw fixation versus casting in treatment of acute Jones fractures, *Am J Sports Med* 33(7):970, 2005.

58. Mulder J: The causative mechanism in Morton's metatarsalgia, *Journal of Bone and Joint Surgery*, 33B:94–95, 1951.

59. Nachazel KMJ: Mechanism and treatment of tendinitis of the flexor hallucis longus in classical ballet dancers, *Athletic Therapy Today* 7(2):13, 2002.

60. Neal B: Foot posture as a risk factor for lower limb overuse injury: A systematic review and meta-analysis, *Journal of Foot and Ankle Research* 7:55, 2014.

61. Neufield S: Plantar fasciitis: Evaluation and treatment, *Journal of the American Academy of Orthopedic Surgeons,* 16(6):338–46, 2008.

62. Newsham K: Strengthening the intrinsic foot muscles, *Athletic Therapy and Training* 15(1): 2010.

63. Nigg, B: Running shoes and running injuries: Myth busting and a proposal for two new paradigms: 'preferred movement path' and 'comfort filter', *British Journal of Sports Medicine* doi:10.1136/bjsports-2015-095054, 2015.

64. Nigg B: Shoe inserts and orthotics for sport and physical activities, *Medicine and Science in Sport and Exercise* 31(7):S421–S428, 1999.

65. Nigg B: The role of impact forces and foot pronation: A new paradigm, *Clinical Journal of Sports Medicine* 11:2–9, 2001.

66. Norris R: Common foot and ankle injuries in dancers. In Solomon R, ed: *Preventing dance injuries*, ed 2, Champaign, IL, 2005, Human Kinetics.

67. Olmsted L: Influence of foot type and orthotics on static and dynamic postural control, *J Sport Rehabil* 13(1):54, 2004.

68. Oloff L: Flexor hallucis longus dysfunction, *J Foot Ankle Surg* 37(2):101–09, 1998.

69. Patla CE, Abbott JH: Tibialis posterior myofascial tightness as a source of heel pain: Diagnosis and treatment, *J Orthop Sports Phys Ther* 30(10):624, 2000.

70. Perkins K: The risks and benefits of running barefoot or in minimalist shoes: A systematic review, *Sports Health* 6(8):475–80, 2014.

71. Perry J: *Gait analysis: Normal and pathological function*, Thorofare, NJ, 2010, Slack.

72. Peterson J: 10 steps for preventing and treating foot problems, *ACSM's Health and Fitness Journal* 6(2):44, 2002.

73. Petrizzi M: Foot injuries. In Birrer R: *Sports medicine for the primary care physician*, ed 3, Boca Raton, FL, 2004, CRC Press.

74. Pfeffer GB: Plantar heel pain. In Porter D, ed: *Baxter's the foot and ankle in sports*, St. Louis, MO, 2007, Mosby.

75. Pommering T: Ankle and foot injuries in pediatric and adult athletes, *Primary Care* 32(1):133–61, 2005.

76. Prentice W, Hunter S, Zinder S: Rehabilitation of foot injuries. In Prentice WE, ed: *Rehabilitation techniques in sports medicine and athletic training,* Thorofare, NJ, 2015, Slack.

77. Roney J: Management strategies for cuboid syndrome, *Athletic Therapy and Training* 15(5): 10–13, 2010.

78. Rose J: Acute orthotic intervention does not affect muscular response times and activation patterns at the knee, *J Athl Train* 37(2):133, 2002.

79. Sandrey J: Rear-foot motion in soccer players with excessive pronation under four experimental conditions, *J Sport Rehabil* 10(2):143, 2001.

80. Sauer L: Considering the intrinsic foot musculature in evaluation and rehabilitation for lower extremity injuries, *Athl Train Sports Health Care* 3:43–47, 2011.

81. Schnirring L: New treatment for plantar fasciitis, *Physician Sportsmed* 29(3):16, 2001.

82. Shea M: Plantar fasciitis: Describing effective treatments, *Physician Sportsmed* 30(7): 21, 2002.

83. Sherman KP: The foot in sport, *British Journal of Sports Medicine* 33(1):6, 1999.

84. Shindle M: Stress fractures about the tibia, foot, and ankle, *Journal of the American Academy of Orthopedic Surgeons* 20(3):167–76, 2012.

85. Simpson M: Tendonopathies of the foot and ankle, *American Family Physician,* 80(10): 1107–14, 2009.

86. Swanik C: Orthotics in sports medicine, *Athletic Therapy Today* 5(1):5, 2000.

87. Tiller R: Prevention of common pes problems, *Athletic Therapy Today* 7(6):52, 2002.

88. Valmassy R: *Clinical biomechanics of the lower extremities*, St. Louis, MO, 1996, Mosby.

89. Wadsworth D: Conservative management of subtle Lisfranc joint injury: A case report, *J Orthop Sports Phys Ther* 35(3):54, 2005.

90. Whittle M: *An introduction to gait analysis*, Waltham, MA, 2007, Butterworth and Heinemann.

## ANNOTATED BIBLIOGRAPHY

Alexander I: Podiatry sourcebook, Detroit, 2007, Omnigraphics.

*Basic consumer health information about foot conditions, disease, and injuries, including bunions, corns, calluses, athlete's foot, plantar warts, hammertoes and claw toes, clubfoot, heel pain, gout, and more, along with facts about foot care, disease prevention, foot safety, choosing a foot care specialist, a glossary of terms, and resource listings for additional information.*

Altchek D: *Foot and ankle sports medicine*, Baltimore, MD, 2012, Wolters Kluwer, Lippincott, Williams and Wilkins.

*More than 40 specialists in orthopedic surgery, podiatry, physiatry, physical therapy, and athletic training contributed to this book's contents making it a comprehensive and practical resource for the treatment of foot and ankle sports injuries.*

Philbin T: *Sports injuries of the foot: Evolving diagnosis and treatment*, New York, 2014, Springer.

*This book focuses on sports injuries of the foot and succeeds both in covering the most common injuries and reviewing the gamut of how to treat these common injuries from office to operating room to rehabilitation.*

Porter D, Schon, L: *Baxter's the foot and ankle in sport,* St. Louis, MO, 2007, Mosby.

*A complete medical text on all aspects of the foot and ankle. It covers common sports syndromes, anatomical disorders in sports, unique problems, shoes, orthoses, and rehabilitation.*

Vonhof J: *Fixing your feet: Prevention and treatment for athletes,* Birmingham, AL, 2012, Wilderness Press.

*This comprehensive resource covers footwear basics, prevention, and treatments along with clear diagrams, photos, and charts that demonstrate techniques and solutions.*

Wolman R, Saifuddin A, Betts A: *Sports injuries: the foot, ankle and lower leg*, CD-ROM, 2003, Primal Picture Ltd.

*Provides a 3-D study of the anatomy of the foot and ankle and discusses a variety of injuries related to the anatomy.*

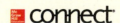

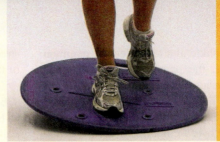

© William E. Prentice

# The Ankle and Lower Leg

## ■ Objectives

*When you finish this chapter you should be able to*

- Identify the major anatomical components of the ankle and lower leg that are commonly injured.
- Accurately assess ankle and lower leg injuries.

- Discuss the etiology, symptoms and signs, and management of injuries occurring to the ankle and lower leg.
- Develop a rehabilitation plan for various injuries to the ankle and lower leg.

## ■ Outline

## ■ Key Terms

syndesmotic joint                    ankle mortise

## ■ Connect Highlights  █ connect

*Visit connect.mcgraw-hill.com for further exercises to apply your knowledge:*

- Clinical application scenarios covering assessment of the ankle and lower leg, etiology, symptoms and signs, and management of ankle and lower leg injuries, and rehabilitation for the ankle and lower leg
- Click-and-drag questions covering structural anatomy of the ankle and lower leg, assessment of ankle and lower leg injuries, and rehabilitation plan for the ankle and lower leg
- Multiple-choice questions covering anatomy, assessment, etiology, management, and rehabilitation of ankle and lower leg injuries
- Selection questions covering rehabilitation plan for various injuries to the ankle and lower leg
- Video identification of special tests for ankle and lower leg injuries, rehabilitation techniques for the ankle and lower leg, taping and wrapping for ankle and lower leg injuries
- Picture identification of major anatomical components of the ankle and lower leg, rehabilitation techniques of the ankle and lower leg, and therapeutic modalities for management

Like the foot, the ankle and lower leg are common sites of injury in the physically active population.[88] Ankle injuries, especially to the stabilizing ligaments, are the most frequent injuries in athletes at all levels, the military, and the performing arts. This chapter focuses on traumatic and overuse injuries in the ankle and lower leg.

# ANATOMY OF THE ANKLE AND LOWER LEG

## Bones

The portion of the lower extremity that lies between the knee and the ankle is defined as the lower leg and contains two bones, the tibia and the fibula. The bones that form the ankle joint (talocrural joint) are the distal portion of the tibia, the distal portion of the fibula, and the talus. The calcaneus also plays a critical role in the function of the ankle joint.

**Tibia** With the exception of the femur, the tibia is the longest bone in the body. It serves as the principal weight-bearing bone of the leg. It is located on the medial side of the lower leg. The tibia is triangular in its upper two-thirds but is rounded and more constricted in the lower third. The most pronounced change occurs in the lower third of the shaft and produces an anatomical weakness that establishes this area as the site of most fractures occurring to the leg. The shaft of the tibia has three surfaces: posterior, medial, and lateral. The posterior and lateral surfaces are covered by muscle; the medial surface is subcutaneous and, as a result, is vulnerable to outside trauma (Figure 19–1).

**Fibula** The fibula is long and slender and is located along the lateral aspect of the tibia, joining it in an arthrodial articulation at the upper end, just below the knee joint, and as a **syndesmotic joint** at the lower end. Both the upper and the lower tibiofibular joints are held in position by strong anterior and posterior ligaments. The main function of the fibula is to provide for the attachment of muscles.

***Tibial and Fibular Malleoli*** The thickened distal ends of both the tibia and the fibula are referred to as the medial malleolus and lateral malleolus, respectively. The lateral malleolus of the fibula extends farther distally, so that the stability created by the bony arrangement at the ankle joint is greater on the lateral aspect of the ankle than on the medial aspect (Figure 19–1).

**Talus** The talus, the second largest tarsal and the main weight-bearing bone of the articulation, rests on the calcaneus and receives the articulating surfaces of the lateral and medial malleoli. The talus forms a link between the lower leg and the foot, or tarsus (Figure 19–2).

**Calcaneus** The calcaneus is one of the tarsal bones and was discussed in Chapter 18. The calcaneus is the bone that forms the heel and to which many of the supporting ligaments of the ankle joint, as well as the Achilles tendon, attach (Figure 19–2).

## Articulations

The ankle complex consists of three articulations: the distal tibiofibular syndesmosis, the talocrural joint, and the subtalar joint. These joints work in concert with one another to permit simultaneous movement in three planes: plantar flexion-dorsiflexion in the sagittal plane, inversion-eversion in the frontal plane, and internal rotation-external rotation in the transverse plane.[41]

**Superior and Inferior Tibiofibular Joints** The tibia and fibula articulate with one another superiorly and inferiorly (tibiofibular joints). The superior tibiofibular joint is diarthrotic, allowing some gliding movements. The articulation is formed by the tibia's lateral condyle and the head

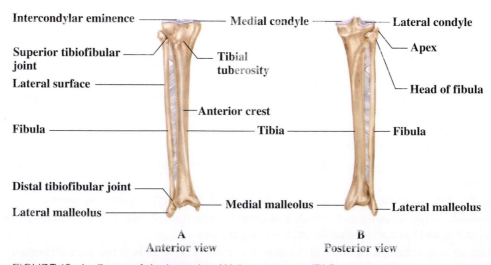

Intercondylar eminence — Medial condyle — Lateral condyle

Superior tibiofibular joint

Lateral surface

Tibial tuberosity

Apex

Head of fibula

Anterior crest

Fibula — Tibia — Fibula

Distal tibiofibular joint

Lateral malleolus — Medial malleolus — Lateral malleolus

A
Anterior view

B
Posterior view

FIGURE 19–1  Bones of the lower leg. **(A)** Anterior view. **(B)** Posterior view.

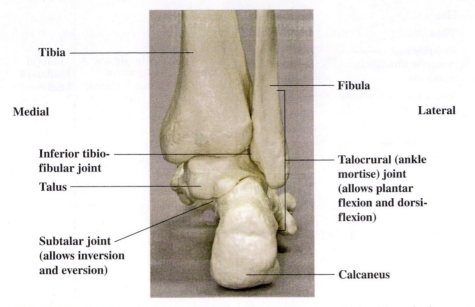

**FIGURE 19–2** The ankle joint is formed by the tibia, fibula, and talus. The subtalar joint is formed by the talus and calcaneus.
© William E. Prentice

Labels on figure:
Tibia
Fibula
Medial
Lateral
Inferior tibio-fibular joint
Talocrural (ankle mortise) joint (allows plantar flexion and dorsiflexion)
Talus
Subtalar joint (allows inversion and eversion)
Calcaneus

of the fibula. It is surrounded by a fibrous capsule reinforced with anterior and posterior ligaments. The superior tibiofibular joint is stronger in front than in back (see Figure 19–1).

The inferior tibiofibular joint is a fibrous articulation or syndesmosis. The articulation is between the lateral malleolus and the distal end of the tibia. The joint is reinforced by the ankle ligaments (Figure 19–2).

**Talocrural Joint** The ankle joint, or talocrural joint, is a hinge joint (ginglymus) that is formed by the articular facet on the distal portion of the tibia, which articulates with the superior articular surface (trochlea) of the talus; the medial malleolus, which articulates with the medial surface of the trochlea of the talus; and the lateral malleolus, which articulates with the lateral surface of the trochlea (Figure 19–2). This bony arrangement is typically referred to as the **ankle mortise**. The ankle movements that occur at the talocrural joint are plantar flexion and dorsiflexion.

**Subtalar Joint** The anatomy and function of the subtalar joint were discussed in Chapter 18. The subtalar joint consists of the articulation between the talus and the calcaneus. The ankle movements that occur at the subtalar joint are inversion, eversion, pronation, and supination (Figure 19–2).

## Stabilizing Ligaments

**Tibiofibular Ligaments** Joining the tibia and fibula is a strong interosseous membrane. The fibers display an oblique downward and outward pattern. The oblique arrangement aids in diffusing the forces placed on the leg. The membrane completely fills the tibiofibular space except for a small area at the superior aspect that is provided for the passage of the anterior tibial vessels. The anterior and posterior tibiofibular

ligaments, which hold the tibia and fibula together and form the distal portion of the interosseous membrane, are sometimes referred to as the syndesmotic ligaments.

**Ankle Ligaments** In addition to the tibiofibular ligaments, the ligamentous support of the ankle consists of three lateral ligaments and the medial, or deltoid, ligament (Figures 19–3 and 19–4).

*Lateral Ligaments* The three lateral ligaments are the anterior talofibular, the posterior talofibular, and the calcaneofibular (Table 19–1).

*Medial Ligaments* The deltoid ligament is triangular. It attaches superiorly to the borders of the medial malleolus; it attaches inferiorly to the medial surface of the talus, to the sustentaculum tali of the calcaneus, and to the posterior margin of the navicular bone. The deltoid ligament is the primary resistance to foot eversion. It, along with the plantar calcaneonavicular (spring) ligament, also helps maintain the inner longitudinal arch. Although it should be considered one ligament, the deltoid ligament includes both superficial and deep fibers (Figure 19–4). Anteriorly are the anterior tibiotalar part and the tibionavicular part. Medially is the tibiocalcaneal part, and posteriorly is the posterior tibiotalar part. The functions of the stabilizing ligaments of the ankle joint complex are summarized in Table 19–1.

## Joint Capsule

A thin articular capsule encases the ankle joint and attaches to the borders of the bone involved. It is somewhat different from most other capsules in that it is thick on the medial aspects of the joint but becomes a thin, gauze-like membrane at the back.

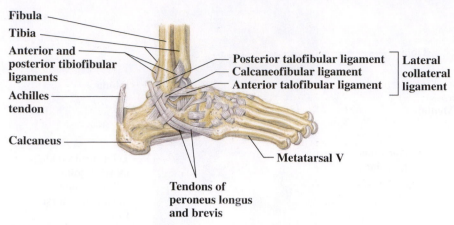

FIGURE 19-3   Lateral ligaments of the ankle.

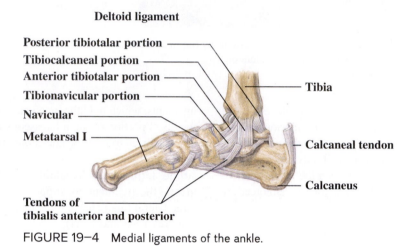

FIGURE 19-4   Medial ligaments of the ankle.

| TABLE 19-1 | Function of Key Ankle Ligaments |
|---|---|
| **Ligament** | **Primary Function** |
| Anterior talofibular | Restrains anterior displacement of talus |
| Calcaneofibular | Restrains inversion of calcaneus |
| Posterior talofibular | Restrains posterior displacement of talus |
| Deltoid | Prevents abduction and eversion of ankle and subtalar joint |
| | Prevents eversion, pronation, and anterior displacement of talus |

## Ankle Musculature

The movements of the talocrural joint are dorsiflexion (flexion) and plantar flexion (extension). Inversion and eversion occur at the subtalar joint. Tendons of muscles passing posterior to the malleoli produce ankle plantar flexion along with toe flexion in the foot. Muscles and their tendons passing anteriorly to the talocrural joint dorsiflex the foot and produce toe extension. The muscles that cross the ankle joint laterally cause eversion, whereas the muscles that cross the ankle joint medially cause inversion (Figure 19–5).

**Muscle Compartments**   The musculature of the lower leg is contained within four distinct compartments, which are bounded by heavy fascia (Figure 19–6). Traumatic or overuse injury to any of these compartments can lead to swelling and neurological motor and sensory deficits.

The *anterior compartment* contains those muscles that dorsiflex the ankle and extend the toes—the tibialis anterior, extensor hallucis longus, and extensor digitorum longus muscles—and contains the anterior tibial nerve and the tibial artery.

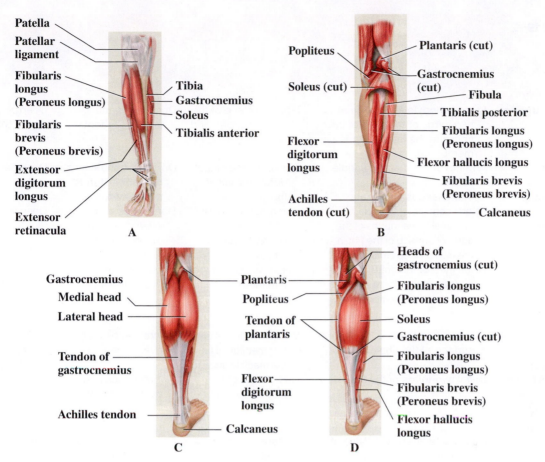

FIGURE 19–5    Muscles of the ankle and lower leg. **(A)** Anterior. **(B)** Lateral. **(C)** Superficial posterior. **(D)** Deep posterior.

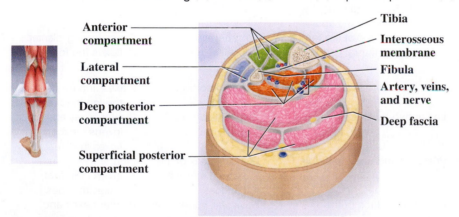

FIGURE 19–6    The four compartments of the lower leg.

The *lateral compartment* contains the fibularis longus and brevis (Peroneus longus and brevis), which evert the ankle; the Fibularis tertius (Peroneus tertius) muscle, which assists in dorsiflexion; and the superficial branch of the peroneal nerve.

The *superficial posterior compartment* contains the gastrocnemius muscle and the soleus muscle. These muscles plantar flex the ankle.

The *deep posterior compartment* contains the tibialis posterior, flexor digitorum longus, and flexor hallucis longus muscles, which invert the ankle, and the posterior tibial artery.

Table 19–2 summarizes the muscles in the ankle and lower leg and their actions.

## Nerve Supply

The lower leg is supplied by the common peroneal nerve anteriorly. The common peroneal branches into the superficial peroneal nerve and the deep peroneal nerve. The tibial nerve runs posteriorly and supplies the ankle and the foot (Figure 19–7).

## Blood Supply

The ankle and lower leg are supplied by the anterior tibial artery and posterior tibial arteries. Blood drains via the peroneal vein, posterior tibial vein, and anterior tibial vein (Figure 19–8).

**TABLE 19–2**     Muscles of the Ankle and Lower Leg

| Muscle | Origin | Insertion | Muscle Action | Nerve/Nerve Root |
|---|---|---|---|---|
| *Anterior compartment* | | | | |
| **Tibialis anterior** | Lateral condyle and proximal two-thirds of the shaft of the tibia and the interosseous membrane | Medial surface of the first cuneiform and first metatarsal | Dorsiflexes and inverts the foot | Deep peroneal (L5, S1) |
| **Extensor hallucis longus** | Anterior surface of the middle of the fibula and the interosseous membrane | Dorsal surface of the distal phalanx of the great toe | Dorsiflexes and inverts the foot; extends the great toe | Deep peroneal (L5, S1) |
| **Extensor digitorum longus** | Lateral condyle of the tibia, proximal three-fourths of the anterior surface of the fibula, and the interosseous membrane | Dorsal surface of the phalanges of the second through fifth toes | Dorsiflexes and everts the foot; extends the toes | Deep peroneal (L5, S1) |
| **Fibularis tertius (peroneus tertius)** | Distal third of the anterior surface of the fibula and the interosseous membrane | Dorsal surface of the fifth metatarsal | Dorsiflexes and everts the foot | Deep peroneal (L5, S1) |
| *Lateral compartment* | | | | |
| **Fibularis longus (peroneus longus)** | Proximal two-thirds of the lateral surface of the fibula | Ventral surface of the first metatarsal and the medial cuneiform | Plantar flexes and everts the foot | Superficial peroneal (L4, L5, S1) |
| **Fibularis brevis (peroneus brevis)** | Distal two-thirds of the fibula | Lateral side of the fifth metatarsal | Plantar flexes and everts the foot | Superficial peroneal (L4, L5, S1) |
| *Superficial posterior compartment* | | | | |
| **Gastrocnemius** | Medial and lateral condyles of the femur | Calcaneus, via the Achilles tendon | Flexes the leg; plantar flexes the foot | Tibial (L5, S1) |
| **Soleus** | Posterior surface of the proximal third of the fibula and the middle third of the tibia | Calcaneus, via the Achilles tendon | Plantar flexes the foot | Tibial (L5, S1) |
| **Plantaris** | Posterior surface of the femur above the lateral condyle | Calcaneus, via the Achilles tendon | Flexes the leg; plantar flexes the foot | Tibial (L5, S1) |
| *Deep posterior compartment* | | | | |
| **Popliteus** | Lateral condyle of the femur | Proximal portion of the tibia | Flexes and rotates the leg medially | Tibial (L5, S1) |
| **Flexor hallucis longus** | Lower two-thirds of the fibula | Distal phalanx of the great toe | Plantar flexes and inverts the foot; flexes the great toe | Tibial (L5, S1) |
| **Flexor digitorum longus** | Posterior surface of the tibia | Distal phalanx of the second through fifth toes | Plantar flexes and inverts the foot; flexes the toes | Tibial (L5, S1) |
| **Tibialis posterior** | Posterior surface of the interosseous membrane, the tibia, and the fibula | Navicular, cuneiforms, cuboid; second through fourth metatarsals | Plantar flexes and inverts the foot | Tibial (L5, S1) |

Movements of the ankle joint.*

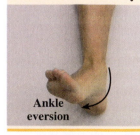

Ankle eversion

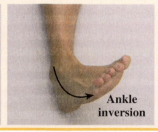

Ankle inversion

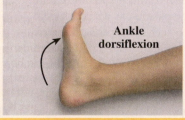

Ankle dorsiflexion

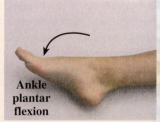

Ankle plantar flexion

*Manual muscle tests and goniometric measurements of range of motion for the ankle joint can be found in Appendix F and Appendix G at the end of the text.

© William E. Prentice

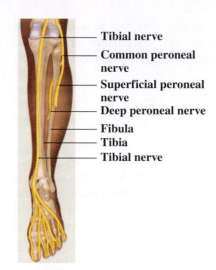

- Tibial nerve
- Common peroneal nerve
- Superficial peroneal nerve
- Deep peroneal nerve
- Fibula
- Tibia
- Tibial nerve

FIGURE 19–7    Nerve supply of the lower leg (posterior view).

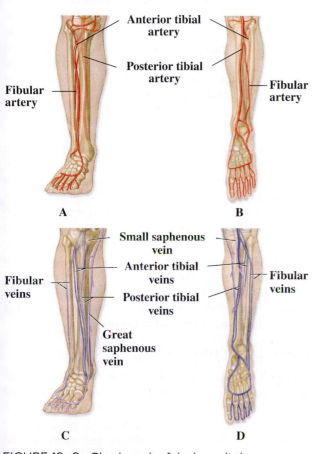

- Anterior tibial artery
- Posterior tibial artery
- Fibular artery (left)
- Fibular artery (right)

A          B

- Small saphenous vein
- Anterior tibial veins
- Posterior tibial veins
- Fibular veins (left)
- Fibular veins (right)
- Great saphenous vein

C          D

FIGURE 19–8    Blood supply of the lower limb.
**(A)** Arteries (anterior view). **(B)** Arteries (posterior view).
**(C)** Veins (anterior view). **(D)** Veins (posterior view).

# FUNCTIONAL ANATOMY

The biomechanical motions occurring at the ankle and rear foot are complex. Anatomically, the ankle is a stable hinge joint in which the dome of the talus articulates with the distal ends of the tibia and fibula. Medial or lateral displacement of the talus is prevented by the malleoli. The arrangement of the ankle ligaments permits flexion and extension at the talocrural joint and limits inversion and eversion at the subtalar joint (see Chapter 18).[41]

> **Because the talus is wider anteriorly than posteriorly, the most stable position of the ankle is with the foot in dorsiflexion.**

The square shape of the talus contributes to ankle stability. Because the talus is wider anteriorly than posteriorly, the most stable position of the ankle is with the foot in dorsiflexion. In this position, the wider anterior aspect of the talus comes in contact with the narrower portion lying between the malleoli, gripping it tightly. By contrast, as the ankle moves into plantar flexion, the wider portion of the tibia is brought in contact with the narrower posterior aspect of the talus, which makes plantar flexion a much less stable position than dorsiflexion.

The degree of motion for the ankle joint ranges from 10 degrees of dorsiflexion to 50 degrees of plantar flexion. Normal gait mechanics require at least 20 degrees of plantar flexion and 10 degrees of dorsiflexion with the knee extended.[55]

Normal ankle function depends on the joints of the rearfoot, the most important of which is the subtalar joint. Supination and pronation occur at the subtalar joint. These movements are triplanar movements, that is, movements that occur in all three planes simultaneously. In weight bearing, the subtalar joint acts as a torque convertor to translate the pronation/supination into leg rotation. The movements of the talus during pronation and supination have profound effects on the lower extremity, both proximally and distally, as discussed in Chapter 18. The ankle joint is a critical link in the kinetic chain. Dysfunction in the ankle can lead to associated dysfunction in the knee and hip joints.

## Surface Anatomy

Figure 19–9A and Figure 19–9B show the surface anatomy with pertinent landmarks for the ankle. Figure 19–10 shows the surface anatomy for the lower leg.

# PREVENTING INJURY TO THE ANKLE AND LOWER LEG

Many ankle and lower leg conditions, especially sprains, can be reduced if an individual engages in the following: Achilles tendon stretching, strength training, neuromuscular control and balance training, proper footwear, and preventive ankle bracing and orthoses.[87,106]

## Achilles Tendon Stretching

It is critical for normal gait that the ankle dorsiflex at least 10 degrees or more. If dorsiflexion ROM is limited, techniques to enhance arthrokinematic and osteokinematic motion for possible prevention of ankle injury should be incorporated.[35]
**SoR:C** A tight

> **Preventing ankle sprains:**
>
> - Achilles tendon stretching
> - Strength training
> - Neuromuscular control and balance training
> - Footwear
> - Bracing and taping

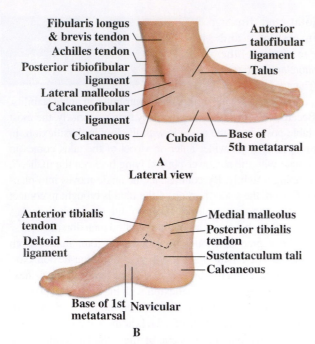

A
Lateral view

B

FIGURE 19–9    The foot (A) Lateral view. (B) Medial view.
© JW Ramsey/McGraw-Hill Education

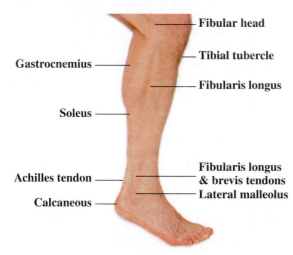

FIGURE 19–10    Lower leg surface anatomy, lateral view.
© JW Ramsey/McGraw-Hill Education

Achilles tendon may limit dorsiflexion and may predispose the individual to ankle injury. Anyone who engages in physical activity, especially with tight Achilles tendons, should routinely stretch before and after activity.[80] To adequately stretch the Achilles tendon complex, stretching should be performed both with the knee extended and then with it flexed 15 to 30 degrees.

## Strength Training

To prevent ankle injury, it is important to achieve both static and dynamic joint stability. A normal range of motion must be maintained, and the muscles and tendons that surround the talocrural joint must be kept strong. Addressing the strength of the lower leg muscles that produce movement at the ankle joint and the hip

extensors and abductors may be an effective ankle injury prevention strategy. Dysfunction of these muscles may result in susceptible positions during movement, thereby causing injury.[58] SoR:C

## Neuromuscular Control and Balance Training

Neuromuscular control and balance are important for the prevention of ankle sprains. They are also important elements for recovery following acute ankle sprains as well as in those with chronic ankle instability.[77] It has been recommended that an injury-prevention program that focuses on balance and neuromuscular control lasting at least 3 months be implemented to reduce the risk of ankle injury. Athletes with a history of ankle injury may benefit more from this type of training.[58,74] SoR:A Neuromuscular control involves adapting to uneven surfaces by controlling motion at the ankle joint while maintaining balance. Ankle neuromuscular control can be enhanced by working on balance training in controlled activities on uneven surfaces or by spending time each day on a BAPS (Biomechanical Ankle Platform System) board, Bosu Balance Trainer, rocker board, or Dynadisc.

## Footwear

As discussed in Chapter 7, proper footwear can be an important factor in reducing injuries to both the foot and the ankle. Shoes should not be used in activities for which they were not intended—for example, running shoes designed for straight-ahead activity should not be used to play tennis, a sport that demands a great deal of lateral movement. Cleats on a shoe should not be centered in the middle of the sole, but should be placed far enough on the border to avoid ankle sprains. High-top shoes, when worn by athletes with a history of ankle sprain, can offer greater support than low-top shoes although it is unclear if they help reduce the risk of ankle sprains.[93]

## Preventive Ankle Bracing and Taping

Chapter 8 discusses the controversy surrounding the benefits of routinely taping ankles that have no history of sprain. There is some indication that tape, properly applied, can provide some prophylactic protection.[40,94] However, tape that is too tight will be uncomfortable and therefore might cause an athlete to alter his or her normal biomechanics. Lace-up supports and semirigid ankle braces are increasingly being used in place of tape.[14] It has been demonstrated that ankle braces are effective in reducing ankle sprains.[75] Although braces alter biomechanics they do not alter performance.[18] The sport-stirrup orthosis has been found to be superior to taping in preventing recurrent ankle sprains (see Figure 7–26). It must be emphasized that wearing a semirigid ankle brace not only alters the biomechanics at the ankle joint but also at the knee joint.[102] Lastly, bracing is a much more cost effective way of reducing ankle sprains relative to taping.[86]

# ASSESSING THE ANKLE AND LOWER LEG

A thorough assessment of injuries to the ankle and lower leg can provide important information relative to the anatomical structures that may be injured in a patient suspected of having an ankle sprain.[58] **SoR:C**

## History

The patient's history may vary depending on whether the problem is the result of sudden trauma or is chronic. The athletic trainer should ask the patient with an acute injury to the ankle or lower leg the following questions:[13,66]

- Have you ever hurt your ankle before?
- How did you hurt your ankle?
- What did you hear when the injury occurred—a crack, snap, or pop?
- How bad was the pain, and how long did it last?
- Is there any sense of muscle weakness or difficulty in walking?
- How disabling was the injury? Could you walk right away, or were you not able to bear weight for a period of time?
- Has a similar injury occurred before?
- Was there immediate swelling, or did the swelling occur later (or at all)?
- Where did the swelling occur?

The patient with a chronic painful condition might be asked the following:

- How much does it hurt?
- Where does it hurt?
- Under what circumstances does pain occur—when bearing weight, after activity, or when arising after a night's sleep?
- What past ankle injuries have occurred?
- What first aid and therapy, if any, were given for these previous injuries?

## Observation

In looking initially at the ankle, the athletic trainer should determine the following:[13,66]

- Are there any postural deviations? (Toeing in may indicate tibial torsion or genu valgum or varum; foot pronation should also be noted.)
- Is there any difficulty in walking?
- Is there an obvious deformity or swelling?
- Are the bony contours of the ankle normal and symmetrical, or is there a deviation, such as a bony deformity?
- Are the color and texture of the skin normal?
- Is there crepitus or abnormal sound in the ankle joint?

- Is heat, swelling, or redness present?
- Is the patient in obvious pain?
- Does the patient have a normal ankle range of motion?
- If the patient is able to walk, is there a normal walking pattern?

## Palpation

The area of injury should be palpated to determine obvious structural deformities, areas of swelling, and points of tenderness.

**Bony Palpation** The following bony landmarks should be palpated:

**Anterior aspect**

- Fibular head
- Fibular shaft
- Lateral malleolus
- Tibial plateau
- Tibial shaft
- Medial malleolus
- Dome of the talus

**Posterior aspect**

- Medial malleolus
- Lateral malleolus
- Dome of the talus
- Calcaneus
- Sustentaculum tali

**Soft-Tissue Palpation** The following soft-tissue structures should be palpated:

**Lateral aspect**

- Lateral compartment
  —Fibularis longus muscle and tendon
  —Fibularis brevis muscle and tendon
  —Fibularis tertius muscle and tendon
- Anterior talofibular ligament
- Calcaneofibular ligament
- Posterior talofibular ligament

**Medial aspect**

- Deep posterior muscles
  —Posterior tibialis muscle and tendon
  —Flexor digitorum longus muscle and tendon
  —Flexor hallucis muscle and tendon
- Deltoid ligament

**Anterior aspect**

- Anterior compartment
  —Anterior tibialis muscle and tendon
  —Extensor hallucis longus muscle and tendon
  —Extensor digitorum longus muscle and tendon
- Anterior tibiofibular ligament

**Posterior aspect**

- Superficial posterior compartment
  —Gastrocnemius muscle
  —Soleus muscle
- Achilles tendon
- Posterior tibiofibular ligament

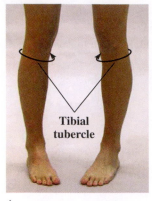
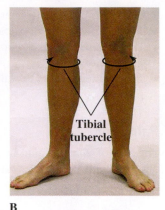

**A**                      **B**

FIGURE 19–11   Malalignment of the lower leg.
**(A)** Internal tibial torsion. **(B)** External tibial torsion.
© William E. Prentice

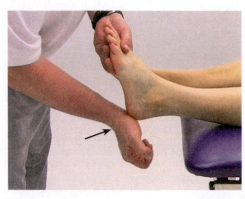

FIGURE 19–12   Percussion (bump) test to check for fractures of the ankle or lower leg.
© William E. Prentice

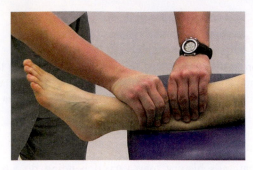

FIGURE 19–13   Compression (squeeze) test to check for fractures of the tibia or fibula.
© William E. Prentice

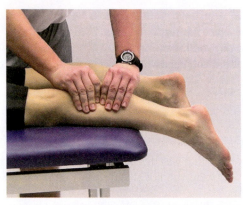

FIGURE 19–14   Thompson test to determine an Achilles tendon rupture by squeezing the calf muscle. A positive result to the test is one in which there is no plantar flexion of the foot.
© William E. Prentice

## Special Tests

Special tests to assess injury to the ankle ligaments, performed soon after injury and before joint effusion has accumulated, may have better diagnostic accuracy than tests performed after effusion has occurred.[58] **SoR:C** However, the diagnostic accuracy of special tests is higher 5 days following injury than at 2 days.[58,101] **SoR:B**

### Lower Leg

***Lower Leg Alignment Tests***  Determining malalignment of the lower leg can reveal the causes of abnormal stresses applied to the foot, ankle, and lower leg as well as the knees and hip. In normal alignment of the lower extremity, anteriorly, a straight line can be drawn from the anterior superior iliac spine of the pelvis, through the patella, and to the web between the first and second toes. Laterally, a straight line can be drawn from the greater trochanter of the femur, through the center of the patella, and to just behind the lateral malleolus. Posteriorly, a straight line can be drawn from the center of the lower leg to the midline of the Achilles tendon and calcaneus.[13] A common malalignment of the lower leg is internal or external tibial torsion (Figure 19–11). In external tibial torsion, the tibial tubercle is laterally

positioned; in internal tibial torsion, the tibial tubercle is medially positioned.

***Percussion (Bump) and Compression (Squeeze) Tests***[25]  When fracture is suspected, a gentle percussive blow can be given to the tibia or fibula below or above the suspected site. Percussion can also be applied upward on the bottom of the heel. Such blows set up a vibratory force that resonates at the fracture, causing pain (Figure 19–12). The use of a tuning fork has also been recommended as an alternative method of providing vibration at the site of a suspected fracture. But although tuning fork tests have some value in ruling out fractures, reliability, or accuracy are insufficient for widespread clinical use.[79]

In a compression or squeeze test, the tibia and fibula are compressed either above or below the fracture site (Figure 19–13). Increased pain over the area of point tenderness may indicate a fracture, and referral should be made for X-rays. **Sn. 0.30 | Sp. 0.94 | +LR 4.60 | -LR 0.75**

***Thompson Test***[68]  The Thompson test is used to determine whether there is a rupture of the Achilles tendon. The Thompson test (Figure 19–14) is performed by squeezing the calf muscle while the leg is extended and the foot is hanging over the edge of the table. A positive Thompson sign is one in which squeezing the calf muscle

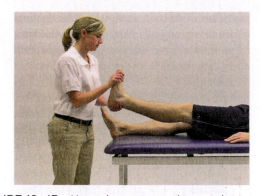

FIGURE 19–15   Homan's sign may indicate a deep vein thrombophlebitis.
© William E. Prentice

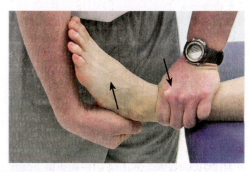

FIGURE 19–16   Anterior drawer test for ankle ligament instability.
© William E. Prentice

does not cause the heel to move or pull upward or causes the heel to move less when compared with the uninjured leg. Sn. 0.96 | Sp. 0.93 | +LR 13.47 | -LR 0.4

**Homan's Sign[36]** The test for Homan's sign has been said to give some indication of the presence of a deep vein thrombophlebitis. But as can be seen from test sensitivity and specificity, it appears to be a relatively useless clinical test. With the patient in a supine position with the knee fully extended, the ankle is passively dorsiflexed so that the calf muscles are stretched. Pain in the calf is a positive sign (Figure 19–15). Swelling and calf pain that doesn't change with position is another excellent diagnostic tool. The patient should be referred immediately to a physician for further diagnosis using doppler ultrasound. Sn. 0.56 | Sp. 0.39 | +LR .15 | -LR .17

### Ankle Stability Tests
**Anterior Drawer Test[43]** The anterior drawer test is used to determine the extent of injury to the anterior talofibular ligament primarily and to the other lateral ligaments secondarily (Figure 19–16). The patient sits on the edge of a treatment table with the ankle at a 90-degree angle. The athletic trainer grasps the lower tibia in one hand and the calcaneus in the palm of the other hand. The tibia is then pushed backward as the calcaneus is pulled forward. A positive anterior drawer sign occurs when the foot slides forward, sometimes making a clunking sound as it reaches

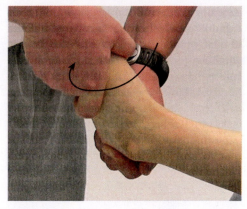

FIGURE 19–17   Talar tilt testing for lateral ankle instability.
© William E. Prentice

its end point, and generally indicates a tear in the anterior talofibular ligament. An ankle arthrometer has

> A positive anterior drawer sign of ankle stability is when the foot slides forward, sometimes making a clunking sound as it reaches its end point.

been used to determine anterior stability of the talocrural joint.[51,63] Sn. 0.58 | Sp. 1.0 | +LR 4.0 | -LR 0.57

**Talar Tilt Test[43]** Talar tilt tests are used to determine the extent of inversion or eversion injuries. With the foot positioned at 90 degrees to the lower leg and stabilized, the calcaneus is inverted. Excessive motion of the talus indicates injury to

> A positive talar tilt occurs when the calcaneofibular ligament is sprained.

the calcaneofibular and possibly the anterior and posterior talofibular ligaments (Figure 19–17).

The deltoid ligament can be tested in the same manner except that the calcaneus is everted. Sn. 0.5 | Sp. 0.88 | +LR Infinity | -LR 0.42

**Kleiger's Test (External Rotation Test)[25]** Kleiger's test is used primarily to determine injury to the structures that support the distal ankle syndesmosis, including the anterior tibiofibular ligament, the posterior tibiofibular ligament, and the interosseous membrane. The patient should be seated with the knee flexed and the legs over the end of the table. The athletic trainer uses one hand to stabilize the lower leg and the other to hold the medial aspect of the foot and rotate it externally. External rotation of the talus applies pressure to the lateral malleolus, causing a widening of the tibiofibular joint. Pain in the the anterolateral ankle may indicate injury to the syndesmosis, whereas pain over the deltoid ligament may indicate a sprain of that structure (Figure 19–18). Sn. 0.20 | Sp. 0.85 | +LR 1.31 | -LR 0.94

**Cotton Test[97]** The Cotton test is performed to determine if there is a sprain to the distal tibiofibular syndesmosis. The patient is seated with the ankle in neutral. The clinician cups the calcaneus and talus and, with the lower leg stabilized, attempts to translate the talus laterally. The test

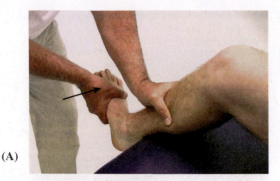

(A)

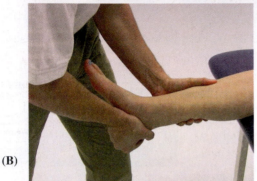

(B)

FIGURE 19–18   Tests for ankle syndesmosis. **(A)** Kleiger's test (external rotation test). **(B)** Cotton test.

© William E. Prentice

is positive if pain is increased and there is excessive lateral translation compared to the opposite side (Figure 19–18B). Sn. 0.25 | Sp. NA | +LR 6.30 | -LR 0.28

***Medial Subtalar Glide Test*[43]**   The medial subtalar glide test is done to determine the presence of excessive medial translation of the calcaneus on the talus in the transverse plane.[43] The athletic trainer uses one hand to hold the talus in subtalar neutral, then glides the calcaneus in a medial direction on the fixed talus (Figure 19–19). In a positive test, there is excessive movement, indicating injury to the lateral ligaments. Sn. 0.58 | Sp. 0.88 | +LR 4.67 | -LR 0.48

**Functional Tests**   Muscle function is important in evaluating the ankle injury (Figure 19–20). Athletic trainers routinely have individuals with traumatic ankle sprains perform these tests. However, these tests should not be done if the patient is unable to bear weight. The following functional tests can be used:

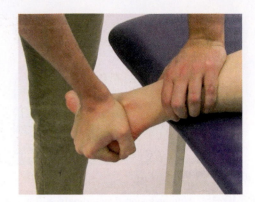

FIGURE 19–19   The medial subtalar glide test looks for excessive medial translation of the calcaneus relative to the talus, indicating injury to the lateral ligaments.

© William E. Prentice

- Walk on toes (tests plantar flexion)
- Walk on heels (tests dorsiflexion)
- Walk on lateral border of feet (tests inversion)
- Walk on medial border of feet (tests eversion)
- Hop on injured ankle

Passive, active, and resistive movements should be manually applied to determine joint integrity and muscle function.

**Clinical Prediction Rules for the Ankle Joint**   There is only a single clinical prediction rule that is commonly used for the ankle joint.

- *Ottawa Ankle Rules*[54] were developed to determine the need for radiographs after acute ankle injury secondary to the risk of fracture.

# RECOGNITION OF SPECIFIC INJURIES

## Ankle Injuries

Ankle sprains are the single most common injury in physically active populations including athletes, the military, and performing arts.[37] Appreciation of the anatomy and mechanics of the ankle joint and the pathomechanics and pathophysiology related to acute and chronic ankle instability is integral to the process of effectively evaluating and treating ankle injuries.[41] It is estimated that up to

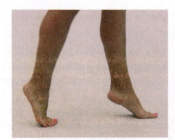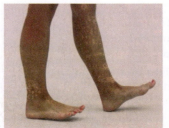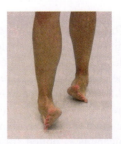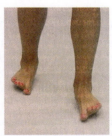

| Toe walking | Heel walking | Lateral walking | Medial walking |

FIGURE 19–20   Evaluating ankle function during walking.

© William E. Prentice

| TABLE 19–3 | Mechanisms of Ankle Sprain and Ligament Injury |
| --- | --- |
| **Mechanisms** | **Structure Injured** |
| Plantar flexion or inversion | Anterior talofibular ligament |
| | Calcaneofibular ligament |
| | Posterior talofibular ligament |
| | Tibiofibular ligament (severe injury) |
| Inversion | Calcaneofibular ligament (along with anterior or posterior talofibular ligament) |
| Dorsiflexion | Tibiofibular ligament |
| Eversion | Deltoid ligament |
| | Tibiofibular ligament (severe injury) |
| | Interosseous membrane (as external rotation increases) |
| | Possible fibular fracture (proximal or distal) |

Modified from from Singer, KM and Jones, DC: Ligament injuries of the ankle and foot. In Nicholas, JA and Hershman, EB (eds): *The lower extremity and spine in sports medicine*, vol. 1, ed. 2, St. Louis: Mosby, 1995

74 percent of patients who sustain an ankle sprain develop chronic ankle instability that results in recurring injury to that ankle and later develops traumatic arthritis.[4,48] Ankle sprains are generally caused by sudden inversion or eversion, often in combination with plantar flexion or dorsiflexion (Table 19–3). Injuries may be classified according to either location or mechanism of injury. The NATA has published a position statement "Conservative management and prevention of ankle sprains in athletes" (www .nata.org/sites/default/files/ankle-sprains.pdf).

**Inversion Ankle Sprains** Inversion ankle sprains represent about 90 percent of all ankle sprains and result in injury to the lateral ligaments. The anterior talofibular ligament is the weakest of the three lateral ligaments. Its major function is to stop forward subluxation of the talus. It is injured in an inverted, plantar flexed, and internally rotated position (Figure 19–21). A complete rupture of the talofibular ligament allows the talus to rotate about it's longitudinal axis in the transverse plane, creating what has been referred to as *rotary ankle instability*.[107] The calcaneofibular and posterior talofibular ligaments may also be injured in inversion sprains as the force of inversion is increased. Increased inversion force is needed to tear the calcaneofibular ligament (Figure 19–22).

Occasionally, an inversion force could be of sufficient magnitude to cause a portion of the bone to be avulsed from the lateral malleolus (Figure 19–23).[88] Also, inversion can cause both an avulsion of the lateral malleolus and a fracture of the medial malleolus. This injury is known as a *bimalleolar fracture* (Pott's fracture).[88] The athletic trainer is often faced with the dilemma of deciding when a patient should be sent to the physician for X-ray to rule out a fracture. The *Ottawa ankle rules* is a valid clinical prediction rule that can be used to decide whether a patient with foot or ankle pain should have a radiograph to diagnose a bone fracture in the malleoli and the midfoot.[34,54,85] SoR:A They are most often used in an emergency room, but the guidelines can be applied by all clinicians.[65] Radiographs are

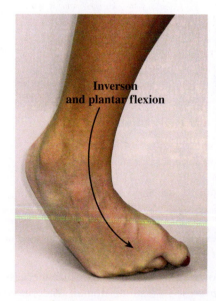

A
Anterolateral view

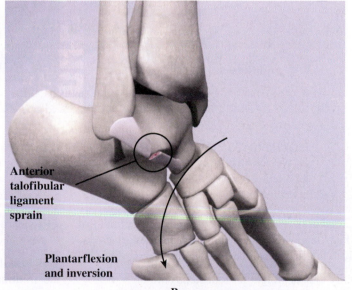

B
Anterolateral view

FIGURE 19–21 A mechanism of injury that involves **(A)** plantar flexion and inversion can cause **(B)** a sprain of the anterior talofibular ligament.
© William E. Prentice

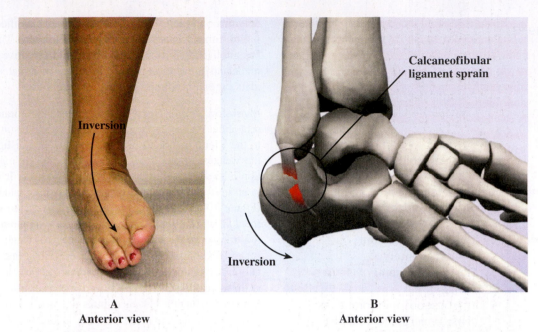

A                          B
Anterior view              Anterior view

FIGURE 19–22   A mechanism of injury that involves **(A)** inversion can cause **(B)** a sprain of the calcaneofibular ligament.

© William E. Prentice

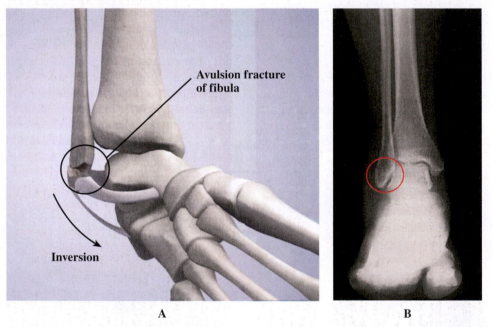

A                                      B

FIGURE 19–23   **(A)** The mechanism that produces an inversion ankle sprain can also cause an avulsion fracture of the fibula. **(B)** X-ray showing fibular avulsion.

(b) Courtesy Jordan B. Renner, MD, Departments of Radiology and Allied Health Sciences, University of North Carolina

only required if there is any pain in the malleolar or midfoot area and any one of the following (note that these rules do *not* apply to injuries more than 10 days old):

- Inability to bear weight for four steps (two on each foot) at the time of injury and at the time of examination
- Tenderness over the inferior or posterior pole of either malleolus, including the distal 6 cm (2.4 inches)

- Tenderness along the base of the fifth metatarsal or navicular bone

The Buffalo modification focuses on tenderness along the midline crest instead of fibular tenderness at the posterior and inferior malleolar edges.[85] However, the Buffalo rules are rarely adopted clinically and the area of point tenderness is very close to those listed for Ottawa.

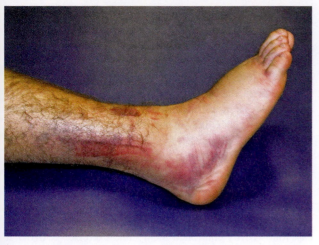

FIGURE 19–24 Typical swelling pattern for an inversion ankle sprain.
© William E. Prentice

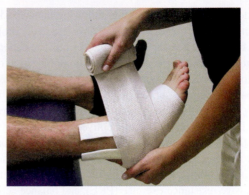

FIGURE 19–25 A horseshoe-shaped pad placed around the malleoleus provides excellent focal compression when held in place by an elastic wrap.
© William E. Prentice

It appears that females are at higher risk for suffering an ankle sprain.[32] A history of ankle sprains is the number one predictor of sustaining an recurrent ankle injury.[49] Patients who have suffered a previous sprain have a decreased risk of reinjury if a brace is worn, and the consensus is that generalized joint laxity and anatomical foot type are not risk factors for ankle sprains. However, the literature is divided on whether height, weight, limb dominance, ankle-joint laxity, and anatomical alignment, muscle strength, and muscle-reaction time are risk factors for ankle sprains.[10] While balance is controversial, the literature is now leaning towards the fact that it is a predictor.[50]

**Grade I Ligament Sprain** The grade 1 ligament sprain is the most common type of sprain. Lateral sprains are probably the most frequent injury in activities in which running and jumping occur.[12]

*Etiology* The severity of ligament sprains is classified according to grades. In each instance, the foot is forcefully inverted, such as when a basketball player jumps and comes down on the foot of another player. Inversion sprains can also occur when an individual is walking or running on an uneven surface or suddenly steps into a hole.

*Symptoms and signs* Mild pain and disability occur. Weight bearing is minimally impaired. Signs are point tenderness and swelling over the ligament with no joint laxity (Figure 19–24).

*Management* Protection, optimal loading, ice, compression, and elevation should be used acutely with ankle injuries to minimize swelling.[11,58] SoR:C POLICE is used for 30 to 60 minutes every 2 hours for 1 to 2 days. Electrical stimulation can also help to minimize swelling during the acute phase.[58] SoR:C Thermotherapy has the potential to exacerbate an injury and should never be used during acute or subacute phases following ankle sprain. The application of a horseshoe pad provides focal compression and may help control edema (Figure 19–25).[89] Some form of immobilization needs to be used to help protect the joint and allow ligament healing to occur.[49] An Air-Stirrup brace with elastic wraps for grade 1 and grade 2 may be the best treatment strategy to prevent long-term pathology.[9] It may be advisable for the patient to limit weight-bearing activities for 1 to 2 days, after which rehabilitation may become more aggressive. Rehabilitation should include comprehensive ROM, flexibility, and strengthening of the surrounding musculature.[10,11,58] SoR:B Early functional rehabilitation has been shown to be more effective than immobilization in managing grades 1 and 2 ankle sprains.[11,58] SoR:A Range of motion exercises and isometric and isotonic strength-training exercises should be included. In the intermediate stage of rehabilitation, a progression of neuromuscular control and balance training exercises should be incorporated, followed by focusing on sport-specific activities to prepare the patient for return to competition. Passive joint mobilizations should be used to specifically increase ankle dorsiflexion and improve function.[58] SoR:B Anterior and posterior mobilization of the talus should begin as soon as tolerable following injury.[20] When the patient returns to weight bearing, application of tape may provide an extra measure of protection.[106] Usually, a patient can return to activity in 7 to 10 days.

**Grade 2 Ligament Sprain** A grade 2 ligament sprain has a high incidence among active individuals and causes a great deal of disability with many days of lost time.[12]

*Etiology* Moderate force on the ankle while it is in a position of inversion, plantar flexion, and/or adduction can cause a grade 2 sprain.

*Symptoms and signs* The patient usually complains of feeling a pop or snap on the lateral side of the ankle. There is moderate pain and disability, weight bearing is difficult, and there is tenderness and edema with blood in the joint. Ecchymosis may occur, as well as a positive talar tilt test. The anterior drawer test elicits slight to moderate abnormal motion.

*Management* POLICE should be used intermittently for at least 72 hours. MRI and CT scans are the most reliable techniques to identify acute ligamentous injuries. Ultrasound is useful, whereas stress radiographs are not reliable.[15,58] SoR:B Anterior and posterior mobilization of the talus should begin as soon as tolerable following injury.[20] The patient should use crutches for 5 to 10 days, gradually progressing to full weight bearing during that period. The patient will need to wear some type of protective immobilization device for 1 to 2 weeks.[12] Plantar flexion and dorsiflexion exercises in a pain-free range should begin 48 hours after the injury occurs. Early movement helps maintain range of motion and normal proprioception. Proprioceptive neuromuscular facilitation (PNF) exercise improves strength, range of motion, and proprioception. Exercise should include isometrics while the ankle is immobilized, followed by range of motion exercises, progressive resistance exercise (PRE), and balance activities to reduce the risk of recurrent ankle sprains lasting at least 4 weeks.[77,90] It has been suggested that protection of healing structures may lead to a more optimal long-term outcome.[23]

Taping using a closed basket weave technique may protect the patient during the early stages of walking (see Figure 8–30). The patient must be instructed to avoid walking or running on uneven surfaces for 2 to 3 weeks after weight bearing has begun. NOTE: The long-term effects of a grade 2 sprain are no more likely to include chronic instability with a recurrence of injury than with any other grade.[42] Over a period of time, this instability can lead to joint degeneration and osteoarthritis. Once a sprain has occurred, the patient must continue to engage in rehabilitative activities to minimize recurrence of injury.[64]

***Grade 3 ligament sprain*** The grade 3 ligament sprain is relatively uncommon. When it does happen, it is extremely disabling. Often, the force causes the ankle to subluxate and then spontaneously reduce.

***Etiology*** The grade 3 sprain is caused by a significant inversion force to the ankle, usually combined with plantar flexion, and adduction. This injury may involve tears to the anterior talofibular, calcaneofibular, or posterior talofibular ligaments as well as the joint capsule.

***Symptoms and signs*** The patient complains of severe pain in the region of the lateral malleolus. Weight bearing is not possible because of the great amount of swelling, with or without pain. Hemarthrosis, discoloration, a positive talar tilt, and a positive anterior drawer test are present.[13] If the anterior talofibular ligament is completely disrupted, rotation of the talus about its long axis in the transverse plane results in what is referred to rotary ankle instability.

***Management*** Normally, POLICE is used intermittently for at least 3 days. Grade 3 sprains should be immobilized for at least 10 days with a rigid stirrup brace or below-knee cast followed by controlled therapeutic exercise.[58] **SoR:B** It is not uncommon for the physician to apply a dorsiflexion cast or weight-bearing walking boot for 3 to 6 weeks, followed by taping for 3 to 6 weeks.[55] Crutches are usually given to the athlete when the cast is removed. Isometric exercise is carried out while the cast is on, followed by range of motion exercises, PRE, and balance exercises. In some cases, surgery is warranted to stabilize the athlete's ankle. NOTE: A grade 3 ankle sprain creates significant joint laxity and instability. Because of this laxity, the ankle joint is prone to degenerative processes. However, chronic ankle instability does not necessarily have a negative effect on functional performance.[23,30]

### Eversion Ankle Sprains

***Etiology*** Eversion ankle sprains represent only about 5 percent to 10 percent of all ankle sprains. The eversion ankle sprain is less common than the inversion ankle sprain, largely because of the bony and ligamentous anatomy (Figure 19–26). As mentioned previously, the fibular

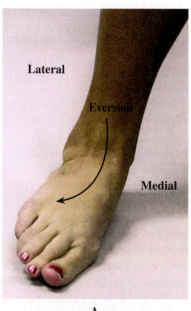
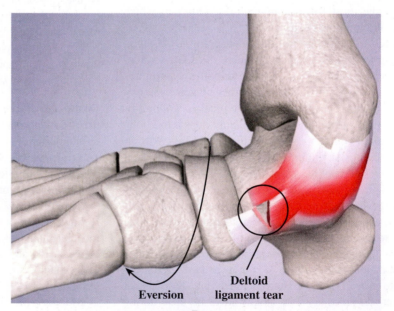

**FIGURE 19–26** A mechanism of injury that involves **(A)** eversion can cause **(B)** a sprain of the deltoid ligament.

(a) © William E. Prentice

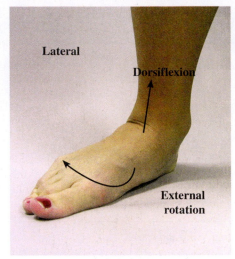

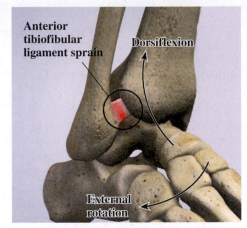

| A | B |
|---|---|
| Anteromedial view | Anterolateral view |

FIGURE 19–27   A mechanism of injury that involves **(A)** hyperdorsiflexion and external rotation of the foot can cause **(B)** a sprain of the anterior tibiofibular ligament.

(a) © William E. Prentice

malleolus extends farther inferiorly than does the tibial malleolus. This protection, combined with the strength of the thick deltoid ligament, prevents excessive eversion. More often, eversion injuries involve an avulsion fracture of the tibia before the deltoid ligament tears.[89] The deltoid ligament may also be contused in inversion sprains due to impingement between the fibular malleolus and the calcaneus. Despite the fact that eversion sprains are less common, they are more severe and may take longer to heal than inversion sprains.

*Symptoms and signs*   Depending on the grade of injury, the patient complains of pain, sometimes severe, that occurs over the foot and lower leg. Usually, the patient is unable to bear weight on the foot. Both abduction and adduction cause pain, but pressing directly upward against the bottom of the foot does not produce pain.

*Management*   X-rays are often necessary to rule out fracture. Initially, POLICE and no weight bearing are recommended. NSAIDs given orally or topically minimize swelling, reduce pain, and improve function following ankle sprain.[73] SoR:A Management of eversion sprain follows the same course as for inversion sprains. The patient engages in a PRE program for the posteromedial ankle muscles, engages in balance activities, and is fitted with an inner heel wedge shoe insert. NOTE: An eversion sprain with a severity of grade 2 or more can produce significant joint instability. Because the deltoid ligament helps support the medial longitudinal arch, a sprain can cause weakness in this area, leading to excessive pronation or a fallen arch.

## Syndesmotic Sprain (High Ankle Sprain)

*Etiology*   Isolated injuries to the distal tibiofibular joint are referred to as syndesmotic sprains,[70,91] or high ankle sprains.[99] The anterior and posterior tibiofibular ligaments are found between the distal tibia and fibula and extend up the lower leg as the interosseous ligament, or syndesmotic ligament. Sprains of the ligaments are more common than has been realized in the past.[33] These ligaments are torn with increased external rotational or forced dorsiflexion and are often injured in conjunction with a severe sprain of the medial and lateral ligament complexes (Figure 19–27).[84] Initial rupture of the ligaments occurs distally at the tibiofibular ligament above the ankle mortise. As the force of disruption is increased, the interosseous ligament is torn more proximally.

*Symptoms and signs*   Evaluation should consist of palpation, functional evaluation, and radiography, with MRI if necessary.[84] SoR:C The patient complains of severe and prolonged pain and loss of function in the ankle region above the talocrural joint, and heterotopic ossification. When the ankle is passively externally rotated or dorsiflexed, there is pain in the lower leg, indicating a syndesmotic sprain or possibly a lateral malleolar fracture. Pain normally occurs along the anterolateral leg.[100]

*Management*   Sprains of the syndesmotic ligaments are extremely hard to treat and often take months to heal.[70] Treatments for this problem are essentially the same as for medial or lateral sprains, with the difference being an extended period of immobilization (nonweight bearing, walking boot, casting, or bracing) for a time period

# MANAGEMENT PLAN

## Grade 2 Inversion Ankle Sprain

**Injury Situation** The patient was crossing the street and stepped off the curb into a pothole, causing a major twist of the left ankle. At the time of injury, the patient felt a severe pain on the lateral aspect of the ankle before he fell to the ground.

**Symptoms and Signs** After the injury, the patient complained of moderate pain on the outside of his left ankle. Initially, it was painful to move the ankle. Walking on the left foot was very difficult. There was moderate tenderness over the lateral aspect of the ankle. Swelling rapidly occurred around the lateral malleoli. The ankle displayed a slight positive talar tilt and a positive anterior drawer test of 4 mm.

---

**Phase 1 Acute Injury**   GOALS: To control hemorrhage, swelling, pain, and spasm.
ESTIMATED LENGTH OF TIME (ELT): 2–3 days.

- **Therapy** Ice packs are applied (20 minutes) intermittently 6 to 8 times daily. X-ray examination rules out fracture. The patient should wear elastic wrap during waking hours and elevate the leg. The leg should also be elevated during sleep. Nonsteroidal antiinflammatory drugs and analgesics should be given. An air splint should be used during this period for support and compression. No weight bearing is allowed. Crutches are used to avoid weight bearing for at least 3 or 4 days or until the patient can walk without a limp with lateral support.
- **Exercise rehabilitation** The patient should begin exercise by toe gripping and spreading if there is no pain (10 to 15 times) every waking hour starting on the second day of injury. General body maintenance exercises should be conducted 3 times a week as long as they do not aggravate the injury.

---

**Phase 2 Repair**   GOALS: To decrease swelling, permit secondary healing to occur, restore full muscle contraction without pain, and restore 50 percent pain-free movement.
ELT: 3 weeks.

- **Therapy** All treatment should be followed immediately by exercise. Ice pack should be used (20 minutes), ice massage (7 minutes), cold whirlpool (60°F, 10 minutes), or massage above and below injury site (5 minutes). When hemorrhage is completely controlled, use whirlpool (90°F to 100°F, 10 to 15 minutes).
- **Exercise rehabilitation** The patient should crutch walk with a toe touch if he or she is unable to walk without a limp while wearing an air cast, tape, or both for 3 weeks. For the first 2 weeks, toe gripping and spreading (10 to 15 times) every waking hour. Active PNF ankle patterns 3 or 4 times daily for a pain-free range of motion. Avoid any exercise that produces pain or swelling. Ankle circumduction (10 to 15 times each direction) 2 or 3 times daily. Achilles tendon stretch from the floor (30 seconds) in each foot position (toe in, toe out, straight ahead) 3 or 4 times daily. Toe raises (10 times, 1 to 3 sets) 3 or 4 times daily. Eversion exercise using a towel or rubber tube or tire resistance 3 or 4 times daily. Shifting body weight between injured and noninjured ankle (up to 20 times 2 or 3 times daily). Wobble board exercise (1 to 3 minutes) 2 or 3 times daily. Progress to straight-ahead short-step walking if it can be done without a limp. General body maintenance exercises are conducted 3 times a week as long as they do not aggravate injury.

---

**Phase 3 Remodeling**   GOALS: To restore symptom-free full range of motion, power, endurance, speed, and agility.
ELT: 3-5 days.

- **Therapy** Therapeutic modalities such as whirlpool (100°F to 105°F) (20 minutes) or ultrasound (0.5 W/cm$^2$ at 100 percent) (5 minutes) should be used symptomatically.
- **Exercise rehabilitation** Achilles tendon stretch using slant board (30 seconds each foot position) 2 or 3 times daily. Toe raises using slant board and resistance (10 repetitions, 1 to 3 sets) 2 or 3 times daily. Resistance ankle device to strengthen anterior, lateral, and medial muscles (starting with 2 lb and progressing to 10 lb) (1 to 3 sets) 2 or 3 times daily. Wobble board for ankle proprioception (begin at 1 minute in each direction; progress to 5 minutes) 3 times daily. Walk-jog routine as long as patient is symptom free: begin with alternate walk-jog-run-walk 25 yards straight ahead, jog 25 yards straight ahead; progress to walk 25 yards in lazy S or to perform 5 figure eights, progress to figure-eight running as fast as possible; progress to run 10 figure eights or Z cuts as fast as possible and to spring up in the air on the injured leg 10 times without pain.

*Criteria for Return to Normal Activity*

1. The ankle is pain free during motion and no swelling is present.
2. The patient has full ankle range of motion and strength.
3. The patient is able to run, jump, and make cutting movements as well as before injury.

sufficient to allow healing and functional return.[3] **SoR:C** Functional activities may be delayed for a longer period of time than for inversion or eversion sprains.[109] It is common for this injury to require surgical fixation in which there is widening of the ankle mortise greater than 2 mm or joint incongruity on standard or stress radiographs.[8] **SoR:C**

**Chronic Ankle Instability** Chronic ankle instability (CAI) develops following about one-third of all acute ankle sprains. A number of instruments, including the Foot and Ankle Ability Measure (FAAM), the Ankle Instability Instrument, and and the Cumberland Ankle Instability Tool (CAIT) have been developed and are used to help identify patients with CAI and quantify the severity of the condition.[29] **SoR:C** A variety of mechanical and neuromuscular factors are thought to contribute to chronic ankle instability.[24,45] Mechanical instability is essentially laxity that physically allows for movement beyond the physiologic limit of the ankle's range of motion. Functional instability is a subjective feeling that the ankle is unstable as a result of recurrent ankle sprains. Functional instability has been attributed to proprioceptive and/or neuromuscular deficits that negatively impact postural control and thus stability and balance.[61] Mechanical and functional deficits may include but are not limited to increased laxity, impaired dorsiflexion ROM, deficient leg and hip strength, diminished postural control, and impaired movement strategies.[58] **SoR:C**

Select manual therapies such as joint mobilization using posterior talar glides have been found to improve postural control.[47,98] Treatment should focus on improving balance, strength, and dynamic movements with changes in direction that can effectively reduce the risk of recurrent ankle sprains in patients with functional deficits.[58,77] **SoR:B**

## Ankle Fracture/Dislocation

*Etiology* There are a number of mechanisms through which an ankle can be fractured or dislocated.[71,89] A foot that is forcibly abducted can produce a transverse fracture of the distal tibia and fibula. In contrast, a foot that is planted in combination with a forced internal rotation of the leg can produce a fracture to the distal and posterior tibia (Figure 19–28).

Avulsion fractures, in which a chip of bone is pulled off by the resistance of a ligament, are common in grades 2 and 3 eversion or inversion sprains.

In a *bimalleolar fracture*, both the medial malleolus of the distal tibia and the lateral malleolus of the distal fibula are fractured.

> A construction worker has a history of numerous lateral ankle sprains.
>
> **?** How can this patient reduce the incidence of these ankle sprains?

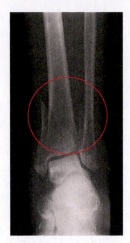

**FIGURE 19–28** Ankle fracture/dislocation.
Courtesy Jordan B. Renner, MD, Departments of Radiology and Allied Health Sciences, University of North Carolina

*Symptoms and signs* In most cases of fracture, swelling and pain are extreme. There may be some or no deformity; however, if a fracture is suspected, splinting is essential.

*Management* POLICE is used as soon as possible to control hemorrhage and swelling. Once swelling is reduced, a walking cast or brace may be applied. Immobilization usually lasts for at least 7 to 9 weeks.[88]

## Osteochondritis Dissecans

*Etiology* Although less common than in the knee, osteochondritis dissecans can occur in the superior medial articular surface of the talar dome. One or several fragments of articular cartilage and its underlying subchondral bone are either partially detached or completely detached and moving within the joint space. The mechanism of injury may be a single trauma, in which case it may be diagnosed as an osteochondral fracture, or it may be due to repeated episodes of ankle sprain.

*Symptoms and signs* Initially, the patient may complain of pain and effusion with signs of progressing atrophy. There may also be complaints of catching, locking, or giving way, particularly if the fragment is detached.

*Management* Diagnosis is usually made by X-ray, although an MRI may also show the articular cartilage overlying the osseous lesion. Incomplete and nondisplaced injuries can be immobilized with early motion and delayed weight bearing until there is evidence of healing.

> A collegiate field hockey player has a history of repeated ankle sprains.
>
> She complains of constant pain and aching and says the ankle feels like it catches when she runs. There also appears to be some mild effusion.
>
> **?** What might the athletic trainer suspect is wrong, and how should this injury be managed?

**19–3 Clinical Application Exercise**

If the fragment is displaced, surgery is recommended to excise the fragment and minimize the risk of nonunion.

## Lower Leg Injuries

### Achilles Tendon Strain

***Etiology*** Achilles tendon strains are common in sports and occur most often after ankle sprains or sudden excessive dorsiflexion of the ankle.

***Symptoms and signs*** The resulting injury may be mild to severe. The most severe injury is a partial or complete avulsion or rupturing of the Achilles tendon. While sustaining this injury, the patient feels acute pain and extreme weakness on plantar flexion.

**19–4 Clinical Application Exercise**

A tennis player sustains a grade 2 ligament sprain of the lateral ankle while making a sudden stop.

**?** Assuming good immediate care was carried out, how should this condition be managed 10 days after injury?

***Management*** Initially, as with other acute conditions, pressure is first applied with an elastic wrap together with the application of cold. Unless the injury is minor, hemorrhage may be extensive, requiring POLICE over an extended period of time. After hemorrhaging has subsided, an elastic wrap should be applied for continued pressure. Because of the tendency for acute Achilles tendon trauma to become a chronic condition, a conservative approach to therapy is required. The patient should begin stretching and strengthening the heel cord complex as soon as possible. A lift should be placed in the heel of each shoe to decrease stretching of the tendon and thus relieve some stress that contributes to chronic inflammation.

### Achilles Tendinopahy

***Etiology*** Achilles tendinopathies may include both tendinitis, tenosynovitis, or tendinosis. Achilles *tendinitis* is an inflammatory condition that involves the Achilles tendon and/or its tendon sheath (the paratenon), in which case the condition is referred to as Achilles *tenosynovitis*. Achilles tendonitis or tenosynovitis cause fibrosis and scarring that can restrict the Achilles tendon's motion within the tendon sheath. Achilles tendonitis or tenosynovitis can occur along with, or lead to, Achilles *tendinosis*. The vast majority of people with Achilles tendon pain have Achilles tendinosis, rather than Achilles

**19–5 Clinical Application Exercise**

A maintenance worker jumps down off a ladder and lands on a hammer, forcing her ankle into dorsiflexion and external rotation.

**?** What type of injury is sustained by this mechanism? What is a characteristic sign of this injury?

tendinitis or tenosynovitis.[2] With Achilles tendinosis, there is no evidence of inflammation, unlike tendinits or tenosynovitis. The injured areas of the Achilles tendon lose their normal appearance, and the collagen fibers that make up the Achilles tendon show that the cells are disorganized, scarred, and degenerated.[2] While many of the symptoms of tendinitis, tenosynovitis, and tendinosis are the same, Achilles tendinosis is a soreness and stiffness that comes on gradually and continues to worsen until treated. Often, the tendon is overloaded because of excessive tensile stress placed on it during movements of a repetitive nature, such as running or jumping. The condition worsens with repetitive weight-bearing activities, such as running or early-season conditioning in which the duration and intensity are increased too quickly with insufficient recovery time. Decreased gastrocnemius and soleus complex flexibility can also increase symptoms.

***Symptoms and signs*** The patient often complains of generalized pain and stiffness about the Achilles tendon region that, when localized, is usually just proximal to the calcaneal insertion. Uphill running or hill workouts usually aggravate the condition. There may be reduced gastrocnemius and soleus muscle flexibility in general that may worsen as the condition progresses. Muscle testing may show a deficit when the patient performs toe raises. Initially, the patient may ignore symptoms that present at the beginning of activity and resolve as the activity progresses. Symptoms may progress to morning stiffness and discomfort with walking after periods of prolonged sitting. The tendon may be warm and painful to palpation as well as thickened, which may indicate the chronicity of the condition. Crepitus may be palpated with active plantar flexion and dorsiflexion, and pain is elicited with passive stretching. Chronic inflammation of the Achilles tendon may lead to thickening when compared with the uninvolved side (Figure 19–29).[46]

***Management*** Achilles tendinosis may be resistant to a quick resolution because of the slower healing response of tendinous tissue. It is important to create a proper healing environment by reducing stress on the tendon. Proper shoeware and foot orthotics should be worn to address structural faults that may be causing the irritation, and flexibility exercises should be performed for the heel cord complex. Modalities such as ice can help reduce pain and inflammation early on, and ultrasound can facilitate an increased blood flow to the tendon in the later stages of rehabilitation. It appears that eccentric exercises have a high level of evidence as a treatment for Achilles

A 35-year-old racquetball player, while moving backward, experiences a sudden snap and pain in the left Achilles tendon.

**?** What type of injury does this mechanism describe, and how should it be examined?

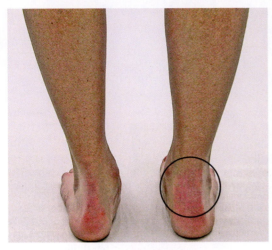

FIGURE 19–29   A thickened Achilles tendon caused by tendinosis.
© William E. Prentice

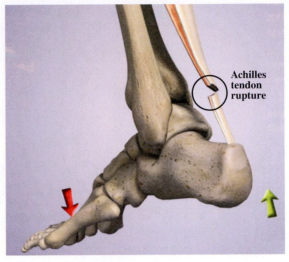

FIGURE 19–30   Achilles tendon rupture involves tearing and separation of fibers.

tendinopathy.[69] Cross-friction massage may be used to break down adhesions that may have formed during the healing response and to further improve the gliding ability of the paratenon. Strengthening of the gastrocnemius-soleus musculature must be progressed carefully so as not to cause a recurrence of the symptoms.[46]

**Achilles Tendon Rupture**   A rupture of the Achilles tendon (Figure 19–30) is possible in activities that require stop-and-go action. Although most common in athletes who are 30 years of age or older, rupture of the Achilles tendon can occur in individuals of any age.[82] It usually occurs in an individual with a history of chronic inflammation and gradual degeneration caused by microtears.[2]

*Etiology*   The initial insult normally is the result of a sudden pushing-off action of the forefoot, with the knee being forced into complete extension.[22]

> A ruptured Achilles tendon may occur because of chronic inflammation.

*Symptoms and signs*   When the rupture occurs, the patient complains of a sudden snap that felt like something kicked him or her in the lower leg. Pain is immediate but rapidly subsides. Point tenderness, swelling, and discoloration are usually associated with the trauma. Toe raising is impossible in an Achilles tendon rupture. The major problem in Achilles tendon rupture is accurate diagnosis, especially in a partial rupture. Any acute injury to the Achilles tendon should be suspected to be a rupture. Signs indicative of a rupture are obvious indentation at the tendon site and a positive Thompson test (see Figure 19–12). An Achilles tendon rupture usually occurs 0.78 to 2.34 inches (2 to 6 cm) proximal to its insertion onto the calcaneus.

*Management*   Usual management of a complete Achilles tendon rupture is surgical repair.[22] Nonoperative treatment consists of POLICE, NSAIDs, and analgesics with a non–weight-bearing cast for 6 weeks, followed by a short-leg walking cast for 2 weeks. With this approach, there is 75 to 80 percent return of normal function.[82] Surgery is usually the choice for serious injuries, providing 75 to 90 percent return of function.[60] Exercise rehabilitation lasts for about 6 months and consists of range of motion exercises, PRE, and the wearing a heel lift in both shoes.[82]

**Fibularis Tendon Subluxation/Dislocation**   The fibularis longus and brevis tendons pass through a common groove located behind the lateral malleolus. The tendons are held in place by the fibularis retinaculum.

*Etiology*   This injury most often occurs in activities that apply dynamic forces to the foot and ankle (e.g., turning and sharply cutting).[46] Wrestling, football, ice skating, skiing, basketball, and soccer have the highest incidence. Another mechanism is a direct blow to the posterior lateral malleolus. A moderate to severe inversion sprain or forceful dorsiflexion of the ankle can tear the fibularis retinaculum, allowing the fibularis tendon to dislocate out of its groove. Occasionally, the fibularis tendon ruptures instead of simply subluxing. As discussed previously, one of the major functions of the fibularis longus muscle is to pull the first metatarsal into plantar flexion.

*Symptoms and signs*   The patient complains that in running or jumping the tendons snap out of the groove and then back in when stress is released. Eversion against manual resistance will often replicate the subluxation. The patient experiences recurrent pain, snapping, and ankle instability. The lateral aspect of the ankle may show ecchymoses, edema, tenderness, and crepitus over the peroneal tendon.

> A volleyball player with a history of repeated ankle sprains complains of a snapping sensation in the right ankle.
>
> ? What procedures should be followed when managing a subluxated peroneal tendon?

19–7 Clinical Application Exercise

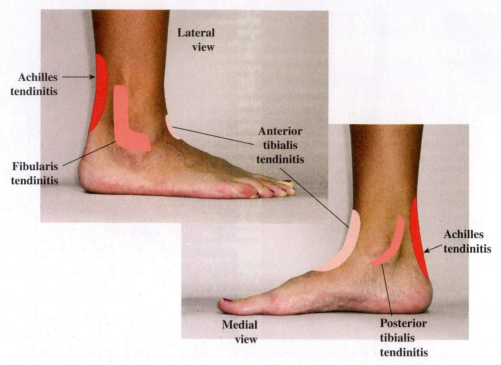

FIGURE 19–31   Common sites of tendinitis around the ankle.
© William E. Prentice

***Management***   A conservative approach should be used first and should include compression with a felt pad cut in a horseshoe-shaped pattern that surrounds the lateral malleolus. This compression can be reinforced with a rigid plastic or plaster splint until acute signs have subsided, and POLICE, NSAIDs, and analgesics are given as needed. The time period for this conservative care is 5 to 6 weeks, followed by a gradual exercise rehabilitation program that includes range of motion exercises, PRE, and balance training. If a conservative approach fails, surgery is required.[46]

### Anterior Tibialis Tendinitis

***Etiology***   Anterior tibialis tendinitis is a common condition in individuals who run downhill for an extended period of time.

***Symptoms and signs***   There is point tenderness over the anterior tibialis tendon (Figure 19–31). The patient complains of pain when the tendon is stretched or when the muscle is contracted.

***Management***   The patient should be advised to rest (or at least decrease running time and distance) and to avoid hills. In more serious cases, ice packs, coupled with stretching before and after running, should help reduce the symptoms. A daily strengthening program also should be conducted. Oral antiinflammatory medications may be required.

### Posterior Tibialis Tendinitis

***Etiology***   Posterior tibialis tendinitis is a common overuse condition among runners with hypermobility or pronated feet. It is a repetitive microtrauma occurring during pronation in movements such as jumping, running, and cutting.[38]

***Symptoms and signs***   The patient complains of pain and swelling in the area of the medial malleolus (Figure 19–31). Inspection reveals edema and point tenderness directly behind the medial malleolus. In serious cases, the pain becomes more intense during resistive inversion and plantar flexion.[38]

***Management***   Initially, POLICE, NSAIDs, and analgesics are given as needed. A non–weight-bearing short-leg cast with the foot in inversion may be used. Management consists of correcting the problem of pronation with LowDye taping or an orthotic device.

### Fibularis Tendinitis

***Etiology***   Although not particularly common, fibularis tendinitis can be a problem in individuals with pes cavus. In pes cavus, the foot tends to supinate excessively, which causes weight bearing on the outside of the foot, placing stress on the peroneal tendon.[46]

***Symptoms and signs***   The patient complains of pain behind the lateral malleolus when rising on the ball of the foot during jogging, running, cutting, or turning activities.

A jogger, after running downhill for an extended period of time, experiences pain in the anterior medial aspect of the left foot. The condition is diagnosed as anterior tibialis tendinitis.

**?** How should this condition be managed?

Tenderness is noted over the tendon located at the lateral aspect of the calcaneus distally to beneath the cuboid bone (Figure 19–31).[46]

*Management* Initially, management consists of POLICE and NSAIDs as required, taping with elastic tape, and appropriate warm-up and flexibility exercises. LowDye taping (see Figure 8–24) or an orthosis to help support the foot and prevent excessive supination may help.

### Shin Contusion

*Etiology* The anterior aspect of the lower leg is often referred to as the shin. The tibia, lying just under the skin, is exceedingly vulnerable and sensitive to blows and bumps. Because of the absence of muscular or adipose padding, the periosteum receives the full force of any impact delivered to the shin. The periosteum is a membrane that surrounds all bony surfaces except articulating surfaces, which are covered by hyaline cartilage. The periosteum is composed of two fibrous layers that adhere closely to the bone and act as a bed for nerves, blood vessels, and bone-forming osteoblasts.

> A forceful blow to an unprotected shin can lead to a severe contusion.

*Symptoms and signs* The patient complains of intense pain when the shin is contused. A hematoma forms rapidly and tends to exhibit a jellylike consistency.[105] There could also be an associated compartment syndrome, particularly in the anterior compartment, as well as a potential tibial fracture.

*Management* POLICE, NSAIDs, and analgesics are administered as needed. Maintaining compression in the area of the hematoma is critical. In some cases, the hematoma may need to be aspirated. The patient should perform range of motion and PRE exercises within pain limitations. The patient should be fitted with a doughnut padding under an orthoplast shell for protection.[46]

An inappropriately managed injury to the periosteum may develop into osteomyelitis, a serious condition that results in the destruction and deterioration of bone (Figure 19–32).

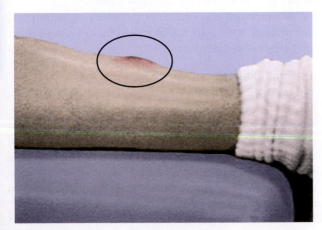

**FIGURE 19–32** A poorly cared-for shin bruise can lead to osteomyelitis.
© William E. Prentice

In sports such as football and soccer, in which the shin is particularly vulnerable, adequate protective padding should be used. All injuries in this area are potentially serious; therefore, even minor shin bruises should never be permitted to go untended.

### Muscle Contusions

*Etiology* Contusions of the leg, particularly in the area of the gastrocnemius muscle, are common in sports. Most often, contusions occur from being kicked in the back of the leg.[46]

*Symptoms and signs* A bruise in this area can produce an extremely handicapping injury for the patient. A bruising blow to the leg causes pain, weakness, and partial loss of the use of the limb. Palpation may reveal a hard, rigid, and somewhat inflexible area because of internal hemorrhage and muscle guarding.

*Management* When this condition occurs, it is advisable to stretch the muscles in the region immediately to prevent spasm and then to apply a compression wrap and ice to control internal hemorrhaging.

If cold therapy or other superficial therapy, such as massage and whirlpool, do not return the athlete to normal activity within 2 to 3 days, the use of ultrasound may be warranted. An elastic wrap or tape support will stabilize the part and permit the athlete to participate without aggravating the injury.

**Leg Cramps and Spasms** Spasms are sudden, violent, involuntary contractions of one or several muscles and may be either clonic or tonic. A *clonic* spasm is identified by intermittent contraction and relaxation. A *tonic* spasm is identified by constant muscle contraction without an intervening period of relaxation. The clonic spasm has a neurological basis and is seen less often in sports.

*Etiology* The specific cause of a muscle cramp is often difficult to determine. Fatigue, excess loss of fluid through sweating, and inadequate reciprocal muscle coordination are some of the factors that predispose an individual to tonic muscle spasm. The gastrocnemius muscle is particularly prone to this condition.[46]

*Symptoms and signs* The patient has considerable muscle cramping and pain with the tonic contraction of the calf muscle.

*Management* Management in such cases includes trying to help the patient relax to relieve the muscle cramp. A firm grasp of the contracted muscle, together with mild, gradual stretching, relieves most acute spasms. An ice pack or gentle ice massage may also be helpful in reducing

**19–9 Clinical Application Exercise**

A football running back receives a hard, low tackle. He hears a loud pop and feels a sharp pain in his right lower leg. Weight bearing is impossible.

? In this situation, what type of injury is suspected?

A gymnast complains of pain in the medial aspect of her right tibia. There is pain before, during, and after activity. Assessment rules out a stress fracture, and the injury is diagnosed as medial tibial stress syndrome (MTSS).

**?** What could be the cause of this condition?

spasm. In cases of recurrent spasm, the athletic trainer should make certain that fatigue or abnormal water or electrolyte loss is not a factor.

### Gastrocnemius Strain

*Etiology* The medial head of the gastrocnemius is particularly susceptible to muscle strain near its musculotendinous attachment. Activities that require quick starts and stops or occasional jumping can cause this gastrocnemius strain. Usually, the patient makes a quick stop with the foot planted flat and suddenly extends the knee, placing stress on the medial head of the gastrocnemius (Figure 19–33). "Tennis leg" is a rupture or tear at the musculotendinous juncture of the gastrocnemius and the Achilles tendon.[46]

*Symptoms and signs* Depending on the grade of injury, there is a variable amount of pain, swelling, and muscle disability. The patient may complain of a sensation of having been "hit in the calf with a stick." Examination reveals edema, point tenderness, and a functional strength loss.[13]

*Management* Initially, POLICE, NSAIDs, and analgesics are given as needed. A grade 1 calf strain should be given a gentle, gradual stretch after muscle cooling. Weight bearing can take place as tolerated. A heel wedge may help reduce stretching of the calf muscle during walking. Appropriate elastic wrap may support the muscle while active. A gradual program of range of motion exercises and PRE should be instituted.

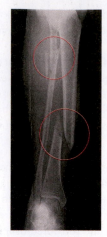

FIGURE 19–34 Midshaft fracture of both the tibia and fibula.

Courtesy Jordan B. Renner, MD, Departments of Radiology and Allied Health Sciences, University of North Carolina

### Acute Leg Fractures

*Etiology* Of all leg fractures, the fibular fracture has the highest incidence. It occurs principally in the middle third, whereas fractures of the tibia occur predominantly in the lower third. Fractures of the shaft of both the tibia and the fibula result from either direct or indirect trauma (Figure 19–34). There may be bony displacement with deformity that results in overriding of the bone ends, particularly if the athlete attempts to move or to stand on the limb after the injury. Crepitus and a temporary loss of limb function are usually present.

*Symptoms and signs* This injury causes soft-tissue insult and hemorrhaging. The patient complains of severe pain and disability. The leg appears hard and swollen, which may indicate the beginning of Volkmann's contracture. Volkmann's contracture is the result of internal tension caused by hemorrhage and swelling within closed fascial compartments, which inhibits the blood supply and results in muscle necrosis and contractures.

*Management* In most cases, fracture reduction and cast immobilization are applied up to 6 weeks, depending on the extent of the injury and any complications.

### Medial Tibial Stress Syndrome

*Etiology* Medial tibial stress syndrome (MTSS) has in the past been referred to as *shinsplints*, which is a catch-all term that indicates pain in the anterior part of the shin (Figure 19–35). Conditions such as stress fractures, muscle strains, and chronic anterior compartment syndromes have all been termed shinsplints.[46] MTSS accounts for approximately 10 to 15 percent of all running injuries and up to 60 percent of all conditions that cause pain in athletes' legs.[50] MTSS is caused by a repetitive microtrauma. It is seen commonly in running and jumping activities. Factors that can contribute to MTSS include weakness of leg muscles, shoes that provide little support or cushioning, and training

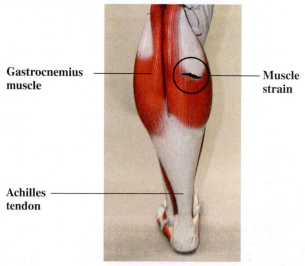

Gastrocnemius muscle

Muscle strain

Achilles tendon

FIGURE 19–33 Gastrocnemius strain.

© William E. Prentice

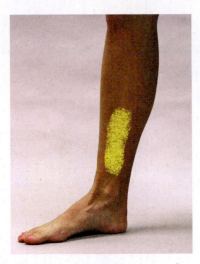

FIGURE 19–35   In medial tibial stress syndrome, the pain is usually located on the medial aspect of the lower leg just posterior to the tibia (shaded area). Pain is most often associated with the posterior tibialis muscle.

© William E. Prentice

errors, such as running on hard surfaces and overtraining.[7] Malalignment problems, such as varus foot, a tight heel cord, a hypermobile pronated foot, or a forefoot supination, can also lead to MTSS.[50]

MTSS involves one of two syndromes: a tibial stress fracture or an overuse syndrome that can progress to an irreversible, exertional compartment syndrome.[7]

***Symptoms and signs***   Four grades of pain can be attributed to medial tibial stress syndrome: grade 1 pain occurring after activity; grade 2 pain occurring before and after activity, but not affecting performance; grade 3 pain occurring before, during, and after activity and affecting performance; and grade 4 pain, so severe that activity is impossible.

***Management***   Management of this condition is difficult, because there are so many factors that can collectively contribute to the development of medial tibial stress syndrome. Physician referral to rule out the possibility of stress fracture via the use of bone scans and X-rays is recommended. Activity modification along with measures to maintain cardiovascular fitness should be set in place immediately. Correction of abnormal pronation during walking and running must also be addressed with shoes and, if needed, custom foot orthotics. Ice massage to the area may be helpful in the reduction of localized pain and inflammation. A flexibility program for the gastrocnemius-soleus musculature should be initiated. Arch taping and circumferential tape applied around the area of pain may also be used.

## Compartment Syndromes

***Etiology***   Compartment syndromes are conditions in which increased pressure within one of the four compartments of the lower leg causes compression of muscular and neurovascular structures within that compartment (see Figure 19–6). The anterior and deep posterior compartments are usually involved.[104]

Compartment syndromes can be divided into three categories: acute compartment syndrome, acute exertional compartment syndrome, and chronic compartment syndrome.[17] *Acute compartment syndrome* occurs secondary to direct trauma to the area, such as being kicked in the anterior aspect of the lower leg. Acute compartment syndrome is considered to be a medical emergency because of the possibility of compression of the arterial and nerve supply, which could result in additional injury to structures distal to the compartment. *Acute exertional compartment syndrome* occurs without any precipitating trauma and can evolve with minimal to moderate activity.[92] *Chronic compartment syndrome* is activity related in that the symptoms arise rather consistently at a certain point in the activity. Chronic compartment syndrome usually occurs during running and jumping activities, and symptoms cease when activity stops.[17,104]

***Symptoms and signs***   Because of the increased intracompartmental pressure associated with compartment syndromes, the athlete complains of a deep, aching pain; tightness and swelling of the involved compartment; and pain with passive stretching of the involved muscles. Reduced circulation and sensory changes can be detected in the foot. Intracompartmental pressure measurements further define the severity of the condition. A compartment syndrome that is not recognized, diagnosed, and treated properly can lead to a poor functional outcome for the patient.[104]

***Management***   Immediate first aid for acute compartment syndrome should include the application of ice and elevation. However, in this situation a compression wrap should not be used to control swelling because there is already a problem with increased pressure in the compartment. Using a compression wrap only increases the pressure.

In the case of both acute compartment syndrome and acute exertional compartment syndrome, measurement of intracompartmental pressures by a physician confirms the diagnosis, with emergency fasciotomy to release the pressure within that compartment being

> Chronic exertional compartment syndrome occurs most commonly in runners, whereas acute compartment syndrome occurs in soccer players.

the definitive treatment. Patients undergoing anterior or deep posterior compartment fasciotomy may not return to full activity for 2 to 4 months postsurgery.[21]

Management of chronic compartment syndrome is initially conservative, with activity modification, icing, and stretching of the anterior compartment musculature and heel cord complex. If conservative measures fail, fasciotomy of the affected compartments has shown favorable results in a patient's return to higher levels of activity.

## Stress Fracture of the Tibia or Fibula

***Etiology***   Stress fractures of the tibia or fibula are a common overuse stress condition, especially among distance runners (Figure 19–36). Stress fractures of the lower leg, like many other overuse syndromes, are more likely

# MANAGEMENT PLAN

## Medial Tibial Stress Syndrome

**Injury Situation** A female college field hockey player at the end of the competitive season began to feel severe discomfort in the medial aspect of the right shin.

**Symptoms and Signs** The patient complained that her shin seemed to ache all the time, but the pain became more intense after practice or a game. During palpation, there was severe point tenderness approximately 2 inches (5 cm) in length, beginning 4½ inches (11.25 cm) from the tip of the medial malleolus. The pain was most severe along the medial posterior edge of the tibia. Further evaluation showed that the athlete had pronated feet. X-ray examination showed no indication of stress fracture.

**Management Plan** The injury was considered to be a medial tibial stress syndrome (shinsplints) involving the long flexor muscle, the great toe, and the posterior tibial muscle.

### Phase 1 Acute Injury
**GOALS:** To reduce inflammation, pain, and point tenderness.
**ESTIMATED LENGTH OF TIME (ELT):** 1–2 weeks.

- **Therapy** Initially POLICE, NSAIDs, and analgesics should be given as needed. The patient should be instructed to rest and avoid weight bearing as much as possible. Ice massage (7 minutes) should be performed, followed by gentle static stretching to the anterior and posterior muscles 2 or 3 times daily. LowDye taping or an orthotic device should be applied to the arch to correct pronation during weight bearing.
- **Exercise rehabilitation** Static stretch of Achilles tendon and anterior part of low leg; stretch is held 30 seconds (2 or 3 times); set should be repeated 3 or 4 times daily. General body maintenance exercises should be conducted 3 times weekly if they do not aggravate injury.

### Phase 2 Repair
**GOALS:** To heal injury, help athlete become symptom free, return athlete to walking, jogging, and, finally, running.
**ELT:** 2–3 weeks.

- **Therapy** Cold application (20 minutes) to shin area before and after walking 1 time daily. Activity should be stopped if there is shin pain. Ultrasound (0.5 to 0.075 W/cm² at 100%) (5 to 10 minutes) 1 or 2 times daily. Transverse friction massage should be given to prevent adhesions. The athlete should wear LowDye taping or orthoses when weight bearing. A counterforce bracing with tape also should be worn 2 to 4 inches (5 to 10 cm) proximal to the malleoli.
- **Exercise rehabilitation** Ankle range of motion exercises plus PRE with rubber tubing to the anterior and posterior leg muscles. Static stretch of lower leg followed by arch and plantar flexion exercises. Towel gathering exercise (10 repetitions, 1 to 3 sets); progress from no resistance to 10 lb of resistance, 3 times daily. Towel scoop exercise (10 repetitions, 1 to 3 sets); progress to 10 lb, 3 times daily. Marble pickup, 3 times daily. General body maintenance exercises should be conducted 3 times weekly if they do not aggravate injury. The patient should engage in a program of progressive weight bearing and locomotion within pain-free limits, starting with slow heel-toe walking, fast walking, jogging, and, finally, running. As pain decreases, activity can increase.

### Phase 3 Remodeling
**GOALS:** To return to full-field hockey activity.
**ELT:** 3–6 weeks.

- **Therapy** The patient should carry out cryokinetics before and after practice. The patient should continue to wear counterforce brace and LowDye taping or orthoses for foot pronation.
- **Exercise rehabilitation** The patient should continue a daily program of lower leg static stretch after ice application before and after activity. The patient should carry out a program of ankle range of motion exercises and lower leg PRE 3 days a week.

#### Criteria for Return to Competitive Field Hockey

1. The leg is symptom free after prolonged activity.
2. The ankle and lower leg have full strength and range of motion.
3. Hyperpronation is controlled to prevent reoccurrence.

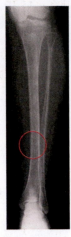

FIGURE 19–36   Tibial stress fracture.

Courtesy Jordan B. Renner, MD, Departments of Radiology and
Allied Health Sciences, University of North Carolina

A soccer player complains of recurrent pain in the anterolateral region of the leg during practice and competition. The pain is described as an ache and a feeling of pressure.

❔ This condition is determined to be an exertional compartment syndrome. How should it be managed?

A novice and poorly conditioned recreational runner with a pes cavus experiences pain and discomfort in the lower third of the left lower leg after 3 weeks of running. The pain and discomfort become more intense immediately after running.

❔ An X-ray shows the beginning of a stress fracture. How should it be managed?

to occur in individuals who have structural deformities of the foot. Individuals who have hypermobile pronated feet are more susceptible to fibular stress fracture, whereas those with rigid pes cavus are more prone to tibial stress fractures. The wider the tibia, the lower the incidence of stress fractures. Runners frequently develop a stress fracture in the lower third of the leg; ballet dancers more commonly acquire one in the middle third. Stress fractures often occur in inexperienced and nonconditioned individuals.[21] Training errors are often the cause.[21] Other causes include amenorrhea and nutritional deficiencies.

*Symptoms and signs*
The patient complains of pain in the leg that is more intense after than during the activity. There is usually point tenderness, but it may be difficult to discern the difference between bone pain and soft-tissue pain. One technique for distinguishing bone pain from soft-tissue pain is bone percussion. The fibula or tibia is tapped firmly above the level of tenderness. Vibration

travels along the bone to the fracture, which may respond with pain. Another percussive technique is to hit the heel upward from below, which causes pain to occur at the fracture site.

Diagnosis of a stress fracture may be extremely difficult. X-ray examination may or may not detect the problem. A bone scan will more accurately assess the presence of a stress fracture but does not clearly distinguish between a stress fracture and periostitis (inflammation of the periosteum).

*Management*   As in medial tibial stress syndrome, because it is not clear exactly what causes a stress fracture, this condition is very difficult to treat. The following regimen may be used for a stress fracture of the tibia or fibula: The patient should discontinue running and other stressful locomotor activities for at least 14 days. When pain is severe, the patient should use a crutch for walking or wear a cast. The patient may resume weight bearing as pain subsides. The patient may bicycle before returning to running. After a pain-free period of at least 2 weeks, the patient can gradually begin running again.[21] Biomechanical foot corrections should be made using orthotics.

# REHABILITATION TECHNIQUES FOR THE ANKLE AND LOWER LEG
## General Body Conditioning

The injured patient should maintain cardiorespiratory conditioning during the entire rehabilitation process. Pedaling a stationary bike or using an upper-extremity ergometer with the hands provides the patient with excellent cardiovascular exercise without placing stress on the lower leg or ankle (Figure 19–37). Swimming and pool running with a float vest are also good cardiovascular exercises.

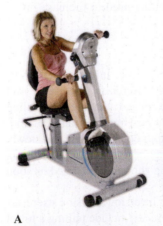
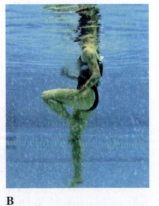

A                                    B

FIGURE 19–37   Non–weight-bearing exercises to maintain cardiorespiratory endurance can be done (A) on an upper-extremity ergometer or (B) in an exercise pool.

(a) Stamina Products, Inc.; (b) © William E. Prentice

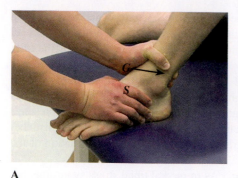 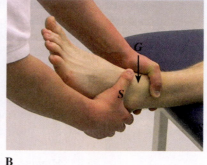 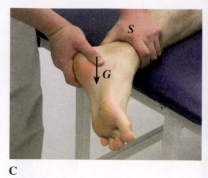

A B C

FIGURE 19–38   Ankle joint mobilization techniques. **(A)** Posterior tibial glides. **(B)** Posterior talar glides. **(C)** Subtalar joint medial and lateral glides. (S = stabilize, G = glide)

© William E. Prentice

## Weight Bearing

During the period of maximum protection immediately following injury, the patient should be either non–weight bearing or partial weight bearing on crutches. Early limited stress following the initial period of inflammation may promote faster and stronger healing.[89] Partial weight bearing with crutches helps control several complications to healing, including muscle atrophy, proprioceptive loss, circulatory stasis, and tendinitis.[72] For these reasons, early ambulation, even if only touch-down weight bearing, is essential.[67] Protected motion facilitates proper collagen reorientation and thus increases the strength of the healing ligament.

## Joint Mobilizations

Movement of an injured joint can be improved by manual joint mobilization techniques (Figure 19–38). Joint mobilizations that concentrate on increasing dorsiflexion and plantar flexion should be started first.[20] Posterior tibial glides and anterior talar glides can be used to improve plantar flexion. Anterior tibial glides and posterior talar glides increase dorsiflexion. Subtalar joint medial and lateral glides can be used to increase inversion and eversion.

## Flexibility

In the early stages of rehabilitation, inversion and eversion should be minimized. Exercises such as towel stretching for the plantar flexors and standing or kneeling stretches for the dorsiflexors can improve range of motion. Patients are encouraged to do these exercises slowly and without pain and to use high repetitions (two sets of 40). Vigorous heel cord stretching should be initiated as soon as possible (Figure 19–39).[110]

As tenderness decreases, inversion-eversion exercises may be initiated.[110] Such exercises include pulling a towel from one side to the other by alternately inverting and everting the foot and drawing the alphabet while the foot is in an ice bath. The alphabet should be done in capital letters to ensure that full range is used.

## Neuromuscular Control

Exercises performed on an unstable surface (BAPS board, wedge board, or Dynadisc) may be beneficial for range of motion and for regaining neuromuscular control.[61] The patient begins these exercises seated and progresses to standing (Figure 19–40). Initially, the patient should start in the seated position and move a wedge board in the sagittal plane (plantar flexion–dorsiflexion). As pain decreases and healing progresses, the board may be turned in the frontal planes (inversion-eversion). When seated exercises are performed with ease, standing balance exercises should be initiated. They may be started with the patient on one leg, standing, without a board. The patient then supports weight with the hands and maintains balance on a wedge board in either the sagittal (plantar flexion–dorsiflexion) or frontal plane (inversion–eversion). Next, hand support may be eliminated while the patient balances on the wedge board. The same sequence is then used on the BAPS board. The BAPS board is initially used with assistance from the hands. Then balance is practiced on the BAPS board unassisted.

Early weight bearing has previously been mentioned as a method of reducing proprioceptive loss. It has been shown that deficits in ankle proprioception can predispose an individual to ankle injury.[26,108] Changes in joint position sense and kinesthesia of a magnitude found in subjects with chronically unstable ankles can lead to an increased risk of lateral ankle sprains. Results from a small number of studies suggest that balance and coordination training can restore the increased uncertainty of joint positioning to normal.[62]

## Balance and Postural Stability

Balance training should be performed throughout rehabilitation and follow-up management to reduce reinjury rates.[58,77] **SoR:A** During rehabilitation, a patient can recoup balance by standing on both feet with eyes closed and progressing to standing on one leg.[96] This exercise may be followed by standing and balancing on a BAPS board, Bosu Balance Trainer, Rocker board, Tremor box, minitramp, or Dynadisc,

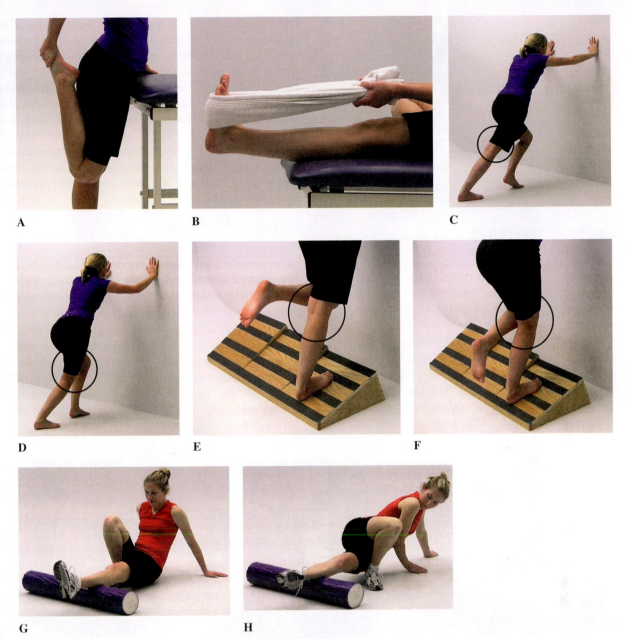

**FIGURE 19–39** Stretching exercises. **(A)** Standing dorsiflexor stretch. **(B)** Gastrocnemius towel stretch (knee straight). **(C)** Gastrocnemius wall stretch (knee straight). **(D)** Soleus wall stretch (knee flexed). **(E)** Gastrocnemius slant board stretch (knee straight). **(F)** Soleus slant board stretch (knee flexed). **(G)** Gastrocnemius myofascial stretch. **(H)** Fibularis myofascial stretch.
© William E. Prentice

which should be done initially with support from the hands (Figure 19–41).[39] As a final exercise, the patient can progress to free standing. Regaining control of balance is key in ankle rehabilitation.[95,96] It is particularly important for patients who have chronic ankle instability.[98] Postural control is significantly impaired with ankle sprain and may require 2 to 4 weeks to return to normal.[42,103] It has been shown that the longer a patient with an ankle sprain continues to do balance exercises the lower the risk of sustaining recurrent sprains.[6]

Other closed kinetic chain exercises may be beneficial. Leg presses and minisquats (Figure 19–42) on the involved leg encourage weight bearing and increase proprioceptive return.[31] Single-leg standing kicks using abduction, adduction, extension, and flexion of the uninvolved side while weight bearing on the affected side increase both balance and proprioception. These kicks may be performed with the patient either standing free or on a machine (Figure 19–43).

### Strengthening

Strengthening techniques should concentrate on achieving a balance in the muscle groups surrounding the ankle.[56] Isometric strengthening exercises may be done

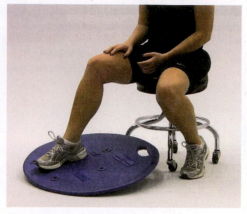

FIGURE 19–40 Seated BAPS board exercises are used for reestablishing neuromuscular control.

© William E. Prentice

in the four major ankle motion planes. They may be accompanied early in the rehabilitative phase by plantar flexion and dorsiflexion isotonic exercises. As healing progresses and range of motion increases, the athlete may begin strengthening exercises in all planes of motion (Figure 19–44).[5] Care must be taken when exercising in inversion and eversion to avoid tibial rotation as a substitute movement. Pain should be the basic guideline for deciding when to start inversion-eversion isotonic exercises.[57] Light resistance with high repetitions has fewer detrimental effects on the ligaments (two to four sets of 10 repetitions). Resistive tubing exercises, ankle weights around the foot, and use of a balance board are excellent methods of strengthening inversion and eversion. Tubing has advantages because it may be used both eccentrically and concentrically. Isokinetics have advantages because the athlete may obtain more functional speeds. PNF strengthening exercises that isolate the desired motions at the talocrural joint can also be used.

## Taping and Bracing

It is most desirable to have the patient return to activity without the aid of ankle support. However, it is common practice for some type of ankle support to be worn initially.[16,19,40] Athletes with a history of previous ankle sprains should wear prophylactic ankle supports in the form of either lace-up and semirigid ankle braces or traditional ankle taping which effectively reduce reoccurrence in practices and games.[58] SoR:B Ankle taping does appear to have a stabilizing effect on unstable ankles without interfering with motor performance.[86] Taping also may help protect the injured ligaments

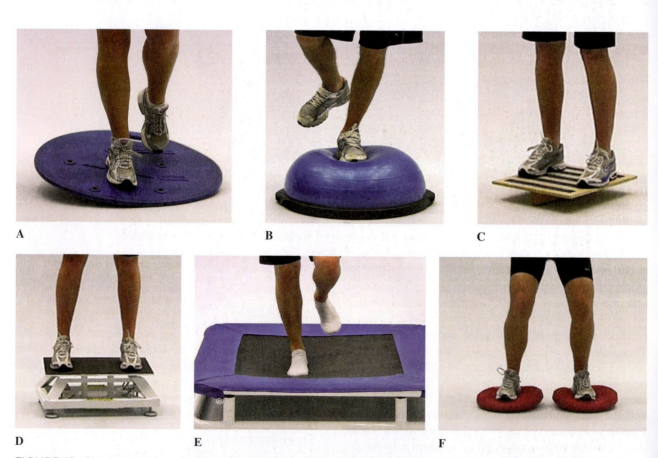

FIGURE 19–41 Activities to enhance both neuromuscular control strengthening and balance. **(A)** BAPS board. **(B)** Bosu Balance Trainer. **(C)** Rocker board. **(D)** Tremor box. **(E)** Ployback. **(F)** Dynadisc.

© William E. Prentice

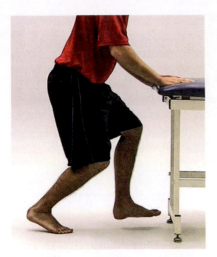

FIGURE 19–42 Both single-leg and double-leg minisquats are helpful both in regaining range of motion and in strengthening.

© William E. Prentice

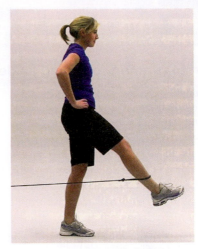

FIGURE 19–43 Single-leg standing kicks can be done in all directions, using cable or tubing resistance.

© William E. Prentice

from excessive loading. However, it appears that taping was much less effective than bracing in reducing the incidence of ankle injuries.[106] The athletic trainer can tape the ankle and tape the shoe onto the foot to make the shoe and ankle function as one unit.[76] It is unclear whether wearing high-topped footwear may further stabilize the ankle.[58] If cleated shoes are worn, cleats should be outset along the periphery of the shoe to provide stability. There is little doubt that ankle bracing prevents both first-time and recurrent ankle sprains.[75] SoR:A Ankle braces have been recommended for improving functional stability, proprioception, postural

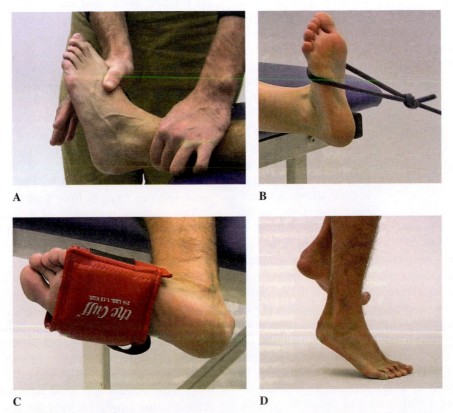

A

B

C

D

FIGURE 19–44 Ankle-strengthening exercises. (A) Manually resisted strengthening exercises can be done in all four directions, as can (B) resisted tubing exercises and (C) exercise with ankle weights. (D) Body weight can serve as a form of resistance.

© William E. Prentice

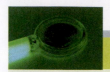

### Return to running following ankle injury functional progression

- Walking
- Jogging on track with walking of curves
- Jogging full track
- Running on track with jogging of curves
- Running full track
- Running for fitness–2 to 3 miles three times per week
- Lunges–90 degrees, pivot, 180 degrees
- Sprints–"W," triangle, 6 sec, 20 yd, 40 yd, 120 yd
- Acceleration/deceleration runs
- Shuffle slides progressing to shuffle run
- Carioca
- Skipping, jumping, hopping

stability, balance, neuromuscular control, and functional performance.[14,19,28,83,103,111] Bracing may help the patient detect movement in the ankle and thus may help reduce injury.[27,52] Bracing is likely more cost effective in the long term than taping.[75,86]

## Functional Progressions

Functional progressions may be as complex or simple as needed. More severe injuries need a more detailed functional progression (see *Focus Box 19–1*: "Return to running following ankle injury functional progression"). The typical progression begins early in the rehabilitation process as the patient becomes partially weight bearing. Full weight bearing should be started when ambulation is performed without a limp.[1]

Running may begin as soon as ambulation is pain free. Pain-free hopping on the affected side may also be a guideline for determining when running is appropriate. Exercising in a pool allows for early running. The patient is placed in the pool in a swim vest that supports the body in water. The patient then runs in place without touching the bottom of the pool. Proper running form should be stressed. Eventually, the patient is moved into shallow water so that more weight is placed on the ankle. The patient then progresses to running on a smooth, flat surface—ideally, a track. Initially, the patient should jog the straights and walk the curves and then progress to jogging the entire track. Speed may be increased to a sprint in a straight line. The cutting sequence should begin with circles of diminishing diameter. Cones may be set up for the patient to run figure eights as the next cutting progression. The crossover or

**19–13 Clinical Application Exercise**

Following a grade 1 ligament sprain of the ankle, a patient is rehabilitating his injury.

? What would be an appropriate progression for him to use to get from non–weight bearing to sprinting?

sidestep is next.[89] The patient sprints to a predesignated spot and cuts or sidesteps abruptly. When this progression is accomplished, the cut should be done without warning on the command of another person. Jumping and hopping exercises should be started on both legs simultaneously and gradually reduced to only the injured side.[44,89]

The patient may perform at different levels for each of these functional sequences. One functional sequence may be done at half speed, whereas another is done at full speed. For example, a patient may run full speed on straights of the track but do figure eights at only half speed. Once the upper levels of all the sequences are reached, the patient may return to limited practice, which may include early training and fundamental drills.[81]

## Return to Play

Functional performance testing should be a primary component of every return-to-play (RTP) decision. Widely used functional performance tests might include single-leg hop for distance, Star Excursion balance test, agility runs, vertical jump, and others. Before the patient returns to sport-specific tasks, the injured limb's functional performance should measure at least 80 percent of the uninjured limb (see Chapter 13).[53] **SoR:B**

The patient's perception of function should be included in any RTP decision. Instruments such as the Lower Limb Task Questionnaire and the Cumberland Ankle Instability Tool (CAIT) can be used to help determine the patient's feelings about his or her readiness to return to play.[58,78] **SoR:C**

The patient should have complete range of motion and at least 80 to 90 percent of preinjury strength before considering a return to normal activity.[89] Finally, if full activity is tolerated without insult to the injured part, the patient may return to competition. Returning to full activity must include a gradual progression of functional activities that slowly increase the stress on the injured structure. The specific demands of each activity dictate the individual drills of this progression.

# SUMMARY

- The portion of the lower extremity that lies between the knee and the ankle is called the lower leg and contains two bones, the tibia and the fibula. The bones that form the ankle joint, or talocrural joint, are the distal portion of the tibia, the distal portion of the fibula, and the talus. The calcaneus also plays a critical role in the function of the ankle joint.
- The ligamentous support of the ankle consists of the tibiofibular ligaments; three lateral ligaments; and the medial, or deltoid, ligament.
- The musculature of the lower leg is contained within four distinct compartments: muscles of the anterior compartment dorsiflex the ankle; muscles of the lateral compartment evert the ankle; muscles of the superficial posterior compartment plantar flex the ankle; and muscles of the deep posterior compartment invert the ankle.
- Individuals can prevent many ankle and lower leg conditions, especially sprains, by stretching the Achilles tendon, strengthening key muscles, engaging in neuromuscular and proprioceptive training, wearing proper footwear, and using taping and ankle support devices appropriately.

- Ankle sprains are the single most common injury in the athletic population. Ankle sprains are classified as inversion, eversion, or syndesmotic injuries. Occasionally, ankle fractures occur along with ankle sprains.
- The Achilles tendon, or heel cord complex, is subject to acute strain that may lead to chronic tendinitis. A rupture of the Achilles tendon is common in the older athlete.
- Tendinitis of the anterior tibialis, posterior tibialis, and peroneal tendons are common around the ankle joint.
- Shin contusions, muscle contusions, muscle cramps, gastrocnemius strains, and fractures of the tibia or fibula are all traumatic injuries that can occur in the lower leg.
- Chronic overuse conditions of the lower leg include medial tibial stress syndrome (shinsplints), compartment syndromes, and stress fractures of the tibia and fibula.
- Perhaps the most important consideration in the rehabilitation of injuries to the ankle and lower leg is to use a gradual progression, beginning with non–weight bearing and subsequently incorporating the appropriate strengthening, range of motion, neuromuscular control, and joint mobilization techniques to facilitate the athlete's return to full activity.

# WEB SITES

**NATA Position, Official and Consensus Statements**

*Conservative Management and Prevention of Ankle Sprains in Athletes:* www.nata.org/sites/default/files /ankle-sprains.pdf

AAOS Online Serivce: Foot and Ankle: http://orthoinfo .aaos.org/menus/foot.cfm
*This site provides answers to a wide range of questions on foot and ankle injuries from the American Academy of Orthopaedic Surgeons.*

American Orthopaedic Foot and Ankle Society: www .aofas.org

American Podiatric Medical Association: www.apma.org
*This site provides a variety of information on foot and ankle injuries from the APMA.*

Cramer First Aider: www.cramersportsmed.com/first -aider.html

The University of Texas Anatomy of the Human Body: www.bartleby.com/107

# SOLUTIONS TO CLINICAL APPLICATION EXERCISES

19–1 The patient most likely has a syndesmotic sprain or sprain of the distal tibiofibular ligaments. This is commonly referred to as a high ankle sprain. This injury may take longer to heal compared with an inversion or eversion ankle sprain.

19–2 The athletic trainer should take a multifaceted approach to reducing ankle sprains. The individual should stretch his Achilles tendon to allow at least 10 degrees of dorsiflexion and should perform strength training on the peroneals, plantar flexors, and dorsiflexors. The individual should also perform proprioceptive training on a balance board. He should wear high-top shoes. Ankle taping with an orthosis can also be employed.

19–3 Based on these symptoms, it is likely that the patient has either an osteochondral fracture or osteochondritis dissecans. The

patient should be referred to a physician for X-rays to confirm this opinion. It is likely that the physician will recommend an arthroscopic procedure to remove these fragments.

19–4 The patient should continue to wear a stirrup brace for 1 to 3 more weeks. Taping at 90 degrees will be conducted for 2 to 4 weeks. The patient should engage in pain-free plantar flexion and dorsiflexion exercises and proprioceptive exercises on a balance board.

19–5 The mechanism describes a syndesmotic ankle sprain. The patient experiences severe pain in the anterolateral leg region when the ankle is externally rotated.

19–6 This injury is a possible partial or complete rupture of the Achilles tendon. The athletic trainer should look for pain that eventually subsides, an inability to perform a toe raise, point tenderness, swelling, discoloration, an obvious indentation at the tendon site, and a positive Thompson test.

19–7 The athletic trainer should apply compression with a horseshoe-shaped felt pad around the lateral malleoleus. This pad should be reinforced by a rigid splint. POLICE, NSAIDs, and analgesics should be given as needed. The patient should follow an exercise program to strengthen, stretch, and enhance balance training.

19–8 The athletic trainer should instruct the patient to rest or reduce the stress of running. The patient should apply ice packs followed by stretching before and after activity. The patient should follow a strengthening program along with treatment by oral antiinflammatory medications as needed.

19–9 The patient has sustained a lower leg fracture. The most common site is in the middle third of the fibula.

19–10 In gymnastics, athletes often run on hard surfaces either barefoot or wearing shoes with little cushioning. This, combined with overtraining and fatigue, could lead to MTSS. Other reasons are a varus or pronated hypermobile foot.

19–11 The conservative approach is to apply POLICE and NSAIDs and rest. With weakness in toe extension and numbness in the dorsal region, surgery may be warranted.

19–12 The runner should avoid stressful locomotor activities for at least 14 days and can engage in bicycling and swimming if pain free. Running can be resumed after a pain-free period of 2 weeks.

19–13 The typical progression begins when the patient becomes partially weight bearing. Full weight bearing should be started when ambulation is performed without a limp. Walking may begin as soon as ambulation is pain free. The patient then progresses to running on a smooth, flat surface—ideally, a track. Initially, the patient should jog the straights and walk the curves and then progress to jogging the entire track. The cutting sequence should begin with circles of diminishing diameter, figure eights, and crossover or side steps. Jumping and hopping exercises should be started on both legs simultaneously and gradually reduced to only the injured side.

## REVIEW QUESTIONS AND CLASS ACTIVITIES

1. Identify and describe the anatomy of the ankle and lower leg.
2. How can ankle injuries be prevented?
3. Demonstrate the steps that should be taken when assessing ankle and lower leg injuries.
4. Describe the three types of ankle sprains.
5. Contrast the management of grades 1, 2, and 3 ligament sprains.
6. What is the usual mechanism for fractures of the ankle?
7. Describe the various injuries that can occur to the Achilles tendon. Indicate their etiology and symptoms and signs.
8. What tendons are most likely to develop tendinitis around the ankle?
9. Discuss the etiology, symptoms and signs, and management of the various acute or traumatic injuries that can occur in the lower leg.
10. What are the possible causes of medial tibial stress syndrome?
11. Contrast the acute anterior compartment syndrome with the chronic type.
12. Describe the various overuse problems that can occur in the lower leg.
13. Describe the appropriate progression of treatment that should be used in the rehabilitation of ankle and lower leg injuries.

## REFERENCES

1. Albensi R: The relationship of body weight and clinical foot and ankle measurements to the heel forces of forward and backward walking, *J Athl Train* 34(4):328, 1999.
2. Alfredson H: Chronic Achilles tendinosis: Recommendations for treatment and prevention, *Sports Med* 29(2):135, 2000.
3. Amendola A: Evidence-based approach to treatment of acute traumatic syndesmosis (high ankle) sprains, *Sports Med Arthroscopy* 14(4):232–36 2006.
4. Anandacoomarasamy A: Long-term outcomes of inversion ankle injuries, *Br J Sports Med* 39(3):e14, 2005.
5. Arnold B: Concentric evertor strength differences and functional ankle instability: A meta-Analysis, *J Athl Train* 44(6):653–62, 2009.
6. Bahr R: A twofold reduction in the incidence of acute ankle sprains in volleyball after the introduction of an injury prevention program: A prospective cohort study, *Scand J Med Sci Sports* 7(3):172–77, 1997.
7. Bartosik K: Anatomical and biomechanical assessments of medial tibial stress syndrome (abstract), *J Athl Train* 40(2 Suppl):S-1, 2005.
8. Beumer A: Effects of ligament sectioning on the kinematics of the distal tibiofibular syndesmosis: A radiostereometric study of 10 cadaveric specimens based on presumed trauma mechanisms with suggestions for treatment, *Acta Orthop* 77(3):531–40, 2006.
9. Beynnon B: A prospective, randomized clinical investigation of the treatment of first time ankle sprains, *American Journal of Sports Medicine* 34(9):1401–02, 2006.
10. Beynnon B: Predictive factors for lateral ankle sprains: A literature review, *J Athl Train* 37(4):376, 2002.
11. Bleakley C: The use of ice in the treatment of acute soft-tissue injury: A systematic review of randomized controlled trials. *Am J Sports Med* 32(1):251–61, 2004.
12. Birrer R: Ankle injuries. In Birrer R, ed: *Sports medicine for the primary care physician,* Boca Raton, FL, 1994, CRC Press.
13. Booher J: *Athletic injury assessment,* ed 4, St. Louis, MO, 2001, McGraw-Hill.
14. Bot S: The effect of ankle bracing and taping on functional performance: A review of the literature, *International Journal of Sports Medicine,* 2011.
15. Breitenseher M: MRI versus lateral stress radiography in acute lateral ankle ligament injuries. *J Comput Assist Tomogr* 21(2):280–85, 1997.
16. Broglio S: The influence of ankle support on postural control. *Journal of Science and Medicine in Sport* 12(3):388–92, 2009.
17. Brown D: Exertional leg pain. In Brown D: *Orthopedic secrets,* Philadelphia, PA, 2003, Hanley and Belfus.
18. Cordova M: Effects of ankle support on lower extremity functional performance: A meta-analysis, *Medicine and Science in Sport and Exercise* 37(4):635–41, 2005.
19. Cordova M: Efficacy of prophylactic ankle support: An experimental perspective, *J Athl Train* 37(4):246, 2002.
20. Cosby N: Immediate effects of anterior to posterior talocrural joint mobilizations following acute lateral ankle sprain, *Journal of Manual and Manipulative Therapy* 19(2):76–83, 2011.
21. Couture CJ: Tibial stress injuries: Decisive diagnosis and treatment of "shin splint," *Physician Sportsmed* 30(6):29, 2002.
22. Davlin C: Traumatic Achilles tendon rupture in a female college basketball player, *J Sport Rehabil* 13(2):151, 2004.
23. Demeritt K: Chronic ankle instability does not affect lower extremity functional performance, *J Athl Train* 37(4):507, 2002.
24. Denegar C: Can chronic ankle instability be prevented? Rethinking management of lateral ankle sprains, *J Athl Train* 37(4):430, 2002.
25. de Cesar P: Comparison of magnetic resonance imaging to physical examination for syndesmotic injury after lateral ankle sprain, *Foot Ankle Int* 32(12):1110–14, 2011.
26. deNoronha M: Do voluntary strength, proprioception, range of motion, or postural sway predict occurrence of lateral ankle sprain? *British Journal of Sports Medicine* 40:824–28, 2006.
27. DesRochers D: Proprioceptive benefit derived from ankle support, *Athletic Therapy Today* 7(6):44, 2002.
28. Dizon J: A systematic review on the effectiveness of external ankle supports in the prevention of inversion ankle sprains among elite and recreational players, *Journal of Medicine and Science in Sport* 13(3), 309–17, 2010.

29. Docherty C: Development and reliability of the ankle instability instrument, *J Athl Train* 41(2):154–58, 2006.

30. Docherty C: Functional-performance deficits in volunteers with functional ankle instability, *J Sport Rehabil* 40(1):30, 2005.

31. Docherty C: Effects of strength training on strength development and joint position sense in functionally unstable ankles, *J Athl Train* 33(4):310, 2000.

32. Doherty C: The incidence and prevalence of ankle sprain injury: A systematic review and meta-analysis of prospective epidemiological studies, *Sports Medicine* 44(1):123–40, 2014.

33. Doughtie M: Syndesmotic ankle sprain in football: A survey of National Football League athletic trainers, *J Athl Train* 34(1):15, 1999.

34. Dowling S: Accuracy of Ottawa Ankle Rules to exclude fractures of the ankle and midfoot in children: a meta-analysis. *Acad Emerg Med* 16(4):277–87, 2009.

35. Drewes L: Dorsiflexion deficit during jogging with chronic ankle instability, *J Sci Med Sport* 12(6):685–87, 2009.

36. Ebell M: Evaluation of the patient with suspected deep vein thrombosis, *J Fam Pract.* 50(2):167–71, 2001.

37. Fong D: A systematic review on ankle injury and ankle sprain in sports, *Sports Med* 37(1):73–94, 2007.

38. Geidman W: Posterior tibial tendon dysfunction, *J Orthop Sports Phys Ther* 30(2):68, 2000.

39. Gribble P: The effects of fatigue and chronic ankle instability on dynamic postural control, *J Athl Train* 39(4):321, 2004.

40. Guskiewicz K: Comparison of three methods of external support for management of acute lateral ankle sprains, *J Athl Train* 34(1):5, 1999.

41. Hertel J: Functional anatomy, pathomechanics, and pathophysiology of lateral ankle instability, *J Athl Train* 37(4):364, 2002.

42. Hertel J: Serial testing of postural control after acute lateral ankle sprain, *J Athl Train* 36(4):363, 2001.

43. Hertel J: Talocrural and subtalar joint instability after lateral ankle sprain, *Med Sci Sports Exerc* 31(11):1501, 1999.

44. Hess D: Effect of a four-week agility-training program on postural sway in the functionally unstable ankle, *J Sport Rehabil* 10(1):24, 2001.

45. Hiller C: Chronic ankle instability: Evolution of the model, *J Athl Train* 46(2):133–41, 2011.

46. Hirth C: Rehabilitation of lower leg injuries. In Prentice W: *Rehabilitation techniques in sports medicine and athletic training,* Thorofare, NJ, 2105, Slack.

47. Hoch M: Two-week joint mobilization intervention improves self-reported function, range of motion, and dynamic balance in those with chronic ankle instability, *Journal of Orthopedic Research* 30(11):1798–1804, 2012.

48. Hockenbury R: Evaluation and treatment of ankle sprains: Clinical recommendations for a positive outcome, *Physician Sportsmed* 29(2): 57, 2001.

49. Hubbard T: Ankle sprain: Pathology, predisposing factors and management strategies, *Open Access Journal of Sports Medicine* 16(1):115–22, 2010.

50. Hubbard T: 2009. Contributing factors to medial tibial stress syndrome: A prospective investigation, *Medicine and Science in Sports and Exercise* 41(3):490–96.

51. Hubbard T: Reliability of intratester and intertester measurements derived from an instrumented ankle arthrometer, *J Sport Rehabil* 12(3):208, 2003.

52. Hubbard T: Kinesthesia is not affected by functional ankle instability status, *J Athl Train* 37(4):481, 2002.

53. Hupperets M: Effect of unsupervised home based proprioceptive training on recurrences of ankle sprain: randomised controlled trial, *British Medical Journal* 339:2684, 2009.

54. Jenkin M: Clinical usefulness of the Ottawa ankle rules for detecting fractures of the ankle and midfoot, *J Athl Train* 45(5):480– 82, 2010.

55. Jepson K: The use of orthoses for athletes. In Birrer R, ed: *Sports medicine for the primary care physician,* Boca Raton, FL, 1994, CRC Press.

56. Kaminski T: Factors contributing to chronic ankle instability: A strength perspective, *J Athl Train* 37(4):394, 2002.

57. Kaminski T: Eversion strength analysis of uninjured and functionally unstable ankles, *J Athl Train* 34(3):239, 1999.

58. Kaminski T, et al.: National Athletic Trainers Association Position Statement: Conservative management and prevention of ankle sprains in athletes, *Journal of Athletic Training* 48(4):528–45, 2013.

59. Kaplan Y: Prevention of ankle sprains in sport: A systematic literature review, *Br J Sports Med* 45:355, 2011.

60. Khan R: Treatment of acute Achilles tendon ruptures, *J Bone Joint Surg* 88(5):1160, 2006.

61. Knapp D: Differential ability of selected postural-control measures in the prediction of chronic ankle instability status, *J Athl Train* 46(3):257–62, 2011.

62. Konradsen L: Factors contributing to chronic ankle instability: Kinesthesia and joint position sense, *J Athl Train* 37(4):381, 2002.

63. Kovaleski J: Instrumented ankle arthrometry, *Athletic Therapy Today* 8(1):44, 2003.

64. Kovaleski J: Functional rehabilitation after lateral ankle injury, *Athletic Therapy Today* 1(3):52, 2006.

65. Leddy J: Implementation of the Ottawa ankle rule in a university sports medicine center, *Med Sci Sports Exerc* 34(1):57, 2002.

66. Lynch S: Assessment of the injured ankle in the athlete, *J Athl Train* 37(4):406, 2002.

67. Madras D: Rehabilitation for functional ankle instability, *J Sport Rehabil* 12(2):133, 2003.

68. Maffulli N: The clinical diagnosis of subcutaneous tears of the Achilles tendon, *Am J Sports Med* 26(2):266–70, 1998.

69. Magnussen R: Nonoperative treatment of midportion Achilles tendinopathy: A systematic review, *Clinical Journal of Sports Medicine* 19(1):54–64, 2009.

70. Mangus B: Management of tibiofibular syndesmosis injuries, *Athletic Therapy Today* 4(5):47, 1999.

71. Mattacola C: Management of talus fractures, *Athletic Therapy Today* 7(1):32, 2002.

72. Mattacola C: Rehabilitation of the ankle after acute or chronic injury, *J Athl Train* 37(4):413, 2002.

73. Mazieres B: Topical ketoprofen patch (100 mg) for the treatment of ankle sprain a randomized, double-blind, placebo-controlled stud, *Am J Sports Med* 33(4):515–23, 2005.

74. McGuine T: The effect of a balance training program on the risk of ankle sprains in high school athletes, *Am J Sports Med* 34(7):1103–11, 2006.

75. McGuine T: The effect of lace-up ankle braces on injury rates in high school football players, *American Journal of Sports Medicine* 40(1):49–57, 2012.

76. McKenzie J: The effects of ankle taping and spatting on the reaction time of the supporting musculature of the ankle after sudden inversion (abstract), *J Athl Train* 39(2 Suppl):S-10, 2004.

77. McKeon P: Systematic review of postural control and lateral ankle instability, part II: Is balance training clinically effective? *Journal of Athletic Training* 42(3):305–15, 2008.

78. McNair P: The lower-limb task questionnaire: An assessment of validity, reliability, responsiveness, and minimal important differences, *Arch Phys Med Rehabil* 88(8):993–1001, 2007.

79. Mugunthan K: Is there sufficient evidence for tuning fork tests in diagnosing fractures? A systematic review, *British Medical Journal Open,* 4(8):e005238, 2014.

80. Muir I: Effect of a static calf-stretching exercise on the resistive torque during passive ankle dorsiflexion in healthy subjects, *J Orthop Sports Phys Ther* 29(2):106, 1999.

81. Munn J: Do functional-performance tests detect impairment in subjects with ankle instability? *J Sport Rehabil* 11(1):40, 2002.

82. Nilsson-Helander K: Acute Achilles tendon rupture: A randomized, controlled study comparing surgical and nonsurgical treatments using validated outcome measures, *American Journal of Sports Medicine* 38(11), 2010.

83. Nishikawa T: Peroneal motoneuron excitability increases immediately following application of a semirigid ankle brace, *J Orthop Sports Phys Ther* 29(3):168, 1999.

84. Norkus S: The anatomy and mechanisms of syndesmotic ankle sprains, *J Athl Train* 36(1):68, 2001.

85. Northrup R: The Ottawa ankle rules and the "Buffalo" rule, Part 2: A practical application, *Athletic Therapy Today* 10(2):68, 2005.

86. Olmsted L: Prophylactic ankle taping and bracing: A numbers needed-to-treat and cost-benefit analysis, *J Athl Train* 39(1):95, 2004.

87. Olmsted-Kramer L: Preventing recurrent lateral ankle sprains: An evidence-based approach, *Athletic Therapy Today* 9(6):19, 2004.

88. Porter D: *Baxter's the foot and ankle in sport,* New York, 2007, Mosby.

89. Prentice W: Rehabilitation of ankle and foot injuries. In Prentice W: *Rehabilitation techniques in sports medicine and athletic training,* Thorofare, NJ, 2015, Slack.

90. Pugia M: Comparison of acute swelling and function in subjects with lateral ankle injury, *J Orthop Sports Phys Ther* 31(7):384, 2001.

91. Ransone J: Syndesmotic ankle sprains, *Athletic Therapy Today* 6(5):48, 2001.

92. Ray T: Exercise-induced shin pain, *Athletic Therapy Today* 10(5):72, 2005.

93. Ricard M: Effects of high-top and low-top shoes on ankle inversion, *J Athl Train* 35(1):38, 2000.

94. Ricard M: Effects of taping and exercise on dynamic ankle inversion, *J Athl Train* 35(1):31, 2000.

95. Riemann B: Is there a link between chronic ankle instability and postural instability? *J Athl Train* 37(4):386, 2002.

96. Rozzi S: Balance training for persons with functionally unstable ankles, *J Orthop Sports Phys Ther* 29(8):478, 1999.

97. Schwieterman B: Diagnostic accuracy of physical examination tests of the ankle/foot complex a systematic review, *Int J Sports Phys Ther* 8(4):416–26, 2013.

98. Silkman C: Balance training for patients with chronic ankle instability, *Athletic Therapy Today,* 15(1):36, 2010.

99. Silvestri PG: Management of syndesmotic ankle sprains, *Athletic Therapy Today* 7(5):48, 2002.

100. Smith A, Bach B: High ankle sprains, *Physician Sportsmed* 32(12):39, 2004.

101. van Dijk C: Physical examination is sufficient for the diagnosis of sprained ankles, *J Bone Joint Surg Br* 78(6):958–62, 1996.

102. Venesky K: Prophylactic ankle braces and knee varus-valgus and internal-external rotation torque, *J Athl Train* 41(3):239, 2006.

103. Wikstrom E: Dynamic postural stability in subjects with braced, functionally unstable ankles, *J Athl Train* 41(3):245, 2006.

104. Wilder R: Exertional compartment syndrome, *Clinics in Sports Medicine,* 29(3):429–35, 2010.

105. Wilder R: Overuse injuries: Tendinopathies, stress fractures, compartment syndrome, and shin splints, *Clin Sports Med* 23(1):55, 2004.

106. Wilkerson G: Biomechanical and neuromuscular effects of ankle taping and bracing, *J Athl Train* 37(4):236, 2002.

107. Wilkerson G: Rotary ankle instability: Overview of pathomechanics and prognosis, *Athletic Therapy Today* 15(4):175, 2010.

108. Willems T: Proprioception and muscle strength in subjects with a history of ankle sprains and chronic instability, *J Athl Train* 37(4):487, 2002.

109. Williams G: Syndesmotic ankle sprains in athletes, *The American Journal of Sports Medicine* 35(7):1197–1207, 2007.

110. Wright I: The effects of ankle compliance and flexibility on ankle sprains, *Med Sci Sports Exerc* 32(2):260, 2000.

111. Zinder S: Ankle bracing and the neuromuscular factors influencing joint stiffness, *J Athl Train* 44(4):363–69, 2009.

## ANNOTATED BIBLIOGRAPHY

Altchek D: *Foot and Ankle Sports Medicine,* Philadelphia, PA, 2012, Lippincott, Williams and Wilkins.

*A comprehensive and practical resource for the treatment of foot and ankle sports injuries.*

Brown DE, Neumann RD, editors: *Orthopedic secrets*, Philadelphia, PA, 2014, Hanley and Belfus.

*Presents an overview of orthopedics in a question-and-answer format. The ankle and lower leg are well presented.*

*Journal of Athletic Training*, 37:4, 2002.

*A special issue that contains articles that discuss various aspects of ankle injury.*

Nyska M, Mann G, editors: *The unstable ankle*, Champaign, IL, 2002, Human Kinetics.

*Covers the basic concepts and practical applications in the diagnosis, treatment, and prevention of acute ankle ligament injury and acute and chronic ankle instability.*

Pfeffer R: *Athletic injuries to the foot and ankle*, Park Ridge, IL, 2000, American Academy of Orthopaedic Surgeons.

*Goes into great detail on a wide variety of injuries that occur in the ankle joint.*

Porter D: *Baxter's the foot and ankle in sport*, New York, 2007, McGraw-Hill.

*A comprehensive text edited by an orthopedist who specializes in foot and ankle injuries.*

Prentice WE, editor: *Rehabilitation techniques in sports medicine and athletic training*, Thorofare, NJ, 2015, Slack Inc.

*Chapters 24 and 25 of this text are dedicated to a discussion of rehabilitation techniques for injuries to the ankle and lower leg. The text first covers the pathomechanics and mechanisms of various injuries and then presents rehabilitation concerns and progressions in specific detail.*

Sammarco GJ: *Rehabilitation of the foot and ankle*, St. Louis, MO, 1995, Mosby.

*Specifically addresses the aspects of rehabilitation directed at both the foot and the ankle.*

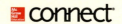

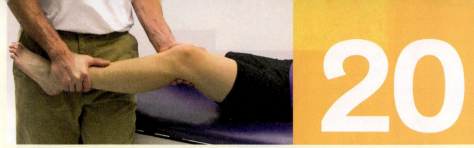

© William E. Prentice

# The Knee and Related Structures

## ■ Objectives

*When you finish this chapter you should be able to*

- Recognize the normal structural and functional knee anatomy.
- Demonstrate the various ligamentous and meniscal stability tests discussed in this chapter.
- Explain how knee injuries can be prevented.
- Compare and contrast male/female differences relative to anterior cruciate ligament (ACL) injuries.

- Discuss etiological factors, symptoms and signs, and management procedures for the injuries to the ligaments and menisci.
- Identify the various etiological factors, symptoms and signs, and management procedures for injuries that occur in the patellofemoral joint and in the extensor mechanism.
- Design appropriate rehabilitation protocols for the injured knee.

## ■ Outline

## ■ Key Terms

patella alta
patella baja
genu valgum
genu varum
genu recurvatum

hemarthrosis
translation
iliotibial band syndrome

## ■ Connect Highlights   connect

*Visit connect.mcgraw-hill.com for further exercises to apply your knowledge:*

- Clinical application scenarios covering assessment and recognition of knee injuries, etiology, symptoms and signs, and management of knee injuries, as well as rehabilitation for the knee
- Click-and-drag questions covering structural anatomy of the knee, assessment of knee injuries, and rehabilitation plan of the knee
- Multiple-choice questions covering anatomy, assessment, etiology, management, and rehabilitation of knee injuries
- Selection questions covering rehabilitation plan for various injuries to the knee
- Video identification of special tests for the knee injuries, rehabilitation techniques for the knee, and taping and wrapping for knee injuries
- Picture identification of major anatomical components of the knee, rehabilitation techniques of the knee, and therapeutic modalities for management

**B**ecause so many activities place extreme stress on the knee, it is one of the most traumatized joints in the physically active population. The knee is commonly considered a hinge joint because its two principal movements are flexion and extension. However, because rotation of the tibia is an essential component of knee movement, the knee is not a true hinge joint. The stability of the knee joint depends primarily on the ligaments, the joint capsule, and the muscles that surround the joint. The knee is designed primarily to provide stability in weight bearing and mobility in locomotion; however, it is especially unstable laterally and medially.

> Muscles and ligaments provide the main source of stability in the knee.

## ANATOMY OF THE KNEE

### Bones

The knee joint complex consists of the femur, the tibia, the fibula, and the patella (Figure 20–1). The distal end of the femur expands and forms the convex lateral and medial condyles, which are designed to articulate with the tibia and the patella. The articular surface of the medial condyle is longer from front to back than is the surface of the lateral condyle. Anteriorly, the two condyles form a hollowed femoral groove, or trochlea, to receive the patella. The proximal end of the tibia, the tibial plateau, articulates with the condyles of the femur. On this flat tibial plateau are two shallow concavities that articulate with their respective femoral condyles and are divided by the popliteal notch. Separating these concavities, or articular facets, is a roughened area where the cruciate ligaments attach and from which a process commonly known as the tibial spine arises.

**Patella** The patella is the largest sesamoid bone in the human body. It is located in the tendon of the quadriceps femoris muscle and is divided into three medial facets and a lateral facet that articulate with the femur (Figure 20–1). The lateral aspect of the patella is wider than the medial aspect. The patella articulates between the concavity provided by the femoral condyles. Tracking within this groove depends on the pull of the quadriceps muscle and patellar tendon, the depth of the femoral condyles, and the shape of the patella.

### Articulations

The knee joint complex consists of four articulations between the femur and the tibia, the femur and the patella, the femur and the fibula, and the tibia and the fibula.

### Menisci

The menisci (Figure 20–2A) are two oval (semilunar) fibrocartilages that deepen the articular facets of the tibia, cushion any stresses placed on the knee joint, and maintain spacing between the femoral condyles and tibial plateau. The consistency of the menisci is much like that of the intervertebral disks. They are located medially and laterally on the tibial plateau, or shelf. The menisci transmit one-half of the contact force in the medial compartment and an even higher percentage of the contact load in the lateral compartment. The menisci help stabilize the knee, especially the medial meniscus, when the knee is flexed at 90 degrees.

**Medial Meniscus** The medial meniscus is a C-shaped fibrocartilage, the circumference of which is attached firmly to the medial articular facet of the tibia and to the joint capsule by the coronary ligaments. Posteriorly, it is also attached to fibers of the semimembranous muscle.

**Lateral Meniscus** The lateral meniscus is more O-shaped and is attached to the lateral articular facet on the superior aspect of the tibia. The lateral meniscus also attaches loosely to the lateral articular capsule and to the popliteal tendon. The ligament of Wrisberg attaches to the posterior horn of the lateral meniscus that projects upward, close to the attachment of the posterior cruciate ligament. The transverse ligament joins the anterior portions of the lateral and medial menisci.

**Meniscal Blood Supply** Blood is supplied to each meniscus by the medial genicular artery. Each meniscus can be divided into three circumferential zones: the red-red zone is the outer, or peripheral, one-third and has a good

> Generally, the meniscus has a poor blood supply.

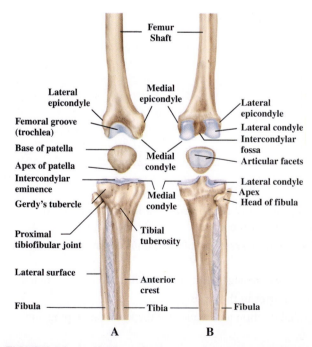

**FIGURE 20–1** The bones of the knee joint. **(A)** Anterior view. **(B)** Posterior view.

Labels (A):
Femur Shaft; Lateral epicondyle; Medial epicondyle; Femoral groove (trochlea); Base of patella; Apex of patella; Intercondylar eminence; Gerdy's tubercle; Medial condyle; Proximal tibiofibular joint; Tibial tuberosity; Lateral surface; Anterior crest; Fibula; Tibia

Labels (B):
Lateral epicondyle; Lateral condyle; Intercondylar fossa; Articular facets; Medial condyle; Lateral condyle; Apex; Head of fibula; Fibula

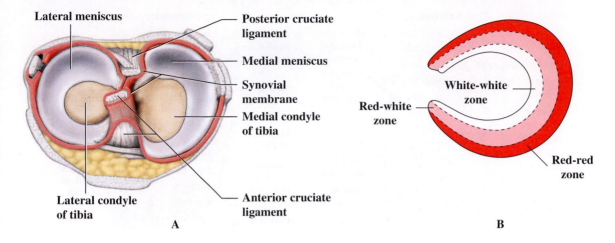

**Lateral meniscus**

**Posterior cruciate ligament**

**Medial meniscus**

**Synovial membrane**

**Medial condyle of tibia**

**Lateral condyle of tibia**

**Anterior cruciate ligament**

**A**

**Red-white zone**

**White-white zone**

**Red-red zone**

**B**

FIGURE 20–2 **(A)** Medial and lateral menisci of the knee. **(B)** The three vascular zones of the meniscus. (A: From Saladin, KS: Anatomy and physiology, ed. 5, Dubuque, IA: McGraw-Hill Higher Education, 2010.)

vascular supply; the red-white zone is the middle one-third and has minimal blood supply; and the white-white zone, on the inner one-third, is avascular (Figure 20–2B).[37]

## Stabilizing Ligaments

The major stabilizing ligaments of the knee are the cruciate ligaments, the collateral ligaments, and the capsular ligaments (Figure 20–3).

**Cruciate Ligaments** The cruciate ligaments account for a considerable amount of knee stability. They are two ligamentous bands that cross one another within the joint capsule of the knee. The anterior cruciate ligament (ACL) attaches below and in front of the tibia; then, passing posteriorly, it attaches laterally to the inner surface of the lateral condyle. The posterior cruciate ligament (PCL), the stronger of the two, crosses from the back of the tibia in an upward, forward, and medial direction and attaches to the anterior portion of the lateral surface of the medial condyle of the femur.

*Anterior Cruciate Ligament* The anterior cruciate ligament comprises three twisted bands: the anteromedial, intermediate, and posterolateral bands. In general, the anterior cruciate ligament prevents the femur from moving posteriorly during weight bearing and limits anterior translation of the tibia in non–weight bearing. It also stabilizes the tibia against excessive internal rotation and serves as a secondary restraint for valgus or varus stress with collateral ligament damage.

When the knee is fully extended, the posterolateral section of the cruciate ligament is most tight. In flexion the posterolateral fibers loosen and the anteromedial fibers tighten.[88] The anterior cruciate ligament works in conjunction with the thigh muscles, especially the hamstring muscle group, to stabilize the knee joint.

*Posterior Cruciate Ligament* Some portion of the posterior cruciate ligament is taut throughout the full range of motion. In general, the posterior cruciate ligament resists internal rotation of the tibia, prevents hyperextension of the knee, limits anterior translation of the femur during weight bearing, and limits posterior translation of the tibia in non–weight bearing.

**Capsular and Collateral Ligaments** Additional stabilization of the knee is provided by the capsular and collateral ligaments. Besides providing stability, they also direct movement in a correct path. Although they move in synchrony, they are divided into the medial and lateral complexes.

*Medial Collateral Ligament* The superficial position of the medial (tibial) collateral ligament (MCL) is separate from the deeper capsular ligament at the joint line. It attaches above the joint line on the medial epicondyle of the femur and below on the tibia, just beneath the attachment of the pes anserinus. The posterior aspect of the ligament blends into the deep posterior capsular ligament and semimembranous muscle. Fibers of the semimembranous muscle go through the capsule and attach to the posterior aspect of the medial meniscus, pulling it backward during knee flexion. Some of its fibers are taut through flexion and extension. Its major purpose is to prevent the knee from valgus and external rotating forces. The medial collateral ligament was thought to be the principal stabilizer of the knee in a valgus position when combined with rotation. It is now known that other structures, such as the anterior cruciate ligament, play an equal or greater part in this function.[88]

*Deep Medial Capsular Ligaments* The deep medial capsular ligament is divided into three parts: the anterior, medial, and posterior capsular ligaments. The anterior capsular ligament connects with the extensor mechanism and the medial meniscus through the coronary ligaments.

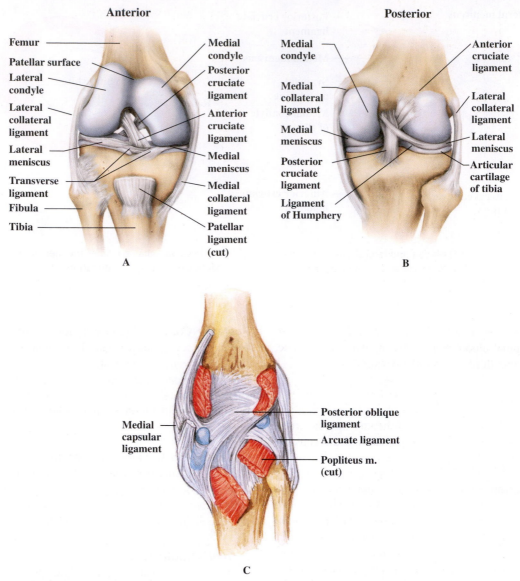

**Anterior**

- Femur
- Patellar surface
- Lateral condyle
- Lateral collateral ligament
- Lateral meniscus
- Transverse ligament
- Fibula
- Tibia
- Medial condyle
- Posterior cruciate ligament
- Anterior cruciate ligament
- Medial meniscus
- Medial collateral ligament
- Patellar ligament (cut)

A

**Posterior**

- Medial condyle
- Medial collateral ligament
- Medial meniscus
- Posterior cruciate ligament
- Ligament of Humphery
- Anterior cruciate ligament
- Lateral collateral ligament
- Lateral meniscus
- Articular cartilage of tibia

B

- Medial capsular ligament
- Posterior oblique ligament
- Arcuate ligament
- Popliteus m. (cut)

C

FIGURE 20–3    The ligaments of the knee. **(A)** Anterior view. **(B)** Posterior view. **(C)** Capsular ligaments, posterior view.

It relaxes during knee extension and tightens during knee flexion. The primary purposes of the medial capsular ligaments are to attach the medial meniscus to the femur and to allow the tibia to move on the meniscus inferiorly. The posterior capsular ligament is sometimes called the posterior oblique ligament and attaches to the posterior medial aspect of the meniscus and intersperses with the semimembranous muscle.[88]

### Lateral Collateral Ligament and Related Structures

The lateral (fibular) collateral ligament (LCL) is a round, fibrous cord that is about the size of a pencil. It is attached to the lateral epicondyle of the femur and to the head of the fibula. The lateral collateral ligament is taut during knee extension but relaxed during flexion and functions as a lateral stabilizer of the knee.

The arcuate ligament is formed by a thickening of the posterior articular capsule. Its posterior aspect attaches to the fascia of the popliteal muscle and the posterior horn of the lateral meniscus.

Other structures that stabilize the knee laterally are the iliotibial band, popliteus muscle, and biceps femoris. The iliotibial band, a tendon of the tensor fasciae latae and gluteus maximus, attaches to the lateral epicondyle of the femur and lateral tibial tubercle (Gerdy's tubercle). It becomes tense during both extension and flexion. The popliteus muscle stabilizes the knee during flexion and, when contracting, protects the lateral meniscus by pulling it posteriorly.

The biceps femoris muscle also stabilizes the knee laterally by inserting into the fibular head, iliotibial band, and capsule.

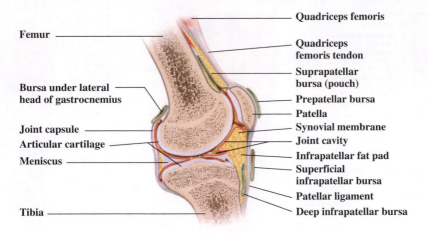

**FIGURE 20–4** Sagittal cross section of the knee, showing the location of bursae and synovial membranes.

## Joint Capsule

The articular surfaces of the knee joint are completely enveloped by the largest joint capsule in the body (Figure 20–4). Anteriorly, the joint capsule extends upward underneath the patella to form the suprapatellar pouch. The inferior portion contains the infrapatellar fat pad and the infrapatellar bursa. Medially, a thickened section of the capsule forms the deep portion of the medial collateral ligament. Posteriorly, the capsule forms two pouches that cover the femoral condyles and the tibial plateau. The capsule thickens medially to form the posterior oblique ligament and laterally to form the arcuate ligament (see Figure 20–3C).

The joint capsule is divided into four regions: the posterolateral, posteromedial, anterolateral, and anteromedial. Each of these four "corners" of the capsule is reinforced by other anatomical structures. The posterolateral corner is reinforced by the iliotibial band, the popliteus, the biceps femoris, the LCL, and the arcuate ligament. The MCL, the pes anserinus tendons, the semimembranosus, and the posterior oblique ligament reinforce the posteromedial corner. The anterolateral corner is reinforced by the iliotibial band, the patellar tendon, and the lateral patellar retinaculum. The superficial MCL and the medial patellar retinaculum reinforce the anteromedial corner.

A tennis player injures her knee during a match. As she hits a forehand stroke, her foot is weight-bearing, her knee is in flexion, and she feels pain in it as she rotates on the follow-through. She feels some diffuse pain around her knee joint and is concerned that she has sprained a ligament.

**?** In a position of full extension, which of the supporting ligaments are most likely to be injured in this position?

Synovial membrane lines the inner surface of the joint capsule, except posteriorly, where it passes in front of the cruciates, making them extrasynovial (Figure 20–4).

## Knee Musculature

For the knee to function properly, a number of muscles must work together in a complex manner. The following is a list of knee actions and the muscles that initiate them (Figure 20–5). Table 20–1 lists all of the muscles that produce movement at the knee.

- Knee flexion is executed by the biceps femoris, semitendinosus, semimembranosus, gracilis, sartorius, gastrocnemius, popliteus, and plantaris muscles.
- Knee extension is executed by the quadriceps muscle of the thigh, consisting of three vasti—the vastus medialis, vastus lateralis, and vastus intermedius—and by the rectus femoris.
- External rotation of the tibia in non-weight-bearing activity is controlled by the biceps femoris. The bony anatomy also produces external tibial rotation as the knee moves into extension.
- Internal rotation of the tibia in non-weight-bearing activity is accomplished by the popliteal, semitendinosus, semimembranosus, sartorius, and gracilis muscles. Rotation of the tibia is limited and can occur only when the knee is in a flexed position. It must be added that when weight bearing, the popliteus externally rotates the femur and pulls the lateral meniscus posteriorly initiating knee flexion.
- The iliotibial band on the lateral side primarily functions as a dynamic lateral stabilizer.

## Bursae

A bursa is composed of pieces of synovial tissue separated by a thin film of fluid. The function of a bursa is to reduce the friction between anatomical structures.

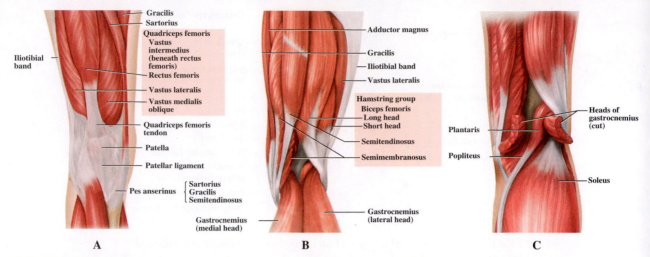

FIGURE 20–5   Muscles of the knee. **(A)** Anterior view. **(B)** Posterior view. **(C)** Deep posterior view.

| TABLE 20–1 | Muscles of the Knee | | | |
|---|---|---|---|---|
| **Muscle** | **Origin** | **Insertion** | **Muscle Action (non–weight bearing)** | **Innervation** |
| **Sartorius** | Anterior superior iliac spine | Proximal medial surface of the tibia, below the tuberosity | Knee flexion and internal rotation | Femoral (L2, L3, L4) |
| **Quadriceps femoris:** | | | | |
| Rectus femoris | Anterior inferior iliac spine and just above the acetabulum of the os coxae | Tibial tuberosity, via the patella and the patellar ligament | Knee extension | Femoral (L2, L3, L4) |
| Vastus lateralis | Greater trochanter and lateral lip of the linea aspera of the femur | | | |
| Vastus medialis | Medial lip of the linea aspera of the femur | | | |
| Vastus intermedius | Anterior surface of the shaft of the femur | | | |
| **Hamstrings:** | | | | |
| Biceps femoris | *Long head:* ischial tuberosity  *Short head:* lateral lip of the linea aspera | Lateral surface of the head of the fibula and the lateral condyle of the tibia | Knee flexion and external rotation | Sciatic (L5, S1, S2) |
| Semitendinosus | Ischial tuberosity | Medial surface of the proximal end of the tibia | Knee flexion and internal rotation | Tibial (S1, S2) |
| Semimembranosus | Ischial tuberosity | Medial surface of the proximal end of the tibia | Knee flexion and internal rotation | Tibial (S1, S2) |
| **Popliteus** | Lateral condyle of the femur | Posterior surface of the tibia below the tibial plateau | Knee flexion and internal rotation | Tibial (L4, L5, S1) |
| **Gastrocnemius** | *Lateral head:* posterior lateral condyle of the femur  *Medial head:* popliteal surface of the femur above medial condyle | Posterior surface of the calcaneous | Knee flexion | Tibial (S1, S2) |

*(Continued)*

**TABLE 20-1**     Muscles of the Knee *(continued)*

| Muscle | Origin | Insertion | Muscle Action (non–weight bearing) | Innervation |
|---|---|---|---|---|
| Plantaris | Lateral supracondylar ridge of the femur | Posterior surface of the calcaneous | Knee flexion | Tibial (L4, L5, S1) |
| Gracilis | Inferior ramus of pubis | Medial surface of the tibia | Knee flexion and internal rotation | Obturator (L3, L4) |

**Movements of the Knee Joint***

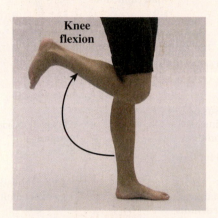
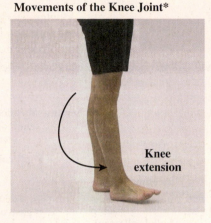
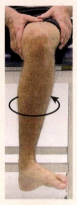
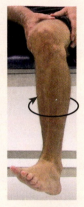

Knee flexion

Knee extension

Tibial external rotation

Tibial internal rotation

*Manual muscle tests and goniometric measurements of range of motion for the knee joint can be found in Appendix F and Appendix G at the end of the text.

© William E. Prentice

Bursae are found between muscle and bone, tendon and bone, tendon and ligament, and so forth. As many as two dozen bursae have been identified around the knee joint. The suprapatellar, prepatellar, infrapatellar, pretibial, and gastrocnemius bursae are perhaps the most commonly injured about the knee joint (see Figure 20–4).

## Fat Pads

There are several fat pads around the knee. The infrapatellar fat pad is the largest. It serves as a cushion to the front of the knee and separates the patellar tendon from the joint capsule. Other major fat pads in the knee include the prepatellar fat pad which lies exposed on the anterior surface of the patella, in addition to the anterior and posterior suprapatellar and the popliteal. Some fat pads occupy space within the synovial capsule (see Figure 20–4).

## Nerve Supply

The tibial nerve innervates most of the hamstrings and the gastrocnemius. The common peroneal nerve innervates the short head of the biceps femoris and then courses through the popliteal fossa and wraps around the proximal head of the fibula. Because the peroneal nerve is exposed at the head of the fibula, contusion of the nerve can cause distal sensory and motor deficits. The femoral nerve innervates the quadriceps and the sartorius muscles (Figure 20–6).

## Blood Supply

The main blood supply to the knee comes from the popliteal artery, which stems from the femoral artery. From the popliteal artery, four branches supply the knee: the medial and lateral superior genicular and medial and lateral inferior genicular arteries (Figure 20–7A&B). Blood drains via the small saphenous vein into the popliteal vein and then to the femoral vein (Figure 20–7C).

## Surface Anatomy

Figure 20–8 shows the pertinent surface anatomy landmarks of the knee joint complex from anterior, posterior, and lateral views.

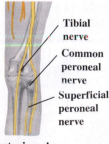

Tibial nerve

Common peroneal nerve

Superficial peroneal nerve

**Posterior view**

**FIGURE 20–6**    Nerve supply to the knee.

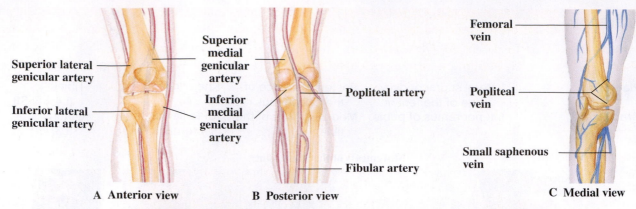

FIGURE 20–7  Blood supply of the knee. **(A)** Anterior arteries. **(B)** Posterior arteries. **(C)** Venous supply.

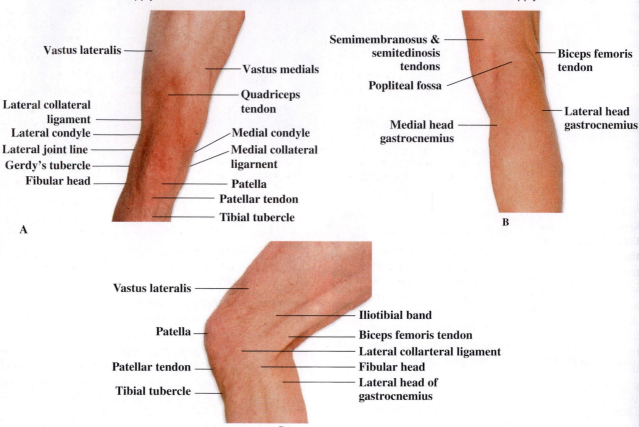

FIGURE 20–8  Surface anatomy of the knee from **(A)** anterior view, **(B)** posterior view, and **(C)** lateral view.

# FUNCTIONAL ANATOMY

Movement between the tibia and the femur involves the physiological motions of flexion, extension, and rotation as well as arthrokinematic motions, including rolling and gliding. As the tibia extends on the stationary femur, the tibia glides and rolls anteriorly. If the femur is extending on the stationary tibia, gliding occurs in a posterior direction, whereas rolling occurs anteriorly.

Axial rotation of the femur relative to the weight-bearing tibia is an important component of knee motion. In the "screw home" mechanism of the knee, in weight bearing with the tibia fixed as the knee extends, the femur must internally rotate to achieve full extension because the medial femoral condyle is larger than the lateral condyle. The rotational component gives a great deal of stability to the knee in full extension. When weight bearing, the popliteus muscle must contract and externally rotate the femur to "unlock" the knee so that flexion can occur.

**Major actions of the knee:**

- Flexion
- Extension
- Rotation
- Rolling
- Gliding

The capsular ligaments are taut during full extension and somewhat more lax during flexion. Relaxation of the more superficial collateral ligaments allows rotation to occur. In contrast, the deeper capsular ligament tightens to prevent excessive rotation of the tibia.[43]

During the last 15 degrees of extension, the tibia externally rotates and the anterior cruciate ligament unwinds. In full extension the posteriolateral portion of anterior cruciate ligament is taut, and it loosens during flexion. As the femur glides on the tibia, the posterior cruciate ligament becomes taut and prevents further gliding. In general, the anterior cruciate ligament stops excessive internal rotation, stabilizes the knee in full extension, and prevents hyperextension. The posterior cruciate ligament prevents excessive internal rotation of the tibia, limits anterior translation of the femur on the fixed tibia, and limits posterior translation of the tibia in non–weight bearing.[43]

In complete flexion, approximately 140 degrees, the range of the knee movement is limited by the extremely shortened position of the hamstring muscles, the extensibility of the quadriceps muscles, and the bulk of the hamstring muscles. In this position, the femoral condyles rest on their corresponding menisci at a point that permits a small degree of internal rotation.

The patella aids the knee during extension by lengthening the lever arm of the quadriceps muscle.[74] It distributes the compressive stresses on the femur by increasing the contact area between the patellar tendon and the femur.[125] It also protects the patellar tendon against friction. During full extension, the patella lies slightly lateral and proximal to the femoral groove, or trochlea. At 20 degrees of knee flexion, there is tibial rotation, and the patella moves into the trochlea. At 30 degrees, the patella is most prominent. At 30 degrees and more, the patella moves deeper into the trochlea. At 90 degrees, the patella again becomes positioned laterally. When knee flexion is 135 degrees, the patella has moved laterally beyond the trochlea.[125]

## The Knee in the Kinetic Chain

The knee is part of the kinetic chain that was discussed in Chapter 16. It is directly affected by motions and forces occurring to and being transmitted from the foot, ankle, and lower leg. In turn, the knee must transmit forces to the thigh, hip, pelvis, and spine. Abnormal forces that cannot be distributed must be absorbed by the tissues. When the foot is in contact with the ground, a closed kinetic chain exists. In a closed kinetic chain, forces must either be transmitted to proximal segments or be absorbed in a more distal joint. The inability of this closed system to dissipate these forces typically leads to a breakdown in some part of the system. As part of the kinetic chain, the knee joint is susceptible to injury resulting from the absorption of these forces.[27]

# ASSESSING THE KNEE JOINT

It is the responsibility of the team physician to provide a medical diagnosis of the severity and exact nature of a knee injury. Although the physician is charged with the final medical diagnosis, the athletic trainer is usually the first person to observe the injury; therefore, he or she is charged with clinical diagnosis and immediate care. The most important aspect of understanding what pathological process has taken place is to become familiar with the traumatic sequence and mechanisms of injury, either through having seen the injury occur or through learning its history (Figure 20–9).[24] Often, the team physician is not present when the injury occurs, and the athletic trainer must relate the pertinent information.[88]

## History

To determine the history and major complaints involved in acute knee injury, the athletic trainer should ask the following questions.

### Current Injury

- What were you doing when the knee was hurt?
- What position was your body in?
- Did the knee collapse?
- Did you hear a noise or feel any sensation at the time of injury, such as a pop or crunch?
- Could you move the knee immediately after the injury? If not, was it locked in a bent or extended position? (Locking could mean a meniscal tear.) After being locked, how did it become unlocked?
- Did swelling occur? If yes, was it immediate, or did it occur later? (Immediate swelling could indicate a cruciate or tibial fracture, whereas later swelling could indicate a capsular, synovial, or meniscal tear.)
- Where was the pain? Was it local, all over, or did it move from one side of the knee to the other?
- Have you hurt the knee before? (Refer to "Recurrent or Chronic Injury," which follows)

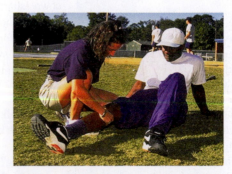

**FIGURE 20–9** It is extremely important that the sequence and mechanism of a knee injury be known before the pathological process can be understood.
© William E. Prentice

When first evaluating the injury, the athletic trainer should observe whether the patient is able to support body weight flatfooted on the injured leg or whether the patient needs to stand and walk on the toes. Toe walking is an indication that the patient is holding the knee in a splinted position to avoid pain or that the knee is being held in a flexed position by a piece of a torn or dislocated meniscus. In first-time acute knee sprains, fluid and blood effusion is not usually apparent until after a 24-hour period. However, in an anterior cruciate ligament sprain, a hemarthrosis may occur during the first hour after injury. Swelling and ecchymosis will occur and are necessary effects of the inflammatory process. Compression and elevation are key immediate treatments that can be used to help limit swelling.

**Recurrent or Chronic Injury**

- What is your major complaint?
- When did you first notice the condition?
- Is there recurrent swelling?
- Does the knee ever lock or catch? (If yes, it may be a torn meniscus or a loose body in the knee joint.)
- Is there severe pain? Is it constant, or does it come and go?
- Do you feel any grinding or grating sensations? (If yes, it could indicate chondromalacia or traumatic arthritis.)
- Does your knee ever feel like it is going to give way, or has it actually done so? (If yes and often, it may be a capsular, cruciate, or meniscal tear; a loose body; or a subluxating patella.)
- What does it feel like to go up and down stairs? (Pain could indicate a patellofemoral pain syndrome or meniscal tear, for example.)
- What past treatment (past surgery, physical therapy, etc.), if any, have you received for this or any other previous lower extremity injury or condition?

## Observation

A visual examination should be performed after the major complaints have been determined. The patient should be observed in a number of situations: walking, half-squatting, and going up and down stairs. The leg also should be observed for alignment and symmetry or asymmetry.

> **If possible, the patient with an injured knee should be observed in the following actions:**
>
> - Walking
> - Half-squatting
> - Going up and down stairs

- Does the patient walk with a limp, or is the walk free and easy? Is the patient able to fully extend the knee during heel strike?
- Can the patient fully bear weight on the affected leg?
- Can the patient perform a half-squat to extension?
- Can the patient go up and down stairs with ease? (If stairs are unavailable, stepping up on a box or stool will suffice.)

- Does the patient have full range of motion (full extension to 0 degrees and 135 degrees of flexion)?
- If movement screens such as the double leg squat, single leg squat, or jump landing (see Chapter 13) are used, what can be observed about knee function?

**Leg Alignment** The patient should be observed for leg alignment. Anteriorly, the patient should be evaluated for genu valgum, genu varum, and the position of the patella. Next, the patient should be observed from the side to ascertain conditions such as the hyperflexed or hyperextended knee.

Deviations in normal leg alignment may be a factor in a knee injury but should always be considered as a possible cause. Like alignment in any other body segment, leg alignment differs from person to person; however, obvious discrepancies could predispose the individual to an acute or chronic injury.

Anteriorly, with the knees fully extended, the following points should be noted:

- Are the patellas level with each other?
- Are the patellas facing inward (squinting patella)?

Looking at the patient's knees from the side, these questions should be answered:

- Are the knees fully extended with only slight hyperextension?
- Are both knees equally extended?

***Leg Alignment Deviations That May Predispose to Injury*** Four major leg deviations could adversely affect the knee and patellofemoral joints: patellar malalignment, genu valgum (knock-knees), genu varum (bowlegs), and genu recurvatum (hyperextended knees).

> **Leg deviations:**
>
> - Patella alta
> - Patella baja
> - Genu valgum
> - Genu varum
> - Genu recurvatum

*Patellar malalignment* In **patella alta**, the patella sets in a more superior position than normal when the patient is standing. The ratio of patellar tendon length to the height of the patella is greater than the normal 1:1 ratio. In patella alta, the length of the patellar tendon is 20 percent greater than the height of the patella. In **patella baja**, the patella sets in a more inferior position than normal and the ratio of patellar tendon length to the height of the patella is less than the normal 1:1 ratio.

A patella that is rotated inward or outward from the center may be caused by a complex set of circumstances. For example, a combination of genu recurvatum, genu varum, and internal rotation, or anteversion, of the hip and internal rotation of the tibia could cause the patella to face inward. Internal rotation of the hip also may be associated with knock-knees, along with external rotation of the tibia, or tibial torsion. Patients who toe-out when they walk may have an externally rotated hip, or retroversion. The normal angulation of

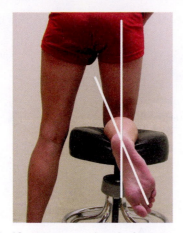

FIGURE 20–10   Measuring for tibial torsion.
© William E. Prentice

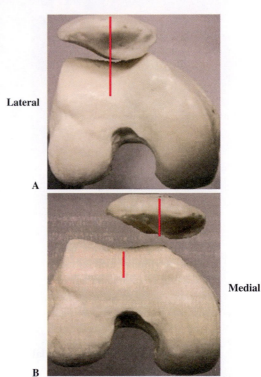

FIGURE 20–11   Glide component. **(A)** Normal. **(B)** Positive medial glide.
© William E. Prentice

the femoral neck after 8 years of age is 15 degrees; an increase of this angle is considered anteversion, and a decrease is considered retroversion. If an abnormal angulation seems to be a factor with the patella, malalignment or tibial torsion angles should be measured.

***Measuring for tibial torsion, femoral anteversion, and femoral retroversion***   Tibial torsion is determined by having the patient kneel on a stool, chair, or bench with the foot relaxed. An imaginary line is drawn along the center of the thigh and lower leg, bisecting the middle of the heel and the bottom of the foot. Another line starts at the center of the middle toe and crosses the center of the heel. The angle formed by the two lines is measured (Figure 20–10); an angle measuring more or less than 15 degrees is a sign of tibial torsion.

Femoral anteversion or retroversion can be determined by the number of degrees the thigh rotates in each direction. As a rule, external rotation and internal rotation added together equal close to 100 degrees. If internal rotation exceeds 70 degrees, there may be anteversion of the hip (see Chapter 21).

Hyperextension of the knee may result in internal rotation of the femur and external rotation of the tibia. Internal rotation at the hip is caused by weak external rotator muscles or foot pronation.

***Patellar orientation***   *Patellar orientation* refers to the positioning of the patella relative to the tibia.[88] Assessment should be done with the patient in supine position. Four components should be assessed when looking at patellar orientation: the glide component, the tilt component, the rotation component, and the anteroposterior tilt component. The *glide* component assesses whether the patella is deviated either laterally or medially to the center of the trochlear groove of the femur (Figure 20–11). Glide should be assessed both statically and dynamically. Patellar *tilt* is determined by comparing the height of the medial patellar border with the lateral patellar border (Figure 20–12). If the medial border is more anterior than the lateral border, a positive lateral tilt exists. Patellar *rotation* is identified by assessing the deviation of the longitudinal axis (line drawn from superior pole to inferior pole) of the patella relative to the

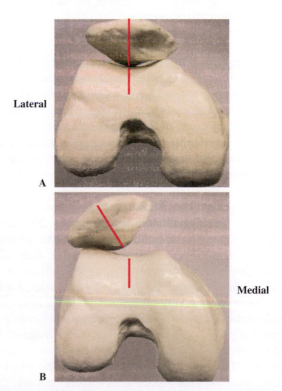

FIGURE 20–12   Tilt component. **(A)** Normal. **(B)** Positive medial tilt.
© William E. Prentice

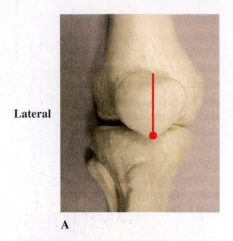

Lateral

A

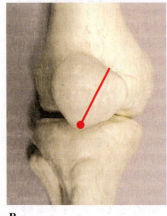

Medial

B

FIGURE 20–13   Rotation component. **(A)** Normal.
**(B)** Positive external rotation.
© William E. Prentice

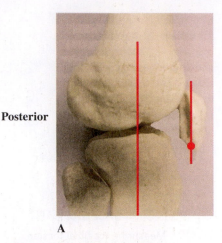

Posterior

A

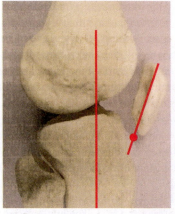

Anterior

B

FIGURE 20–14   Anteroposterior tilt (lateral view).
**(A)** Normal. **(B)** Positive inferior anteroposterior tilt.
© William E. Prentice

femur (Figure 20–13). The point of reference is the inferior pole. Thus, if the inferior pole is more lateral than the superior pole, a positive external rotation exists. The *anteroposterior tilt* component must be assessed laterally to determine if a line drawn from the inferior patellar pole to the superior patellar pole is parallel to the long axis of the femur (Figure 20–14). If the inferior pole is posterior to the superior pole, the patient has a positive anteroposterior tilt component.[88]

*Genu valgum*   The causes of **genu valgum**, or knock-knees, can be multiple (Figure 20–15A). Normally, toddlers and very young children display knock-knees. When the legs have strengthened and the feet have become positioned more in line with the pelvis, the condition is usually corrected. Commonly associated with genu valgum are excessively pronated feet. Genu valgum places chronic tension on the ligamentous structures of the medial part of the knee, abnormal compression of the lateral aspect of the knee surface, and abnormal tightness of the iliotibial band. One or both legs may be affected, and the hip's external rotator muscles may be weak.[86]

*Genu varum*   The two types of **genu varum**, or bow-legs, are structural and functional (Figure 20–15B). The structural type, which is seldom seen in young patients,

reflects a deviation of the femur and tibia. The more common functional, or postural, type usually is associated with knees that are hyperextended and femurs that are internally rotated. Often, correcting genu recurvatum also corrects genu varum.

*Genu recurvatum*   **Genu recurvatum** (Figure 20–15C), or hyperextended knees, commonly occurs as a compensation for lordosis, or swayback (see Figure 25–14).[70] There is notable weakness and stretching of the hamstring muscles. Chronic hyperextension can produce undue anterior pressure on the knee joint and posterior ligaments and tendons.

**Knee Symmetry**   The athletic trainer must establish whether both of the patient's knees look the same:

• Do the knees appear symmetrical?
• Is one knee obviously swollen?
• Is muscle atrophy apparent?

**Leg-Length Discrepancy**   Discrepancies in leg length can occur as a result of many causes, either anatomical or functional (see Chapter 21 for a detailed discussion). True anatomical leg length can be measured from the anterior superior iliac spine (ASIS) to the medial malleolus.

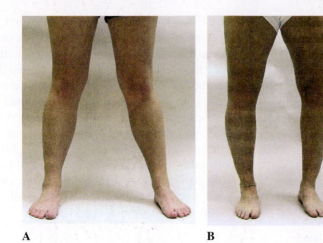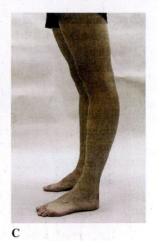

FIGURE 20–15   Leg alignment. **(A)** Genu valgum. **(B)** Genu varum. **(C)** Genu recurvatum.
© William E. Prentice

Functional leg length can be measured from the umbilicus to the medial malleolus.

Anatomical differences in leg length can cause problems in all weight-bearing joints. Functional differences can be caused by rotations of the pelvis or malalignments of the spine.

## Palpation

**Bony Palpation**  The bony structures of the knee are palpated for pain and deformities that might indicate a fracture or dislocation. The patient sits on the edge of the treatment table or a bench. With the patient's knee flexed to 90 degrees, the athletic trainer palpates the following bony structures:

### Medial Aspect
- Medial tibial plateau
- Medial femoral condyle
- Medial epicondyle
- Adductor tubercle

### Lateral Aspect
- Lateral tibial plateau
- Lateral femoral condyle
- Lateral epicondyle
- Head of the fibula
- Gerdy's tubercle

### Anterior Aspect
- Patella
- Tibial tuberosity

### Patella
- Superior patellar border (base)
- Inferior patellar border (apex)
- Around periphery with the knee relaxed
- Around periphery with the knee in full extension

### Soft-Tissue Palpation
The following soft-tissue structures should be palpated:

### Anterior
- Vastus medialis
- Vastus lateralis
- Rectus femoris
- Quadriceps tendon
- Sartorius
- Medial patellar plica
- Patellar tendon
- Anterior joint capsule

### Medial
- Medial collateral ligament, superficial portion
- Medial collateral ligament, capsular portion
- Pes anserinus insertion (sartorius, gracilis, semitendinosus)
- Medial joint capsule

### Posterior
- Semitendinosus
- Popliteus
- Medial and lateral heads of the gastrocnemius
- Biceps femoris
- Posterior oblique ligament

### Lateral
- Lateral collateral ligament
- Iliotibial band
- Lateral joint capsule
- Arcuate complex

**Palpation of Swelling Patterns**  Palpation of joint effusion and associated swelling patterns are critical in assessing knee injury (Figure 20–16). Swelling may be *intracapsular* (inside the joint capsule) or *extracapsular* (outside the joint capsule). Intracapsular swelling may also be referred to as a *joint effusion*. A moderate amount of swelling that occurs immediately following injury and that is caused by synovial fluid and by blood in the joint is called a **hemarthrosis**. A hemarthrosis can only be identified by having the team physician aspirate the joint with a needle. With intracapsular

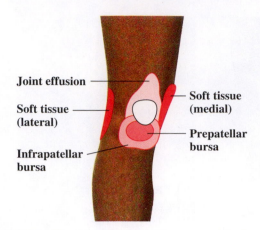

**FIGURE 20–16**  Typical swelling sites around the knee.
© William E. Prentice

Labels on figure:
Joint effusion
Soft tissue (lateral)
Infrapatellar bursa
Soft tissue (medial)
Prepatellar bursa

joint effusion, the fluid in the joint can be moved manually from one side of the joint to the other. In a *sweep maneuver*, pressure applied from superior to the patella downward moves fluid into the center of the joint capsule; then pressure from the medial side of the joint line will cause a bulging laterally. Joint effusion can also cause what has been referred to as a *ballotable patella*. With the knee in full extension and the quadriceps relaxed, a release of downward pressure on the patella sitting on top of the joint capsule causes the patella to bounce back to its normal position.

Extracapsular swelling from bursitis, tendinitis, or injury to one of the collateral ligaments tends to localize over the injured structure and then gradually migrate downward toward the foot and ankle because of the effects of gravity.

### Special Tests for Assessment of Knee Joint Instability

Both traumatic and overuse injury to the knee can produce ligamentous instability. It is advisable that the injured knee's stability be evaluated as soon after injury as possible. The injured knee and uninjured knee are tested and contrasted to determine any differences in their stability.

Determination of the degree of instability is made by feeling the endpoint during stability testing. As stress is applied to a joint, there will be some motion, which is limited by an intact ligament. In a normal joint, the endpoint will be abrupt with little or no give and no reported pain. With a grade 1

sprain, the endpoint will still be firm with little or no instability, and some pain will be indicated. With a grade 2 sprain, the endpoint will be soft with some instability present and a moderate amount of pain. In a grade 3 complete rupture, the endpoint will be very soft with marked instability, and pain will be severe initially, then mild.[86]

The use of magnetic resonance imaging (MRI) as a diagnostic tool has aided tremendously in the classification of ligamentous sprains. Despite its expense, MRI is being widely used by physicians to detect ligament injuries.

Table 20–2 provides a summary of the various tests and what a positive test indicates in terms of the injured structures.

**Classification of Knee Joint Instabilities**  A good deal of controversy exists over the most appropriate terminology for classifying instabilities in the knee joint.[103] For years, the American Orthopedic Society for Sports Medicine has classified knee laxity as either a straight or a rotatory instability. *Straight instability* implies laxity in a single direction—medial, lateral, anterior, or posterior. *Rotatory instability* refers to excessive rotation of the tibial plateau relative to the femoral condyles and is identified as anterolateral, anteromedial, posterolateral, or, rarely, posteromedial. It is not unusual to see combined instabilities, depending on the structures that have been injured. This classification system is still the most widely used and accepted by athletic trainers (Table 20–3).

The concept of tibial translation has been proposed.[103]  **Translation** refers to the amount of gliding of the medial tibial plateau as compared with the lateral tibial plateau relative to the femoral condyles. For example, in anterolateral rotatory instability, the anterior translation of the lateral tibial plateau would be much greater than the more stable medial tibial plateau. The amount of anterior translation is determined by the integrity of the anatomical restraints that normally restrict excessive translation. More ligamentous, tendinous, and capsular structures will be damaged as the severity of the injury increases.

**Collateral Ligament Stress Tests**  Valgus and varus stress tests are intended to reveal laxity of the medial and lateral stabilizing complexes, especially the collateral ligaments. The patient lies supine with the leg extended.

***Valgus Stress Test***[60]  To test the medial side, the athletic trainer holds the ankle firmly with one hand while placing the other hand over the head of the fibula. The athletic trainer then places a force inward in an attempt to open the side of the knee. This valgus stress is applied with the knee fully extended, or at 0 degrees, and at 30 degrees of flexion (Figure 20–17A&B). The examination in full extension tests the MCL, posteromedial capsule, and cruciates. At 30 degrees of flexion, the MCL is isolated. Sn. 0.56 | Sp. 0.91 | +LR 6.4 | -LR 0.5

## TABLE 20–2  Knee Stability Tests

| Test | If Positive |
| --- | --- |
| Valgus stress test at 0° | Torn MCL and possibly ACL, PCL, PMC |
| Valgus stress test at 20°/30° | Torn MCL (if grade 3 check ACL, PCL, PMC) |
| Varus stress test at 0° | Torn LCL and possibly ACL, PCL, PLC |
| Varus stress test at 20°/30° | Torn LCL (if grade 3 check ACL, PCL, PLC) |
| Lachman drawer test (20°/30° flexion) | Torn ACL, PCL (positive more often than anterior drawer because hamstrings are relaxed and medial meniscus/collateral ligaments do not block anterior displacement at 20°) |
| Anterior drawer test (neutral) | Torn ACL |
| Anterior drawer test (15° ER) | Torn PMC, ACL, and possibly MCL |
| Anterior drawer test (30° IR) | Torn PLC, ACL |
| Pivot-shift tests (Galaway and McIntosh) | Torn ACL, ALC |
|   Extension/IR/valgus (tibia subluxated) → flexion (tibia reduces at 20°) | |
| Slocum's test | Torn ACL, ALC |
|   Side-lying extension/IR/valgus (tibia subluxated) → flexion (tibia reduces at 20°) | |
| Jerk test (Hughston) | Torn ACL, ALC |
|   Flexion/IR/valgus (tibia reduced) → extension (tibia subluxates at 20°) | |
| Losee test | Torn ACL, ALC |
|   45° flexion/ER/valgus (tibia subluxated anteriorly) → extension (tibia reduces at 20°) | |
| Flexion-rotation drawer test | Torn ACL |
|   45° flex (tibia subluxated anteriorly/femur ER) → flexion (tibia reduces posteriorly/femur IR) | |
| Posterior drawer test 90° | Torn PCL |
| External rotation recurvatum test (tibia ER) | Torn PCL, PLC |
| Posterior sag test 90° | Torn PCL |
| Reverse pivot-shift test (Jakob) | Torn PCL |
|   Extension (tibia reduced) → flexion (tibia subluxated posteriorly with ER) | |
| McMurray's test | |
|   (IR) | Torn LM |
|   (ER) | Torn MM |
| Apley's grinding test | Torn MM |
| Thessaly's Test | Torn LM or MM |

ACL = anterior cruciate ligament; ALC = anterior lateral corner; ER = external rotation; IR = internal rotation; LCL = lateral collateral ligament; LM = lateral meniscus; MCL = medial collateral ligament; MM = medial meniscus; PCL = posterior cruciate ligament; PLC = posterior lateral corner; PMC = posterior medial corner.

A football running back is hit on the lateral surface of his knee by an opponent making a tackle. He has significant pain and some immediate swelling on the medial surface of his knee. The athletic trainer suspects that the athlete has sustained a sprain of the MCL.

? What are the most appropriate tests that the athletic trainer should do to determine the exact nature and extent of the injury?

**Varus Stress Test**[76]
The athletic trainer reverses hand positions and tests the lateral side with a varus force on the fully extended knee and then with 30 degrees of flexion (Figure 20–17C&D). With the knee extended, the LCL and posterolateral capsule are examined. At 30 degrees of flexion, the LCL is isolated.[86] NOTE: The lower limb should be in a neutral position with no internal or external rotation. Sn. 0.25 | Sp. 0.99 | +LR 17.3 | -LR 0.76

**Apley Distraction Test**[44]  With the patient in the same position as for the Apley compression test, the athletic trainer applies traction to the lower leg while rotating it back and forth (Figure 20–18). This maneuver distinguishes collateral ligamentous tears from capsular and meniscal tears. If the

## TABLE 20–3  Classification of Instabilities

| Straight Instabilities | Rotatory Instabilities |
| --- | --- |
| Medial | Anterolateral |
| Lateral | Anteromedial |
| Anterior | Posterolateral |
| Posterior | |

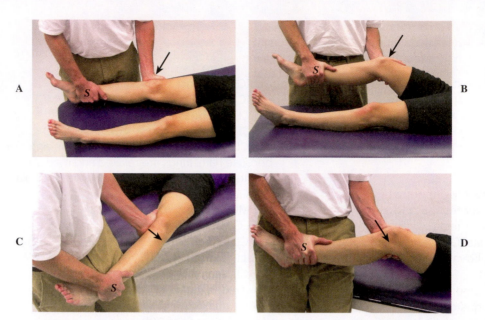

FIGURE 20–17   Valgus and varus knee stress tests. **(A)** Valgus at 0 degrees.
**(B)** Valgus at 30 degrees. **(C)** Varus at 0 degrees. **(D)** Varus at 30 degrees. (S = stabilize)
© William E. Prentice

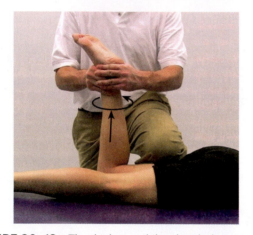

FIGURE 20–18   The thigh is stabilized with the examiner's knee while the lower leg is distracted and rotated.
© William E. Prentice

capsule or ligaments are affected, pain will occur; if the meniscus is torn, no pain will occur from the traction and rotation.[86] Sn. 0.60 | Sp. 0.70 | +LR 2.0 | -LR 0.57

**Anterior Cruciate Ligament Tests**   A number of tests are used to establish the integrity of the cruciate ligaments.[103] They are the drawer test at 90 degrees of flexion, the Lachman drawer test, the pivot-shift test, the jerk test, and the flexion-rotation drawer test.

***Drawer Test at 90 Degrees of Flexion*[62]**   The patient lies on the treatment table with the injured leg flexed. The athletic trainer stands facing the anterior aspect of the patient's leg, with both hands encircling the upper portion of the leg immediately below the knee joint. The athletic trainer positions his or her fingers in the popliteal space of the affected leg, with the thumbs on the medial and lateral joint lines (Figure 20–19). The athletic trainer places his or her index

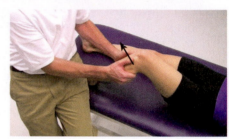

FIGURE 20–19   Anterior drawer test for cruciate laxity. With the knee flexed to 90 degrees, apply an anterior force first with the foot pointing straight. Slocum's test is performed with the knee at 90 degrees and the leg internally rotated, then with the knee at 90 degrees and the leg externally rotated.
© William E. Prentice

fingers on the hamstring tendon to ensure that it is relaxed before the test is administered.[62] If the tibia slides forward from under the femur, this is considered a positive anterior drawer sign.[87] Slocum's test should be performed with the patient's leg rotated internally 30 degrees and externally 15 degrees (Figure 20–19). Anterior translation of the tibia when the leg is externally rotated is an indication that the posteromedial aspect of the joint capsule, the anterior cruciate ligament, or possibly the medial collateral ligament is torn. Movement when the leg is internally rotated indicates that the anterior cruciate ligament and posterolateral capsule may be torn. Anterior translation of ½ inch, ½ to ¾ inch, and ¾ inch or more (1.25 cm, 1.25 to 1.9 cm, and 1.9 cm or more) corresponds to grades 1, 2, and 3, respectively.[62] Sn. 0.41 | Sp. 0.95 | +LR 8.2 | -LR 0.62

***Lachman Drawer Test*[62]**   The Lachman drawer test is considered to be a better test than the drawer test at 90 degrees of flexion (Figure 20–20).[112] This preference is especially true for examinations immediately after injury. One reason for

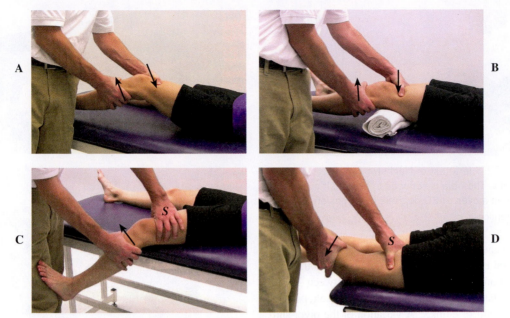

FIGURE 20–20   Lachman drawer test for anterior cruciate laxity. **(A)** Standard Lachman drawer test. **(B)** Alternative technique one. **(C)** Alternative technique two. **(D)** Prone Lachman drawer test. (S = stabilize)
© William E. Prentice

using it immediately after an injury is that it does not force the knee into the painful 90-degree position but tests it at a more comfortable 20 to 30 degrees. Another reason for its increased popularity is that it reduces the restriction created by the hamstring muscles.[83] That contraction causes a secondary knee-stabilizing force that tends to mask the real extent of injury. The Lachman drawer test is administered by positioning the knee in approximately 30 degrees of flexion. The athletic trainer uses one hand to stabilize the leg by grasping the distal end of the thigh and the other hand to grasp the proximal aspect of the tibia and attempts to move it anteriorly. One problem with the Lachman test is that, if the patient is very large or if the athletic trainer has small hands, it is difficult to perform this test efficiently.[52] Several alternative methods may be used. First, a tightly rolled towel or other support can be placed under the femur and the athletic trainer can use one hand to stabilize the femur and the other to anteriorly translate the tibia (Figure 20–20B). A second alternative is to slide the lower leg off the edge of the examining table with the knee and femur supported by the edge

of the table. Again, one hand should be used to stabilize the femur and the other to anteriorly translate the tibia (Figure 20–20C). Finally, the patient may be placed prone with the knee and lower leg just off the edge of the table. This position minimizes any posterior sag of the tibia that can mask a positive test.[83] Using the table to stabilize the femur, the athletic trainer can anteriorly translate the tibia (Figure 20–20D). A positive Lachman test indicates damage to the anterior cruciate. Sn. 0.68 | Sp. 0.94 | +LR 11.3 | -LR 0.39

***Pivot-Shift Test***[62]   The pivot-shift test is designed to determine anterolateral rotary instability (Figure 20–21A). It is most often used in chronic conditions and is a sensitive test when the anterior cruciate ligament has been torn. The patient lies supine. The athletic trainer uses one hand to press against the head of the fibula and the other to grasp the patient's ankle. To start, the lower leg is internally rotated and the knee is fully extended. The thigh is then flexed 30 degrees at the hip while the knee is also flexed, and the athletic trainer applies a simultaneous valgus force and axial load with his

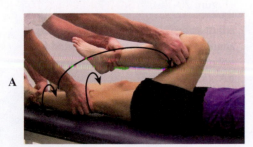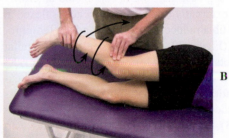

FIGURE 20–21   **(A)** Pivot-shift test (Gallaway and McIntosh) for anterolateral rotary instability. The tibia is subluxated in extension. It reduces at 20 degrees of flexion. **(B)** Slocum's knee test is exactly the same but done in a side-lying position.
© William E. Prentice

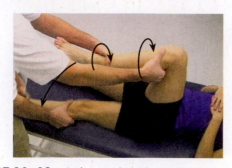

FIGURE 20–22  Jerk test of Hughston for anterolateral rotary instability. The tibia is reduced in flexion. It subluxates as the knee moves to 20 degrees of extension.
© William E. Prentice

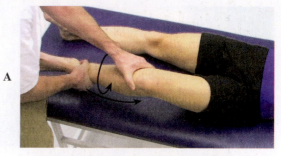

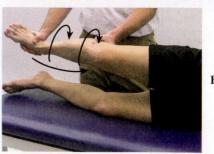

FIGURE 20–23  **(A)** Flexion-rotation drawer test. The leg is externally rotated and moved from extension to flexion. **(B)** Losee's test is similar but is done with the patient side-lying.
© William E. Prentice

or her upper hand. If the anterior cruciate ligament is damaged, the lateral tibial plateau will be subluxated in the fully extended position. As the knee is flexed to between 20 and 40 degrees, the lateral tibial plateau will reduce itself, producing a palpable shift or clunk.[86] A variation of the pivot-shift test is Slocum's test, which is done in a side-lying position (Figure 20–21B).[86] Sn. 0.82 | Sp. 0.98 | +LR +41 | -LR 0.18

**Jerk Test**  The jerk test reverses the direction of the pivot-shift test.[86] The position of the knee is identical to that for the pivot-shift test except that the knee is moved from a position of flexion into extension with the lateral tibial plateau in a reduced position. If there is anterior cruciate insufficiency, as the knee moves into extension the tibia will subluxate at about 20 degrees of flexion, once again producing a palpable shift or clunk (Figure 20–22).

**Flexion-Rotation Drawer Test[3]**  With this test, the lower leg is cradled with the knee flexed between 15 and 30 degrees. At 15 degrees, the tibia is subluxated anteriorly with the femur externally rotated. As the knee is flexed to 30 degrees, the tibia reduces posteriorly and the femur rotates internally (Figure 20–23A).[103] Losee's test is similar to the flexion-rotation drawer test, but it is done in a side-lying position. It begins at 45 degrees of flexion with external tibial rotation and the tibia subluxated anteriorly. As the knee is extended, the tibia reduces at about 20 degrees (Figure 20–23B). Sn. 0.38 | Sp. 0.96 | +LR 9.5 | -LR 0.65

**Posterior Cruciate Ligament Tests**  Tests for posterior cruciate ligament instability include the posterior drawer test, the external rotation recurvatum test, and the posterior sag test.

**Posterior Drawer Test[100]**  The posterior drawer test is performed with the knee flexed at 90 degrees and the foot in neutral. Force is exerted in a posterior direction at the proximal tibial plateau. A positive posterior drawer test indicates damage to the posterior cruciate ligament (Figure 20–24). Sn. 0.90 | Sp. 0.99 | +LR +90 | -LR -0.10

**External Rotation Recurvatum Test[100]**  The athletic trainer grasps the great toe and lifts the leg off the table. If the tibia externally rotates and slides posteriorly, there may be injury to the posterior cruciate ligament and posterolateral corner of the joint capsule, creating posterolateral instability (Figure 20–25).[103] Sn. 0.90 | Sp. 0.99 | +LR NA | -LR NA

**Posterior Sag Test (Godfrey's Test)[100]**  With the patient supine, both knees are flexed to 90 degrees. Observing laterally on the injured side, the tibia will appear to sag posteriorly when compared with the opposite extremity if the posterior cruciate ligament is damaged (Figure 20–26).[103] Sn. 0.79-1.0 | Sp. 1.0 | +LR NA | -LR NA

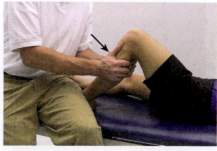

FIGURE 20–24  Posterior drawer test.
© William E. Prentice

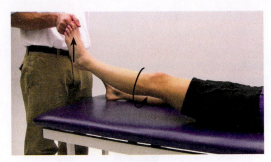

**FIGURE 20–25** External rotation recurvatum test.
© William E. Prentice

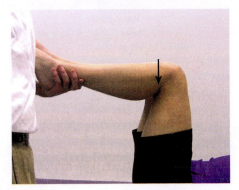

**FIGURE 20–26** Posterior sag test (Godfrey's test).
© William E. Prentice

**Instrument Assessment of Cruciate Laxity**[100] Several ligament-testing devices called arthrometers are currently available that objectively quantify the anterior or posterior displacement of the knee joint, thus reducing much of the subjectivity associated with the previously described tests.[88] The KT-2000 knee arthrometer, the Stryker knee laxity tester, and the Genucom are three such testing devices (Figure 20–27).

Measurements taken postoperatively and at periodic intervals throughout the rehabilitation process provide an objective indication to the athletic trainer about the effectiveness of the treatment program in maintaining or reducing anterior or posterior translation.[103]
Sn. 0.76–0.90 | Sp. 0.98–0.96 | +LR NA | -LR NA

**Meniscal Tests** Determining a torn meniscus can be difficult. The three most commonly used tests are McMurray's meniscal test, the Apley compression test, and the Thessaly test.

***McMurray's Meniscal Test***[30] McMurray's meniscal test (Figure 20–28) is used to determine the presence of a displaceable meniscal tear within the knee. The patient is positioned faceup on the table with the injured leg fully flexed. The athletic trainer places one hand on the foot and one hand over the top of the knee, fingers touching the medial joint line. The ankle hand scribes a small circle and pulls the leg into extension. As this occurs, the hand on the knee feels for a clicking response. Medial meniscal tears can be detected when the lower leg is externally rotated, and internal rotation allows the detection of lateral tears.
Sn. 0.16 | Sp. 0.98 | +LR 8.0 | -LR 0.86

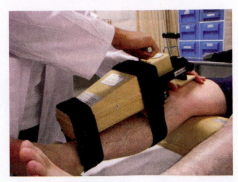

**FIGURE 20–27** Knee arthrometer for measuring knee laxity objectively.
Lam, Mak-Ham et al. "Knee Stability Assessment on Anterior Cruciate Ligament Injury: Clinical and Biomechanical Approaches." Sports Medicine, Arthroscopy, Rehabilitation, Therapy, and Technology : SMARTT 1: 20 (2009). *PMC*. © 2009 by Lam, Mak-Ham et al. All rights reserved. Used with Permission.

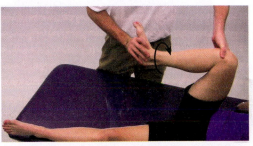

**A**

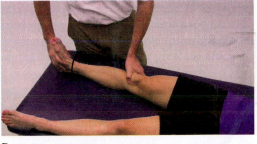

**B**

**FIGURE 20–28** McMurray's meniscal test. **(A)** The clinician flexes the knee and laterally rotates the tibia, then **(B)** extends the knee while palpating the medial joint line. Next, the clinician flexes the knee and medially rotates the tibia, then extends the knee while palpating the lateral joint line.
© William E. Prentice

***Apley Compression Test***[21] The Apley compression test (Figure 20–29) is performed with the patient lying facedown and the affected leg flexed to 90 degrees. While stabilizing the thigh, the athletic trainer applies a hard, downward pressure to the leg and rotates the leg back and forth. If pain results, a meniscal injury has occurred. A medial meniscal tear is noted by external rotation, and a lateral meniscal tear is noted by internal rotation of the lower leg. Sn. 0.97 | Sp. 0.87 | +LR 7.46 | -LR 0.03

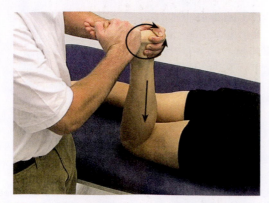

FIGURE 20–29   Apley compression test.
© William E. Prentice

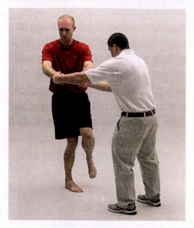

FIGURE 20–30   Thessaly's test performed at both 5 degrees and 20 degrees of knee flexion.
© William E. Prentice

**Thessaly Test**[59]   In the Thessaly test, the patient stands flatfooted on the floor (Figure 20–30).[59] The clinician stands in front of and supports the patient by holding his or her outstretched hands. The patient then rotates his or her knee and body, internally and externally, three times, keeping the knee in 5 degrees of flexion. This procedure is repeated with the knee flexed at 20 degrees. In a positive test, the patient reports medial or lateral joint-line discomfort and may have a sense of locking or catching. With this maneuver, the knee with a meniscal tear is subjected to excessive loading conditions. The test is always performed first on the normal knee, so that the patient can compare the Normal with the injured knee.[59]

Medial Meniscus: Sn. 0.89 | Sp. 0.92 | +LR +29.67 | -LR 0.11
Lateral Meniscus: Sn. 0.97 | Sp. 0.96 | +LR +23 | -LR -0.083

**Girth Measurement**   A knee injury is almost always accompanied by an eventual decrease in the girth of the thigh musculature. The muscles most affected by disuse are the quadriceps group, which are

> Because the musculature of the knee atrophies so readily after an injury, girth measurements must be taken routinely.

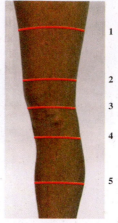

1. 8 to 10 cm
   above joint line
2. 2 cm above patella
3. Joint line (tibial plateau)
4. Tibial tubercle
5. Belly of gastrocnemius

FIGURE 20–31   Five sites for girth measurement.
© William E. Prentice

antigravity muscles and assist humans in maintaining an erect, straight-leg position. They are in constant use in effecting movement. Atrophy results when a lower limb is favored and is not used to its potential. Measurement of the circumference of both thighs can often detect former leg injuries or determine the extent of exercise rehabilitation. Five sites have been suggested for girth measurement: the joint line (tibial plateau), 8 to 10 cm above the tibial plateau; the level of the tibial tubercle; the belly of the gastrocnemius muscle measured in centimeters from the tibial tubercle; and 2 cm above the superior border of the patella recorded in centimeters above the tibial tubercle (Figure 20–31).[86]

**Subjective Rating Scales**   Subjective rating scales, such as the Lysholm Knee Scoring Scale, the Cincinnati Knee Scale, the International Knee Documentation Committee (IKDC) Scale, the Knee Outcome Survey, and the Knee Injury and Osteoarthritis Outcome Score (KOOS) are widely used to determine the patient's perception of how well the injured knee is doing relative to pain, stability, and functional performance.[16] The information obtained from these rating scales can be combined with findings from stability testing to help with an initial diagnosis or evaluation of progress in rehabilitation (*Focus Box 20–1*: "Lysholm knee scoring scale").

## Functional Examination

It is important that the patient's knee also be tested for function. It must be added that not only do patients need to be able to do these functional tests, but do them correctly without altered movements/compensations. The patient must be able to bear weight prior to attempting functional testing. The patient should be observed walking and, if possible, running, turning, performing figure eights,

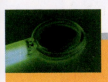

## Lysholm knee scoring scale

1. Please check the statement that best describes the way you walk.
_____ I never walk with a limp.
_____ I rarely walk with a limp or I walk with a slight limp.
_____ I walk with a constant and severe limp.

2. Which of the following do you presently use as a support while you walk?
_____ I can walk without crutches or a cane.
_____ I can put some weight on my leg, but I need at least one crutch or a cane to walk.
_____ I cannot put any weight on my leg when walking.

3. Do you experience LOCKING of your knee?
_____ No, never.
_____ My knee catches, but does not lock.
_____ Yes, my knee locks occasionally.
_____ Yes, my knee locks frequently.
_____ Yes, my knee is locked all the time.

4. Do you experience slipping or giving way of your knee?
_____ No, never.
_____ Yes, rarely during sporting activities or other severe exertion.
_____ Yes, frequently during sporting activities or other severe exertion.
_____ Yes, occasionally during daily activities.
_____ Yes, frequently during daily activities.
_____ Yes, on every step.

5. Which of the following best describes your level of pain?
_____ I have no pain in my knee.
_____ I have occasional pain, which is slight and present only after severe exertion.

_____ I have marked pain during severe exertion.
_____ I have marked pain after walking more than 2 miles.
_____ I have marked pain after walking less than 2 miles.
_____ I have constant pain.

6. Which of the following best describes swelling in your knee?
_____ I have no swelling.
_____ I have swelling only after severe exertion.
_____ I have swelling after ordinary exertion.
_____ I have constant swelling.

7. Which of the following best describes your ability to climb stairs?
_____ I have no problems on stairs.
_____ I am only slightly impaired on stairs.
_____ I can negotiate stairs, but only one at a time.
_____ I cannot go up or down stairs.

8. Can you get into a full squat position?
_____ Yes, no problems.
_____ No, but I am only slightly impaired.
_____ No, I cannot squat with my knee past 90 degrees.
_____ No, I cannot squat at all.

THANK YOU FOR TAKING TIME TO COMPLETE THIS QUESTIONNAIRE.

Tegner Y, Lysholm J: Rating systems in the evaluation of knee ligament injuries, *Clin Orthop* 198:43, 1985.

---

backing up, and stopping. The cocontraction test, vertical jump, and single-leg hop test are also useful functional tests. If the patient can do a deep knee bend or duck walk without discomfort, it is doubtful that there is a meniscal tear. The resistive strength of the hamstring and quadriceps muscles should be compared with the strength of the uninjured knee (Figure 20–32). The patient should be able to perform these tests at full speed, without limping or favoring the injured knee. If baseline testing was done prior to injury, the baseline results should be used to compare with postinjury test results to determine if the patient is able to perform at preinjury levels.

### Patellar Examinations

Any knee evaluation should include inspection of the patella. Numerous evaluation procedures are associated with the patella and its associated structures. The following evaluation procedures can provide valuable information about possible reasons for knee discomfort and problems in functioning.[22,34]

**The Q Angle** The Q angle is created when lines are drawn from the middle of the patella to the anterosuperior spine of the ilium and from the tubercle of the tibia through the center of the patella (Figure 20–33A). It should be measured with the knee fully extended and with the knee flexed at 30 degrees. The normal Q angle is 10 degrees for males and 15 degrees for females. Q angles that exceed 20 degrees are considered excessive and could lead to a pathological condition associated with improper patellar tracking in the femoral groove.[109]

> A Q angle greater than 20 degrees could predispose the athlete to patellar femoral pathology.

**The A Angle** The A angle measures the patellar orientation to the tibial tubercle. It is created by the intersection of a line that bisects the patella longitudinally and a line from the tibial tubercle to the apex of the inferior pole of the patella (Figure 20–33B).[88] An A angle of 35 degrees or

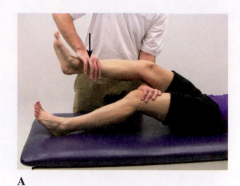

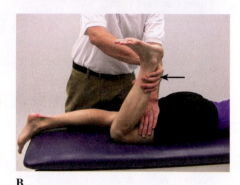

**A**

**B**

FIGURE 20–32  **(A)** Testing quadriceps strength.
**(B)** Testing hamstring strength.
© William E. Prentice

greater has been correlated with patellofemoral pathomechanics that seem to result in constant patellofemoral pain. The A angle serves as a quantitative measure of patellar realignment after rehabilitative intervention.

**Palpation of the Patella** With the patient's quadriceps muscle fully relaxed, the examiner palpates the patella for pain sites around its periphery and under its sides (Figure 20–34).

**Patellar Compression, Patellar Grinding[75], and Apprehension Tests[1]** With the knee held to create approximately 20 degrees of flexion, the *patellar compression test* forces the patella downward into the femoral groove; it is then moved forward and backward as the patient flexes and extends the knee. A positive test causes pain and/or crepitus (Figure 20–35).

If the patient feels pain or if a grinding sound is heard during the *patellar grind test*, a pathological condition is probably present.[34] With the knee still flexed, the patella is forced downward and is held in this position as the athlete contracts the quadriceps (Figure 20–36). A positive *Clarke's sign* is present when the patient experiences pain and grinding.
Sn. NA | Sp. NA | +LR 1.94 | -LR 0.69

Another test that indicates whether the patella can easily be subluxated or dislocated is known as the *Fairbank's patellar apprehension test* (Figure 20–37). With the knee and patella in a relaxed position, the examiner pushes the patella laterally. The patient will express sudden apprehension at the point at which the patella begins to dislocate.[34] Sn. 1.00 | Sp. 0.88 | +LR NA | -LR NA

**Clinical Prediction Rules** The following clinical prediction rules are currently used for the knee joint:

- *Manipulation for Patellofemoral Pain Syndrome*[54]— Identifies patients with patellofemoral pain syndrome (PFPS) who will likely have a positive immediate response to lumbopelvic manipulation.
- *Orthotics for Patellofemoral Pain Syndrome*[117]— identifies patients with patellofemoral pain who are more likely to benefit from foot orthoses.
- *Patellar Taping for Patellofemoral Pain Syndrome*[68]— identifies patients presenting with patellofemoral pain syndrome who will likely respond favorably to patellar taping.

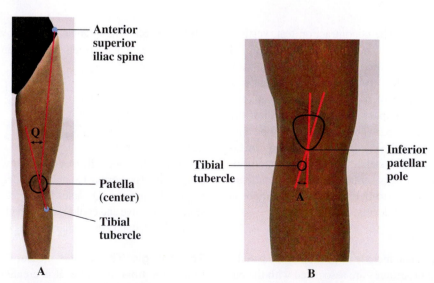

**A** Anterior superior iliac spine — Q — Patella (center) — Tibial tubercle

**B** Tibial tubercle — Inferior patellar pole — A

FIGURE 20–33  **(A)** Measuring the Q angle of the knee.
**(B)** Determining the A angle.
© William E. Prentice

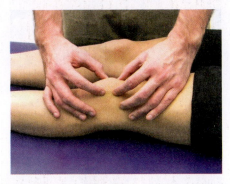

FIGURE 20–34   Palpating the periphery of the patella while the quadriceps muscle is fully relaxed.
© William E. Prentice

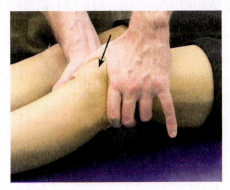

FIGURE 20–35   Patellar compression test. The patella is pressed downward in the femoral groove and moved forward and backward to elicit pain or crepitus.
© William E. Prentice

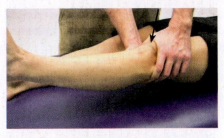

FIGURE 20–36   Patellar grind test. While the knee is flexed, the patella is forced forward; the patient then actively contracts the quadriceps. The test reveals a positive Clarke's if the athlete feels pain or grinding.
© William E. Prentice

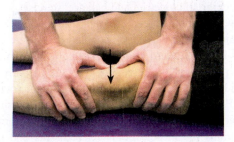

FIGURE 20–37   Fairbanks patellar apprehension test for the easily subluxated or dislocated patella.
© William E. Prentice

- *Medial Collateral Ligament Pathology*[60]—identifies patient characteristics indicative of a medial collateral ligament injury.
- *Meniscal Pathology*[71]—identifies patients who likely have meniscal pathology based on specific patient characteristics and examination findings.
- *Ottawa Knee Rules*[6]—developed to determine the need for radiographs after acute knee injury secondary to the risk of fracture.
- *Pittsburgh Knee Rules*[19]—developed to determine the need for radiographs after acute knee injury secondary to the risk of fracture.

# PREVENTION OF KNEE INJURIES

Preventing knee injuries in sports is a complex problem. Physical conditioning, rehabilitation and skill development, and shoe type are important factors. The routine use of protective bracing may be a questionable practice.

## Physical Conditioning and Rehabilitation

To avoid knee injuries, an athlete should be well conditioned, which means total body conditioning that includes strength, neuromuscular control, flexibility, cardiovascular and muscle endurance, agility, speed, and balance.[88] Specifically, the muscles surrounding the knee joint must be strong and flexible. The joints and soft tissue that make up the kinetic chain of which the knee is a part must also be considered sources of knee injury and therefore must be specifically conditioned for strength and flexibility.[61] Athletes should acquire a strength ratio between the quadriceps and hamstring muscle groups. For example, the hamstring muscles of football players should have 60 percent to 70 percent of the strength of the quadriceps muscles.[88] The gastrocnemius muscle should also be strengthened to help stabilize the knee. Although maximizing muscle strength may prevent some injuries, it fails to prevent rotatory-type injuries.

Avoiding abnormal contraction of the muscles through flexibility exercises is a necessary protection for the knee. Gradual stretching of the knee musculature helps the muscle fibers become more extensible and elastic.[88] Of special concern in preventing knee injuries is the extensibility of the hamstrings, erector spinae, groin, quadriceps, and gastrocnemius muscles.

Knees that have been injured must be properly rehabilitated. Repeated minor injuries to a knee make it susceptible to a major injury. (See the section on knee joint rehabilitation later in this chapter.)

## Interventions for Decreasing the Risk of ACL Injury

Even though the exact mechanisms of ACL injury have not been scientifically confirmed and agreed upon, the numerous theories concerning biomechanical and neuromuscular aspects of ACL injury have provided the foundation for success in the early development of ACL injury prevention programs.[88,93] An integrated preventive training program consisting of a combination of flexibility, agility, strengthening, plyometric, and balance exercises in combination with technique feedback and instruction can reduce ACL injuries in a variety of populations.[63,118] A proprioceptive balance board training program performed during the preseason has been shown to significantly reduce the incidence of ACL injuries in professional soccer athletes.[88] Prevention strategies that incorporate high-intensity plyometrics reduce ACL risk. The plyometric component which trains the muscles, connective tissue, and nervous system and that focuses on proper technique and body mechanics, appears to reduce ACL injuries.[48] A program involving a combination of weight training, landing instructional cues, stretching, balance and plyometric training has been successfully used to influence jump-landing kinematics and kinetics in adolescent athletes.[26]

An intervention program consisting of strength, balance, and technique training was designed to influence an athlete's ability to jump and land properly, to potentially reduce acute and chronic noncontact lower-extremity injuries.[31,88] The premise of this program is based on the following concepts: jump-landing occurring in all functions (e.g., running, pivoting, and jumping), prehabilitation or the intervention of establishing ability prior to injury occurrence, and a single-leg concept of athletic movement that states that most athletic tasks are performed during a single-leg stance. The jump-landing technique is the main focus of the training program and is based on the use of verbal cues, observational modeling, videotape feedback, and physical practice. Four verbal cues are stressed during the program: soft knees (landing with knee flexion to absorb impact forces), load hips (hip flexion to aid in impact absorption), quiet sound (try not to make a sound when landing), and toe-to-heel (landing on forefoot and rolling into heel contact).[84,85]

## Shoe Type

Noncontact knee injury commonly occurs when the shoe "sticks" to the ground, placing abnormal stress on the knee. The risk of knee injury, particularly ruptures of the anterior cruciate ligament, is increased when the shoe remains firmly planted on the ground.[58] This is called *traction* and there are two types. Translational

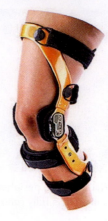

**FIGURE 20–38** Prophylactic knee brace.
Courtesy Dj Global

traction is involved in forward, straight-line running, and rotational traction which occurs in pivoting or making a cut (see Chapter 7).[119] In sports that involve running and cutting, better traction of the shoe on the playing surface can significantly enhance performance. But from an injury prevention perspective, shoes that don't stick when cutting or changing direction (rotational traction) seem to be the safest compared to shoes that grip the playing surface when sprinting forward (translational traction).[36] Thus, the ideal shoe would find a balance between maximizing performance while minimizing the chance of injury. The incidence of injury is similar on both synthetic turf and natural grass playing surfaces.[119]

## Functional and Prophylactic Knee Braces

Functional and prophylactic knee braces are discussed in Chapter 7. These braces have been designed to prevent or reduce the severity of knee injuries.[126] Prophylactic knee braces are worn on the lateral surface of the knee to protect the medial collateral ligament.[126] Functional knee braces are used to protect grade 1 or 2 sprains of the ACL or, most commonly, a surgically reconstructed ACL. These braces are custom-molded and are designed to control rotational stress or tibial translation. The effectiveness of protective knee braces is controversial at best (Figure 20–38).[38] It is generally accepted that they have little or no effect on functional performance measures.[38]

# RECOGNITION AND MANAGEMENT OF SPECIFIC INJURIES

## Ligament Injuries

The major ligaments of the knee can be torn in isolation or in combination. Depending on the application of forces, injury can occur from a direct straight-line or single-plane force, from a rotary force, or from a combination of the two.[44]

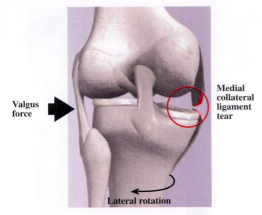

FIGURE 20–39   A valgus force with the tibia in lateral rotation injures the medial collateral and capsular ligaments, the medial meniscus, and sometimes the anterior cruciate ligament.

## Medial Collateral Ligament Sprain

*Etiology*   Most knee sprains affect the MCL from either a direct blow from the lateral side in a medial direction (valgus force) or from lateral tibial rotation.[56] Greater injury results from medial sprains than from lateral sprains because of their more direct relation to the articular capsule and the medial meniscus (Figure 20–39). Medial and lateral sprains occur in varying degrees, depending on knee position, previous injuries, the strength of the muscles crossing the joint, the force and angle of the trauma, fixation of the foot, and the conditions of the playing surface.

The position of the knee is important in establishing its vulnerability to traumatic sprains. Any position of the knee, from full extension to full flexion, can result in injury if there is sufficient force. Full extension tightens both lateral and medial ligaments. Flexion affords a loss of stability to the lateral ligament but maintains stability in various portions of the medial capsular ligament.[56] Medial collateral ligament sprains result most often from adduction and internal rotation. The most prevalent mechanism of a lateral collateral ligamentous or capsular sprain is one in which the foot is everted and the knee is forced laterally into a varus position.

The cumulative effects of several mild to moderate sprains leave the knee unstable and thus vulnerable to additional internal derangements. Torn menisci seldom happen as a result of an initial trauma; most occur after the collateral ligaments have been stretched by repeated injury. The strength of the muscles crossing the knee joint is important in helping the ligaments support the articulation. These muscles should be strengthened to minimize the possibility of injury. Athletes can help protect themselves from knee injuries by developing muscular strength through proper conditioning.

The force and angle of the trauma usually determine the extent of injury that takes place. Even after an athletic trainer witnesses the occurrence of a knee injury, it is difficult to predict the amount of tissue damage. The most

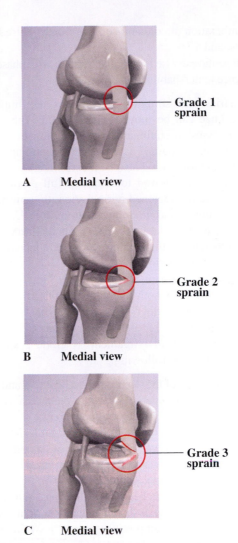

**A**      Medial view

**B**      Medial view

**C**      Medial view

FIGURE 20–40   Medial collateral ligament sprain: **(A)** Grade 1. **(B)** Grade 2. **(C)** Grade 3.

revealing time for testing joint stability is immediately after injury before effusion masks the extent of derangement.

*Grade 1 medial collateral ligament sprain*   A grade 1 MCL injury of the knee has the following characteristics (Figure 20–40A):

- A few ligamentous fibers are torn and stretched.
- The joint is stable during valgus stress tests.
- There is little or no joint effusion.
- There may be some joint stiffness and point tenderness just below the medial joint line.
- Even with minor stiffness, there is almost full passive and active range of motion.

*Management*   Immediate care consists of POLICE for at least 24 hours. After immediate care, the following procedures should be undertaken:

- Crutches are used if the patient is unable to walk without a limp.
- Follow-up care may involve cryokinetics, including 20 minutes of ice pack treatment before exercise or

a combination of cold and compression or pulsed ultrasound.

- Therapeutic exercise is essential, starting with phase 1 of the knee joint rehabilitation procedures.

Isometrics and straight-leg exercises are important until the knee can be moved without pain. The patient then progresses to stationary bicycle riding or a high-speed isokinetic program. Exercises for regaining neuromuscular function should also be incorporated.

The patient is allowed to return to full participation when the knee has regained normal strength, power, flexibility, endurance, and neuromuscular control. Usually, a period of 1 to 3 weeks is necessary for recovery. When returning to activity, the patient may require tape or brace support for a short period.

***Grade 2 medial collateral ligament sprain*** Grade 2 MCL knee sprain indicates both microscopic and gross disruption of ligamentous fibers (Figure 20–40B). The only structures involved are the medial collateral ligament and the medial capsular ligament. A grade 2 sprain is characterized by the following:

- A complete tear of the deep capsular ligament and a partial tear of the superficial layer of the medial collateral ligament or a partial tear of both areas
- No gross instability but minimum or slight laxity during full extension; however, at 30 degrees of flexion when the valgus stress test is performed, laxity may be greater
- Moderate swelling unless the meniscus or anterior cruciate ligament has been torn; additional injuries, such as a subluxated or dislocated patella or an osteochondral fracture, can produce extensive swelling and hemarthrosis
- Moderate to severe joint tightness with an inability to fully, actively extend the knee; the patient is unable to place the heel flat on the ground
- Definite loss of passive range of motion
- Pain in the medial aspect, with general weakness and instability

***Management*** Management consists of the following:

- POLICE should be applied for 48 to 72 hours.
- The patient should use crutches with a three-point gait until the acute phase of injury is over and he or she can walk without a limp.
- Depending on the severity and possible complications, a posterior splint or postoperative knee-immobilizing splint (Figure 20–41) may be used for 2 to 5 days, after which range of motion exercises are begun.
- Modalities should be used two or three times daily to modulate pain and to control inflammation.
- Isometric exercise emphasizing quadriceps strengthening (quad sets, straight-leg lifts) should progress to active resisted full-range exercise as soon as possible.
- Closed kinetic chain exercises, such as cycling on a stationary bike, stair climbing, and resisted flexion and extension, should be used as early as possible.

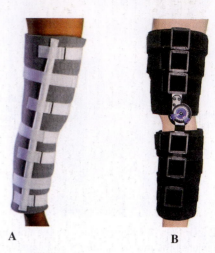

**A**　　　　　　　　　　**B**

FIGURE 20–41　Knee immobilizer used after a ligamentous injury. **(A)** Soft posterior splint. **(B)** Postoperative/rehabilitation brace.

(a) Courtesy DJO Global; (b) Courtesy Air A Med

- Functional progression activities should be incorporated early in the rehabilitation program.
- The patient should be encouraged to use a hinged brace when he or she tries to return to running activities.

Conservative care of the grade 2 medial collateral ligament sprain has been successful. Studies show that there can be spontaneous ligament and capsular healing because other structures, such as the anterior cruciate ligament, also protect the knee against valgus and rotary movement.[56]

***Grade 3 medial collateral ligament sprain*** Grade 3 MCL sprain means a complete tear of the supporting ligaments (Figure 20–40C). Major symptoms and signs include

- Complete loss of medial stability
- Minimum to moderate swelling
- Immediate, severe pain followed by a dull ache
- Loss of motion because of effusion and hamstring guarding
- A valgus stress test that reveals some joint opening in full extension and significant opening at 30 degrees of flexion

Isolated grade 3 sprains of the MCL occur most often when the mechanism of injury involves a direct valgus force with the foot fixed and loaded. MCL tears resulting from rotation combined with valgus stress with the foot fixed but not loaded virtually always result in ACL and occasionally PCL tears. Thus, testing must include evaluation of ACL and PCL integrity.[103]

***Management*** POLICE should be used for at least 72 hours. Conservative nonoperative treatment is recommended for isolated grade 3 MCL sprains. The question of repair or nonoperative management of MCL tears with associated ACL or PCL tears remains controversial. Recovery times and long-term results regarding knee function and stability appear to be better than with surgical repair. It is necessary to rule out ACL damage before beginning conservative treatment.

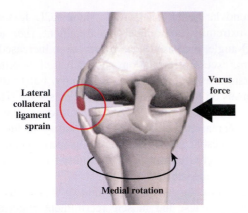

FIGURE 20–42   A varus force with the tibia medially rotated injures the lateral collateral ligament; in some cases both the cruciate ligaments and the attachments of the iliotibial band and biceps muscle of the thigh may be torn.

Conservative treatment usually involves limited immobilization in a hinged rehabilitation brace set to allow 30 to 90 degrees of motion and progressive weight bearing for 2 to 3 weeks, with motion increased to 0 to 90 degrees for another 2 to 3 weeks. The rehabilitation program would be similar to that for grade 1 and 2 sprains, although recovery time would be longer.

**Lateral Collateral Ligament Sprain**   Sprain of the lateral collateral ligament of the knee is much less prevalent than sprain of the medial collateral ligament.

*Etiology*   The force required to tear this ligament is varus, often with the tibia internally rotated (Figure 20–42).

> A lateral collateral ligament sprain can be caused by a varus force when the tibia is internally rotated.

In skiing, the LCL can be injured when the skier fails to hold a snowplow and the tips cross, throwing the body weight to the outside edge of the ski. If the force or blow is severe enough, both cruciate ligaments, the attachments of the iliotibial band, and the biceps muscle may be torn. The same mechanism could also disrupt the lateral and even the medial meniscus. If the force is great enough, bony fragments can be avulsed from the femur or tibia. An avulsion can also occur through the combined pull of the lateral collateral ligament and biceps muscle on the head of the fibula.

*Symptoms and signs*   The major signs are the following:

- Pain and tenderness over the LCL; with the knee flexed and internally rotated, the defect may be palpated
- Swelling and effusion over the LCL
- Some joint laxity with a varus stress test at 30 degrees; if laxity exists in full extension, ACL and possibly PCL injury should be evaluated
- The greatest pain with grade 1 and grade 2 sprains; in grade 3 sprains, pain may be intense initially and then will become a dull ache

An injury can also occur to the peroneal nerve, causing temporary or permanent palsy. The common peroneal nerve originates from the sciatic nerve. It lies behind the head of the fibula and winds laterally around the neck of the fibula, where it branches into deep and superficial peroneal nerves (see Figure 20–6). Tears or entrapment of this nerve can produce varying weaknesses and paralysis of the lateral aspect of the lower leg. Injury of the peroneal nerve requires immediate medical attention.

*Management*   Management of the lateral collateral ligamentous injury should follow procedures similar to those for medial collateral ligamentous injuries.

### Anterior Cruciate Ligament Sprain

*Etiology*   The anterior cruciate ligament sprain is generally considered to be the most serious ligament injury in the knee.[87] There has been considerable discussion on the specific mechanisms that are responsible for injury to the ACL.[107] To date there is no agreement on one single injury mechanism. However, there is agreement that the ACL may be injured either by a noncontact mechanism, by direct contact, or by indirect contact. Noncontact mechanisms are approximately 80% more likely to cause an ACL injury.[39]

It has become clear that a noncontact injury involves a combination of multiple biomechanical forces collectively acting on the knee joint.[12,20] Most typically, the athlete is decelerating from a jump or forward running[31,85] (Figure 20–43). The foot contacts the ground with the heel, or in a flat-foot

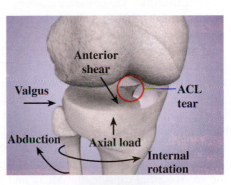

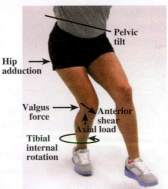

FIGURE 20–43   The primary mechanism of noncontact injury to the ACL involves an axial load with the knee close to extension, a valgus force, anterior shear, and internal rotation of the tibia, and adduction of the hip.
(b) © William E. Prentice

position, with little plantar flexion. Weight-bearing creates an axial force with the knee near full extension and abducted or in knee valgus.[12] The axial and valgus forces in combination with a contraction of the quadriceps group, produces both an anterior shear and an internal rotation subluxation of the lateral tibia on the femur.[106] This position imposes a substantial strain on the ACL thus increasing it's risk of injury. It should be added that while internal rotation creates greater loading forces on the ACL, external rotation has also produced tears of the ACL.[106]

Most recently it has become apparent the position of the hips also has a substantial impact on the incidence of ACL injury.[88] It appears that if the hip is adducted relative to the pelvis the chances of ACL injury are significantly increased. Additionally, in ACL injuries the pelvis on the opposite (non-weight-bearing) side drops into a Trendelenberg position thus further increasing hip adduction on the weight-bearing side and forcing the knee into a more varus position increasing the chance of ACL injury even further.[88]

In a direct contact injury, the athlete is decelerating and usually changing directions. The foot is planted on the ground with the knee abducted. There is contact from another athlete most often from lateral and posterior direction that forces the knee into a valgus and internally rotated position with anterior shear. Once again in this position the ACL is at risk of being injured.[107]

A third mechanism, indirect contact, occurs concurrently with contact by another player to a part of the body other than the lower extremity.[22] Perturbations resulting from that contact could potentially shift the individual's center of mass causing a loss of balance or an unanticipated directional alteration in lower extremity movement creating kinematic forces that can collectively result in injury to the ACL.

Tears of the ACL combined with injury to other supporting structures in the knee can produce rotatory instabilities. Anterolateral rotatory instability may involve injury to the anterolateral joint capsule, the LCL, and possibly the PCL and structures in the posterolateral corner. Anteromedial rotatory instability usually involves injury to the anteromedial capsule, the MCL, and possibly the PCL and posteromedial corner.[4]

Hyperextension from a force to the front of the knee with the foot planted can tear the ACL and, if severe enough, can sprain the MCL.

Females are much more likely than males to suffer noncontact ACL injuries, especially in activities that require running, jumping, and cutting.[5,55] A number of factors generally classified as either extrinsic or intrinsic have been investigated as plausible explanations for this difference.[15,50] Extrinsic factors include level of conditioning, skill acquisition, playing style, amount of preparation and practice, environmental considerations, and types of equipment (e.g., knee braces) used. These factors may be somewhat controllable.[49,50]

Intrinsic factors are the individual physiological and psychological factors that are more difficult to control. There is a great amount of information on femoral intercondylar notch size, ACL size, ACL laxity, and lower-extremity anatomical malalignment (i.e., excessive Q-angle, increased knee recurvatum, increased genu valgum, excessive pronation, and increased external tibial torsion) as they relate to ACL injury, but to date no consensus on their role in ACL injury exists.[53,107] There is also no consensus that sex-specific hormones play a role in the increased incidence of ACL injury in females.[49] Thus, at present, there is no reason to recommend modification of activity or restriction from sport for females at any time during the menstrual cycle.[45,108,116]

Neuromuscular factors (e.g., joint stiffness, muscle activation latencies, and muscle recruitment patterns) are important contributors to the increased risk of ACL injuries in females and appear to be the most important reason for the differing ACL injury rates between males and females.[49] It also appears that strong quadriceps activation during eccentric contraction is a major factor in ACL injury.[99]

***Symptoms and signs*** The patient with a torn ACL will often experience a pop followed by immediate disability and will complain that the knee feels like it is shifting. Anterior cruciate ligament tears produce rapid swelling at the joint line. The patient with an isolated ACL tear will exhibit a positive anterior drawer sign and a positive Lachman's sign. The pivot-shift test, jerk test, and flexion-rotation drawer test may be positive even with an isolated ACL tear. Proprioception is also decreased in the anterior cruciate–deficient knee.[98]

***Management*** Even with the application of proper first aid and immediate POLICE, swelling begins within 2 hours and becomes a notable hemarthrosis within 6 hours.[44] The patient typically cannot walk without help. If a clinical evaluation is inconclusive, an arthroscopic examination may be warranted to make a proper diagnosis.

Anterior cruciate ligamentous injury can lead to serious knee instability; an intact anterior cruciate ligament is necessary for a knee to function in high-performance situations.[115] Controversy exists among physicians about how best to treat an acute anterior cruciate ligamentous rupture and when surgery is warranted.[120] It is well accepted that an unsatisfactorily treated anterior cruciate ligamentous rupture will eventually lead to major joint degeneration.[53] Therefore, a decision for or against surgery must be based on the patient's age, the type of

A soccer player has suffered an isolated grade 2 sprain of his anterior cruciate ligament. At this point, the physician feels that surgery is not required and decides to try to rehabilitate the athlete and have him return to practice. It is likely that, when the patient returns to full activity, he will experience some feeling of instability when stopping, starting, and cutting.

**?** What can the athletic trainer recommend to the patient to help him minimize feelings of instability and to prevent the occurrence of additional injury to the ACL?

## Surgical Repair of Anterior Cruciate Ligament

**Injury Situation** A female college soccer player injured her right knee while cutting to her left with her right foot planted. There was no contact.

**Symptoms and Signs** She stated that she felt a pop and severe pain immediately. A few minutes later she felt that she could walk on it; however, it gave way as she put weight on it. Swelling was apparent at the joint line and over the medial aspect of the knee. Stability tests demonstrated positive anterior drawer, Lachman, pivot-shift, flexion-rotation drawer, and valgus stress tests at 0 and 30 degrees.

**Management Plan** She was diagnosed as having torn the ACL, MCL, and possibly the medial meniscus. Surgical repair was performed using an intraarticular ACL repair with a bone–patellar tendon–bone graft.

**Preoperative Phase (3 to 6 Weeks after Injury)** The goal during this phase is resolution of postinjury swelling and pain and restoration of full range of motion. The patient should begin strengthening exercises through a full pain-free range of motion as soon as she can tolerate them. The patient should be psychologically prepared for surgery during this phase.

---

### Phase 1 Acute Injury

**GOALS:** To minimize swelling, pain, and hemorrhage afer surgery; establish and maintain full knee extension; achieve good quardriceps control; begin working on regaining knee flexion; and regain neuromuscular control.
**ESTIMATED LENGTH OF TIME (ELT):** 1 week.

- **Therapy** POLICE during the entire first week 3 or 4 times per day to control swelling. Electrical muscle stimulation to control pain and elicit muscle contraction. Constant passive motion machine.
- **Exercise rehabilitation** Achieve full extension by end of first week. Weight shifting on crutches. Early quadriceps activity is important. Perform straight-leg raises and multiangle submaximal isometrics at 90, 60, and 40 degrees. Hip exercises, especially adduction, for VMO function. Active isotonic hamstring contractions to achieve 90 degrees of flexion by end of second week. Mobilize patella. Weight bearing as tolerated with brace locked in full extension.

---

### Phase 2 Repair

**GOALS:** To achieve a normal gait pattern; maintain full extension, strengthen quadriceps and hamstrings, increase knee flexion, maintain cardiorespriratory endurance, improve neuromuscular control, and begin light functional activities.
**ELT:** 1 to 6 weeks.

- **Therapy** Electrical muscle stimulation; POLICE to control swelling initially and after each treatment session. The amount of swelling will determine the athlete's ability to contract the quadriceps. Electrical muscle stimulation to facilitate muscle contraction and for reeducation. Ultrasound to increase blood flow.
- **Exercise rehabilitation** Ambulation with brace locked in full extension initially, although this is very surgeon dependent. Patient should progressively increase range of motion in brace as tolerated. Remove brace by week 3 or 4. Full weight bearing without a limp at the end of 4 weeks. Patient should attain full range of motion before she engages in intense strength training. Patient should concentrate on hamstring strengthening and should use closed kinetic chain activities and cocontractions as much as possible as well as strengthening exercises, such as minisquats, step-ups, hamstring and hip leg presses, and standing knee flexion and extension using surgical tubing. Multidirection patellar mobilization should be used to mobilize the tibia. A stationary bike should be used as soon as range of motion permits, as well as proprioceptive activities on BAPS board. Instrument assessment of cruciate laxity should be performed every 2 weeks for up to 12 weeks.[84] Patient should continue bicycling and use step climbing.

---

### Phase 3 Remodeling

**GOALS:** To concentrate on functional progressions and return to high-demand activity.
**ELT:** 7 weeks to 6 months.

- **Therapy** Electrical muscle stimulation to facilitate contraction. Ultrasound to facilitate blood flow. Massage to decrease scar. Mobilization techniques as needed.
- **Exercise rehabilitation** Isokinetic testing. High-speed training using rubber tubing. Patient should begin hop training and work on balance, always emphasizing the quality of movement with each activity. Functional activities should be incorporated. Patient should begin returning to running program at about 4 months. Patient should return to sport activity with injury maintenance.

*Continued*

## Surgical Repair of Anterior Cruciate Ligament, *continued*

*Criteria for Return to Competitive Soccer*

1. Knee is symptom free.
2. Appropriate isokinetic evaluation.
3. Appropriate arthrometer measurement.
4. Appropriate performance in functional tests that emphasize the quality of movement.
5. Patient is psychologically prepared for return.

stress applied to the knee, and the amount of instability present, as well as the techniques available to the surgeon.[81,114] A simple surgical repair of the ligament may not establish the desired joint stability.[81]

Surgery may involve joint reconstruction, which uses a graft from either the patellar tendon, hamstring tendon, or less commonly the quadriceps tendon that will roughly follow the course of the ACL and will functionally replace the ACL. Techniques for reconstructive surgery for the ACL continue to evolve and the choice of a particular technique is most often based on the surgeon's preference and expertise.[88] This type of surgery involves a brief hospital stay, a week of protection for healing wounds,[77] 3 to 5 weeks in braces, and 4 to 6 months of rehabilitation.[10,92,113,120] A detailed rehabilitation program for an ACL reconstruction is provided in the accompanying management plan. It has been suggested that it may take up to 2 years for a patient to regain normal quadriceps muscle function following ACL reconstruction.[97]

Little scientific evidence exists to support the use of functional knee braces, yet many physicians feel that the braces can provide some protection during activity.[11]

**Posterior Cruciate Ligament Sprain** The PCL has been called the most important ligament in the knee, providing a central axis for rotation.[102] The PCL provides about 95 percent of the total restraining force to straight posterior displacement of the tibia.

***Etiology*** The PCL is most at risk when the knee is flexed to 90 degrees. A fall with full weight on the anterior aspect of the bent knee with the foot in plantar flexion or receipt of a hard blow to the front of the bent knee can tear the PCL (Figure 20–44).[124] A PCL has also been referred to as a "dashboard injury," relating to a motor vehicle accident in which the driver's or passenger's knee hits the dashboard, forcing the tibia posteriorly and injuring the PCL. In addition, it can be injured by a rotational force, which also affects the medial or lateral side of the knee.[102]

> Simple surgical repair of the torn anterior cruciate ligament may not establish proper stability.

***Symptoms and signs*** The patient will report feeling a pop in the back of the knee. Tenderness and relatively little swelling will be evident in the popliteal fossa. Laxity will be demonstrated in a posterior sag test. The posterior drawer test is fairly reliable; however, an abduction stress test that is positive both at 30 degrees and in full extension is considered to be a definitive test for a torn PCL.

***Management*** POLICE should be initiated immediately. If clinical evaluation is inconclusive, arthroscopic evaluation may be warranted.

Nonoperative rehabilitation of grade 1 and grade 2 injuries should focus on quadriceps strengthening. As with isolated tears of the ACL, there is controversy over whether

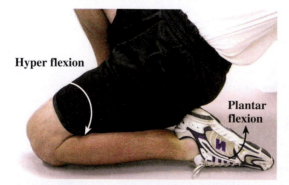
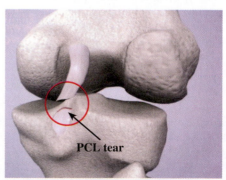

**FIGURE 20–44** The primary mechanism of a PCL tear is falling on the knee and forcing it into hyperflexion when the ankle is plantar flexed.

(a) © William E. Prentice

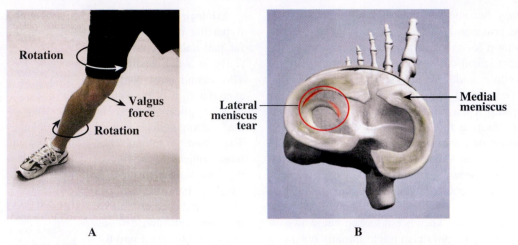

**FIGURE 20–45** **(A)** The primary mechanism for a meniscus tear is rotation from a cutting maneuver creating a valgus force. **(B)** This often results in a tear of the meniscus.

(a) © William E. Prentice

tears to the PCL should be treated nonoperatively or with surgical intervention.[89,102] Satisfactory outcomes achieved by nonoperative means have been reported.[57,96,105] Although techniques for repairing the torn PCL are technically difficult, surgery is occasionally recommended.[127] Rehabilitation after surgery generally involves 6 weeks of immobilization in extension with full weight bearing on crutches. Range of motion exercises are begun at 6 weeks, progressing to the use of PRE at 4 months.[88]

## Meniscal Lesions

The medial meniscus has a much higher incidence of injury than does the lateral meniscus because the coronary ligament attaches the medial meniscus peripherally to the tibia and to the capsular ligament. The lateral meniscus does not attach to the capsular ligament and is more mobile during knee movement. Because of the attachment to the medial structures, the medial meniscus is prone to disruption from valgus and torsional forces.

***Etiology*** A valgus force can adduct the knee, often tearing and stretching the medial collateral ligament; meanwhile, its fibers twist the medial meniscus outward.[9] Repeated mild sprains reduce the strength of the knee to a state favorable for a cartilaginous tear by lessening its normal ligamentous stability. The most common mechanism is weight bearing combined with a rotary force while the knee is extended or flexed.[9] If an individual makes a cutting

> A maintenance worker stepped down off a ladder and hurt his knee. He is diagnosed by a physician as having a torn medial meniscus. On evaluation, McMurray's test was positive, and a subsequent MRI revealed a longitudinal bucket-handle tear in the posterior horn of the medial meniscus.
>
> **?** What are the typical mechanisms of injury that can result in a tear of a meniscus?

motion while running, it can distort the medial meniscus. Stretching of the anterior and posterior horns of the meniscus can produce a vertical-longitudinal, or "bucket-handle" tear (Figure 20–45). Another way that a longitudinal tear occurs is if the knee is forcefully extended from a flexed position while the femur is internally rotated. During extension, the medial meniscus is suddenly pulled back, causing the tear (Figure 20–45B). In contrast, the lateral meniscus can sustain an oblique tear by a forceful knee extension with the femur externally rotated.[9] These oblique tears are sometimes referred to as "parrot beak" tears and occur in the inner periphery of the meniscus. A large number of medial meniscus lesions are the outcome of a sudden, strong internal rotation of the femur with a partially flexed knee while the foot is firmly planted. The force of this action pulls the meniscus out of its normal bed and pinches it between the femoral condyles.

Meniscal lesions can be longitudinal, oblique, or transverse. Because of the blood supply of a meniscus, tears in the outer one-third of the meniscus may heal over time if stress in the area is a minimized.[46] Tears that occur within the midsubstance of the meniscus often fail to heal because of lack of adequate blood supply.[46]

***Symptoms and signs*** An absolute diagnosis of meniscal injury is difficult. To determine the possibility of such an injury, the athletic trainer should obtain a complete history that consists of information about past knee injuries and an understanding of how the present injury occurred. Diagnosis of meniscal injuries should be made immediately after the injury has occurred and before muscle spasm and swelling obscure the normal shape of the knee.

A meniscal tear may or may not result in the following: effusion developing gradually over forty-eight to 72 hours; joint-line pain and loss of motion; intermittent locking and giving way of the knee; and pain when the patient squats.

Once a meniscal tear occurs, the ruptured edges harden and may eventually atrophy. Portions of the meniscus may become detached and wedge themselves between the articulating surfaces of the tibia and femur, thus imposing a locking, catching, or giving way of the joint. Chronic meniscal lesions may also display recurrent swelling and obvious muscle atrophy around the knee. The patient may complain of a sense of the knee collapsing, of a popping sensation, or of an inability to perform a full squat or to change direction quickly without pain when running. Such symptoms and signs usually warrant surgical intervention. NOTE: Symptomatic meniscal tears can eventually lead to serious articular degeneration with major impairment and disability.

***Management*** If the knee is not locked but shows indications of a tear, the physician might initially obtain an MRI. A diagnostic arthroscopic examination may also be performed.

The knee that is locked by a displaced meniscus may require unlocking with the patient under anesthesia, so that a detailed examination can be conducted. If discomfort, disability, and locking of the knee continue, arthroscopic surgery may be required to remove a portion of the meniscus.

Surgical management of meniscal tears should make every effort to minimize loss of any portion of the meniscus.[17] The menisci are critical in preventing degenerative joint disease. Healing of the torn meniscus depends on where the tear has occurred. Tears in the red-red or the red-white zone may heal well after surgical repair because those cones have a good vascular supply. Tears in the inner white-white zone will have to be resected because they are unlikely to heal, even with surgical repair, due to avascularity (see Figure 20–2B). Resection, or a partial menisectomy, involves removing as little as possible of the meniscus through an arthroscope. Partial menisectomy of a torn meniscus is much more common than meniscal repair.

Postsurgical management for a partial menisectomy does not require bracing and allows partial to full weight bearing on crutches as quickly as can be tolerated for about 2 weeks. It is not uncommon for an athlete to return to full activity in as little as 6 days.

A repaired meniscus requires immobilization in a rehabilitative brace for 5 to 6 weeks. The patient should be on crutches, progressing from partial to full weight bearing at 6 weeks. During immobilization, the patient can perform active ROM exercises between 0 and 90 degrees. At 6 weeks, full ROM resistive exercises can begin.

## Joint Injuries

**Knee Plica** A fetus has three synovial knee cavities whose internal walls, at 4 months, are gradually absorbed to form one chamber; however, in 20 percent of all individuals, the knee fails to fully absorb these cavities.[34] In adult life, these septa form synovial folds known as plicae.

***Etiology*** The most common synovial fold is the infrapatellar plica, which originates from the infrapatellar fat pad and extends superiorly in a fanlike manner. The second most common synovial fold is the suprapatellar plica, located in the suprapatellar pouch. The least common, but most subject to injury, is the mediopatellar plica, which is bandlike and begins on the medial wall of the knee joint and extends downward to insert into the synovial tissue that covers the infrapatellar fat pad.[34] Because most synovial plicae are pliable, most are asymptomatic; however, the mediopatellar plica may be thick, nonyielding, and fibrotic, causing a number of symptoms. The mediopatellar plica is associated with chondromalacia of the medial femoral condyle and patella (Figure 20–46).[34]

***Symptoms and signs*** The patient may have a history of knee injury. If symptoms are preceded by trauma, it is usually from blunt force, such as a fall on the knee, or from a twist with the foot planted. A major complaint is recurrent episodes of painful pseudolocking of the knee when the patient has been sitting for a period of time. As the knee passes 15 to 20 degrees of flexion, a snap may be felt or heard. Such characteristics of locking and snapping could be misinterpreted as a torn meniscus. The patient complains of pain while ascending or descending stairs or when squatting. Unlike meniscal injuries, there is little or no swelling and no ligamentous laxity.

> A female patient with no history of knee injury comes to the athletic trainer, complaining of knee pain. She has pain while ascending or descending stairs and when squatting. Her major complaint is recurring episodes of painful pseudolocking of the knee when she sits for a period of time. There is little or no swelling and no ligamentous laxity. A palpable tenderness begins on the medial wall of the knee joint and extends downward into the infrapatellar fat pad. As the knee passes 15 to 20 degrees of flexion, a snap may be felt or heard.
>
> **?** Based on the findings of the evaluation, what might be causing these symptoms and signs?

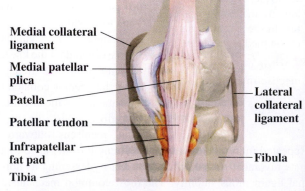

**FIGURE 20–46** Medial patellar plica.
© William E. Prentice

**Management**  A knee plica that becomes inflamed as a result of trauma is usually treated conservatively with rest, anti-inflammatory agents, and local heat. If the condition recurs, causing a chondromalacia of the femoral condyle or patella, the plica will require surgical excision.

## Osteochondral Knee Fractures

**Etiology**  Osteochondral fracture of articular cartilage and underlying bone on the weight-bearing surface of the femur, tibia, or under the patella creates fragments of bone and/or cartilage that vary in size and depth (Figure 20–47). Osteochondral fractures typically result from either rotation or direct trauma that compresses the articular cartilage between the medial or lateral femoral condyles and the tibial plateau.[104] Usually, an osteochondral fracture is localized to a single area, but occasionally more than one occurs at the time of injury. This injury, which occurs primarily in children, adolescents, and those 30 and older, can lead to the development of osteoarthritis.[122] Osteoarthritis is discussed in detail in Chapter 9.

> Knee plicae that have become thick and hard are often mistaken for meniscal injuries.

**Symptoms and signs**  The patient commonly complains of diffuse pain along the joint line. Symptoms include immediate joint effusion and crepitus and pain with weight bearing when standing or walking.[104]

**Management**  The athletic trainer should refer the patient to a physician. The physician will usually order a computed tomography (CT) scan or magnetic resonance imaging (MRI) to diagnose an osteochondral fracture. Treatment depends on the stability of the fracture. If the fracture fragment is still attached to the bone, the knee may be casted. If the fragment is loose within the joint, it may be either reattached (within

10 days of the injury) or removed arthroscopically. A microfracture procedure is used to repair a defect in the bone surface about the size of a dime or smaller by drilling the bone to cause a small amount of bleeding, which stimulates the growth of fibrocartilage.[104] An alternative is to transplant cartilage from another non-weight-bearing area of the articular surface.

If the microfracture is on the femoral condyles, the patient should be non–weight bearing or light touch-down weight bearing for 6 to 8 weeks, then gradually progressed over time. If the fracture occurs on the patella or within the femoral groove, the patient should be in a brace locked in full extension but weight bearing as tolerated for 8 weeks. Range of motion is usually initiated early on after surgery. Active strengthening exercises should be stressed after 6 weeks. It may be 3 to 6 months before the patient can return to full activity.

## Osteochondritis Dissecans

**Etiology**  Osteochondritis dissecans is a painful condition involving partial or complete separation of a piece of articular cartilage and subchondral bone.[90] Both teenagers and adults can have this condition. These fragments are referred to as loose bodies or "joint mice." However, loose bodies can also stem from menisci, pieces of synovial tissue, or pieces of torn cruciate ligament.[90] The vast majority of fragments, more than 85 percent, occur in the lateral portion of the medial femoral condyle.[65] Clinically, osteochondral detachments are seen wherever there is osteochondritis dissecans. Typically, the lesion results in normal articular cartilage with dead subchondral bone underneath, separated by a layer of fibrous tissue.

The exact cause of osteochondritis dissecans is unknown. It usually has a very slow onset. Possible etiological factors include direct or indirect trauma, association with certain familial skeletal or endocrine abnormalities, a prominent tibial spine impinging on the medial femoral condyle, or a facet of the patella impinging on the medial femoral condyle.

**Symptoms and signs**  The patient with osteochondritis dissecans complains of a knee that aches, swells recurrently, and occasionally may catch or lock. There may be atrophy of the quadriceps muscle and point tenderness.

> A knee that locks and unlocks during activity may indicate a torn meniscus.

**Management**  For children, rest and immobilization using a cylinder cast are usually prescribed. This management affords proper resolution of the injured cartilage and normal ossification of the underlying bone. Like many other osteochondroses, osteochondritis dissecans may take as long as 1 year to resolve. This condition in the teenager and adult may warrant surgery, such as multiple drilling in the area to stimulate healing, pinning of loose fragments, or bone grafting.

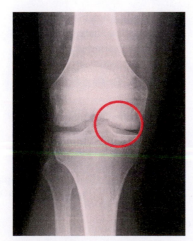

**FIGURE 20–47**  Osteochondral fracture with osteochondritis dissecans.
Courtesy Jordan B. Renner, MD, Departments of Radiology and Allied Health Sciences, University of North Carolina

## Joint Contusions

***Etiology*** A blow struck against the muscles crossing the knee joint can result in a disabling condition. One of the muscles frequently involved is the vastus medialis of the quadriceps group, which is primarily involved in locking the knee in a position of full extension.

***Symptoms and signs*** Bruises of the vastus medialis produce all the appearances of a knee sprain, including severe pain, loss of movement, and signs of acute inflammation. Such bruising is often manifested by swelling and discoloration caused by the tearing of muscle tissue and blood vessels. If adequate first aid is given immediately, the knee will usually return to functional use 24 to 48 hours after the trauma.

Bruising of the capsular tissue that surrounds the knee joint is often associated with muscle contusions and deep bone bruises. A traumatic force delivered to capsular tissue may cause capillary bleeding, irritate the synovial membrane, and result

> Because the knee joint and patella are poorly padded, they are prone to bruising.

in profuse fluid effusion into the joint cavity and surrounding spaces, thereby producing intraarticular swelling. Effusion often takes place slowly and almost imperceptibly. The patient should not engage in further activity for at least 24 hours after he or she receives a capsular bruise. Activity causes an increase in circulation and may cause extensive swelling and hematoma at the knee joint. Scar tissue develops wherever internal bleeding with clot organization is present. If this condition is repeated time after time, chronic synovitis or an arthritic sequela may develop.

***Management*** Care of a bruised knee depends on many factors. However, management principally depends on the location and severity of the contusion. Apply compression bandages and cold until resolution has occurred. Prescribe inactivity and rest for 24 hours. If swelling occurs, continue cold application for 72 hours. If swelling and pain are intense, refer the patient to the physician. Once the acute stage has ended and there is little or no swelling, conduct cold application with active ROM exercises within a pain-free range. If a gradual use of heat is elected, use great caution to prevent swelling. Allow the patient to return to normal activity, with protective padding, when pain and the initial irritation have subsided. If swelling is not resolved within a week, a chronic condition of either synovitis or bursitis may exist, indicating the need for rest and medical attention.

## Peroneal Nerve Contusion

***Etiology*** Compression of the peroneal nerve as it crosses directly behind the underlying neck of the fibula most commonly occurs from a kick or direct blow.

***Symptoms and signs*** Immediately following the impact, the patient experiences local pain from the contusion and pain (likened to an electric shock) radiating down the anterior leg into the dorsum of the foot. Numbness and paresthesia in the cutaneous distribution of the nerve may also be present. Locally, there may be skin abrasions or ecchymosis with tenderness of the underlying peroneal nerve. Local pressure may exacerbate the tingling. Usually, numbness, paresthesia, and tingling last only a few seconds or minutes, but, if the injury is severe, the hypesthesia and weakness of the peroneals and dorsiflexors persist, and the patient can develop a drop foot. However, most of the time the contusion of the nerve is minor, and usually the athlete recovers within 2 days following injury.

***Management*** Initially, the injury is managed with POLICE. The patient may return to normal activity as soon as the symptoms abate and there is no weakness of the peroneals or dorsiflexors. Protective padding over the fibular head area should be used to protect the nerve for a few weeks. An orthosis for a drop foot is rarely necessary.

**Bursitis** Bursitis in the knee can be acute, chronic, or recurrent. Although any one of the numerous knee bursae can become inflamed, anteriorly the prepatellar, deep infrapatellar, and suprapatellar bursae have the highest incidence of irritation (see Figure 20–4).

> The knee has many bursae; the prepatellar, deep infrapatellar, and suprapatellar bursae are most often irritated.

***Etiology*** The prepatellar bursa often becomes inflamed from placing pressure on the front of the knee while kneeling, and the deep infrapatellar bursa becomes irritated from overuse of the patellar tendon.

***Symptoms and signs*** Prepatellar bursitis results in localized swelling above the knee that is ballotable. Swelling is not intraarticular, and there may be some redness and increased temperature. Swelling in the popliteal fossa could be a sign of a Baker's cyst (Figure 20–48).

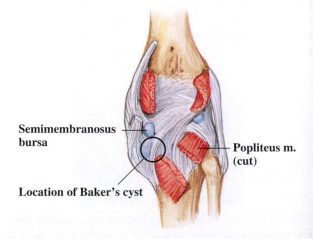

Semimembranosus bursa

Popliteus m. (cut)

Location of Baker's cyst

FIGURE 20–48  Location of a Baker's cyst in the popliteal fossa.

A Baker's cyst is associated with the semimembranosus bursa and occurs under the medial head of the gastrocnemius muscle. It is connected directly to the joint, and it swells because of a problem in the joint, not because of bursitis. A Baker's cyst is commonly painless, causing no discomfort or disability. Some inflamed bursae may be painful and disabling because of the swelling and should be treated accordingly.

*Management* Management usually follows a pattern of eliminating the cause, prescribing rest, and reducing inflammation. Perhaps the two most important techniques for controlling bursitis are the use of elastic compression wraps and anti-inflammatory medication. When the bursitis is chronic or recurrent and the synovium has thickened, the use of aspiration and a steroid injection may be warranted.

## Patellar Conditions

Patellofemoral disorders are likely the most common knee pathology the athletic trainer encounters.[33] In fact, they may be among the most common musculoskeletal conditions the athletic trainer sees.[72] Traditionally, there has been difficulty in classifying specific patellofemoral disorders because of the similarity among the reported symptoms.[33]

### Patellar Fracture

*Etiology* Fractures of the patella can be caused by either direct or indirect trauma (Figure 20–49). Most patellar fractures are a result of indirect trauma in which a severe pull of the patellar tendon occurs against the femur when the knee is semiflexed. This position subjects the patella to maximum stress from the quadriceps tendon and the patellar ligament. Forcible muscle contraction may then fracture the patella at its lower half. Direct injury most often produces fragmentation with little displacement. Falling, jumping, or running may result in a fracture of the patella. NOTE: Approximately 3 percent of the population has a bipartite patella, meaning there are two portions of the patella. This condition can be misdiagnosed as a patellar fracture.

*Symptoms and signs* The fracture causes hemorrhage and joint effusion, resulting in generalized swelling. Indirect fracture causes capsular tearing, separation of bone fragments, and possible tearing of the quadriceps tendon. Direct fracture involves little bone separation.

*Management* Diagnosis is accomplished through use of the history, palpation of separated fragments, and an X-ray confirmation. As soon as the examiner suspects a patellar fracture, a cold wrap should be applied, followed by an elastic compression wrap and splinting. The athletic trainer should then refer the patient to the physician. Normally, the patient will be immobilized for 2 to 3 months.

### Acute Patellar Subluxation or Dislocation

*Etiology* When an individual plants his or her foot, decelerates, and simultaneously cuts in an opposite direction from the weight-bearing foot, the thigh rotates internally while the lower leg rotates externally, causing a forced knee valgus. The quadriceps muscle attempts to pull in a straight line and, as a result, pulls the patella laterally—a force that may dislocate the patella. As a rule, displacement takes place laterally, with the patella resting on the lateral condyle (Figure 20–50).

> **Knees that give way or catch have a number of possible pathological conditions:**
>
> - Subluxating patella
> - Meniscal tear
> - Anterior cruciate ligamentous tear
> - Hemarthrosis

With this mechanism, the patella is forced to slide laterally into a partial or full dislocation. Some patients are more predisposed to this condition because of the following anatomical structures:[88]

- A wide pelvis with anteverted hips
- Genu valgum, which increases the Q angle
- Shallow femoral grooves
- Flat lateral femoral condyles
- High-riding and flat patellas
- Vastus medialis and ligamentous laxity with genu recurvatum and externally rotated tibias
- Pronated feet
- Externally pointing patellas

A patella that subluxates repeatedly places abnormal stress on the patellofemoral joint and the medial restraints. The knee may be swollen and painful. Pain is a result of swelling but also results because the medial capsular tissue has been stretched and torn. Because of the associated swelling, the knee is restricted in flexion and extension. There may also be a palpable tenderness over the adductor tubercle where the medial retinaculum (patellofemoral) attaches.

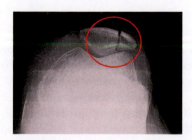

FIGURE 20–49 Patellar fracture (sunrise view).
Courtesy Jordan B. Renner, MD, Departments of Radiology and Allied Health Sciences, University of North Carolina

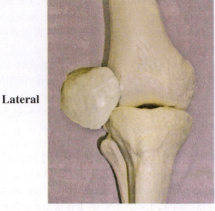

**Lateral**

FIGURE 20–50   Laterally dislocated patella.
© William E. Prentice

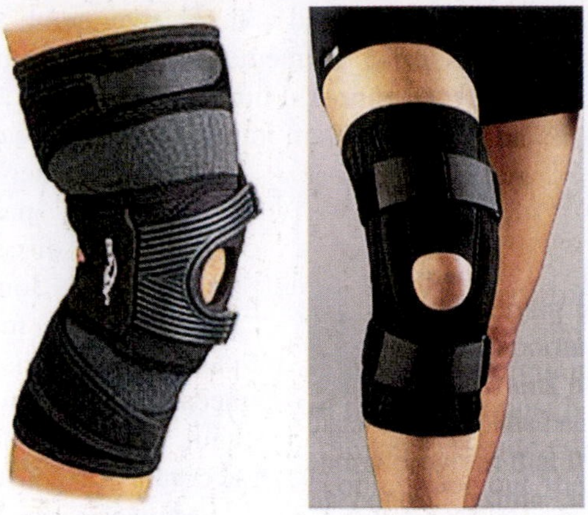

FIGURE 20–51   Special pads for the dislocated patella.
Courtesy DJ Global

An acute patellar dislocation is often associated with sudden twisting of the body while the foot or feet are planted and is associated with a painful giving-way episode, creating injury to the ACL, PCL, or P/ACL.[78]

***Symptoms and signs***   The patient experiences pain, swelling, and a complete loss of knee function, and the patella rests in an abnormal position. The physician immediately reduces the dislocation by applying mild pressure on the patella with the knee extended as much as possible. If a period of time has elapsed before reduction, a general anesthetic may have to be used. After aspiration of the joint hematoma, ice is applied, and the joint is splinted. A first-time patellar dislocation is sometimes associated with a chondral or osteochondral fracture. X-ray evaluation is performed before and after reduction.

***Management***   To reduce a dislocation, the hip is flexed and the patella is gently moved medially as the knee is slowly extended. (Reductions should be done only by a physician.) After reduction, the knee is immobilized in extension for 4 weeks or longer, and the patient is instructed to use crutches when walking. During immobilization, the patient should perform isometric exercises at the knee joint. After immobilization, the patient should wear a horseshoe-shaped felt pad that is held in place around the patella by an elastic wrap or sewn into an elastic sleeve that is worn while the patient runs or performs an activity. Commercial braces are also available (Figure 20–51).

Muscle rehabilitation should focus on all the musculature of the knee, thigh, and hip. Knee exercise should be confined to straight-leg raises.

If surgery is performed, it is usually to release constrictive ligaments or to reconstruct the patellofemoral joint. It is important to strengthen and to balance the strength of all musculature associated with the knee joint. Postural malalignments must be corrected as much as possible. Shoe orthotic devices may be used to reduce foot pronation, tibial internal rotation, and subsequent stress to the patellofemoral joint.

### Injury to the Infrapatellar Fat Pad

The two most important fat pads of the knee are the infrapatellar fat pad and the suprapatellar fat pad. The infrapatellar fat pad lies between the synovial membrane on the anterior aspect of the joint and the patellar tendon, and the suprapatellar fat pad lies between the anterior surface of the femur and the suprapatellar bursa. Of the two pads, the infrapatellar is more often injured, principally as a result of its large size and particular vulnerability during activity.

***Etiology***   The infrapatellar fat pad may become wedged between the tibia and the patella, irritated by chronic kneeling pressures, or traumatized by direct blows.

***Symptoms and signs***   Repeated injury to the fat pad produces capillary hemorrhaging and swelling of the fatty tissue; if the irritation continues, scarring and calcification may develop. The patient may complain of pain below the patellar ligament, especially during knee extension, and the knee may display weakness, mild swelling, and stiffness during movement.

***Management***   Care of acute fat pad injuries involves rest from irritating activities until inflammation has subsided, heel elevation of ½ to 1 inch (1.25 to 2.5 cm), and the therapeutic use of cold. Heel elevation prevents added irritation during full extension; the application of hyperextension taping may also be necessary to prevent full extension.

### Patellofemoral Pain Syndrome

*Patellofemoral pain syndrome or patellofemoral arthralgia* is a catchall term that refers to any type of pain that occurs in or around the patellofemoral joint.[69] The patella, in relation to the femoral groove, can be subject to direct trauma or disease that leads to chronic pain and disability.[111] Of primary concern are those conditions that stem from abnormal patellar tracking within the femoral groove, of which the two most common are chondromalacia patella and patellofemoral stress syndrome.[7,23]

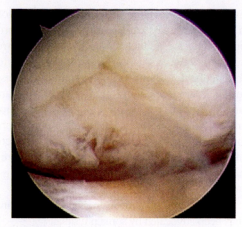

FIGURE 20–52 Arthroscopic image of the posterior surface of the patella, showing degeneration and fissures of the articular cartilage. Normally, the cartilage is very smooth, as is the superior aspect of the patella.

Chu, Constance R et al. "Early Diagnosis to Enable Early Treatment of Pre-Osteoarthritis." *Arthritis Research & Therapy* 14.3: 212 (2012). *PMC*. © 2012 by Chu, Constance R et al. All rights reserved. Used with permission.

## Chondromalacia Patella

***Etiology*** Chondromalacia patella is a softening and deterioration of the articular cartilage on the back of the patella (Figure 20–52). Chondromalacia undergoes three stages:

- Stage 1—swelling and softening of the articular cartilage
- Stage 2—fissuring of the softened articular cartilage
- Stage 3—deformation of the surface of the articular cartilage caused by fragmentation

The exact cause of chondromalacia is unknown. As indicated previously, abnormal patellar tracking could be a major etiological factor; however, individuals with normal tracking have acquired chondromalacia, and some individuals with abnormal tracking are free of it.[7] Abnormal patellofemoral tracking can be produced by genu valgum, external tibial torsion, foot pronation, femoral anteversion, a quadriceps Q angle greater than 20 degrees, patella alta, a shallow femoral groove, a shallow articular angle of the patella, an abnormal articular contour of the patella, or laxity of the quadriceps tendon.[65]

***Symptoms and signs*** The patient may experience pain in the anterior aspect of the knee while walking, running, ascending and descending stairs, or squatting. There may be recurrent swelling around the patella and a grating sensation when flexing and extending the knee.

The patella displays crepitation during the patellar grind test. During palpation, there may be pain on the inferior border of the patella or when the patella is compressed within the femoral groove while the knee is passively flexed and extended. The patient has one or more lower-limb alignment deviations.

Degenerative arthritis occurs on the medial facet of the patella, which makes contact with the femur when the patient performs a full squat.[7] Degeneration first occurs in the deeper portions of the articular cartilage, followed by blistering and fissuring that stems from the subchondral bone and appears on the surface of the patella.[7]

***Management*** In some cases, chondromalacia patella is initially treated conservatively, as follows:

- Avoidance of irritating activities, such as stair climbing and squatting
- Isometric exercises that are pain free to strengthen the quadriceps and hamstring muscles
- Oral anti-inflammatory agents, including small doses of aspirin
- A neoprene knee sleeve
- An orthotic device to correct pronation and reduce tibial torsion

If conservative measures fail to help, surgery may be the only alternative. Some of the following surgical measures may be indicated:[7]

- Moving the insertion of the vastus medialis muscle forward through realignment procedures, such as lateral release of the retinaculum
- Shaving and smoothing the irregular surfaces of the patella, femoral condyle, or both
- Elevating the tibial tubercle
- As a last resort, completely removing the patella

## Patellofemoral Stress Syndrome

***Etiology*** Patellofemoral stress syndrome results from lateral deviation of the patella as it tracks in the femoral groove (Figure 20–53). This tendency toward lateral tracking may be the result of several factors:[13,42]

- Tightness of the hamstrings and gastrocnemius
- Tightness of the lateral retinaculum, which compresses the lateral facet of the patella against the lateral femoral condyle
- Increased Q angle
- Tightness of the iliotibial band
- Pronation of the foot
- Patella alta (the patellar tendon is longer than the patella)

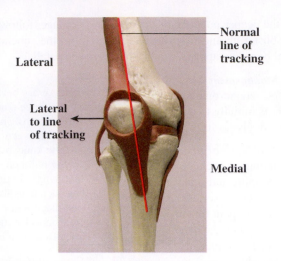

FIGURE 20–53 Lateral patellar tracking. The patella tends to move laterally when the knee goes into full extension.
© William E. Prentice

- Vastus medialis oblique (VMO) insufficiency caused by imbalance with the strength of the vastus lateralis (VL) or by inhibition resulting from the presence of 20 to 30 milliliters of effusion in the knee[10]
- Weak hip adductors to which the VMO is attached

***Symptoms and signs*** There will be tenderness of the lateral facet of the patella and some swelling associated with irritation of the synovium, as well as reports of a dull ache in the center of the knee. Patellar compression will elicit pain and crepitus. The athlete will be apprehensive when the patella is forced laterally.

***Management*** The causes of patellofemoral pain as identified during evaluation should provide the basis for treatment.[34] There is good evidence that proximal strengthening and neuromuscular reeducation are critical in many patients. The rehabilitation program should focus on improving neuromuscular control and strengthening of the hip and core musculature to reduce the knee abduction moment, which is associated with developing patellofemoral pain syndrome.[29] The patient must engage in a program for strengthening the adductor muscles and for correcting the imbalance between the VMO and the VL through the use of biofeedback techniques.[14,64] Stretching exercises for the hamstrings, gastrocnemius, and iliotibial band are also necessary.[68] Orthotics can be used to correct pronation and other malalignments.[2] The McConnell taping technique (see Chapter 8) has been demonstrated to be effective in regaining proper patellar alignment and thus a more symmetrical loading on the lower extremity.[2,18,47] Taping is designed to correct the orientation of the patella.[47,91]

If conservative treatment measures fail, lateral retinacular release has been advocated by some physicians.

## Extensor Mechanism Injuries

Many extensor mechanism problems can occur in the physically active individual. They can occur in the immature adolescent's knee or as a result of jumping and running.

### Larsen-Johansson Disease and Osgood-Schlatter Disease

***Etiology*** Two conditions common to the immature adolescent's knee are Larsen-Johansson disease and Osgood-Schlatter disease (Figure 20–54A&B). Osgood-Schlatter disease is an apophysitis characterized by pain at the attachment of the patellar tendon to the tibial tubercle. This condition most often represents an avulsion fracture of the tibial tubercle. This fragment is cartilaginous initially, but, with growth, a bony callus forms and the tuberosity enlarges. This condition usually resolves when the patient reaches approximately age eighteen. The only remnant is an enlarged tibial tubercle.

| Conditions that may be mistaken for one another: |
| --- |
| • Osgood-Schlatter disease |
| • Larsen-Johansson disease |
| • Jumper's or kicker's knee |

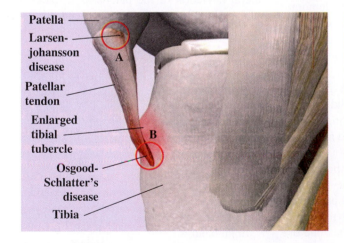
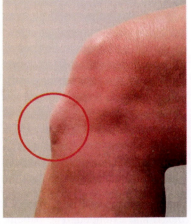

FIGURE 20–54 Two conditions of the immature extensor mechanism. **(A)** Larsen-Johansson disease. **(B)** Osgood-Schlatter disease. **(C)** An enlarged tibial turbercle.
(b) © William E. Prentice

# MANAGEMENT PLAN

## Patellofemoral Pain

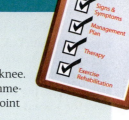

**Injury Situation** A 16-year-old high school basketball player complains of pain in her left anterior knee. She has been experiencing this pain for several weeks. At first, pain was present only during and immediately after practice, but lately her knee seems to ache all the time. Her pain has increased to the point that she now has difficulty completing a practice session.

**Symptoms and Signs** The patient complains of pain in the anterior aspect of the knee while walking, running, ascending and descending stairs, and squatting. Pain is increased during the patellar grind test. During palpation, there is pain on the inferior border of the patella or when the patella is compressed within the femoral groove while the knee is passively flexed and extended. She has tightness of the hamstrings, an increased Q angle, excessive pronation in her left foot, and weakness in her vastus medialis obliques (VMO).

**Management Plan** The goal is to reduce pain initially and then to identify and correct faulty biomechanics that may collectively contribute to her anterior knee pain.

---

*Phase* **1** *Acute Injury*    **GOALS:** To modulate pain and begin appropriate strengthening exercises.
**ESTIMATED LENGTH OF TIME (ELT):** 1 to 4 days.

- **Therapy** Use ice and electrical stimulation to decrease pain. If there appears to be inflammation, anti-inflammatory medications may be helpful. McConnell taping should be used to try to correct any patellar malalignment. The patient may need to sit out of practice for a couple of days to remove the source of irritation.

- **Exercise rehabilitation** An orthotic insert should be constructed to correct the excessive pronation that occurs during gait. Quadriceps strengthening begins with isometric exercises–specifically, quad sets. Isometric contractions may be done at several positions throughout the range from 90 degrees of flexion to full extension.

---

*Phase* **2** *Repair*    **GOALS:** Increase VMO strength and improve hamstring flexibility.
**ELT:** 5 days to 2 weeks.

- **Therapy** Ice and electrical stimulation may be continued. McConnell taping technique should also be continued, with day-to-day reassessment of its effectiveness. The use of biofeedback may help the athlete learn to contract the VMO.

- **Exercise rehabilitation** The effectiveness of the orthotic should be reassessed, with appropriate correction adjustments. Aggressive hamstring stretching exercises should be used. Quadriceps-strengthening exercises should concentrate on the VMO and should progress from isometrics to full-range isotonics as soon as full range of motion resisted exercise no longer causes pain. Closed kinetic chain exercises, particularly minisquats and lateral step-ups, should be recommended. The patient may resume practice; however, activities that seem to increase pain should be modified or replaced with alternative activities. Fitness levels must be maintained by either stationary cycling or aquatic exercise.

---

*Phase* **3** *Remodeling*    **GOALS:** To completely eliminate pain and fully return to activity.
**ELT:** 2 weeks to full return.

- **Therapy** The patient gradually can be weaned from McConnell taping. She may find it helpful to wear a neoprene sleeve during activity.

- **Exercise rehabilitation** The patient must continue quadriceps-strengthening and hamstring-stretching exercises. The athlete should now be accustomed to the orthotic insert. It may be necessary to continue to use alternative fitness activities indefinitely.

### Criteria for Return to Competitive Basketball

1. Pain is eliminated in squatting and in ascending or descending stairs.
2. The patient has good hamstring flexibility.
3. Quadriceps strength, particularly VMO strength, is good.

The most commonly accepted cause of Osgood-Schlatter disease is repeated avulsion of the patellar tendon at the apophysis of the tibial tubercle. Complete avulsion of the patellar tendon is a major complication of Osgood-Schlatter disease.

Larsen-Johansson disease is similar to Osgood-Schlatter disease, but it occurs at the inferior pole of the patella. Like the cause of Osgood-Schlatter disease, the cause of Larsen-Johansson disease is believed to be excessive repeated strain on the patellar tendon. Swelling, pain, and point tenderness characterize Larsen-Johansson disease. Later, degeneration can be noted during X-ray examination.

***Symptoms and signs*** Repeated irritation causes swelling, hemorrhage, and gradual degeneration of the apophysis as a result of impaired circulation. The patient complains of severe pain when kneeling, jumping, and running. There is point tenderness over the anterior proximal tibial tubercle (Figure 20–54C).

***Management*** Management is usually conservative and includes the following:[8]

- Decrease stressful activities until the epiphyseal union occurs, within 6 months to 1 year.
- Use a cylindrical cast in severe cases.
- Apply ice to the knee before and after activities.
- Perform isometric strengthening of the quadriceps and hamstring muscles.

## Patellar Tendinopathy (Jumper's Knee)

***Etiology*** Jumper's knee occurs when chronic inflammation develops in the patellar tendon either at the superior patellar pole (usually referred to as quadriceps tendinitis), the tibial tubercle, or most commonly at the distal pole of the patella (patellar tendinitis), often the result of overuse.[40] It usually develops in athletes from mechanical overloading of the tendon with activities that require rapid acceleration and deceleration, as in repetitive jumping and landing; hence the name. Following injury, an acute tendinitis with active inflammation develops that may become chronic lasting 3 to 6 weeks.[101] As chronic inflammation persists, degenerative changes occur in the tendon, which is more correctly referred to as patellar tendinosis.

***Symptoms and signs*** Point tenderness with palpation on the posterior aspect of the inferior pole of the patella is the hallmark of patellar tendinopathy. This condition is felt to be related to the shock-absorbing function (an eccentric contraction) that the quadriceps provides upon landing from a jump. The patient initially complains of a dull aching pain after jumping or running following repetitive jumping activities. There may be thickening of the tendon, but there is little or no effusion. Pain usually disappears with rest but returns with activity. Pain becomes progressively worse until the patient is unable to continue. There are also reports of difficulty in stair climbing and squatting, and an occasional feeling of "giving way."

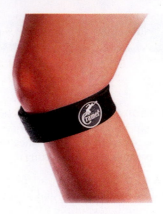

**FIGURE 20–55** Patellar tendon tenodesis braces or straps for patellofemoral pain.
Courtesy Cramer

***Management*** Many approaches to initial treatment of patients with acute inflammation associated with patellar tendinitis have been reported, including the use of ice, phonophoresis, iontophoresis, ultrasound, and various forms of superficial heat modalities, such as whirlpool, together with a program of exercise.[35,123] A patellar tendon tenodesis brace or strap may also be used (Figure 20–55).

Deep transverse friction massage has been used successfully for treating patellar tendinitis.[110] Friction is created by firm massage of the patellar tendon at the inferior patellar pole perpendicular to the direction of the fibers. Friction massage is used to increase the inflammatory process, so that healing may progress to the fibroblastic phase. When transverse friction massage is used, other techniques for reducing inflammation should not be used. If chronic inflammation persists, the focus of treatment will eventually shift to treating tendon degeneration and not inflammation. It has been suggested that a graded program of eccentric stress will stimulate tendon healing.[25] Treatment of patellar tendinosis should concentrate on eccentric exercise using squats, which has been demonstrated to be safe and effective. Performing squats on a 25-degree decline board has been demonstrated to be more effective for eccentric strengthening of the quadriceps when compared to standard squats (Figure 20–59J).[101]

## Patellar Tendon Rupture

***Etiology*** A sudden, powerful contraction of the quadriceps muscle with the weight of the body applied to the affected leg can cause a rupture.[33] The rupture may occur to the quadriceps tendon or to the patellar tendon. Usually, rupture does not occur unless there has been tendon degeneration over a period of time in the region of the knee extensor mechanism, causing tissue degeneration. A rupture seldom occurs in the middle of the tendon; usually, the tendon is torn from its attachment. The quadriceps tendon ruptures from the superior pole of the patella,

A ballet dancer has been diagnosed as having patellar tendinitis. In 3 weeks, she has two performances and wants to know what she can do to get rid of the problem as soon as possible.

**?** What options does the athletic trainer have in treating the dancer?

whereas the patellar tendon ruptures from the inferior pole of the patella.

***Symptoms and signs*** The patella moves upward toward the thigh, and the defect can be palpated. The patient cannot extend the knee. There is considerable swelling with significant pain initially, followed by a feeling that the injury may not be serious.

***Management*** A rupture of the patellar tendon usually requires surgical repair. Proper conservative care of patellar tendinitis can minimize the chances of patellar tendon rupture. Patients who use anti-inflammatory drugs, such as steroids, must avoid intense exercise involving the knee. Steroids injected directly into these tendons weaken collagen fibers and mask pain.[72]

### Runner's Knee (Iliotibial Band Syndrome and Pes Anserinus Tendinitis or Bursitis)

***Etiology*** *Runner's knee* is a general expression for many repetitive and overuse conditions. Many runner's knee problems can be attributed to malalignment and structural asymmetries of the foot and lower leg, including leg-length discrepancy. Common are patellar tendinitis and patellofemoral problems that may lead to chondromalacia. Two conditions that are prevalent among joggers, distance runners, and some cyclists are iliotibial band friction syndrome and pes anserinus tendinitis or bursitis.

*Iliotibial band syndrome* Iliotibial band syndrome is an overuse condition commonly occurring in runners and cyclists who have genu varum and pronated feet.[66] It has been proposed that since the iliotibial band is actually not a discrete structure, but instead a thickened part of the fascia lata which envelops the thigh. Irritation develops at the band's insertion not by frictional forces created by moving forward and backward over the epicondyle during flexion and extension of the knee, but rather by compression of the loose connective tissue over the lateral femoral condyle.[32] Ober's test (see Chapter 21) will cause pain at the point of irritation. Treatment includes stretching the iliotibial band and reducing inflammation.[95]

*Pes anserinus tendinitis or bursitis* The pes anserinus is where the sartorius, gracilis, and semitendinosus muscles join to the tibia (see Figure 20–5). Associated with pes anserinus tendinitis is pes anserinus bursitis. Inflammation results from excessive genu valgum and weakness of the vastus medialis muscle. This condition is commonly produced by running on a slope with one leg higher than the other.

***Management*** Management of runner's knee involves correction of foot and leg alignment problems. Therapy includes cold packs or ice massage before and after activity, proper warm-up and stretching, and avoidance of activities that aggravate the problem, such as running on inclines. Other management tools include anti-inflammatory medications and orthotic shoe devices to reduce leg conditions, such as genu varum.

## KNEE JOINT REHABILITATION

Rehabilitation of the injured knee joint presents a challenge to the athletic trainer who is overseeing the rehabilitation process.[82] The goal of every rehabilitation program is to achieve return to normal activity. For the athlete, "normal" activity involves psychological and physiological stresses that are at a considerably higher level than those experienced by the average person in the population. The athletic trainer must assume the responsibility for rehabilitating the whole athlete and not just the injured knee.

Every injured patient must be treated individually. The athletic trainer who attempts to use a cookbook approach to rehabilitation protocols will become frustrated because a rehabilitation program needs the flexibility to be altered based on the specific needs of the individual athlete.[88]

It is difficult for anyone supervising rehabilitation programs to stay abreast of the newest techniques and philosophies, which are constantly being updated or altered. This difficulty is perhaps truer for injuries involving the knee joint than any other body part. Rapid advances in technology and surgical techniques, along with an ever-increasing understanding of the physiological, biomechanical, and neural components of knee function, have drastically and repeatedly changed the approach to knee rehabilitation in recent years.

### General Body Conditioning

The patient must work hard to maintain levels of cardiorespiratory endurance. Full return to activity will be delayed if endurance levels must be improved after the injured knee is rehabilitated. The patient can engage in non-weight-bearing activities, such as using an upper-extremity ergometer, aquatic exercising, and, if range of motion permits, riding a stationary bicycle (see Figure 4–7). It is essential for the patient to concentrate on maintaining existing levels of strength, flexibility, and proprioception in all other areas of the body throughout the rehabilitation process.

### Weight Bearing

Generally, it is best for the patient to go non–weight bearing on crutches for at least 1 day after acute injury to the knee. This precaution will allow the healing process to progress well into the inflammatory stage before the patient does anything that may interfere with healing. Frequently, the patient will be allowed to progress gradually to weight bearing while continuing to wear a rehabilitative brace. The patient should then progress to touch-down weight bearing, three-point gait, four-point gait, and finally full weight bearing as soon as the healing constraints of

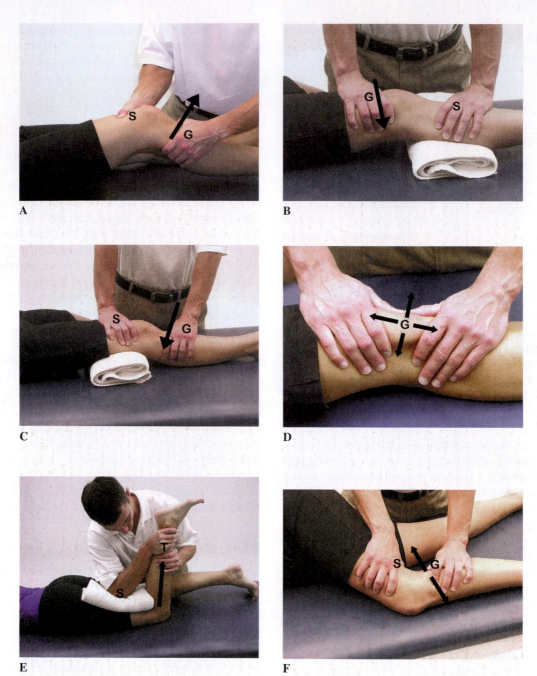

FIGURE 20–56   Knee mobilization techniques. **(A)** Anterior tibial glides. **(B)** Posterior femoral glides. **(C)** Posterior tibial glides. **(D)** Patellar glides. **(E)** Tibiofemoral joint traction. **(F)** Fibular head glides. (S = stabilize, G = glide)

© William E. Prentice

the particular injury allow. Injured structures in the knee joint will not heal fully until they are subjected to normal tensile forces and strains.

## Knee Joint Mobilization

Mobilization techniques should be incorporated as early as possible to reduce the arthrofibrosis that normally occurs with immobilization.[88] After surgery, patellar mobility is generally considered to be one of the keys to regaining normal knee motion. Patellar mobilizations that include medial, lateral, superior, and inferior glides should be used

along with anterior and posterior tibial glides to ensure the return of normal joint arthrokinematics (Figure 20–56).

## Flexibility

Regaining full range of motion after knee injury is one of the most critical aspects of a knee rehabilitation program. Regardless of whether an injury is treated conservatively or surgically, efforts toward achieving full range of motion are begun on the first day. The athletic trainer should emphasize active ROM exercises throughout the rehabilitation program. Once normal movement of the knee joint has been achieved, efforts should be directed toward maintaining or improving the flexibility of each of the muscle groups surrounding the knee joint through stretching. PNF stretching techniques are the most effective.[88]

## Muscular Strength

Strengthening generally follows a progression from isometric exercise (e.g., straight-leg raises, quad setting) (Figure 20–57) to isotonic exercise stressing both concentric and eccentric components, to isokinetic exercise, to plyometric exercise. It is essential to concentrate on strengthening all the muscle groups that have some function at the knee joint, including the quadriceps, hamstrings, abductors, adductors, and gastrocnemius.[88]

Eccentric muscle contraction should be routinely incorporated into strengthening programs through both isotonic and isokinetic exercise. Eccentric contraction of the quadriceps is necessary for deceleration of the lower leg during running. Conversely, the hamstrings must contract eccentrically to decelerate the lower leg in a kicking motion.[121] Plyometric exercises used during the later phases of rehabilitation use a quick, eccentric muscle contraction to facilitate a concentric contraction.

It is important also to emphasize closed kinetic chain exercises, in which the foot is in contact with the ground.[80]

Closed kinetic chain activities are more functional and eliminate many of the stress and shearing forces associated with an open-lever system. Thus, they are safer than open kinetic chain exercises. Minisquats, step-ups onto a box,[80] leg presses on a machine, and the use of stationary bicycles, stair climbing machines, and exercise tubing are examples of closed kinetic chain activities (Figure 20–58).[121] These exercises also emphasize and facilitate cocontraction of antagonistic muscle groups (e.g., quadriceps and hamstrings). This cocontraction aids in providing appropriate neuromuscular control of opposing muscle groups and thus promotes stability about the joint.[88] Strengthening exercises should also incorporate balance and postural control activities.[79]

PNF strengthening techniques using D1 and D2 lower-extremity patterns allow the athletic trainer to work on coordinated movement patterns and, in particular, emphasize the tibial rotation component of knee motion (see Figure 16–12A–H).[88]

## Neuromuscular Control

Regaining neuromuscular control of joint motion after injury is also important. The patient quickly "forgets" how to contract a muscle after injury. Loss of neuromuscular control usually occurs because of pain inhibition or swelling. Arthrogenic muscle inhibition (AMI) is a reflex inhibition of musculature surrounding a joint following damage and subsequent swelling. AMI slows gains in strength and proprioception during rehabilitation, thus increasing susceptibility to further injury. However, it is clear that early active exercise combined with cryotherapy and transcutaneous electric nerve stimulation (TENS) helps control AMI and safely increases strength and neuromuscular control essential for decreased healing time during joint rehabilitation.[51] Efforts directed

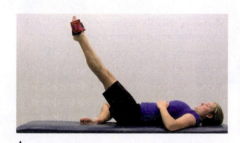
A

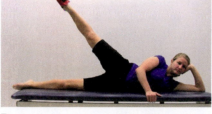
B

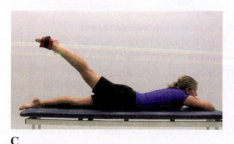
C

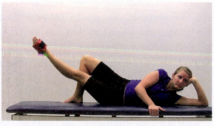
D

FIGURE 20–57 Straight-leg raising. **(A)** Hip flexion. **(B)** Hip abduction. **(C)** Hip extension. **(D)** Hip adduction.
© William E. Prentice

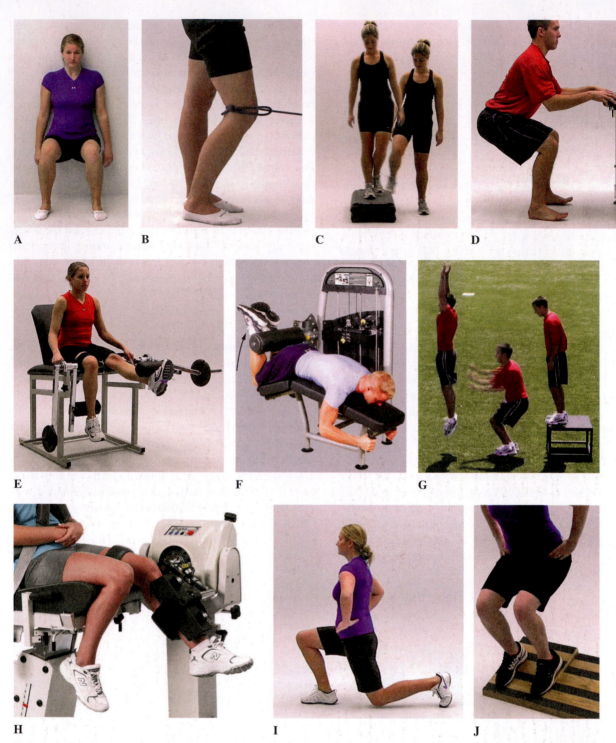

FIGURE 20–58   Knee-strengthening exercises. **(A)** Wall slides. **(B)** Terminal knee extension using tubing. **(C)** Step-ups. **(D)** Mini squats. **(E)** Open kinetic chain knee extensions. **(F)** Open kinetic chain knee flexion. **(G)** Plyometric depth jumping. **(H)** Isokinetic knee extension. **(I)** Forward lunges. **(J)** Eccentric squat on a 25-degree incline board.

(a–e, g) © William E. Prentice; (h) Photo courtesy Biodex Medical Systems, Inc.; (i, j) © William E. Prentice

toward proprioceptive control are begun immediately after injury to the knee with weight-shifting exercises on crutches, straight-leg lifts, and quad sets. The strengthening and flexibility exercises mentioned previously will help facilitate the return of proprioception. The BAPS board, Bosu Balance trainer rocker board, tremor box, mini-tramp, and Dynadisc (see Figure 19–39A–F) can all be used to improve proprioception and balance, as can the balance shoes (see Figure 18–44). It is essential to challenge the patient with exercises designed to improve neuromuscular control in the injured knee (Figure 20–59).

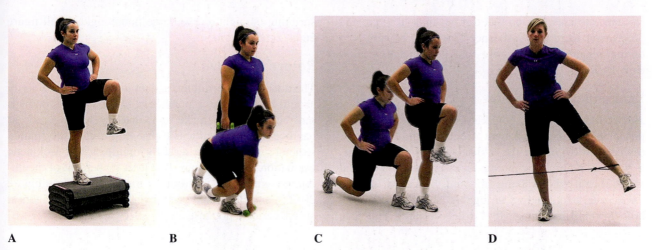

A                    B                    C                    D

FIGURE 20–59   Exercises to reestablish neuromuscular control. **(A)** Step-up to single-leg balance. **(B)** Single-leg squat dumbell touch-down. **(C)** Lunge to single-leg balance. **(D)** Single-leg tubing kicks.

© William E. Prentice

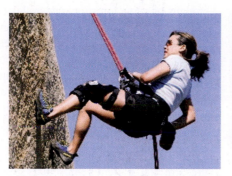
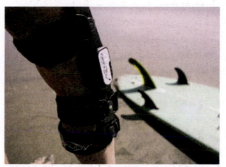

FIGURE 20–60   Functional knee braces provide support to the injured knee on return to activity.

Courtesy DJO Global

## Bracing

Rehabilitative knee braces have been designed to allow protected motion of either operative or nonoperative knees.[94] Braces enclose the thigh and calf with fabric fasteners, are lightweight, and are hinged so that motion can be limited within a specific degree range (see Figure 20–41B). Depending on the specific injury or the surgical technique used, the knee must be protected in limited ranges for some period of time. The braces are removed during rehabilitation sessions to allow the athlete to work in the greatest range of motion possible. Rehabilitative braces are typically worn for 3 to 6 weeks after surgery.

Functional knee braces are worn to provide support to the unstable knee on return to activity.[94] All functional braces are custom-fitted to some degree and use hinges and posts for support. Some braces use custom-molded thigh and calf enclosures to hold the brace in place, whereas others rely on straps for suspension (Figure 20–60). Braces are designed to improve the stability of the ACL-deficient knee by preventing full extension. Some braces attempt to control rotation or varus force. Functional knee braces alone do not seem to be able to control pathological laxity associated with ACL deficiency. However, if combined with an appropriate rehabilitation program,

these braces have been shown to restrict anterior-posterior translation of the tibia at low loads.

Functional resistance braces have been designed for use in individuals who have patellofemoral pain syndrome (Figure 20–61). These braces provide variable

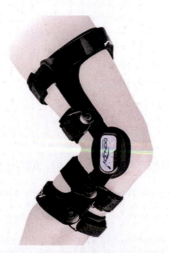

FIGURE 20–61   Functional resistance brace.

Courtesy DJO Global

resistance to knee flexion that can be adjusted to provide progressive increasing resistance. The brace is worn both during rehabilitative exercise and during activities of daily living.[28]

## Functional Progression

Activity-specific skills should be broken down into component parts, and the patient should be gradually reintroduced to them. For the athlete with an injured knee, a gradual return to running is essential. The patient should begin with walking (forward, backward, straight line, curve) and progress to jogging (straight, curve, uphill, downhill), running (forward, backward), and then sprinting (straight, curve, large figure eight, small figure eight, zigzag, carioca).[73]

## Return to Activity

The decision to permit the patient to return to full activity should be based on a number of criteria.[88] It is perhaps most important to make sure that the healing process has been given a sufficient chance to repair the injured structure. Objective criteria for return include isokinetic evaluation (torque values of at least 90 percent of the uninjured extremity), arthrometer measurement (see Figure 20–27), and functional performance tests (figure eights at speed, carioca, hop test, etc.).[27] (See Chapter 16.)

## SUMMARY

- The knee is a hinge joint that also glides and has some rotation; it is also one of the most traumatized joints. Three types of structures are most often injured: the medial and lateral collateral capsules and ligaments, the menisci, and the cruciate ligaments.
- Knee injuries may be avoided if individuals maximize muscle strength and wear appropriate shoes. The use of protective knee bracing is questionable.
- Ligamentous and capsular sprains occur frequently to the medial aspect of the knee and less often to the lateral aspect. The most common ligamentous injury occurs to the anterior cruciate ligament.
- A meniscus can be injured in a variety of ways, including a rotary force to the knee with the foot planted, a sudden valgus or varus force, or sudden flexion or extension of the knee. There may be severe pain and loss of motion, locking of the knee, and pain in the area of the tear.
- The patella and its surrounding area can develop a variety of injuries. Some of these injuries are fracture, dislocation, and chronic articular degeneration, such as chondromalacia. Other conditions in the region include Larsen-Johansson disease, Osgood-Schlatter disease, patellar tendinitis, and patellar tendon rupture.
- The goal of the knee rehabilitation program is to restore the patient's muscular strength, power, endurance, flexibility, neuromuscular control, and functional capability. The program varies according to the patient's level of activity.

## WEB SITES

Knee1.com: www.knee1.com
*This is a complete, free knee resource. Find healing technology/rehabilitation for knee pain, ACL injuries, osteoarthritis, other diseases, and knee replacements. Talk online to surgeons and patients.*

Knee surgery information:
www.arthroscopy.com

MEDLINEplus: Knee Injuries and Disorders:
www.nlm.nih.gov/medlineplus/kneeinjuries anddisorders.html
*This site is from the National Institutes of Health for research on knee injuries and disorders.*

Wheeless' Textbook of Orthopaedics:
www.wheelessonline.com

## SOLUTIONS TO CLINICAL APPLICATION EXERCISES

20-1 When the patient is weight bearing with the knee in flexion and the femur is internally rotated relative to the tibia the most likely injury is either to the anterior cruciate ligament or the meniscus or both.

20-2 During the evaluation, the athletic trainer should look for tightness of the hamstrings or gastrocnemius, tightness of the lateral retinaculum, increased Q angle, tightness of the iliotibial band, pronation of the foot, patella alta, vastus medialis oblique (VMO) insufficiency, inhibition resulting from the presence of effusion in the knee, and weak hip adductors to which the VMO is attached.

20-3 A valgus stress test should be used to test the MCL. The examination in full extension tests the MCL, posteromedial capsule, and cruciates. At 30 degrees of flexion, the MCL is isolated. If some instability is present with the knee in full extension, the athletic trainer should closely evaluate the integrity of the cruciate ligaments.

20-4 This mechanism is typical for a sprain of the anterior cruciate ligament, although other ligamentous, capsular, and meniscal structures may be injured as well. Appropriate stability tests for the ACL include the anterior drawer test done in neutral, internal, and external rotation; the Lachman test; the pivot-shift test; the jerk test; and the flexion-rotation drawer test.

20-5 If the officer still is concerned about his knee not being ready to return to active duty, then he is not ready, regardless of whether he is wearing a knee brace. The athletic trainer should design a series of functional progression activities that will help the patient gain confidence in his abilities while continuing to work on strengthening and neuromuscular control exercises. If the patient feels strongly about wearing a brace, the athletic trainer should make every effort to provide him with one, despite the fact that the literature supporting the use of functional knee braces is unclear.

20-6 It is important to understand that, once a ligament has been sprained, the inherent stability provided to the joint by that ligament has been lost and will never be totally regained. Thus, the patient must rely on the other structures that surround the joint—the muscles and their tendons—to help provide stability. It is essential for the athlete to work hard at strengthening all the muscle groups that play a role in the function of the knee joint.

20-7 The most common mechanism the weight bearing combined with a rotary force while the knee is extended or flexed. A large number of medial meniscus lesions are the outcome of a sudden, strong internal rotation of the femur with a partially flexed knee while the foot is firmly planted. Another way a longitudinal tear occurs is by forceful extension of the knee from a flexed position while the femur is internally rotated. During extension, the medial meniscus is suddenly pulled back, causing the tear.

20-8 It is likely that the patient has an inflamed or irritated mediopatellar plica. The mediopatellar plica may be thick, nonyielding, and fibrotic, which can cause a number of symptoms. The presence of an inflamed mediopatellar plica is sometimes associated with chondromalacia of the medial femoral condyle and patella.

20-9 The injury is most likely prepatellar bursitis due to the extracapsular swelling pattern, redness, and the mechanism of injury. A possible fracture should be ruled out as well. Ballotable patella or a sweep maneuver can be used to evaluate the swelling pattern to determine whether the swelling is intracapsular or extracapsular.

20-10 The athletic trainer should recommend that the patient reduce the length of her training sessions—in particular, limiting the running phase of training. Pain-free isometric exercises to strengthen the quadriceps and hamstring muscles can be used initially, and the patient can progress to closed kinetic chain strengthening exercises. Oral anti-inflammatory agents may also be helpful. A neoprene knee sleeve may also help modulate pain. Use of an orthotic device to correct pronation and reduce tibial torsion can sometimes help eliminate pain.

20-11 It is likely that this patient has chondromalacia patella. The athletic trainer should recommend avoiding irritating activities, such as stair climbing and squatting. The athletic trainer should recommend use of a neoprene sleeve and isometric exercises that are pain free to strengthen the quadriceps and hamstring muscles. If conservative measures fail to help, surgery may be the only alternative.

20-12 A conservative approach would be to use the normal techniques to reduce inflammation, such as rest, ice, ultrasound, and anti-inflammatory medications. An alternative and more aggressive technique would be to use a deep transverse friction massage technique to increase the inflammatory response, which will ultimately facilitate healing. If successful, the more aggressive treatment may allow a quicker return to full activity.

20-13 Closed kinetic chain strengthening exercises, such as mini-squats, lateral or forward step-ups onto a box, leg presses on a machine, terminal knee extensions using exercise tubing, and use of stationary bicycles, stair climbing machines, and stepping machines are all appropriate exercises that can be used safely and effectively almost immediately after surgery. Limited range of motion secondary to pain and swelling may restrict the athlete's ability to perform these strengthening exercises.

# REVIEW QUESTIONS AND CLASS ACTIVITIES

1. Describe the major structural and functional anatomical features of the knee.
2. Explain how a knee injury can best be prevented. What injuries are most difficult to prevent?
3. Demonstrate the steps that should be taken when assessing a knee injury.
4. Describe the symptoms, signs, and management of knee contusions and bursitis.
5. Distinguish collateral ligament sprains from cruciate sprains.
6. What is the difference between a meniscal lesion and a knee plica?
7. Explain how different fractures (e.g., patellar and epiphyseal fractures) may occur in the knee.
8. Describe the relationship of loose bodies within the knee to osteochondral fractures.
9. How do the patella fracture and the patellar dislocation occur?
10. Compare the causes of patellofemoral pain syndrome.
11. What types of injuries can occur to the extensor mechanism in a physically immature athlete?
12. Describe and compare the iliotibial band friction syndrome and pes anserinus tendinitis or bursitis.
13. What causes the knee to collapse?
14. Describe knee rehabilitation after conservative treatment of a grade 2 medial collateral sprain and after surgical repair of a torn anterior cruciate ligament.

# REFERENCES

1. Ahmad C: The moving patellar apprehension test for lateral patellar instability, *Am J Sports Med* 37(4):791–96, 2009.
2. Aminaka N: Patellar taping, patellofemoral pain syndrome, lower extremity kinematics and dynamic postural control, *J Athl Train* 43(1): 21–28, 2008.
3. Anderson A: Clinical analysis of the pivot shift tests: Description of the Pivot drawer test, *Am J Knee Surg* 13(1):19–23, 2000.
4. Arangio G: Incidence of associated knee lesions with torn anterior cruciate ligament: Retrospective cohort assessment, *J Sport Rehabil* 7(1): 1, 1998.
5. Arendt E: Anterior cruciate ligament injury patterns among collegiate men and women, *J Athl Train* 34(2):86, 1999.
6. Bachmann L: The accuracy of the Ottawa Knee Rule to rule out knee fractures: A systematic review, *Ann Intern Med* 140:121–24, 2004.
7. Baker M: Patellofemoral pain syndrome in the female athlete, *Clin Sports Med* 19(2):315, 2000.
8. Bedigrew S: Inexpensive Osgood-Schlatter management, *Athletic Therapy Today* 8(3):54, 2003.
9. Bernstein J: Meniscal tears of the knee: Diagnosis and individualized treatment, *Physician Sportsmed* 28(3):83, 2000.
10. Beynnon B: Accelerated versus nonaccelerated rehabilitation after anterior cruciate ligament reconstruction, *American Journal of Sports Medicine* 39(12):2536–48, 2011.
11. Birmingham T: Knee bracing after ACL reconstruction: Effects on postural control and proprioception, *Med Sci Sports Exerc* 33(8):1253, 2001.
12. Boden B: Non-contact ACL ligament injury: Mechanism and risk factors, *Journal American Academy of Orthopedic Surgeons*, 18(9):520–27, 2010.
13. Boling M: A prospective investigation of biomechanical risk factors for patellofemoral pain syndrome. The joint undertaking to monitor and

prevent ACL injury (JUMP-ACL) cohort, *Am J Sports Med* 37(11):2108–16, 2009.

14. Boling M: Rehabilitation alters VL and VMO recruitment, decreases pain, and increases function in patients with patellofemoral pain syndrome (abstract), *J Athl Train* 40(2 Suppl):S-68, 2005.

15. Bonci C: Assessment and evaluation of predisposing factors to anterior cruciate ligament injury, *J Athl Train* 34(2):155, 1999.

16. Borsa P: Sport specificity of knee scoring systems to assess disability in anterior cruciate ligament deficient athletes, *J Sport Rehabil* 7(1):44, 1998.

17. Brindle T: The meniscus: Review of basic principles with application to surgery and rehabilitation, *J Athl Train* 36(2):160, 2001.

18. Callaghan MJ: The effects of patellar taping on knee joint proprioception, *J Athl Train* 37(1):19, 2002.

19. Cheung T: Diagnostic accuracy and reproducibility of the Ottawa Knee Rule vs the Pittsburgh Decision Rule, *Am J Emerg Med* 31(4):641–45, 2013.

20. Chmielewski T: Biomechanical evidence supporting a differential response to acute ACL injury, *Clinical Biomechanics* 16(7):586–91, 2001.

21. Cleland J: *Orthopedic clinical examination: An evidence-based approach for physical therapists*, Carlstadt, NJ, 2005, Icon Learning Systems.

22. Cochrane J: Characteristics of anterior cruciate ligament injuries in Australian football, *Journal of Science and Medicine in Sport* 10(2):96–104, 2007.

23. Collado H: Patellofemoral pain syndrome, *Clinics in Sports Medicine* 29(3):379–98, 2010.

24. Curtis N: Evidence-based knee evaluation and rehabilitation, *Athletic Therapy Today* 11(2):36, 2006.

25. Curwin S: *Tendinitis: Its etiology and treatment*. New York, 1984, Collamore Press.

26. DiStefano L: Influence of age, sex, technique, and exercise program on movement patterns after an anterior cruciate ligament injury prevention program in youth soccer players, *Am J Sports Med* 37(3):495–505, 2009.

27. Dolan M: Open kinetic chain versus closed kinetic chain exercise after ACL injury, *Athletic Therapy Today* 15(3):376, 2010.

28. Earl J, Piazza S, Hertel J: The protonics brace unloads the quadriceps muscle in healthy subjects, *J Athl Train* 39(1):44, 2004.

29. Earl-Boehm J: A proximal strengthening program improves pain, function, and biomechanics in women with patellofemoral pain syndrome, *American Journal of Sports Medicine* 39(1):154–63, 2011.

30. Evans P: Prospective evaluation of the McMurray Test, *Am J Sports Med* 21(4):604–8, 1993.

31. Fagenbaum R: Jump landing strategies in male and female college athletes and the implications of such strategies for anterior crucial ligament injuries, *Am J Sports Med* 31(2):233, 2003.

32. Faircolugh J: Is iliotibial band syndrome really a friction syndrome? *J Sci Med Sport* 10(2): 77–78, 2007.

33. Faltus J: Effective management of patellofemoral joint dysfunction, *Athletic Therapy Today* 14(6): 235, 2009.

34. Fredrickson M: Physical examination and patellofemoral pain syndrome, *American Journal of Physical Medicine and Rehabilitation* 85(3):234–43, 2006.

35. Gaida J: Treatment options for patellar tendinopathy: Critical review, *Current Sports Medicine Reports* 10(5):255–70, 2011.

36. Gehring D: Effect of soccer shoe cleats on knee joint loads, *International Journal of Sports Medicine*, 28:1030–34, 2007.

37. Gray JC: Neural and vascular anatomy of the menisci of the human knee, *J Orthop Sports Phys Ther* 29(1):23, 1999.

38. Greene DL, et al.: Effects of protective knee bracing on speed and agility, *Am J Sports Med* 28(4):453, 2000.

39. Griffin L: Understanding and preventing non-contact anterior cruciate ligament injuries: A review of the Hunt Valley II meeting, *Am J Sports Med* 34(9):1513, 2006.

40. Hale S: Etiology of patellar tendinopathy in athletes (review), *J Sport Rehabil* 14(3):258, 2005.

41. Harilainen A: Evaluation of knee instability in acute ligamentous injuries, *Ann Chir Gynaecol* 76:269–73, 1987.

42. Harrison A: An evidence-based approach for patients with patellofemoral-pain syndrome, *Athletic Therapy Today* 11(2):6, 2006.

43. Harner C: Anatomical and biomechanical considerations of the PCL, *J Sport Rehabil* 8(4):260, 1999.

44. Hegedus E: Physical examination tests for assessing a torn meniscus in the knee: A systematic review with meta-analysis, *Journal of Orthopaedic and Sports Physical Therapy* 37(9):541–50, 2007.

45. Heitz N: Hormonal changes throughout the menstrual cycle and increased anterior cruciate ligament laxity in females, *J Athl Train* 34(2):144, 1999.

46. Henning C: Vascularity for healing of meniscus repairs, Arthroscopic and related surgery, 26(10):1368–69, 2010.

47. Herrington L: The effect of patellar taping on patellar position measured using ultrasound scanning, *The Knee* 17(2):132–34, 2010.

48. Hewett T: Anterior cruciate ligament injuries in female athletes: Mechanics and risk factors, *The American Journal of Sports Medicine* 34(2):299–311, 2006.

49. Hewett T: Neuromuscular and hormonal factors associated with knee injuries in female athletes: Strategies for intervention, *Sports Med* 29(5):313, 2000.

50. Hewett T: Anterior cruciate ligament injuries in female athletes, Parts 1 and 2: A meta-analysis of neuromuscular interventions aimed at injury prevention, *Am J Sports Med* 34(3):490, 2006.

51. Hopkins T: Cryotherapy and TENS decrease arthrogenic muscle inhibition of the vastus medialis after knee joint effusion, *Journal of Athletic Training* 37(1):25–31, 2002.

52. Hurley WL: Influences of clinician technique on performance and interpretation of the Lachman test, *J Athl Train* 38(1):34, 2003.

53. Ireland ML: Anterior cruciate ligament injury in female athletes: Epidemiology, *J Athl Train* 34(2):150, 1999.

54. Iverson C: Lumbopelvic manipulation for the treatment of patients with patellofemoral pain syndrome: Development of a clinical prediction rule, *J Orthop Sports Phys Ther* 38(6):297–312, 2008.

55. Jacobs C: Sex differences in eccentric hip-abductor strength and knee joint kinematics when landing from a jump, *J Sport Rehabil* 14(4):346, 2005.

56. Jacobson K: Evaluation and treatment of medial collateral ligament and medial-sided injuries of the knee, *Sports Med Arthroscopy Review* 14(2):58, 2006.

57. Janousek A: Posterior cruciate ligament injuries of the knee joint, *Sports Med* 28(6):429, 1999.

58. Kaili R: Influence of modern studded and bladed soccer boots and sidestep cutting on knee loading during match play conditions, *American Journal of Sports Medicine* 35:1528–36, 2007.

59. Karachalios T: Diagnostic accuracy of a new clinical test (the Thessaly test) for early detection of meniscal tears, *Bone Joint Surg* 87:955, 2005.

60. Kastelein M: Assessing medial collateral ligament knee lesions in general practice, *American Journal of Medicine* 121(11): 982–88, 2008.

61. Kelly A: Anterior cruciate ligament injury prevention, *Current Sports Medicine Reports* 7(5):255–62, 2008.

62. Katz J: The diagnostic accuracy of ruptures of the anterior cruciate ligament comparing the Lachman test, the anterior drawer sign, and the pivot shift test in acute and chronic knee injuries, *Am J Sports Med* 14:88–91, 1986.

63. Labella C: Effect of neuromuscular warm-up on injuries in female soccer and basketball athletes in urban public high schools: Cluster randomized controlled trial, *JAMA Pediatrics* 165(11):1033–40, 2011.

64. Laprade J: Comparison of five isometric exercises in the recruitment of the vastus medialis oblique in persons with and without patellofemoral pain syndrome, *J Orthop Sports Phys Ther* 27(3):197, 1998.

65. Lathinghouse L: Effects of isometric quadriceps activation on the Q-angle in women before and after quadriceps exercise, *J Orthop Sports Phys Ther* 30(4):211, 2000.

66. Lavine R: Iliotibial band friction syndrome, *Current Reviews in Musculoskeletal Medicine* 3(4):18–22, 2010.

67. Learmonth D: Incidence and diagnosis of anterior cruciate injuries in the accident and emergency department, *Injury* 22:287–90, 1991.

68. Lesher J: Development of a clinical prediction rule for classifying patients with patellofemoral pain syndrome who respond to patellar taping, *J Orthop Sports Phys Ther* 36(11):854–66, 2006.

69. Loudon J: Intrarater reliability of functional performance tests for subjects with patellofemoral pain syndrome, *J Athl Train* 37(3):256, 2002.

70. Loudon J: Genu recurvatum syndrome, *J Orthop Sports Phys Ther* 27(5):361, 1998.

71. Lowery D: A clinical composite score accurately detects meniscal pathology, *Arthroscopy* 22(11): 1174–79, 2006.

72. Lynch A: Non-operative treatment of patellofemoral pain: Role of physical therapy. In Zaffagnini S: *Patellofemoral pain, instability and arthritis*, New York, 2010, Springer.

73. MacLean C: Functional rehabilitation for the PCL-deficient knee, *Athletic Therapy Today* 6(6):32, 2001.

74. Mae T: Biomechanics of the patellofemoral joint, *Journal of Joint Surgery*, 25(11):1146–52, 2006.

75. Magee DJ: *Orthopedic physical assessment*, Philadelphia, PA, 2008, Saunders.

76. Malanga G: Physical examination of the knee: A review of the original test description and scientific validity of common orthopedic tests, *Arch Phys Med Rehab* 84(4):592–603, 2003.

77. Martin M: Problematic external wound healing after ACL-reconstructive surgery, *Athletic Therapy Today* 7(3):36, 2002.

78. Matheny M: Acute, traumatic rupture of the PCL, ACL, and MCL with patellar dislocation, *Athletic Therapy Today* 6(3):52, 2001.

79. Mattacola C: Strength, functional outcome, and postural stability after anterior cruciate ligament reconstruction, *J Athl Train* 37(3):262, 2002.

80. Mesfar W: Knee joint biomechanics in open kinetic chain flexion exercises, *Clinical Biomechanics* 23(4):477–82, 2008.

81. Moksnes H: Performance-based functional evaluation of non-operative and operative treatment after anterior cruciate ligament injury, *Scandinavian Journal of Medicine and Science in Sports* 19(3):345–55, 2009.

82. Mullin M: Functional rehabilitation of the knee, *Athletic Therapy Today* 5(2):28, 2000.

83. Norkus S: Advantages of the prone Lachman test, *Athletic Therapy Today* 7(2):52, 2002.

84. Onate J: Non-contact knee injury prevention plan (NC-LEIPP). Workshop presented at National Athletic Trainers' Association 52nd annual meeting, Los Angeles, CA, June 2001.

85. Onate J: Augmented feedback reduces jump-landing forces, *J Orthop Sports Phys Ther* 31(9):511, 2001.

86. Orndorff D: Physical examination of the knee, *Current Sports Medicine Reports* 4(5):243–48, 2005.

87. Ostrowski J: Accuracy of three diagnostic tests for anterior cruciate ligament tears, *J Athl Train* 41(1):120, 2006.

88. Padua D: Rehabilitation of knee injuries. In Prentice W, ed: *Rehabilitation techniques in sports medicine and athletic training*, Thorofare, NJ, 2015, Slack.

89. Pepe M: Assessment and surgical decision making for PCL injuries in athletes, *Athletic Therapy Today* 6(6):9, 2001.

90. Peters T: Osteochondritis dissecans of the patellofemoral joint, *Am J Sports Med* 28(1):63, 2000.

91. Piva S: Predictors of pain and function outcome after rehabilitation in patients with patellofemoral pain syndrome, *Journal of Rehabilitation Medicine* 41(8):604–12, 2009.

92. Pizzari T: Adherence to anterior cruciate ligament rehabilitation: a qualitative analysis, *J Sport Rehabil* 11(2):90, 2002.

93. Powers C: Mechanisms underlying ACL injury-prevention training: The brain-behavior relationship, *J Athl Train* 45(5):513–15, 2010.

94. Powers C: Effect of bracing on patellar kinematics in patients with patellofemoral joint pain, *Med Sci Sports Exerc* 31(12):1714, 1999.

95. Racioppi E: Iliotibial band friction syndrome, *Athletic Therapy Today* 4(5):9, 1999.

96. Reinold M: Rehabilitation after PCL reconstruction, *Athletic Therapy Today* 6(6):23, 2001.

97. Risberg M: Prospective study of changes in impairments and disabilities after anterior cruciate ligament reconstruction, *J Orthop Sports Phys Ther* 29(7):400, 1999.

98. Roberts D: Proprioception in people with anterior cruciate ligament–deficient knees: Comparison of symptomatic and asymptomatic patients, *J Orthop Sports Phys Ther* 29(10):587, 2000.

99. Rosene J: Anterior tibial translation in collegiate athletes with normal anterior cruciate ligament integrity, *J Athl Train* 34(2):93, 1999.

100. Rubinstein D: The accuracy of the clinical examination in the setting of posterior cruciate ligament injuries, *Am J Sports Med* 22:550–57, 1994.

101. Rutland M: Evidence-supported rehabilitation of patellar tendinopathy. *North American Journal of Sports Physical Therapy* 5(3):166–78, 2010.

102. Safran M: Effects of injury and reconstruction of the posterior cruciate ligament on proprioception and neuromuscular control, *J Sport Rehabil* 8(4):304, 1999.

103. Scott N: *Install and Scott surgery of the knee*, Philadelphia, PA, 2005, Elsevier Health Sciences.

104. Sgaglione N: Update on the treatment of osteochondral fractures and osteochondritis dissecans of the knee, *Sports Med Arthroscopy Review* 1(4):222, 2003.

105. Shelbourne D: Natural history study of athletes with PCL-deficient knees, *J Sport Rehabil* 8(4):279, 1999.

106. Shimokochi Y: Mechanisms of non-contact ACL injury, *J Athl Train* 43(4):396–408, 2008.

107. Shultz S, et al.: ACL research retreat VI: An update on ACL injury risk and prevention, *Journal of Athletic Training* 47(5):591–603, 2012.

108. Slauterbeck J: The menstrual cycle, sex, hormones, and anterior cruciate ligament injury, *J Athl Train* 37(3):275, 2002.

109. Smith T: The reliability and validity of the Q-angle: Systematic review, *Knee Surgery, Sports Traumatology, Arthroscopy* 16(12):1068–79, 2008.

110. Stasinopoulos D: Comparison of effects of exercise programme, pulsed ultrasound and transverse friction in the treatment of chronic patellar tendionopathy, *Clinical Rehabilitation* 18(4):347–52, 2004.

111. Thomee R: Patellofemoral pain syndrome: A review of current issues, *Sports Med* 28(4):245, 1999.

112. Toy B: Anatomy of the ACL: Influence on anterior drawer and Lachman test, *Athletic Therapy Today* 4(2):54, 1999.

113. Trulock S: Modifying postsurgical ACL rehabilitation for associated pathology, *Athletic Therapy Today* 7(4):34, 2002.

114. Udry E: Psychological readiness for anterior cruciate ligament surgery: Describing and comparing the adolescent and adult experiences, *J Athl Train* 38(2):176, 2003.

115. Urabe Y: Changes in isokinetic muscle strength of the lower extremity in recreational athletes with anterior cruciate ligament reconstruction, *J Sport Rehabil* 11(4):252, 2002.

116. Van Lunen B: Association of menstrual-cycle hormone changes with anterior cruciate laxity measurements, *J Athl Train* 38(4):298, 2003.

117. Vicenzino B: A clinical prediction rule for identifying patients with patellofemoral pain who are likely to benefit from foot orthoses: A preliminary determination, *Br J Sports Med* 44(12): 862–66, 2010.

118. Walden M: Prevention of acute knee injuries in adolescent female football players: Cluster randomized controlled trial, *British Medical Journal* 344:e3042, 2012.

119. Wannop J: Footwear traction and lower extremity non-contact injury, *Medicine and Science in Sports and Exercise* 45(11):2137–43, 2013.

120. Wilk K: Recent advances in the rehabilitation of ACL injuries. In Provencher M: *ACL Surgery: How to get it right the first time and what to do if it fails*, Thorofare, NJ, 2010, Slack.

121. Wilk K: Rehabilitation after anterior cruciate ligament reconstruction in the female athlete, *J Athl Train* 34(2):177, 1999.

122. Wilkerson G: Quadriceps strength and knee osteoarthritis, *Athletic Therapy Today* 8(1):25, 2003.

123. Wilson J: A comparison of rehabilitation methods in the treatment of patellar tendinitis, *J Sport Rehabil* 9(4):304, 2000.

124. Wind W: Evaluation and treatment of posterior cruciate ligament injuries: Revisited, *Am J Sports Med* 32(7):1765, 2004.

125. Woo S: Biomechanics of knee ligaments: Injury, healing and repair, *Journal of Biomechanics* 39(1):1–20, 2006.

126. Wu G: Effects of knee bracing on the functional performance of patients with anterior cruciate ligament reconstruction, *Arch Phys Med Rehabil* 82(2):282, 2001.

127. Yasuda K: The effect of PCL injury on muscle performance, *J Sport Rehabil* 8(4):322, 1999.

# ANNOTATED BIBLIOGRAPHY

DeCarlo M: *Knee rehabilitation*, Philadelphia, PA, 2004, Taylor and Francis.

*A complete guide to the most commonly encountered problems in sports medicine.*

Ellenbecker T: *Knee ligament rehabilitation*, Philadelphia, PA, 2000, Churchill-Livingston.

*Provides data to diagnose and rehabilitate knee ligament injuries. Includes protocols for nonoperative and postoperative rehabilitation.*

Fanelli G: *The multiple ligament injured knee*, New York, 2004, Springer-Verlag.

*A review of the most recent and advanced knowledge needed to successfully diagnose and treat knee ligament injuries.*

Fulkerson J, Buuck D, Post W: *Disorders of the patellofemoral joint*, Baltimore, MD, 2004, Lippincott, Williams and Wilkins.

*Explains such aspects of patellofemoral joint conditions as normal anatomy, biomechanics, nonarthritic anterior knee pain, dysplasias, patellar dislocation, nonoperative and surgical treatments, and chronic pain.*

Grelsamer R, McConnell J: *The patella: a team approach*, Austin, TX, 2004, PRO-ED.

*A comprehensive discussion that concentrates specifically on the patella from both a physician's and a physical therapist's perspective.*

Mascarenhas R: *The knee: Current concepts in kinematics, injury types, and treatment options*, Hauppauge, NY, 2012, Nova Science Publishers.

*This book provides an overview of current research examining knee injury mechanisms, prevention, and treatment options.*

Prentice W: *Rehabilitation techniques in sports medicine and athletic training*, ed 6, Thorofare, NJ, 2015, Slack.

*A comprehensive, well-illustrated text on the rehabilitation techniques used in sports medicine. Chapter 23 deals specifically with rehabilitation of the knee and provides up-to-date recommendations for a rehabilitation program.*

Rodriguez-Merchan C: *Traumatic injuries of the knee,* New York, 2013, Springer Milan.

*This book reviews the most important traumatic injuries that occur around the knee joint, providing detailed information on mechanisms of injury, diagnosis, and treatment.*

Scott N: *Insall and Scott surgery of the knee*, Philadelphia, PA, 2005, Elsevier Health Sciences.

*Built on a solid foundation of basic anatomy, pathology, and diagnostic techniques; offers comprehensive coverage of value to anyone involved in the diagnosis and treatment of knee disorders.*

Special Issue: Anterior cruciate ligament injury in the female athlete, *J Athl Train* 34(2):1999.

*An entire issue devoted to a discussion of various aspects of ACL injury in female athletes.*

Zaffagnini D: *Patellofemoral Pain, and Arthritis: Clinical Presentation, Imaging and Treatment,* New York, 2010, Springer.

*This book adopts an evidence-based approach to assess patellofemoral pain, instability, and arthritis.*

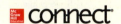

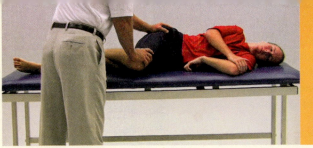

# 21

# The Thigh, Hip, Groin, and Pelvis

## ■ Objectives

*When you finish this chapter you should be able to*

- Recognize the normal structural anatomy of the thigh.
- Conduct an assessment of the injured thigh.
- Correctly recognize the various injuries that can occur to the anatomical structures in the thigh.
- Review the anatomy of the hip, groin, and pelvic region.

- Accurately evaluate injuries that occur in or around the hip, groin, and pelvis.
- Outline the etiology, symptoms and signs, and management procedures for the injuries that occur in the hip, groin, and pelvis.
- Develop a generalized rehabilitation plan for dealing with injuries to the thigh, hip, groin, and pelvis.

## ■ Outline

## ■ Connect Highlights    connect

*Visit connect.mcgraw-hill.com for further exercises to apply your knowledge:*

- Clinical application scenarios covering assessment and recognition of thigh, groin, hip, and pelvis injuries, etiology; symptoms and signs, and management of thigh, groin, hip, and pelvis injuries; and rehabilitation for the thigh, groin, hip, and pelvis
- Click-and-drag questions covering structural anatomy of the thigh, groin, hip, and pelvis; assessment of thigh, groin, hip, and pelvis injuries; and rehabilitation plan of the thigh, groin, hip, and pelvis
- Multiple-choice questions covering anatomy, assessment, etiology, management and rehabilitation of thigh, groin, hip, and pelvis injuries
- Selection questions covering rehabilitation plan for various injuries to the thigh, groin, hip, and pelvis
- Video identification of special tests for the thigh, groin, hip, and pelvis injuries; rehabilitation techniques for the thigh, groin, hip, and pelvis, taping; and wrapping for thigh, groin, hip, and pelvis injuries
- Picture identification of major anatomical components of the thigh, groin, hip, and pelvis; rehabilitation techniques of the thigh, groin, hip, and pelvis; and therapeutic modalities for management

lthough the thigh, hip, groin, and pelvis have relatively lower incidences of injury than the knee and ankle, they are subject to considerable trauma from a variety of activities.[22]

# ANATOMY OF THE THIGH

The thigh is generally considered that part of the leg between the hip and the knee. Several important anatomical units must be considered in terms of their relationship to injury: the shaft of the femur, the musculature, the nerves and blood vessels, and the fascia that envelops the thigh.

## Bones

The femur (Figure 21–1) is the longest and strongest bone in the body and is designed to permit maximum mobility and support during locomotion. The cylindrical shaft is bowed anterior and lateral to accommodate the stresses placed on it during bending of the hip and knee and during weight bearing. The proximal head of the femur articulates with the pelvis to form the hip joint, and the distal femoral condyles articulate with the tibia at the knee joint.

## Musculature

The muscles of the thigh may be categorized according to their location: anterior, posterior, and medial (Table 21–1).

**Anterior Thigh Muscles** The anterior thigh muscles consist of the sartorius muscle and the quadriceps femoris group. The sartorius (Figure 21–2) is a narrow band that is superficial throughout its length. It stems from the anterosuperior iliac spine and crosses obliquely downward

and medially across the anterior aspect of the thigh, where it attaches to the anteromedial aspect of the tibial head. It helps flex the thigh at the hip joint, abducts and outwardly rotates the thigh at the hip joint, and inwardly rotates the flexed knee. When the legs are stabilized, the sartorius flexes the pelvis on the thigh. When the sartorius muscle contracts, the pelvis is laterally rotated.

The quadriceps femoris muscle group (Figure 21–2) consists of four muscles: the rectus femoris, vastus medialis, vastus lateralis, and vastus intermedius. These four muscles form a common tendon that attaches distally at the superior border of the patella and indirectly into the patellar ligament, which attaches to the tibial tuberosity. The rectus femoris muscle is attached superiorly to the anterior inferior iliac spine and the ilium above the acetabulum and inferiorly to the patella and patellar ligament. The vastus medialis and vastus lateralis muscles originate from the lateral and medial linea aspera of the femur. The vastus intermedius muscle originates mainly from the anterior and lateral portion of the femur. Inferiorly, the three vastus muscles are attached to the rectus femoris muscle and to the lateral and proximal aspects of the patella. Of particular importance is the vastus medialis muscle, which serves as a stabilizer for patellar tracking.

**Posterior Thigh Muscles** The posterior thigh muscles are the popliteus and the hamstring muscles. The function of the popliteus muscle was discussed in Chapter 20. It externally rotates the femur in weight bearing to unlock the knee, so that flexion can occur (see Figure 20–6C). Located posteriorly, the hamstring muscle group (Figure 21–2) consists of three muscles: the biceps femoris, semimembranosus, and semitendinosus muscles.

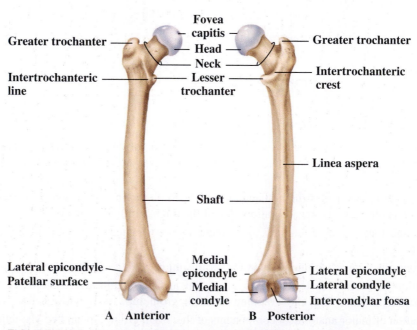

FIGURE 21–1   The femur. **(A)** Anterior view. **(B)** Posterior view.

| TABLE 21–1 | Muscles of the Thigh* | | | |
|---|---|---|---|---|
| Muscle | Origin | Insertion | Muscle Action (non–weight bearing) | Innervation |
| **Anterior compartment** | | | | |
| Sartorius | Anterior superior iliac spine | Proximal medial surface of the tibia, below the tuberosity | Flexes the thigh and the leg and laterally rotates the thigh | Femoral (L2, L3) |
| **Quadriceps femoris** | | | | |
| Rectus femoris | Anterior inferior iliac spine and just above the acetabulum of the os coxae | Tibial tuberosity, via the patella and the patellar ligament | Extends the leg; the rectus femoris also flexes the thigh | Femoral (L2, L3) |
| Vastus lateralis | Greater trochanter and lateral lip of the linea aspera of the femur | | | |
| Vastus medialis | Medial lip of the linea aspera of the femur | | | |
| Vastus intermedius | Anterior surface of the shaft of the femur | | | |
| **Posterior compartment** | | | | |
| **Hamstrings** | | | | |
| Biceps femoris | *Long head:* ischial tuberosity *Short head:* lateral lip of the linea aspera | Lateral surface of the head of the fibula and the lateral condyle of the tibia | Flexes the leg; the long head extends the thigh | Sciatic (L5, S1, S2, S3) |
| Semitendinosus | Ischial tuberosity | Medial surface of the proximal end of the tibia | Flexes the leg and extends the thigh | Tibial (L4, L5, S1) |
| Semimembranosus | Ischial tuberosity | Medial surface of the proximal end of the tibia | Flexes the leg and extends the thigh | Tibial (L4, L5, S1) |
| Popliteus | Lateral condyle of the femur | Posterior tibia | Flexes the leg and medially rotates the tibia | Tibial (L4, L5, S1) |
| **Medial compartment** | | | | |
| Adductor magnus Adductor longus Adductor brevis Pectineus | These muscles act only on the femur. | | Adducts and laterally rotates the thigh | Obturator (L3, L4) |
| Gracilis | Symphysis pubis and the pubic arch | Medial surface of the tibia just below the condyle | Adducts the thigh and flexes the leg | Obturator (L3, L4) |

*Manual muscle tests and goniometric measurements of range of motion for the thigh and hip joint can be found in Appendix F and Appendix G at the end of the text.

The biceps femoris muscle, as its name implies, has two heads. Its long head originates with the semitendinosus at the medial aspect of the ischial tuberosity. Its short head is attached to the linea aspera inferior to the gluteus maximus attachment on the femur and medial to the attachment of the vastus lateralis. Both muscle heads attach with a common tendon to the head of the fibula.

The semitendinosus muscle originates at the medial aspect of the ischial tuberosity along with the biceps femoris muscle. Together with the semimembranosus muscle, the semitendinosus muscle attaches to the medial aspect of the proximal tibia. This attachment is just posterior to the sartorius and gracilis muscles, which all together form the pes anserinus tendon. The tibial branch of the sciatic nerve supplies this muscle.

The semimembranosus muscle originates from the lateral aspect of the upper half of the ischial tuberosity. Moving distally, it attaches into the medial femoral

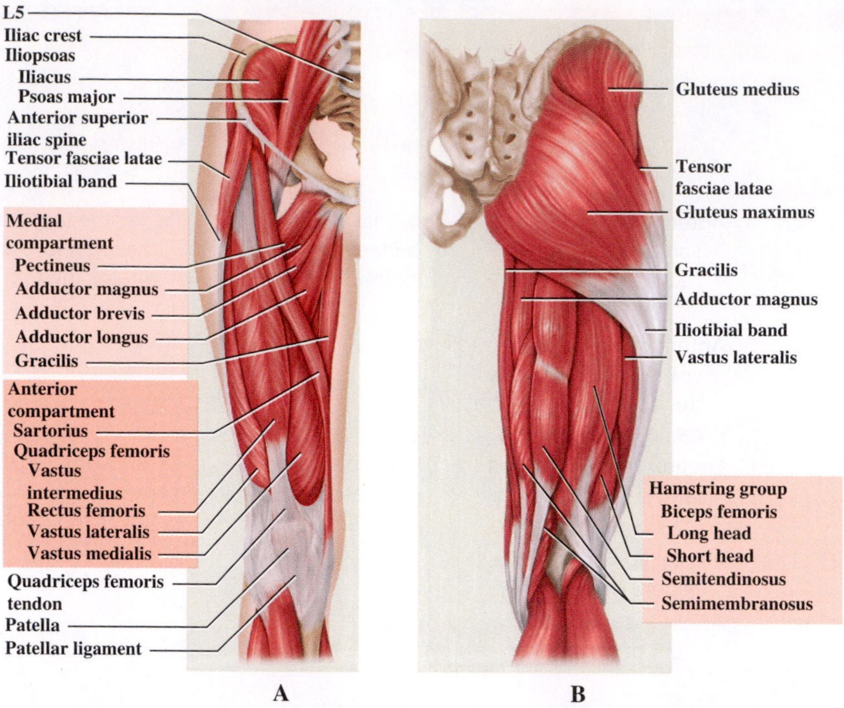
L5
Iliac crest
Iliopsoas
Iliacus
Psoas major
Anterior superior iliac spine
Tensor fasciae latae
Iliotibial band
Medial compartment
Pectineus
Adductor magnus
Adductor brevis
Adductor longus
Gracilis
Anterior compartment
Sartorius
Quadriceps femoris
Vastus intermedius
Rectus femoris
Vastus lateralis
Vastus medialis
Quadriceps femoris tendon
Patella
Patellar ligament
A
Gluteus medius
Tensor fasciae latae
Gluteus maximus
Gracilis
Adductor magnus
Iliotibial band
Vastus lateralis
Hamstring group
Biceps femoris
Long head
Short head
Semitendinosus
Semimembranosus
B

FIGURE 21–2 Muscles of the hip and thigh. **(A)** Anterior view. **(B)** Posterior view.

condyle. It also attaches to the medial side of the tibia, the popliteus muscle fascia, and the posterior capsule of the knee joint. The tibial branch of the sciatic nerve supplies this muscle.

**Medial Thigh Muscles** The medial thigh muscles include the gracilis, sartorius, pectineus, and three adductor muscles. All act as adductors and lateral rotators of the thigh at the hip joint (Figure 21–2). These muscles collectively make up a part of the anatomical region on the inner thigh referred to as the *groin*.

The gracilis muscle is attached superiorly to the body of the inferior ramus of the pubis and inferiorly to the medial aspect of the proximal tibia. It is a relatively narrow-appearing muscle that adducts the thigh at the hip and flexes and medially rotates the leg at the knee joint. The anterior branch of the obturator nerve serves this muscle.

The pectineus muscle arises from the pectineal crest of the pubis and attaches distally on the pectineal line of the femur. As one of the adductors, it also flexes and outwardly rotates the thigh.

The adductor longus, brevis, and magnus muscles originate at the ramus of the pubis and attach inferiorly on the linea aspera of the femur. The muscles adduct the thigh at the hip and outwardly rotate the thigh. All these muscles assist in the flexion of the thigh.

### Nerve Supply

Among the nerves that emerge from the sacral plexus are the tibial and common peroneal nerves, which in the thigh form the largest nerve in the body, the greater sciatic nerve. The sciatic nerve supplies the muscles of the thigh and lower leg (see Figure 21–14A).

### Blood Supply

The main arteries that supply the thigh are the medial circumflex femoral, deep femoral, and femoral arteries. The two main veins are the superficial great saphenous and the femoral veins (see Figure 21–15).

### Fascia

The fascia lata femoris is that part of the deep fascia that invests the thigh musculature. It is relatively thick anteriorly, laterally, and posteriorly but thin on the medial side where it covers the adductors. On its most lateral part, the iliotibial track, an attachment is provided for the tensor fascia lateral and greater aspect of the gluteus maximus.

### Surface Anatomy

Figure 21–3 shows the surface anatomy for the thigh from both the anterior view, which shows the quadriceps muscle group, and the posterior view, which shows the hamstrings.

## FUNCTIONAL ANATOMY OF THE THIGH

The quadriceps inserts by a common tendon to the proximal patella. The rectus femoris is the only quadriceps muscle that crosses the hip joint. It not only extends the knee but also flexes the hip. This is very important in differentiating hip flexor strains (i.e., iliopsoas versus

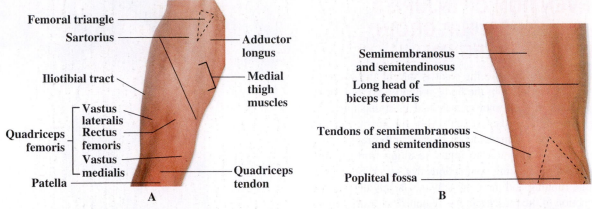

**FIGURE 21–3** Thigh and Knee. **(A)** An anterior view of the right thigh reveals the quadriceps femoris and patella, while **(B)** a posterior view illustrates the hamstrings.
© JW Ramsey/McGraw-Hill Education

rectus femoris) and the ensuing treatment and rehabilitation programs.[23]

The hamstrings all cross the knee joint posteriorly, and all except the short head of the biceps cross the hip joint. These biarticular muscles produce forces that depend on the position of both the knee joint and the hip joint. The position of the hip and knee during movement and the injury mechanism provide important information for preventing and rehabilitating hamstring injuries.[73]

# ASSESSMENT OF THE THIGH

## History

The athletic trainer should ask the following questions:

- Was the onset sudden or slow?
- Has this injury occurred before?
- How was the thigh injured?
- Can the athlete describe the intensity or duration of the pain?
- Is the pain constant? If not, when does it occur?
- Can the athlete specify exactly where the pain is?
- What type of pain is there? (Muscle pain is dull, achy, and hard to localize. Vascular pain is sharp, bright, and sometimes burning. Bone pain feels deep, penetrating, and highly localized.)
- Is there neural pain (tingling, numbness, paresthesia)?

## Observation

The athletic trainer should compare the thighs:

- Are they symmetrical?
- Is there obvious deformity?
- Are both the same size? Is there swelling?
- Are the skin color and texture normal?
- Is the athlete in obvious pain?
- Is the athlete willing to move the thigh?

## Palpation

Both thighs should be palpated for comparison while the patient is as relaxed as possible.

**Bony Palpation** The following bony landmarks should be palpated:

- Medial femoral condyle
- Lateral femoral condyle
- Greater trochanter
- Lesser trochanter
- Anterior superior iliac spine.
- Ischial tuberosity

**Soft-Tissue Palpation** The following soft-tissue structures should be palpated:

*Anterior*
- Sartorious
- Rectus femoris
- Vastus lateralis
- Vastus medialis

*Posterior*
- Semimembranosus
- Semitendinosus
- Biceps femoris
- Popliteus

*Medial*
- Adductor brevis
- Adductor longus
- Adductor magnus
- Gracilis
- Pectineus

*Lateral*
- Iliotibial band
- Gluteus medius
- Tensor fasciae latae

## Special Tests

NOTE: If a fracture is suspected, the following tests should not be performed.

- Passive range of motion. Beginning in extension, the knee is passively flexed. A normal muscle will elicit full range of motion that is pain free. A muscle that has swelling or spasm will have restricted passive motion.
- Active range of motion. Active movement from flexion to extension that is strong and painful may indicate muscle strain. A movement that is weak and pain free may indicate a grade 3 or partial muscle rupture.[46]
- Muscle weakness against an isometric resistance may indicate a nerve injury or a muscle injury.

# PREVENTION OF INJURIES TO THE THIGH, HIP, GROIN, AND PELVIC REGION

Despite the fact that the hip joint is one of the strongest and most stable joints in the body, primarily because of its strong ligaments and joint capsule and its strong musculature, many injuries can occur.[29] Although many muscles produce a variety of movements throughout this region, they are extremely vulnerable to injury resulting from the dynamic power-producing contractions that occur. Success in dynamic running and jumping activities largely depends on the function of the muscles in this region. The same muscles working in conjunction with the pelvis and the hip with its ligaments and capsule provide a base of core stability on which the extremities function. Core strength ensures proper hip alignment and prevention of muscle injuries due to misalignment and changes in length-tension relationships.

To prevent or at least minimize the chance of injury, it is essential to maintain the strength and flexibility of the muscles of the thigh, hip, and pelvis. Because flexibility ensures mobility, individuals should concentrate on a dynamic stretching program that focuses on the quadriceps, hamstrings, hip flexors, gluteal muscles, iliotibial band, tensor fascia latae, and groin muscles. Muscle strains in any of these muscle groups can have long-term consequences for healing and can be disabling. Strengthening exercises should routinely include open and closed chain movements, paying attention to both concentric and eccentric movement patterns to develop proper muscle strength. Closed chain exercises can include squats, lunges, and leg presses and are typically more functional in nature. Open chain exercises allow for exercise choices that focus on specific muscle groups in isolation. Core strengthening exercises assist with maintaining stability of the pelvis and preventing misalignments that could adversely affect the muscles of the thigh and hip (see Chapter 4).

> Flexibility and strengthening of the muscles in this region are the keys to preventing injury.

Proper running mechanics can play a big role in injury prevention as it assists in dissipating force through the entire lower extremity.

# RECOGNITION AND MANAGEMENT OF THIGH INJURIES

Injuries to the thigh muscles are among the most common in sports. Contusions and strains occur most often, with the former having the higher incidence.[15]

## Quadriceps Contusions

***Etiology*** The quadriceps group is continually exposed to traumatic impact in a variety of activities. Contusions

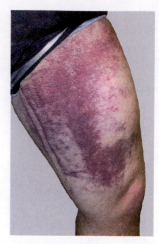

**FIGURE 21–4**  Quadriceps contusion.
Courtesy Chris Bartlett, Central Davidson High School, Lexington, NC

usually develop as a result of a severe impact to the relaxed thigh that compresses the muscle against the underlying femur. The extent of the force and the degree of thigh relaxation determine the depth of the injury and the amount of structural and functional disruption that takes place.[77]

***Symptoms and signs***  Contusions of the quadriceps display all the classic symptoms of most muscle bruises (Figure 21–4). Pain, a transitory loss of function, and immediate capillary bleeding usually occur at the instant of trauma. The patient usually describes having been hit by a sharp blow to the thigh, which produces intense pain and weakness. Immediate control of hemorrhage is critical in effecting a fast recovery. Palpation may reveal a circumscribed swollen area that is painful to the touch.

The grade 1 quadriceps contusion is a superficial intramuscular bruise that produces mild hemorrhage, little pain, no swelling, and mild point tenderness at the site of the trauma. There is no restriction of the range of motion. The grade 2 contusion is deeper than grade 1 and produces mild pain, mild swelling, and point tenderness, with the patient unable to flex the knee more than 90 degrees. The grade 3 contusion causes moderate pain, swelling, and a range of knee flexion that is 90 to 45 degrees and an obvious limp. The severe, or grade 4, contusion represents a major disability. A blow may have been so intense as to split the fascia, allowing the muscle to protrude (muscle herniation). A characteristic deep intramuscular hematoma with an intermuscular spread is present (Figure 21–4). Pain is severe, and swelling may lead to hematoma. Movement of the knee is severely restricted, with 45 degrees or less flexion and a decided limp.

***Management***  The knee should be placed immediately in flexion, with an ice pack, to stretch the muscle and prevent shortening (Figure 21–5). Placing and holding the knee in 120 degrees of flexion immediately following a quadriceps contusion appears to shorten the time to return to unrestricted full athletic activities.[4] POLICE and analgesics are used as needed. NSAIDs should be limited in

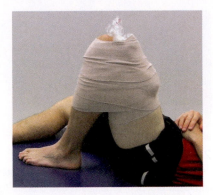

FIGURE 21–5    Immediate care of the thigh contusion, including POLICE and a constant stretch of the quadriceps muscle.

© William E. Prentice

the initial acute injury phase. Crutches may be warranted in grade 2 and grade 3 contusions. A hematoma that develops may have to be aspirated.[41] Considerable bleeding may occur in the anterior thigh. The patient should be placed on crutches. After exercise or reinjury, POLICE must be routinely applied to the thigh. Follow-up care consists of range of motion (ROM) exercises and progressive resistance exercises (PRE) within a pain-free limitation. Heat, massage, and ultrasound should be avoided initially to prevent the possibility of myositis ossificans (Figure 21–6).

Generally, the rehabilitation of a thigh contusion should be handled conservatively. Cold packs combined with gentle stretching may be the preferred treatment. If heat therapy is used, it should not be initiated until the acute phase of the injury has clearly passed. An elastic bandage should be worn to provide constant pressure and mild support to the quadriceps area. An open/closed chain strengthening progression should be used to

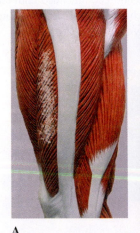
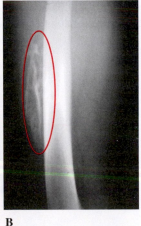

A                         B

FIGURE 21–6    (A) Myositis ossificans is likely to develop in the anterior thigh following repeated contusion (see shaded area). (B) X-ray view.

(a) © William E. Prentice; (b) Courtesy Jordan B. Renner, MD, Departments of Radiology and Allied Health Sciences, University of North Carolina

ensure the quadriceps have regained proper function and symmetrical strength compared with the opposite side. Exercise should be graduated from mild stretching of the quadriceps in the early stages of the injury to swimming, and then to jogging and running. Exercise should be avoided if it produces pain.

Medical care of a quadriceps contusion may include surgical repair of a herniated muscle or aspiration of a hematoma. Some physicians have recommended administering enzymes either orally or through injection to help dissolve a hematoma, but it is unclear if this is effective.[34]

Once a patient has sustained a severe quadriceps contusion, he or she must take great care to avoid sustaining another contusion. An injured athlete should routinely wear a protective pad held in place by an elastic wrap while engaging in sports activity.

### Heterotrophic Ossification (Myositis Ossificans)

*Etiology*    A severe blow or repeated blows to the thigh, usually to the quadriceps muscle, can lead to heterotrophic ossification, or myositis ossificans.[41] This condition commonly follows bleeding into the quadriceps muscle and a hematoma. The contusion to the muscle causes disruption of the muscle fibers, capillaries, fibrous connective tissue, and periosteum of the femur. Acute inflammation follows the resolution of hemorrhage. The irritated tissue may then produce calcified formations that resemble cartilage or bone. Areas of calcification may be noted during X-ray examination 2 to 6 weeks after the injury. If the injury is to a muscle belly, complete absorption or a decrease in the size of the formation may occur. This decrease is less likely if calcification is at a muscle origin or insertion. In terms of bone attachment, some calcifications are completely free of the femur, some are stalklike, and some are broadly attached (Figure 21–6).

> **Myositis ossificans can occur from:**
> - A single severe impact
> - Repeated impact to soft tissue
> - Improper care of a contusion

As mentioned earlier, improper care of a thigh contusion can lead to myositis ossificans. The following can initially cause the condition or, once present, can aggravate it, causing it to become more pronounced:

- Failure to aggressively control initial bleeding
- Too-vigorous treatment of a contusion—for example, massage directly over the contusion, ultrasound therapy, or superficial heat to the thigh

> **21–1 Clinical Application Exercise**
>
> A rodeo cowboy gets kicked in the anterior thigh after being thrown off a bull.
>
> **?** What is the most important thing that an athletic trainer can do to allow this cowboy to continue to compete?

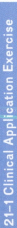

***Symptoms and signs*** The patient complains of pain, muscle weakness, soreness, swelling, and decreased muscle function. On examination, there is tissue tension and point tenderness along with a decreased ROM.

***Management*** Once myositis ossificans is apparent, treatment should be extremely conservative. Treatment is focused on regaining full pain-free range of motion, progressive return to activity or sport based on symptoms, strength, and function. A recent case study reported use of phonophoresis with acetic acid significantly decreased patient signs, symptoms, and the size of the calcification on diagnostic ultrasound in most patients at a 4-week post diagnosis mark.[5] If the condition is painful and restricts motion, the calcification may be surgically removed.

## Quadriceps Muscle Strain

***Etiology*** A quadriceps strain usually occurs because of a sudden, violent, forceful contraction of the hip and knee into flexion, with the hip initially extended.[23,33] An overstretch of the quadriceps, with the hip in extension and the knee flexed (especially coupled with an eccentric muscle contraction), can also cause a quadriceps strain. A strain can be very disabling, especially when the rectus femoris muscle is involved due to its involvement at two joints. The quadriceps muscles, like the hamstrings, produce a great deal of force and contract in a rapid fashion. Most strains occur at the musculotendinous junctions. Rectus femoris involvement is more disabling than a strain to any of the other quadriceps muscles.[33]

***Symptoms and signs*** A strain shows acute pain, possibly after a workout has been completed, swelling to a specific area, and loss of knee flexion. If the rectus femoris is involved, knee flexion range of motion lying prone (hip in extended position) is severely limited and painful.

A patient with a grade 1 quadriceps strain may complain of tightness in the front of the thigh, ambulate with a normal gait cycle, and present with a history of the thigh feeling fatigued and tight. Swelling might not be present, and the patient usually has very mild discomfort on palpation.

A patient with a grade 2 quadriceps strain may have an abnormal gait cycle. The knee may be splinted in extension. The patient may have felt a sudden twinge and pain down the length of the rectus femoris during activity. Swelling may be noticeable, and palpation may produce pain. A defect in the muscle may also be evident in a grade 2 strain. Resistive knee extension, both when sitting and when lying supine, may reproduce pain. With a quadriceps strain, any decrease in knee flexion range of motion should classify the injury as a grade 2 or 3 strain.

A patient with a grade 3 quadriceps strain may be unable to ambulate without the aid of crutches and is in severe pain, with a noticeable defect in the quadriceps muscle. Palpation is usually not tolerated, and swelling is present almost immediately. The patient may not be able to extend the knee actively and against resistance. An isometric contraction is painful and may produce a bulge or defect in the quadriceps muscle, especially the rectus femoris (Figure 21–7).[23]

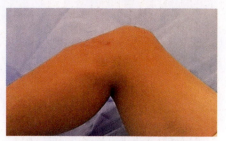

**FIGURE 21–7** Rupture of the rectus femoris.

***Management*** A patient with a grade 1 quadriceps strain should start ice, compression, pain-free active range of motion, and isometric quadriceps exercises immediately. Pain-free quadriceps progressive resistive strengthening exercises may be performed within 2 days. Compression using a neoprene sleeve (Figure 21–8) should be used at all times until the patient is free of pain and no longer complaining of tightness.

With a grade 2 quadriceps strain, the patient should use ice for 24 hours and compression and crutches for the first 3 to 5 days. Passive flexion should be progressed symptomatically allowing pain to guide the process. Knee range of motion progresses to actual quad stretching once the muscle has healed enough to allow for pain-free movement. At approximately the third day, the patient may perform quadriceps isometric exercises and pain-free quadriceps active range of motion exercises. Ice in conjunction with active range of motion exercises may be helpful in regaining motion and strengthening the quadriceps muscles without pain. Passive stretching exercises are not recommended until later phases because a passive stretch might have been the cause of the strain. Rehabilitation may take 14 to 21 days.

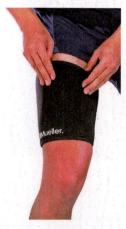

**FIGURE 21–8** A neoprene sleeve may be worn for soft-tissue support.

Courtesy Mueller Sports Medicine

A patient with a grade 3 quadriceps strain should be on crutches for 7 to 14 days or longer to allow for rest and normal gait before walking without crutches. Twenty-four-hour compression, ice, and electrical muscle stimulation modalities should be used immediately. Quadriceps stretching exercises are not performed until later phases. When pain free, the patient may begin quadriceps isometric exercises and gentle quadriceps active range of motion exercises that avoid overstretching the quadriceps muscles. Weight may be added after days 10 to 14. The patient may need 12 weeks to return to full activity.[23]

## Hamstring Muscle Strains

*Etiology* Hamstring injuries are one of the most common muscle injuries in athletics and are also an injury with a relatively high recurrence rate.[53] The exact cause of hamstring strain is not known. Eccentric contraction of the hamstring as it moves into hip flexion and knee extension places the muscle in a lengthened position. Asymmetrical alignment (rotation) of the pelvis creates an imbalance in the length-tension relationship affecting proper muscle function. A delay in firing of the gluteus maximus relative to the biceps femoris may predispose the biceps femoris to injury due to increased demand.[19,48] Possible reasons include muscle fatigue, faulty posture, leg-length discrepancy, tight hamstrings, improper form, adverse neural tension,[52,72] and an imbalance of strength between hamstring muscle groups. NOTE: Hamstring muscles function as decelerators of leg swing and commonly become injured when an individual suddenly changes direction or starts too slowly. In most individuals, the hamstring muscle group should have a strength 60 percent to 70 percent of that of the quadriceps group.[62]

*Symptoms and signs* Hamstring strain can involve the muscle belly or bony attachment. The extent of injury can vary from the pulling apart of a few muscle fibers to a complete rupture or an avulsion fracture (Figure 21–9).[48]

Capillary hemorrhage, pain, and immediate loss of function vary according to the degree of trauma. Discoloration may occur a day or two after injury.

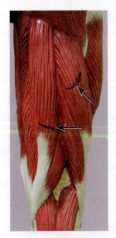

FIGURE 21–9 A hamstring strain results in separation or tearing of muscle fibers.
© William E. Prentice

Grade 1 hamstring strain usually is evidenced by muscle soreness during movement, accompanied by point tenderness. These strains are often difficult to detect when they first occur. Irritation and stiffness do not become apparent until the athlete has cooled down after activity. The soreness of the mild hamstring strain in most instances can be attributed to muscle spasm rather than to the tearing of tissue.

A grade 2 hamstring strain represents a partial tearing of muscle fibers, identified by a sudden snap or tear of the muscle accompanied by severe pain and a loss of function during knee flexion. Fewer than 70 percent of fibers are torn in a grade 2 hamstring tear.

A grade 3 hamstring strain constitutes the rupturing of tendinous or muscular tissue and involves major hemorrhage and disability. With more than 70 percent of fibers torn, there is severe edema, tenderness, loss of function, ecchymosis, and a palpable mass or palpable gap in the muscle.[44]

*Management* Initially, POLICE, NSAIDs, and analgesics are given as needed. Activity should be reduced until soreness has been completely alleviated. The strategy for rehabilitation should incorporate neuromuscular control exercises and eccentric strength training, which are critical for safe return to play but also for minimizing the risk of reinjury.[28] A patient with a grade 1 hamstring strain, as with the other grades of strain, should not be allowed to resume full activity until complete function of the injured part is restored.

Grades 2 and 3 strains should be treated extremely conservatively. For grade 2 strains, POLICE should be used for 24 to 48 hours; for grade 3 strains, for 48 to 72 hours. After the early inflammatory phase of injury has stabilized, a treatment regimen of isometric exercise, cryotherapy, and ultrasound may be of benefit. In later stages of healing, gentle stretching within pain limits, jogging, stationary cycling, and isokinetic exercise at high speeds may be used. It is essential to incorporate closed kinetic chain eccentric exercises such as squats, lunges, and multiplanar movements. After the elimination of soreness, the athlete may begin isotonic knee curls. Full recovery may take from 1 month to a full season.[23]

Strains are always a problem for the patient because they tend to recur as a result of the inelastic, fibrous scar tissue that sometimes forms during the healing process. The higher the incidence of strains at a particular muscle site, the greater the amount of scar tissue and the greater the likelihood of further injury. For some individuals, the fear of another pulled muscle becomes almost an obsession, which is often more disabling than the injury itself.

### Femoral Fractures

*Etiology*  Femoral fractures are rare in the adolescent patient, occur more often in middle-age patients, and are relatively common in elderly individuals with osteoporosis.[44] A significant trauma is necessary to cause a femoral fracture in the young population. Even though femoral fractures are relatively rare in young patients, the potential complications of this injury are significant.[55] Due to a limited blood supply in the region of the femoral head, there is a high incidence of avascular necrosis, which is an important consideration until the patient becomes skeletally mature and collateral blood supply has been well established. The prognosis of the fracture is dependent on the specific location of the injury and the degree to which the blood supply is compromised. Fractures that occur across the epiphysis have the highest likelihood of developing avascular necrosis.[1]

*Symptoms and signs*  After injury, the patient complains of significant pain and generally cannot stand or walk. The patient is muscle guarding and resists any attempts to move. The hip is usually externally rotated and slightly adducted. Shortening of the limb may also be evident.

*Management*  The patient must be immediately immobilized and transported for medical care. The physician will perform either an open or a closed reduction with some type of rigid internal fixation using multiple pins or plates.[55] Following surgery, the athlete must be immobilized with a hinged brace. Rehabilitation requires a slow progression that may require as long as 7 and 13 months.[65]

### Femoral Stress Fractures

*Etiology*  Stress fractures of the femoral neck are fairly uncommon, and femoral shaft stress fractures are rare. They occur most often in endurance athletes (e.g., triathlon, marathon) and thus the primary mechanism of injury is attributed to overuse.[24] These injuries are more likely in females who are amenorrheic.[6]

> Femoral stress fractures are becoming more prevalent because of the increased popularity of repetitive, sustained activities, such as distance running.

*Symptoms and signs*  Onset of symptoms may occur several weeks after increasing the intensity of a training program. The patient with a stress fracture complains of pain in the groin or anterior thigh, which increases during activity and may persist after activity.[75] Pain may be referred to the knee and is relieved with longer periods of rest. Eventually, the pain becomes constant, even with no activity. The patient walks with an antalgic gait using an abduction lurch-type movement.[54] There is also a positive Trendelenburg's sign (see Figure 21–22). Early X-rays may not show any clear signs.

*Management*  Initial treatment requires complete rest with no running. The prognosis varies according to the location of the stress fracture. Stress fractures on the medial side of the femoral neck tend to heal well with conservative management. Stress fractures on the lateral side of the femoral neck are more likely to displace eventually and cause additional complications. Stress fractures of the femoral shaft usually heal with conservative management but, in rare cases, can progress to failure of cortical bone. If a fracture does occur, surgery may be indicated, and the time required for fracture healing and remodeling can be as long as 12 months.[75] In fractures not requiring surgery healing will require approximately 21 weeks.[78]

## ANATOMY OF THE HIP, GROIN, AND PELVIC REGION

The hip and pelvis are part of the kinetic chain that transmits a load from the foot to the spine and vice versa in all three planes of movement.[50]

### Bones

The pelvis, or pelvic girdle, is a bony ring formed by the left and right innominate bones, the sacrum, and the coccyx (Figure 21–10). Each innominate bone is composed of an ilium, an ischium, and a pubis (Figure 21–11). The functions of the pelvis are to support the spine and trunk and to transfer their weight to the lower limbs. In addition to providing skeletal support, the pelvis serves as a place of attachment for the trunk and thigh muscles and as protection for the pelvic viscera. The basin formed by the pelvis is separated into a false and a true pelvis. The false pelvis is composed of the wings of the ilium. The true pelvis is composed of the coccyx, sacrum, the ischium, and the pubis.

The innominate bones are three bones that ossify and fuse early in life. They include the ilium, which is positioned superiorly and posteriorly; the pubis, which forms the anterior part; and the ischium, which is located inferiorly. Lodged between the innominate bones is the wedge-shaped sacrum, composed of five fused vertebrae.

### Articulations

**Sacroiliac Joint and Coccyx**  The sacrum is joined to other parts of the pelvis by strong ligaments, forming the sacroiliac joint. A small backward-forward movement is present at the sacroiliac junction. The coccyx is composed of four or five small, fused vertebrae that articulate with the sacrum. The sacroiliac joint is discussed in detail in Chapter 25.

**Hip Joint**  The hip joint is formed by articulation of the femur with the innominate or hip bone. The articulating, spherical head of the femur fits into a deep socket in the innominate bone called the acetabulum, which is padded at

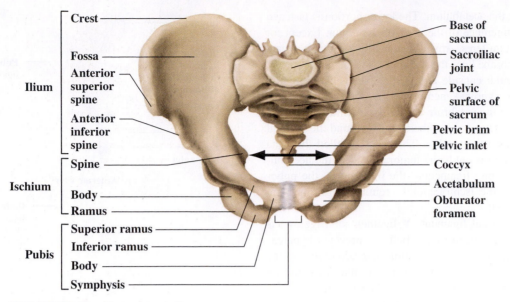

FIGURE 21–10   The pelvic girdle.

Crest

Fossa

Ilium

Anterior superior spine

Anterior inferior spine

Spine

Ischium

Body

Ramus

Superior ramus

Inferior ramus

Pubis

Body

Symphysis

Base of sacrum

Sacroiliac joint

Pelvic surface of sacrum

Pelvic brim

Pelvic inlet

Coccyx

Acetabulum

Obturator foramen

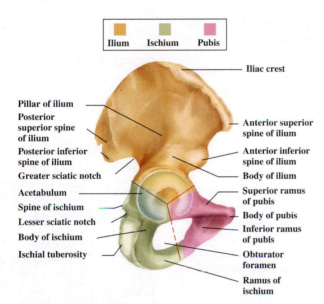

| Ilium | Ischium | Pubis |

Iliac crest

Pillar of ilium

Posterior superior spine of ilium

Posterior inferior spine of ilium

Greater sciatic notch

Acetabulum

Spine of ischium

Lesser sciatic notch

Body of ischium

Ischial tuberosity

Anterior superior spine of ilium

Anterior inferior spine of ilium

Body of ilium

Superior ramus of pubis

Body of pubis

Inferior ramus of pubis

Obturator foramen

Ramus of ischium

FIGURE 21–11   Each innominate bone consists of an ilium, an ischium, and a pubis.

its center by a mass of fatty tissue, ligaments, and capsule. The acetabulum forms an incomplete bony ring that is interrupted by a notch on the lower aspect of the socket. The ring is completed by the transverse ligament that crosses the notch. The socket faces anteriorly, inferiorly, and laterally. The femoral head is a sphere that fits into the acetabulum in a medial, proximal, and slightly anterior direction.

## Ligaments, Joint Capsule, and Synovial Membrane

Surrounding the rim of the acetabulum is a fibrocartilage known as the acetabular labrum. A loose sleeve of articular tissue is attached to the circumference of the acetabulum above and to the neck of the femur below. The capsule is lined by an extensive synovial membrane, and the iliofemoral, pubocapsular, and ischiocapsular ligaments give it strong reinforcement. Hyaline cartilage completely covers the head of the femur, with the exception of the fovea capitis, a small area in the center to which the ligamentum teres is attached. The ligamentum teres gives little support to the hip joint; its main function is the transport of nutrient vessels to the head of the femur. Because of its bony, ligamentous, and muscular arrangements, many consider this joint to be the strongest articulation in the body.

The synovial membrane is a vascular tissue enclosing the hip joint in a tubular sleeve, with the upper portion surrounding the acetabulum. The lower portion is fastened to the circumference of the neck of the femur. Except for the ligamentum teres, which lies outside the synovial cavity, the membrane lines the acetabular socket.

The articular capsule is a fibrous, sleevelike structure covering the synovial membrane; its upper end attaches to the cartilaginous labrum and its lower end to the neck of the femur. The circular fibers that surround the femoral neck serve as a tight collar. This area is called the zona orbicularis, and it holds the femoral head in the acetabulum. Many strong ligaments—the iliofemoral, the pubofemoral, and the ischiofemoral—reinforce the hip joint (Figure 21–12).

The iliofemoral ligament (Y ligament of Bigelow) is the strongest ligament of the body. It prevents hyperextension, controls external rotation and adduction of the thigh, and limits the pelvis during any backward rolling of the femoral head during weight bearing. It reinforces the anterior aspect of the capsule and is attached to the anterior iliac spine and the intertrochanteric line on the anterior aspect of the femur.

The pubofemoral ligament prevents excessive abduction of the thigh and is positioned anterior and inferior to the pelvis and femur.

The ischiofemoral ligament prevents excessive internal rotation and adduction of the thigh and is located posterior and superior to the articular capsule.

## Hip Musculature

The muscles of the hip can be divided into anterior and posterior groups (Table 21–2). The anterior group includes the iliacus and psoas major and minor muscles (see Figure 21–2A). The posterior group's muscles include the tensor fasciae latae, gluteus maximus, gluteus medius, and gluteus minimus and the six deep outward rotators—the piriformis, gemellus superior, gemellus inferior, obturator internus, obturator externus, and quadratus femoris (see Figure 21–2B, and Figure 21–13).

**Anterior Hip Muscles** The iliacus and psoas muscles are anterior hip muscles. The tensor fasciae latae muscle is located on the upper anterior aspect of the lateral thigh. It is attached superiorly to the iliac crest just posterior to the anterior superior iliac spine and it inserts inferiorly into the iliotibial tract. Its primary action is flexion and medial rotation of the thigh. It is innervated by the superior gluteal nerve. The triangular iliacus is contained within the iliac fossa within the abdomen. Its tendon merges with the psoas major muscle, forming a common tendon called the iliopsoas. The iliopsoas attaches on the iliac fossa and part of the inner surface of the sacrum proximally, and it attaches distally on the lesser trochanter of the femur. The psoas major and minor muscle attaches proximally on the transverse processes and bodies of the lumbar vertebrae. Their distal attachment is on the lesser trochanter. The iliopsoas muscle flexes the thigh at the hip joint and tends to rotate the thigh outwardly and to adduct the thigh when

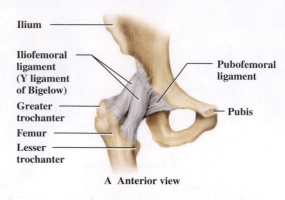

A  Anterior view

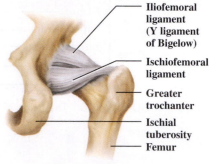

B  Posterior view

FIGURE 21–12   Ligaments of the hip. **(A)** Anterior view. **(B)** Posterior view.

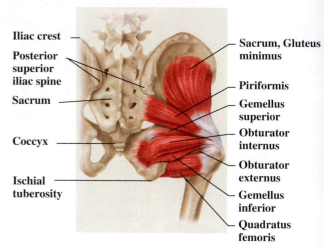

FIGURE 21–13   The six deep muscles of the hip.

free to move. When fixed, the iliopsoas assists in flexing the trunk and hip.

**Posterior Hip Muscles** The posterior muscles of the hip consist of the tensor fasciae latae, the three gluteal muscles, and the six deep outward rotators (see Figure 21–2B and Figure 21–13).

The gluteus maximus muscle forms the buttocks in the hip region. Lateral to and underneath the gluteus maximus are the gluteus medius and the gluteus minimus muscles (see Figure 21–2B and Figure 21–13). The gluteus maximus muscle is attached above to the posterior aspect of

TABLE 21–2   Muscles of the Hip*

| Muscle | Origin | Insertion | Muscle Action (non–weight bearing) | Innervation/ Nerve Root |
|---|---|---|---|---|
| *Iliopsoas* | | | | |
| Psoas major and psoas minor | Transverse processes and bodies of the last thoracic and all the lumbar vertebrae | Lesser trochanter of the femur | Flexes the thigh and the trunk on the femur | Femoral and first lumbar (L1–L4) |
| Iliacus | Iliac crest and fossa | | | |
| Tensor fasciae latae | Anterior portion of the iliac crest and the anterior superior iliac spine | Iliotibial band of the fasciae latae | Tenses the fasciae latae and assists in flexion, abduction, and medial rotation of the thigh | Superior gluteal (L4, L5, S1) |
| Gluteus maximus | Posterior gluteal line of the ilium and the posterior surface of the sacrum and the coccyx | Gluteal tuberosity of the femur; iliotibial band | Extends and laterally rotates the thigh | Inferior gluteal (L5, S1, S2) |
| Gluteus medius | Outer surface of the ilium between the posterior and the anterior gluteal lines | Lateral surface of the greater trochanter of the femur | Abducts and medially rotates the thigh | Superior gluteal (L4, L5, S1) |
| Gluteus minimus | Outer surface of the ilium between the anterior and the inferior gluteal lines | Anterior surface of the greater trochanter of the femur | Abducts and medially rotates the thigh | Superior gluteal (L4, L5, S1) |
| Piriformis | Anterior surface of the sacrum | Superior border of the greater trochanter of the femur | Laterally rotates the thigh and assists in extending and abducting the thigh | Second sacral (S2) |
| Superior gemellus | Ischial spine | Greater trochanter of the femur | Laterally rotates the thigh | Fifth lumbar and first and second sacral (L5, S1, S2) |
| Inferior gemellus | Ischial tuberosity | Greater trochanter of the femur | Laterally rotates the thigh | Fourth and fifth lumbar and first sacral (L4, L5, S1) |
| Obturator internus | Inner surface of the obturator membrane and the bony margins of the obturator foramen | Greater trochanter of the femur | Laterally rotates the thigh | Fifth lumbar and first and second sacral (L5, S1, S2) |
| Obturator externus | Outer surface of the obturator membrane and the bony margins of the obturator foramen | Trochanteric fossa of the femur | Laterally rotates the thigh | Obturator (L3, L4) |

*Continued*

**TABLE 21–2** **Muscles of the Hip (continued)**

| Muscle | Origin | Insertion | Muscle Action (non–weight bearing) | Innervation/ Nerve Root |
|---|---|---|---|---|
| Quadratus femoris | Ischial tuberosity | Shaft of the femur just below the greater trochanter | Laterally rotates the thigh | Fourth and fifth lumbar (L4, L5) |

**Hip Joint Movements***

Hip abduction — Hip adduction

Hip extension — Hip flexion

Hip external rotation — Hip internal rotation

*Manual muscle tests and goniometric measurements of range of motion for the hip joint can be found in Appendix F and Appendix G at the end of the text.

© William E. Prentice

the iliac crest, the sacrum, and the coccyx, as well as to the fascia in the area. Distally, this muscle attaches to the iliotibial tract and into the gluteal tuberosity of the femur between the linea aspera and greater trochanter. The gluteus maximus muscle acts as a lateral rotator of the thigh at the hip joint and allows the body to rise from a sitting to a standing position. Through its attachment to the iliotibial tract, the muscle helps extend the flexed knee. The inferior gluteal nerve supplies this muscle. The gluteus medius muscle is located lateral to the hip. It is attached superiorly to the lateral aspect of the ilium and inferiorly to the lateral aspect of the "greater" trochanter of the femur. The gluteus maximus muscle covers this muscle posteriorly, and it is covered anteriorly by the tensor fasciae latae. The gluteus medius muscle acts primarily as a thigh abductor at the hip, with some flexion and medial rotation occurring from its anterior aspect and some extension and lateral rotation occurring from its posterior aspect. It is innervated by the superior gluteal nerve. The gluteus minimus muscle originates above the lateral aspect of the ilium and attaches inferiorly to the anterior aspect of the greater trochanter of the femur. Its main action is to cause medial rotation at the hip joint; its secondary action is abduction of the thigh at the hip joint. It is innervated by the superior gluteus nerve.

Underneath these larger muscles are much smaller muscles that, along with the gluteus maximus, laterally rotate the hip: the piriformis, the quadratus femoris, the obturator internus and externus, and the gemellus superior and inferior (Figure 21–13). Collectively, they stabilize the head of the femur in the acetabulum.

## Bursae

The hip joint has many bursae. Clinically, the most important of them are the iliopsoas bursa and the deep trochanteric bursa. The iliopsoas bursa is located between the articular capsule and the iliopsoas muscle on the anterior aspect of the joint. The deep trochanteric bursa lies between the greater trochanter and the deep fibers of the gluteus maximus muscle.

## Nerve Supply

The lumbar plexus is created by the intertwining of the fibers stemming from the first four lumbar nerves (see Chapter 25). The femoral nerve, a major nerve emerging from this plexus, later divides into many branches to supply the thigh and lower leg. Nerve fibers from the fourth and fifth lumbar nerves and the first, second, and third sacral nerves form the sacral plexus within the pelvic cavity, anterior to the piriformis muscle (see Chapter 25.) Along with other nerves, the tibial and common peroneal nerves emerge from the sacral plexus and form the large sciatic nerve in the thigh (Figure 21–14).

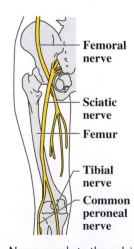

Femoral nerve

Sciatic nerve

Femur

Tibial nerve

Common peroneal nerve

FIGURE 21–14  Nerve supply to the pelvis, hip, and thigh.

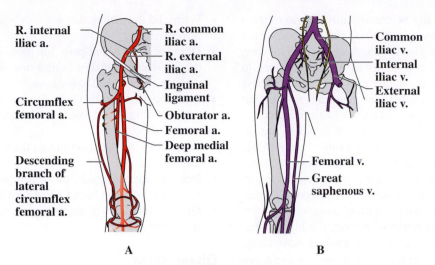

FIGURE 21–15    **(A)** Arterial blood supply and **(B)** veins of the hip, pelvis, and thigh.

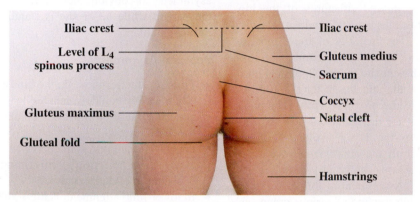

FIGURE 21–16    Posterior view of the surface anatomy for the hip and buttocks.
© JW Ramsey/McGraw-Hill Education

## Blood Supply

**Arteries**  At the level of the fourth lumbar vertebra, the aorta divides to become the two common iliac arteries (Figure 21–15A). They in turn pass downward to divide, opposite the sacroiliac joint, into the internal and external iliac arteries. Most of the branches of the internal iliac artery supply blood to the pelvic viscera. The external iliac artery is the primary artery to the lower limb.

**Veins**  Three major veins are found in the region of hips, groin, and pelvis (Figure 21–15B). The first is the common iliac vein, which stems from the inferior vena cava on both sides draining the lower body. The second is the internal iliac vein, which ascends behind its iliac artery to the brim of the true pelvis, where it joins the external vein to form the common iliac vein. Its tributaries drain the pelvis and adjoining area. Third is the external iliac vein, which passes upward from the femoral vein behind the inguinal ligament and follows the brim of the true pelvis, where it joins the internal iliac vein.

## Surface Anatomy

Figure 21–16 shows the pertinent surface anatomy in a posterior view of the hip and buttocks.

# FUNCTIONAL ANATOMY OF THE HIP, GROIN, AND PELVIC REGION

The pelvis and hip are made up of the pelvic girdle and the articulation of the femoral head to the bony socket of the pelvic girdle, the acetabulum, forming a ball-in-socket joint. This joint connects the lower extremity to the pelvic girdle. The pelvis itself moves in three directions, anteroposterior tilting, lateral tilting, and rotation. The iliopsoas muscle and other hip flexors, as well as extensors of the lumbar spine, perform anterior tilting in the sagittal plane and facilitate lumbar lordosis. The gluteus maximus and hamstrings, along with the rectus abdominus and the obliques, posteriorly tilt the pelvis and cause a decrease in lumbar lordosis. During lateral tilting in the frontal plane, the hip joint acts as the center of rotation. Hip abduction or adduction is a result of pelvic lateral tilting. The hip abductors control lateral tilting by contracting isometrically or eccentrically. Pelvic rotation occurs in the transverse plane, using the hip joint as the axis of rotation. The gluteal muscles, external rotators, adductors, pectineus, and iliopsoas all act together to perform this movement in the transverse plane. These movements of the pelvis play an important role in gait analysis, injury evaluation, and correct gait education.[64]

The hip joint is a true ball-in-socket joint and has intrinsic stability not found in other joints. This intrinsic stability does not prevent the hip joint from retaining great mobility. During normal gait, the hip joint moves in all three planes, sagittal, frontal, and transverse. To participate in athletic activities, a greater range of motion is needed. With its great range of motion, the hip is capable of performing many different combined movements. Forces at the hip joint have been increased to five times the body weight during running. These forces can also contribute to injuries, both muscular and bony.[40]

The most frequently injured structures of the hip, groin, and pelvis are the muscles and tendons that perform the movements.[79] The majority of these muscles originate on the pelvis or the proximal femur. The iliac crest serves as the attachment site for the abdominal muscles, the ilium serves as the attachment for the gluteals, and the gluteals insert to the proximal femur. The pubis serves as the attachment for the adductors, and the iliopsoas inserts distally to the lesser trochanter of the proximal femur. Due to all the attachments in a small area, injury to these structures can be very disabling and difficult to distinguish.[23] Assessment of this area is also complicated due to the intersection of various organ systems, nerves from the lumbar spine in addition to the musculoskeletal system.

# ASSESSMENT OF THE HIP, GROIN, AND PELVIS

The hip, groin, and pelvis form the body's core. The body's center of gravity is located just in front of the upper part of the sacrum. Injuries to the hip, groin, or pelvis cause the patient disability in the lower limb, trunk, or both.[2,15]

Because of the close proximity of the hip and pelvis to the low back region, many evaluative procedures overlap (see Chapter 25).

## History

The athletic trainer should determine the following information:

- Is there any history of previous injury?
- What was the mechanism of injury?
- Was the onset acute or did it develop over time?
- Are there any asymmetries or obvious deformities?
- Where exactly is the pain located?
- What are the patient's symptoms (e.g., weakness, disability, pain)?

- When did the patient first notice a problem with the hip or pelvis?
- Describe the types of pain (hip pain is felt mainly in the groin and medial or frontal side of thigh; hip pain may also be referred to the knee).
- Describe the sacroiliac pain. Does it radiate in the posterior thigh, iliac fossa, or buttock on the affected side?
- When does the pain occur (e.g., during activity, while turning in bed)?
- Note the age and gender of the patient (e.g., boys 3 to 12 years old can have Legg-Calvé-Perthes disease; distance-running amenorrheic girls may develop a hip stress fracture).

## Observation

The athletic trainer should check the patient for postural asymmetry or obvious deformities and should observe the patient while he or she is standing on one leg and during ambulation.

### Postural Asymmetry

- From an anterior view, do the hips look even? A laterally tilted hip could mean a leg-length discrepancy or abnormal muscle contraction on one side of the hip or low back region.
- From a lateral view, is the pelvis abnormally tilted anteriorly or posteriorly? This tilting may indicate lordosis or flat back, respectively.
- In lower-limb alignment, is there an indication of genu valgum, genu varum, foot pronation, or genu recurvatum? The patella should also be noted for relative position and alignment.
- The posterior superior iliac spines, represented by the skin depressions above the buttocks and the anterior superior iliac spines, should be horizontal to one another. Uneven depressions could indicate that one side of the pelvis is rotated.

**Standing on One Leg**  Standing on one leg may produce pain in the hip, abnormal movement of the symphysis pubis, or a fall of the pelvis on the opposite side as a result of abductor weakness (see Figure 21–22).

**Ambulation**  The patient should be observed during walking and sitting. Pain in the hip and pelvic region will normally be reflected in abnormal movements.

## Palpation

The following bony landmarks should be palpated:

- Iliac crest
- Anterior superior iliac spine
- Anterior inferior iliac spine
- Greater trochanter
- Femoral neck

- Lesser trochanter
- Symphysis pubis
- Ischial tuberosity
- Posterior inferior iliac spine
- Posterior superior iliac spine
- Medial epicondyle
- Lateral epicondyle

**Soft-Tissue Palpation** The soft-tissue sites of major concern are in the regions of the groin, femoral triangle, sciatic nerve, and major muscles. Groin pain could result from swollen lymph glands, indicating an infection, or from an adductor muscle strain.

The following soft-tissue structures should be palpated:

*Anterior*
- Rectus femoris
- Sartorius
- Iliopsoas
- Inguinal ligament

*Medial*
- Gracilis
- Adductor magnus
- Adductor longus
- Adductor brevis
- Pectineus

*Posterior*
- Gluteus maximus
- Piriformis
- Hamstrings

*Lateral*
- Gluteus medius
- Gluteus minimus
- Tensor fasciae latae
- Iliotibial band

## Special Tests

Few of the current diagnostic tests used to evaluate the hip are of substantial diagnostic accuracy to dictate clinical decision making. The special tests that have good-to-excellent accuracy include FADDIRs, Flexion and Internal Rotation, Patellar-Pubic Percussion Test, Trendelenberg's, and Resisted Abduction.[60,69]

## Tests for Labral Pathologies

**Flexion-Adduction-Internal Rotation Test (FADDIR)[60]**
The patient lies supine with the legs extended. Standing on the side of the leg to be tested the clinician passively flexes the hip and knee to 90 degrees, then passively adducts and internally rotates the leg to end range applying overpressure. A positive test produces pain and locking, clicking or catching indicating injury to the labrum (Figure 21–17).
Sn. 0.94 | Sp. 0.08 | +LR 1.02 | -LR 0.48

**Flexion-Abduction-External Rotation Test (FABER)[68]**
In a FABER test (flexion, abduction, external rotation of the hip) or Patrick's test, the patient lies supine on the examining table. The foot on the side of the painful sacroiliac is placed on the opposite extended knee. Pressure is then applied downward on the bent knee. Any pain that is felt in the hip may indicate injury to the labrum (Figure 21–18).
Sn. 0.57 | Sp. 0.71 | +LR 1.19 | -LR 0.61

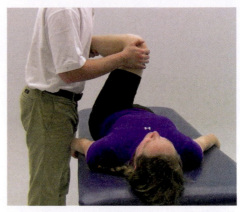

FIGURE 21–17   Flexion-Adduction-Internal Rotation (FADDIR) test for labral tears.
© William E. Prentice

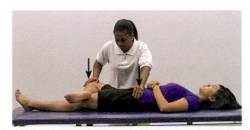

FIGURE 21–18   The Patrick test or FABER test for a pathological condition of the hip and sacroiliac joint.
© William E. Prentice

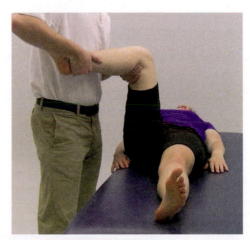

FIGURE 21–19   Flexion Internal Rotation test for labral tears.
© William E. Prentice

**Flexion Internal Rotation Test[60]** The patient is supine with legs extended. Standing on the side of the leg to be tested the clinician passively flexes the hip and knee to 90 degrees while simultaneously internally rotating the leg. A positive test produces groin pain, and any locking, clicking, or catching indicates injury to the labrum (Figure 21–19).
Sn. 0.96 | Sp. 0.17 | +LR 1.12 | -LR 0.27

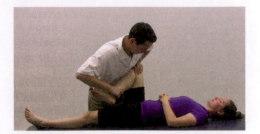

FIGURE 21–20    Scour test for labral tears.
© William E. Prentice

**Scour Test**[68] The patient lies supine with the examiner standing on the involved side. The hip is passively flexed and adducted and the knee is in full flexion. A downward force is applied along the shaft of the femur while passively adducting and externally rotating the hip. A positive test is any pain, apprehension, or unusual movements that may indicate a labrum tear, osteoarthritis, or impingement (Figure 21–20). Sn. 0.62 | Sp. 0.75 | +LR 2.4 | -LR 0.51

## Tests for Femoral Fracture/Stress Fracture

**Patellar-Pubic Percussion**[60] The patient is supine with legs extended. Standing on the side of the leg to be tested the clinician places a stethoscope over the pubic tubercle, then taps the patella on the near leg side. In a positive test the sound is diminished when compared to the contralateral side (Figure 21–21).[70] Sn. 0.95 | Sp. 0.86 | +LR 6.11 | -LR 0.07

## Tests for Gluteal Tendinopathies

**Trendelenberg's Test**[60] While the patient stands, the foot on the unaffected side is lifted so that the hip flexes. Normally, in this position, the iliac crest on the unaffected

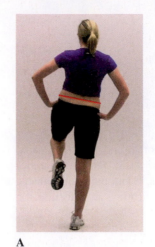 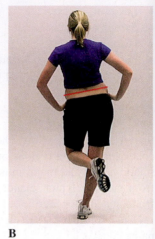

A                                                                  B

FIGURE 21–22    Trendelenburg's test. **(A)** Normal. **(B)** Positive.
© William E. Prentice

side is higher than on the affected side. If the iliac crest on the affected side is higher than on the unaffected side, the test is positive, indicating weakness in the hip abductors, particularly the gluteus medius (Figure 21–22).[80] Sn. 0.61 | Sp. 0.92 | +LR 6.83 | -LR 0.25

**Resisted Hip Abduction Test**[60] The patient is lying supine. The leg is flexed to 30 degrees. Then the patient is asked to abduct the leg and hold against resistance from the clinician. A positive finding is a complaint of pain at the greater trochanter (Figure 21–23). Sn. 0.71 | Sp. 0.84 | +LR 5.50 | -LR 0.37

## Tests for Hip Flexor Tightness

Contractures of the hip flexors are major causes of lordosis and susceptibility to groin pain and discomfort. Two tests can be used: the Kendall test and the Thomas test.

**Kendall Test** The patient lies supine on a table with one knee flexed on the chest and the back completely

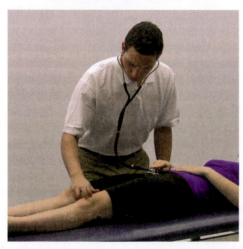

FIGURE 21–21    Patellar-Pubic Percussion for femoral fractures or stress fractures.
© William E. Prentice

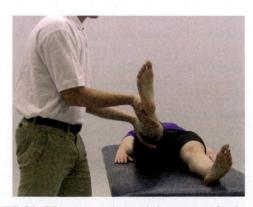

FIGURE 21–23    Resisted Hip Abduction test for femoral fractures or stress fractures.
© William E. Prentice

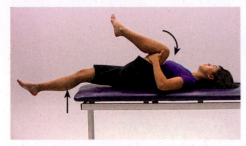

FIGURE 21–24   Kendall test for hip flexor tightness.
© William E. Prentice

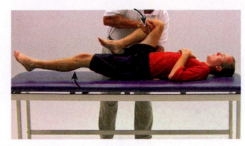

FIGURE 21–26   Thomas test for hip contractures.
© William E. Prentice

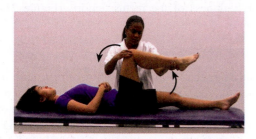

FIGURE 21–25   Demonstrating tight hip flexors.
© William E. Prentice

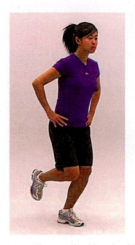

FIGURE 21–27   Renne's test for iliotibial band tightness.
© William E. Prentice

A young gymnast has a history of moderate groin pain. She is susceptible to strains in that region. The patient also appears to have an exaggerated lumbar lordotic curve.

**?** What tests should be given to evaluate the tightness of the groin region?

flat (Figure 21–24). The other knee is flexed over the table's end. Normal extensibility of the hip flexors allows the thigh to touch the table with the knee flexed approximately 70 degrees. Tight hip flexors are revealed by the inability of the thigh to lie flat on the table. If only the rectus femoris muscle is tight, the thigh will touch the table, but the knee will extend more than 70 degrees (Figure 21–25).

**Thomas Test[60]** The Thomas test indicates whether hip contractures are present (Figure 21–26). The patient lies supine on a table, arms across the chest, legs together and fully extended. The athletic trainer places one hand under the patient's lumbar curve; one thigh is brought to the chest, flattening the spine. In this position, the extended thigh should be flat on the table. If not, there is a hip contracture. When the patient fully extends the leg again, the curve in the low back returns. Sn. 0.89 | Sp. 0.92 | +LR 11.1 | -LR 0.12

## Testing the Tensor Fasciae Latae and Iliotibial Band

Three tests can be used to discern iliotibial band tightness and inflammation of the bursa overlying the

lateral femoral epicondyle or direct irritation of the iliotibial band and periosteum: Renne's test, Nobel's test, and Ober's test.[46]

**Renne's Test** The patient stands and supports his or her full weight on the affected leg with the knee bent at 30 degrees to 40 degrees. A positive response of fasciae latae tightness occurs when pain is felt at the lateral femoral condyle (Figure 21–27).[38]

**Nobel's Test** The patient lies supine, the hip and knee flexed to 90 degrees, and pressure is applied to the lateral femoral epicondyle while the knee is gradually extended. A positive response occurs when severe pain is felt at the lateral femoral epicondyle with the knee at 30 degrees of flexion (Figure 21–28).[46]

**Ober's Test[59]** The patient lies on the unaffected side. Beginning with the knee flexed at 90 degrees, the affected hip is passively abducted and extended with the knee flexed to 90 degrees With the pelvis stabilized, the abducted thigh is then relaxed and allowed to drop into adduction with the knee flexed. A tight tensor fasciae latae or iliotibial band will keep the thigh in an abducted position,

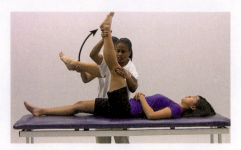

FIGURE 21–28   Nobel's test for iliotibial band tightness.
© William E. Prentice

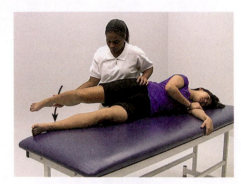

FIGURE 21–29   Ober's test for iliotibial band tightness.
© William E. Prentice

not allowing it to fall into adduction (Figure 21–29).[59]
Sn. 0.90 | Sp. 0.91 | +LR NA | -LR NA

## Other Hip Tests

**Piriformis Test[26]** The patient lies on the unaffected side with the affected leg in 60 degrees of hip flexion and the knee relaxed. The pelvis is stabilized and pressure is applied downward on the knee, rotating the hip internally. Tightness or pain is indicative of piriformis tightness (Figure 21–30). Sn. 0.88 | Sp. 0.83 | +LR 5.2 | -LR 0.14

**Ely's Test[47]** While the patient lies in a prone position, the pelvis is stabilized and the knee on the affected side is flexed. If the hip on that side flexes the knee is flexed,

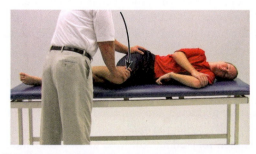

FIGURE 21–30   Piriformis tightness test.
© William E. Prentice

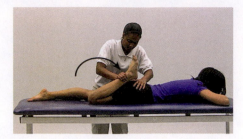

FIGURE 21–31   Ely's test for tightness of the rectus femoris
© William E. Prentice

there is tightness of the rectus femoris (Figure 21–31).
Sn. 0.59 | Sp. 0.85 | +LR NA | -LR NA

## Femoral Anteversion and Retroversion

The patient with a painful hip problem may have a discrepancy in the relationship between the neck of the femur and the shaft of the femur. The normal angle of the femoral neck is 8 to 15 degrees relative to the long axis of the shaft of the femur (Figure 21–32C). Individuals who walk in a pronounced toe-out manner may be displaying a condition in which the femoral neck is less than 8 degrees posterior to the long axis of the femur (femoral retroversion) (Figure 21–32A and B). In contrast, individuals who walk in a toe-in manner may be reflecting a hip deformity in which the femoral neck is greater than 15 degrees anterior to the normal long axis of the femur (femoral anteversion) (Figure 21–32D and E).

Toeing in or out can also be caused by tibial torsion (see Chapter 20). Femoral anteversion or retroversion is almost always symmetrical, and tibial torsion is usually symmetrical.

**Craig's Test** The patient is prone with the knee of the affected leg at 90 degrees of flexion. The clinician locates the posterior aspect of the greater trochanter then passively rotates the hip laterally and medially until the greater trochanter is at its most lateral position. Using a goniometer, if the angle between the vertical axis from the treatment table and the longitudinal axis of the lower leg is greater than 15 degrees, the test is positive for femoral anteversion, and if the angle is less than 8 degrees, it is positive for femoral retroversion (Figure 21–33).[66]

## Measuring Leg-Length Discrepancy

In individuals who are not physically active, leg-length discrepancies of more than 1 inch may produce symptoms; however, shortening of as little as ⅛ inch (3 mm) may cause symptoms in highly active athletes. Such discrepancies can cause cumulative stresses to the lower limbs, hip, and pelvis or the low back.[13]

There are three types of leg-length discrepancy: (1) true, or anatomical, shortening; (2) apparent shortening; and (3) functional shortening. X-ray examination is the most valid means of measurement. It is difficult to be

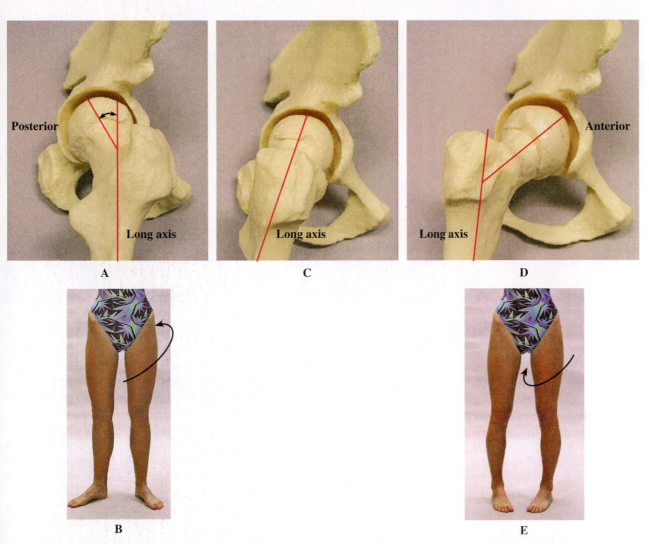

FIGURE 21–32    (A) Femoral retroversion: The femoral neck is posterior to the long axis of the femur and (B) the feet toe out. (C) Normal femoral neck and long axis alignment. (D) Femoral anteversion: The femoral neck is anterior to the long axis of the femur and (E) the feet toe in.

© William E. Prentice

completely accurate with clinical evaluation of leg length because of mobility of the soft tissue over bony landmarks (Figure 21–34A).[56]

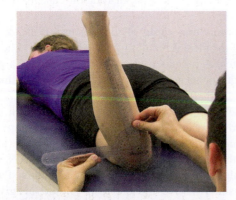

FIGURE 21–33    Craig's test for measuring femoral anteversion and retroversion.

© William E. Prentice

**Anatomical Discrepancy**

In an anatomical discrepancy, shortening may be equal throughout the lower limb or localized within the femur or lower leg. The patient lies supine and fully extended on the table. Measurement is taken between the medial malleoli and the anterior superior iliac spine of each leg (Figure 21–34B).

**Apparent Discrepancy**

In an apparent discrepancy, leg shortening can occur as a result of lateral pelvic tilt (obliquely) or from a flexion or adduction deformity.

**21–4 Clinical Application Exercise**

During a gait evaluation, an athletic trainer notices that the patient walks with a swinging hip—one side of the pelvis drops to the side during single-leg stance.

? What could be a cause of this movement?

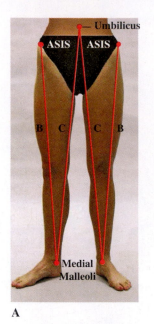

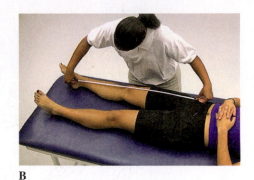

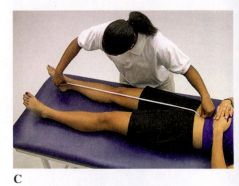

FIGURE 21–34 **(A)** Measuring for leg-length discrepancy. **(B)** Anatomical discrepancy. **(C)** Functional discrepancy.
© William E. Prentice

**Functional Discrepancy** In a functional discrepancy, there is a deformity (such as a valgus knee) that, unlike an apparent discrepancy, cannot be treated or "fixed." Measurement of a functional deformity is taken from the umbilicus to the medial malleoli of each ankle (Figure 21–34C).[46]

## Clinical Prediction Rules

The following clinical prediction rules are currently used for the hip joint:

- *Hip osteoarthritis*[68]–identifies patients likely to be presenting with hip osteoarthritis.
- *Hip mobilization for knee osteoarthritis*[21]–identifies patients presenting with knee osteoarthritis who will respond favorably to hip mobilization.

# RECOGNITION AND MANAGEMENT OF SPECIFIC HIP, GROIN, AND PELVIC INJURIES

## Hip Joint

### Adductor/Hip Flexor Strain (Groin Strain)

*Etiology*   The groin is the region that lies on the medial and anterior aspect of the upper thigh. The musculature of this area includes the iliopsoas, the rectus femoris, and the adductor group (the gracilis, pectineus, adductor brevis, adductor longus, and adductor magnus). Groin pain is one of the more difficult problems to diagnose, especially if it is chronic.[49]

> Leg-length discrepancy in an athlete can lead to stress-related physical injuries.

Any one of the muscles in the region of the groin can be injured during activity and elicit what is commonly

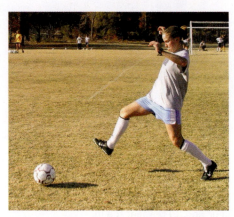

FIGURE 21–35   Many sports that require stretch of the hip region can cause an adductor/hip flexor strain.
© William E. Prentice

considered a "groin strain" (Figure 21–35). The adductor longus muscle is most often strained.[49] Running, jumping, or twisting with external rotation can produce such injuries.

*Symptoms and signs*   The adductor/hip flexor strain is one of the most difficult injuries to care for.[16] The strain can be felt as a sudden twinge or sensation of a pop or tearing during an active movement, or the patient may not notice it until after the termination of activity.[17] Like most tears, the adductor/hip flexor strain produces pain, weakness, and internal hemorrhage.

*Management*   If it is detected immediately after it occurs, the strain should be treated by POLICE, NSAIDs, and analgesics as needed for 48 to 72 hours. Passive, active, and resistive muscle tests should be given to ascertain the exact muscle or muscles that are involved.

The athletic trainer frequently encounters difficulty when attempting to care for an adductor/hip flexor

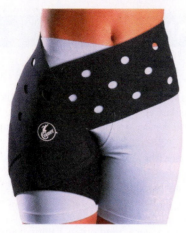

FIGURE 21–36  Groin and thigh braces can help provide support for hip adductor/flexor strains.

Courtesy Cramer

strain. Rest has been the best treatment. Daily whirlpool therapy, cryotherapy, or ultrasound have been used. Exercise should be delayed until the groin is pain free. Exercise rehabilitation should emphasize gradual stretching and restoration of the normal range of motion. Strength progressions should include open chain or closed chain exercises. These progressive multiplanar strength training exercises begin in the sagittal plane and progress to frontal and transverse planes as strength and symptoms allow. Until normal flexibility and strength are developed, a protective spica bandage or a commercial brace should be applied (Figure 21–36).[32]

## Trochanteric Bursitis

*Etiology*  Trochanteric bursitis is a relatively common condition of the greater trochanter of the femur. Although commonly called bursitis, the condition also can be an inflammation at the site where the gluteus medius muscle inserts or the iliotibial band passes over the trochanter.[41]

*Symptoms and signs*  The patient complains of pain in the lateral hip. Pain may radiate down to the knee, causing a limp. Palpation reveals tenderness over the lateral aspect of the greater trochanter. The athletic trainer should perform tests for tensor fasciae latae and iliotibial tightness.

*Management*  Therapy initially includes POLICE, NSAIDs, and analgesics as needed. ROM exercises and PRE directed toward hip abductors and external rotators should follow. Soft tissue mobilization of the tensor fascia latae, the gluteus maximus, and the IT Band using a foam roller, manual or instrument-assisted soft tissue mobilization may be done to ensure proper tissue length. Phonophoresis may be added if the patient does not respond in three to 4 days. The patient's return to running should be cautious; the patient should avoid running on inclined or uneven surfaces. Faulty running form, leg-length

An increased Q angle or a leg-length discrepancy can lead to trochanteric bursitis in women runners.

discrepancy, and faulty foot biomechanics must be taken into consideration. The condition is most common among women runners who have an increased Q angle or a leg-length discrepancy.

### Sprains of the Hip Joint

*Etiology*  The hip joint, the strongest and best-protected joint in the human body, is seldom seriously injured during sports activities.[10] The hip joint is substantially supported by the ligamentous tissues and muscles that surround it, so any unusual movement that exceeds the normal range of motion may result in tearing of tissue. Such an injury may occur as a result of a violent twist, produced by an impact force delivered by another participant, forceful contact with another object, or a situation in which the foot is firmly planted and the trunk is forced in an opposing direction.[1]

*Symptoms and signs*  A hip sprain displays all the signs of an acute injury but is best revealed through the patient's inability to circumduct the thigh. There is significant pain in the hip region. Hip rotation increases pain.

*Management*  X-rays or an MRI should be done to rule out fracture; POLICE, NSAIDs, and analgesics should be given as needed. Depending on the grade of sprain, weight bearing should be restricted. Crutch walking is used for grade 2 and 3 sprains. ROM exercises and PRE should be delayed until acute inflammation has subsided and a pain-free arc of motion can be achieved.

21–5 Clinical Application Exercise

A construction worker jumps down off a ladder. Landing off balance, he violently twists his right hip.

**?** From the information provided, what type of injury could he have sustained?

### Dislocated Hip Joint

*Etiology*  Dislocation of the hip joint rarely occurs in sports and then usually only as a result of traumatic force directed along the long axis of the femur.[51] Such dislocations are produced when the knee is flexed. The most common displacement is one posterior to the acetabulum, with the femoral shaft adducted and flexes.

*Symptoms and signs*  The injury presents a picture of a flexed, adducted, and internally rotated thigh (Figure 21–37). Palpation will reveal that the head of the femur has

21–6 Clinical Application Exercise

A sedentary office assistant has been determined to have a Q angle of 22 degrees. Her left leg is ¾ inch shorter than her right leg. She complains of pain at the point just over the left greater trochanter when she walks.

**?** Based on the information provided, what might the condition be?

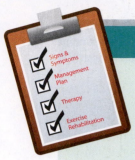

## Acute Groin Strain

**Injury Situation** A ballet dancer had a history of tightness in her groin. During a performance, she suddenly rotated her trunk while stretching to the right side. The dancer experienced a sudden, sharp pain and a sense of "giving way" in the left side of the groin that caused her to stop immediately and limp offstage.

**Symptoms and Signs** As the dancer described it to the athletic trainer, there was severe pain when rotating her trunk to the right and flexing her left hip. Inspection revealed the following:

1. There was major point tenderness in the groin, especially in the region of the adductor magnus muscle.
2. There was no pain during passive movement of the hip, but severe pain did occur during both active and resistive motion.
3. When muscle was tested for injury, the illiopsoas and rectus femoris muscles were ruled out as having been injured; however, when the dancer adducted the hip from a stretch position, it caused her extreme discomfort.

**Management Plan** Based on the athletic trainer's inspection, with findings confirmed by the physician, it was determined that the dancer had sustained a grade 2 strain of the groin, particularly to the adductor magnus muscle.

---

*Phase* 1 *Acute Injury*   GOALS: To stop hemorrhage, reduce pain, and stop muscle spasms.
ESTIMATED LENGTH OF TIME (ELT): 2 to 3 days.

- **Therapy** Careful physical examination plus MRI to rule out conditions other than a strain. IMMEDIATE CARE: POLICE (20 min) intermittently, 6 to 8 times daily. When weight bearing, the dancer should wear a 6-inch elastic hip spica.
- **Exercise rehabilitation** No exercise–as much complete rest as possible.

---

*Phase* 2 *Repair*   GOALS: To reduce pain, control spasm, and restore full ability to contract and stretch the adductor longus muscle. To maintain cardiorespiratory fitness.
ELT: 2 to 3 weeks.

- **Therapy** Ice massage (1 min) 3 or 4 times daily followed by hip ROM movements. Muscle electrical stimulation using the surge current at 7 or 8, depending on patient's tolerance, together with ultrasound, set at 1 W/cm² (7 min), once daily. Cold therapy in the form of ice massage (7 min) or ice packs (10-15 min) followed by exercise, 2 or 3 times daily.
- **Exercise rehabilitation** Proprioceptive neuromuscular facilitation hip patterns 2 or 3 times daily after cold application, progressing to PRE using pulley, isokinetic, or free weights (10 repetitions, 3 sets) once daily. Jogging in chest-level water (10 to 20 min) 1 or 2 times daily for first exercise rehabilitation week followed by flutter kick swimming (pain free) once daily during subsequent weeks. General body maintenance exercises 3 times a week as long as they do not aggravate the injury.

---

*Phase* 3 *Remodeling*   GOALS: To restore full power, endurance, and muscle extensibility. The patient gradually returns to practice and finally performs, wearing a groin restraint.
ELT: 3 to 6 weeks.

- **Therapy** If symptom free, precede exercise with ice massage (7 min) or ice pack (5-15 min).
- **Exercise rehabilitation** Progressively increase practice time and concentrate on active, pain-free range stretching and strengthening.

*Criteria for Return to Dancing*

1. As measured by an isokinetic dynamometer, the dancer's injured hip should have strength equal to that of the uninjured hip.
2. The hip has full range of motion.
3. The dancer is able to run figure eights at full speed around obstacles set 5 feet apart.

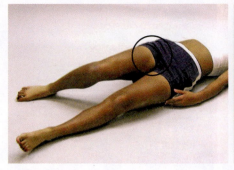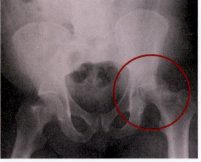

**A**                                              **B**

FIGURE 21–37   Dislocated hip. **(A)** Typical position for a hip dislocation: slightly flexed, adducted, and internally rotated. **(B)** X-ray of a hip dislocation.

(a) © William E. Prentice; (b) Courtesy of Jordan B. Renner, MD, Departments of Radiology and Allied Health Sciences, University of North Carolina

moved to a position posterior to the acetabulum. A hip dislocation causes serious pathology by tearing capsular and ligamentous tissue. A fracture is often associated with this injury, accompanied by possible damage to the sciatic nerve and disruption of the blood supply to the femoral head.

***Management***   A dislocation requires immediate medical attention. Muscle contractures may complicate the reduction. Immobilization usually consists of 2 weeks of bed rest and the use of a crutch for walking for a month or longer. After the crutches are discontinued, rehabilitation should include progressive ROM in a pain-free arc, open chain exercises progressing to closed chain exercises, followed by running, cutting, and the return to sport.

***Complications***   Complication of the posterior hip dislocation is likely, with such possibilities as a palsy of the sciatic nerve and later the development of osteoarthritis. Hip dislocation also can lead to disruption of the blood supply to the head of the femur, which eventually leads to the degenerative condition known as avascular necrosis.[51]

### Avascular Necrosis

***Etiology***   Avascular necrosis results from the temporary or permanent loss of the blood supply to the proximal femur.[18] Without blood, the bone tissue dies and causes degeneration and deformity of the joint surface. Avascular necrosis has several causes. Loss of blood supply to the bone can be caused by an injury such as a hip dislocation (trauma-related avascular necrosis) in which the blood vessels are damaged, thus interfering with the blood circulation to the bone. In a hip dislocation, the lateral circumflex artery, which supplies most of the blood to the femoral head, can be compromised. If this condition is not rectified quickly, the chances of developing avascular necrosis are markedly increased. Certain other risk factors, such as the use of some medications (e.g., steroids), blood coagulation disorders, or excessive alcohol use, create increased pressure within the bone, causing the blood vessels to narrow and making it hard for the vessels to deliver enough blood to the bone cells.

***Symptoms and signs***   In the early stages of avascular necrosis, the patient may not have any symptoms. As the disease progresses, however, most individuals experience joint pain—at first, only when weight bearing on the affected joint, and then even when resting. Pain usually develops gradually and may be mild or severe. If avascular necrosis progresses and the bone and surrounding joint surface collapse, pain may develop or increase dramatically. Pain may be severe enough to limit the patient's range of motion in the affected joint. Osteoarthritis may develop. The period of time between the first symptoms and loss of joint function is different for each individual, ranging from several months to more than a year.

***Management***   In cases of suspected avascular necrosis, the patient should be referred to a physician for an MRI, an X-ray, or a CT scan. The goals in treating avascular necrosis are to improve the patient's use of the affected joint, stop further damage to the bone, and ensure bone and joint survival. Several conservative treatments are available that can help prevent further bone and joint damage and reduce pain. Range of motion exercises may be used to maintain or improve joint range of motion. Electrical bone stimulation has been recommended to induce bone growth. If avascular necrosis is diagnosed early, the physician may begin treatment by having the patient be non–weight bearing. When combined with medication to reduce pain, non–weight bearing can be an effective way to avoid or delay surgery. The use of medications to reduce fatty substances (lipids) that increase with corticosteroid treatment or to reduce blood clotting in the presence of clotting disorders is also recommended. Most patients will eventually require surgery to repair the joint permanently.[18]

### Hip Labral Tear

***Etiology***   The socket of the hip joint (acetabulum) is lined by articular cartilage called the labrum (Figure 21–38). This cartilage provides stability and cushioning for the hip joint, permitting the head of the femur to move smoothly and painlessly in the acetabulum. A hip

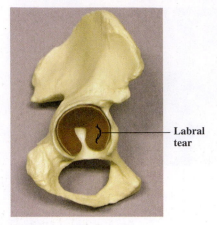

FIGURE 21–38   Hip labral tear.
© William E. Prentice

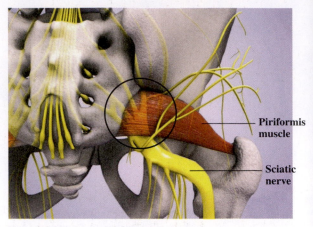

FIGURE 21–39   In piriformis syndrome, the sciatic nerve is irritated as it courses either under or through the piriformis muscle, causing pain in the buttocks that perhaps radiates down the back of the thigh.

labral tear most often results from deep hip flexion such as squats below 90 degrees that increase hip joint stresses, or from repetitive movements, such as running or pivoting of the hip, that cause degeneration and breakdown of the labrum. It may also be caused by an acute injury, such as a dislocation.

***Symptoms and signs***   Most commonly, a hip labral tear is asymptomatic. Occasionally, however, a hip labral tear causes a catching, locking, or clicking sensation in the hip joint; pain in the hip or groin; and a feeling of stiffness or limited motion.

***Management***   Treatment for a hip labral tear may consist of exercises to maximize hip range of motion, hip strengthening and stability exercises, and avoidance of movements that place stress on the hip joint. Pain medications may also help and a physician may choose to inject a corticosteroid. If pain persists more than 4 weeks, surgery may be indicated, either to remove a piece of the torn labrum or to repair the tear using sutures.

### Sciaticia/Piriformis Syndrome

***Etiology***   The sciatic nerve is a continuation of the sacral plexus as it passes through the greater sciatic notch and descends deeply through the back of the thigh. Hip and buttock pain is often diagnosed as sciatic nerve irritation. *Sciatica* is a term used to describe any pain produced by irritation of the sciatic nerve, but there are many potential causes of this irritation. The sciatic nerve can be irritated by a disk problem in the low back, direct trauma, or trauma from surrounding structures such as the piriformis muscle, in which case sciatic nerve irritation is also called piriformis syndrome (Figure 21–39).[23] It has been proposed that piriformis syndrome results from overstretching of the muscle due to femoral adduction and internal rotation during gait.[71] Piriformis syndrome is seen more in women than men, and the cause of this condition is typically attributed to a tight piriformis muscle as the nerve passes underneath the muscle or to an anatomical variation in which the sciatic nerve passes through the piriformis muscle. In approximately 15 percent of the population, the sciatic nerve passes through the piriformis muscle, separating it in two.[71]

***Symptoms and Signs***   To differentiate low back problems (disk disease) from piriformis syndrome as the cause of sciatica, determine whether the patient has low back pain with radiation into the extremity. Back pain is most likely midline, exacerbated by trunk flexion and relieved by rest. Coughing and straining may also increase back pain and possibly the radiation. Muscle weakness and sensory numbness may also be found in a patient with disk disease.[37]

In the case of piriformis syndrome, the patient might report a deep pain in the buttock, without low back pain, and possibly radiating pain in the back of the thigh, lateral calf, and foot, also indicating sciatica. Palpation in the sciatic notch also produces pain. It is possible that pain is associated with an active myofascial trigger point in the piriformis.[23]

***Management***   Severe sciatica caused by piriformis syndrome can keep the patient out of competition for 2 to 3 weeks or longer. If the sciatic nerve is irritated and the patient complains of radiating pain in the buttocks or down the back of the leg, the first 3 to 5 days should consist of rest and modalities to decrease the pain associated with sciatica.[37]

After the acute pain has been controlled, stretching exercises can be used to treat piriformis syndrome. The hip is internally rotated while the patient sits on a plyoball positioned over the lesser sciatic notch (Figure 21–44K). Piriformis strengthening should focus on weak hip abductors and external rotators to improve pain, strength, and kinematics using a step-down task. In cases where piriformis syndrome becomes chronic, injection with a corticosteroid may provide temporary relief.[23]

## Hip Joint Problems in the Young Athlete

The athletic trainer working with a child or an adolescent should understand three major problems. They are

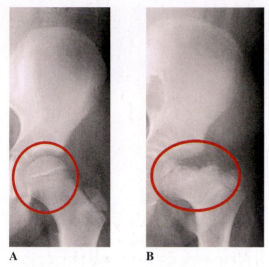

A                B

FIGURE 21–40  Legg-Calvé-Perthes disease.
**(A)** Normal femoral head X-ray. **(B)** Femoral head with avascular necrosis.
Courtesy Jordan B. Renner, MD, Departments of Radiology and Allied Health Sciences, University of North Carolina

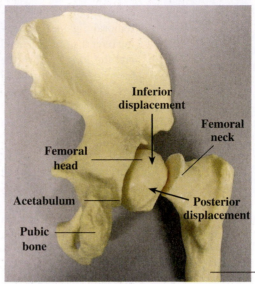

**Anterior View**

FIGURE 21–41  Slipped capital femoral epiphysis (anterior view).
© William E. Prentice

Legg-Calvé-Perthes disease, a slipped capital femoral epiphysis, and a snapping hip.

## Legg-Calvé-Perthes Disease

*Etiology*  Legg-Calvé-Perthes disease is avascular necrosis of the femoral head (Figure 21–40). It occurs in children ages four to ten and in boys more often than in girls. For the most part, this condition is not clearly understood. Trauma accounts for 25 percent of the cases seen.[76] It is listed under the broad heading of osteochondrosis. Because of a disruption of circulation at the head of the femur, articular cartilage becomes necrotic and flattens.[40]

*Symptoms and signs*  The young patient commonly complains of pain in the groin, which sometimes is referred to the abdomen or knee.[35] Limping is also typical. The condition can have a rapid onset, but more often it comes on slowly over a number of months. Examination may show limited hip movement and pain.

> A young individual complaining of pain in the groin, abdomen, or knee and walking with a limp may display signs of Legg-Calvé-Perthes disease or a slipped capital femoral epiphysis.

*Management*  Care of this condition could mean complete bed rest to alleviate synovitis.[76] The athlete may have to wear a special brace to avoid direct weight bearing on the hip. If treated in time, the head of the femur will revascularize and reossify.

*Complications*  If the condition is not treated early enough, the head of the femur will become deformed, creating problems of osteoarthritis in later life.[74]

## Slipped Capital Femoral Epiphysis

*Etiology*  The problem of a slipped capital femoral epiphysis (Figure 21–41) is found mostly in boys between the ages of ten and seventeen who are characteristically tall and thin or obese.[45] Although idiopathic, it may be related to the effects of a growth hormone. One-quarter of the cases seen have the condition in both hips. Trauma accounts for 25 percent of cases.[8] X-ray examination may show femoral head slippage posteriorly and inferiorly.

*Symptoms and signs*  Like Legg-Calvé-Perthes disease, a slipped capital femoral epiphysis causes groin pain that comes on suddenly as a result of trauma or over weeks or months as a result of prolonged stress. In the early stages of this condition, signs may be minimal.[31] In its most advanced stage, however, there is hip and knee pain during passive and active motion; limitations of abduction, flexion, and medial rotation; and a limp.[45]

*Management*  In minor slippage, rest and non–weight bearing may prevent further slipping. Major displacement usually requires corrective surgery.

*Complications*  If the slippage goes undetected or if surgery fails to restore normal hip mechanics, severe hip problems may occur in later life.[74]

## Snapping Hip

*Etiology*  Excessive repetitive movement has been linked to a snapping hip in dancers, gymasts, hurdlers, and sprinters—a muscle imbalance develops. A snapping hip can have several causes. The most common causes of the "snapping," when muscle is involved, are the iliotibial band moving over the greater trochanter, resulting in trochanteric bursitis, and the iliopsoas tendon moving over the iliopectineal eminence.[25] Other extraarticular causes of

A 15-year-old football player complains of pain in his hip off and on during the season. There is increasing hip and knee pain during movement. The athlete has a restriction of hip abduction, flexion, and medial rotation. He is beginning to walk with a limp.

**?** What should the athletic trainer be concerned about in this 15-year-old, and what steps should be taken?

the snapping are the iliofemoral ligaments moving over the femoral head and the long head of the biceps femoris moving over the ischial tuberosity. Extraarticular causes commonly occur when the hip is externally rotated and flexed. Other causes are anatomical structures that can predispose an individual to a snapping hip, including a narrow pelvis, abnormal increases in abduction range of motion, and lack of range of motion into external rotation or tight internal rotators. Intraarticular causes are loose bodies, acetabulum labral tears, and subluxation of the hip joint itself.[30]

***Symptoms and signs*** Due to the extraarticular causes, the hip joint capsule, ligaments, and muscles become loose and allow the hip to become unstable. The patient will complain of a snapping, possibly accompanied by severe pain and disability with each snap.

***Management*** The key to treating and rehabilitating the snapping hip is to decrease pain and inflammation with ice, antiinflammatory medication, and other modalities, such as ultrasound.[36] This could significantly decrease the pain initially, so that the patient can begin a stretching and strengthening program.

## Pelvic Conditions

Individuals who perform activities that involve jumping, running, and violent collisions can sustain serious acute and overuse injuries to the pelvic region.[7] In running the pelvis rotates along a longitudinal axis proportionate to the amount of arm swing. It also tilts up and down as the leg engages in support and nonsupport. This combination of motion causes shearing at the sacroiliac joint and symphysis pubis. Tilting of the pelvis also produces both a decrease and an increase in lumbar lordosis, depending on the slant of the running surface. Running downhill increases lumbar lordosis, and running uphill decreases it.[14]

### Contusion (Hip Pointer)

***Etiology*** Iliac crest contusion and contusion of the abdominal musculature, commonly known as a hip pointer, occurs most often in contact sports (Figure 21–42). The hip pointer results from a blow to an inadequately protected iliac crest. The hip pointer is considered one of the most disabling injuries and one that is difficult to manage. A direct force to the unprotected iliac crest causes severe pinching action to the soft tissue of that region.

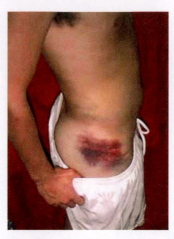

**FIGURE 21–42** A blow to the iliac crest can cause a bruise and hematoma known as a hip pointer.
Courtesy Scott Barker

***Symptoms and signs*** A hip pointer produces immediate pain, spasms, and transitory paralysis of the soft structures. As a result, the patient is unable to rotate the trunk or to flex the thigh without pain.

***Management*** POLICE should be applied immediately after injury and should be maintained intermittently for at least 48 hours. In severe cases, bed rest for 1 to 2 days will speed recovery. The mechanisms for the hip pointer are the same as those for an iliac crest fracture or epiphyseal separation.

A young patient complains to the athletic trainer that her hip snaps when she stands on one leg.

**?** What is the possible cause of this snapping hip?

The patient must be referred to a physician and an X-ray examination performed. A variety of treatment procedures can be used for this injury. Ice massage and ultrasound have been found to be beneficial. Initially, the injury may be injected with a steroid. Later, oral antiinflammatory agents may be used. Recovery time usually ranges from 1 to 3 weeks.

### Osteitis Pubis

***Etiology*** Because the popularity of distance running has increased, a condition known as osteitis pubis has become more prevalent. It is also seen in soccer, football, and wrestling. Restricted motion at the sacroiliac joint or hips has been shown to increase motion at the pubic symphysis. Repetitive stress on the symphysis pubis and adjacent bony structures, caused by the pull of muscles in the area, creates a chronic inflammatory condition.

***Symptoms and signs*** The patient has pain in the groin region and in the area of the symphysis pubis. There is point tenderness on the pubic tubercle, and the patient experiences pain while running, doing sit-ups, and doing squats. Acute osteitis pubis may occur as a result of pressure from a bicycle seat.

*Management*  Treatment should focus on mobility of the joints above and below the pubic symphysis. Follow-up care usually consists of rest, an oral antiinflammatory agent, and a gradual return to activity.

## Athletic Pubalgia

*Etiology*  The term *pubalgia* is a catchall term that generally refers to chronic pubic region or inguinal pain. It may be caused by repetitive stress to the symphysis pubis from kicking and twisting or cutting at high speeds, such as occurs in soccer and ice hockey.[61] Forceful hip adduction from a hyperextended position creates shear forces that are transmitted through the symphysis pubis to the common insertion of the rectus abdominus, the hip adductors, and the conjoined tendon at the pubic tubercle. These forces may result in microtears of the transversalis abdominis fascia or the aponeurosis of the internal and external obliques or in a defect or weakness at the conjoint tendon. These factors collectively can create a weakness in the anterior wall of the inguinal canal, although there is no direct or indirect hernia present.[58]

*Symptoms and signs*  Chronic pain, often occurring only during exertion, may persist for several months. Sharp, burning pain localizes to the lower abdominal and inguinal region initially and later radiates to the adductors and testicles. There is point tenderness at the pubic tubercle. Pain is increased with resisted hip flexion, internal rotation, and abdominal muscle contraction. Pain also occurs with resisted hip adduction, although the adductors are not tender, which differentiates this condition from an adductor strain.[20]

*Management*  Conservative treatment is rarely effective and pain often returns with activity. Nevertheless, conservative treatment should be attempted, beginning initially with deep-tissue massage of the affected structures. After a week, stretching of the hip flexors, adductors and rotators,

> A soccer player complains of a sharp, burning pain in his groin and his testicles whenever he kicks the ball. He has palpable tenderness over his pubic tubercle and indicates there is also pain on resisted adduction. The athlete is concerned that he has a hernia.
>
> **?** What might the athletic trainer suspect is wrong with this athlete?

> A football player who was not wearing hip pads receives a hard, compressive hit to his left iliac crest region.
>
> **?** What injury has this patient sustained? What are the expected symptoms and signs?

hamstrings, and low back muscles can be incorporated. At 2 weeks, strengthening of the abdominals and hip adductors and flexors should begin. At three to 4 weeks, running can begin, followed as tolerated by jumping and kicking. If conservative treatment is not effective, cortisone injection may be used cautiously. Surgical intervention to tighten the pelvic floor may be necessary if more conservative measures fail.[23]

## Pelvic Floor Dysfunction

*Etiology*  *Pelvic floor dysfunction* is a term applied to a wide variety of clinical conditions that are common for the female in all patient populations at all ages. Pelvic floor dysfunction most often occurs in athletes engaging in sports involving high impact activities such as gymnastics, track and field, or sports that involve jumping.[11]

*Symptoms and Signs*  In the female athlete, pelvic floor dysfunction is most likely to result in urinary incontinence, prolapse of the pelvic organs, or complaints of chronic pelvic pain.[11] Although urinary incontinence and prolapse of the pelvic organs has been associated with weakness and neuromuscular inefficiency of the pelvic floor muscles primarily in females, chronic pelvic pain has been attributed to the existence of active myofascial trigger points located in the pelvic floor muscles or the hip muscles in both female and male athletes.[3]

*Management*  A stiff, strong pelvic floor may be crucial in counteracting the increases in abdominal pressure that occur during high-impact activities. Strength training of the pelvic floor muscles has been shown to be effective in treating stress urinary incontinence in females in the general population.[11] Electrical stimulation has also been recommended to help retrain the pelvic floor muscles to contract. Myofascial trigger point release and relaxation training has been recommended for treating chronic pelvic pain.[3]

## Stress Fractures

*Etiology*  Stress fractures in the pelvic area are seen mostly in distance runners. Repetitive cyclical forces created by ground reaction forces can produce stress fractures in the pelvis and the proximal femur. They constitute approximately 16 percent of all stress fractures and are more common in women than in men. The most common sites are the inferior pubic ramus and the femoral neck and subtrochanteric area of the femur.

*Symptoms and signs*  Commonly, the patient complains of groin pain along with an aching sensation in the thigh that increases with activity and decreases with rest. Standing on one leg may be impossible for the patient. Deep palpation will cause severe point tenderness. Pelvic stress fracture has a tendency to occur during intensive interval training or competitive racing. For the ischium and the pubis, crutch walking is recommended.[8]

*Management*  Rest is usually the treatment of choice for 2 to 5 months. Normally, a bone scan will pick up

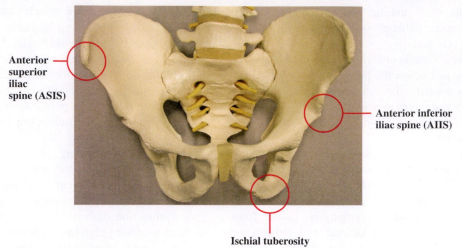

**Anterior superior iliac spine (ASIS)**

**Anterior inferior iliac spine (AIIS)**

**Ischial tuberosity**

FIGURE 21–43   Potential avulsion fractures to the pelvic apophyses.
© William E. Prentice

osteoclastic activity early.[8] Swimming can be performed for aerobic exercise. The breast stroke must be avoided.

### Avulsion Fractures and Apophysitis

*Etiology*   An apophysis, or traction epiphysis, is a bony outgrowth and is contrasted to pressure epiphyses, which are the growth plates for long bones. The pelvis has a number of apophyses where major muscles make their attachments. The three most common sites for avulsion fractures and apophysitis in the pelvic region are the ischial tuberosity and the hamstring attachment, the anterior inferior iliac spine and the rectus femoris muscle attachment, and the anterior superior iliac spine where the sartorius muscle makes its attachment (Figure 21–43). In some sports, such as football, soccer, and basketball, sudden acceleration or deceleration can cause a convulsion, a fracture, or an apophysitis.[12]

*Symptoms and signs*   The patient complains of a sudden, localized pain with limited movement. There is swelling and point tenderness. Muscle testing increases pain.

*Management*   X-ray examination is routinely given with apophyseal pain. Uncomplicated conditions can be treated with POLICE and crutches, with toe-touch weight bearing for 1 to 2 months. After the control of pain and inflammation (2 to 3 weeks), a gradual stretch program should begin. When 80 degrees of range of motion have been returned, a PRE program should be instituted.[2] When

full range of motion and strength have been regained, the athlete can return to competition.

## THIGH AND HIP REHABILITATION TECHNIQUES

### General Body Conditioning

As with other sports injuries, the athlete must maintain cardiorespiratory endurance, muscular endurance, and strength of the total body. If weight bearing is painful or if the patient is not capable of performing functional activities while fully weight bearing, fitness can be maintained by engaging in aquatic exercise, riding a stationary bike, or using an upper body ergometer.[39]

### Flexibility

In the rehabilitation of injuries in the hip and thigh region, regaining pain-free range of motion is a primary concern.[27] Muscle injuries, particularly of the quadriceps, hamstrings, and groin muscles, can significantly restrict motion, thus limiting function. Likewise, injuries to the strong ligamentous and capsular structures of the hip can limit motion. Stretching exercises usually progress from gentle passive stretching to static stretching to proprioceptive neuromuscular facilitation stretching, all within pain-free limits.[67] A complete rehabilitation program must include stretching exercises for those muscles that produce internal and external rotation, adduction, abduction, extension, flexion, and circumduction (Figure 21–44).

### Mobilization

If limitations in motion are caused by injury and subsequent tightness in the ligaments and capsule surrounding the hip, joint mobilization techniques should be incorporated to regain normal arthrokinematic movements at

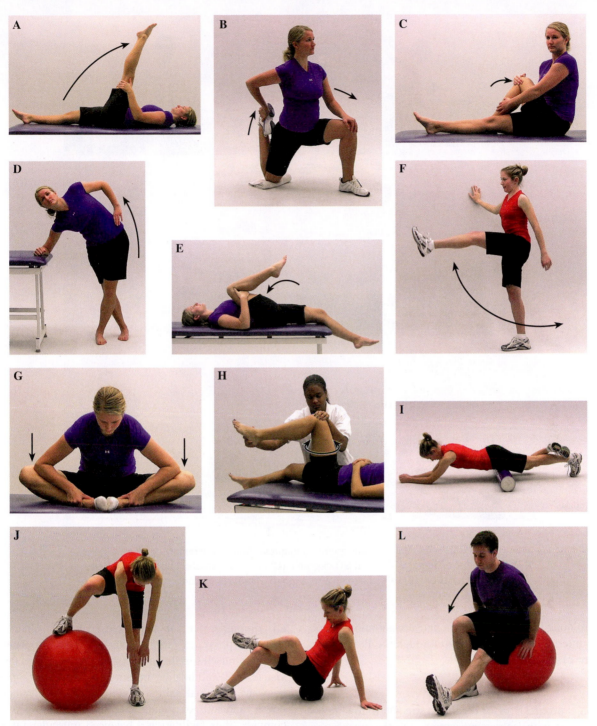

FIGURE 21–44   Stretching exercises for the thigh and hip. **(A)** Supine static hamstring stretch. **(B)** Kneeling quadriceps and hip flexor stretch. **(C)** Sitting piriformis stretch. **(D)** Standing hip abductor stretch. **(E)** Supine gluteal stretch. **(F)** Dynamic forward hip swing gluteal stretch. **(G)** Sitting abductor stretch. **(H)** Supine hip internal and external torator stretch. **(I)** Quadriceps myofascial stretch. **(J)** Standing adductor stretch on stability ball. **(K)** Piriformis myofascial stretch on plyoball. **(L)** Hamstring stretch on stability ball.
© William E. Prentice

the hip.[57] The basic joint mobilization techniques may include, but are not limited to, the following techniques. Inferior femoral glides at 90 degrees of hip flexion are used to increase abduction and flexion. With the patient supine, a posterior femoral glide can be done by stabilizing underneath the pelvis and using the body weight applied through the femur to glide posteriorly. Posterior glides are used to increase hip flexion. Anterior femoral glides increase extension and are accomplished by using some support to stabilize under the pelvis and applying an anterior glide posteriorly on the femur. Medial femoral rotations may be used for increasing medial rotation

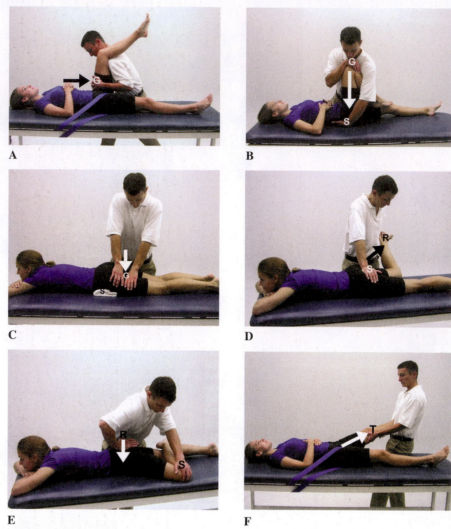

FIGURE 21–45    Joint mobilization techniques. **(A)** Inferior femoral glides. **(B)** Posterior femoral glides at 90 degrees. **(C)** Anterior femoral glides. **(D)** Medial femoral rotation. **(E)** Lateral femoral rotation. **(F)** Femoral traction.

© William E. Prentice

and are done by stabilizing the opposite innominate bone while internally rotating the hip through the flexed knee (Figure 21–45).[57]

## Strength

A typical progression for regaining strength following injury begins with isometric exercise until the muscle can be fully contracted, followed by active isotonic contraction, then isotonic progressive-resistive exercise, and finally isokinetic exercise. Proprioceptive neuromuscular facilitation strengthening techniques that use both knee and hip patterns are also effective functional strengthening techniques. Active exercises done within a pain-free range of motion should begin as soon as safely possible after injury, without exacerbating the condition. Figure 21–46 shows examples of various strengthening exercises for the muscles of the hip and thigh.

It is becoming more apparent that a dynamic core stabilization training program is an important component of all comprehensive functional closed kinetic chain rehabilitation programs (see Chapters 16 and 25). The core includes muscles in the lumbar spine, the hip, and the pelvis. A core stabilization training program is designed to help an individual gain strength, neuromuscular control, power, and muscular endurance in the lumbo-pelvic-hip complex, thus facilitating a balanced muscular functioning of the entire kinetic chain. Key hip muscles in the core include the psoas, gluteus medius, gluteus maximus, and hamstrings.[63] The goal of core stabilization should be to develop optimal levels of functional strength and dynamic stabilization. Figure 21–47 shows several core stabilization exercises that involve the key hip and pelvis muscles (also see Figures 4–11 and 16–2).

## Neuromuscular Control

Neuromuscular control is established by the appropriate combination of postural alignment and stability strength. If the neuromuscular system is not efficient, it will be

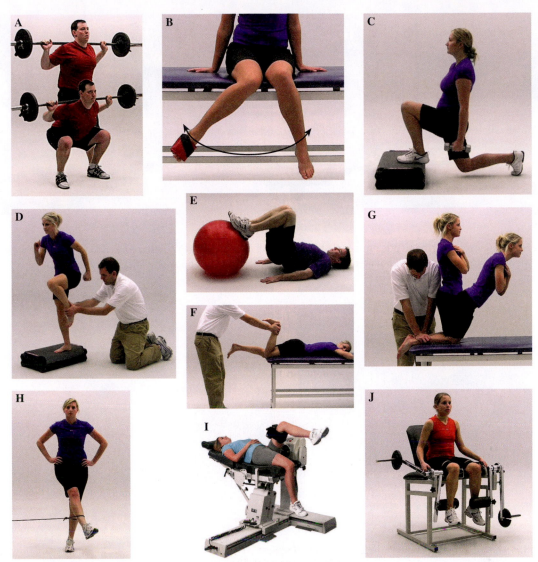

FIGURE 21–46   Examples of hip and thigh strengthening exercises. **(A)** Barbell squat. **(B)** Cuff weight-resisted hip internal and external rotation. **(C)** Weight-resisted lunge. **(D)** Standing hip flexor–resisted running pattern. **(E)** Hamstring curls on stability ball. **(F)** Manually resisted hamstring curls. **(G)** Hamstring forward leans. **(H)** Tubing-resisted hip adduction. **(I)** Isokinetic hip flexion and extension. **(J)** NK table hamstring curls and quadriceps extensions.

(a–h, j) © William E. Prentice; (i) Photo courtesy Biodex Medical Systems, Inc

A waitress who stands a lot in her job sustains a stress fracture to the right subtrochanter.

❓ As the stress fracture heals, what should be the neuromuscular control concerns?

unable to respond to the demands placed on it during functional activities. As the efficiency of the neuromuscular system decreases, the ability of the kinetic chain to maintain appropriate forces and dynamic stabilization decreases significantly. This decreased neuromuscular efficiency leads to compensation and substitution patterns as well as poor posture during

functional activities. In turn, this leads to increased mechanical stress on the contractile and noncontractile tissue, leading to repetitive microtrauma, abnormal biomechanics, and injury.

In maintaining or restoring neuromuscular control to the thigh or hip region, there should be a focus on balance and closed kinetic chain exercises. For balance, the patient can engage in weight bearing on just the affected leg, using both stable and unstable surfaces. Closed kinetic chain exercises include single-leg squats and wall slides (Figure 21–48).

Balance shoes have been used to activate the lumbo-pelvic-hip musculature, especially the gluteus medius and gluteus maximus (see Figure 18–42A). Balance shoes essentially use platform sandals with a dense rubber

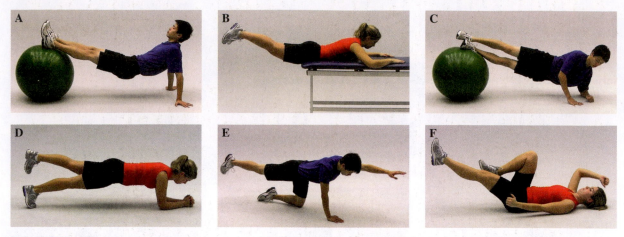

FIGURE 21–47   Core strengthening exercises. **(A)** Stability ball pike-ups. **(B)** Prone hip extensions. **(C)** Stability ball side-lying hip lift. **(D)** Human arrow with single-leg extension. **(E)** Alternating opposite arm-opposite leg lifts. **(F)** Dying bug.

© William E. Prentice

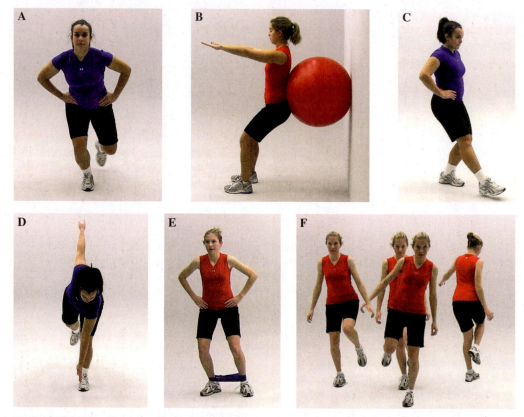

FIGURE 21–48   Exercises for balance. **(A)** Single-leg squat. **(B)** Stability ball wall slides. **(C)** Single-leg balance reach. **(D)** Single-leg windmill. **(E)** Monster walks using Theraband. **(F)** Multiplanar single-leg hops.

© William E. Prentice

half-sphere attached to the sole at the approximate center of gravity in the middle of the undersole. When the athlete walks over a short distance on an unstable surface, such as that created by the design of the balance shoe, muscles used for postural control and stabilization are activated subconsciously, developing enhanced neuromuscular control of the gluteals and thus improving pelvic stabilization (Figure 21–49).[9] Once the pelvis has been stabilized by the gluteal muscles, distal lower-extremity stability is enhanced.

## Functional Progressions

The functional progression might begin in a pool, where non–weight-bearing running can be performed. Depending on the injury and the nature of the sport, the weight-bearing progression might consist of walking, jogging, slow running, zigzag running, figure-eight running, and sprinting.

## Return to Activity

Before returning to activity and competition, the patient must demonstrate full pain-free function of the thigh and hip region. The athlete must have full range of motion, strength, balance, and agility.

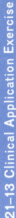

**21–13 Clinical Application Exercise**

An athlete has successfully completed the rehabilitation process after a hip injury.

? What are the criteria for this athlete's return to activity?

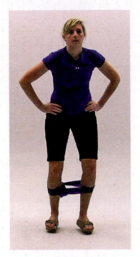

FIGURE 21–49   Standing and walking in balance shoes is effective in strengthening and improving neuromuscular control in the gluetus medius, especially when using Theraband.

© William E. Prentice

## SUMMARY

- The thigh comprises the femoral bone, musculature, nerves, blood vessels, and fascia that envelops the soft tissue. The thigh is considered that part of the leg between the hip and the knee. The quadriceps contusion and the hamstring strain represent the most common sports injuries to the thigh; the quadriceps contusion has the highest incidence. Early detection and the avoidance of internal bleeding are of major importance in acute thigh contusions. One major complication of repeated contusions is myositis ossificans.

- Jumping or falling on a bent knee can strain the quadriceps muscle. A more common strain is that of the hamstring muscle; however, it is not clearly known why hamstring muscles become strained. Strain occurs most often to the short head of the biceps femoris muscle.

- The femur can sustain both acute fractures and stress fractures. Acute fractures occur most often to the femoral shaft, usually from a direct blow. Femoral stress fractures are most common in the femoral neck.

- The groin is the depression that lies between the thigh and the abdominal region. Groin strain can occur to any one of a number of muscles located in this region. Running, jumping, or twisting can produce a groin strain.

- A common problem among women runners is trochanteric bursitis. An irritation occurs in the region of the greater trochanter of the femur.

- The hip joint, the strongest and best-protected joint in the human body, has a low incidence of acute injuries. More common are conditions stemming from an immature hip joint. They include Legg-Calvé-Perthes disease, slipped capital femoral epiphysis, and snapping hip.

- A common problem in the pelvic region is the hip pointer. This condition results from a blow to an inadequately protected iliac crest. The contusion causes pain, spasm, and malfunction of the muscles in the area. The pelvis can also sustain overuse conditions, such as osteitis pubis and athletic pubalgia, as well as acute fractures and stress fractures.

## WEB SITES

American Orthopaedic Society for Sports Medicine: www.sportsmed.org

Cramer First Aider: www.cramersportsmed.com/first -aider.html

Hip, Knee, Ankle, and Foot Conditions: www.uihealthcare .org/content.aspx?id=245078

*This site discusses biomechanics of the knee-thigh-hip complex injuries.*

Wheeless' Textbook of Orthopaedics: www .wheelessonline.com

# SOLUTIONS TO CLINICAL APPLICATION EXERCISES

21–1 It is critical that the athletic trainer construct a protective thigh pad that can be worn to prevent another contusion to the injured area. Repeated contusions may result in the development of myositis ossificans.

21–2 Initially, activity should be significantly reduced. Isometric exercise should be carried out after the early inflammatory phase. In later stages of healing, pain-free exercise such as gentle stretching, jogging, stationary cycling, and high-speed isokinetics may be employed.

21–3 The two tests that can be used for hip flexion tightness are the Kendall and Thomas tests. The Kendall test evaluates the athlete's ability to place her thigh flat on the table while the other leg is flexed on her chest. The Thomas test evaluates whether the athlete can lie on the table with her legs fully extended and keep her lumbar spine flat.

21–4 This movement is considered a positive Trendelenburg's test, indicating weakness in the gluteus medius.

21–5 The off-balanced dismount could have created a sprain of the hip joint.

21–6 This condition could be an inflammation of the gluteus medius muscle or iliotibial band, or it could be trochanteric bursitis caused by the increased Q angle and short leg.

21–7 Because of the athlete's age, the athletic trainer should consider the possibility of a growth problem, most likely a slipped capital femoral epiphysis. The athletic trainer must refer this athlete immediately to a physician for X-rays.

21–8 A likely cause of this problem is a strength imbalance of the muscles that help stabilize the hip joint while flexing and rotating. There also could be a structurally narrow pelvis, greater than usual ROM of hip abduction, or a restricted ROM during lateral rotation.

21–9 It is likely that he has athletic pubalgia, which is essentially groin pain caused by a weakness in the anterior wall of the inguinal canal. This condition is not associated with either a direct or an indirect hernia.

21–10 This patient has sustained a hip pointer, or contusion to the skin and musculature in the region of the iliac crest. The patient most likely will experience severe pain, muscle spasm, and an inability to rotate his trunk or flex his hip without pain.

21–11 This patient's complaints represent a number of possible conditions: osteitis pubis, stress fracture of the inferior pubic ramus, a possible avulsion apophysis fracture, or an apophysitis.

21–12 As the stress fracture heals, the patient must maintain and restore neuromuscular control of the thigh and hip region. The focus should be on balance and closed kinetic chain exercises. Balance board exercises and affected leg weight-bearing activities can also be conducted. Minisquats, leg presses, and stair climbing and stepping are other possible closed kinetic chain exercises.

21–13 The patient must demonstrate pain-free movement of the thigh and hip. There must be full ROM, strength, balance, and agility, along with a preinjury level of cardiorespiratory endurance.

# REVIEW QUESTIONS AND CLASS ACTIVITIES

1. How does the function of the rectus femoris muscle differ from that of the other quadriceps muscles?
2. What is the greatest concern for an individual who suffers repeated contusions to the anterior thigh?
3. What can be done to prevent injuries to the hip, thigh, and groin region?
4. How can the athletic trainer differentiate among grades 1, 2, and 3 quadriceps strains?
5. Explain how the musculature in the hip, thigh, and groin contribute to core stability.
6. What is the difference between femoral anteversion and retroversion, and how do they manifest clinically?
7. What is the difference between anatomical apparent and functional leg length discrepancies.
8. What does the groin region consist of?
9. How are avascular necrosis of the femoral head and Legg-Calvé-Perthes disease related?
10. What is the difference between osteitis pubis and athletic pubalgia?
11. Design a rehabilitation protocol for a patient with a dislocated hip.

# REFERENCES

1. Adkins S: Hip pain in athletes, *Am Fam Physician* 61(7):2109, 2000.
2. Anderson K: Hip and groin injuries in athletes, *Am J Sports Med* 29(4):521, 2001.
3. Anderson R: Integration of myofascial trigger point release and paradoxical relaxation training treatment of chronic pelvic pain in men, *J Urol* 174(1):155–60, 2005.
4. Aronen J: Quadriceps contusions: Clinical results of immediate immobilization in 120 degrees of knee flexion, *Clinical J Sports Med* 16(5):383–87, 2006.
5. Bagnulo A: Treatment of myositis ossificans with acetic acid phonophoresis: A case series, *Can Chiropr Assoc* 58(4):253–60, 2014.
6. Barrack M: Higher incidence of bone stress injuries with increasing female athlete triad-related risk factors: A prospective multisite study of exercising girls and women, *Am J Sports Med* 42(4):949–58, 2014.
7. Bickham D: Relationship between a lumbopelvic stabilization strength test and pelvic motion in running, *J Sport Rehabil* 9(3):219, 2000.
8. Bielak K: Injuries of the pelvis and hip. In Birrer P, ed: *Sports medicine for the primary care physician,* ed 2, Boca Raton, FL, 2004, CRC Press.
9. Blackburn T: Exercise sandals increase lower extremity electromyographic activity during functional activities, *J Athl Train* 38(3):198, 2003.
10. Blankenbaker D: Hip injuries in athletes, *Radiologic clinics of North America* 48(6):1155–78, 2010.
11. Bo K: Urinary incontinence, pelvic floor dysfunction, exercise and sport, *Sports Medicine* 34(7):451–64, 2004.
12. Bolgla L: Hip pain in a high school football player: A case report, *J Athl Train* 36(1):81, 2001.
13. Brady R: Limb length inequality: Clinical implications for assessment and intervention, *J Orthop Sports Phys Ther* 33(5):221, 2003.
14. Browning K: Hip and pelvis injuries in runners: Careful evaluation and tailored management, *Physician Sportsmed* 29(1):23, 2001.
15. Bruckner P: Hip and groin pain. In Bruckner P, ed: *Bruckner and Kahn's clinical sports medicine,* Sydney, 2011, McGraw-Hill.
16. Brumm L: Looking beyond the soft tissue: Illustrative case studies of groin injuries, *Athletic Therapy Today* 6(4):24, 2001.
17. Brumm L: Structural evaluation and manual medicine treatment of groin injuries: Looking beyond the soft tissue, *Athletic Therapy Today* 6(4):15, 2001.
18. Chacko P: The importance of differential diagnosis of hip pain: A case of non-traumation avascular necrosis, *J Orthop Sports Phys Ther* 35(1):A15, 2005.
19. Chance-Larsen K: Prone hip extension with lower abdominal hollowing improves the relative timing of gluteus maximus activation in relation to biceps femoris, *Manual Therapy* 15(1):61–65, 2010.
20. Copperhite K: Athletic pubalgia, Part 1: Anatomy and diagnosis, *Athletic Therapy Today* 15(5):4–6, 2010.
21. Currier L: Development of a clinical prediction rule to identify patients with knee pain and clinical evidence of knee osteoarthritis who demonstrate a favorable short-term response to hip mobilization, *Physical Therapy* 87(9): 1106–19, 2007.
22. Curtis N: Evaluation and management of hip injuries, *Athletic Therapy Today* 9(4):36, 2004.
23. DePalma B, Halvorsen, D: Rehabilitation of groin, hip, and thigh injuries. In Prentice W, ed: *Rehabilitation techniques in sports medicine and athletic training,* ed 6, Thorofare, NJ, 2015, Slack.
24. Dugan D: Femoral-neck stress fracture in an amenorrheic runner, *Athletic Therapy Today* 6(4):40, 2001.
25. Ferber R: Normative and critical criteria for iliotibial band and iliopsoas muscle flexibility, *J Athl Train* 45(4):344–48, 2010.
26. Fishman L: Piriformis syndrome: Diagnosis, treatment and outcome—a 10 year study, *Arch Phys Med Rehabil* 283:295–301, 2002.
27. Griffin K: Rehabilitation after hip arthroscopy, *J Sport Rehabil* 9(1):77, 2000.
28. Heiderscheit B: Hamstring strain injuries: Recommendation for diagnosis, rehabilitation and injury prevention, *JOSPT* 40(2):67–81, 2010.

29. Hocutt J: General types of injuries. In Birrer R, ed: *Sports medicine for the primary care physician,* ed 2, Boca Raton, FL, 2004, CRC Press.

30. Idjadi J: Symptomatic snapping hip, *Physician Sportsmed* 32(1):25, 2004.

31. Iwinski H: Slipped capital femoral epiphysis, *Current Opinion in Orthopedics* 17(6):511–16, 2006.

32. Jansen J: Treatment of long standing groin pain in athletes: A systematic review, *Scandinavian Journal of Medicine and Science in Sports* 18(3):263–74, 2008.

33. Kary J: Diagnosis and management of quadriceps strains and contusions, *Current Reviews in Musculoskeletal Medicine* 3(1–4):26–31, 2010.

34. Kerkhoffs G: A double-blind, randomised, parallel group study on the efficacy and safety of treating acute lateral ankle sprain with oral hydrolytic enzymes, *Br J Sports Med* 38:431–35, 2004.

35. Kerr H: Thoracoabdominal injuries. In Micheli L, ed: *The adolescent athlete: A practical approach,* New York, 2007, Springer.

36. Keskula D: Snapping iliopsoas tendon in a recreational athlete: A case report, *J Athl Train* 34(4):382, 1999.

37. Kirshner J: Piriformis syndrome, diagnosis and treatment, *Muscle and Nerve* 40(1):10–18, 2009.

38. Konin J: Incorporating the Renne test into the learning-over-time model, *Athletic Therapy Today* 7(4):12, 2002.

39. Konin J: Rehabilitation of soft-tissue injuries to the hip, *Athletic Therapy Today* 9(4):15, 2004.

40. Kurl M: Acute non-traumatic hip pathology in children: Incidence and presentation in family practice, *Family Practice* 27(2):166–70, 2010.

41. Larson C: Evaluating and managing muscle contusions and myositis ossificans, *Physician Sportsmed* 30(2):41, 2002.

42. Larson C: Evaluation and management of hip pain, *Physician Sportsmed* 33(10):26, 2005.

43. Leibold M: Concurrent criterion-related validity of physical examination tests for hip labral lesions: a systematic review, *J Man Manip Ther* 16(2):E24–41, 2008.

44. Levandowski R: Thigh injuries. In Birrer RB, ed: *Sports medicine for the primary care physician,* ed 2, Boca Raton, FL, 2004, CRC Press.

45. Loder R: Atypical and typical idiopathic slipped capital femoral epiphysis, *J Bone Joint Surg* 88(7):1574, 2006.

46. Magee D: *Orthopedic physical assessment,* Philadelphia, PA, 2007, Elsevier Health Sciences.

47. Marks M: Clinical utility of the Duncan-Ely test for rectus femoris dysfunction during the swing phase of gait, *Dev Med Child Neurology* 45(11):763–68, 2003.

48. Mason D: Rehabilitation for hamstring injuries, *Scandinavian Journal of Medicine and Science in Sports* 17(2):191–92, 2007.

49. Mens J: A new view on adduction-related groin pain, *Cl J Sports Med* 16(1):15, 2006.

50. Meyers W: Anatomic basis for evaluation of abdominal and groin pain in athletes, *Operative Techniques in Sports Medicine* 13(1):55, 2005.

51. Moorman C: Traumatic posterior hip subluxation in American football, *J Bone Joint Surg* 85(7):1190, 2003.

52. Newsham K: The role of neural tension in minor and recurrent hamstring injury, Part 1: Evaluation, *Athletic Therapy Today* 1(4):54, 2006.

53. Orchard J: Epidemiology of injuries in the Australian Football League, seasons 1997–2000, *Br J Sports Med* 36: 39–44, 2002.

54. Owens C: Femoral shaft stress fracture in a female recreational runner, *Athletic Therapy and Training* 16(1):21–23, 2011.

55. Parr K: Fractured femur in a middle distance sprinter, *Athletic Therapy Today* 6(1):50, 2001.

56. Petrone M: The accuracy of the palpation meter (PALM) for measuring pelvic crest height difference and leg length discrepancy, *J Orthop Sports Phys Ther* 33(6):319, 2003.

57. Prentice WE: Mobilization and traction techniques in rehabilitation. In Prentice WE, ed: *Rehabilitation techniques in sports medicine and athletic training,* ed 6, Thorofare, NJ, 2015, Slack.

58. Rabe S: Athletic pubalgia: Recognition, treatment and prevention, *Athletic Training and Sports Health Care* 2(1):25–30, 2010.

59. Reese N: Use of an inclinometer to measure flexibility of the iliotibial band using the Ober test and the modified Ober test: Differences in magnitude and reliability of measurements, *J Orthop Sports Phys Ther* 33(6):226, 2003.

60. Reiman M: Diagnostic accuracy of clinical tests of the hip: a systematic review with meta-analysis, *British Journal of Sports Medicine* 49(6):357–61, 2015.

61. Rodriguez C: Osteitis pubis syndrome in the professional Soccer athlete: A case report, *J Athl Train* 36(4):437, 2001.

62. Rosene J: Isokinetic hamstrings: Quadriceps ratios in Intercollegiate athletics, *J Athl Train* 36(4):378, 2001.

63. Schmitz R: Gluteus medius activity during isometric closed-chain hip rotation, *J Sport Rehabil* 11(3):179, 2002.

64. Seidenberg P: *The hip and pelvis in sports medicine and primary care,* New York, 2010, Springer.

65. Sikka R: Femur fractures in professional athletes: A case series, *J Ath Train* 50(4):442–48, 2015.

66. Souza R: Concurrent criterion-related validity and reliability of a clinical test to measure femoral anteversion, *J Orthop Sports Phys Ther* 39(8):586–92, 2009.

67. Spernoga S: Duration of maintained hamstring flexibility after a 1-time modified hold-relax stretching protocol, *J Athl Train* 36(1):44, 2001.

68. Sutlive T, et al.: Development of a clinical prediction rule for diagnosing hip osteoarthritis in individuals with unilateral hip pain, *J Orthop Sport Phys Ther* 38: 542–50, 2008.

69. Tijssen M: Diagnostics of femoroacetabular impingement and labral pathology of the hip: A systematic review of the accuracy and validity of physical tests, *Arthroscopy* 28(6):860–71, 2012.

70. Tiru M: Use of percussion as a screening tool in the diagnosis of occult hip fractures, *Singapore Med J* 43:467–69, 2002.

71. Tonley J: Treatment of an individual with piriformis syndrome focusing on hip muscle strengthening and movement reeducation: A case report, *J Orthop Sports Phys Ther* 40(2): 103–11, 2010.

72. Turl S: Adverse neural tension: A factor in repetitive hamstring strain? *J Orthop Sports Phys Ther* 27(1):16, 1998.

73. Tyler T: The role of hip muscle function in the treatment of patellofemoral pain, *Am J Sports Med* 34(4):630–36, 2006.

74. Waite B: Examination and treatment of pediatric injuries of the hip and pelvis, *Physical Medicine and Rehabilitation Clinics of North America* 19(2):305–18, 2008.

75. Weisharr M: Management of a midshaft femoral stress fracture in a direct-access physical therapy setting, *J Orthop Sports Phys Ther* 34(1):A16, 2004.

76. Wise S: Current management and rehabilitation in Legg-Calve-Perthes disease, *Athletic Therapy Today,* 15(4):76, 2010.

77. Wissen W: An aggressive approach to managing quadriceps contusions, *Athletic Therapy Today* 5(1):36, 2000.

78. Wood A: Incidence and time to return to training for stress fractures during military basic training, *J Sports Med* 2014(282980):1–5, 2014.

79. Woolf J: Pathoanatomy of the painful hip. In *Proceedings, National Athletic Trainers' Association 51st annual meeting and clinical symposia,* Champaign, IL, 2000, Human Kinetics.

80. Youdas J: Usefulness of the Trendelenburg test for identification of patients with hip joint osteoarthritis, *Physiother Theory Pract* 26: 184–94, 2010.

## ANNOTATED BIBLIOGRAPHY

Busconi B: Sports-related injuries of the hip, An Issue of *Clinics in Sports Medicine,* Philadelphia, PA, 2011, Saunders.
*Discusses sports-related injuries of the hip, including broad topics such as clinical diagnosis of hip pain, historical perspective of hip injuries, and radiology of hip injuries, as well as specific ones on certain injuries.*

Guanche C: Hip and pelvis injuries in sports medicine, Philadelphia, PA, 2011, Lippincott, Williams and Wilkins.
*A comprehensive clinical reference that covers the diagnosis and treatment of hip and pelvis injuries seen in sports medicine practice. Detailing the physical examination and radiology of the hip and pelvis, it describes techniques for treating all the important problems encountered in athletes.*

Knopf K: *Healthy hips handbook: Exercises for treating and preventing common hip joint injuries,* 2010, Ulysses Press.

*Outlines the causes for common hip conditions, including snapping hip, IT band fasciitis, osteoarthritis, and sciatica.*

Seidenberg P: *The hip and pelvis in sports medicine and primary care,* New York, 2010, Springer.
*A resource for improving the management of hip and pelvis injuries that presents a spectrum of functional therapeutic interventions.*

Tile M, Helfet D, Kellam J: *Fractures of the pelvis and acetabulum: Principles of Management,* Philadelphia, PA, 2003, Lippincott, Williams and Wilkins.
*Discusses anatomy, biomechanics, pathoanatomy, and aspects of trauma and examines diagnosis, treatment, and management options.*

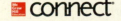

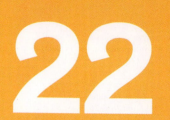
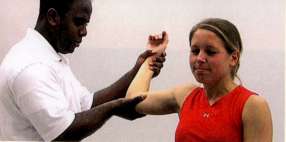

© William E. Prentice

# The Shoulder Complex

## ■ Objectives

*When you finish this chapter you should be able to*

- Point out the critical anatomical features of the four articulations in the shoulder complex.
- Perform an in-depth evaluation of the shoulder complex.
- Recognize the steps that can be taken to minimize the chances of injury to the shoulder complex.
- Explain how shoulder stability is maintained by the joint capsule, ligaments, and muscles.

- Summarize the anatomical and functional relationship between shoulder stability and shoulder impingement.
- Identify the etiology and recognize the symptoms and signs of specific injuries that occur around the shoulder joint, and discuss plans for management.
- Formulate a general plan that may be effectively incorporated into a rehabilitation program for treating a variety of injuries in the shoulder complex.

## ■ Outline

## ■ Key Terms

external rotation gain (ERG)        glenohumeral internal
                                      rotation deficit (GIRD)

## ■ Connect Highlights    Mc Graw Hill Education **connect**

*Visit connect.mcgraw-hill.com for further exercises to apply your knowledge:*

- Clinical application scenarios covering assessment and recognition of shoulder injuries, etiology, symptoms and signs, and management of shoulder injuries, and rehabilitation for the shoulder
- Click-and-drag questions covering structural anatomy of the shoulder, assessment of shoulder injuries, and rehabilitation plan of the shoulder
- Multiple-choice questions covering anatomy, assessment, etiology, management, and rehabilitation of shoulder injuries
- Selection questions covering rehabilitation plans for various injuries to the shoulder
- Video identification of special tests for the shoulder injuries, rehabilitation techniques for the shoulder, and taping and wrapping for shoulder injuries
- Picture identification of major anatomical components of the shoulder, rehabilitation techniques of the shoulder, and therapeutic modalities for management

The shoulder complex, as the name implies, is an extremely complicated region of the body. Because of its anatomical structure, the shoulder complex has a great degree of mobility. This mobility requires some compromise in stability, and thus the shoulder is highly susceptible to injury. Many overhead activities—in particular, those that involve repetitive overhead movements—place a great deal of stress on the supporting structures (Figure 22–1). Consequently, injuries related to overuse in the shoulder are commonplace. Some understanding of the anatomy and mechanics of this joint is essential for the athletic trainer.

# ANATOMY OF THE SHOULDER

## Bones

The bones that make up the shoulder complex and shoulder joint are the clavicle, sternum, scapula, and humerus (Figure 22–2).

**Clavicle** The clavicle is a slender, S-shaped bone approximately 6 inches (15 cm) long. It supports the anterior portion of the shoulder, keeping it free from the thoracic cage. It extends from the sternum to the tip of the shoulder, where it joins the acromion process of the scapula. The shape of the medial two-thirds of the clavicle is primarily circular, and its lateral third assumes a flattened appearance. The medial two-thirds bends convexly forward, and the lateral third is concave. The point at which the clavicle changes shape and contour presents a structural weakness, and the largest number of fractures to the bone occur at this point. Lying superficially with no muscle or fat protection makes the clavicle subject to direct blows.

**Sternum** The sternum, also referred to as the breastbone, is divided into three parts: the manubrium, the body, and the xiphoid process. It provides an attachment for the clavicle at the sternoclavicular joint, which is the only axial skeleton attachment for the entire upper extremity. It also serves as a site of attachment for the ribs via costal cartilage.

**Scapula** The scapula is a flat, triangular bone that serves mainly as an articulating surface for the head of the humerus. It is located on the dorsal aspect of the thorax and has three prominent projections: the spine, the acromion, and the coracoid process. The spine divides the posterior aspect unequally. The superior dorsal aspect is a deep depression called the supraspinous fossa, and the area below, a more shallow depression, is called the infraspinous fossa. The acromion is a process at the lateral tip of the spine. A hooklike projection called the coracoid process arises anteriorly from the scapula. It curves upward, forward, and outward in front of the glenoid fossa, which is the articulating cavity for the reception of the humeral head. The glenoid cavity is situated laterally on the scapula below the acromion and is relatively shallow. However, the presence of the fibrocartilaginous glenoid labrum increases the depth of articulation. The scapula serves as a site of attachment for many of the muscles that move the shoulder complex.

**Humerus** The head of the humerus is spherical, with a shallow, constricted neck; it faces upward, inward, and backward, articulating with the scapula's shallow glenoid fossa. Circumscribing the humeral head is a slight groove called the anatomical neck, which is the attachment for the articular capsule of the glenohumeral joint. The greater and lesser tubercles are located adjacent and immediately inferior to the head. The lesser tubercle is

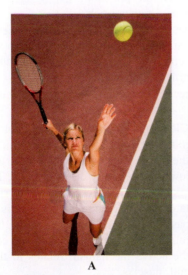
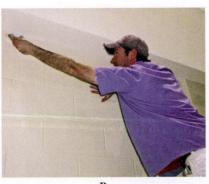

FIGURE 22–1   Vigorous and/or repetitive overhead activities, such as **(A)** serving in tennis or **(B)** painting, can result in a variety of shoulder injuries.

(a) © moodboard/Corbis; (b) © William E. Prentice

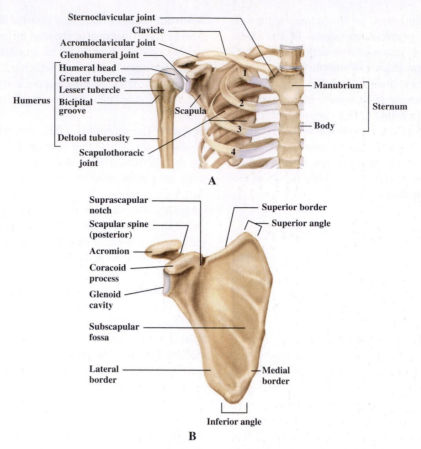

FIGURE 22–2 **(A)** Skeletal anatomy of the shoulder complex. **(B)** Anatomy of the scapula.

positioned anteriorly and medially, with the greater tubercle placed somewhat higher and laterally. Lying between the two tubercles is a deep groove called the bicipital groove, which retains the long tendon of the biceps brachii muscle.

## Articulations

Four major articulations are associated with the shoulder complex: the sternoclavicular joint, the acromioclavicular joint, the glenohumeral joint, and the scapulothoracic joint (Figure 22–2).

**Sternoclavicular Joint** The clavicle articulates with the manubrium of the sternum to form the sternoclavicular (SC) joint, the only direct connection between the upper extremity and the trunk. The sternal articulating surface is larger than the sternum, causing the clavicle to rise much higher than the sternum. A fibrocartilaginous disk is interposed between the two articulating surfaces. It functions as a shock absorber against the medial forces and helps prevent any displacement upward. The articular disk is placed so that the clavicle moves on the disk and the disk in turn moves separately on the sternum. The clavicle is permitted to move up and down, forward and backward, in combination, and in rotation.

**Acromioclavicular Joint** The acromioclavicular (AC) joint is a gliding articulation of the lateral end of the clavicle with the acromion process. It is a rather weak junction. A fibrocartilaginous disk separates the two articulating surfaces. A thin, fibrous capsule surrounds the joint.

> **Shoulder complex articulations:**
> - Sternoclavicular
> - Acromioclavicular
> - Glenohumeral
> - Scapulothoracic

**Glenohumeral Joint** The glenohumeral joint (shoulder joint) is an enarthrodial, or ball-and-socket, joint in which the round head of the humerus articulates with the shallow glenoid cavity of the scapula. The cavity is deepened slightly by a fibrocartilaginous rim called the glenoid labrum. The glenohumeral joint is maintained by both a passive and an active mechanism; the passive mechanism relates to the glenoid labrum and capsular ligaments, and the active mechanism relates to the deltoid and rotator cuff muscles.

**Scapulothoracic Joint** The scapulothoracic joint is not a true joint; however, the movement of the scapula on the wall of the thoracic cage is critical to shoulder

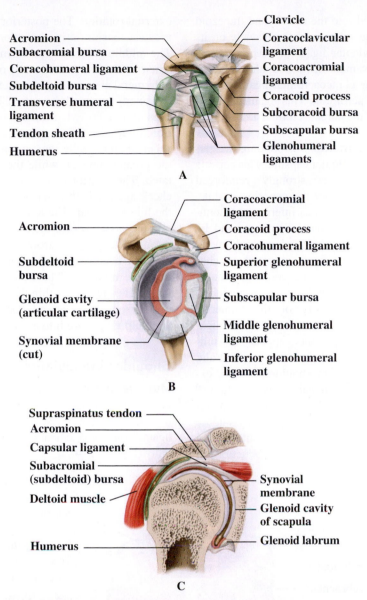

**FIGURE 22–3** Shoulder complex articulations, ligaments, and bursae. **(A)** Anterior view. **(B)** Lateral view. **(C)** Frontal section.

Figure labels (A):
Acromion
Subacromial bursa
Coracohumeral ligament
Subdeltoid bursa
Transverse humeral ligament
Tendon sheath
Humerus
Clavicle
Coracoclavicular ligament
Coracoacromial ligament
Coracoid process
Subcoracoid bursa
Subscapular bursa
Glenohumeral ligaments

Figure labels (B):
Acromion
Subdeltoid bursa
Glenoid cavity (articular cartilage)
Synovial membrane (cut)
Coracoacromial ligament
Coracoid process
Coracohumeral ligament
Superior glenohumeral ligament
Subscapular bursa
Middle glenohumeral ligament
Inferior glenohumeral ligament

Figure labels (C):
Supraspinatus tendon
Acromion
Capsular ligament
Subacromial (subdeltoid) bursa
Deltoid muscle
Humerus
Synovial membrane
Glenoid cavity of scapula
Glenoid labrum

joint motion. Contraction of the scapular muscles, which attach the scapula to the axial skeleton, is critical in stabilizing the scapula and thus in providing a base on which a highly mobile joint can function. The scapula serves as the origin for the muscles of the rotator cuff, and the scapulothoracic joint allows for upward/downward rotation, internal/external rotation, and anterior/posterior tilting.[57,67]

## Ligaments

Figure 22–3 shows the ligamentous arrangement of the shoulder complex.

**Sternoclavicular Joint Ligaments** The sternoclavicular joint is extremely weak because of its bony arrangement, but it is held securely by strong ligaments that

tend to pull the sternal end of the clavicle downward and toward the sternum—in effect, anchoring it. The main ligaments are the anterior sternoclavicular, which prevents upward displacement of the clavicle; the posterior sternoclavicular, which also prevents upward displacement of the clavicle; the interclavicular, which prevents lateral displacement of the clavicle; and the costoclavicular, which prevents lateral and upward displacement of the clavicle.

**Acromioclavicular Joint Ligaments** The acromioclavicular ligament consists of anterior, posterior, superior, and inferior portions. In addition to the acromioclavicular ligament, the coracoclavicular ligament joins the coracoid process and the clavicle and helps maintain the position of the clavicle relative to the acromion. The coracoclavicular ligament is further divided into the conoid and trapezoid ligaments. Because of the rotation of the clavicle on its long axis, the coracoclavicular ligament develops some slack, which permits movement of the scapula at the acromioclavicular joint. The coracoacromial ligament connects the coracoid to the acromion. This ligament, along with the acromion, forms the coracoacromial arch.

**Glenohumeral Joint Ligaments** Surrounding the glenohumeral joint is a loose, articular capsule. This capsule is strongly reinforced by the superior, middle, and inferior glenohumeral ligaments and by the tough coracohumeral ligament, which attaches to the coracoid process and to the greater tuberosity of the humerus. The glenohumeral ligaments appear to produce a major restraint in shoulder flexion, extension, and rotation.[103] The anterior glenohumeral ligament is tense when the shoulder is in extension, abduction, or external rotation. The posterior glenohumeral ligament's greatest tension is in abduction and internal rotation.[103] The middle glenohumeral ligament is in greatest tension when in flexion and external rotation. The inferior glenohumeral ligament is most tense when the shoulder is abducted, extended, or externally rotated. The posterior capsule is tense when the shoulder is in flexion, abduction, internal rotation, or any combination of these. The superior and middle segment of the posterior capsule has the greatest tension while the shoulder is internally rotated. The inferior glenohumeral ligament is primarily a check against both anterior and posterior dislocation of the humeral head. The long tendon of the biceps brachii muscle passes across the head of the humerus and then through the bicipital groove. In the anatomical position, the long head of the biceps moves in close relationship with the humerus. The transverse ligament retains the long biceps tendon within the bicipital groove by passing over it from the lesser and greater tuberosities, converting the bicipital groove into a canal.

## Shoulder Musculature

**Muscles Acting on the Glenohumeral Joint** The muscles that cross the glenohumeral joint produce dynamic motion and establish stability to compensate for a bony and ligamentous arrangement that allows for a great deal of mobility (Figure 22–4).

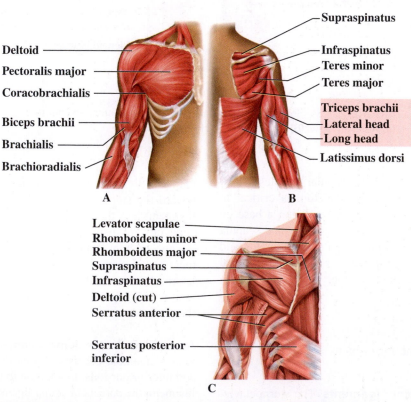

Deltoid
Pectoralis major
Coracobrachialis
Biceps brachii
Brachialis
Brachioradialis

A

Supraspinatus
Infraspinatus
Teres minor
Teres major
Triceps brachii
Lateral head
Long head
Latissimus dorsi

B

Levator scapulae
Rhomboideus minor
Rhomboideus major
Supraspinatus
Infraspinatus
Deltoid (cut)
Serratus anterior
Serratus posterior inferior

C

FIGURE 22–4    Shoulder musculature. **(A)** Anterior muscles. **(B)** Posterior muscles. **(C)** Scapular muscles.

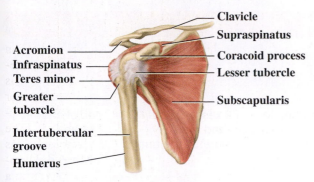

FIGURE 22–5    Rotator cuff muscles.

Movements at the glenohumeral joint include flexion, extension, abduction, adduction, horizontal adduction/abduction, internal/external rotation, and circumduction. The muscles acting on the glenohumeral joint may be separated into two groups. The first group consists of muscles that originate on the axial skeleton and attach to the humerus and includes the latissimus dorsi and the pectoralis major. The second group originates on the scapula and attaches to the humerus and includes the deltoid, the teres major, and the coracobrachialis. Additionally, the subscapularis, supraspinatus, infraspinatus, and teres minor muscles constitute the short rotator muscles, commonly called the rotator cuff, whose tendons adhere to the articular capsule and serve as reinforcing structures (Figure 22–5). The biceps and triceps muscles attach on the glenoid and effect elbow motion (Table 22–1).

| Glenohumeral joint movements: |
| --- |
| • Flexion |
| • Extension |
| • Abduction |
| • Adduction |
| • Horizontal adduction |
| • Horizontal abduction |
| • Internal rotation |
| • External rotation |
| • Circumduction |

**Scapular Muscles** A third group of muscles attaches the axial skeleton to the scapula and includes the levator scapulae, the trapezius, the rhomboids, and the serratus anterior and posterior. The scapular muscles are important in providing dynamic stability to the shoulder complex (Table 22–1).

| Rotator cuff muscles: |
| --- |
| • Subscapularis |
| • Supraspinatus |
| • Infraspinatus |
| • Teres minor |

## Bursae

Several bursae are located around the shoulder joint, the most important of which is the subacromial bursa (see Figure 22–3), located between the coracoacromial arch and the glenohumeral capsule and reinforced by the

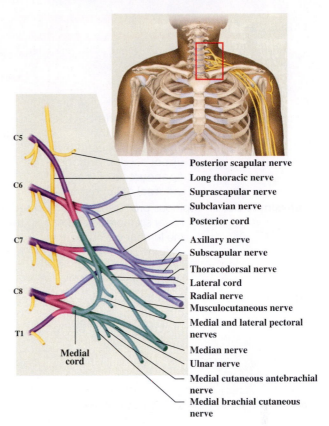

FIGURE 22–6    The brachial plexus and nerve supply of the shoulder.

supraspinous tendon. The subacromial bursa is easily subjected to trauma when the humerus is in the overhead position because it becomes compressed under the coracoacromial arch.

## Nerve Supply

The spinal nerve roots from the fifth cervical vertebra through the first thoracic vertebra to create the complex nerve network called the brachial plexus (Figure 22–6), which is discussed in Chapter 25. Stemming from this plexus are the peripheral nerves that innervate the muscles of the upper extremity, including the axillary (C5, C6), the musculocutaneous (C5–C7), the subscapular (C5, C6), the suprascapular (C5, C6), the dorsal scapular (C5), the pectoral (C5–T1), and the radial (C5–T1) nerves.[1]

## Blood Supply

The subclavian artery, which lies distal to the sternoclavicular joint, arches upward and outward, passes the anterior scalene muscle, and then moves downward laterally behind the clavicle and in front of the first ribs (Figure 22–7). The subclavian artery continues on to become the axillary artery at the outer border of the first rib and to become the brachial artery in the region of the teres major muscle in the upper arm.

**TABLE 22–1**     Muscles of the Shoulder Complex

| Muscle | Origin | Insertion | Muscle Action | Innervation/ Nerve Root |
|---|---|---|---|---|
| **Muscles acting on humerus** | | | | |
| **Pectoralis major** | Medial half of the clavicle, the sternum, the costal cartilages of the upper six ribs, and the aponeurosis of the external oblique muscle | Greater turbercle of the humerus | Flexes, adducts, and medially rotates the arm | Medial and lateral pectoral (C5–C8, T1) |
| **Latissimus dorsi** | Spinous processes of the lower six thoracic and the lumbar vertebrae, the sacrum, and the posterior iliac crest—all via the lumbodorsal fascia | Medial margin of the intertubercular groove of the humerus | Extends, adducts, and medially rotates the arm; pulls the shoulder downward | Thoracodorsal (C6–C8) |
| **Deltoid** | Lateral third of the clavicle, the acromion process, and the spine of the scapula | Deltoid tuberosity of the humerus | Abducts the arm; anterior fibers flex and medially rotate the arm; posterior fibers extend and laterally rotate the arm | Axillary (C5, C6) |
| **Supraspinatus** | Supraspinatus fossa of the scapula | Greater tubercle of the humerus | Abducts the arm; slight lateral rotation | Suprascapular (C5, C6) |
| **Infraspinatus** | Infraspinatus fossa of the scapula | Greater tubercle of the humerus (posterior to the supraspinatus) | Laterally rotates the arm; slight adduction | Suprascapular (C5, C6) |
| **Subscapularis** | Subscapular fossa of the scapula | Lesser tubercle of the humerus | Medially rotates the arm | Subscapular (C5, C6) |
| **Teres major** | Dorsal surface of the interior angle of the scapula | Lesser tubercle of the humerus | Adducts, extends, and medially rotates the arm | Subscapular (C5, C6) |
| **Teres minor** | Axillary border of the scapula | Greater tubercle of the humerus (posterior to the infraspinatus) | Laterally rotates the arm | Axillary (C5, C6) |
| **Coracobrachialis** | Coracoid process of the scapula | Middle of the humerus, medial surface | Flexes and adducts the arm | Musculocutaneous (C5, C6) |
| **Muscles acting on scapula** | | | | |
| **Trapezius** | Occipital bone, the ligamentum nuchae, and the spinous processes of the seventh cervical and all the thoracic vertebrae | Lateral third of the clavicle, the acromion process, and the spine of the scapula | Elevates (upper portion) or depresses (lower portion), rotates, adducts, and stabilizes the scapula | Spinal accessory (cranial nerve XI) |
| **Rhomboideus major** | Spinous processes of the seventh cervical and first thoracic vertebrae | Vertebral border of the scapula, below the spine of the scapula | Adduct, stabilize, and rotate the scapula, lowering its lateral angle | Dorsal scapular (C5) |
| **Rhomboideus minor** | Spinous processes of the second through the fifth thoracic vertebrae | Vertebral border of the scapula, at the base of the spine of the scapula | | |

*(continued)*

| TABLE 22–1 | Muscles of the Shoulder Complex (*continued*) |

| Muscle | Origin | Insertion | Muscle Action | Innervation/ Nerve Root |
|---|---|---|---|---|
| *Muscles acting on scapula* | | | | |
| **Levator scapulae** | Transverse processes of the upper four cervical vertebrae | Vertebral border of the scapula, above the spine of the scapula | Elevates the scapula and bends the neck laterally when the scapula is fixed | Dorsal scapular (C5) |
| **Pectoralis minor** | Anterior surface of the third through fifth ribs | Coracoid process of the scapula | Draws the scapula anteriorly and downward | Medial pectoral (eight cervical and first thoracic) (C8, T1) |
| **Serratus anterior** | Outer surface of the first nine ribs | Entire length of the ventral surface of the vertebral border of the scapula | Stabilizes, abducts, and rotates the scapula | Long thoracic (C5–C7) |

**Shoulder Joint Movements***

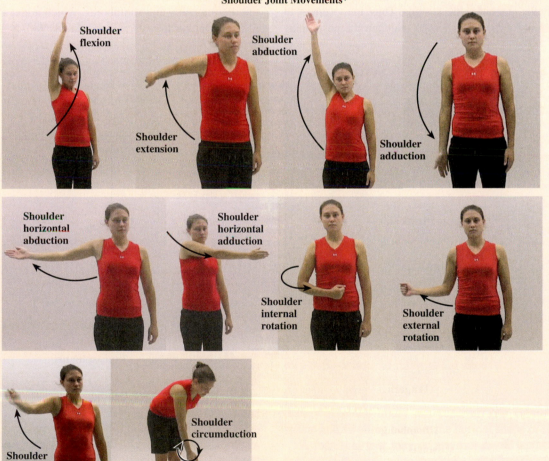

Shoulder flexion

Shoulder extension

Shoulder abduction

Shoulder adduction

Shoulder horizontal abduction

Shoulder horizontal adduction

Shoulder internal rotation

Shoulder external rotation

Shoulder scaption

Shoulder circumduction

*Manual muscle tests and goniometric measurements of range of motion for the shoulder joint complex can be found in Appendix F and Appendix G at the end of the text.

© William E. Prentice

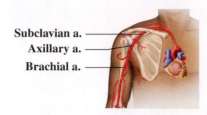

Subclavian a.
Axillary a.
Brachial a.

FIGURE 22–7  Blood supply of the shoulder complex.

## Surface Anatomy

Figure 22–8 shows the surface anatomy that is pertinent to the shoulder complex from anterior, lateral, and posterior views.

# FUNCTIONAL ANATOMY

The anatomy of the shoulder complex allows for a great degree of mobility.[110] To achieve this mobility, stability of the complex is sometimes compromised. Instability of the shoulder frequently leads to injury, particularly in those activities that involve overhead movement. In the glenohumeral joint, the rounded humeral head articulates with a relatively flat glenoid on the scapula. Thus, in movement of the shoulder joint, it is critical to maintain the positioning of the humeral head relative to the glenoid. The muscles of the rotator cuff—the subscapularis, infraspinatus, supraspinatus, and teres minor—along with the long head of the biceps provide dynamic stability, control position, and prevent excessive displacement of the humeral head relative to the position of the glenoid.[43] The supraspinatus compresses the humeral head into the glenoid, while cocontraction of the infraspinatus, teres minor, and subscapularis depresses the humeral head during overhead movements.[24]

The glenohumeral joint capsule also helps control humeral head movement. The tendons of the rotator cuff blend into the glenohumeral joint capsule. As the muscles contract, they dynamically tighten the joint capsule, which helps center the humeral head relative to the glenoid.[102]

Dynamic movement, as well as stabilization of the shoulder complex, requires integrated functioning of not only the glenohumeral joint but also of the scapulothoracic, acromioclavicular, and sternoclavicular joints.[22] The muscles that produce movement of the scapula on the thorax help maintain the position of the glenoid relative to the moving humerus and include the levator scapulae and upper trapezius, which elevate the scapula; the middle trapezius and rhomboids, which adduct the scapula; the lower trapezius, which adducts and depresses the

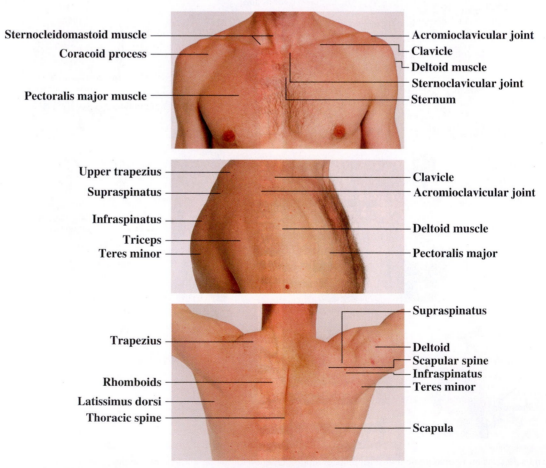

Sternocleidomastoid muscle
Coracoid process
Pectoralis major muscle

Acromioclavicular joint
Clavicle
Deltoid muscle
Sternoclavicular joint
Sternum

Upper trapezius
Supraspinatus
Infraspinatus
Triceps
Teres minor

Clavicle
Acromioclavicular joint
Deltoid muscle
Pectoralis major

Trapezius

Rhomboids
Latissimus dorsi
Thoracic spine

Supraspinatus
Deltoid
Scapular spine
Infraspinatus
Teres minor
Scapula

FIGURE 22–8  Surface anatomy of the shoulder complex.
© JW Ramsey/McGraw-Hill Education

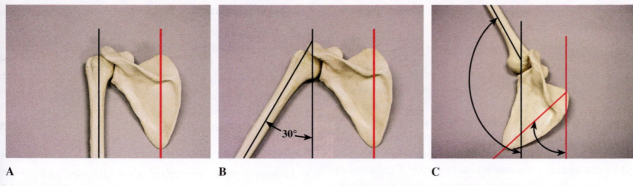

FIGURE 22–9    Scapulohumeral rhythm. **(A)** Starting position. **(B)** Setting phase. **(C)** Full elevation.
© William E. Prentice

scapula; and the serratus anterior, which abducts and up-wardly rotates the scapula.[41,74,106]

## Scapulohumeral Rhythm

Scapulohumeral rhythm describes the movement of the scapula relative to the movement of the humerus throughout a full range of abduction (Figure 22–9). As the humerus elevates to 30 degrees, there is no movement of the scapula. This phase is referred to as the setting phase, during which a stable base is being established on the thoracic wall. After the setting phase, there is a 2:1 ratio of glenohumeral to scapulothoracic movement.[105]

For the scapula to abduct and upwardly rotate throughout 180 degrees of humeral abduction, clavicular movement must occur at both the sternoclavicular and the acromioclavicular joints.[68] The clavicle must elevate approximately 20 degrees and must rotate in a posterior direction at least 35 degrees.[56]

## PREVENTION OF SHOULDER INJURIES

Proper physical conditioning is important in preventing many shoulder injuries. Like all preventive conditioning programs, the shoulder program should be directed toward general body development and the development of specific body areas for a given activity. If an activity places extreme, sustained demands on the arms and shoulders or if the shoulder is at risk for sudden traumatic injury, an individual should extensively strengthen that area. Strengthening through a full range of motion of all the muscles involved in movement of the shoulder complex is essential.

Anyone involved in overhead activities (athletes, construction workers, etc.) should perform a proper warm-up gradually before attempting explosive arm movements. This warm-up includes a general increase in body temperature, followed by sport-specific stretching of selected muscles.

Throwing athletes commonly use rubber-tubing resistance exercises as part of a warm-up before throwing. The following seven exercises are beneficial for throwers during their warm-up routine:

- External rotation at 90 degrees of abduction
- Throwing deceleration
- Humeral flexion
- Humeral extension
- Low scapular rows
- Throwing acceleration
- Scapular punch

These exercises collectively exhibit moderate activation in each muscle of the rotator cuff, the primary humeral movers, and the scapular stabilizer muscles, which are important to the throwing motion.[82]

All athletes in collision and contact sports should be instructed and drilled on how to fall properly. They must be taught not to try to catch themselves with an outstretched arm. Performing a shoulder roll is a safer way to absorb the shock of a fall. Specialized protective equipment, such as shoulder pads, must be properly fitted to help prevent shoulder injuries in tackle football.

To avoid overuse shoulder injuries, it is essential that athletes be taught the appropriate techniques of throwing, spiking, overhead smashing, overhand serving, tackling and blocking, and the proper swimming strokes.

## ASSESSMENT OF THE SHOULDER COMPLEX

The shoulder complex is one of the most difficult regions of the body to evaluate.[81] One reason for this difficulty is that the biomechanical demands placed on these structures during overhand accelerations and decelerations are not yet clearly understood.[5]

## History

It is essential that the athletic trainer understand the patient's major complaints and the possible mechanism of an injury.[44] It is also necessary to know whether the condition was produced by a sudden trauma or was of slow onset. If the injury was sudden, the athletic trainer must determine whether the precipitating cause was external and direct trauma or some resistive force.[5] Decisions as to how to best treat a specific existing injury or condition must be based on the best available evidence.[33] The following questions can help the athletic trainer determine the nature of the injury:

- What happened to cause this pain?
- Has the patient ever had this problem before?
- What are the duration and intensity of the pain?
- Where is the pain located?
- Is there crepitus during movement, numbness, or distortion in temperature, such as a cold or warm feeling?
- Is there a feeling of weakness or a sense of fatigue?
- What shoulder movements or positions seem to aggravate or relieve the pain?
- If therapy has been given before, what, if anything, offered pain relief (e.g., cold, heat, massage, or analgesic medication)?

## Observation

The patient should be generally observed while walking and standing. Observation during walking can reveal an asymmetrical arm swing or a lean toward the painful shoulder. Next, the patient should be observed from the front, side, and back while in a standing position. The athletic trainer should look for any postural asymmetries, bony or joint deformities, or muscle spasm or guarding patterns.

### Anterior Observation

- Are both shoulder tips even with one another, or is one depressed?
- Is one shoulder held higher because of muscle spasm or guarding?
- Is the lateral end of the clavicle prominent (indicating a step deformity caused by acromioclavicular sprain or dislocation)?
- Is one lateral acromion process more prominent than the other (indicating a possible glenohumeral dislocation)?
- Does the clavicular shaft appear deformed (indicating possible fracture)? Is there loss of the normal lateral deltoid muscle contour (indicating glenohumeral dislocation)?
- Is there an indentation in the upper biceps region (indicating rupture of the biceps tendon)?
- Are the deltoid muscles symmetrical?

### Lateral Observation

- Is there thoracic kyphosis, or shoulders slumped forward (indicating weakness of the erector muscles of the spine and tightness in the pectoral region)?
- Is the position of the head normal or is it forward?
- Is there forward or backward arm hang (indicating possible scoliosis)?

### Posterior Observation

- Is there asymmetry, such as a low shoulder, and are the scapulae even? (One scapula being unusually high may indicate *Sprengel's deformity*, which is a congenital deformity in which the scapula does not descend.)
- Is the scapula protracted because of constricted pectoral muscles?
- Is there a distracted, or winged, scapula on one or both sides? (A winged scapula on both sides could indicate a general weakness of the serratus anterior muscles; if only one side is winged, the long thoracic nerve may be injured. Winging of only one scapula may indicate scoliosis.)
- Is there normal scapulohumeral rhythm?

## Palpation

**Bony Palpation**  Palpation of the bony structures should be done with the athletic trainer standing in front of and then behind the patient. The athletic trainer should palpate both shoulders at the same time for pain sites and deformities.

### Anterior Structures
- Sternoclavicular joint
- Clavicular shaft
- Acromioclavicular joint
- Coracoid process
- Acromion process
- Humeral head (axilla)
- Greater tuberosity of the humerus
- Lesser tuberosity of the humerus
- Bicipital groove

### Posterior Structures
- Scapular spine
- Scapular vertebral border
- Scapular lateral border
- Scapular superior angle
- Scapular inferior angle

**Soft-Tissue Palpation**  Palpation of the soft tissue of the shoulder detects pain sites, abnormal swelling or lumps, muscle spasm or guarding, and trigger points. Trigger points are commonly found in the following muscles: levator scapulae, lesser rhomboid, supraspinous, infraspinous, scalene, deltoid, subscapular, teres major, trapezius, serratus anterior, and pectoralis major and minor. The shoulder is palpated anteriorly and posteriorly.

### Anterior Palpation

- Sternoclavicular ligament
- Acromioclavicular ligament
- Coracoclavicular ligament
- Anterior and middle deltoid muscle
- Rotator cuff tendons
- Subacromial bursa
- Pectoralis major muscle
- Sternocleidomastoid muscle
- Biceps muscle and tendon
- Coracoacromial ligament
- Glenohumeral joint capsule

### Posterior Palpation

- Posterior deltoid
- Rhomboids
- Latissimus dorsi
- Serratus anterior
- Levator scapulae
- Trapezius
- Supraspinatus
- Infraspinatus
- Teres major and minor

## Special Tests

A number of special tests can help determine the nature of an injury to the shoulder complex.

**Test for Sternoclavicular Joint Instability** With the patient sitting, pressure is applied anteriorly, then superiorly, and then inferiorly to the proximal clavicle to determine any instability or increased pain associated with a sprain (Figure 22–10A). Pressure applied to the tip of the shoulder in a medial direction may increase pain.[26]

**Test for Acromioclavicular Joint Instability** The patient with AC lesions typically complains of pain on the top of the shoulder near the AC joint.[13] The acromioclavicular joint is first palpated to determine whether there is any displacement of the acromion process and the distal head of the clavicle. Next, pressure is applied to the distal clavicle in all four directions to determine stability and any associated increase in pain (Figure 22–10B). Pressure is applied to the tip of the shoulder, which compresses the acromioclavicular joint and may increase pain.[52]

### Tests for Glenohumeral Instability
#### *Glenohumeral Translation (Load and Shift Test)*[15]
This test may be done with the patient either sitting or supine. First, the athletic trainer places one hand over the shoulder to stabilize the scapula (Figure 22–11). With the other hand, he or she grasps the humeral head between the thumb and index finger. A stress load is applied and translation of the humerus is assessed in both an anterior and a posterior direction.

With stress, the humeral head may be felt to ride up the glenoid rim. This test is said to not only assess the amount of translation but also provide an idea of the adequacy of the

| Tests for glenohumeral instability: |
| --- |
| • Load and shift test |
| • Anterior drawer test |
| • Posterior drawer test |
| • Sulcus test |
| • Clunk test |
| • O'Brien's test |
| • Apprehension test |
| • Relocation test |

glenoid lip. Excessive translation of greater than ⅜ inch (1 cm) is an indication of anterior and/or posterior instability and likely injury to the glenohumeral ligament. The athletic trainer should compare both shoulders to appreciate their similarities or differences in translation.[26]
Sn. 0.90 | Sp. 0.85 | +LR 6.0 | -LR .12

***Anterior and Posterior Drawer Tests*** The anterior drawer test checks for anterior glenohumeral instability. The patient lies supine with the arm abducted 45 degrees, horizontally adducted 10 degrees, and externally rotated 10 degrees. The scapula is stabilized, and the humeral head is glided anteriorly while slight distraction is applied to the glenohumeral joint (Figure 22–12A). A positive test

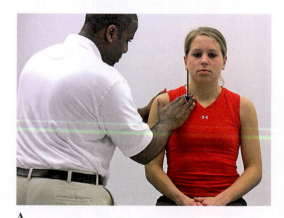

A

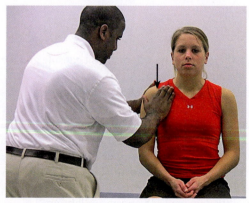

B

FIGURE 22–10    **(A)** Assessing sternoclavicular joint stability. **(B)** Assessing acromioclavicular joint stability.

© William E. Prentice

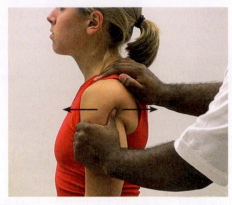

FIGURE 22-11   The load and shift test assesses anterior-posterior translation.
© William E. Prentice

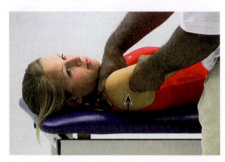

**A**

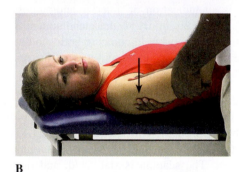

**B**

FIGURE 22-12   **(A)** Anterior drawer test. **(B)** Posterior drawer test.
© William E. Prentice

indicates insufficiency of the anterior joint capsule and the integrity of the anterior labrum.

The posterior drawer test checks for posterior glenohumeral instability. The patient lies supine with the arm abducted 90 degrees and horizontally adducted 20 degrees, the elbow flexed at 90 degrees. The scapula is stabilized, and the humerus is internally rotated as the humeral head is glided posteriorly (Figure 22-12B). A positive test indicates insufficiency of the posterior capsule and possible damage to the posterior labrum.[52]

***Sulcus Test***[83]  The athletic trainer grasps the elbow and applies traction in an inferior direction. With excessive inferior translation, a depression occurs just below the

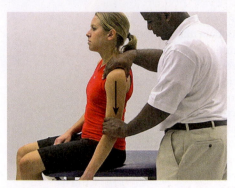

FIGURE 22-13   Sulcus test.
© William E. Prentice

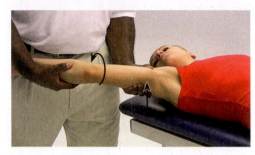

FIGURE 22-14   Clunk test.
© William E. Prentice

acromion. The appearance of this sulcus is a positive sign (Figure 22-13).[26] Sn. 0.17 | Sp. 0.93 | +LR 2.5 | -LR 0.90

***Clunk Test***[83]  While the patient lies supine, the athletic trainer grasps the elbow with one hand and places the other hand on the posterior humerus. The arm is passively abducted and externally rotated with an anterior force applied to the humeral head. The arm is then circumducted while the athletic trainer feels for a clunking sensation. A positive test may indicate the presence of a tear in the glenoid labrum (Figure 22-14).[52] Sn. 0.44 | Sp. 0.68 | +LR 1.38 | -LR 0.82

***O'Brien's Test (Active Compression Test)***[84]  With the patient sitting, the glenohumeral joint is flexed to 90 degrees and horizontally adducted 15 degrees from the sagittal plane. The humerus is fully internally rotated with the forearm pronated (Figure 22-15). The athletic trainer applies downward pressure over the distal forearm. The test is repeated with the humerus externally rotated and the forearm supinated. If pain is present when the humerus is internally rotated but decreases in external rotation, and if there is clicking within the glenohumeral joint, this may indicate an anteroposterior tear in the superior glenoid labrum, which is called a superior labrum anterior posterior (SLAP) lesion. Pain in the acromioclavicular joint with this test may indicate AC joint pathology.[84] Sn. 0.99 | Sp. 0.98 | +LR 61.1 | -LR 0.0

***Apprehension Test (Crank Test)***[34] *and* ***Relocation Test***[34]  With the arm abducted 90 degrees, the shoulder is slowly and gently externally rotated as far as the patient

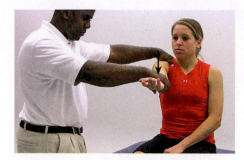

FIGURE 22–15   O'Brien's test, done with both the forearm supinated and pronated and the humerus internally rotated.
© William E. Prentice

will allow. The patient with a history of anterior glenohumeral instability will show great apprehension, reflected by a facial grimace before an endpoint can be reached. At no time should the athletic trainer force this movement (Figure 22–16A). Sn. 0.39 | Sp. 0.67 | +LR 1.23 | -LR 0.90

Posterior instability also can be determined through a *posterior apprehension test*. With the patient in a supine position, the shoulder is flexed to 90 degrees and the arm is horizontally adducted and internally rotated while a force is applied through the long axis of the humerus (Figure 22–16B). Sn. 0.4 | Sp. 0.73 | +LR 1.48 | -LR 0.82

The *relocation test* is done with the patient lying supine, the shoulder at 90 degrees and the elbow at 90 degrees. As the shoulder is externally rotated, pressure is applied posteriorly to stabilize the humeral head, which allows for a greater degree of external rotation than does the apprehension test (Figure 22–16C).[100] The test is positive if apprehension or pain is relieved with this maneuver. Sn. 0.36 | Sp. 0.63 | +LR 1.0 | -LR 1.0

### Tests for Shoulder Impingement

*Neer's Test*[83] In Neer's test, forced flexion of the humerus in the overhead position may cause impingement of soft-tissue structures between the humeral head and the coracoacromial arch (Figure 22–17A).[42] Sn. 0.33 | Sp. 0.60 | +LR 0.8 | -LR 1.1

*Hawkins-Kennedy Test*[50] The Hawkins-Kennedy test involves horizontal adduction with forced internal rotation of the humerus, which produces impingement (Figure 22–17B). A positive sign is indicated if the patient feels pain and reacts with a grimace.[42] Sn. 0.72 | Sp. 0.39 | +LR 1.2 | -LR 0.70

### Tests for Supraspinatus Muscle Weakness

*Drop Arm Test*[11] The drop arm test is designed to determine tears of the rotator cuff, primarily of the supraspinatus muscle. The patient abducts the arm as far as possible and then slowly lowers it to 90 degrees. From this position the patient with a torn supraspinatus muscle will be unable to lower the arm farther with control (Figure 22–18A). If the patient can hold the arm in a 90-degree position, pressre on the wrist will cause the arm to fall.[11] Sn. 0.78 | Sp. 0.97 | +LR 2.79 | -LR 0.95

*Empty Can Test*[40] The empty can test for supraspinatus muscle strength has the patient bring the arm into 90 degrees of forward flexion and 30 degrees of horizontal abduction (Figure 22–18B). In this position, the arm is internally rotated as far as possible, thumb pointing downward. The athletic trainer then applies a downward pressure. Weakness and pain can be detected in this position.[40] Sn. 0.65 | Sp. 0.70 | +LR 1.99 | -LR 0.43

> **Tests for supraspinatus weakness:**
> - Drop arm test
> - Empty can test
> - Rent test

*Rent Test*[113] With the patient seated with the arm relaxed the examiner palpates anterior to the anterior edge of the acromion with one hand while holding the patient's flexed elbow with the other. The shoulder is passively extended while slowly rotating the shoulder into external and internal rotation. The greater tuberosity will be prominent and a depression of about one finger width will be felt if a rotator cuff tear is present (Figure 22–18C). Sn. 0.96 | Sp. 0.97 | +LR 32 | -LR 0.04

**Test for Serratus Anterior Muscle Weakness** The patient performs a push-up movement against a wall.

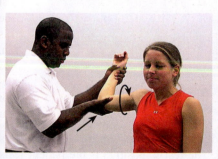
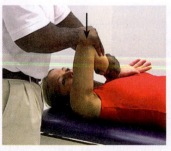
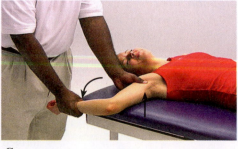

A                                B                                C

FIGURE 22–16   **(A)** Shoulder apprehension test. **(B)** Posterior apprehension test. **(C)** Relocation test.
© William E. Prentice

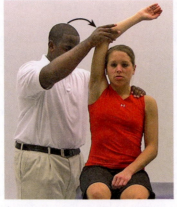
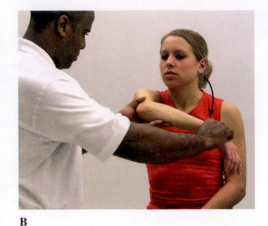

**A**    **B**

FIGURE 22–17   Shoulder impingement tests. **(A)** Neer's test—the humerus is in forced flexion in an overhead position. **(B)** Hawkins-Kennedy test—the humerus is forced into horizontal adduction and internal rotation.
© William E. Prentice

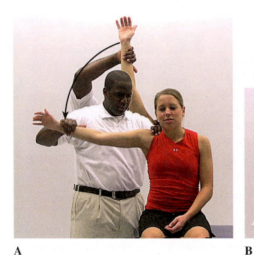
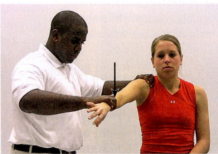
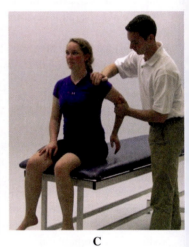

**A**                          **B**                                    **C**

FIGURE 22–18   Supraspinatus tests. **(A)** Drop arm test. **(B)** Empty can test. **(C)** Rent test.
© William E. Prentice

Winging of the scapula indicates weakness of the serratus anterior muscle. Winging of only one scapula could indicate an injury to the long thoracic nerve (Figure 22–19).[52]

### Tests for Biceps Tendon Irritation

***Yergason's Test***[39]   This test involves keeping the elbow at 90 degrees with the forearm pronated while the athlete attempts to actively supinate against the resistance of the athletic trainer as the humerus is also being pulled downward (Figure 22–20A). Pain indicates biceps tendon irritation.[39] Sn. 0.43 | Sp. 0.79 | +LR 2.05 | -LR 0.72

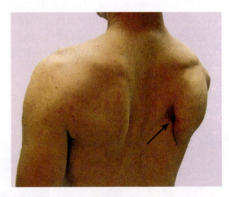

FIGURE 22–19   Winged scapula.
© William E. Prentice.

***Speed's Test***[39]
This test is performed with the patient's elbow extended, the forearm supinated, and

| Tests for biceps tendon irritation: |
|---|
| • Yergason's test |
| • Speed's test |
| • Ludington's test |

resistance applied as the humerus elevates to 60 degrees (Figure 22–20B). The test is positive if the patient feels pain in the region of the bicipital groove. If there is instability, the tendon may subluxate out of its groove.[39]
Sn. 0.32 | Sp. 0.75 | +LR 1.28 | -LR 0.91

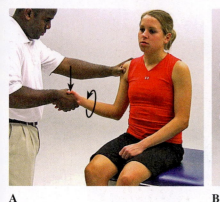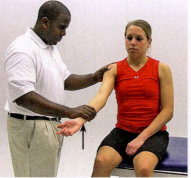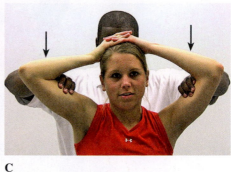

**A**        **B**        **C**

FIGURE 22–20    Biceps tendon irritation tests. **(A)** Yergason's test. **(B)** Speed's test. **(C)** Ludington's test.
© William E. Prentice

**Ludington's Test**[75] This test is performed with the patient in a seated position with hands clasped behind the head. The biceps muscles are alternately contracted and relaxed. The athletic trainer palpates the biceps muscles; if no contraction is felt on one side, there is likely a rupture (Figure 22–20C).[75] Sn. 0.81 | Sp. 0.91 | +LR* 3.24 | -LR* 0.21

An assembly line worker comes into the athletic training clinic, complaining of paresthesia and pain extending down the arm, of a sensation of cold, impaired circulation in the fingers, and muscle weakness. During the evaluation, it also becomes apparent that the patient has some muscle atrophy in the affected extremity. The athletic trainer suspects that the patient has thoracic outlet compression syndrome.

**?** What specific tests should the athletic trainer do to determine whether thoracic outlet compression syndrome is present, and what do those tests indicate?

**Circulatory Assessment** It is essential that patients with shoulder complaints be evaluated for impaired circulation. Pulse rates are routinely obtained over the axillary, brachial, and radial arteries. The axillary artery is found in the axilla against the shaft of the humerus. The brachial artery is a continuation of the axillary artery and follows the medial border of the biceps brachii muscle toward the elbow. The radial pulse is found at the anterior lateral aspect of the wrist over the radius. Taking the radial pulse indicates the total circulation the shoulder and arm.

Skin temperature is subjectively assessed by a comparison of the backs of the patient's hands. A cold temperature can be an indication of blood vessel constriction.

**Tests for Thoracic Outlet Compression Syndrome**
**Anterior Scalene Syndrome Test (Adson's Test)**[59] The purpose of this test is to determine whether the subclavian artery is being compressed as it enters the outlet

canal that lies between the heads of the anterior and middle scalene muscles. Compression can also occur between the cervical rib and the anterior scalene muscle. This maneuver is performed with the patient seated on a stool, with one hand resting on the thigh. The athlete's radial pulse is taken, first with the arm relaxed and then extended, while the patient elevates the chin, turns the face toward the extended hand, and holds the breath (Figure 22–21A). A positive test is one in which the pulse is depressed or stopped completely in the testing position.[85] Sn. 0.53 | Sp. 0.94 | +LR* 8.83 | -LR* 0.5

> **Tests for thoracic outlet compression syndrome:**
> • Adson's test
> • Allen test
> • Military brace position test
> • Roo's test

**Hyperabduction Syndrome Test (Allen Test)**[62] In a patient with hyperabduction syndrome, the subclavian and axillary vessels and the brachial plexus are compressed as they move behind the pectoralis minor muscle and beneath the coracoid process. To test for this syndrome, the patient's radial pulse is taken while the elbow is flexed to 90 degrees and the shoulder is extended horizontally and rotated laterally. The patient is asked to rotate the head away from the affected arm. If the pulse disappears, the test is positive (Figure 22–21B).[62] Sn. 0.73 | Sp. 0.97 | +LR* 24.3 | -LR* 0.28

**Military Brace Position Test**[88] The military brace position test indicates costoclavicular compression of the subclavian artery. While the patient stands, the shoulders are retracted as if coming to attention. The arm is abducted to 30 degrees and extended, and the head is turned to the opposite shoulder (Figure 22–21C). If the test is positive, the radial pulse disappears. Sn. 0.95 | Sp. 0.53 | +LR* 2.02 | -LR* 0.09

**Costoclavicular Syndrome Test (Roo's Test)**[53] This test indicates whether the subclavian artery is being compressed between the first rib and the clavicle. While the patient is in

*Calculated from sensitivity and specificity.

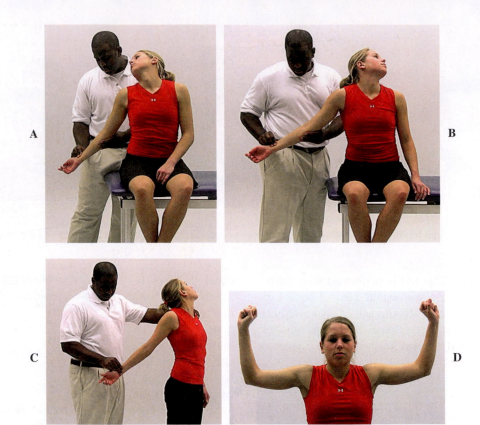

FIGURE 22–21  Thoracic outlet compression syndrome tests. **(A)** Anterior scalene syndrome test (Adson's test). **(B)** Hyperabduction syndrome test (Allen test). **(C)** Military brace position test. **(D)** Costoclavicular syndrome test (Roo's test).
© William E. Prentice

a sitting position, both arms are abducted to 90 degrees and externally rotated (Figure 22–21D). The patient opens and closes the hands and fingers, making fists for 3 minutes. Loss of strength in the hands or loss of sensation in the upper extremity are indicative of thoracic outlet compression syndrome.[53] Sn. 0.84 | Sp. 0.30 | +LR* 1.2 | -LR* 0.53

**Sensation Testing**  When there is injury to the shoulder complex, a routine test of cutaneous sensation should be performed.[89] Dermatome levels are tested for pain and light pressure (see Figure 13–5).

*Clinical Prediction Rules*  The following clinical prediction rules are currently used for the knee joint:

- *Rotator cuff pathology*[55]—identifies patients who likely have a full-thickness rotator cuff tear based on specific physical examination findings.
- *Subacromial impingement*[86]—identifies patients who likely have subacromial impingement based on specific physical examination findings.
- *Anterior shoulder instability*[29]—identifies patients likely to present with anterior shoulder instability due to a traumatic incident.

*Calculated from sensitivity and specificity.

- *Cervicothoracic manipulation for shoulder pain*[77]—identifies individuals with shoulder pain who are likely to experience immediate improvement in pain and disability following cervical and thoracic spine manipulation.

### Subjective Shoulder Scale Assessment

The American Shoulder and Elbow Surgeons (ASES) Subjective Shoulder Scale contains both a patient-derived subjective assessment and a physician-derived objective assessment.[51] It is widely used for outcomes assessment in patients with shoulder instability, rotator cuff disease, and glenohumeral arthritis. The subjective patient self-report section consists of two domains, pain and function. Pain is recorded on an ordinal scale, ranging from 0 to 10, and accounts for 50 percent of the overall ASES score. Function is also recorded on an ordinal scale, ranging from 0 to 10 in difficulty; it accounts for the other 50 percent of the overall score and is based on 10 questions:

- Putting on a coat
- Sleeping on the affected side
- Washing the back or putting on a bra
- Managing toileting
- Combing hair
- Reaching a high shelf

- Lifting 10 pounds (4.5 kg) above the shoulder
- Throwing a ball overhead
- Participating in work
- Participating in sports

# RECOGNITION AND MANAGEMENT OF SPECIFIC INJURIES

## Clavicular Fractures

***Etiology*** Clavicular fractures are among the most frequent fractures in sports. Fractures of the clavicle result from a fall on the outstretched arm, a fall on the tip of the shoulder, or a direct impact (Figure 22–22A). The majority of clavicle fractures occur in the middle third of the bone from a direct impact. In young patients, these are usually greenstick fractures.[90]

***Symptoms and signs*** The patient with a fractured clavicle usually supports the arm on the injured side and tilts his or her head toward that side, with the chin turned to the opposite side. During inspection the injured clavicle appears slightly lower than the unaffected side (Figure 22–22B). Palpation may also reveal swelling, point tenderness, and mild deformity.

***Management*** The clavicular fracture is cared for immediately by applying a sling and swathe bandage and by treating the patient for shock, if necessary. If X-ray examination reveals a fracture (Figure 22–22C), the physician should attempt a closed reduction followed by immobilization with a figure-eight brace (Figure 22–22D). Immobilization should be maintained for 6 to 8 weeks. After this period of immobilization, gentle isometric and mobilization exercises should begin while the patient wears a sling for an additional 3 to 4 weeks to provide protection. Occasionally, clavicle fractures require operative management.[18]

## Scapular Fractures

***Etiology*** Fracture of the scapula is an infrequent injury (Figure 22–23). Although the scapula appears extremely vulnerable to trauma, it is well protected by a heavy outer bony border and a cushion of muscle above and below. Those fractures that do occur happen as a result of a direct impact or when the force is transmitted through the humerus to the scapula. Fractures may occur to the body, the glenoid, the acromion, and the coracoid.[10]

***Symptoms and signs*** A scapular fracture may cause the patient to have pain during shoulder movement, as well as swelling and point tenderness.

***Management*** When this injury is suspected, the patient should be given a supporting sling and sent directly to the physician for X-rays. The arm should be supported in a sling for 3 weeks, with overhead strengthening exercises beginning at week 1.

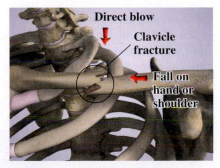

A

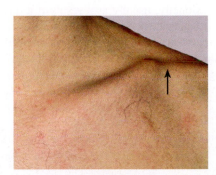

B

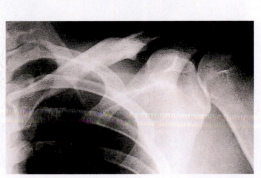

C

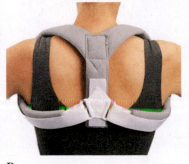

D

FIGURE 22–22 **(A)** Mechanisms of clavicular fracture. **(B)** Typical appearance of a clavicular fracture with obvious bone deformity. **(C)** X-ray of a comminuted clavicular fracture. **(D)** Protective sling for clavicular fracture.

(b–c) © William E. Prentice; (d) Courtesy DJO Global

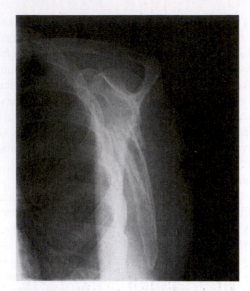

FIGURE 22–23  Fractures of the scapula are infrequent in sports.

Courtesy Jordan B. Renner, MD, Departments of Radiology and Allied Health Sciences, University of North Carolina

**Fractures of the Humerus** Fractures can occur to the humeral shaft, the proximal humerus, and the head of the humerus (epiphyseal fracture).[92]

*Etiology* The etiology of a fracture of the humerus varies with the type of fracture.

*Humeral shaft* Fractures of the humeral shaft (Figure 22–24A) happen occasionally, usually as a result of a direct blow or a fall on the arm. The type of fracture is usually comminuted or transverse, and a deformity is often produced because the bone fragments override each other as a result of strong muscular pull. The pathological process is characteristic of most uncomplicated fractures, except that there may be a tendency for the radial nerve, which encircles the humeral shaft, to be severed by jagged bone edges, resulting in radial nerve paralysis and causing wrist drop and an inability to perform forearm supination.

*Proximal humerus* Fractures of the proximal humerus (Figure 22–24B) pose considerable danger to the nerves and vessels of that area. Fractures of the humerus can result from a direct blow, a dislocation, or the impact received by falling onto the outstretched arm. Various parts of the end of the humerus may be involved, such as the anatomical neck, tuberosities, or surgical neck. This fracture may be mistaken for a shoulder dislocation. Most fractures take place at the surgical neck.[92]

*Epiphyseal fracture* In young patients, epiphyseal fracture of the head of the humerus (Figure 22–24C) is much more common than is a bone fracture. An epiphyseal injury in the shoulder region occurs most frequently in individuals 10 years of age and younger. It is caused by a direct blow or by an indirect force traveling along the length of the axis of the humerus. This condition causes shortening of the arm, disability, swelling, point tenderness, and pain. There also may be a false joint (immature cartilagenous joint). This type of injury should be suspected when the aforementioned signs appear in young athletes.

*Symptoms and signs* It may be difficult to recognize a fracture of the humerus by visual inspection alone; therefore, X-ray examination gives the only positive proof. Some of the more prevalent signs that may be present are pain, inability to move the arm, swelling, point tenderness, and discoloration of the superficial tissue. Because of the proximity of the axillary blood vessels and the brachial plexus, a fracture to the upper end of the humerus may result in severe hemorrhaging or paralysis.

*Management* Recognition of humeral shaft fractures requires immediate application of a splint, treatment for

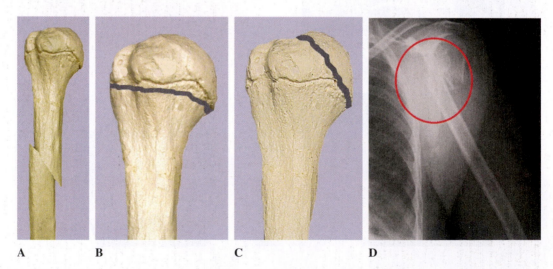

A          B          C          D

FIGURE 22–24  Humeral fractures. **(A)** Upper shaft fracture. **(B)** Proximal humeral fracture. **(C)** Epiphyseal fracture. **(D)** X-ray of proximal humeral fracture.

(a–c) © William E. Prentice; (d) Courtesy Jordan B. Renner, MD, Departments of Radiology and Allied Health Sciences, University of North Carolina

shock, and referral to a physician. The patient with a fracture to the humeral shaft will be out of competition for 3 to 4 months.

A suspected fracture of the proximal humerus warrants immediate support with a sling and swathe bandage and referral to a physician. Incapacitation may last for 2 to 6 months.

Initial treatment for epiphyseal fractures should include splinting and immediate referral to a physician. Healing is initiated rapidly; immobilization is necessary for only approximately 3 weeks. The main danger of this injury lies in the possibility of damage to the epiphyseal growth centers of the humerus.[92]

## Sternoclavicular Sprain

*Etiology*   A sternoclavicular sprain (Figure 22–25) is a relatively uncommon occurrence, but occasionally this sprain results from one of the various traumas affecting the shoulder complex. The mechanism of injury can be initiated by an indirect force transmitted through the humerus of the shoulder joint; by direct violence, such as a blow that strikes the poorly padded clavicle; or by torsion of a posteriorly extended arm.[35] Depending on the direction of force, the medial end of the clavicle can be displaced upward and forward, slightly anteriorly.

*Symptoms and signs*   Trauma resulting in a sprain to the sternoclavicular joint can be described in three grades. A grade 1 sprain is characterized by little pain and disability, with some point tenderness but no joint deformity. A grade 2 sprain displays subluxation of the sternoclavicular joint with visible deformity, pain, swelling, point tenderness, and an inability to abduct the shoulder in full range or to bring the arm across the chest, indicating disruption of stabilizing ligaments.

A grade 3 sprain, which is the most severe, presents a picture of complete dislocation with gross displacement of the clavicle at its sternal junction, swelling, and disability, indicating complete rupture of the sternoclavicular and costoclavicular ligaments. If the clavicle is displaced posteriorly, pressure may be placed on the blood vessels, esophagus, or trachea, causing a life-or-death situation.

*Management*
POLICE should be used immediately after injury. Care of this condition is based on reducing a displaced clavicle to its original position, which is done by a physician, and immobilizing it at that point, so that healing can take place. A deformity, primarily caused by the formation of scar tissue at that point, is usually apparent after healing is completed. There is no loss of function. Immobilization is usually maintained for 3 to 5 weeks, followed by graded reconditioning exercises. There is a high incidence of recurrence of sternoclavicular sprains.[35]

## Acromioclavicular Sprain

*Etiology*   The acromioclavicular joint is extremely vulnerable to sprains among active sports participants, especially in collision sports (Figure 22–26).[7] The mechanism of an acromioclavicular sprain is most often a direct impact to the tip of the shoulder, forcing the acromion process downward, backward, and inward while the clavicle is pushed down against the rib cage. Injury may also occur when an upward force is exerted against the long axis of the humerus by a fall on an outstretched arm. The position of the arm during indirect injury is one of adduction and partial flexion.[7] Depending on the extent of ligamentous involvement, the acromioclavicular sprain may be classified as a grade 1 through a grade 6 (Figure 22–27).[2] Direct impact injuries usually cause more severe injury.

A program of prevention should entail proper fitting of protective equipment, conditioning to provide a balance of strength and flexibility to the entire shoulder complex, and education on the proper techniques of falling and the use of the arm in sports.

*Contusion to the distal end of the clavicle*   Contusions of this type are often called shoulder pointers and cause a bone bruise and subsequent irritation to the periosteum. During initial inspection, this injury may be mistaken for a grade 1 acromioclavicular sprain. In most cases, these conditions are self-limiting. When the athlete is able to move the shoulder freely, he or she can return to sports activities.

*Symptoms and signs*   The grade 1 acromioclavicular sprain reflects point tenderness and discomfort during movement at the junction between the acromion process and the outer end of the clavicle. There is no disruption of the acromioclavicular joint, indicating only mild stretching of the acromioclavicular and coracoclavicular ligaments (Figure 22–27A).

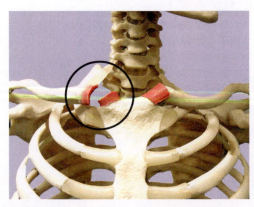

FIGURE 22–25   Sternoclavicular sprain and dislocation.
© William E. Prentice

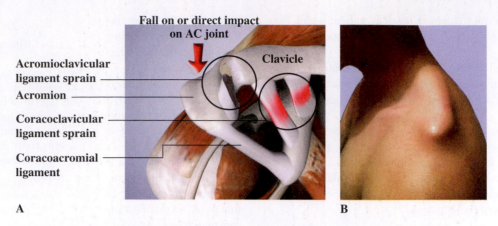

FIGURE 22–26   Acromioclavicular sprain. **(A)** Direct impact is a primary mechanism.
**(B)** The acromioclavicular ligament is disrupted, and the clavicle may be displaced.

(b) Courtesy Cody Malley, PA, ATC, Duke Orthopedics

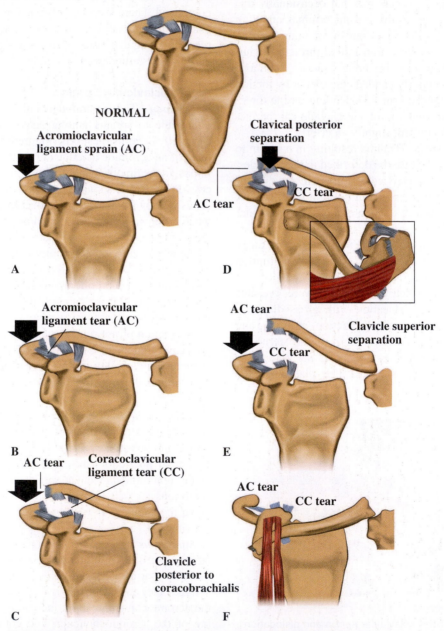

FIGURE 22–27   Classification of acromioclavicular sprains. **(A)** Grade 1.
**(B)** Grade 2. **(C)** Grade 3. **(D)** Grade 4. **(E)** Grade 5. **(F)** Grade 6.

A grade 2 sprain indicates tearing or rupture of acromioclavicular ligaments, with associated stretching of the coracoclavicular ligament. There is partial displacement and prominence of the lateral end of the clavicle when compared with the unaffected side, especially when the acromioclavicular stress test is initiated. In this moderate sprain, there is point tenderness during palpation of the injury site, and the athlete is unable to fully abduct through a full range of motion or to bring the arm completely across the chest (Figure 22–27B).

Although it occurs less frequently, a grade 3 sprain involves complete rupture of the acromioclavicular and coracoclavicular ligaments (Figure 22–27C).

A grade 4 sprain exhibits posterior separation of the clavicle, with complete disruption of the acromioclavicular ligament (Figure 22–27D). In some grade 4 sprains, the coracoclavicular ligaments may remain intact.

In a grade 5 sprain, there is complete loss of both the acromioclavicular and the coracoclavicular ligaments, in addition to tearing of the trapezius and deltoid attachment to the clavicle and acromion. Such an injury reflects gross deformity and prominence of the distal clavicle, severe pain, loss of movement, and instability of the shoulder complex (Figure 22–27E).

A grade 6 injury is very rare and involves the clavicle being displaced inferior to the coracoid behind the coracobrachialis tendon (Figure 22–27F).

*Management*   Immediate care of the acromioclavicular sprain involves three basic procedures: (1) application of cold and pressure to control local hemorrhage, (2) stabilization of the joint by a sling and swathe bandage, and (3) referral to a physician for definitive diagnosis and treatment.

A grade 1 sprain requires use of a sling for 3 or 4 days. A grade 2 sprain requires 10 to 14 days of protection in a sling. The current recommended management for a grade 3 sprain is nonoperative with approximately 2 weeks of protection in a sling. Grades 4 through 6 require surgical intervention using open reduction with internal fixation.[2] If there is posterior displacement of the clavicle, surgical reduction and fixation will be necessary. With all grades, an aggressive rehabilitation program involving joint mobilization, flexibility exercises, and strengthening exercises should begin immediately after the recommended period of protection. Progression should be as rapid as the patient can tolerate without increased pain or swelling. The joint should also be protected with appropriate padding until a pain-free, full range of motion returns.[2]

### Glenohumeral Joint Sprain

*Etiology*   The mechanism of this injury is similar to that which produces dislocations and strains. Anterior capsular sprains occur when the arm is forced into abduction (e.g., when making an arm tackle in football). Sprains can also occur from external rotation of the arm. A direct blow to the shoulder can also result in a sprain. The pathological process of a sprain to the glenohumeral joint often involves the rotator cuff muscles.[65]

The infraspinatus–teres minor muscle group is the most effective in controlling external rotation of the humerus and in reducing ligamentous injury.[69] The posterior capsule can be sprained by a forceful movement of the humerus posteriorly when the arm is flexed.

*Symptoms and signs*   The patient complains of pain during arm movement, especially when the sprain mechanism is reproduced. There may be decreased range of motion and pain during palpation.

*Management*   Care after acute trauma to the shoulder joint requires the use of a cold pack for 24 to 48 hours, elastic or adhesive compression, rest, and immobilization by a sling. After hemorrhage has subsided, a program of cryotherapy or ultrasound and massage may be added, and mild passive and active exercise is advocated for regaining full range of motion. Once the patient can execute full shoulder range of motion without signs of pain, a resistance exercise program should be initiated. Any traumatic injury to the shoulder joint can lead to a subacute and chronic condition of either synovitis or bursitis, which, in the absence of shoulder movement, allows muscle contractures, adhesions, and atrophy to develop, resulting in an ankylosed (stiffened or fixed) shoulder joint.[65]

### Acute Dislocations and Subluxations   Shoulder dislocations account for up to 50 percent of all dislocations. The extreme range of mobility in the normal shoulder creates an inherent instability in the joint, which is susceptible to dislocation. The most common kind of displacement is that occurring anteriorly. Posterior dislocations account for 1 to 4.3 percent of all shoulder dislocations. Inferior dislocations are extremely rare. Of dislocations caused by direct trauma, 85 to 90 percent recur.[65]

*Etiology*

*Subluxations*   With glenohumeral subluxations, there is excessive translation of the humeral head without complete separation of the joint surfaces. Subluxation is a brief, transient occurrence in which the humeral head quickly returns to its normal position relative to the glenoid. Subluxation can occur anteriorly, posteriorly, or inferiorly.

*Anterior/Inferior glenohumeral dislocation*   An anterior/inferior glenohumeral dislocation may result from direct

A football player has suffered an anterior dislocation of the glenohumeral joint while making a tackle. He is really concerned about missing the remainder of the season and is the type of athlete who wants to know everything there is to know about the injury. He asks the athletic trainer to explain to him exactly what has happened and what other problems might exist along with this injury.

**?** What should the athletic trainer tell this player about the possible ramifications of this injury?

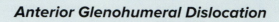

# MANAGEMENT PLAN

## Anterior Glenohumeral Dislocation

**Injury Situation** An army infantry soldier was training on an obstacle course. While attempting to scale a wall, the soldier fell and injured his shoulder. When he landed on the ground, the shoulder was forced into a position of abduction, external rotation, and extension. He was taken to the infirmary, where he was evaluated by a civilian athletic trainer.

**Symptoms and Signs** The patient felt his shoulder give way and felt a pop and a tearing sensation with intense pain. There was a flattened deltoid contour. Palpation of the axilla revealed prominence of the humeral head. The dislocated arm was in slight abduction and external rotation, and the patient was unable to touch the opposite shoulder with the hand of the affected arm.

**Management Plan** The athletic trainer immediately immobilized the dislocated shoulder, without attempting reduction. The patient was then referred to a physician for reduction after X-rays ruled out fracture. After the dislocation was reduced and immobilized, muscle reconditioning was initiated as soon as possible.

---

*Phase* 1 *Acute Injury*   **GOALS:** To control pain and swelling and to begin to regain range of motion.
**ESTIMATED LENGTH OF TIME (ELT):** 1 to 5 days.

- **Therapy** POLICE should be applied immediately and should continue to be used for the next several days. Initial management of an anterior shoulder dislocation requires immediate immobilization in a position of comfort, using a sling with a folded towel or small pillow placed under the arm. Protective sling immobilization should continue for approximately 1 week after reduction. In anterior dislocations, the arm should be maintained in a relaxed position of adduction and internal rotation.
- **Exercise rehabilitation** While the shoulder is immobilized, the patient is instructed to perform isometric exercises for strengthening the internal and external rotator muscles. Codman's pendulum exercises and sawing exercises (see Figure 22–34A) can help the patient regain range of motion as pain allows.

---

*Phase* 2 *Repair*   **GOALS:** To achieve full range of motion and increase strength.
**ELT:** 5 to 12 days.

- **Therapy** Ice and electrical stimulation should be used to modulate pain. Low-intensity ultrasound may also be used to facilitate healing. The patient may continue to wear the sling but should be progressively weaned from it as pain allows.
- **Exercise rehabilitation** Range of motion exercises using a T-bar can be instituted as early as tolerated. Wall climbing and rope-and-pulley exercises can also be used to regain motion. The strengthening program should progress from isometrics to resistive rubber tubing exercises and then to dumbbells and other resistance devices as quickly as can be tolerated. Exercises should concentrate on strengthening the rotator cuff. Weight shifting with the hands on the ground can help the patient begin strengthening the scapular stabilizers and reestablishing neuromuscular control.

---

*Phase* 3 *Remodeling*   **GOALS:** To regain normal strength and return to full activity.
**ELT:** 12 days to 3 weeks.

- **Therapy** Electrical stimulation can be used for muscle reeducation. Ultrasound can be used for deep heating to increase blood flow to clean up the injured area. Ice should be used after exercise.
- **Exercise rehabilitation** Strengthening exercises should progress from resisted isotonics to isokinetics at greater speeds. Functional D1 and D2 PNF strengthening patterns should be used, adjusting resistance to the patient's capabilities. Plyometric activities using weighted balls can be used to work on more dynamic control. Closed kinetic chain exercises using weight shifting on a ball or balance device improves neuromuscular control. Functional progressions use various activities that require overhead motion and throwing.

### Criteria for Return to Activity

1. The shoulder should have full range of motion and be pain free.
2. Shoulder strength should be nearly normal.
3. Throwing and catching activities should not produce pain.
4. Protective shoulder braces may be worn to help limit shoulder motion.

impact to the posterior or posterolateral aspect of the shoulder. The most common mechanism is forced abduction, external rotation, and extension that forces the humeral head out of the glenoid cavity (Figure 22–28).[65] An arm tackle in football or rugby or abnormal forces created in executing a throw can produce a sequence of events resulting in dislocation.

In an anterior/inferior glenohumeral dislocation, the head of the humerus is forced out of its articular capsule in an anterior direction past the glenoid labrum and then downward to rest under the coracoid process. The scope of the pathological process is extensive, with torn capsular and ligamentous tissue, possibly tendinous avulsion of the rotator cuff muscles or long head of the biceps, possibly injury to the brachial plexus, and profuse hemorrhage.

A tear, or detachment, of the glenoid labrum may occur and is considered the essential lesion in shoulder instability.[12,54] Healing is usually slow, and the detached labrum and capsule can produce a permanent anterior defect on the labrum called a *Bankart lesion*.[19] A moderately frequent occurrence resulting from instability in primary and recurrent dislocations would be a bony Bankart lesion. This would potentially necessitate early surgical intervention.[50] Another defect that can occur after dislocation is found on the posterior lateral aspect of the humeral head and is referred to as a *Hill-Sachs lesion*. It is caused by the compression of the cancellous bone of the head of the humerus against the anterior glenoid rim that creates a divot in the humeral head. A *superior labrum anterior/posterior (SLAP) lesion* is another defect in the

labrum.[19] It is caused by an injury to the superior aspect of the labrum that begins posteriorly, extends anteriorly, and affects the attachment of the long head of the biceps to the superior labrum.

Additional complications may arise if the head of the humerus comes in contact with and injures the brachial nerves and vessels. Rotator cuff tears may also occur with anterior dislocations. The bicipital tendon may also be subluxated from its canal as a result of a rupture of its transverse ligament.[76]

***Posterior glenohumeral dislocation*** The mechanism of injury is usually forced adduction and internal rotation of the shoulder or a fall on an extended and internally rotated arm. As with anterior dislocations, posterior dislocations exhibit significant soft-tissue damage. Tears of the posterior glenoid labrum are common in posterior dislocation. A fracture of the lesser tuberosity may occur as the subscapularis tendon avulses its attachment. A *reverse Hill-Sachs lesion* defect can occur on the anteromedial portion of the humeral head following a posterior shoulder dislocation.

***Symptoms and signs*** The patient with an anterior dislocation displays a flattened deltoid contour. Palpation of the axilla reveals prominence of the humeral head. The patient carries the affected arm in slight abduction and external rotation and is unable to touch the opposite shoulder with the hand of the affected arm. There is often moderate pain and disability.

Posterior glenohumeral dislocation produces severe pain and disability. The arm is often held in adduction and internal rotation. The anterior deltoid muscle is flattened, the acromion and coracoid processes are prominent, and the head of the humerus also may be seen posteriorly. There is limited external rotation and elevation.

***Management*** Initial management of the shoulder dislocation requires immediate immobilization in a position of comfort, using a sling with a folded towel or small pillow placed under the arm; immediate reduction by a physician; and control of the hemorrhage by cold packs. Physicians generally agree that a first-time dislocation

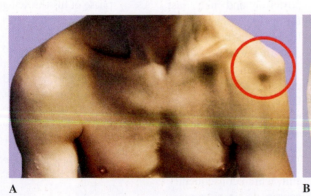
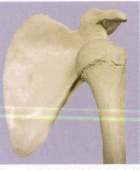
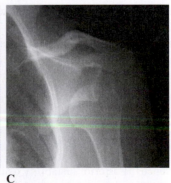

A                                    B                                    C

FIGURE 22–28  Glenohumeral dislocation. **(A)** Appearance of an anterior/inferior dislocation. **(B)** The humeral head is anterior and inferior to the glenoid. **(C)** X-ray view.

(a) Courtesy Dave Haygarth; (b) © William E. Prentice; (c) Courtesy Jordan B. Renner, MD, Departments of Radiology and Allied Health Sciences, University of North Carolina

may be associated with a fracture and therefore should not be reduced by the athletic trainer. Ideally, X-rays should be taken before the physician attempts to reduce the dislocated shoulder.[25]

Often, a physician will attempt an immediate reduction of anterior dislocations on the field, using the *Milch technique*, which is a method of elevation and external "derotation" of the arm placed in minimal traction. If unsuccessful, the physician may suggest other methods that use a muscle relaxant. Recurrent dislocations do not present the same complications or attendant dangers as the acute type. However, risk is always involved. Reducing the anterior dislocation usually can be accomplished by applying traction to the abducted and flexed arm.

Reduction of a posterior dislocation may have to be performed with the patient under anesthesia. The procedure usually involves traction on the arm with the elbow bent, followed by adduction of the arm, with posterior pressure being applied to the humeral head anteriorly. While in traction, the arm is slowly externally rotated and then internally rotated.

After the dislocation has been reduced and immobilized, muscle reconditioning should be initiated as soon as possible.[80] Protective sling immobilization should continue for approximately 3 weeks after reduction.[108] In anterior dislocations, the arm should be maintained in a relaxed position of adduction and internal rotation. In posterior dislocations, the shoulder is immobilized in a position of external rotation and slight abduction. While immobilized, the patient should perform isometric exercises for strengthening the internal and external rotator muscles. The strengthening program should progress from isometrics to resistive rubber tubing exercises, then to dumbbells and other resistance devices as quickly as pain will allow. A major criterion for the patient's return to activity is that internal and external rotation strength equals to 20 percent of the patient's body weight. Protective shoulder braces may help limit shoulder motion (see Figure 22–32).[108]

**Recurrent Instabilities of the Shoulder** Recurrent shoulder instabilities can occur after acute subluxation or dislocation. Recurrent instabilities may be anterior, posterior, inferior, or multidirectional. Anterior instability accounts for 95 percent of all recurrent instabilities and usually results after an acute anterior dislocation. With anterior instability, repeated episodes of anterior dislocation have a high probability of occurrence.[69] Posterior instability usually recurs as a subluxation rather than a dislocation. Shoulders that have either an anterior or a posterior instability may also subluxate or dislocate inferiorly.[64] If this occurs, a multidirectional instability exists in which there is instability in more than one plane of motion. Multidirectional instabilities most

> Recurrent instabilities may be anterior, posterior, inferior, or multidirectional.

often involve a combination of anteroinferior or posteroinferior laxity but can involve all three directions.[17] It is also possible for a shoulder to dislocate in one direction and subluxate in another.[65]

***Etiology*** The causes of shoulder instabilities may be traumatic (macrotraumatic), atraumatic, microtraumatic (repetitive use), congenital, or neuromuscular.[37] As discussed earlier, traumatic episodes occur from one or more traumatic situations that cause a complete or partial joint displacement. Atraumatic episodes occur in a patient who either voluntarily or involuntarily displaces the shoulder joint because of inherent ligamentous laxity.[64]

> Shoulder instabilities may be attributed to traumatic (macrotraumatic), atraumatic, microtraumatic (repetitive use), congenital, or neuromuscular causes.

Microtraumatic episodes are created by repetitive use of the shoulder, usually involving some faulty biomechanics, that leads to soft-tissue laxity. Sports activities such as baseball pitching, tennis serving, and freestyle swimming may produce anterior shoulder instabilities; swimming the backstroke or hitting a backhand stroke in tennis can produce posterior instability. As the supporting tissue becomes increasingly lax, more mobility of the glenohumeral head is allowed, eventually damaging the glenoid labrum. Increased laxity of the supportive capsular and tendinous structures leads to more instability and increases the likelihood of recurrent subluxations and dislocations.

***Symptoms and signs***
***Recurrent anterior instability*** Recurrent anterior instability may cause the athlete who throws to complain of pain or clicking or to experience what is described as a dead arm syndrome in the cocking phase of the overhead throwing motion.[96] Pain is often posterior and may last for several minutes, followed by extreme weakness of the entire arm.[69] Anterior instability may permit excessive translation of the humeral head on the glenoid.[69] This translation can produce repetitive compression of the rotator cuff, which consequently causes an impingement of soft tissues under the coracoacromial arch. Tests for apprehension may be positive. Range of motion should be assessed because of the possible decrease in external rotation.

> A baseball pitcher comes to the athletic trainer complaining of pain and a clicking feeling in his shoulder in the cocking phase of his throwing motion. He also indicates that he feels like his arm is "dead." His pain seems to be posterior and lasts for several minutes, followed by extreme weakness of the entire arm. On examination, he exhibits a positive apprehension sign.
>
> **?** What is likely the cause of this problem?

A javelin thrower has been forced to cease his training activity because of pain in his shoulder. He also feels that his shoulder is very unstable. He has been diagnosed by the physician as having both shoulder impingement syndrome and a multidirectional instability.

**?** Often, impingement and instability are thought of as being completely unrelated, when, in fact, it is common to find that athletes who engage in overhead motions exhibit signs and symptoms of both problems. How are impingement and instability related to one another?

*Recurrent posterior instability* A recurrent posterior instability may cause pain to occur posteriorly, anteriorly, or both as a result of subluxation. Joint laxity in a posterior instability, as in an anterior instability, can produce impingement, which is often more of a problem than the subluxation. Crepitation may also be noted on certain movements. There may be a loss of internal rotation when the arm is positioned at 90 degrees of abduction. Stress applied with the arm at 90 degrees of abduction and at 90 degrees of forward flexion, along with abduction and internal rotation, will allow the degree of posterior humeral head translation to be graded.

*Multidirectional instability* Multidirectional instability causes some inferior laxity, which exhibits a positive sulcus sign.[117] There is usually some pain and clicking when the arm is held by the side. Any of the symptoms and signs associated with anterior and posterior recurrent instability may be present with multidirectional instability.[17]

*Management* Recurrent instabilities may be managed either conservatively or surgically. The initial choice is almost always conservative. Strengthening of all the muscles surrounding the glenohumeral joint, as well as the muscles acting on the scapula, is critical to the success of the rehabilitative program. In particular, strengthening exercises should concentrate on the rotator cuff muscles, which provide dynamic stability in the glenohumeral joint, as well as on the scapular stabilizing muscles. With anterior instability, strengthening should focus on the internal rotators and the long head of the biceps; the external rotators should be strengthened with posterior instability; with multidirectional instability, the internal or external rotators and the biceps should be strengthened. Joint mobilization and flexibility exercises should be avoided regardless of the type of recurrent instability. Various types of shoulder harnesses and restraints may be used to limit shoulder motion.[14,65]

Surgical stabilization may be necessary if the strengthening program fails to improve shoulder function and comfort.[110] Strengthening exercises should be continued for a reasonable period of time before surgery is considered. A physician may choose a variety of surgical techniques or procedures to enhance shoulder stability.[8,87]

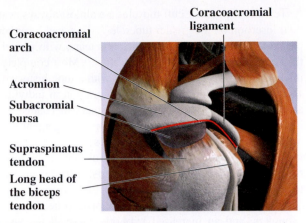

FIGURE 22–29 Shoulder impingement compresses the subacromial bursa, the supraspinatus tendon, and the long head of the biceps under the coracoacromial arch during humeral elevation.

## Shoulder Impingement

*Etiology* Shoulder impingement involves a mechanical compression of the supraspinatus tendon, the subacromial bursa, and the long head of the biceps tendon, all of which are located under the coracoacromial arch (Figure 22–29).[111] This mechanical compression is due to a decrease in space under the coracoacromial arch. Repetitive compression eventually leads to irritation and inflammation of these structures. Impingement most often occurs in repetitive overhead activities.[111]

Shoulder impingement is closely related to shoulder instability.[17] Individuals involved with overhead activities often exhibit hypermobility and significant capsular laxity.[42,115] Failure by the rotator cuff muscles to maintain the position of the humeral head relative to the glenoid in overhead activities allows for excessive translation of the humeral head.[56] Eventually, this repetitive stress leads to inflammation of the structures under the coracoacromial arch. Prolonged inflammation causes decreased muscular efficiency, and a progressively worsening cycle is created, which can ultimately result in rupture of the supraspinatus or biceps tendons.[71]

> Shoulder impingement involves a mechanical compression of the supraspinatus tendon, the subacromial bursa, and the long head of the biceps tendon under the coracoacromial arch.

A volleyball player consistently experiences pain when serving the ball overhead. She also indicates that, most of the time when she spikes a ball at the net, she experiences pain. During an evaluation, the athletic trainer observes that when the humerus is flexed and internally rotated the pain is worse.

**?** What is most likely causing this athlete's pain when her shoulder is placed in the overhead position?

22–9 Clinical Application Exercise

Tears of the rotator cuff muscles are almost always near their insertion on the greater tubercle.[114] They can be either partial-thickness or complete-thickness tears, with partial-thickness tears occurring twice as often.[71] Most complete-thickness tears appear in individuals with a long history of shoulder injury and are relatively uncommon in individuals under the age of 40 years.[58] The primary mechanism of injury is usually either acute trauma or impingement.[20] A rotator cuff tear nearly always involves the supraspinatus muscle.[111] A tear or complete rupture of one of the other rotator cuff tendons—the subscapularis, infraspinatus, or teres minor—is extremely rare.

Postural malalignment, such as a forward head, round shoulders, and an increased kyphotic curve, that causes the scapular glenoid to be positioned such that the space under the coracoacromial arch is decreased can also contribute to impingement.[109] Individuals who have a hook-shaped acromion are more likely to have problems with impingement.[63]

***Symptoms and signs*** Patients complain of diffuse pain around the acromion and may not complain of stiffness. Palpation of the subacromial space increases the pain. Overhead activities also increase pain.[98] Range of motion and rotator cuff strength are important physical exam findings.[79] Total range of motion in both internal and external rotation is a key in predicting injury. Swimmers and throwers demonstrate significantly increased glenohumeral external rotation, referred to as **external rotation gain (ERG)** and significantly decreased glenohumeral internal rotation, referred to as **glenohumeral internal rotation deficit (GIRD)**, in the throwing arm.[101] The external rotators are generally weaker than the internal rotators.[38] There is usually a positive impingement sign (see Figure 22–29), and both the empty can test and the drop arm test may increase pain.

Neer has described a series of progressive stages of shoulder impingement.[63] Stage I occurs in patients less than 25 years of age. An initial injury to the supraspinatus or long head of the biceps tendon produces aching after activity, point tenderness over the supraspinatus or biceps tendons, pain during abduction that becomes worse at 90 degrees, pain during straight-arm full flexion or resisted supination with external rotation, no palpable muscle defect, inflammation with edema, temporary thickening of the rotator cuff and the subacromial bursa, and possible atrophy and constriction of muscles in the region of the shoulder joint.

Stage II involves a permanent thickening and fibrosis of the supraspinatus and biceps tendons and at times the subacromial bursa. Symptoms include aching during activity that becomes worse at night, some restriction of arm movement, and no obvious muscle defect.

Stage III occurs in patients between the ages of 25 and 40. In this stage, the patient has a long history of shoulder problems, shoulder pain during activity with increased pain at night, a tendon defect of $\frac{3}{8}$ inch (1 cm) or less, a possible partial muscle tear, and permanent thickening of the rotator cuff and the acromial bursa with scar tissue.

Stage IV occurs in patients over the age of 40. In this stage, there is obvious infraspinatus and supraspinatus wasting, a great deal of pain when the arm is abducted to 90 degrees, a tendon defect greater than $\frac{3}{8}$ inch (1 cm), limited active and full passive range of motion, weakness during abduction and external rotation, and possible degeneration of the clavicle.

***Management*** Management of stages I and II impingement involves restoring normal biomechanics to the shoulder joint in an effort to maintain space under the coracoacromial arch during overhead activities.[31] Specific goals in the rehabilitation program should be based on the information obtained from a thorough evaluation.[78] Exercises should concentrate on strengthening the rotator cuff muscles, which compress and depress the humeral head relative to the glenoid. The muscles that abduct, elevate, and upwardly rotate the scapula and the external rotators should also be strengthened.[47] Strengthening of the lower-extremity and trunk muscles to reduce the strain placed on the shoulder and arm is also important for the throwing athlete. Posterior and inferior glenohumeral joint mobilizations should be done to reduce tightness in the posterior and inferior joint capsule.[16] Initially, POLICE and electrical stimulating currents can be used to modulate pain. Ultrasound and antiinflammatory medications should be used to reduce inflammation. The activity that caused the problem in the first place should be modified, so that there is some initial control over the frequency and level of the activity, with a gradual and progressive increase in intensity.[27]

Stages III and IV may require immobilization and complete rest. A patient who wants to continue activity may require surgical intervention.[97] Most typically, surgical intervention involves subacromial decompression.

## Scapular Dyskinesis

***Etiology*** Scapular dyskinesis is abnormal movement of the scapula. The term *SICK scapula* is a mnemonic that describes several factors that contribute to scapular dyskinesis: *s*capular malposition, *i*nferior medial scapular winging, *c*oracoid tenderness, and *k*inesis abnormalities of the scapula.[67] This occurs due to adaptive changes from the repetitive use of the shoulder, particularly in throwing athletes. These changes are detrimental to normal function of the shoulder and can increase the chances of injury.

***Symptoms and signs*** The patient tends to hold the affected shoulder lower than the other and rotated forward in what appears to be a slouched position. The inferior medial border of the scapula tends to be prominent, particularly in the cocking phase of the throwing motion. This is due to anterior tightness of the pectoralis major and minor muscles and weakness of the posterior lower trapezius and serratus anterior muscles. Posterior tipping of the scapula is responsible for functional narrowing of the subacromial space during the overhead motion, leading to pain

A painter is complaining of shoulder pain, particularly when his arm is in the overhead position when painting a ceiling. He has been diagnosed as having an impingement syndrome, and the physician has referred him to the athletic trainer for rehabilitation.

**?** What general considerations must the athletic trainer take into account when treating shoulder impingement syndrome?

in abduction and external rotation.[48] Winging of the entire medial border of the scapula at rest, which becomes more prominent in the cocking phase after repetitive elevation of the upper extremity, is caused by fatigue of the scapular stabilizing muscles, particularly the trapezius and rhomboids.[9] Winging of the superior medial border of the scapula is likely due to impingement and rotator cuff injury.[76]

*Management* Exercises should be incorporated into the treatment plan to stretch the posterior shoulder capsule, strengthen the scapular stabilizers, and stretch the pectoralis minor, coracobrachialis, and short head of the biceps. Throwing athletes should not return to throwing until there is some evidence of improvement in scapular positioning.

## Shoulder Bursitis

*Etiology* The shoulder joint is subject to chronic inflammatory conditions resulting from trauma or overuse. Inflammation may develop from a direct impact, a fall on the tip of the shoulder, or shoulder impingement. The bursa that is most often inflamed is the subacromial bursa. The pathological process in this condition involves fibrous buildup and fluid accumulation developing from a constant inflammatory state.[36]

*Symptoms and signs* The patient has pain when trying to move the shoulder, especially in abduction or with flexion, adduction, and internal rotation. There is also tenderness to palpation in the subacromial space. Impingement tests are positive.

*Management* The use of cold, ultrasound, and antiinflammatory medications to reduce inflammation is necessary. If impingement is the primary mechanism precipitating bursitis, the measures described in the previous section should be taken to correct it. The patient must maintain a consistent program of exercise that emphasizes maintaining a full range of motion, so that muscle contractures and adhesions do not immobilize the joint.

## Adhesive Capsulitis (Frozen Shoulder)

*Etiology* Adhesive capsulitis, or frozen shoulder, is a condition more characteristic of an older person, but occasionally it occurs in the younger patient. The exact cause of adhesive capsulitis is unclear. However, it involves a contracted and

Adhesive capsulitis is also called a frozen shoulder.

thickened joint capsule that is tight around the humeral head, with little synovial fluid.[93] There is also chronic inflammation with some fibrosis. The rotator cuff muscles are also contracted and inelastic. Constant, generalized inflammation causes pain on both active and passive motion. Thus, the individual will progressively resist moving the joint because of pain. The result is a stiff, or frozen, shoulder.[28]

*Symptoms and signs* Pain is reported in all directions of movement about the shoulder, with restriction or limitation of both active and passive movement.

*Management* The objectives are to relieve discomfort and restore motion. Treatment usually involves aggressive joint mobilization and stretching of tight muscles. Electrical stimulating currents may be used to reduce pain. Ultrasound is useful in providing penetrating heat to the area.

## Thoracic Outlet Compression Syndromes

*Etiology* Thoracic outlet compression syndromes involve compression of the brachial plexus, subclavian artery, and subclavian vein (neurovascular bundle) in the neck and shoulder.[91] Neurovascular compression can occur as a result of the following conditions:

- Compression of the neurovascular bundle in the narrowed space between the first rib and the clavicle (costoclavicular syndrome)
- Compression between the anterior and middle scalene muscles
- Compression by the pectoralis minor muscle as the neurovascular bundle passes beneath the coracoid process or between the clavicle and first rib
- The presence of a cervical rib (an abnormal rib originating from a cervical vertebra and the thoracic rib)

*Symptoms and signs* Abnormal pressure on the subclavian artery, subclavian vein, and brachial plexus produces a variety of symptoms, including paresthesia and pain, a sensation of cold, impaired circulation in the fingers, muscle weakness, muscle atrophy, and radial nerve palsy. Four tests, described earlier in this chapter, can be used to determine thoracic outlet compression syndromes: the anterior scalene syndrome test, the hyperabduction syndrome test, the military brace position test, and the costoclavicular syndrome test.[85]

*Management* A conservative approach should be taken with early and mild cases of thoracic outlet compression syndromes. Conservative treatment is favorable in 50 to 80 percent of cases.[91] It involves correcting the anatomical condition that is responsible for these syndromes with a series of stretching and strengthening exercises. Exercises should be done to strengthen the trapezius, the rhomboids, the serratus anterior, and the erector muscles of the spine. Stretching exercises for the pectoralis minor and the scalene muscles should also be used. If conservative treatment fails, it may be necessary to surgically release the anterior scalene muscle or possibly remove the first rib.

## Shoulder Impingement

**Injury Situation** A 24-year-old female middle-distance swimmer is in the third week of her preseason training program. She has significantly increased the distance she has been swimming during the last 3 weeks. Her workouts have increased to twice a day, and she has been swimming all freestyle. She is complaining of an aching pain in her left shoulder.

**Symptoms and Signs** The swimmer complains of diffuse pain around the acromion, with point tenderness over the supraspinatus or biceps tendons. Palpation of the subacromial space increases the pain. Overhead activities also increase the pain. There is an achy feeling when she finishes her workout. The external rotators are generally weaker than the internal rotators. There is tightness in the posterior and inferior joint capsule. There is a positive impingement sign, and both the empty can test and the drop arm test increase pain.[21]

**Management Plan** Management involves restoring normal biomechanics to the shoulder joint in an effort to maintain space under the coracoacromial arch during her swimming workout.

*Phase* 1 *Acute Injury*  GOALS: To control pain and inflammation.
ESTIMATED LENGTH OF TIME (ELT): 1 to 6 days.

- **Therapy** POLICE and electrical stimulating currents can be used to modulate pain initially. Ultrasound and anti-inflammatory medications should be used to reduce inflammation.
- **Exercise rehabilitation** Her aggressive swimming workout, which caused the problem in the first place, should be modified, so that there is some initial control over the frequency and the duration of the workout, with a gradual and progressive increase in distance. It may be necessary to keep her out of the pool during phase 1 to allow the inflammation to subside. To maintain her level of fitness, she should substitute running or exercising on a stationary bike for her swimming workout. She may continue her strengthening program, but she must discontinue any strengthening exercise using her sore shoulder.

*Phase* 2 *Repair*  GOALS: To alter joint biomechanics to reduce the likelihood of impingement.
ELT: 1 to 2 weeks.

- **Therapy** Continue using electrical stimulation and ice to modulate pain. Ultrasound is also helpful in reducing inflammation. Continue antiinflammatory medication.
- **Exercise rehabilitation** She may now get back into the pool and begin with a short kicking only workout initially and then gradually increase the duration and intensity, using increased pain or stiffness as a guide for progression. Exercises should concentrate on strengthening the rotator cuff and the muscles that abduct, elevate, and upwardly rotate the scapula. The external rotators should also be strengthened. It may be necessary to limit strengthening exercises in flexion or abduction. Any exercise that places the shoulder in impingement should be avoided. Posterior and inferior glenohumeral joint mobilizations should be done to reduce tightness in the posterior and inferior joint capsule.

*Phase* 3 *Remodeling*  GOALS: To return to unrestricted activity.
ELT: 2 weeks to full return.

- **Therapy** Use ultrasound before the workout and ice after completing the workout. Continue antiinflammatory medication.
- **Exercise rehabilitation** Strengthening exercises should progress to full-range overhead activities. PNF D1 and D2 strengthening patterns may be used with either manual or surgical tubing resistance. She must continue to work on strengthening the appropriate scapular muscles, as she did in phase 2. Exercises designed to stretch the inferior and posterior capsule should also be continued.

*Criteria for Return to Competitive Swimming*

1. The gradual program that has been used to increase the duration and intensity of the workout has allowed her to complete a workout without pain.
2. She exhibits improved strength in the rotator cuff and the scapular muscles.
3. She no longer has a positive impingement sign, drop arm test, or empty can test.
4. She can discontinue the use of antiinflammatory medications without a return of pain.

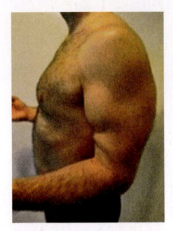

FIGURE 22–30    Biceps brachii rupture.

Blønd, Lars, and Bo Kaewkongnok. "Reconstruction of Delayed Diagnoses Simultaneous Bilateral Distal Biceps Tendon Ruptures Using Semtendinosus and Quadriceps Tendon Autografts." SpringerPlus 4: 117 (2015). PMC. © 2015 by Blønd, Lars, and Bo Kaewkongnok. All rights reserved. Used with permission.

### Biceps Brachii Ruptures

***Etiology***    Ruptures of the biceps brachii (Figure 22–30) can occur in any individual who is performing a powerful concentric or eccentric contraction of the muscle. The rupture commonly occurs near the origin of the muscle in the bicipital groove.[66]

***Symptoms and signs***    The patient usually hears a resounding snap and feels a sudden, intense pain at the point of injury. A bulge may appear near the middle of the biceps. When asked to flex the elbow joint of the injured arm and supinate the forearm, the patient displays a definite weakness.

***Management***    Treatment should include immediately applying a cold pack to control hemorrhage, placing the arm in a sling, and referring the patient to the physician. In some instances, the patient with a ruptured bicep will have surgery to repair it. But surgery is not always required and is sometimes deferred in overhead athletes. Older individuals may not require surgical repair because the brachialis muscle is the primary flexor of the elbow joint, and the majority of patients are able to function without their biceps.[95]

### Bicipital Tenosynovitis

***Etiology***    Tenosynovitis of the long head of the biceps muscle is common among individuals engaged in overhead activities. The repeated stretching of the biceps in highly ballistic activities may eventually cause an irritation of both the tendon and its synovial sheath as it passes under the transverse humeral ligament in the bicipital groove. Complete rupture of the transverse ligament, which holds the biceps in its groove, may take place, or a constant inflammation may result in degenerative scarring or a subluxated tendon.

***Symptoms and signs***    There will be tenderness in the anterior upper arm over the bicipital groove. There may also be some swelling, increased warmth, and crepitus because of the inflammation. The patient may complain of pain when performing dynamic overhead throwing-type activities.

***Management***    Bicipital tenosynovitis is best cared for by complete rest for several days, with daily applications of cryotherapy or ultrasound to reduce inflammation. Antiinflammatory medications are also beneficial in reducing inflammation. After the inflammation is controlled, a gradual program of strengthening and stretching for the biceps should be initiated.

### Contusions of the Upper Arm

***Etiology***    Contusions of the upper arm are common. Although any muscle of the upper arm is subject to bruising, the area most often affected is the lateral aspect, primarily the brachialis muscle and portions of the triceps and biceps muscles. Repeated contusions to the lateral aspect of the upper arm can lead to myositis ossificans, more commonly known as "linebacker's arm" or "blocker's exostosis." Myositis ossificans is a condition in which calcifications, or bone fragments, occur in a muscle or in soft tissues adjacent to bone.

***Symptoms and signs***    Bruises to the upper arm area can be particularly disabling, especially if the radial nerve is contused through forceful contact with the humerus, which produces transitory paralysis and consequent inability to use the extensor muscles of the forearm.

***Management***    POLICE should be applied for a minimum of 24 hours after injury. In most cases, this condition responds rapidly to treatment, usually within a few days. The key to treatment is to protect the contused area to prevent repeated episodes, which increase the likelihood of myositis ossificans. It is also important to maintain a full range of motion by stretching the contused muscle.

### Peripheral Nerve Injuries

***Etiology***    Injuries about the shoulder can produce and cause serious nerve injuries.[1] Injuries to shoulder nerves commonly stem from blunt trauma or a stretch type of injury. Nerve injury must be considered when there is constant pain, muscle weakness, paralysis, or muscle atrophy.[94]

***Symptoms and signs***    Peripheral nerve injuries can result in muscle weakness. Table 22–2 lists the peripheral nerves that can be injured and the muscles that are affected.

***Management***    If the injury results from blunt trauma, there may also be associated contusion. Thus, POLICE should be applied immediately. In many instances, muscle weakness is transient with a relatively quick return to normal function.[23] If muscle weakness persists or if there is any muscle wasting or atrophy, referral to a physician is essential.[94]

## THROWING MECHANICS

Throwing activities account for a considerable number of acute and chronic injuries to the shoulder joint. Throwing is a unilateral action that subjects the arm to repetitive

**TABLE 22–2    The Peripheral Nerves**

| Peripheral Nerves | Muscles Affected |
|---|---|
| Suprascapular | Supraspinatus and infraspinatus |
| Superior subscapular | Subscapularis |
| Inferior subscapular | Subscapularis and teres minor |
| Thoracodorsal | Latissimus dorsi |
| Medial pectoral | Pectoralis major and minor |
| Lateral pectoral | Pectoralis major |
| Axillary | Deltoid and teres minor |
| Dorsal scapular | Rhomboids major and minor and levator scapulae |
| Long thoracic | Serratus anterior |
| Spinal accessory | Trapezius |
| Musculocutaneous | Biceps, coracobrachialis, brachialis |
| Radial | Triceps and muscles of the forearm and hand |
| Median | Muscles of the forearm and hand |
| Ulnar | Muscles of the forearm and hand |

stresses of great intensity, particularly in repetitive overhead motions in activities such as throwing a baseball or football, throwing a javelin, serving or spiking a volleyball, and serving or hitting an overhead smash in tennis. If the thrower uses faulty technique, the joints are affected by atypical stresses that result in trauma to the joint and its surrounding tissues.[112]

Throwing is a sequential pattern of movements in which each part of the body must perform a number of carefully timed and executed acts.[70] For example, throwing a ball or javelin uses one particular pattern of movements; hurling the discus or hammer makes use of a similar pattern, but one in which centrifugal force is substituted for linear force and the type of terminal movements used in release are different. Putting the shot—a pushing rather than a throwing movement—has in its overall pattern a number of movements similar to those used in throwing.

In the act of throwing, momentum is transferred from the thrower's body to the object that is thrown. Basic physics dictates that the greater and heavier the mass, the greater the momentum needed to move it. Hence, as the size and weight of the object increase, more parts of the body are used to effect the summation of forces needed to accomplish the throw. The same is true with respect to the speed of the object: The greater the speed, the more body parts that must come into play to increase the body's momentum. Timing and sequence of action are of the utmost importance.[116] They improve with correct practice.

In throwing, the arm acts as a sling or catapult, transferring and imparting momentum from the body to the ball. There are various types of throwing; the overhand, sidearm, and underarm styles are the most common. The act of throwing is fairly complex and requires considerable coordination and timing to be successful.

In throwing, the most powerful muscle groups are brought into play initially, and the emphasis progresses ultimately to the least powerful but the most coordinated (i.e., the legs, trunk, shoulder girdle, arm, forearm, and hand).[70] The body's center of gravity is transported in the direction of the throw as the leg opposite the throwing arm is first elevated and then moved forward and planted on the ground, thus stopping the forward movement of the leg and permitting the body weight to be transferred from the supporting leg to the moving leg. Initially, the trunk rotates backward as the throwing arm and wrist are cocked, then rotates forward, continuing its rotation beyond the planted foot as the throwing arm moves forcibly from a position of extreme external rotation, abduction, and extension through flexion to forcible and complete extension in the terminal phase of the delivery, bringing into play the powerful internal rotators and adductors. These muscles exert a tremendous force on the distal and proximal humeral epiphysis and over a period of time create cumulative microtraumas that can result in shoulder problems.[45]

Relative to the shoulder complex, throwing or pitching involves five distinct phases: windup, cocking, arm acceleration, arm deceleration, and follow-through (Figure 22–31).[3,4]

**The throwing mechanism consists of five phases:**

- Windup
- Cocking
- Acceleration
- Deceleration
- Follow-through

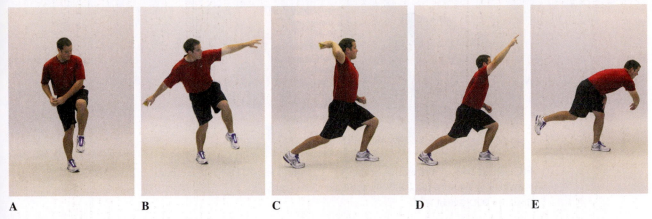

FIGURE 22–31   Phases of throwing from left to right: **(A)** Wind-up. **(B)** Cocking. **(C)** Acceleration. **(D)** Deceleration. **(E)** Follow-through.

© William E. Prentice

## Windup Phase

The windup, or preparation, phase lasts from the first movement until the ball leaves the gloved opposite hand. During this phase, the lead leg strides forward. Both shoulders abduct, externally rotate, and horizontally abduct.

## Cocking Phase

The cocking phase begins when the hands separate and ends when maximum external rotation of the humerus has occurred. During this phase, the lead foot comes in contact with the ground.

## Acceleration Phase

The acceleration phase lasts from maximum external rotation until ball release. The humerus abducts, horizontally abducts, and internally rotates at velocities approaching 7,000 degrees per second, with a force approaching 800 Newtons.[116] The scapula elevates, abducts, and rotates upward.

## Deceleration Phase

The deceleration phase lasts from ball release until maximum shoulder internal rotation. During this phase, the external rotators of the rotator cuff contract eccentrically to decelerate the humerus. The rhomboids contract eccentrically to decelerate the scapula.

## Follow-Through Phase

The follow-through phase lasts from maximum shoulder internal rotation until the end of the motion, when the athlete is in a balanced position.

# REHABILITATION OF THE SHOULDER COMPLEX

Rehabilitation of the shoulder joint after injury requires that the athletic trainer have a sound understanding of the complex anatomical and biomechanical functions of the shoulder complex.[30] As emphasized earlier, the shoulder is capable of a wide range of movement and consequently sacrifices some degree of stability for the sake of mobility.[46] Achieving the necessary balance between the two is essential, especially in patients who are high-performance athletes.

In recent years, the shoulder joint, like the knee joint, has received considerable attention within the athletic training community. The philosophy of and approach to treatment, management, and rehabilitation continue to change rapidly.[49] Attempts by athletic trainers to use cookbook approaches to rehabilitation protocols sometimes fail to allow for essential alteration of those protocols in response to the specific needs of the individual patient.[80] The athletic trainer should be creative when designing shoulder rehabilitation programs. There are a variety of exercises to choose from, and it is not necessary to use a lot of expensive equipment to achieve good results.[32]

A baseball pitcher is throwing a fastball. To execute this motion effectively, the pitcher must develop significant velocity in glenohumeral internal rotation during the acceleration phase. During the follow-through phase, this high-velocity internal rotation must quickly decelerate.

**?** Which muscles actively internally rotate the glenohumeral joint during the acceleration phase, and which muscles decelerate internal rotation during follow-through?

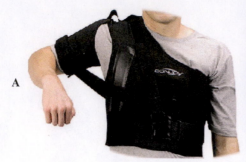 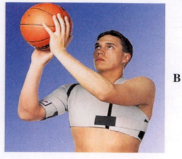

FIGURE 22–32   Protective braces for the shoulder. **(A)** DonJoy shoulder stabilizer (Sawa brace). **(B)** Sully shoulder stabilizer.
Courtesy DJO Global

## Immobilization after Injury

Rehabilitation programs should be tailored to the individual patient's needs. The length of the immobilization period varies depending on the structures injured, the severity of the injury, and whether the injury is treated conservatively or surgically by the physician. Regardless of the injury, the injured patient usually begins to exercise isometrically while wearing an immobilization device (Figure 22–32).[20] For certain injuries, it may be unnecessary to wear a sling or brace at all. Other injuries may require that a sling be worn 24 hours a day and removed only for rehabilitative exercises. Certain injuries may require that a sling be worn only at night in the early stages of healing, that a motion-limiting brace be worn during activity only, or that no sling or brace be worn after the first couple of weeks but that motion above 90 degrees be limited for a certain number of weeks. Progression in range of motion and strengthening techniques should be dictated by an understanding of the physiological process of healing and is generally determined by a lack of pain and swelling with increased activity.[46]

## General Body Conditioning

It is essential for the athlete to maintain a high level of cardiorespiratory endurance throughout the rehabilitation process. For shoulder joint injuries, activities such as running, speed walking, and riding an exercise bike may be used to maintain cardiorespiratory endurance. Because many athletic activities involve some running, engaging in such training for a shoulder injury is more useful than, for example, swimming for the rehabilitation of an ankle sprain. Patients engaged in sports that require upper-extremity endurance, such as swimming and throwing, should be progressed to these activities as soon as they can tolerate these activities. Training and conditioning activities may be modified, so that the patient can continue to maintain strength, flexibility, and neuromuscular control in the rest of the body during shoulder rehabilitation. Even though weight bearing is not a consideration in rehabilitation of the upper extremity, aquatic exercise can still be a useful tool, because it can help with both maintaining cardiorespiratory endurance and strengthening the shoulder complex.[104]

## Shoulder Joint Mobilization

Normal joint arthrokinematics must be maintained for the patient to regain normal full-range physiological movement. Mobilization techniques should be used whenever there is some limitation in motion that can be attributed to tightness of the joint capsule or surrounding ligaments rather than to tightness of the musculotendinous units.[80] Mobilization techniques, including inferior, anterior, and dorsal humeral glides, anterior/posterior and inferior/superior glides of the clavicle at both the acromioclavicular and sternoclavicular joints, and generalized scapulothoracic mobilizations can be incorporated into the early stages of rehabilitation as needed (Figure 22–33).

## Flexibility

Regaining a full, nonrestricted, pain-free range of motion is one of the most important aspects of shoulder rehabilitation. Because the shoulder consists of four joints that must all function together, the athletic trainer must make certain that normal movement occurs at each joint individually and that the patient eventually regains normal scapulohumeral rhythm. Gentle ROM exercises, such as Codman's circumduction exercise (Figure 22–34A) and a sawing motion (Figure 22–34B) should be started immediately. Exercises that stretch the joint capsule should also be incorporated (Figure 22–34E,F,G). Exercises can be progressed to a series of active assisted ROM exercises that use a T-bar and are done in a pain-free arc for all the cardinal plane movements (Figure 22–34H&I). Cardinal plane movements at the shoulder include flexion, extension, abduction, adduction, internal and external rotation, and horizontal adduction and abduction. Rope-and-pulley exercises (Figure 22–34D) and wall-climbing exercises (Figure 22–34C) are particularly effective in regaining flexion and abduction. Exercises that stretch the scapular stabilizers must also be integrated into the rehabilitation program

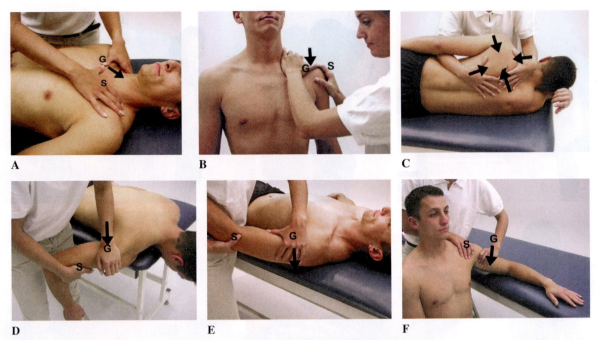

FIGURE 22–33 Shoulder complex joint mobilization. **(A)** Sternoclavicular posterior glides. **(B)** Acromioclavicular inferior glides. **(C)** Scapular mobilizations. **(D)** Anterior humeral glides. **(E)** Posterior humeral glides. **(F)** Inferior humeral glides.

© William E. Prentice

(Figure 22–34J–M) Postoperative progressive ROM exercise combined with rotator cuff and scapular strengthening is effective in improving strength in internal and external rotation.[80]

## Muscular Strength

Strengthening exercises in the shoulder generally follow a progression from positional isometrics, to full-range isotonics that concentrate on both eccentric and concentric contractions, to isokinetics, to plyometrics. Gentle isometrics should begin immediately after injury or after surgery while the arm is still immobilized at the side.

Athletic trainers should give particular attention to strengthening the scapular stabilizers by incorporating exercises to resist scapular abduction, adduction, elevation, depression, upward rotation, downward rotation, protraction, and retraction (Figure 22–35).[61] Strengthening exercises for the scapular stabilizers may also be done on a physioball and include Y, W, and T exercises (Figure 22–36). Strengthening the muscles that control the stability of the scapula helps provide a base for the function of the highly mobile glenohumeral joint.[107] An inertial training system can significantly increase shoulder joint stability.[80]

Isotonic exercise may be incorporated with the use of different types of resistance, including dumbbells and barbells, surgical tubing or Theraband (Figure 22–37), or manual resistance techniques, including PNF strengthening techniques.[6,82] Resistance exercises should include all cardinal plane movements.

Isokinetic exercises are used to exercise the muscles of the shoulder complex at varying speeds (Figure 22–38). The maximum angular velocities currently available on isokinetic devices (approximately 600 degrees per second) do not approach functional speeds of the throwing shoulder; the latter may be as great as 7,000 degrees per second of internal rotation.

Isotonic and isokinetic training should both emphasize concentric and eccentric components. Eccentric contraction of the external rotators is essential during the deceleration phase of throwing.[99] Plyometric exercises incorporated into the later stages of a rehabilitation program use a quick, eccentric stretch of a muscle to facilitate a concentric contraction. Plyometric exercises for the upper extremity can be done with a weighted ball (Figure 22–39).[61]

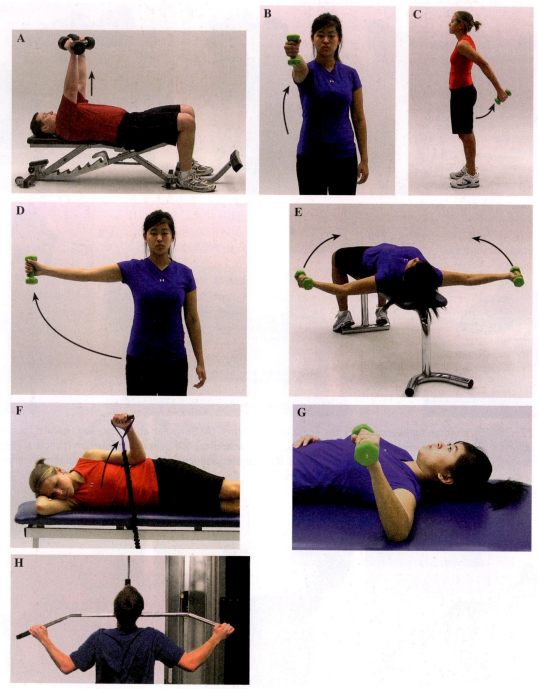

FIGURE 22–37   Isotonic exercises. **(A)** Chest press (pectoralis major, triceps). **(B)** Flexion to 90 degrees (anterior deltoid, coracobrachialis, deltoid pectoralis major, biceps). **(C)** Extension (latissimus dorsi, teres major, posterior deltoid). **(D)** Abduction to 90 degrees (middle deltoid, supraspinatus, anterior deltoid). **(E)** Horizontal adduction (pectoralis major, anterior deltoid). **(F)** External rotation (infraspinatus, teres minor, posterior deltoid). **(G)** Internal rotation (subscapularis, pectoralis major, latissimus dorsi, teres minor, anterior deltoid). **(H)** Lat pull-downs (latissimus dorsi).
© William E. Prentice

## Functional Progressions

Functional progressions usually incorporate some activity-specific skill that involves overhead motions. Strengthening activities should make use of the D2 upper-extremity PNF pattern, which closely resembles overhead throwing and serving motions (see Chapter 16).[6] Attaching surgical tubing to a baseball or tennis racket and having the patient move through the throwing or serving motion helps increase the patient's strength, both concentrically and eccentrically

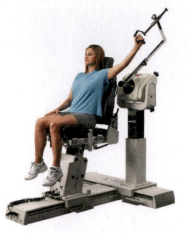

FIGURE 22–38   Isokinetic exercises may be incorporated into the later stages of a rehabilitation program.
Photo courtesy Biodex Medical Systems, Inc.

(Figure 22–41). Throwing and serving motions require high-speed angular velocities. Thus, functional progressions should concentrate on a gradual and progressive increase in these angular velocities. Throwing programs, for example, should increase the throwing distance and the throwing velocity through a series of progressive

stages. Progression to a more advanced stage is dictated by lack of pain and swelling at the previous stage.[3,4] See *Focus Box 22–1:* "Throwing progression" for an example of a program for a return to throwing.

## Return to Activity

Decisions to return a patient to full activity should be based on pre-established criteria that can be clearly demonstrated by functional performance. Isokinetic testing can provide at least some objective measure of strength. The athletic trainer must have a clear understanding of the healing process and the general time frames required for rehabilitation. Return to full activity should be based on mutual agreement among the athlete, team physician, athletic trainer, and coach.

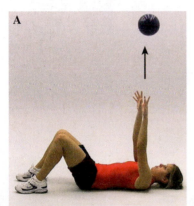
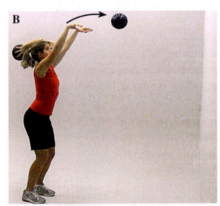
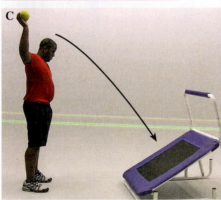
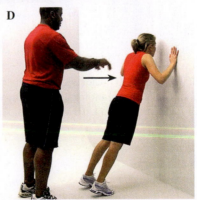

FIGURE 22–39   Plyometric exercises. **(A)** Supine weighted ball toss. **(B)** Standing weighted ball soccer throw against wall. **(C)** Weighted ball toss to plyoback. **(D)** Push into wall.
© William E. Prentice

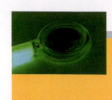

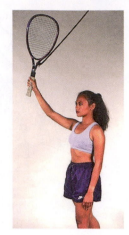

FIGURE 22-41   Surgical tubing attached to a tennis racket may be used as a functional progression for strengthening overhead motions.
© William E. Prentice

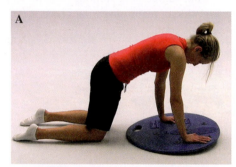
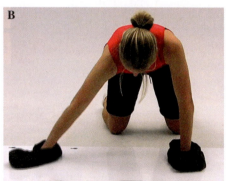
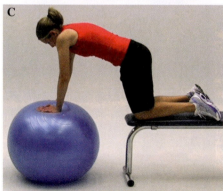

FIGURE 22-40   Closed kinetic chain activities such as weight shifting may be functionally important for certain patients. **(A)** On a BAPS board. **(B)** On a slide board. **(C)** On a stability ball. **(D)** In a 2-point kneeling position.
© William E. Prentice

## SUMMARY

- The shoulder complex has a great degree of mobility. This mobility, however, requires some compromise in stability, and thus the shoulder is highly susceptible to injury. Many sport activities that involve repetitive overhead movements place a great deal of stress on the shoulder joint.

- Four major articulations are associated with the shoulder complex: the sternoclavicular joint, the acromioclavicular joint, the glenohumeral joint, and the scapulothoracic joint. The muscles that act on the shoulder joint consist of those that originate on the axial skeleton and attach to the humerus, those that originate on the scapula and attach to the humerus, and those that attach the axial skeleton to the scapula.

- Dynamic movement and stabilization of the shoulder complex require integrated functions of the rotator cuff muscles, the joint capsule, and the muscles that stabilize and position the scapula. In movement of the shoulder joint, it is critical to maintain the positioning of the humeral head relative to the glenoid.
- The athletic trainer, when evaluating injuries to the shoulder complex, must take into consideration all four joints. A number of special tests can provide insight into the nature of a particular injury.
- Fractures can occur to the clavicle, scapula, and humerus. Sprains can occur at the sternoclavicular, acromioclavicular, and glenohumeral joints.
- Shoulder dislocations and subluxations are relatively common, with an anterior dislocation and posterior subluxation being the most likely to occur. After a dislocation has been reduced and immobilized, muscle reconditioning should be initiated as soon as possible.
- Recurrent shoulder instability can occur after acute subluxation or dislocation. Recurrent instabilities may be anterior, posterior, inferior, or multidirectional. The causes of shoulder instabilities may be traumatic

(macrotraumatic), atraumatic, microtraumatic (repetitive use), congenital, or neuromuscular.

- Shoulder impingement is closely related to shoulder instability. Patients involved with overhead activities often exhibit hypermobility and significant capsular laxity. Shoulder impingement involves a mechanical compression of the supraspinatus tendon, the subacromial bursa, and the long head of the biceps tendon under the coracoacromial arch.
- A number of injuries, including subacromial bursitis, contusions, bicipital tenosynovitis, adhesive capsulitis, peripheral nerve injuries, and thoracic outlet compression syndromes, are common injuries of the shoulder complex.
- Rehabilitation after injury to the shoulder joint may require a brief period of immobilization. Joint mobilization, flexibility, and strengthening exercises should be initiated as soon as possible after injury. Progression in range of motion and strengthening techniques should be dictated by a lack of pain and swelling associated with increased activity. Activities that stress closed kinetic chain function emphasize cocontraction of antagonistic muscle groups and thus provide neuromuscular control of opposing muscle groups and promote stability about the shoulder joint. For the patient with an injured shoulder joint, functional progressions usually incorporate some activity-specific skill that involves overhead motions.

## WEB SITES

Cramer First Aider: www.cramersportsmed.com/first-aider .html

Wheeless' Textbook of Orthopaedics: www.wheelessonline.com

American Orthopaedic Society for Sports Medicine: www .sportsmed.org

OrthoNet: www.orthonet.on.ca

## SOLUTIONS TO CLINICAL APPLICATION EXERCISES

22–1 The athletic trainer should point out to the patient that, regardless of the strengthening exercises, there is still a high probability that a recurrent dislocation will occur. The dynamic stabilizers of the glenohumeral joint include the subscapularis, infraspinatus, teres minor, and supraspinatus. It is perhaps just as important to strengthen the scapular muscles.

22–2 Normal scapulohumeral rhythm exhibits no movement of the scapula as the humerus elevates to 30 degrees. Overall, the scapula should abduct and upwardly rotate 1 degree for every 2 degrees of humeral elevation.

22–3 Thoracic outlet compression syndromes involve compression of the brachial plexus, subclavian artery, and subclavian vein. The anterior scalene syndrome test, or Adson's test, tests for compression by the heads of the anterior and middle scalene muscles or between the cervical rib and the anterior scalene muscle. The costoclavicular syndrome tests (Roo's test or the military brace position test) test for compression between the first rib and the clavicle. The hyperabduction syndrome test, or Allen test, tests for compression behind the pectoral muscle and beneath the coracoid process.

22–4 Falling on the tip of the shoulder is a typical mechanism of injury for a sprain of both the acromioclavicular and sternoclavicular joints. It is also possible that a clavicular fracture has occurred.

22–5 In an anterior glenohumeral dislocation, the head of the humerus is forced out of its articular capsule in an anterior direction past the glenoid labrum and then downward to rest under the coracoid process. Torn capsular and ligamentous tissue, a possible tendinous avulsion of the rotator cuff muscles or long head of the biceps, a possible tear or detachment of the glenoid labrum, a possible injury to the brachial plexus, and profuse hemorrhage are all potential problems.

22–6 A dislocation can cause a variety of injuries within the glenohumeral joint, including a Bankart lesion, a Hill-Sachs lesion, and a SLAP lesion. A Bankart lesion is a defect of the anterior labrum, whereas a Hill-Sachs lesion is a defect on the posterior lateral aspect of the humeral head. A SLAP lesion involves a tear of the superior labrum that may also involve the biceps tendon.

22–7 It is most likely that the pitcher has some anterior instability that is allowing for excessive translation of the humeral head on the glenoid. During throwing, this can create a repetitive compression of the rotator cuff, consequently causing impingement of soft tissues under the coracoacromial arch.

22–8 If the dynamic stabilizers (rotator cuff) and the static stabilizers (joint capsule) of the glenohumeral joint cannot maintain the position of the humeral head relative to the glenoid, there will be excessive translation of the humeral head. Excessive translation of the humerus in the overhead position can result in mechanical impingement of those structures under the coracoacromial arch. If the scapular muscles do not maintain the position of the glenoid relative to the humerus, impingement can result.

22–9 Her pain is probably due to mechanical impingement or compression of the supraspinatus tendon, the subacromial bursa, or the long head of the biceps under the coracoacromial arch as the arm moves into a fully abducted or flexed position. The space under the arch becomes even more compressed as the humerus is internally rotated, as would occur during the follow-through.

22–10 Restoring normal biomechanics to the shoulder joint in an effort to maintain space under the coracoacromial arch during overhead activities is critical. The athletic trainer should use techniques that strengthen the rotator cuff muscles, which compress and depress the humeral head relative to the glenoid, and strengthen the scapular muscles, which abduct, elevate, and upwardly rotate the scapula. The athletic trainer should also

incorporate posterior and inferior glenohumeral joint mobilizations to reduce tightness in the posterior and inferior joint capsule.

22–11 The subscapularis, pectoralis major, latissimus dorsi, teres major, and anterior deltoid must all contract concentrically to produce internal rotation during the acceleration phase. The infraspinatus, teres minor, and posterior deltoid must contract eccentrically during the follow-through to decelerate internal rotation.

22–12 Efforts toward regaining neuromuscular control should begin immediately in the rehabilitation program. Closed kinetic chain exercises emphasize cocontraction of antagonistic muscle groups, which provides neuromuscular control of opposing muscle groups and promotes stability about the shoulder joint. Activities that stress closed kinetic chain function include weight shifting on the hands or on a ball and push-ups. Biofeedback techniques can help the athlete regain control of specific muscle actions.

22–13 Because the patient is having difficulty regaining active range of motion, the athletic trainer might try using diagonal 1 and 2 upper-extremity PNF patterns with rhythmic initiation. This technique involves a progression from passive to active assisted to active contraction throughout a functional range. The trainer should also use joint mobilization techniques for not only the acromioclavicular joint but also the sternoclavicular, glenohumeral, and scapulothoracic joints if needed.

## REVIEW QUESTIONS AND CLASS ACTIVITIES

1. Explain why a full range of motion of the shoulder joint requires motion at all four joints in the shoulder complex.
2. Explain how the positioning of the humeral head is maintained relative to the glenoid in overhead throwing motions.
3. What is the relationship between shoulder instability and shoulder impingement?
4. What are the mechanisms of an anterior dislocation and a posterior dislocation?
5. How do recurrent instabilities develop?
6. What can be done to minimize the chances of a baseball pitcher developing shoulder impingement?
7. What is myositis ossificans, and how can its development be prevented?
8. How may an individual acquire bicipital tenosynovitis? How does this condition lead to a ruptured biceps tendon?
9. Describe the tests for thoracic outlet compression syndromes.
10. Discuss the mechanics involved in throwing a baseball.
11. Explain why closed kinetic chain exercises are useful in the rehabilitation of shoulder injuries.
12. Develop an exercise rehabilitation program for a rotator cuff injury, a glenohumeral dislocation, and an acromioclavicular sprain.

## REFERENCES

1. Allen J: Recognizing, managing, and treating an axillary-nerve dysfunction, *Athletic Therapy Today* 7(2):28, 2002.
2. Axe M: Acromioclavicular joint injuries in the athlete, *Sports Med Arthroscopy Review* 8(2):182, 2000.
3. Axe M: Data-based interval throwing programs for baseball position players from age 13 to college level, *J Sport Rehabil* 10(4):267, 2001.
4. Axe M: Data-based interval throwing programs for collegiate softball players, *J Athl Train* 37(2):194, 2002.
5. Baker C: Clinical evaluation of the athlete's shoulder, *J Athl Train* 35(3):256, 2000.
6. Barry D: Proprioceptive neuromuscular facilitation for the scapula, *Athletic Therapy Today* 10(3):51, 2005.
7. Beim G: Acromioclavicular joint injuries, *J Athl Train* 35(3):261, 2000.
8. Blackburn T: Rehabilitation after ligamentous and labral surgery of the shoulder: Guiding concepts, *J Athl Train* 35(3):373, 2000.
9. Borsa P: Scapular positioning patterns during humeral elevation in nonimpaired shoulders, *J Athl Train* 38(1):12, 2003.

10. Butters K: The scapula. In Rockwood C, ed: *Rockwood and Masten's the shoulder,* Philadelphia, PA, 2009, Saunders.
11. Calis M, et al.: Diagnostic values of clinical diagnostic tests in subacromial impingement syndrome, *Ann Rheum Dis* 59(1):44–47, 2012.
12. Chan R: Glenoid labrum lesion in an elite tennis player: A clinical challenge in diagnosis, *J Sport Rehabil* 15(2):168, 2006.
13. Chronopoulus E: Diagnostic value of physical tests for isolated chronic AC lesions. *Am J Sports Med* 32(3): 655–61, 2004.
14. Chu J : The effect of a neoprene shoulder stabilizer on active joint reposition sense in subjects with stable and unstable shoulders, *J Athl Train* 37(2):141, 2002.
15. Cleland J: *Orthopedic clinical examination: An evidence-based approach for physical therapists,* Carlstadt, NJ, 2005, Icon Learning Systems.
16. Conroy D: The effect of joint mobilization as a component of comprehensive treatment for primary shoulder impingement syndrome, *J Orthop Sports Phys Ther* 28(1):3, 1998.

17. Cordasco F: Understanding multidirectional instability of the shoulder, *J Athl Train* 35(3):278, 2000.
18. Craig E: Fractures of the clavicle. In Rockwood C, Masten F, eds: *Rockwood and Masten's the shoulder*, Philadelphia, PA, 2009, Saunders.
19. D'Alessandro D: Superior labral lesions: Diagnosis and management, *J Athl Train* 35(3):286, 2000.
20. Donatelli R: *Physical therapy of the shoulder*, ed 4, St. Louis, MO, 2011, Churchill-Livingstone.
21. Dover G: Assessment of shoulder proprioception in the female softball athlete, *Am J Sports Med* 31(3):43, 2003.
22. Dover G: Reliability of joint position sense and force production measures during internal and external rotation of the shoulder, *J Athl Train* 38(4):304, 2003.
23. Duralde X: Neurologic injuries in the athlete's shoulder, *J Athl Train* 35(3):316, 2000.
24. Durall C: The effects of training the humeral rotators on arm elevation in the scapular plane, *J Sport Rehabil* 10(2):79, 2001.
25. Eachempati K: The external rotation method for reduction of acute anterior dislocations and

fracture dislocations of the shoulder, *J Bone Joint Surg* 86(11):2431, 2004.

26. Ellenbecker T: *Clinical examination of the shoulder*, Philadelphia, PA, 2004, Elsevier Health Sciences.

27. Ellenbecker T: Rehabilitation of shoulder impingement syndrome and rotator cuff injuries: An evidence-based review, *British Journal of Sports Medicine* 44:319–27, 2010.

28. Ewald A: Adhesive capsulitis: A review, *American Family Physician* 83(4):417–22, 2011.

29. Farber A: Clinical assessment of three common tests for traumatic anterior shoulder instability, *Journal of Bone and Joint Surgery* 88A(7):1467–74, 2006.

30. Faltus J: Optimal therapeutic management of chronic shoulder dysfunction, *Athletic Therapy and Training* 16(6):4–7, 2010.

31. Fleming J: Exercise protocol for the treatment of rotator cuff impingement syndrome, *J Athl Train* 45(5):483–85, 2010.

32. Floyd R: Innovative tools for shoulder rehabilitation, *Athletic Therapy Today* 4(4):47, 1999.

33. Flynn T: *User's guide to the musculoskeletal examination: Fundamentals for the evidence-based clinician*, Buckner, KY, 2008, Evidence in Motion.

34. Guanche C: Clinical testing for tears of the glenoid labrum, *Arthroscopy*, 19:517–23, 2003.

35. Groh G: Management of traumatic sternoclavicular joint injuries, *Journal of the American Academy of Orthopedic Surgeons* 19(1):1–7, 2011.

36. Harrison A: Subacromial impingement syndrome, *Journal of the American Academy of Orthopedic Surgeons* 19(11):701–08, 2011.

37. Hayes K: Shoulder instability: Management and rehabilitation, *J Orthop Sports Phys Ther* 32(10):497, 2002.

38. Henry T: The effect of muscle fatigue on muscle force-couple activation of the shoulder, *J Sport Rehabil* 10(42):24, 2001.

39. Holtby R: Accuracy of the speed's and Yergason's test in detecting biceps pathology and SLAP lesions: Comparison with arthroscopic findings, *Arthroscopy: The Journal of Arthroscopic and Related Surgery* 20(3):231–36, 2004.

40. Itoi E: Which is more useful, the "full can test" or the "empty can test," in detecting the torn supraspinatus tendon? *Am J Sports Med* 27:65–68, 1999.

41. Janwantanakul P: Characteristics of shoulder-position sense: Effects of mode of movement, scapular support, and arm orientation, *J Sport Rehabil* 11(3):157, 2002.

42. Jobe C: Evaluation of impingement syndromes in the overhead-throwing athlete, *J Athl Train* 35(3):293, 2000.

43. Joshi M: Posterior rotator cuff fatigue affects scapular muscle activation during a diagonal movement task, *J Orthop Sports Phys Ther* 36(1):A70, 2006.

44. Keskula D: Defining and measuring functional limitations and disability in the athletic shoulder, *J Sport Rehabil* 10(3):221, 2001.

45. Kibler B: Pathomechanics of the throwing shoulder, *Sports Medicine and Arthroscopy Review* 20(1):22–29, 2012.

46. Kibler B: Rehabilitation of the athlete's shoulder, *Clinics in Sports Medicine* 27(4):821–31, 2008.

47. Kibler B: The role of the scapula in athletic shoulder function, *Am J Sports Med* 26(2):325, 1998.

48. Kibler B: Scapular dysfunction, *Athletic Therapy Today* 11(5):6, 2006.

49. Kibler B: Shoulder rehabilitation strategies, guidelines, and practice, *Operative Techniques in Sports Medicine* 8(4):258, 2000.

50. Kim D: Prevalence comparison of accompanying lesions between primary and recurrent anterior dislocation in the shoulder, *Am J Sports Med* 38(10):2071–76, 2010.

51. Kocher M: Reliability, validity, and responsiveness of the American Shoulder and Elbow Surgeons Subjective Shoulder Scale in patients with shoulder instability, rotator cuff disease, and glenohumeral arthritis, *J Bone Joint Surg* 87:2006, 2005.

52. Krishnan S: *The shoulder and the overhead athlete*, Baltimore, MD, 2004, Lippincott, Williams and Wilkins.

53. Lee J: Thoracic outlet syndrome, *Physical Medicine and Rehabilitation* 2(1):64–70, 2010.

54. Line L: Labral tears: Diagnosis, treatment and rehabilitation, *Athletic Therapy Today* 4(4):18, 1999.

55. Litaker D: Returning to the bedside: Using the history and physical examination to identify rotator cuff tears, *J Am Geriatr Soc* 48(12):1633–37, 2000.

56. Ludewig P: Motion of the shoulder complex during multiplanar humeral elevation, *J Bone Joint Surg Am* 91(2):378–89, 2009.

57. Ludewig P: Translations of the humerus in persons with shoulder impingement symptoms, *J Orthop Sports Phys Ther* 32(6):248, 2002.

58. Lyons A: Clinical diagnosis of tears of the rotator cuff, *J Bone Joint Surg Br* 74:414–15, 1992.

59. Malanga G: *Musculoskeletal physical examination: An evidence-based approach*, Philadelphia, PA, 2006, Elsevier Health Sciences.

60. Manske R: Electromyographically assessed exercises for the scapular muscles, *Athletic Therapy Today* 11(5):19, 2006.

61. Manske R, Davies G: Post-rehabilitation outcomes of muscle power (torque/acceleration energy) in patients with selected shoulder dysfunctions, *J Sport Rehabil* 12(3):181, 2003.

62. Martin A, et al.: Reliability of Allen's test in selection of patients for radial artery harvest: The society of thoracic surgeons, *Ann Thorac Surg* 70:1362–65, 2000.

63. Masten F: Subacromial impingement. In Rockwood C, ed: *Rockwood and Masten's the shoulder*, Philadelphia, PA, 2009, Saunders.

64. Matsen F: Principles for the evaluation and management of shoulder instability, *J Bone Joint Surg* 88(3):648, 2006.

65. Matsen F: Glenohumeral instability. In Rockwood C, ed: *Rockwood and Masten's the shoulder*, Philadelphia, PA, 2009, Saunders.

66. Mazzocca A: Distal biceps rupture, *Orthopedic Clinics of North America* 39(2):237–49, 2008.

67. McClure P: A clinical method for identifying scapular dyskinesis, Parts 1 and 2, *J Athl Train* 44(2):160–75, 2009.

68. McClure P: Direct 3-dimensional measurement of scapular kinematics during dynamic movements in vivo, *J. Shoulder Elbow Surg* 10(3):269–77, 2001.

69. McCluskey G: Pathophysiology of anterior shoulder instability, *J Athl Train* 35(3):268, 2000.

70. McFarland E: Examination of the shoulder in the overhead throwing athlete, *Clinics in Sports Medicine* 27(4):553–78, 2008.

71. McFarland E: Clinical evaluation of impingement: What to do and what works, *J Bone Joint Surg* 88(2):432, 2006.

72. McLoda T: Functional effects of inertial training of the upper extremity, *J Sport Rehabil* 12(3):229, 2003.

73. McMullen J: A kinetic chain approach for shoulder rehabilitation, *J Athl Train* 35(3):329, 2000.

74. Meininger A: Scapular winging: An update, *Journal of the American Academy of Orthopedic Surgeons* 19(8):453–62, 2011.

75. Milano G: *Shoulder arthroscopy: Principles and practice*, New York, 2013, Springer Science.

76. Millett P: Open operative treatment for anterior shoulder instability: When and why? *J Bone Joint Surg* 87(2):419, 2005.

77. Mintken P: Some factors predict successful short-term outcomes in individuals with shoulder pain receiving cervicothoracic manipulation: A single-arm trial, *Phys Ther* 90(1):26–42, 2010.

78. Myers J: Conservative management of shoulder impingement syndrome in the athletic population, *J Sport Rehabil* 8(3):230, 1999.

79. Myers J: Glenohumeral range of motion deficits and posterior shoulder tightness in throwers with pathologic internal impingement, *Am J Sports Med* 34:385, 2006.

80. Myers J: Rehabilitation of shoulder injuries. In Prentice W, ed: *Rehabilitation techniques in sports medicine and athletic training*, Thorofare, NJ, 2015, Slack.

81. Myers J: The role of the sensorimotor system in the athletic shoulder, *J Athl Train* 35(3):351, 2000.

82. Myers J: On-the-field resistance-tubing exercises for throwers: An electromyographic analysis, *J Athl Train* 40(1):15, 2005.

83. Nakagawa S: Forced shoulder abduction and elbow flexion test: A new simple clinical test to detect superior labral injury in the throwing shoulder, *Arthroscopy*, 21:1290–95, 2005.

84. 84. O'Brien S: The active compression test: A new and effective test for diagnosing labral tears and acromioclavicular joint abnormality, *Am J Sports Med* 26(5):610–13, 1998.

85. Ozcakar L: Quantification of the weakness and fatigue in thoracic outlet syndrome with isokinetic measurements, *British Journal of Sports Medicine* 39(3):178, 2005.

86. Park H: Diagnostic accuracy of clinical tests for the different degrees of subacromial impingement syndrome, *J Bone Joint Surg Am* 87(7):1446–55, 2005.

87. Perkins S: Patient satisfaction after thermal shrinkage of the glenohumeral joint capsule, *J Sport Rehabil* 10(3):157, 2001.

88. Placzek D: *Orthopedic physical therapy secrets*, New York, 2008, Elsevier Health Sciences.

89. Pujalte G: Stingers and burners, *Athletic Therapy and Training* 17(1):24–28, 2012.

90. Rabe S: Clavicular fracture in a collegiate football player: A case report of rapid return to play, *J Athl Train* 46(1):107–11, 2011.

91. Richardson A: Thoracic outlet syndrome in aquatic athletes, *Clin Sports Med* 18(2):361, 1999.

92. Rockwood C: *Rockwood and Green's fractures in adults*, Philadelphia, PA, 2009, Lippincott.

93. Rookmoneea M: The effectiveness of interventions in the management of patients with primary frozen shoulder, *Journal of Bone and Joint Surgery* 92(9):1267–72, 2010.

94. Rosenfield J: Peripheral nerve injuries and repair in the upper extremity, *Bulletin of the NYU Hospital for Joint Diseases* 60(3):155, 2004.

95. Ryu J: Rehabilitation of biceps tendon disorders in athletes, *Clinics in Sports Medicine* 29(2):229–46, 2010.

96. Satterwhite Y: Evaluation and management of recurrent anterior shoulder instability, *J Athl Train* 35(3):273, 2000.

97. Sauers B: Effectiveness of rehabilitation for patients with subacromial impingement syndrome, *J Athl Train* 40(3):221, 2005.

98. Scibek J: Rotator cuff tear pain and tear size and scapulohumeral rhythm, *J Athl Train* 44(2): 148–59, 2009.

99. Smith D: Incorporating kinetic-chain integration, Part 2: Functional shoulder rehabilitation, *Athletic Therapy Today* 11(5):63, 2006.

100. Speer K: An evaluation of the shoulder relocation test, *Am J Sports Med* 22:177–83, 1994.

101. Spigelman T: Identifying and assessing glenohumeral internal-rotation deficit, *Athletic Therapy Today* 11(3):23, 2006.

102. Terry G: Functional anatomy of the shoulder, *J Athl Train* 35(3):248, 2000.

103. Terry G: The stabilizing function of passive shoulder restraints, *American Journal of Sports Medicine* 19(1):26–34, 1991.

104. Thein J: Aquatic-based rehabilitation and training for the shoulder, *J Athl Train* 35(3):382, 2000.

105. Thigpen C: Scapulohumeral rhythm for anteriorposterior tipping during dynamic humeral rotation, *J Athl Train* 39(2 Suppl):S-41, 2004.

106. Uhl T: Shoulder musculature activation during upper extremity weight-bearing exercise, *J Orthop Sports Phys Ther* 33(3):109, 2003.

107. Voight M: The role of the scapula in the rehabilitation of shoulder injuries, *J Athl Train* 35(3):364, 2000.

108. Weise K: Effectiveness of glenohumeral joint stability braces in limiting active and passive shoulder range of motion in collegiate football players, *J Athl Train* 39(2):151, 2004.

109. Weldon E: Upper extremity overuse injuries in swimming: A discussion of swimmer's shoulder, *Clin Sports Med* 20(3):423, 2001.

110. Wilk K: Current concepts: The stabilizing structures of the glenohumeral joint, *J Orthop Sports Phys Ther* 25(6):364, 1997.

111. Williams G: Management of rotator cuff and impingement injuries in the athlete, *J Athl Train* 35(3):300, 2000.

112. Wolf B: Throwing injuries: Biomechanics, injury mechanisms and rehabilitation, *Current Orthopedic Practice* 21(5):467–71, 2010.

113. Wolf E: Transdeltoid palpation (the rent test) in the diagnosis of rotator cuff tears, *J Shoulder Elbow Surg* 10:470–73, 2001.

114. Wolin P: Rotator cuff injury: Addressing overhead overuse, *Physician Sportsmed* 25(6):54, 1997.

115. Yanai T: Shoulder impingement in front-crawl swimming: I. A method to identify impingement, *Med Sci Sports Exerc* 32(1):21, 2000.

116. Zheng N: Biomechanics and injuries of the shoulder during throwing, *Athletic Therapy Today* 4(4):6, 1999.

117. Ziaks L: Severe multidirectional instability of the glenohumeral joint, *Athletic Therapy Today* 51(1):37–39, 2010.

## ANNOTATED BIBLIOGRAPHY

Andrews J, Wilk K: *The athlete's shoulder*, New York, 2008, Churchill-Livingstone.

*Concentrates on both conservative and surgical treatment of shoulder injuries that occur specifically in the athletic population.*

Donatelli, R: *Physical therapy of the shoulder,* Philadelphia, PA, 2011, Churchill Livingstone.

*Clinical reference on shoulder rehabilitation, for physical therapists and rehabilitation professionals.*

Ellenbecker T: *Clinical examination of the shoulder*, Philadelphia, PA, 2004, Elsevier Health Sciences.

*Devoted solely to the musculoskeletal examination of the shoulder joint. Presents a combination of clinical tests, functional evaluation parameters, throwing, and interval sport return/evaluation procedures.*

Iannotti JP, Williams GR: *Disorders of the shoulder: Diagnosis and management*, Baltimore, MD, 2013, Lippincott, Williams and Wilkins.

*Presents the basic concepts of diagnosis and management of the common shoulder disorders.*

Kirshnan S, Hawkins R: *The shoulder and the overhead athlete*, Philadelphia, PA, 2004, Lippincott, Williams and Wilkins.

*Written by a multidisciplinary team of expert shoulder surgeons, athletic trainers, and physical therapists. Delivers comprehensive and up-to-date information on the evaluation, treatment, rehabilitation, and prevention of shoulder injuries in athletes who throw and use other overhead movements.*

Lippitt S, Rockwood C, Masten, F: *Rockwood and Masten's the shoulder*, Philadelphia, PA, 2009, Elsevier Science.

*A two-volume set that covers every subject relative to the shoulder complex.*

Porterfield J, DeRosa C: *Mechanical shoulder disorders,* Philadelphia, PA, 2008, Elsevier Health Sciences.

*A clinical reference that provides a thorough discussion of the shoulder from the normal and abnormal perspectives with an emphasis on the anatomical and mechanical foundations of shoulder disorders.*

Special Issue: Evaluation and management of shoulder injuries in the athlete, *J Athl Train* 35(3), 2000.

*An entire issue dedicated to research articles dealing with injuries to the shoulder joint.*

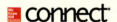

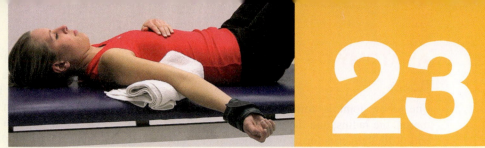
© William E. Prentice

# 23

# The Elbow

*When you finish this chapter you should be able to*

- Recall the structural and functional anatomy of the elbow, and relate it to overuse and traumatic injuries.
- Explain the process for assessing the injured elbow.

- Demonstrate proper immediate and follow-up management of elbow injuries.
- Devise appropriate rehabilitation techniques that can be used following injury to the elbow.

■ **Outline**

■ **Connect Highlights**    McGraw Hill Education **connect**

*Visit connect.mcgraw-hill.com for further exercises to apply your knowledge:*

- Clinical application scenarios covering assessment and recognition of elbow injuries, etiology, symptoms and signs, management of elbow injuries, and rehabilitation for the elbow
- Click-and-drag questions covering structural anatomy of the elbow, assessment of elbow injuries, and rehabilitation plan of the elbow
- Multiple-choice questions covering anatomy, assessment, etiology, and management and rehabilitation of elbow injuries
- Selection questions covering rehabilitation plan for various injuries to the elbow
- Video identification of special tests for the elbow injuries, rehabilitation techniques for the elbow, and taping and wrapping for elbow injuries
- Picture identification of major anatomical components of the elbow, rehabilitation techniques of the elbow, and therapeutic modalities for management

# ANATOMY OF THE ELBOW JOINT

## Bones

The elbow joint is composed of three bones: the humerus, the radius, and the ulna (Figure 23–1). The distal end of the humerus forms two articulating condyles. The lateral condyle is the capitulum, and the medial condyle is the trochlea. The convex capitulum articulates with the concave head of the radius. The trochlea, which is spool-shaped, fits into an articulating groove, the semilunar notch, which is provided by the ulna between the olecranon and coronoid processes. Above each condyle is a projection called the epicondyle. The structural design of the elbow joint permits flexion and extension through the articulation of the trochlea with the trochlear notch of the ulna. Forearm pronation and supination are made possible because the head of the radius rotates against the capitulum freely without any bone limitations.[20]

## Articulations

The elbow complex consists of three separate joints: the humeroulnar joint, the humeroradial joint, and the proximal radioulnar joint (Figure 23–2). The humeroulnar joint is the articulation between the distal humerus medially and the proximal ulna. When the elbow is in flexion, the ulna slides forward until the coronoid process of the ulna stops in the floor of the coronoid fossa of the humerus. In extension, the ulna slides backward until the olecranon process of the ulna makes contact with the olecranon fossa of the humerus posteriorly. The humeroradial joint is the articulation of the lateral distal humerus and the capitulum. In flexion, the radius is in contact with the radial fossa of the distal humerus. The radiocapitellar joint narrows with

elbow valgus and forearm pronation. In full flexion, the radial head comes in contact with the radial fossa of the distal humerus.[35] The proximal radioulnar joint is the articulation between the radial notch of the proximal lateral aspect of the ulna and the radial head. The proximal and distal radioulnar joints are important in supination and pronation. The proximal and distal aspects of this joint cannot function without each other.

## Capsule and Ligaments

The capsule of the elbow, both anteriorly and posteriorly, is relatively thin and is covered by the brachialis muscle in front and the triceps brachii behind. The capsule is reinforced by the ulnar and radial collateral ligaments (Figure 23–2). The ulnar collateral ligament (medial collateral ligament) is composed of a strong anterior band with weaker transverse and posterior bands. The radial collateral ligament (lateral collateral ligament) does not attach to the radius, which is free to rotate. The radius rotates in the radial notch of the ulna and is stabilized by a strong annular ligament. The annular ligament is attached to the anterior and posterior margins of the radial notch and encircles the head and neck of the radius. The radial collateral ligament (lateral collateral ligament) originates from the lateral epicondyle and inserts on the annular ligament, instead of on the radius itself. This allows the radial head to rotate freely in the radial notch on the ulna during forearm pronation and supination.[2]

Valgus elbow stability depends mainly on the integrity of the ulnar collateral ligament. Lateral elbow stability depends on two factors: the integrity of the lateral collateral ligament and stabilization by the annular ligament, which maintains the relationship of the radial head to the

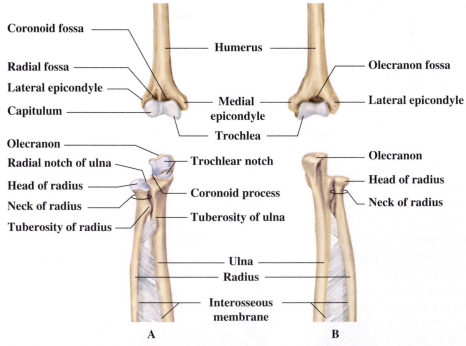

FIGURE 23–1 Bones of the elbow joint. (**A**) Anterior view. (**B**) Posterior view.

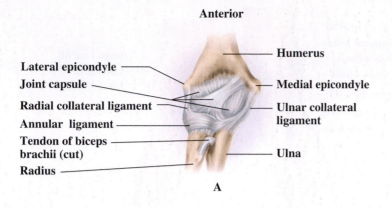

Anterior

Humerus

Lateral epicondyle

Joint capsule

Radial collateral ligament

Annular ligament

Tendon of biceps
brachii (cut)

Radius

Medial epicondyle

Ulnar collateral
ligament

Ulna

A

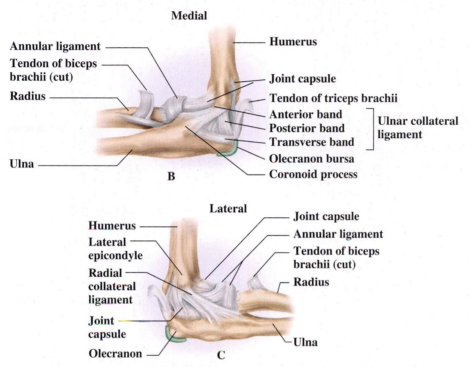

Medial

Annular ligament

Tendon of biceps
brachii (cut)

Radius

Humerus

Joint capsule

Tendon of triceps brachii

Anterior band

Posterior band        Ulnar collateral
                      ligament
Transverse band

Olecranon bursa

Coronoid process

Ulna

B

Lateral

Joint capsule

Annular ligament

Tendon of biceps
brachii (cut)

Radius

Humerus

Lateral
epicondyle

Radial
collateral
ligament

Joint
capsule

Olecranon

Ulna

C

FIGURE 23–2    Joint capsule and ligaments of the elbow. **(A)** Anterior. **(B)** Medial. **(C)** Lateral.

proximal radioulnar joints. The ulnar collateral ligament plays a key role in maintaining elbow stability against valgus torque. The integrity of this ligament is of major importance in activities that produce forceful valgus and/or flexion-supination movements. Integrity of the radial collateral ligament and the annular ligament that stabilizes the proximal radioulnar joint are crucial to maintaining the lateral elbow stability. While these ligaments provide significant stability to the joint, additional support from the congruity of the humeroulnar and radiocapitellar joints, and dynamic support from the muscle tendons are necessary to achieve adequate elbow joint stability.

## Synovium and Bursae

A common synovial membrane invests the elbow and the superior radioulnar articulations, lubricating the deeper structures of the two joints; a sleevelike capsule surrounds the entire elbow joint. The most important bursae

in the area of the elbow are the bicipital and olecranon bursae. The bicipital bursa lies in the anterior aspect of the bicipital tuberosity and cushions the tendon when the forearm is pronated. The olecranon bursa lies between the olecranon process and the skin (Figure 23–2B).

## Elbow Musculature

The elbow flexors are the biceps brachii, brachialis, and brachioradialis muscles (Figure 23–3). The biceps brachii originates via two heads proximally at the shoulder: the long head from the supraglenoid tuberosity of the scapula and the short head from the coracoid process of the scapula. The insertion is from a common tendon at the radial tuberosity. The biceps brachii flexes the elbow and supinates the forearm. The brachialis originates from the lower two-thirds of the anterior humerus and inserts on the coronoid process and the tuberosity of the ulna. It flexes the elbow. The brachioradialis, which originates

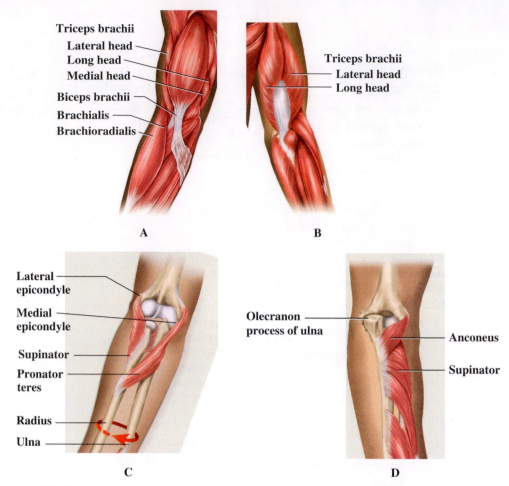

FIGURE 23–3    Muscles of the elbow joint. **(A)** Anterior view. **(B)** Posterior view. **(C)** Deep pronator teres and supinator muscles (anterior view). **(D)** Anconeus and supinator muscles (posterior view).

from the lower two-thirds of the lateral humerus and attaches to the lateral styloid process of the distal radius, functions as an elbow flexor, pronator, and semisupinator.

The elbow extensors are the triceps brachii and the anconeus muscles. The triceps brachii consists of long, medial, and lateral heads. The long head originates at the infraglenoid tuberosity of the scapula. The lateral and medial heads originate at the posterior aspect of the humerus. The insertion is via the common tendon posteriorly at the olecranon process. The triceps and the anconeus muscle cause extension of the elbow complex.

The pronator teres (Figure 23–4C) at the elbow joint and pronator quadratus at the distal aspect of the wrist (see Figure 24–2A) cause pronation of the forearm. Supination is caused by a combined action of the biceps brachii and the supinator muscle. With both supination and pronation, the radius moves on the ulna.

In addition to the movers of the elbow, many of the muscles that move the wrist cross the elbow joint. The wrist flexors and pronator teres originate from a common tendon from the medial epicondyle. Similarly, the wrist extensors originate from a common tendon from the lateral epicondyle.[52]

## Nerve Supply

Musculoskeletal, radial, ulnar, and median nerves that stem from the brachial plexus (C5-T1) control elbow movement (Table 23–1). The radial and median nerves run anterior to the elbow, while the ulnar nerve runs through the groove between the medial epicondyle and olecranon process (cubital tunnel) (Figure 23–4A).

## Blood Supply

The subclavian artery becomes an axillary artery and then the brachial artery, whose branches supply the elbow (Figure 23–4B). The deep brachial, ulnar recurrent, and radial recurrent arteries eventually anastomose with the brachial to supply the radial and ulnar arteries of the forearm. The medial cubital, basilic, cephalic, and brachial veins collectively drain blood from the elbow region into the axillary vein (Figure 23–4C).

## Surface Anatomy

Figure 23–5 shows the pertinent surface anatomy of the elbow joint from lateral, anterior, and posterior views.

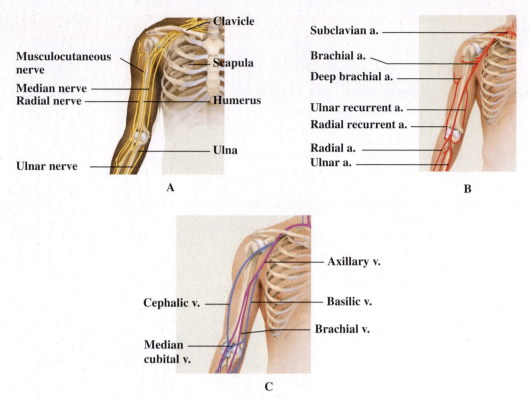

FIGURE 23–4    (A) Nerves. (B) Arteries. (C) Veins supplying the elbow joint.

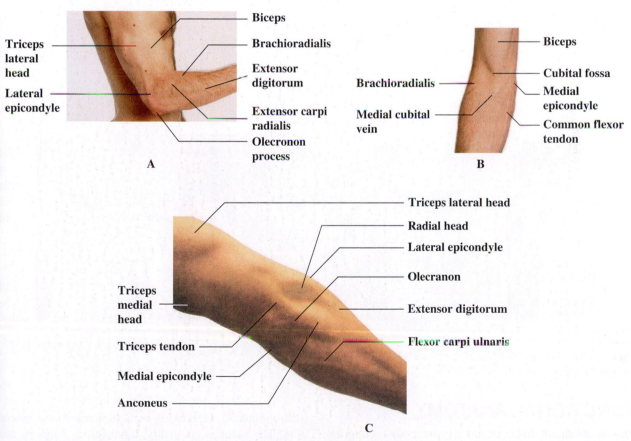

FIGURE 23–5    Surface anatomy of the elbow. (A) Lateral view. (B) Anterior view. (C) Posterior view.

TABLE 23–1    Muscles Acting on the Elbow Joint

| Muscle | Origin | Insertion | Muscle Action | Innervation/ Nerve Root |
|---|---|---|---|---|
| **Biceps brachii** | *Long head:* Supraglenoid tuberosity of the scapula *Short head:* Coracoid process of the scapula | Tuberosity of the radius | Flexes the elbow and the shoulder; supinates the forearm | Musculocutaneous (C5, C6) |
| **Brachialis** | Anterior surface of the distal half of the humerus | Coronoid process of the ulna | Flexes the elbow | Musculocutaneous (C5, C6) and radial (C7, C8) |
| **Brachioradialis** | Lateral supracondular ridge of the humerus | Styloid process of the radius | Flexes the elbow | Radial (C7, C8) |
| **Triceps brachii** | *Long head:* Infraglenoid tuberosity of the scapula *Lateral head:* Posterior surface of the humerus above the radial groove *Medial head:* Posterior surface of the humerus below the radial groove | Olecranon process of the ulna | Extends the elbow and the arm | Radial (C7, C8) |
| **Supinator** | Lateral epicondyle of the humerus | Proximal end of the lateral surface of the shaft of the radius | Supinates the elbow | Radial (C7, C8) |
| **Pronator teres** | Medial epicondyle of the humerus and the coronoid process of the ulna | Middle of the lateral surface of the shaft of the radius | Pronates the elbow | Median (C6, C7) |
| **Anconeus** | Lateral epicondyle of the humerus | Lateral surface of the olecranon process of the ulna | Extends the elbow | Radial (C7, C8) |

**Elbow Joint Movements***

*Manual muscle tests and goniometric measurements of range of motion for the elbow joint can be found in Appendix F and Appendix G at the end of the text.

© William E. Prentice

# FUNCTIONAL ANATOMY

The anatomical arrangement of the elbow complex allows for flexion, extension, pronation, and supination. The elbow has approximately 145 degrees of flexion and 90 degrees of both supination and pronation. The osseous congruity, ligamentous support, and muscular stability at the elbow help protect it from overuse and traumatic injury.[2] Because of the more

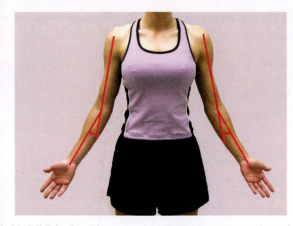

FIGURE 23–6  Observing for elbow carrying angle and the extent of cubitus valgus and cubitus varus.

© William E. Prentice

distal projection of the humerus medially, the elbow complex demonstrates a carrying angle that is an abducted position of the elbow in the anatomical position (Figure 23–6).[20] The normal carrying angle in females is 10 to 15 degrees and in males, 5 to 10 degrees. In the athletic environment, the elbow complex can be subjected to forces ranging from overhead throwing activities to blunt trauma that can cause various injuries.

The elbow is a critical link in the kinetic chain of the upper extremity. Alteration of elbow movement due to joint instability, pain, or muscle tightness can affect the movement and stress at the shoulder and wrist joints. On the other hand, movement alteration at the shoulder complex can affect elbow joint function.[14]

## Prevention of Elbow Injuries

The elbow is vulnerable to a variety of both acute traumatic injuries as well as chronic overuse-type injuries. Acute injuries usually occur either from a direct blow or falling on an outstretched hand.[21]

The chances of developing chronic overuse injuries that typically occur in the elbow may be reduced by using several strategies.[40] The athlete should limit the number of repetitions in throwing a baseball or hitting a tennis ball. Taking adequate recovery time between practices/games and using cross training to take a break from sports for a few months out of the year is also recommended. This is especially true with young baseball pitchers who need to limit their pitch count so that they are not putting too much stress on the elbow joint as they become fatigued.[9] Make certain that the mechanics of the throwing or hitting techniques being used are correct and are not creating unnecessary stresses and strains.[10] Select and use equipment that is appropriate for a specific skill level (e.g., a tennis racket with

the appropriate grip size). The athlete should maintain appropriate levels of strength and endurance in the muscles surrounding the scapula, shoulder, and elbow. by engaging in strength training. He or she should routinely stretch the muscles in the upper extremity, to make certain that they have the necessary flexibility to allow fluid joint motion. If a chronic overuse problem seems to be developing, the athlete should take some time off and give the injury a chance to heal before it gets worse.[54]

# ASSESSMENT OF THE ELBOW

## History

An elbow injury requires the athletic trainer first to understand the possible mechanism of injury. The athletic trainer should ask the following questions when evaluating the elbow:

- Is the pain or discomfort caused by a direct trauma, such as falling on an outstretched hand (FOOSH) or landing on the tip of a bent elbow (the most common mechanism for a variety of elbow injuries)?[29]
- Can the problem be attributed to sudden overextension of the elbow or to repeated overuse?[8]

> **FOOSH** falling on outstretch hand.

- What are the location and duration of the pain? Elbow pain or discomfort could be from internal organ dysfunction or referred from a nerve root irritation or nerve impingement.[8]
- Are there movements or positions of the arm that increase or decrease the pain?
- Has a previous elbow injury been diagnosed or treated?
- Is there a feeling of locking or crepitation during movement?

## Observation

The patient's elbow should be observed for obvious deformities and swelling. The carrying angle of the elbow should be observed.[8] If the carrying angle is abnormally increased, a cubitus valgus is present; if it is abnormally decreased, a cubitus varus is present (Figure 23–6). The patient is next observed for the extent of elbow flexion and extension. Both elbows are compared (Figure 23–7). A decrease in normal flexion, an inability to extend fully, or extension beyond normal (cubitus recurvatus) could be precipitating reasons for joint problems (Figure 23–8). Normal elbow range of motion is 0 degrees to 140 degrees of flexion. Next, the elbow is bent to a 45-degree angle and observed from the rear to determine whether the two epicondyles and olecranon process form an isosceles triangle (Figure 23–9).

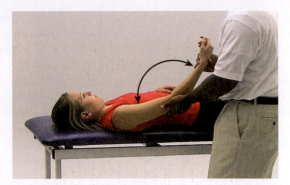

FIGURE 23–7   Testing for elbow flexion and extension.
© William E. Prentice

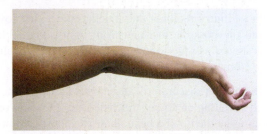

FIGURE 23–8   Testing for cubitus recurvatus (elbow hyperextension).
© William E. Prentice

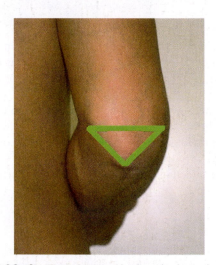

FIGURE 23–9   Determining whether the lateral and medial epicondyles, along with the olecranon process, form an isosceles triangle.
© William E. Prentice

## Palpation

**Bony Palpation** The following bony landmarks should be palpated:

- Medial epicondyle
- Lateral epicondyle
- Olecranon process
- Radial head
- Radius
- Ulna

**Soft-Tissue Palpation** The following soft tissue structures should be palpated:

### Anterior
- Biceps brachii
- Brachialis
- Brachioradialis
- Pronator teres

### Posterior
- Triceps
- Supinator

### Medial
- Ulnar collateral ligament
- Wrist flexor muscles
- Ulnar nerve

### Lateral
- Radial collateral ligament
- Annular ligament
- Wrist extensor muscles

## Special Tests

**Elbow-Extension Test[3]** The seated patient, with exposed and supinated arms, is asked to flex his or her shoulders to 90 degrees and then to fully extend and lock both elbows. Injured and uninjured sides are compared visually, and those with equal extension are recorded as full extension. In a positive test there is an inability to fully straighten the elbow, or the pain worsens or does not improve (Figure 23–10).[15]
Sn. 0.97 | Sp. 0.49 | +LR NA | -LR 0.03

**Valgus and Varus Stress Tests** A valgus stress test checks for sprain of the ulnar collateral ligament. A varus stress test checks for sprain or instability of the radial collateral ligament. For the valgus stress test, the athletic

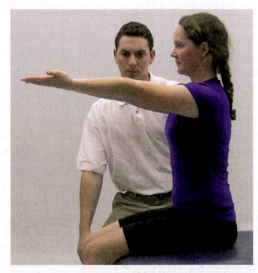

FIGURE 23–10   Elbow-extension test.
© William E. Prentice

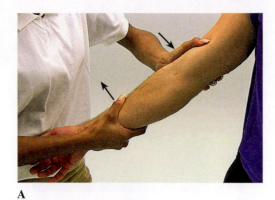

**A**

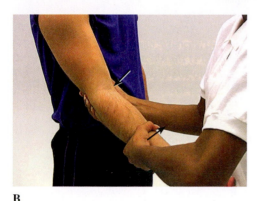

**B**

FIGURE 23–11 Collateral ligament test of the elbow.
**(A)** Ulnar collateral ligament. **(B)** Radial collateral ligament.
© William E. Prentice

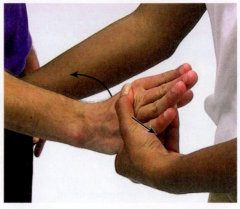

FIGURE 23–12 Lateral epicondylitis test or Cozen's test.
© William E. Prentice

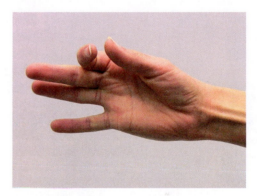

FIGURE 23–13 Pinch grip test.
© William E. Prentice

trainer grasps the patient's forearm with one hand and places the other hand over the lateral aspect of the elbow. The patient's elbow should be slightly flexed. Using the hand placed over the lateral elbow as a fulcrum, use the other hand to rotate the forearm into valgus (Figure 23–11).

For the varus stress test, the hand is placed over the medial aspect of the elbow, and the forearm is rotated into varus. The athletic trainer should note whether there is gapping at the joint line.

> A patient sustains a serious injury to the left elbow.
>
> ❓ What tests and basic examination procedures should be performed to determine the nature of this injury?

**Lateral (Cozen's Test) and Medial Epicondylitis Tests[49]** Keeping the patient's elbow flexed to 45 degrees, the clinician resists wrist extension (referred to as Cozen's test) and then flexion. Pain in lateral epicondyle when wrist extension is resisted indicates lateral epicondylitis. Pain in medial epicondyle when wrist flexion is resisted indicates medial epicondylitis (Figure 23–12). Sn. 0.84 | Sp. 0.0 | +LR 0.84 | -LR Infinity

**Pinch Grip Test** The patient is instructed to pinch the tips of the thumb and index finger together. An inability to touch the thumb and index finger indicates entrapment of the anterior interosseous nerve between the two heads of the pronator muscle (Figure 23–13).

**Pronator Teres Syndrome Test** The athletic trainer resists forearm pronation. Increased pain proximally over the pronator teres indicates possible entrapment and compression of the median nerve by the pronator teres (Figure 23–14).

**Moving Valgus Stress Test[38]** With the patient sitting, the shoulder is adducted to 90 degrees and the elbow fully flexed to apply valgus stress; move the elbow to 30 degrees of flexion (Figure 23–15). A positive test produces medial elbow pain and may indicate an injury to the ulnar collateral ligament. Sn. 1.00 | Sp. 0.75 | +LR 4.00 | -LR 0.00

**Functional Evaluation** The joint and muscles are evaluated for pain sites and weakness through passive, active, and resistive motions consisting of elbow flexion and extension (see Figure 23–7), forearm pronation and supination (Figure 23–16A) and wrist flexion and extension (Figure 23–16B). Wrist flexion and extension must also

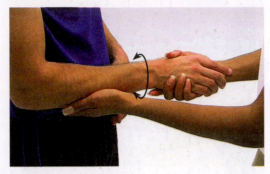

FIGURE 23–14  A positive pronator teres syndrome test indicates compression of the median nerve.
© William E. Prentice

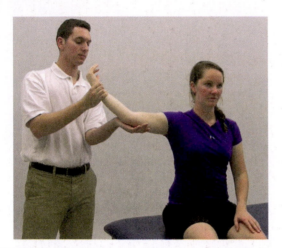

FIGURE 23–15  Moving valgus stress test. Medial elbow pain may indicate injury to the ulnar collateral ligament.
© William E. Prentice

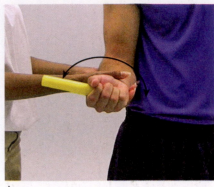

A

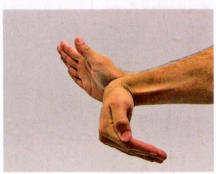

B

FIGURE 23–16  Functional evaluation tests should include **(A)** pronation and supination, and **(B)** wrist flexion and extension.
© William E. Prentice

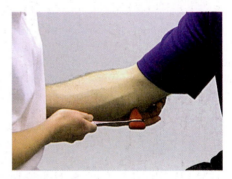

FIGURE 23–17  Tinel's test.
© William E. Prentice

be evaluated, considering that wrist extensors and flexors cross the elbow joint.

**Circulatory and Neurological Evaluation**  With an elbow injury, a pulse should routinely be taken at the brachial artery and at the radial artery at the wrist. Alteration of skin sensation also should be noted, as it can indicate nerve root compression or irritation in the cervical or shoulder region or in the elbow itself. Additional nerve evaluation is made through active and resistive muscle tests (see Table 23–1).

***Tinel's Sign*[5]**  Tinel's test is designed to determine ulnar nerve compromise. The patient is seated with the elbow in slight flexion. The athletic trainer stands and grasps the patient's wrist and, with the other hand, taps the cubital notch between the olecranon process and medial epicondyle with a reflex hammer or the index finger. A positive Tinel's sign is when the patient complains of a tingling sensation along the forearm, hand, and fingers (Figure 23–17).[5] Sn. 0.62 | Sp. 0.53 | +LR 0.77 | -LR 0.30

# RECOGNITION AND MANAGEMENT OF INJURIES TO THE ELBOW

The elbow is subject to injury because of its range of motion, weak lateral bone arrangement, and relative exposure to soft-tissue damage.[33] Many activities place excessive stress on the elbow joint.[21]

## Contusions

***Etiology***  Because of its lack of padding and its general vulnerability, the elbow often becomes contused. Bone bruises arise from a deep penetration or a succession of blows to the sharp projections of the elbow.

***Symptoms and signs*** A contusion of the elbow may swell rapidly after an irritation of the olecranon bursa or the synovial membrane.

***Management*** The contused elbow should be treated immediately with cold and pressure for at least 24 hours. If injury is severe, the patient should be referred to a physician for X-ray examination to determine whether a fracture exists.

## Olecranon Bursitis

***Etiology*** The olecranon bursa, lying between the end of the olecranon process and the skin, is the most frequently injured bursa in the elbow (Figure 23–18).[27] Its superficial location makes it prone to acute or chronic injury, particularly as a result of direct blows.[53]

***Symptoms and signs*** The inflamed bursa produces pain, severe swelling, and point tenderness. Occasionally, swelling will appear almost spontaneously and without the usual pain and heat.

***Management*** If the condition is acute, POLICE should be applied for at least 1 hour. Chronic olecranon bursitis requires a program of conservative treatment primarily involving compression. If swelling fails to resolve, in some cases aspiration will hasten healing. Although seldom serious, olecranon bursitis can be annoying and should be well protected by padding while the patient is engaged in competition.

## Strains

***Etiology*** The acute mechanisms of muscle strain associated with the elbow joint are usually excessive resistive motions, such as a fall on the outstretched hand with the elbow in extension, which forces the joint into hyperextension. Repeated microtears that cause chronic injury are discussed in the section on epicondylitis.[46]

The biceps, brachialis, and triceps muscles should be tested through active and resistive movement. The muscles of pronation and supination are also tested. Rupture of the distal biceps brachii at its radial attachment is the most common muscle rupture in the upper extremity.[51]

***Symptoms and signs*** During active or resistive movement, the patient complains of pain. There is usually point tenderness in the muscle, tendon, or myotendinous junction.

***Management*** Immediate care includes POLICE as well as sling support for the most severe cases. Follow-up management may include cryotherapy, ultrasound, and rehabilitative exercises. Conditions that cause moderate to severe loss of elbow function should routinely be referred for X-ray examination. It is important to rule out the possibility of an avulsion or epiphyseal fracture.

## Ulnar Collateral Ligament Injuries

***Etiology*** The ulnar collateral ligament is most often injured as a result of repetitive valgus loading on the elbow, which occurs in the late cocking and early acceleration phases of throwing, during a forehand stroke in tennis, and in the trailing arm during an improper golf swing. The valgus torque on the elbow increases tension in medial elbow structures, including ulnar collateral ligament, ulnar nerve, and wrist flexor tendons that originates from the medial elbow.[44] For that reason, the same mechanism can result in ulnar nerve inflammation or tendinosis at the medial elbow (medial epicondylitis).[36] It is not uncommon to see these conditions present along with the ulnar collateral ligament sprain. The injuries can vary from mild irritation of the ulnar collateral ligament to a complete rupture of the ligament.

***Symptoms and signs*** On examination, the patient typically complains of pain along the medial aspect of the elbow. There is tenderness over the ulnar collateral ligament, usually at the distal insertion and occasionally in a more diffuse distribution. In some cases, the patient describes associated paresthesias in the distribution of the ulnar nerve with a positive Tinel's sign.[12] When valgus stress is applied to the elbow at 20 to 30 degrees of flexion, local pain, tenderness, and endpoint laxity are

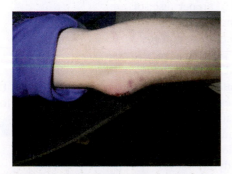

**FIGURE 23–18** Olecranon bursitis.
Courtesy Tom Anderson

assessed. On standard X-ray, hypertrophy of the humeral condyle and posteromedial aspect of the olecranon, marginal osteophytes (bony outgrowths) of the ulnohumeral or radiocapitellar joints, calcification within the ulnar collateral ligament, and loose bodies in the posterior compartment may be present.[1]

**Management** Conservative treatment of patients with chronic ulnar collateral ligament injury should begin with rest and NSAIDs. With resolution of symptoms, rehabilitation should be instituted with an emphasis on strengthening. The athletic trainer, along with the coach, should analyze the athlete's throwing mechanics, which may include video assessment, to correct any existing faulty mechanics. If periods of rest and rehabilitation fail to resolve the symptoms, surgical intervention may be necessary.

Operative management consists of repair or reconstruction, which is fairly common, particularly among higher-level baseball players.[18] Reconstruction usually consists of using a palmeris longus autograft and occasionally transposition of the ulnar nerve. In the case of an acute rupture, surgical repair can be considered; however, the indications are extremely limited.[4] In baseball players, surgical repair of the ulnar collateral ligament has been referred to as a "Tommy John" procedure. Generally, the athlete can begin throwing about 22 to 26 weeks after surgery,[47] although it is likely that full recovery will take 18 to 24 months.[22]

**Lateral Epicondylitis** Lateral epicondylitis is a degenerative condition of the wrist extensor tendons at the lateral epicondyle. The injury is commonly associated with occupational or sports activities that involve repetitive wrist extension and forearm supination such as tennis, and fencing.[52]

**Etiology** Lateral epicondylitis is one of the most common problems of the elbow.[25] The cause of lateral epicondylitis is repetitive microtrauma with overuse of the extensor muscles.[57] It usually involves the extensor carpi radialis brevis and extensor digitorum communis laterally (Figure 23–19).[6] Microtrauma or overuse can occur in an activity that involves repetitive wrist extension, or supination or repetitive heavy lifting. Whether there is inflammation is debatable. However, it is likely that there is *tendinosis* in which there is a degeneration of the tendon without inflammation.[37] *Tennis elbow* is another name for

> **Lateral epicondylitis is also called tennis elbow.**

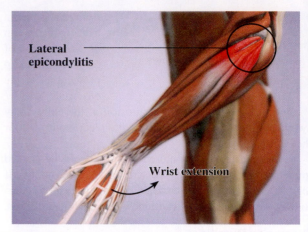

Lateral epicondylitis

Wrist extension

**FIGURE 23–19** Lateral epicondylitis occurs with repeated forceful hyperextension of the wrist.

lateral epicondylitis; it stems from a backhand stroke involving wrist overextension.[16]

**Symptoms and signs** The patient complains of an aching pain in the region of the lateral epicondyle during and after activity. The pain gradually becomes worse, and weakness develops in the hand and wrist. Inspection reveals tenderness at the lateral epicondyle and pain on resisted extension of the wrist and full extension of the elbow. The elbow has decreased range of motion.[41]

**Management** Treatment includes the immediate use of POLICE, NSAIDs, and analgesics as needed. Rehabilitation includes ROM exercises, PRE, deep friction massage, hand grasping while in supination, and avoidance of pronation movements.[50] Use of prolotherapy and injection of platelet-rich plasma and autologous blood are also incorporated in the treatment.[48] Mobilization and stretching may be used within pain-free limits. The patient may wear a counterforce or neoprene elbow sleeve for 1 to 3 months.[31] The patient must be taught proper skill techniques and the proper use of equipment to avoid recurrence of the injury.[27]

**Medial Epicondylitis**

**Etiology** Medial epicondylitis is a condition that involves degenerative changes in the tendons that originate from the medial epicondyle. Medial epicondylitis may involve the pronator teres, flexor

> **Medial epicondylitis:**
> - Pitcher's elbow
> - Racquetball elbow
> - Golfer's elbow
> - Javelin-thrower's elbow

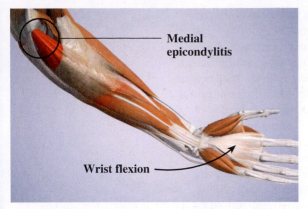

Medial
epicondylitis

Wrist flexion

FIGURE 23–20   Medial epicondylitis occurs from repeated forceful wrist flexion.

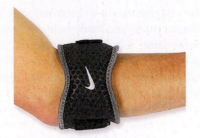

FIGURE 23–22   Counterforce brace for treatment of elbow epicondylitis.

Courtesy NIKE, Inc.

carpi radialis, and ulnaris and the palmaris longus tendons. There also may be an associated neuropathy of the ulnar nerve, producing pain radiating to the medial forearm and fingers (Figure 23–20). Pitcher's elbow, racquetball elbow, golfer's elbow, and javelin-thrower's elbow are other names for medial epicondylitis.[28] Young baseball pitchers learning to throw a curveball or screwball tend to use excessive wrist flexion when imparting a spin on the baseball (Figure 23–21A).[56] A forehand stroke in racquetball requires an explosive wrist flexion at impact to achieve maximum velocity. Golfers may use too much wrist flexion on the trailing arm on follow-through (Figure 23–21B).[19] Throwing the javelin requires powerful wrist flexion at release (Figure 23–21C).

***Symptoms and signs***   Pain around the medial epicondyles of the humerus can be produced during forceful wrist flexion and pronation. The pain may be centered at the medial epicondyle, or it may radiate down the arm. There is usually point tenderness and, in some cases, mild swelling. Passive movement of the wrist into extension seldom elicits pain, although active flexion does.

***Management***   Conservative management of moderate to severe epicondylitis usually includes the use of sling rest, cryotherapy, or heat through the application of ultrasound. Analgesics and antiinflammatory agents may be prescribed. A curvilinear brace applied just below the bend of the elbow is highly beneficial in reducing elbow stress. This brace provides a counterforce, disseminating stress over a wide area and relieving the concentration of forces directly on the bony muscle attachments (Figure 23–22). For more severe cases, elbow splinting and complete rest for 7 to 10 days may be warranted.[23]

### Elbow Osteochondritis Dissecans

***Etiology***   Although osteochondritis dissecans is more common in the knee, it also occurs in the elbow. Its cause is unknown; however, impairment of the blood supply to the anterior

> A golfer is complaining of pain on the medial aspect of the trailing arm during follow-through on the golf swing. When not playing golf, the patient constantly has an aching feeling.
>
> **?** What is the most likely cause of this medial elbow pain?

> Osteochondritis dissecans in the elbow is similar to that in the knee but is less common.

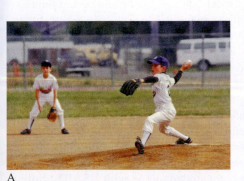

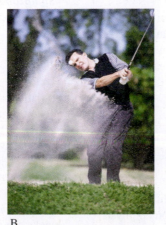

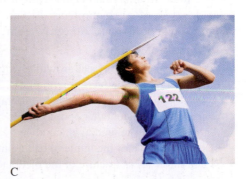

A                                B                                C

FIGURE 23–21   Activities that involve repeated forceful wrist flexion can cause medial epicondylitis at the elbow.
**(A)** Baseball. **(B)** Golf. **(C)** Javelin throw.

(a) © Corbis RF; (b) © Stockbyte/Getty Images; (c) © Image Source

surfaces leads to fragmentation and separation of a portion of the articular cartilage and bone, which creates loose bodies within the joint.[7] Elbow osteochondritis dissecans is seen in the young patient 10 to 15 years of age who throws or engages in racquet sports.[24] A repetitive micro-trauma in the movements of elbow rotation, extension, and valgus stress leads to a compression of the radial head and shearing of the radiocapitular joint.[25] Osteochondritis in children younger than ten is usually referred to as *Panner's disease*.[61]

Some confusion exists as to whether there is any difference between osteochondritis dissecans and Panner's disease. Although Panner's disease might just be a part of the spectrum of osteochondritis dissecans, it is probably better to limit the diagnosis of Panner's disease to children age 10 or younger at the time of onset.[61] Panner's disease is an osteochondrosis of the capitellum in which there is a localized avascular necrosis, leading to the loss of the subchondral bone of the capitellum, which can cause softening and fissuring of articular surfaces of the radiocapitellar joint.[7] If loose bodies develop, Panner's disease will produce osteochondritis dissecans.

***Symptoms and signs*** The child or young adolescent patient usually complains of sudden pain and locking of the elbow joint.[13] Range of motion returns slowly over a few days. Swelling, pain, and crepitation may also occur. There is a decreased ROM, especially in full extension, and tenderness at the radiohumeral joints. There may be a grating sensation on pronation or supination. X-ray examination shows a flattening of the capitellum, a crater in the capitellum, and loose bodies.[24]

***Management*** In the beginning stage of this condition, activity is restricted for 6 to 12 weeks, and NSAIDs are administered.[28] With increased degeneration, activity is restricted, and a splint or cast is applied along with treatment. If there are loose bodies with repeated locking, fragments are removed surgically.[7]

### Little League Elbow

***Etiology*** Little League elbow occurs in 10 percent to 25 percent of young pitchers.[40] It is caused by repetitive microtrauma that occurs from throwing and not from the type of pitch thrown.[12] Little League elbow includes many disorders of growth in the pitching elbow:[26,30,39]

- An accelerated apophyseal growth region plus a delay in the medial epicondylar growth plate
- A traction apophysitis with a possible fragmentation of the medial epicondylar apophysis
- An avulsion of the medial epicondyle
- Osteochondrosis of the humeral capitellum
- A nonunion stress fracture of the olecranon epiphysis

***Symptoms and signs*** Injury onset is usually slow. In the beginning, the patient may have a flexion contracture, which includes a tightness of the anterior joint capsule and a weakness of the triceps muscle.[11] The patient may complain of a locking or catching sensation. There is decreased ROM of forearm pronation and supination.

***Management*** Initially, POLICE, NSAIDs, and analgesics are given as needed.[25] Throwing is stopped until pain is resolved and full ROM is returned. Gentle stretching and triceps strengthening are carried out. Surgical removal of loose bodies may be required.[7] Throwing under guidance and with good technique is essential in preventing elbow injuries in adolescents (see Figure 22–32).[45,59]

### Cubital Tunnel Syndrome

***Etiology*** Because of the exposed position of the medial humeral condyle, the ulnar nerve is subject to a variety of problems. The patient with a pronounced cubitus valgus may develop a friction problem. The ulnar nerve can also become recurrently dislocated because of a structural deformity. The ulnar nerve can become impinged by the arcuate ligament during flexion activities.[23] In a problem of the ulnar nerve seen in sports such as baseball, tennis, racquetball, and javelin throwing, fascial bands forming the roof of the cubital tunnel compress the ulnar nerve.[23]

Normally, four factors can lead to cubital tunnel syndrome: traction injury from a valgus torque, irregularities within the tunnel, subluxation of the ulnar nerve because of a lax ligament, and a progressive compression of the ligament on the nerve.[23]

***Symptoms and signs*** The patient complains of pain on the medial aspect of the elbow that may be referred proximally or distally. Palpation indicates tenderness in the cubital tunnel, primarily on hyperflexion. There is intermittent paresthesia reflected by burning and tingling in the fourth and fifth fingers.[23]

***Management*** Initially, rest and immobilization for 2 weeks are recommended, along with NSAIDs. Splinting or surgical decompression or transposition of a subluxating ulnar nerve may be necessary. The patient must avoid elbow hyperflexion and valgus stresses.[25]

A Little League pitcher complains of pain, swelling, and grating in the pitching elbow.

**?** What might this condition be?

A javelin-thrower with a pronounced elbow cubitus valgus places abnormal pressure on the ulnar nerve.

**?** What nerve involvement could occur from this situation?

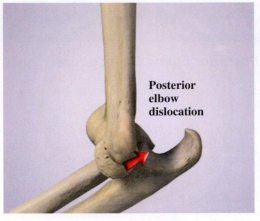
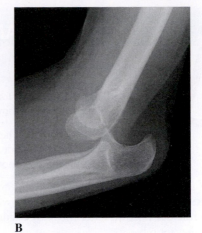

**A**

**B**

Posterior
elbow
dislocation

FIGURE 23–23   **(A)** A fall on the outstretched hand, with the elbow flexed, can produce an elbow dislocation and/or fracture. **(B)** Posterior dislocation X-ray.
(b) Courtesy Jordan B. Renner, MD, Departments of Radiology and Allied Health Sciences, University of North Carolina

## Dislocation of the Elbow

***Etiology***   Dislocation of the elbow (Figure 23–23) occurs most often either by a fall on the outstretched hand with the elbow in a position of hyperextension or by a severe twist while the elbow is in a flexed position.[32] The bones of the ulna and radius may be displaced backward, forward, or laterally. By far the most common dislocation is one in which both the ulna and the radius are forced backward.[55] The forward-displaced humerus appears deformed. The olecranon process extends posteriorly, well beyond its normal alignment with the humerus. The athletic trainer can distinguish this dislocation from the supracondylar fracture by observing that the lateral and medial epicondyles are normally aligned with the shaft of the humerus.

***Symptoms and signs***   Elbow dislocations involve rupturing and tearing of most of the stabilizing ligamentous tissue, accompanied by profuse hemorrhage and swelling. There is severe pain and disability. The complications of such traumas are injury to the median and radial nerves and the major blood vessels and arteries as well as myositis ossificans. Elbow dislocation is often associated with a radial head fracture.[32]

***Management***   The primary responsibility is to apply cold and pressure immediately, then a sling, and to refer the patient to a physician for reduction. The neurovascular status of the brachial artery and the median and ulnar nerves

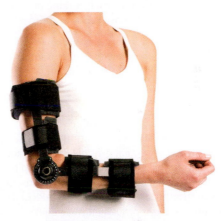

FIGURE 23–24   Advance Dynamic ROM splint for the reduction of elbow flexion contraction.
Courtesy DJ Global

must be evaluated before and after reduction.[46] Only a physician should reduce an elbow dislocation. It must be performed as soon as possible to prevent prolonged derangement of the soft tissue.[32] In most cases, the physician administers an anesthetic before reduction to relax muscle spasms. After reduction, the physician often immobilizes the elbow in a position of flexion and applies a sling suspension, which should be used for approximately 3 weeks (Figure 23–24). The length of immobilization should be minimized if the ulnar collateral ligament is intact and stable.[55] While the arm is maintained in flexion, the patient should execute hand gripping and shoulder exercises. Once initial healing has occurred, heat and gentle, passive exercise may be applied to help regain a full range of motion. Above all, the patient should avoid massage and joint movements that are too strenuous before complete healing has occurred because of the high probability of myositis ossificans. The patient should follow both range of

A firefighter sustains a posterior elbow dislocation from falling off a ladder.

**?** What is the proper management of this injury, and what are the possible consequences of delayed treatment?

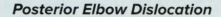

# MANAGEMENT PLAN

## *Posterior Elbow Dislocation*

**Injury Situation** A professional bull rider was thrown from a bull during a rodeo and landed on his outstretched left hand. The elbow was forced into hyperextension, dislocating the radial head posteriorly.

**Symptoms and Signs** The patient complained of extreme pain in the elbow region and numbness in the forearm and hand. From the side, the forearm appeared shortened. An obvious deformity was that the radial head stuck out beyond the posterior aspect of the elbow. The neurovascular status was assessed and found to be normal.

**Management Plan** The patient was referred immediately to a physician, who performed an X-ray examination of the elbow to rule out fracture. After the X-ray examination, the physician reduced the elbow and placed it in a cast and sling at 60 degrees for 6 weeks.

---

### Phase 1 *Acute Injury*

**GOAL DURING IMMOBILIZATION PHASE:** To maintain wrist and hand strength and shoulder range of motion while the elbow is immobilized.
**ESTIMATED LENGTH OF TIME (ELT):** 6 weeks.

- **Exercise rehabilitation** Ball squeeze (10 to 15 repetitions) each waking hour. Shoulder circles in all directions (10 to 15 repetitions) each waking hour. General body maintenance exercises should be conducted 3 times a week as long as they do not aggravate injury.

---

### Phase 2 *Repair*

**GOAL AFTER CAST IS REMOVED:** To increase range of motion 50 percent and both strength and coordination 50 percent.
**ELT:** 4 to 6 weeks.

- **Therapy** Ice (5 to 15 minutes) before and after exercise, electrical stimulation to modulate pain, and low-intensity ultrasound to facilitate healing.
- **Exercise rehabilitation** Continue exercises during immobilization phase, 3 or 4 times daily. Isometric exercise (2 or 3 times) every waking hour. Pain-free active flexion and extension and forearm pronation and supination (10 to 15 repetitions) every waking hour; avoid forcing movements. Proprioceptive neuromuscular facilitation (PNF) also can be beneficial. Isokinetic exercise or isotonic exercise against dumbbell resistance, once daily, using daily adjustable progressive resistance exercise (DAPRE). General body maintenance exercises should be conducted 3 times a week as long as they do not aggravate injury.

---

### Phase 3 *Remodeling*

**GOALS:** To restore 90 percent of elbow ROM and strength, including power, endurance, and neuromuscular control, and to reenter competition.
**ELT:** 3 to 6 weeks.

- **Therapy** Electrical stimulation for muscle reeducation. Ultrasound or massage to increase blood flow in the area. Follow exercise with cryotherapy.
- **Exercise rehabilitation** Continue phase 2 exercises, and add isotonic machine resistance or free-weight barbell exercises; bar dips and chin-ups (10 repetitions), 3 or 4 times a week, can be added to routine. Return to daily training within pain-free limits. If elbow becomes symptomatic in any way, such as pain, swelling, or decreased range of motion, the patient should return to phase 2 exercises.

*Criteria for Return to Competition*

1. Extend and flex the elbow to at least 95 percent of the extent of the uninjured elbow.
2. Pronate and supinate the forearm to at least 95 percent of the extent of the uninjured arm.
3. Perform an elbow curl 10 times, for 3 sets, against a resistance equal to or greater than that which the uninjured elbow can handle (this resistance could be measured by an isokinetic testing device).
4. Perform an elbow extension 10 times, for 3 sets, against a resistance equal to or greater than that which the uninjured elbow can handle (this resistance also can be measured by an isokinetic testing device).
5. Pronate and supinate the forearm against a resistance equal to or greater than that which the uninjured forearm can handle.
6. Perform 10 full bar dips.
7. Perform 10 chin-ups.

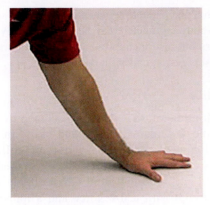

FIGURE 23–25   A fall on the outstretched hand can produce an elbow fracture.
© William E. Prentice

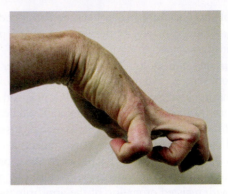

FIGURE 23–26   Volkmann's contracture. The wrist is flexed and the muscles in the forearm that flex and extend the fingers are involved.
© William E. Prentice

movement and strength programs but should avoid forced stretching.[61]

## Fractures of the Elbow

*Etiology*   An elbow fracture is usually caused by a fall on the outstretched hand or the flexed elbow or by a direct blow to the elbow (Figure 23–25). Children and young individuals have a much higher rate of this injury than do adults. A fracture can take place in any one or more of the bones that compose the elbow.[8]

A fall on the outstretched hand often fractures the humerus above the condyles, the condyles proper, or the area between the condyles.[60] A condylar fracture at the elbow may cause a *gunstock deformity*, in which the forearm, when extended, creates an angle with the upper arm relative to the long axis of the upper arm that resembles a gunstock. The ulna and radius also may receive trauma, and direct force delivered to the olecranon process of the ulna or a force transmitted to the head of the radius may cause a fracture.[60]

*Symptoms and signs*   An elbow fracture may or may not result in visible deformity. There is usually hemorrhage, swelling, and muscle spasm in the injured area.

*Management*   Like a dislocation, an elbow fracture can be associated with certain complications. One major complication is decreased ROM. The neurovascular status of the injury must be continually monitored. Surgery is used to stabilize an adult unstable elbow fracture and is followed by early ROM exercises. Stable fractures do not require surgery. Removable splints are used for 6 to 8 weeks.[8]

## Volkmann's Contracture

*Etiology*   Volkmann's contracture is a type of forearm ischemic contracture resulting from brachial artery injury, usually associated with supracondylar fracture of the humerus.[42] There may also be loss of motor and sensory function; however, classic involvement is with the median nerve. Contracture results from insufficient arterial perfusion and venous stasis followed by ischemic

degeneration of the muscle (Figure 23–26). Irreversible muscle necrosis begins after 4 to 6 hours. The resulting edema impairs circulation, which propagates progressive muscle necrosis. Muscle degeneration is most effected at the middle third of the muscle belly and is most severe closer to the bone. Necrosis of the muscle with secondary fibrosis may develop, followed by calcification in its final phase. It is essential that patients who sustain a serious elbow injury have their brachial or radial pulse monitored periodically to rule out the possibility of a Volkmann's contracture.[42]

*Symptoms and signs*   Such a contracture can become permanent. The first indication of this problem is pain in the forearm that becomes greater when the fingers are passively extended. This pain is followed by cessation of the brachial and radial pulses.[42]

> Volkmann's contracture is a major complication of a serious elbow injury.

*Management*   Management of the patient with beginning signs of tissue pressure reflected by pain, coldness, and decreased motion includes removing elastic wraps or casts and elevating the part. The patient must be closely monitored.

## Pronator Teres Syndrome

*Etiology*   Pronator teres syndrome involves entrapment of the median nerve either at or just above the elbow or in the pronator teres muscle itself where the median nerve passes between the superficial and deep heads of the muscle.[34] It can become entrapped due to edema and hypertrophy (enlargement) of the pronator teres muscle.

***Symptoms and signs*** Neuropathies at either site involve both sensory and motor deficits on the flexor side of the forearm. Numbness, tingling, and/or pins and needles sensations occur in the thumb, index and middle fingers, and half the ring finger. Motor deficits include loss of flexion and opposition of the thumb and fingers involved. If there is entrapment above the pronator teres, pronation will also be weak. Symptoms are reproduced by gripping tightly with resisted pronation of the arm from the elbow to full extension.

***Management*** Treatments include antiinflammatories, rest, modification of daily activities, TENS for pain reduction, and splinting. If these treatments are not helpful, decompression surgery may be considered. The results of decompressive surgery have been variable.

# REHABILITATION OF THE ELBOW

Rehabilitation of the elbow depends on the type of injury incurred, the specific sport played, and whether conservative or postsurgical care is involved. In general, the entire upper-arm kinetic chain, as well as the trunk and lower extremities, must be considered.

## General Body Conditioning

While the elbow is being rehabilitated, the patient should perform general body exercises to maintain preinjury fitness level. The patient should begin some activity (for example, using a stationary bicycle, a stair climber, or an elliptical trainer) that allows him or her to maintain cardiorespiratory conditioning while protecting the elbow. Once the patient regains pain-free range of motion, an upper-body ergometer may be used not only to maintain fitness but also to improve muscular endurance, thus accomplishing two goals with one exercise.

## Flexibility

Early initiation of the wrist and elbow ROM helps nourish the articular cartilage and assist in the synthesis, alignment, and organization of collagen tissue.[58] A variety of approaches can be applied as long as they do not force the joint. One example is a slow passive stretch with a low force and a long duration. Active assistive stretching can follow passive stretching, and PNF exercise aids in restoring a normal ROM (Figure 23–27).

After a severe injury, such as a dislocation, or after a surgical procedure, initial rehabilitation is directed toward regaining or maintaining normal range of motion. After surgery, a continuous passive movement can be used.

## Joint Mobilizations

An elbow that has been injured—particularly one that has been immobilized for any length of time—will likely lose range of motion due to restrictions in the arthrokinematic movements around the joint.[43] This can be attributed to arthrofibrosis, adhesive capsulites, or calcific tendinitis. It is therefore important that early ROM and mobilizations be instituted. Mobilization and traction techniques increase joint mobility and decrease pain by restoring accessory movements.[43] Humeroulnar traction increases elbow flexion and extension (Figure 23–28A). With patient's elbow flexed to 90 degrees, the ulna is grasped and glided inferiorly. Humeroradial inferior glides increase the joint space and improve flexion and extension. One hand stabilizes the humerus above the elbow; the other grasps the distal forearm and glides the radius inferiorly (Figure 23–28B). Proximal anterior/posterior radial glides use the thumbs and index fingers to glide the radial head. Anterior glides increase flexion, whereas posterior glides increase extension (Figure 23–28C). Medial and lateral ulnar oscillations increase flexion and extension.

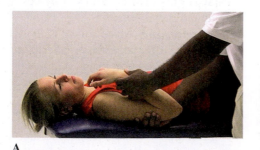
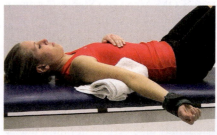

**A**                                           **B**

FIGURE 23–27 Stretching exercises. **(A)** Stretching of triceps (medial and lateral head) and anconeus. **(B)** Cuff weight supported elbow extension hang.
© William E. Prentice

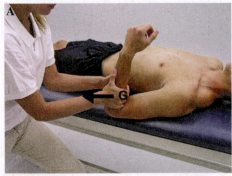
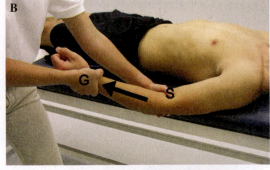
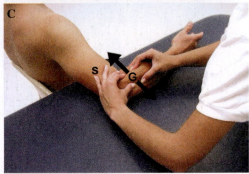
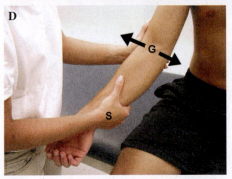

FIGURE 23–28   Elbow joint mobilization techniques. **(A)** Humeroulnar inferior glides.
**(B)** Humeroradial inferior glides. **(C)** Proximal anterior/posterior radial glides. **(D)** Medial and
lateral ulnar oscillations.
© William E. Prentice

Valgus and varus forces are used with a short lever arm
(Figure 23–28D).

## Strength

Beginning strengthening is achieved by low-resistance,
high-repetition exercise of the biceps brachialis, triceps,
pronators, supinators, wrist flexors, and wrist extensors.[61]
Grip and shoulder exercises are also performed to increase strength and range of motion. All activities must be
pain free.[59]

Two procedures may be used to maintain elbow mobility following surgery: the use of the continuous passive
machine immediately after surgery, followed by the use
of a dynamic splint. The initial stage of the rehabilitation
should include subpain-
ful submaximal isomet-
ric exercises to facilitate
voluntary activation of
muscle and retarding
muscular atrophy.[58] Maintaining the strength of
these articulations will
speed the recovery of the
elbow.[61] As the elbow
regains passive ROM,
strengthening exercises
should be performed to
improve active ROM.
PNF exercises are valu-
able in improving active

ROM and strength in the early and intermediate active state
of rehabilitation. A graded, progressive resistive exercise
program using either rubber tubing, weights, or manual
resistance should be initiated that includes flexion, extension, pronation, and supination exercises (Figure 23–29).
Isokinetic exercise may be used for regaining strength.[17] A
plyoback and weighted ball can be used to improve both
concentric and eccentric strength in the muscles surrounding the wrist and elbow (Figure 23–30).

Closed kinetic chain exercises help provide both static
and dynamic stability to the elbow. Proprioceptive conditioning of the elbow must be considered (Figure 23–31).

## Functional Progressions

Functional activities that enhance the healing and performance of the elbow include PNF patterns, swimming, and the use of pulley machines or rubber tubing
to simulate sports activity. An example of a functional
progression for throwing for the elbow should include
the following steps. First the patient must be instructed
in and complete a proper warm-up. During the warm-up,
the patient should practice the throwing motion at a slow
velocity and with low stress. The activity can then progress through increasingly difficult stages as follows:

- Functional activity with assisted PNF techniques
- Rubber tubing exercises simulating PNF patterns and/
  or sports motions
- Swimming
- Push-ups

A landscaping contractor
is rehabilitating her elbow
following a posterior
dislocation.

**?** What exercises
should this patient
do to strengthen the
musculature around the
elbow joint?

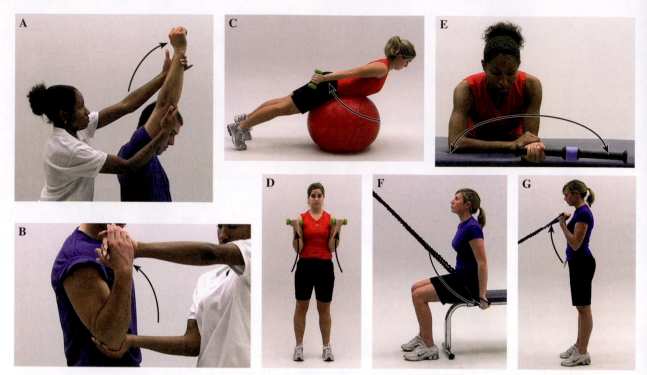

FIGURE 23–29 Examples of elbow strengthening exercises. **(A)** Manually resisted elbow extension. **(B)** Manually resisted elbow flexion. **(C)** Prone triceps extensions on stability ball. **(D)** Standing dumbbell biceps curls. **(E)** Resisted forearm pronation and supination. **(F)** Seated triceps extensions using tubing or cable. **(G)** Standing biceps curls using tubing or cable.
© William E. Prentice

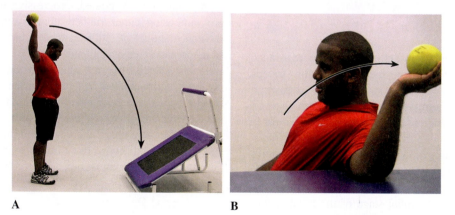

A                                              B

FIGURE 23–30 **(A)** A plyoback can be used for plyometric strengthening of the muscles surrounding the elbow joint. **(B)** Single-arm weighted ball catch and throw.
© William E. Prentice

- Sports drills—interval throwing program (45-foot (14 m) phase) (see Chapter 22)

Any upper-extremity injury can benefit from one of these programs or can be exercised in similar fashion using any equipment needed for the particular sport.[61]

## Return to Activity

The patient may return to full activity when specific criteria have been met. Range of motion in flexion, extension, supination, and pronation should be within normal limits. Strength should be at least equal to that of the uninvolved elbow, and the patient should not complain of pain in the elbow while performing a progression of activity in normal conditions. The return to activity progresses with the use of restrictions that can be helpful in objectively measuring activity and progression. The throwing progression for the elbow shows a gradual increase in activity in terms of time, repetitions, duration, and intensity.

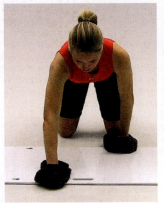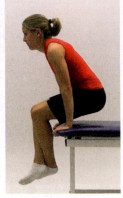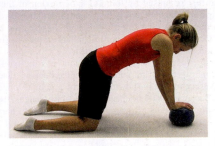

**A**           **B**           **C**

FIGURE 23–31  Closed kinetic chain strengthening exercises. **(A)** Slide board exercises. **(B)** Sitting push-ups. **(C)** Weight shifting on a ball.

© William E. Prentice

## SUMMARY

- The elbow is anatomically one of the more complex joints in the human body. The elbow joint allows the movements of flexion and extension, and the radioulnar joint allows forearm pronation and supination.
- Osteochondritis dissecans affects the lateral aspect of the elbow. It is associated with a loose body in the joint and in young patients is called Panner's disease.
- The repetitive valgus loading from overhead throwing can result in ulnar collateral ligament injuries, medial epicondylitis, osteochondritis dissecans, Little League elbow, ulnar neuritis, and cubital tunnel syndrome.
- Epicondilitis is a degenerative condition of the tendons that attach to the medial and lateral elbow epicondyle. Repetitive wrist flexion and pronation can result in

medial epicondylitis, and repetitive wrist extension and supination can result in lateral epicondylitis.
- Elbow dislocations result from elbow hyperextension. The typical injury is a fall on an extended arm that dislocates the radius and ulna posteriorly. The degree of stability present determines the course of rehabilitation. If the elbow is stable, a brief period of immobilization is followed by rehabilitation.
- Fractures in the elbow may occur from a direct blow or from falling on an outstretched hand. They may be treated by casting or, in some cases, by surgical reduction and fixation.
- Rehabilitation of the elbow should include early restoration of joint mobility, progressive strengthening exercises, and sports-specific functional activities.

## WEB SITES

Braces and Supports for Tennis Elbow and Elbow Pain: www.advancedbrace.com/ortho-catalog/elbow

MEDLINEplus: Elbow Injuries and Disorders: www.nlm .nih.gov/medlineplus/elbowinjuriesanddisorders.html

Tennis Elbow Central: www.tennis-elbow.net

Wheeless' Textbook of Orthopaedics: www.wheelessonline .com

## SOLUTIONS TO CLINICAL APPLICATION EXERCISES

23–1  The athletic trainer should perform tests for ligamentous and capsular stability. Pulses should be taken at the wrist and antecubital fossa. Changes of skin sensation and the patient's pain reaction to passive, active, and resistive exercise should be noted.

23–2  Swelling in the region of the olecranon process following irritation may indicate olecranon bursitis. This condition is best treated with a compression wrap and antiinflammatory medications.

23–3  It is most likely that this patient has a sprain of the ulnar collateral ligament due to valgus forces created during throwing. He should be referred to a physician for X-rays and then treated

conservatively with NSAIDs and activity modification. It is likely that he will ultimately require surgical reconstruction if he is to continue to perform at a high level.

23–4  It is likely that this tennis player has an inflammation of the lateral epicondyle, which is typically called tennis elbow. Tennis elbow occurs from repeated and forceful hyperextension of the wrist. It is best treated using rest, ice, compression, and antiinflammatory medications.

23–5  Immediate care consists of POLICE and NSAIDs. More definitive management can include ROM exercises, PRE, friction massage, and hand grasping exercises while the elbow is in supination. Pronation movements should be avoided. Mobilization and stretching can also be used within pain-free limits.

23–6 This injury is most likely an inflammation of the medial epicondyle that is caused by forceful hyperflexion of the wrist. Often called golfer's elbow, this condition almost always occurs in the trailing arm (for a right-handed golfer, the trailing arm is the right arm). Rest, antiinflammatory medication, and ice should be used to treat this problem.

23–7 The young pitcher's condition indicates the possibility of elbow osteochondritis dissecans, sometimes called Panner's disease.

23–8 This javelin thrower is showing signs of a cubital tunnel syndrome. Because of a pronounced elbow cubitus valgus, the ulnar recurrently subluxates. Ligamentous laxity leads to nerve impingement and compression.

23–9 Immediate treatment is critical for an elbow dislocation because of the tissues involved. Ice should be applied and the elbow should be immobilized until a physician is able to reduce the dislocation. If treatment is delayed, the soft tissue can be seriously damaged and the neurovascular supply can be compromised. Due to their close proximity to the joint, the brachial artery and the radial and median nerves are subject to injury. Fractures and ligamentous ruptures may also be present and need to be evaluated before and after reduction.

23–10 The athletic trainer should be concerned that this injury can cause a Volkmann's ischemic contracture. The brachial and radial pulses must be monitored for the possibility of a decrease in normal circulation.

23–11 This patient must have regained full ROM in flexion, extension, pronation, and supination and must have regained full strength in these muscles.

23–12 This landscape contractor should do bicep curls to strengthen the biceps brachii, brachialis, and brachioradial muscles, all of which in some way act in flexion: tricep extensions to strengthen the triceps muscle; supination to strengthen the biceps brachii and supinator muscles; and pronation to strengthen the pronator teres and pronator quadratus.

## REVIEW QUESTIONS AND CLASS ACTIVITIES

1. Describe the procedures for assessing an elbow injury.
2. Describe the mechanism and management of elbow strains and sprains.
3. Describe how and why the elbow becomes chronically strained from throwing mechanisms.
4. Describe a dislocated elbow—its cause, appearance, and care.
5. How does the elbow sustain epicondylitis? Describe its appearance and management.
6. Compare elbow osteochondritis dissecans and knee osteochondritis dissecans. How does each occur?
7. What are the symptoms and signs of elbow osteochondritis dissecans?
8. What causes a Volkmann's contracture? How may it be detected early?
9. Discuss the many aspects of elbow exercise rehabilitation.

## REFERENCES

1. Ahmad C: Valgus extension overload syndrome and stress injury of the olecranon, *Clin Sports Med* 23(4):665, 2004.
2. Alcid J: Elbow anatomy and structural biomechanics, *Clin Sports Med* 23(4):503, 2004.
3. Appleboam A: Elbow extension test to rule out elbow fracture: Multicentre prospective validation and observational study of diagnostic accuracy in children, *British Medical Journal* 37:a2428, 2008.
4. Azar F: Operative treatment of ulnar collateral ligament injuries of the elbow in athletes, *Am J Sports Med* 28(1):16, 2000.
5. Beekman R: The diagnostic value of provocative clinical tests in ulnar neuropathy at the elbow is marginal, *J Neurology, Neurosurgery, Psychiatry* 80(12):1369, 2009.
6. Benjamin S, et al: Normalized forces and active range of motion in unilateral radial epicondylalgia (tennis elbow), *J Orthop Sports Phys Ther* 29(11):668, 1999.
7. Bradley J: Osteochondritis dissecans of the humeral capitellum: Diagnosis and treatment, *Clin Sports Med* 20(3):565, 2001.
8. Brukner P: Elbow and forearm pain. In Brukner P, ed: *Bruckner and Kahn's clinical sports medicine,* ed 2, Sydney, 2011, McGraw-Hill.
9. Buettner C: Prevention and treatment of elbow injuries in adolescent pitchers, *Athletic Therapy Today* 5(3):19, 2000.
10. Cain E: Elbow injuries in throwing athletes: A current concept review, *Am J Sports Med* 31(4):621, 2003.
11. Cain E: History and examination of the thrower's elbow, *Clin Sports Med* 23(4):553, 2004.
12. David T: Medial elbow pain in the throwing athlete, *Orthopedics* 26(1):94, 2003.
13. de Villiers R: Osteochondritis dissecans in adolescence, *J Sports Med* 2(5):1, 2001.
14. Dines J: Glenohumeral internal rotation deficits in baseball players with ulnar collateral ligament insufficiency, *Am J Sports Med* 37(3):566–70, 2009.
15. Docherty M: Can elbow extension be used as a test of clinically significant injury? *Southern Medical Journal* 95(5):539–41, 2003.
16. Ekstrom R: Examination and intervention for a patient with chronic lateral elbow pain with signs of nerve entrapment, *Phys Ther* 82(11):1077, 2002.
17. Ellenbecker T: Isokinetic profile of elbow flexion and extension strength in elite junior tennis players, *J Orthop Sports Phys Ther* 33(2):79–84, 2003.
18. Field L: Surgical treatment of ulnar collateral ligament injuries, *Athletic Therapy Today* 5(3):25, 2000.
19. Fincher A: Managing epicondylitis in the golfer, *Athletic Therapy Today* 5(6):38, 2000.
20. Fornalski S: Anatomy and biomechanics of the elbow joint, *Sports Med Arthroscopy Review* 11(1):1, 2003.
21. Frostick S: Sport injuries of the elbow, *British Journal of Sports Medicine* 33(5):301, 1999.
22. Gibson B: Ulnar collateral ligament reconstruction in major league baseball pitchers. *Am J Sports Med* 35(4):575–81, 2007.
23. Grana W: Medial epicondylitis and cubital tunnel syndrome in the throwing athlete, *Clin Sports Med* 20(3):541, 2001.
24. Hall T: Osteochondritis dissecans of the elbow: Diagnosis, treatment, and prevention, *Physician Sportsmed* 27(2):75, 1999.
25. Halpern BC: Elbow and arm injuries. In Birrer RB, ed: *Sports medicine for the primary care physician,* ed 2, Boca Raton, FL, 2004, CRC Press.
26. Harada M: Risk factors for elbow injuries among young baseball players, *Journal of Shoulder and Elbow Surgery* 19(4):502–07, 2010.
27. Hocutt J: General types of injuries. In Birrer RB, ed: *Sports medicine for the primary care physician,* Boca Raton, FL, 2004, CRC Press.
28. Hughes P: Little Leaguer's elbow, medial epicondyle injury, and osteochondritis dissecans, *Sports Med Arthroscopy Review* 11(1):30, 2003.
29. Kaminski T: Differential assessment of elbow injuries, *Athletic Therapy Today* 5(3):6, 2000.
30. Klingele K: Little League elbow: Valgus overload injury in the paediatric athlete, *Sports Med* 32(15):1005, 2003.
31. Knebel P: Effects of the forearm support band on wrist extensor muscle fatigue, *J Orthop Sports Phys Ther* 29(11):677, 1999.
32. Kuhn M: Acute elbow dislocations, *Orthopedic Clinics of North America* 39(2):155–61, 2008.
33. Loftice J: Biomechanics of the elbow in sports, *Clin Sports Med* 23(4):519, 2004.
34. McCulloch R: Median nerve compression secondary to a high insertion of pronator teres, *Shoulder and Elbow*, 2(2):124–26, 2010.
35. Mihata T: Biomechanical characteristics of osteochondral defects of the humeral capitellum, *Am J Sports Med* 41(8):1909–14, 2013.
36. Namdari S: *Orthopsedic secrets,* Philadelphia, 2014, Saunders.
37. Nirschl R: Elbow tendinopathy: Tennis elbow, *Clin Sports Med* 22(4):813, 2003.

38. O'Driscoll S: The "moving valgus stress test" for medial collateral ligament tears of the elbow, *Am J Sports Med* 33(2):231-239, 2005.

39. Olsen S: Risk factors for shoulder and elbow injuries in adolescent baseball pitchers, *Am J Sports Med* 34(6):905, 2006.

40. Patel D: *Overuse injuries of the elbow, forearm, wrist, and hand, pediatric practice: Sports medicine*, New York, 2009, McGraw-Hill.

41. Peters T: Lateral epicondylitis, *Clin Sports Med* 20(3):549, 2001.

42. Prasarn M: Acute compartment syndrome of the upper extremity, *Journal of the American Academy of Orthopedic Surgeons* 19(1):49–58, 2011.

43. Prentice W: Mobilization and traction techniques. In Prentice WE, ed: *Rehabilitation techniques in sports medicine and athletic training*, Thorofare, NJ, 2015, Slack.

44. Rahman R: Elbow medial collateral ligament injuries, *Current Reviews in Musculoskeletal Medicine* 1(3):197–204, 2008.

45. Reinold M : Biomechanics and rehabilitation of elbow injuries during throwing, *Athletic Therapy Today* 5(3):12, 2000.

46. Rettig A: Traumatic elbow injuries in the athlete, *Orthopedic Clinics of North America* 33(3):509, 2002.

47. Safran M: Injury to the ulnar collateral ligament: Diagnosis and treatment, *Sports Med Arthroscopy Review* 11(1):15, 2003.

48. Sims S: Non-surgical treatment of lateral epicondylitis: A systematic review of randomized controlled trials, *Hand (NY)*, 9(4):419–46, 2014.

49. Saroja G:Diagnostic accuracy of provocative tests in lateral epicondylitis, *International, J of Physiotherapy and Research* 2(6):815–23, 2014.

50. Struijis P: Conservative treatment of lateral epicondylitis, *Am J Sports Med* 32(2):462–69, 2004.

51. Thompson K: Rupture of the distal biceps tendon in a collegiate football player: A case report, *J Athl Train* 33(1):62, 1998.

52. Tosti R: Lateral epicondylitis of the elbow, *Am J Med.* Apr 126(4):357 e351–56, 2013.

53. Tyrdal S: Acute elbow injuries. In Bahr R, ed: *Clinical guide to sports injuries*, Champaign, IL, 2004, Human Kinetics.

54. Tyrdal S: Elbow overuse injuries. In Bahr R, ed: *Clinical guide to sports injuries*, Champaign, IL, 2004, Human Kinetics.

55. Uhl T: Uncomplicated elbow dislocation rehabilitation, *Athletic Therapy Today* 5(3):31, 2000.

56. Wassinger C: Reported mechanisms of shoulder injury during the baseball throw, *Physical Therapy Reviews*, 16(5):305–09, 2011.

57. Whaley A: Lateral epicondylitis, *Clin Sports Med* 23(4):677, 2004.

58. Wilk K: Rehabilitation of the overhead athlete's elbow, *Sports Health* 4(5):404–14, 2012.

59. Wilk K: Rehabilitation of the thrower's elbow, *Clin Sports Med* 23(4):765, 2004.

60. Wong A: Elbow fractures: Distal humerus, *The Journal of Hand Surgery* 34(1):176–90, 2009.

61. Zulia P: Rehabilitation of elbow injuries. In Prentice W, ed: *Rehabilitation techniques in sports medicine and athletic training*, Thorofare, NJ, 2015, Slack.

## ANNOTATED BIBLIOGRAPHY

Altchek D, Andrews J: *The athlete's elbow*, Baltimore, MD, 2001, Lippincott, Williams and Wilkins.

*Based on the work of leading authorities on elbow injuries in athletes; provides information on the biomechanics and anatomy of the elbow, as well as guidelines for the evaluation and treatment of injury to the joint.*

Bahr R, *editor: Clinical guide to sports injuries*, Champaign, IL, 2004, Human Kinetics.

*An outstanding guide to the diagnosis, treatment, and rehabilitation of sports injuries. Covers injuries to the elbow.*

Ellenbecker T, Mattalino A: *The elbow in sports*, Champaign, IL, 1997, Human Kinetics.

*Intended for physical therapists, athletic trainers, and sports medicine specialists, a comprehensive guide to the anatomy, biomechanics, musculoskeletal evaluation, and surgical techniques involved in sport-related elbow injuries.*

Morrey B: *The elbow and its disorders*, Philadelphia, PA, 2008, WB Saunders.

*A text primarily for orthopedic surgeons and residents; includes evaluation, diagnosis, children's conditions, adult trauma, sports and overuse injuries, reconstruction, and septic and nontraumatic conditions.*

Safran M: The athlete's elbow. An issue of *Clinics in Sports Medicine*, Philadelphia, PA, 2010, Saunders.

*This issue of* Clinics in Sports Medicine *is dedicated to athlete's elbow and covers topics on imaging, pediatric considerations, rehabilitation, and various injuries and conditions.*

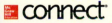

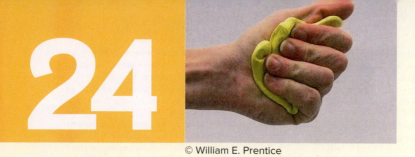

© William E. Prentice

# 24

# The Forearm, Wrist, Hand, and Fingers

## ■ Objectives

*When you finish this chapter you should be able to*

- Review the structural and functional anatomy of the forearm, wrist, hand, and fingers.
- Outline the process of assessment for injuries to the forearm, wrist, hand, and fingers.

- Incorporate management techniques for dealing with injuries to the forearm, wrist, hand, and fingers.
- Implement the appropriate rehabilitation techniques for dealing with injuries to the forearm, wrist, hand, and fingers.

## ■ Outline

## ■ Connect Highlights **connect**

*Visit connect.mcgraw-hill.com for further exercises to apply your knowledge:*

- Clinical application scenarios covering assessment and recognition of forearm, wrist, hand, and finger injuries; etiology, symptoms and signs, and management of forearm, wrist, hand, and finger injuries; and rehabilitation for the forearm, wrist, hand, and finger
- Click-and-drag questions covering structural anatomy of the forearm, wrist, hand, and finger; assessment of forearm, wrist, hand, and finger injuries; and rehabilitation plan of the forearm, wrist, hand, and finger
- Multiple-choice questions covering anatomy, assessment, etiology, management, and rehabilitation of forearm, wrist, hand, and finger injuries
- Selection questions covering rehabilitation plan for various injuries to the forearm, wrist, hand, and finger
- Video identification of special tests for the forearm, wrist, hand, and finger injuries; rehabilitation techniques for the forearm, wrist, hand, and finger; taping and wrapping for forearm, wrist, hand, and finger injuries
- Picture identification of major anatomical components of the forearm, wrist, hand, and finger; rehabilitation techniques of the forearm, wrist, hand, and finger; and therapeutic modalities for management

# ANATOMY OF THE FOREARM

## Bones

The bones of the forearm are the ulna and the radius (Figure 24–1). The ulna, which may be thought of as a direct extension of the humerus, is long, straight, and larger proximally than distally. The radius, considered an extension of the hand, is thicker distally than proximally.

## Articulations

The forearm has three articulations: the superior, middle, and distal radioulnar joints. The superior radioulnar articulation is a pivot joint that moves in a ring formed by the ulna and the annular ligament.

The middle radioulnar joint, which is the junction between the shafts of the ulna and the radius, is held together by an oblique ligamentous cord and the interosseous membrane. The oblique cord is a small band of ligamentous fibers that are attached to the lateral side of the ulna and pass downward and laterally to the radius. The interosseous membrane is a thin sheet of fibrous tissue that runs downward between the radius and the ulna and transmits forces directly through the hand from the radius to the ulna. The middle radioulnar joint provides a surface for muscle attachments, and there are openings for blood vessels at the upper and lower ends.

The distal radioulnar joint is a pivot joint formed by the articulation of the head of the ulna with a small notch on the radius. It is held securely by the anterior and posterior radioulnar ligaments. The inferior ends of the radius and ulna are bound by an articular, triangular disk that allows radial movement of 180 degrees into supination and pronation.

## Forearm Musculature

The forearm muscles consist of flexors and pronators that are positioned anteriorly and extensors and supinators that lie posteriorly. The flexors of the wrist and fingers are separated into superficial muscles and deep muscles (Figure 24–2). The deep flexors arise from the ulna, the radius, and the interosseous tissue anteriorly, and the superficial flexors come from the internal humeral condyle. The extensors of the wrist and fingers originate on the posterior aspect and the external condyle of the humerus (Table 24–1).

## Nerve and Blood Supply

Except for the flexor carpi ulnaris and half of the flexor digitorum profundus, most of the flexor muscles of the forearm are supplied by the median nerve. The majority of the extensor muscles are controlled by the radial nerve. The major blood supply stems from the brachial artery, which divides into the radial and ulnar arteries in the forearm. (See Figure 23–4.)

## Surface Anatomy

Figure 24–3 shows the pertinent surface anatomy landmarks for the forearm from both an anterior and posterior view.

# ASSESSMENT OF THE FOREARM

## History

The following questions should be asked to determine forearm injuries:

- What caused the injury (e.g., blunt trauma, throwing, or chronic overuse)?
- What were the symptoms at the time of injury? Did symptoms occur later?
- Were symptoms localized or diffused?
- Was there swelling or discoloration?
- Was there immediate loss of function?
- What treatment was given?
- How does the forearm feel now?
- Have you ever had this injury before?
- Have you ever previously injured your forearm?

## Observation

The entire forearm, including the wrist and elbow, is first visually inspected for obvious deformities, swelling, and skin defects. If a deformity is not present, the patient then is observed pronating and supinating the forearm.

## Palpation

The injured forearm is palpated at distant sites as well as at the point of injury. Palpation can reveal tenderness, edema, fracture deformity, change in skin temperature, a false joint, bone fragments, or a lack of continuity between bones.

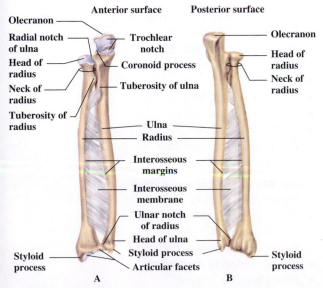

FIGURE 24–1 Bony anatomy of the forearm. **(A)** Anterior view. **(B)** Posterior view.

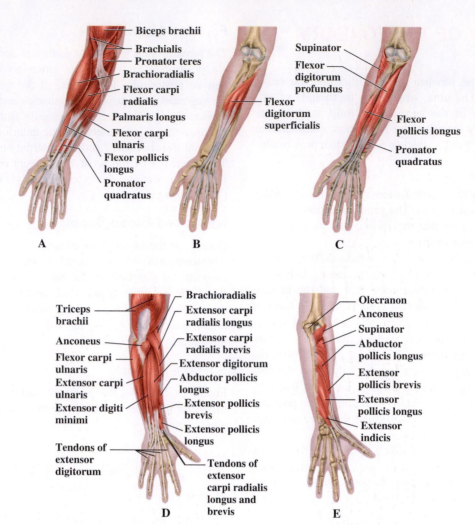

FIGURE 24–2    Muscles of the forearm. **(A)** Superficial flexors. **(B)** The flexor digitorum superficialis, deep to the muscles in A but also classified as a superficial flexor. **(C)** Deep flexors. **(D)** Superficial extensors. **(E)** Deep extensors.

**Bony Palpation** The following bony landmarks should be palpated:

- Proximal radial head
- Olecranon process
- Radial shaft
- Ulnar shaft
- Distal radius
- Radial styloid process
- Ulnar head
- Ulnar styloid

**Soft-Tissue Palpation** The following soft-tissue structures should be palpated:

*Articulations*
- Distal radioulnar joint
- Radiocarpal joint
- Extensor retinaculum (posterior wrist)
- Flexor retinaculum (anterior wrist)

*Extensor Muscles (Posterolateral)*
- Extensor carpi radialis longus
- Extensor carpi radialis brevis
- Extensor carpi ulnaris
- Brachioradialis
- Extensor pollicis longus
- Extensor pollicis brevis
- Abductor pollicis longus
- Extensor indicus supinator

*Flexor Muscles (Anteromedial)*
- Flexor carpi radialis
- Flexor carpi ulnaris
- Palmaris longus
- Flexor digitorum superficialis
- Flexor digitorum profundus
- Flexor pollicis longus
- Pronator quadratus
- Pronator teres

| Muscle | Origin | Insertion | Action | Innervation/ Nerve Root |
|---|---|---|---|---|
| **Flexor carpi radialis** | Medial epicondyle of the humerus | Ventral surface of the second and third metacarpals | Flexes the wrist and abducts the hand; aids in flexion of the elbow and pronation | Median (C6, C7) |
| **Palmaris longus** | Medial epicondyle of the humerus | Palmar aponeurosis | Flexes the wrist | Median (C6, C7) |
| **Flexor carpi ulnaris** | Medial epicondyle of the humerus, olecranon process, and the proximal two-thirds of the posterior surface of the ulna | Pisiform, hamate, and fifth metacarpal | Flexes the wrist and adducts the hand | Ulnar (C8, T1) |
| **Flexor digitorum superficialis** | Medial epicondyle of the humerus, coronoid process of the ulna, and the anterior of the radius | Ventral surface of the middle phalanges of the second through the fifth fingers | Flexes the wrist and the phalanges | Median (C7, C8, T1) |
| **Flexor digitorum profundus** | Medial epicondyle and the coronoid process of the humerus, the interosseus membrane, and the ventral surface of the ulna | Ventral surface of the base of the distal phalanges of the second through the fifth fingers | Flexes the wrist and the phalanges | Median and ulnar (C8, T1) |
| **Flexor pollicis longus** | Ventral surface of the radius and the interosseus membrane | Ventral surface of the base of the distal phalanx of the thumb | Flexes the thumb and aids in flexing the wrist | Median (C8, T1) |
| **Pronator quadratus** | Distal ventral surface of the ulna | Distal ventral surface of the radius | Pronates the hand | Median (C8, T1) |
| **Extensor carpi radialis longus** | Lateral supracondylar ridge of the humerus | Dorsal surface of the base of the second metacarpal | Extends the wrist and abducts the hand | Radial (C6, C7) |
| **Extensor carpi radialis brevis** | Lateral epicondyle of the humerus | Dorsal surface of the base of the third metacarpal | Extends the wrist and abducts the hand | Radial (C6, C7) |
| **Extensor digitorum communis** | Lateral epicondyle of the humerus | Dorsal surface of the phalanges of the second through the fifth fingers | Extends the fingers and the wrist | Radial (C6–C8) |
| **Extensor digiti minimi** | Tendon of the extensor digitorum communis | Tendon of the extensor digitorum communis on the dorsum of the little finger | Extends the little finger | Radial (C6–C8) |
| **Extensor carpi ulnaris** | Lateral epicondyle of the humerus | Base of the fifth metacarpal | Extends the wrist and adducts the hand | Radial (C6–C8) |
| **Abductor pollicis longus** | Posterior surface of the middle of the radius and ulna and the interosseus membrane | Base of the first metacarpal | Abducts the thumb and the hand | Radial (C6, C7) |

*(continued)*

| Muscle | Origin | Insertion | Action | Innervation/ Nerve Root |
|---|---|---|---|---|
| **Extensor pollicis brevis** | Posterior surface of the middle of the radius and the interosseus membrane | Base of the first phalanx of the thumb | Extends the wrist and adducts the hand | Radial (C6, C7) |
| **Extensor pollicis longus** | Posterior surface of the middle of the ulna and the interosseus membrane | Base of the last phalanx of the thumb | Extends the thumb and abducts the hand | Radial (C6–C8) |
| **Extensor indicis** | Posterior surface of the distal end of the ulna and the interosseus membrane | Tendon of the extensor digitorum communis to the index finger | Extends the index finger | Radial (C6–C8) |

**Joint Movements of the Wrist and Hand***

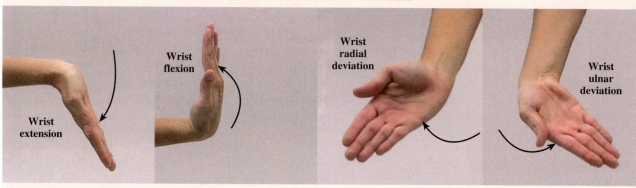

*Manual muscle tests and goniometric measurements of range of motion for the wrist, hand, and finger joints can be found in Appendix F and Appendix G at the end of the text.

© William E. Prentice

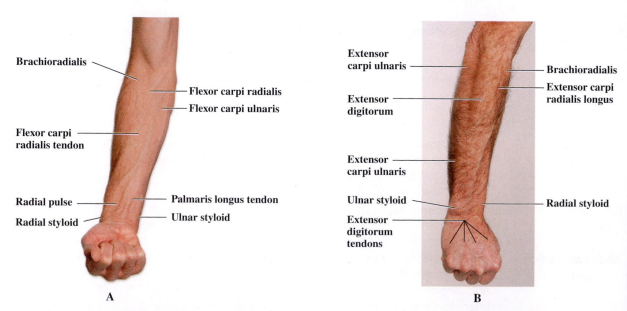

FIGURE 24–3    Surface anatomy landmarks for the forearm from both an anterior and posterior view.
© JW Ramsey/McGraw-Hill Education

# RECOGNITION AND MANAGEMENT OF INJURIES TO THE FOREARM

The forearm, lying between the elbow joint and the wrist, is indirectly influenced by injuries to these areas; however, direct injuries can also occur.

## Contusions

***Etiology*** The forearm is constantly exposed to bruising in contact sports, such as football. The ulnar side receives the majority of blows in arm blocks and, consequently, a greater amount of bruising. Bruises to this area may be classified as acute or chronic. The acute contusion can result in a fracture, but this happens only rarely.

***Symptoms and signs*** Most often, a muscle or bone develops varying degrees of pain, swelling, and hematoma. The chronic contusion develops from repeated blows to the forearm with attendant multiple irritations. Heavy fibrosis may take the place of the hematoma, and a bony callus has been known to arise out of this condition.

***Management*** Care of the contused forearm requires proper attention in the acute stages through the application of POLICE, followed the next day by cryotherapy. Protection of the forearm is important for patients who are prone to this condition. The best protection consists of a full-length sponge rubber pad for the forearm early in the season.

## Forearm Splints

***Etiology*** Forearm strain can occur in a variety of activities from a static contraction. Forearm splints, like medial tibial stress syndrome (shinsplints), are difficult to manage.[30]

> Forearm splints, like shinsplints, commonly occur either early or late in the sports season.

***Symptoms and signs*** The main symptom is a dull ache between the extensor muscles, which cross the back of the forearm. There also may be weakness and extreme pain during muscle contraction. Palpation reveals an irritation of the interosseous membrane and surrounding tissue. The cause of this condition is uncertain. Isometric contraction causes minute tears in the area of the interosseous membrane.[39]

***Management*** Care of forearm splints is symptomatic. The patient should concentrate on increasing the strength of the forearm through resistance exercises. If the condition persists, emphasis should be on rest and cryotherapy or heat and use of a supportive wrap during activity.

> A rower complains of a chronic injury to the posterior lateral portion of the middle forearm resulting in a constant dull ache and pain with weakness during active contraction when the wrist is extended.
>
> ? What fairly common injury, often seen in this sport, should the athletic trainer expect in this rower?

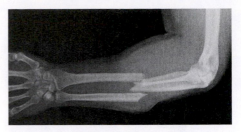

**FIGURE 24–4** A radiograph of mid-shaft fractures of the radius and ulna of the forearm.
Courtesy Jordan B. Renner, MD, Departments of Radiology and Allied Health Sciences, University of North Carolina

The forearm can also sustain an acute or chronic exertional compartment syndrome, although this condition is much less common than in the lower leg. It can occur from muscle avulsion, distal radius fracture, or a crushing injury. The deep forearm compartment containing the flexor digitorum profundus, flexor pollicus longus, and pronator quadratus is most susceptible to changes of muscle and nerve ischemia. Detection and management of this condition are the same as for the lower leg condition.

## Forearm Fractures

***Etiology*** Fractures of the forearm (Figure 24–4) are particularly common among active children and youths and occur as a result of a blow or a fall on the outstretched hand.[30] Fractures to the ulna or the radius alone are much rarer than simultaneous fractures to both. A direct blow to the forearm usually results in a fracture to the shaft of the ulna. The forearm break usually presents all the features of a long-bone fracture: pain, swelling, deformity, and a false joint. If the break is in the upper third, the pronator teres muscle has a tendency to pull the forearm into an abduction deformity, whereas fractures of the lower portion of the arm are often in a neutral position. The older the patient, the greater the danger of extensive damage to soft tissue and the greater the possibility of paralysis from Volkmann's contractures (see Chapter 23).

***Symptoms and signs*** The patient experiences an audible pop or crack followed by moderate to severe pain, swelling, and disability. There is localized tenderness, edema, and ecchymosis with possible crepitus.[30]

***Management*** Initially, POLICE is applied, followed by splinting until definitive care is available. Definitive care consists of a long-arm plaster or fiberglass cast followed by a program of rehabilitation.

## Colles' Fractures

***Etiology*** Colles' fractures are among the most common types of forearm fractures and involve the lower end of the radius (Figure 24–5).[19] The mechanism of injury is usually a fall on the outstretched hand, forcing the radius backward and upward (hyperextension). Much less common is the reverse Colles' fracture, which is more commonly known as a *Smith fracture*. It is a transverse fracture of the distal radial metaphysis, with anterior displacement of the distal fracture fragment. If the fracture is intraarticular, it is

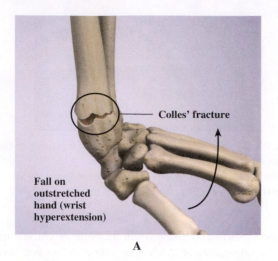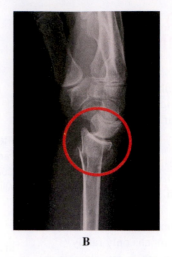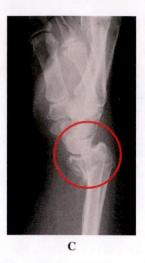

A                    B                    C

FIGURE 24–5   **(A)** Common appearance of the forearm in a Colles' fracture. **(B)** Radiograph of a Colles' fracture showing posterior displacement of the radial styloid. **(C)** Radiograph of a Smiths' fracture showing anterior displacement of the radial styloid.

(b, c) Courtesy Jordan B. Renner, MD, Departments of Radiology and Allied Health Sciences, University of North Carolina

called a *Barton fracture*. The mechanism of this fracture is the result of a fall on the back of the hand.[7]

***Symptoms and signs*** In most cases, there is forward displacement of the radius that causes a visible deformity to the wrist, which is commonly called a *dinner fork* deformity. Sometimes no deformity is present, and the injury may be passed off as a bad sprain—to the detriment of the patient. Bleeding is profuse in this area, and the extravasated fluids can cause extensive swelling in the wrist and, if unchecked, in the fingers and forearm. Ligamentous tissue is usually unharmed, but tendons may be torn and avulsed, and there may be median nerve damage.[19]

***Management*** The main responsibility is to apply a cold compress, splint the wrist, put the limb in a sling, and then refer the patient to a physician for X-ray examination and immobilization. Severe sprains should always be treated as possible fractures. What appears to be a Colles' fracture in children and youths is often a lower epiphyseal separation.[46]

## Madelung Deformity

***Etiology*** Madelung deformity is a developmental abnormality of the wrist. It is characterized by anatomical changes in the radius, ulna, and carpal bones, leading to palmar and ulnar wrist subluxation (Figure 24–6). It is more common in females and is usually present bilaterally.

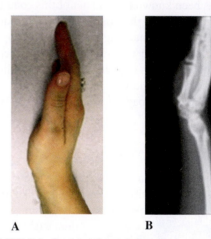

A            B

FIGURE 24–6   Madelung deformity.

Gatta, Valentina et al. "Spectrum of Phenotypic Anomalies in Four Families with Deletion of the SHOX Enhancer Region." BMC Medical Genetics 15: 87 (2014). PMC. © 2014 by Gatta, Valentina et al. All rights reserved. Used with permission.

The deformity usually becomes evident clinically between the ages of 6 and 13. Epiphyseal plate changes in the distal radius and closure of the plate as a result of loading the wrist and forearm produce a skeletal deformity in which the carpus is wedged between the radius and the ulna. There is a concomitant bowing to the radius that is evident on radiograph.[6]

***Symptoms and signs*** Madelung deformity can result in wrist pain and loss of forearm rotation, leading to decreased function of the wrist and hand. There may be palmar subluxation with prominence of the radial and ulnar styloid processes.

***Management*** The deformity is treated with therapeutic modalities and nonsteroidal antiinflammatory medication for pain. The wrist should be taped or the athlete should wear a commercially available wrist brace to prevent end-range wrist extension. Although rare, Madelung deformity is typically corrected surgically in patients with chronic pain and disability.[6]

# ANATOMY OF THE WRIST, HAND, AND FINGERS

## Bones

The wrist, or carpus, is the region that connects the distal forearm to the hand. It is formed by the distal aspect of the radius and the ulna, with a proximal row of four and a distal row of four carpal bones that articulate with five metacarpals. Appearing in order from the radial to the ulnar side in the first, or proximal, row of carpal bones are the scaphoid (navicular), lunate, triquetral, and pisiform bones; the distal row consists of the greater multangular (trapezium), lesser multangular (trapezoid), capitate, and hamate bones (Figure 24–7).

The concave surfaces of the lower ends of the radius and ulna articulate with the convex surfaces of the first row of carpal bones, with the exception of the pisiform, which articulates with the triangular fibrocartilage complex (TFCC) interposed between the head of the ulna and the triquetral bone (Figure 24–8).

## Articulations

**Radiocarpal Joints** The radiocarpal joint is a condyloid joint and permits flexion, extension, abduction, and circumduction. Its major strength is drawn from the great number of tendons that cross it rather than from its bone structure or ligamentous arrangement. The articular capsule is a continuous cover formed by the merging of the radial and the ulnar, volar radiocarpal, and dorsal radiocarpal ligaments (see Figure 24–7).

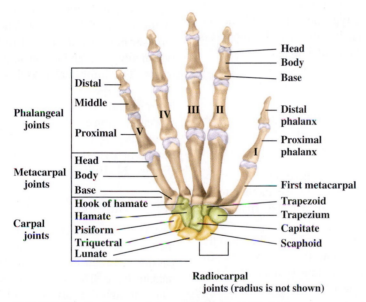

FIGURE 24–7   Bones of the wrist, hand, and fingers.

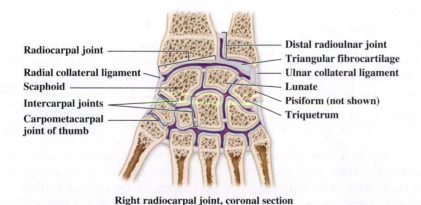

**Right radiocarpal joint, coronal section**

FIGURE 24–8   Cross-sectional view of the bones in the wrist, showing the location of the radial and ulnar collateral ligaments and the triangular fibrocartilage.

**Carpal Joints** The carpal bones articulate with one another in arthrodial, or gliding, joints and combine their movements with those of the radiocarpal joint and the carpometacarpal articulations. They are stabilized by anterior, posterior, and connecting interosseous ligaments (see Figure 24–7).

**Metacarpal Joints** The five metacarpal bones join the carpal bones above and the phalanges below, forming metacarpophalangeal (MCP) articulations of a condyloid type and permitting flexion, extension, abduction, adduction, and circumduction. The thumb varies slightly at its carpometacarpal joint and is classified as a saddle joint, which allows rotation on its long axis in addition to the other metacarpophalangeal movements (see Figure 24–7).

**Phalangeal Joints** Each phalangeal joint, like the carpal joints, has an articular capsule that is reinforced by collateral and accessory volar ligaments. The interphalangeal articulations are of the hinge type, permitting only flexion and extension. Their ligamentous and capsular support is basically the same as that of the MCP joints.

## Ligaments

There are many wrist, hand, and finger ligaments; however, only those most likely to be injured in sports are discussed here.

**Ligaments of the Wrist** The wrist is composed of many ligaments that bind the carpal bones to one another, to the ulna and radius, and to the proximal metacarpal bones. The medial ligaments extend from the tip of the styloid process of the ulna to the pisiform bone and the triquetral bone. The lateral ligaments extend from the styloid process to the radius to the navicular bone (scaphoid). Crossing the volar aspect of the carpal bones is the transverse carpal ligament. This ligament serves as the roof of the carpal tunnel, in which the median nerve is often compressed (Figure 24–8).

**Ligaments of the Phalanges** The proximal interphalangeal (PIP) joints have the same design as the distal interphalangeal (DIP) joints. They comprise the collateral ligaments, palmar fibrocartilages, and a loose posterior capsule or synovial membrane protected by an extensor expansion (Figure 24–9).

## Musculature

Several muscles of the forearm have long tendons that cross the metacarpophalangeal (MCP) joints and move the fingers. On the flexor surface, the flexor digitorum superficialis flexes the proximal interphalangeal (PIP) joint, and the flexor digitorum profundus flexes the distal interphalangeal (DIP) joint (Figure 24–9). Dorsally, as the

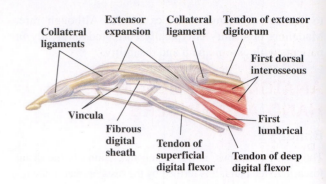

**FIGURE 24–9** Ligamentous and muscular anatomy of the fingers.

extensor digitorum longus tendons cross the MCP joints, they expand into a tendinous aponeurosis called the *extensor expansion*, which extends the PIP and DIP joints of the fingers.

There are a number of muscles that are intrinsic to the hand (Table 24–2). The dorsal and palmar interossei muscles are lateral to the MCP joints and are responsible for abduction and adduction of the MCP joints. The lumbrical muscles are volar to the axis of rotation of the MCP joint, but then they insert into the lateral bands and are dorsal to the PIP and DIP joints. Their function is MCP joint flexion and IP joint extension. The three thenar muscles act on the thumb, and the three hypothenar muscles act on the little finger (Figure 24–10).

## Nerve Supply

The two major nerves of the hand are the ulnar and median nerves. The ulnar nerve comes to the hand by passing between the pisiform bone and the hook of the hamate bone. The median nerve enters the palm of the hand through the carpal tunnel (Figure 24–11). The median nerve supplies three of the four thenar muscles, and the radial two lumbricals and the ulnar nerve supply the rest of the instrinsic muscles of the hand.

## Blood Supply

The wrist and hand are supplied by the radial and ulnar arteries. The radial artery supplies the muscles on the radial side of the forearm and wrist. The ulnar artery supplies the muscles on

> Circulation impairment must be noted as soon as possible in any wrist or hand injury.

the ulnar side of the forearm and wrist. These two arteries form the superficial and deep palmar arches, which in turn supply the digital arteries (Figure 24–12A).

The dorsal venous arch on the back of the hand is cutaneous and anastamoses with deep veins that drain into the basilic and cephalic veins (Figure 24–12B).

## TABLE 24–2  Intrinsic Muscles of the Hand

| Muscle | Origin | Insertion | Action | Innervation/Nerve Root |
|---|---|---|---|---|
| **Palmar muscles** | | | | |
| **Lumbricales** | Tendons of the flexor digitorum profundus | Tendons of the extensor digitorum communis | Flexes the metacarpophalangeal joints and extends the interphalangeal joints | Median and ulnar (C6–C8) |
| **Dorsal interossei (4)** | Adjacent sides of all of the metacarpals | Proximal phalanx of the second, third, and fourth fingers | Abducts the fingers from the middle finger | Ulnar (C8, T1) |
| **Palmar interossei (3)** | Medial side of the second metacarpal and lateral side of the fourth and fifth metacarpals | Proximal phalanx of the same finger | Adducts the fingers toward the middle finger | Ulnar (C8, T1) |
| **Thenar muscles** | | | | |
| **Abductor pollicis brevis** | Flexor retinaculum, scaphoid, and trapezium | Proximal phalanx of the thumb | Abducts the thumb | Median (C6, C7) |
| **Opponens pollicis** | Flexor retinaculum and trapezium | Lateral border of the metacarpal of the thumb | Pulls the thumb in front of the palm to meet the little finger | Median (C6, C7) |
| **Flexor pollicis brevis** | Flexor retinaculum, trapezium, and first metacarpal | Base of the proximal phalanx of the thumb | Flexes and adducts the thumb | Median (C6–T1) |
| **Adductor pollicis** | Capitate and second and third metacarpals | Proximal phalanx of the thumb | Adducts the thumb | Ulnar (C8, T1) |
| **Hypothenar muscles** | | | | |
| **Palmaris brevis** | Flexor retinaculum | Skin on the ulnar border of the hand | Pulls the skin toward the middle of the palm | Ulnar (C8) |
| **Abductor digiti minimi** | Pisiform and the tendon of the flexor carpi ulnaris | Base of the proximal phalanx of the little finger | Abducts the little finger | Ulnar (C8, T1) |
| **Flexor digiti minimi brevis** | Flexor retinaculum and hamate | Base of the proximal phalanx of the little finger | Flexes the little finger | Ulnar (C8, T1) |
| **Opponens digiti minimi** | Flexor retinaculum and hamate | Metacarpal of the little finger | Brings the little finger out to meet the thumb | Ulnar (C8, T1) |

### Joint Movements of the Fingers and Thumb

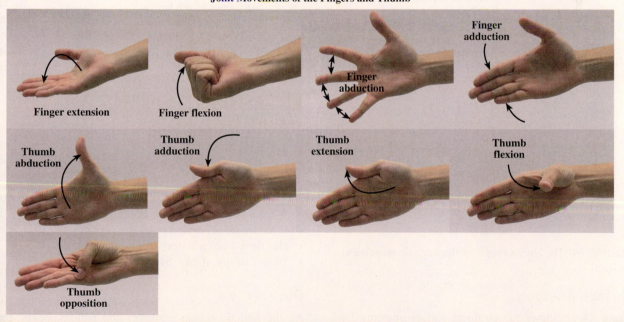

Finger extension
Finger flexion
Finger abduction
Finger adduction
Thumb abduction
Thumb adduction
Thumb extension
Thumb flexion
Thumb opposition

Manual muscle tests and goniometric measurements of range of motion for the hand and fingers can be found in Appendix F and Appendix G at the end of the text.

© William E. Prentice

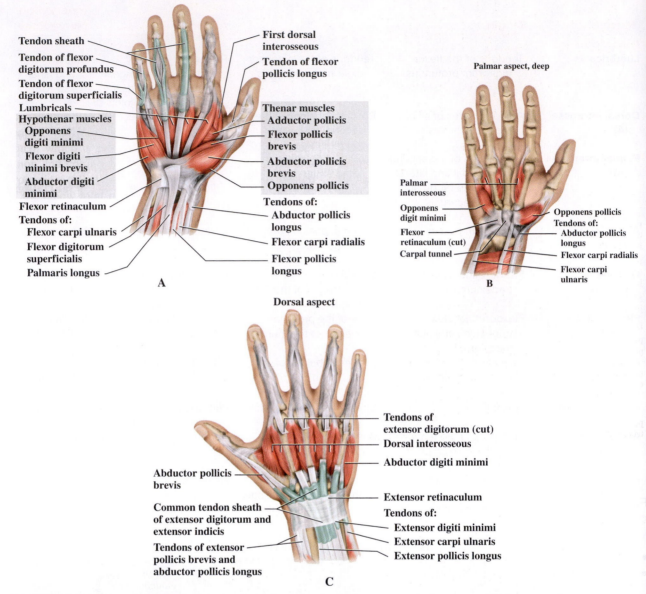

Tendon sheath
Tendon of flexor digitorum profundus
Tendon of flexor digitorum superficialis
Lumbricals
Hypothenar muscles
Opponens digiti minimi
Flexor digiti minimi brevis
Abductor digiti minimi
Flexor retinaculum
Tendons of:
  Flexor carpi ulnaris
  Flexor digitorum superficialis
  Palmaris longus

First dorsal interosseous
Tendon of flexor pollicis longus
Thenar muscles
Adductor pollicis
Flexor pollicis brevis
Abductor pollicis brevis
Opponens pollicis
Tendons of:
  Abductor pollicis longus
  Flexor carpi radialis
  Flexor pollicis longus

A

Palmar aspect, deep

Palmar interosseous
Opponens digit minimi
Flexor retinaculum (cut)
Carpal tunnel

Opponens pollicis
Tendons of:
  Abductor pollicis longus
  Flexor carpi radialis
  Flexor carpi ulnaris

B

Dorsal aspect

Tendons of extensor digitorum (cut)
Dorsal interosseous
Abductor digiti minimi

Abductor pollicis brevis

Extensor retinaculum
Tendons of:

Common tendon sheath of extensor digitorum and extensor indicis

Extensor digiti minimi
Extensor carpi ulnaris
Extensor pollicis longus

Tendons of extensor pollicis brevis and abductor pollicis longus

C

FIGURE 24–10   Intrinsic muscles of the hand. **(A)** Superficial muscles, anterior (palmar) view. **(B)** Deep muscles, anterior view. **(C)** Superficial muscles, posterior (dorsal) view.

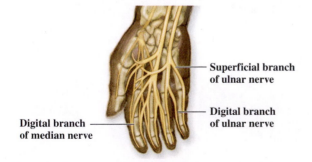

Superficial branch of ulnar nerve
Digital branch of ulnar nerve
Digital branch of median nerve

FIGURE 24–11   Nerve supply of the intrinsic muscles of the hand.

## Surface Anatomy

Figure 24–13 shows the pertinent surface anatomy landmarks for the wrist and hand from a dorsal and a palmer view.

# ASSESSMENT OF THE WRIST, HAND, AND FINGERS

## History

The athletic trainer should ask these questions about the location and type of pain:

- What was the mechanism of injury?
- What increases or decreases the pain?
- Has there been a history of trauma or overuse?
- What therapy, if any, has been given in the past?

## Observation

As the athletic trainer observes the patient, he or she should note arm and hand asymmetries:

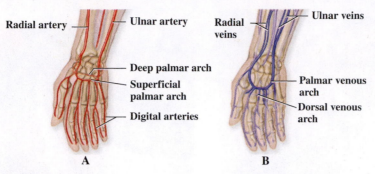

FIGURE 24–12  Blood supply of the hand. **(A)** Arteries. **(B)** Veins.

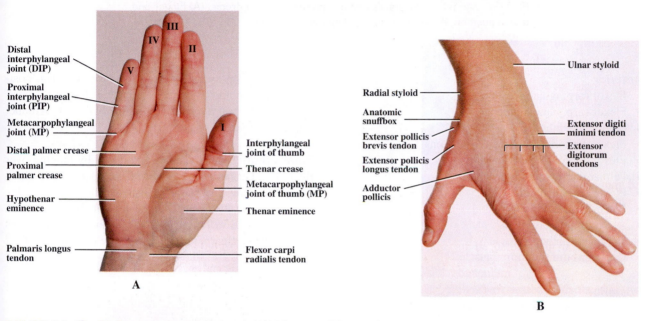

FIGURE 24–13  Surface anatomy of the hand. **(A)** Volar view. **(B)** Dorsal view.

© JW Ramsey/McGraw-Hill Education

- Are there any postural deviations?
- Does the patient hold the part in a stiff or protected manner?
- Is the wrist or hand swollen?

Hand usage, such as writing or unbuttoning a shirt, should be noted. The general attitude of the hand should be observed. When the patient is asked to open and close the hand, the athletic trainer should note whether this movement can be performed fully and rhythmically. Another general functional activity is to have the patient touch the tip of the thumb to each fingertip several times. The last factor to be observed is the color of the fingernails. Nails that are very pale instead of pink may indicate a problem with blood circulation.

## Palpation

**Bony Palpation** The following bony landmarks should be palpated:

- Scaphoid
- Trapezoid

- Trapezium
- Lunate
- Capitate
- Triquetral
- Pisiform
- Hamate (hook of the hamate)
- Metacarpals 1–5
- Proximal, middle, and distal phalanges of the fingers
- Proximal and distal phalanges of the thumb

**Soft-Tissue Palpation** The following soft-tissue structures should be palpated:

*General*
- Triangular fibrocartilage
- Ligaments of the carpal bones
- Carpometacarpal joints and ligaments
- Metacarpophalangeal joints and collateral ligaments
- Proximal interphalangeal joints and collateral ligaments
- Distal interphalangeal joints and collateral ligaments

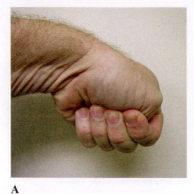
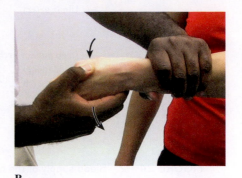

A                                    B

FIGURE 24–14   Finkelstein's test for deQuervain's syndrome. **(A)** Finger and thumb position. **(B)** Wrist is deviated into ulnar flexion.
© William E. Prentice

### Anterior

- Flexor carpi radialis tendon
- Flexor carpi ulnaris tendon
- Lumbricale muscles
- Flexor digitorum superficialis tendons
- Flexor digitorum profundus tendons
- Palmar interossei muscles
- Flexor pollicis brevis
- Flexor pollicis longus tendon
- Abductor pollicis brevis
- Opponens pollicis muscle
- Opponens digiti minimi muscle

### Posterior

- Extensor carpi radialis longus tendon
- Extensor carpi radialis brevis tendon
- Extensor carpi ulnaris tendon
- Extensor digitorum tendons
- Extensor indicis tendon
- Extensor digiti minimi tendon
- Dorsal interossei muscles
- Extensor pollicis brevis tendon
- Extensor pollicis longus tendon
- Abductor pollicis longus tendon

## Special Tests

**Finkelstein's Test[3]** Finkelstein's test is a test for deQuervain's syndrome (discussed later in this chapter) (Figure 24–14). The patient makes a fist with the thumb tucked inside. The wrist is then deviated into ulnar flexion. Sharp pain is evidence of stenosing tenosynovitis. Pain over the carpal tunnel could mean a carpal tunnel syndrome affecting the median nerve. On occasion, the flexor tendons also become trapped, making finger flexion difficult. Sn. 0.81 | Sp. 0.50 | +LR 1.62 | -LR 0.38

**Phalen's Test[32]** Any symptoms of carpal tunnel syndrome are an indication for testing, using Tinel's sign and Phalen's test.[1] In Phalen's test, the patient is instructed to flex both wrists as far as possible and press them together. This position is held for approximately 1 minute. If this test is positive, pain will be produced in the region of the carpal tunnel (Figure 24–15).[1] Sn. 0.77 | Sp. 0.40 | +LR 1.3 | -LR 0.58

**Tinel's Sign[24]** Tinel's sign is produced by tapping over the transverse carpal ligament of the carpal tunnel, which causes tingling and paresthesia over the thumb, index finger, middle finger, and lateral half of the ring finger. This sensory distribution of the median nerve indicates the presence of carpal tunnel syndrome (Figure 24–16).[24] Sn. 0.59 | Sp. 0.67 | +LR 1.8 | -LR 0.6

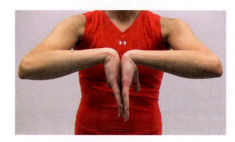

FIGURE 24–15   Wrist press test for carpal tunnel syndrome (Phalen's test).
© William E. Prentice

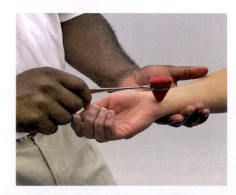

FIGURE 24–16   Tinel's sign at the wrist.
© William E. Prentice

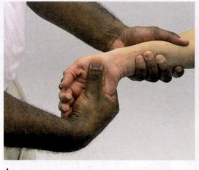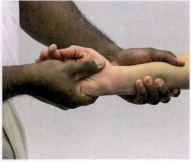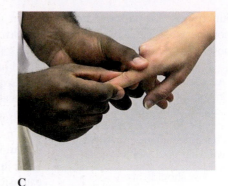

A                          B                          C

FIGURE 24–17   **(A)** Varus stress test produces ulnar deviation at the wrist. **(B)** Valgus stress test produces radial deviation. **(C)** Valgus and varus stress tests can also be done at the interphalangeal joints.
© William E. Prentice

## Valgus/Varus and Glide Stress Tests for Wrist, Metacarpophalangeal, and Interphalangeal Joints

A series of tests can be done to stress the ligamentous integrity of the joints in the wrist, hand, and fingers. Applying valgus and varus stress as well as anterior and posterior glides collectively determines whether a sprain has occurred to one of the many ligaments that connect the carpal bones (Figure 24–17A&B). Valgus/varus stress to the interphalangeal joints of the fingers stress the collateral ligaments, whereas anterior/posterior glides stress the joint capsule (Figure 24–17C). Increased pain or instability with any of these tests usually indicates a ligament sprain.[1]

**Lunotriquetral Ballotment Test**[44] This test requires the examiner to stabilize the lunate with thumb and index finger while sliding the triquetrum anteriorly and posteriorly to look for laxity, pain, and crepitus. A positive test indicates instability of the lunotriquetral joint, which often results in dislocation of the lunate (Figure 24–18). Sn. 0.64 | Sp. 0.44 | +LR 1.2 | -LR 0.8

**Circulatory and Neurological Evaluation** The athletic trainer should inspect the patient's hands to determine whether circulation is being impeded. The hands should be felt for their temperature. A cold hand or portion of a hand is a sign of decreased circulation. Pinching the fingernails can also help detect circulatory problems. Pinching blanches the nail, and on release there should be rapid return of a pink color. Another objective test is Allen's test.

**Allen's Test**[33] Allen's test is used to determine the function of the radial and ulnar arteries supplying the hand. The patient is instructed to squeeze the hand tightly into a fist and then open it fully three or four times. While the patient is holding the last fist, the athletic trainer places firm pressure over each artery. The patient is then instructed to open the hand. The palm should now be blanched. One of the arteries is then released; if normal, the hand will instantly become red. The same process is repeated with the other artery (Figure 24–19).[33] Sn. 0.73 | Sp. 0.97 | +LR 25.1 | -LR 0.27

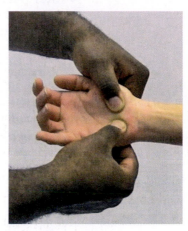

FIGURE 24–18   Lunotriquetral ballotment test.
© William E. Prentice

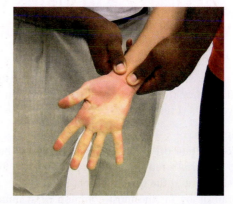

FIGURE 24–19   Testing the radial and ulnar arteries of the hand (Allen's test).
© William E. Prentice

The hand is next evaluated for sensation alterations, especially in cases of suspected tunnel impingements. Nerve involvements will be further evaluated when active and resistive movements are initiated.

**Functional Evaluation** Range of motion is noted in all movements of the wrist and fingers. Active and resistive movements are then compared with those of the uninjured wrist and hand.[26] The following sequence should be conducted:

- Wrist: flexion, extension, radial and ulnar deviation
- MCP joint: flexion, extension
- PIP and DIP joints: flexion, extension
- Fingers: abduction, adduction
- MCP, PIP, and DIP joints of the thumb: flexion, extension

- Thumb: abduction, adduction, opposition
- Fifth finger: opposition

Passive, active, and resistive movements are performed in the wrist and hand. Manual Muscle Tests and Goniometric Measurements of Range of Motion for the wrist, hand and finger joints can be found in Appendix F and Appendix G at the end of the text.

**Clinical Prediction Rules** There is only one clinical prediction rule that is currently used for the hand.

- *Carpal tunnel syndrome*[53]—identifies patients who likely have carpal tunnel syndrome based on specific patient characteristics.

# RECOGNITION AND MANAGEMENT OF INJURIES TO THE WRIST, HAND, AND FINGERS

## Wrist Injuries

Injuries to the wrist usually occur from a fall on the outstretched hand or from repeated flexion, extension, or rotary movements (Figure 24–20).[22,56]

### Wrist Sprains

*Etiology* It is often difficult to distinguish between injury to the wrist's muscle tendons and injury to the supporting structure of the carpal region.[10,17]

A sprain is by far the most common wrist injury and is often poorly managed. It can arise from any abnormal, forced movement of the wrist.[17]

Falling on the hyperextended wrist is the most common cause of wrist sprain, but violent flexion or torsion will also tear supporting tissue.[16] Because the main support of the wrist is derived from the posterior and anterior ligaments that transport the major nutrient vessels to the carpal bones and stabilize the joint, repeated sprains may disrupt the blood supply and, consequently, circulation to the carpal bones.

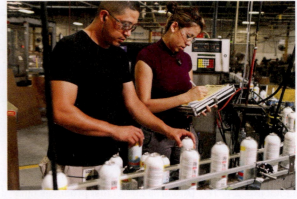

FIGURE 24–20 Injuries to the wrist, hand, and fingers are common not only in sport activities but also in repetitive industrial or manufacturing work.
© DreamPictures/Shannon Faulk/Getty Images

*Symptoms and signs* The patient complains of pain, swelling, and difficulty moving the wrist. On examination, there is tenderness, swelling, and limited ROM. All patients having severe sprains should be referred to a physician for X-ray examination to determine possible fractures. A wrist sprain is often misdiagnosed as a scaphoid fracture.

*Management* Mild and moderate sprains should initially be given POLICE, splinting, and analgesics. It is desirable to have the patient start hand-strengthening exercises almost immediately after the injury has occurred. Taping for support can benefit healing and help prevent further injury (see Figures 8–44 and 8–45).

### Triangular Fibrocartilage Complex (TFCC) Injury

*Etiology* The TFCC is a fibrous and cartilaginous structure that separates the radiocarpal and inferior radioulnar joints of the wrist (see Figure 24–8). It is the major ligamentous stabilizer of the distal radioulnar joint and the ulnar carpus. It provides a flexible mechanism for stable rotational movements of the radiocarpal unit around the ulnar axis and cushions the forces transmitted through the ulnocarpal axis.[36] The TFCC functions like the meniscus in the knee. The TFCC is also prone to cartilage tears that can cause symptoms of wrist pain and clicking or catching sensations. The athlete most often injures the TFCC when swinging a bat or a racquet that creates a violent twist, or torque, of the wrist. Injury to the TFCC can also occur through forced hyperextension of the wrist, as in falling on an outstretched hand, that compresses the TFCC between the radioulnar joint and the proximal row of carpal bones. TFCC injury is often associated with sprain of the ulnar collateral ligament.[36]

***Symptoms and signs*** It is common for the patient not to immediately report this injury. There is pain along the ulnar side of the wrist. Wrist extension is difficult and painful, especially on the ulnar side of the wrist. There is a clicking sound or a catching sensation when moving the wrist. There is considerable swelling around the wrist, although there may not be much swelling initially.

***Management*** The patient with TFCC injury should be referred to a physician for treatment. If it is not properly managed, permanent loss of motion and disability can occur.[36,41] The wrist should be immobilized for 4 weeks, after which range of motion and strengthening exercises should begin. Surgical management is indicated if conservative treatment fails.

## Tenosynovitis

***Etiology*** Wrist tenosynovitis occurs to the extensor carpi radialis longus or brevis.[16] Movements that cause wrist tenosynovitis are those that require the patient to perform repetitive wrist accelerations and decelerations. The cause of tenosynovitis is the repetitive use and overuse of the wrist tendons and their sheaths.[48]

***Symptoms and signs*** The patient complains of pain with use or pain in passive stretching. There is tenderness and swelling over the tendon.

***Management*** Acute pain and inflammation are managed by ice massage for 10 minutes four times a day for the first 48 to 72 hours, NSAIDs, and rest. When swelling has subsided, range of motion is promoted. Ultrasound or phonophoresis can be used for their antiinflammatory effects. When pain and swelling have subsided, PRE can be instituted.[16]

## Tendinitis

***Etiology*** Tendinitis of the flexor carpi radialis and the flexor ulnaris is common in activities that require repetitive wrist flexion. Activities that place prolonged pressure on the palms, such as cycling, can cause flexor digitorum tendinitis. The primary cause of tendinitis is overuse of the wrist.[58]

***Symptoms and signs*** The patient complains of pain on active use or passive stretching of the involved tendon. Isometric resistance to the involved tendon produces pain, weakness, or both.[58]

***Management*** Acute pain and inflammation are managed with ice massage for 10 minutes four times daily for 48 to 72 hours, NSAIDs, and rest. A wrist splint may protect the injured tendon. After swelling has subsided, ROM exercises can be begun. When the patient is pain free, a high-repetition, low-resistance PRE program can be instituted.

## Nerve Compression, Entrapment, Palsy

***Etiology*** Because of the narrow spaces that some nerves must travel through the wrist to the hand, compression neuropathy, or entrapment, can occur. The two most common entrapments are of the median nerve, which travels through the carpal tunnel, and the ulnar nerve, which is compressed in the tunnel of Guyon between the pisiform bone and the hook of the hamate bone.[12] Nerve palsy occurs because of direct trauma to the nerves. The radial and median nerves are most likely to exhibit nerve palsy.

***Symptoms and signs*** Such compression causes a sharp or burning pain that is associated with an increase or decrease in skin sensitivity or with paresthesia. A characteristic deformity of the hand, known as a *benediction* deformity or a *bishop's* deformity, results from damage to the ulnar nerve that affects the hypothenar and intrinsic muscles of the ring and little fingers (Figure 24–21). Compression of both the median and ulnar nerves causes a *claw hand* deformity (Figure 24–22).[12]

A palsy of the radial nerve produces a *drop wrist* deformity, which is caused by paralysis of the extensor muscles such that the wrist and fingers cannot be extended (Figure 24–23). Palsy of the median nerve can cause an *ape hand,* in which the thumb is pulled backward in line with the other fingers by the extensor muscles (Figure 24–24).[12]

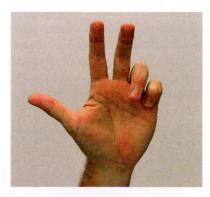

**FIGURE 24–21** Benediction, or bishop's deformity, results from injury to the ulnar nerve.
© William E. Prentice

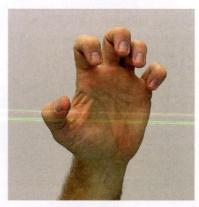

**FIGURE 24–22** A claw hand deformity results from compression of the median and ulnar nerves.
© William E. Prentice

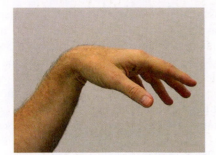

FIGURE 24–23   Drop wrist results from palsy of the radial nerve.
© William E. Prentice

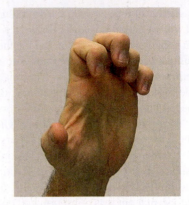

FIGURE 24–24   Ape hand results from palsy of the median nerve.
© William E. Prentice

**Management**   If the possibility exists that chronic entrapment will cause irreversible nerve damage and if conservative treatment is unsuccessful, surgical decompression may be necessary.

### Carpal Tunnel Syndrome

**Etiology**   The carpal tunnel is located on the anterior aspect of the wrist. The floor of the carpal tunnel is formed by the carpal bones and the roof by the transverse carpal ligament (Figure 24–25). A number of anatomical structures course through this limited space, including eight long finger flexor tendons, their synovial sheaths, and the median nerve.[35] Carpal tunnel syndrome results from an inflammation of the tendons and synovial sheaths within this space, which ultimately leads to compression of the median nerve.[12] Carpal tunnel syndrome most often occurs in athletes who engage in activities that require repeated

wrist flexion, although it can also result from direct trauma to the anterior aspect of the wrist.

**Symptoms and signs**   Compression of the median nerve usually results in both sensory and motor deficits. Sensory changes could result in tingling, numbness, and paresthesia in the arc of median nerve innervation over the thumb, index and middle fingers, and palm of the hand. The median nerve innervates the lumbrical muscles of the index and middle fingers and three of the thenar muscles. Thus, weakness in thumb movement is associated with this condition.[35]

**Management**   Initially, conservative treatment involving rest, immobilization, and nonsteroidal antiinflammatory medication is recommended. If the syndrome

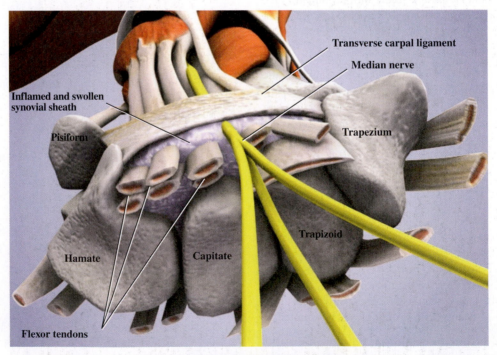

FIGURE 24–25   Cross section of the wrist shows the carpal tunnel that lies under the transverse carpal ligament, with the flexor tendons, an inflamed and swollen synovial sheath, and a compressed median nerve.

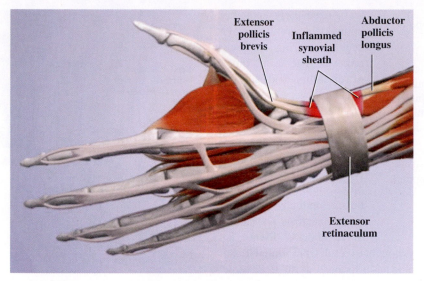

FIGURE 24–26   deQuervain's syndrome is an inflammation of the synovial sheath that surrounds the extensor pollicis brevis and the abductor pollicis longus tendons under the extensor retinaculum.

persists, injection with a corticosteroid and possible surgical decompression of the transverse carpal ligament may be necessary.

### deQuervain's Syndrome

*Etiology*   deQuervain's syndrome (also called Hoffman's disease) is a stenosing tenosynovitis in the thumb. The first tunnel of the wrist becomes contracted and narrowed as a result of inflammation of the synovial lining. The tendons that go through the first tunnel are the extensor pollicis brevis and abductor pollicis longus, which move through the same synovial sheath (Figure 24–26). Because the tendons move through a groove of the radiostyloid process, constant wrist movement can be a source of irritation.[2]

*Symptoms and signs*   Patients who use a great deal of wrist motion are prone to deQuervain's syndrome. Its primary symptom is an aching pain, which may radiate into the hand or forearm. Movements of the wrist tend to increase the pain, and there is a positive Finkelstein's test (see Figure 24–14). There is point tenderness and weakness during thumb extension and abduction, and there may be a painful snapping and catching of the tendons during movement.

*Management*   Management of deQuervain's syndrome involves immobilization, rest, cryotherapy, and antiinflammatory medication. Ultrasound and ice massage are also beneficial. Joint mobilization techniques have been recommended for helping maintain range of motion.[2]

### Dislocation of the Lunate Bone

*Etiology*   Dislocations in the wrist are infrequent. Most occur from a forceful hyperextension of the wrist. Dislocation of the lunate (Figure 24–27) is considered the most common dislocation of a carpal bone.[55] Dislocation

occurs as a result of a fall on the outstretched hand, which forces open the space between the distal and proximal carpal bones. When the stretching force is released, the lunate bone is dislocated anteriorly (palmar side).[38]

*Symptoms and signs*   The primary signs of this condition are pain, swelling, and difficulty in executing wrist and finger flexion. There also may be numbness or even paralysis of the flexor muscles because of lunate pressure on the median nerve.[55]

*Management*   This condition should be treated as acute, and the patient should be sent to a physician for reduction of the dislocation. If the dislocation is not

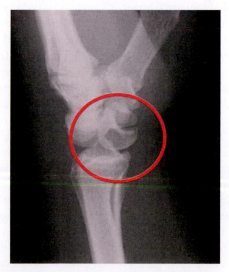

FIGURE 24–27   Dislocation of the lunate bone.
Courtesy Jordan B. Renner, MD, Departments of Radiology and Allied Health Sciences, University of North Carolina

A student-athlete who spends a significant amount of time on her laptop is complaining of feeling tingling, numbness, and paresthesia in the thumb, index, and middle fingers and palm of the right hand.

**?** What condition is this patient likely developing?

recognized early enough, bone deterioration may occur, requiring surgical removal. The usual time of disability and subsequent recovery is 1 to 2 months.

### Kienböck's Disease

*Etiology*   Kienböck's disease involves a loss of blood supply to the lunate bone, eventually resulting in osteonecrosis The cause of Kienböck's disease is unknown. It is generally thought to result from a fall. Often, the patient thinks he or she has a sprained wrist.[15]

*Symptoms and signs*   As the disease progresses, the patient may develop a painful and sometimes swollen wrist, limited range of motion in the affected wrist (stiffness), decreased grip strength in the hand, tenderness directly over the bone (on the top of the hand at about the middle of the wrist), and pain or difficulty in turning the hand upward.[15]

*Management*   The treatment for Kienböck's disease depends on the stage. Early treatment is usually focused on immobilization with a cast and the use of NSAIDs. If Kienböck's disease is more advanced, or if conservative approaches have failed, operative treatment will be needed. Early operative treatments decrease the pressure on the lunate bone by shortening the forearm bone. Fusion of the wrist bones, or removal of some of these bones, may be necessary in the advanced stages of Kienböck's disease.[15]

### Scaphoid Fracture

*Etiology*   The scaphoid bone is the most frequently fractured of the carpal bones.[18] The injury is usually caused by a force on the outstretched hand, which compresses the scaphoid bone between the radius and the second row of carpal bones.[25] This condition is often mistaken for a severe sprain; as a result, the required complete immobilization is not performed.[18] Without proper splinting, the scaphoid fracture often fails to heal because of an inadequate supply of blood; thus, degeneration and necrosis occur.[51] This condition is called Preiser's disease, which is an avascular necrosis of the scaphoid bone. It is necessary to try, in every way possible, to distinguish between a wrist sprain and a fracture of the scaphoid bone because a fracture necessitates immediate referral to a physician.[5]

*Symptoms and signs*   The signs of a recent scaphoid fracture include swelling in the area of the carpal bones, severe point tenderness of the scaphoid bone in the anatomical snuffbox (Figure 24–28A), and scaphoid pain that is elicited by upward pressure exerted on the long axis of the thumb and by radial flexion and ulnar deviation. Absence of the ability to provoke pain by applying pressure

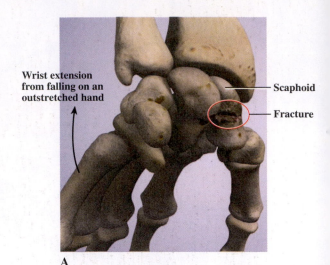

A

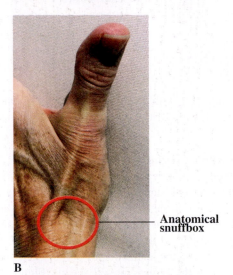

B

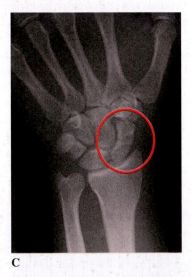

C

FIGURE 24–28   **(A)** A fall on an outstretched hand causes a fracture of the scaphoid that **(B)** results in point tenderness in the anatomical snuffbox. **(C)** X-ray of a fractured scaphoid.

(b) © William E. Prentice; (c) Courtesy Jordan B. Renner, MD, Departments of Radiology and Allied Health Sciences, University of North Carolina

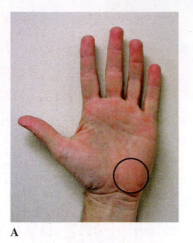

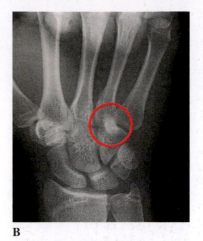

A                                    B

FIGURE 24–29   Hook of the hamate fracture **(A)** Surface location. **(B)** X-ray view.
(a) © William E. Prentice; (b) Courtesy Jordan B. Renner, MD, Departments of Radiology
and Allied Health Sciences, University of North Carolina

in the anatomical snuffbox is perhaps the best way to distinguish a scaphoid fracture from a wrist sprain.

***Management***   With these signs present, cold should be applied, the area splinted, and the patient referred to a physician for X-ray study and casting (Figure 24–28B). In most cases, cast immobilization lasts for approximately 6 weeks and is followed by strengthening exercises coupled with protective taping. Immobilization is discontinued for rehabilitation. The wrist needs protection against impact loading for an additional 3 months.[25] If the fracture extends completely through the scaphoid and it is unstable, a physician will likely choose to insert a screw into the two fractured pieces to make healing more likely. Otherwise the fracture may become a non-union fracture significantly extending the time it may take for the injury to heal.

## Hamate Fracture

***Etiology***   A fracture of the hamate bone—in particular, of the hook of the hamate—can occur from a fall but more commonly occurs from contact while the athlete is holding a sports implement, such as a tennis racket, baseball bat, lacrosse stick, hockey stick, or golf club (Figure 24–29).[13,34]

> A carpenter trips over a ladder and falls on the outstretched left hand, causing a compression force to the scaphoid bone between the radius and the second row of the carpal bones.
>
> **?** What wrist injury is most likely to have occurred

***Symptoms and signs***   The patient experiences wrist pain and weakness and point tenderness. Pull of the muscular attachments can cause nonunion.[13]

***Management***   Casting of the wrist is usually the treatment of choice.[31] The hook of the hamate can be protected by a doughnut-type pad that takes pressure off the area.

## Wrist Ganglion

***Etiology***   The wrist ganglion, which is a synovial cyst, is often seen in sports (Figure 24–30). It is considered by many to be a herniation of the joint capsule or of the synovial sheath of a tendon; others believe it to be a cystic structure.[7] The wrist ganglion usually appears slowly, after a wrist strain, and contains a clear, mucinous fluid. The ganglion most often appears on the back of the wrist but can appear at any tendinous point in the wrist or hand.

***Symptoms and signs***   The patient complains of occasional pain with a lump at the site. Pain increases with use. There is a cystic structure that may feel soft, rubbery, or very hard.[29]

***Management***   An old method of treatment was to first break down the swelling through digital pressure and then

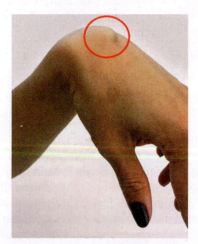

FIGURE 24–30   A wrist ganglion usually occurs in the dorsal aspect of the wrist.
© William E. Prentice

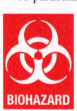
**24–7 Clinical Application Exercise**

A golfer is hitting a ball out of the woods and there are a lot of tree roots near his ball. As he is attempting to strike the ball, he accidentally hits a root and feels immediate pain in his wrist on the lateral side.

**?** What injury might an athletic trainer suspect that he has sustained?

apply a felt pressure pad for a period of time to encourage healing. A newer approach is a combination of aspiration and chemical cauterization, with subsequent application of a pressure pad. Neither of these methods prevents the ganglion from recurring. Ultrasound can be used to reduce the size of the ganglion cyst. Surgical removal is the most effective of the various methods of treatment.

## Hand and Finger Injuries

The hand is one of the most commonly injured sites, yet it is probably the most poorly managed.[21] Immediate evaluation must be afforded to avoid any delay in proper management. When it comes to improper care, the hand is notoriously unforgiving.[21]

### Contusions and Pressure Injuries of the Hand and Phalanges

***Etiology*** The hand and phalanges, having an irregular bony structure combined with little protective fat and muscle padding, are prone to contusion.

***Symptoms and signs*** This condition is easily identified from the history of trauma and the pain and swelling of soft tissues.

***Management*** Cold and compression should be applied immediately until hemorrhage has ceased and is followed by gradual warming of the part in whirlpool or immersion baths. Soreness may still be present, and protection should be given by a sponge rubber pad (see Figure 8–45).

A particularly common contusion of the finger is bruising of the distal phalanx, which results in a subungual hematoma (contusion of the fingernail). This extremely painful condition occurs because of the accumulation of blood underneath the fingernail. The patient should place the finger in ice water until the hemorrhage ceases, and the pressure of blood should then be released (Figure 24–31A). See *Focus Box 24–1:* "Releasing blood from beneath the fingernail."[49]

### Trigger Finger or Thumb

***Etiology*** Repeated movement can cause the tendons of the wrist and hand to sustain irritation that results in tenosynovitis. An inflammation of the tendon sheath leads to swelling, crepitus, and painful movement. Most commonly affected are the extensor tendons of the wrist: the extensor carpi ulnaris, extensor pollicis longus, extensor pollicis brevis, and abductor pollicis longus.[46]

The trigger finger or thumb is an example of stenosing tenosynovitis.[8] It most commonly occurs in a flexor tendon

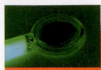

### Releasing blood from beneath the fingernail

The following are two common methods for releasing the pressure of a subungual hematoma.

MATERIALS NEEDED: Small-gauge drill or high-temperature cautery, antiseptic
POSITION OF PATIENT: The patient sits with the injured hand palm downward on the table.

***TECHNIQUE 1***

1. The injured finger should first be coated with an antiseptic solution.
2. The tip of a high-temperature cautery is placed on the surface of the nail with moderate pressure, resulting in melting a hole through the nail to the site of the bleeding (Figure 24–31C).

***TECHNIQUE 2***

1. The injured finger should first be coated with an antiseptic solution.
2. A small-gauge drill is used to penetrate the injured nail through a rotary action (Figure 24–31B).

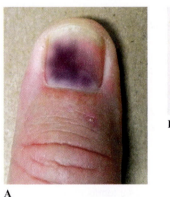
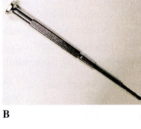
A

B

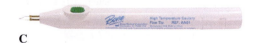
C

FIGURE 24–31 **(A)** Subungual hematoma. **(B)** Manual fingernail drill. **(C)** High-temperature cautery.
(a) © William E. Prentice; (b) © William E. Prentice; (c) Courtesy Bovie Medical Corporation

that runs through a common sheath with other tendons. Thickening of the sheath or tendon can occur, which constricts the sliding tendon. A nodule in the synovium of the sheath adds to the difficulty of gliding.[20] The cause of trigger finger or thumb is nonspecific overuse.

***Symptoms and signs*** The patient complains that when the finger or thumb is flexed, there is resistance to reextension, producing a snapping that is both palpable and audible. During palpation, tenderness is produced, and a lump can be felt at the base of the flexor tendon sheath.

***Management*** Treatment initially is the same as for deQuervain's syndrome; however, if treatment is unsuccessful, steroid injections may produce relief. If steroid injections do not provide relief, splinting the tendon sheath is the last option.

## Extensor Tendon Avulsion (Mallet Finger)

***Etiology*** The mallet finger is sometimes called baseball finger or basketball finger. It is caused by a blow from an object that strikes the tip of the finger, jamming and avulsing the extensor tendon from its insertion, along with a piece of bone.[28]

> A baseball catcher receives a pitch that jams and avulses the extensor tendon of the distal interphalangeal joint of the second finger.
>
> **?** How should this condition be managed?

***Symptoms and signs*** The patient complains of pain at the distal interphalangeal joint. X-ray examination may show a bony avulsion from the dorsal proximal distal phalanx. The patient is unable to extend the finger, carrying it at approximately a 30-degree angle. There is also point tenderness at the site of the injury, and the avulsed bone often can be palpated (Figure 24–32A).[28]

***Management*** POLICE is given for the pain and swelling. If there is no fracture, the distal phalanx should immediately be splinted in a position of extension for 6 to 8 weeks (Figure 24–32B).

## Boutonniere Deformity

***Etiology*** The boutonniere, or buttonhole, deformity is caused by a rupture of the extensor tendon dorsal to the middle phalanx.[11] Trauma occurs to the tip of the finger, which forces the DIP joint into extension and the PIP joint into flexion.[57] The extensor expansion tears over the PIP joint, and the two sides slide down below the axis of volation of the PIP joint. The PIP articulation then pops through the extensor expansion tear, much as a button would through a buttonhole—hence the name of this injury.

***Symptoms and signs*** The patient complains of severe pain and an inability to extend the DIP joint. There is swelling, point tenderness, and an obvious deformity (Figure 24–33).

***Management*** Management of the boutonniere deformity includes cold application followed by splinting of the PIP joint in extension. NOTE: If this condition is inadequately splinted, the classic boutonniere deformity will become permanent. Splinting is continued for 5 to 8 weeks. While the finger is splinted, the patient is encouraged to flex the distal phalanx (Table 24–3).

## Flexor Digitorum Profundus Rupture (Jersey Finger)

***Etiology*** Jersey finger is a rupture of the flexor digitorum profundus tendon from its insertion on the distal phalanx.[11] This condition most often occurs in the ring finger when the athlete tries to grab the jersey of an opponent and either ruptures the tendon or avulses a small piece of bone.[49]

***Symptoms and signs*** Because the tendon is no longer attached to the distal phalanx, the DIP joint cannot be flexed, and the finger is in an extended position (Figure 24–34). There is pain and point tenderness over the distal phalanx.

***Management*** If the tendon is not surgically repaired, the patient will never be able to flex the DIP joint, causing

> A snow skier falls, holding her skipoles, and injures her right thumb. She describes a hyperextension with abduction mechanism of injury. The thumb is point tender over the ulnar side of the metacarpophalangeal joint, and there is mild swelling.
>
> **?** What is this injury? What special test can be used to evaluate this injury?

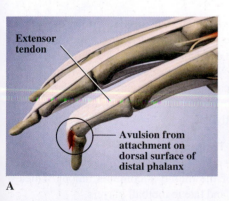
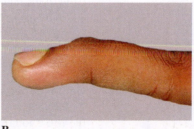
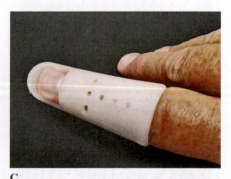

Extensor tendon

Avulsion from attachment on dorsal surface of distal phalanx

A

B

C

**FIGURE 24–32** Mallet finger occurs from **(A)** rupture of the extensor tendon from the distal phalanx, which **(B)** causes the patient to be unable to extend the distal phalanx. **(C)** The distal phalanx can be splinted using a stack splint.

(b, c) © William E. Prentice

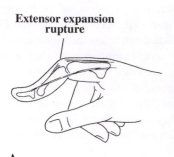

Extensor expansion rupture

**A**

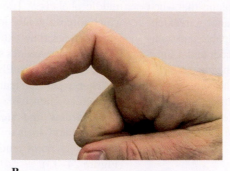

**B**

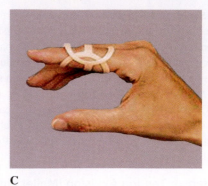

**C**

FIGURE 24–33   **(A&B)** A boutonniere deformity occurs from rupture of the extensor expansion dorsal to the PIP joint. **(C)** Splinting using an Oval-8 splint.

(b, c) © William E. Prentice

| TABLE 24–3 | Conservative Treatment and Splinting of Finger Injuries |  |  |  |
|---|---|---|---|---|
| Injury | Constant Splinting | Begin Motion | Additional Splinting during Competition | Joint Position |
| Mallet finger | 6–8 wk | 6–8 wk | 6–8 wk | Slight DIP hyperextension |
| Collateral ligament sprains | 3 wk | 2 wk | 4–6 wk | 30-degree flexion |
| PIP and DIP dislocations | 3 wk | 3 wk | 3 wk | 30-degree flexion |
| Phalangeal fractures | 4–6 wk | 4–6 wk | 3 wk | N/A |
| PIP and DIP fractures | 9–11 wk | 3 wk | 3 wk | 30-degree flexion |
| Pseudoboutonniere volar plate injuries | 5 wk | 3 wk | 3 wk | 20- to 30-degree flexion |
| Boutonniere deformity | 6–8 wk | 6–8 wk | 6–8 wk | PIP in extension; DIP and MCP not included |
| MCP fractures | 3 wk | 3 wk | 4–6 wk | 30-degree flexion |
| Flexor digitorum profundus repair | 5 wk | 3 wk | 3 wk | Depends on repair |

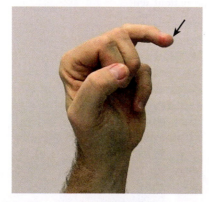

FIGURE 24–34   A Jersey finger involves rupture of the flexor tendon and a loss of ability to flex the finger.

© William E. Prentice

weakness in grip strength; otherwise, function will be relatively normal. If surgery is done, the course of rehabilitation requires about 12 weeks, and there is often poor gliding of the tendon with the possibility of rerupture.[49]

### Dupuytren's Contracture

***Etiology***   The cause of Dupuytren's contracture is unknown. Nodules develop in the palmar aponeurosis that limit finger extension and eventually cause a flexion deformity.[50]

***Symptoms and signs***   A flexion deformity most often develops in which the ring or little finger moves into the palm of the hand and cannot be extended (Figure 24–35).

***Management***   A flexion contracture deformity of this type can significantly interfere with normal hand function. The tissue nodules causing the contracture must be removed surgically.[50]

### Gamekeeper's Thumb

***Etiology***   A sprain of the ulnar collateral ligament of the MCP joint of the thumb is common among athletes, especially skiers and tackle football players.[47]

The mechanism of injury is usually a forceful abduction of the proximal phalanx, which is occasionally combined with hyperextension (Figure 24–36).[8]

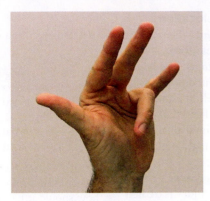

FIGURE 24–35   Dupuytren's contracture is a flexion deformity of the ring or little finger.
© William E. Prentice

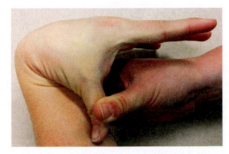

FIGURE 24–36   A gamekeeper's thumb is a sprain of the ulnar collateral ligament at the MCP joint of the thumb.
© William E. Prentice

***Symptoms and signs***   The patient complains of pain over the ulnar collateral ligament in addition to a weak and painful pinch. Inspection demonstrates tenderness and swelling over the medial aspect of the thumb.[48]

***Management***   Because the stability of pinching can be severely deterred, proper, immediate, and follow-up care must be performed. If there is instability in the joints, the patient should be immediately referred to an orthopedist. If the joint is stable, X-ray examination should be performed to rule out fracture. A thumb splint should be applied for protection for 3 weeks or until the thumb is pain free.[37] The splint, extending from the end of the thumb to above the wrist, is applied with the thumb in a neutral position. After the splint is removed, thumb spica taping should be worn during sports participation (see Figure 8–48). If there is a complete tear of the ligament, surgical repair is necessary to allow a return to normal function.

### Sprains of the Interphalangeal Joints of the Fingers

***Etiology***   Interphalangeal finger sprains can include the PIP joint or the DIP joint. Injury can range from minor to complete tears of the collateral ligament, a volar plate tear, or a central extensor expansion tear.[20] A collateral ligament sprain of the interphalangeal joint is common in sports such as basketball, volleyball, and football. A common cause is an axial force that produces a jammed finger.

This mechanism places valgus or varus stress on the interphalangeal joint.

***Symptoms and signs***   The patient complains of pain and swelling at the involved joint. There is severe point tenderness at the joint site, especially in the region of the collateral ligaments. There may be a lateral or medial instability when the joint is in 150 degrees of flexion. Collateral ligamentous injuries may be evaluated by the application of a valgus and varus joint stress test.

***Management***   Management includes POLICE for the acute stage, X-ray examinations, and splinting. Splinting of the PIP joint is usually at 30 to 40 degrees of flexion for 10 days. If the sprain is to the DIP joint, splinting a few days in full extension assists in the healing process. If the sprains are minor, taping the injured finger to a noninjured one will provide protective support. Later, a protective checkrein can be applied for either thumb or finger protection (see Figure 8–49).

### Swan Neck and Pseudoboutonniere Deformities

***Etiology***   The volar plate of the PIP joint is most commonly injured from a severe hyperextension force. A distal tear of the volar plate from the middle phalanx may cause a *swan neck deformity* (Figure 24–37).[9] An avulsion of the volar plate from the proximal phalanx may cause a *pseudoboutonniere deformity*.

***Symptoms and signs***   There is pain and swelling at the PIP joint, and it displays varying degrees of hyperextension. Tenderness is over the volar aspect of the PIP. A major indication of a tear is that the PIP joint can be passively hyperextended in comparison with other PIP joints.

A volleyball player, going up to block a spike, receives an axial force to the middle finger, which causes a valgus force.

**?** What soft-tissue injuries would be expected with such a force?

24-10 Clinical Application Exercise

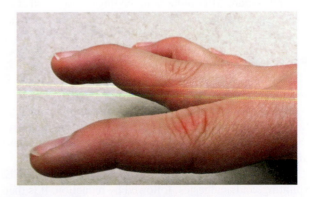

FIGURE 24–37   Swan neck deformity.
© William E. Prentice

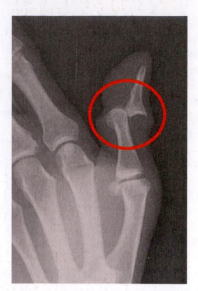

FIGURE 24–38  X-ray showing open dislocation of the interphalangeal joint of a thumb.

Courtesy Jordan B. Renner, MD, Departments of Radiology and Allied Health Sciences, University of North Carolina

*Management*  Initially, the patient is treated with POLICE and analgesics as required. Management consists of splinting at 20 to 30 degrees of flexion for 3 weeks, followed by buddy taping and then PRE.

### PIP Dorsal Dislocation

*Etiology*  Dislocations of the phalanges have a high rate of occurrence (Figure 24–38).[27] Dislocations can occur at a number of joints—for example, PIP dorsal dislocation, PIP palmar dislocation, and MCP dislocation. The mechanism that produces a PIP dislocation is hyperextension that produces a disruption of the volar plate at the middle phalanx. The volar pate is a thick, fibrocartilaginous ligament that is part of the anterior joint capsule. It forms floor of the PIP joint and separates the joint space from the flexor tendons.

*Symptom and signs*  The patient complains of pain and swelling over the PIP. There is an obvious avulsion deformity and disability.

*Management*  Initially, the patient is treated with POLICE, splinting, and analgesics, followed by reduction by a physician. After reduction, the finger is splinted at 20 to 30 degrees of flexion for 3 weeks. After splint removal, buddy taping is used.

### PIP Palmar Dislocation

*Etiology*  The cause is a twist of a finger while it is semiflexed.

*Symptoms and signs*  The patient complains of pain and swelling over the PIP. There is point tenderness over the PIP, primarily on the dorsal side. The finger displays an angular or rotational deformity.[4]

*Management*  The finger is treated with POLICE, splinting, and analgesics, followed by reduction. It is then splinted in full extension for 4 to 6 weeks, after which it is protected for 6 to 8 weeks during activity.

### MCP Dislocation

*Etiology*  The cause of the MCP dislocation is a twisting or shear force.

*Symptoms and signs*  The patient complains of pain, swelling, and stiffness at the MCP joint. The proximal phalanx is dorsally angulated at 60 to 90 degrees.[45]

*Management*  Initially, the injury is treated with POLICE, splinting, and analgesics. It is then reduced, buddy taped, and given early ROM exercise.[45]

During spring break in Florida, a college student gets into a fistfight and injures his right hand through an axial force to the fifth metacarpal bone.

**?** What type of injury should be suspected, and how should it be managed?

### Metacarpal Fracture

*Etiology*  The cause of metacarpal fractures is commonly a direct axial force or a compressive force, such as being stepped on (Figure 24–39). Fractures of the fifth metacarpal are associated with boxing and the martial arts and are usually called a *boxer's fracture*.[40]

*Symptoms and signs*  The patient complains of pain and swelling. The injury may appear to be an angular or rotational deformity.

*Management*  Initially, POLICE and analgesics are given, followed by X-ray examinations. Deformity is reduced, followed by splinting. A splint is worn for 4 weeks, after which early ROM exercises are carried out.[46]

### Bennett's Fracture

*Etiology*  A Bennett's fracture occurs in the first metacarpal just distal to the carpometacarpal (CMC) joint of the thumb as a result of an axial and abduction force to the thumb.[8]

*Symptoms and signs*  The patient complains of pain and swelling over the base of the thumb. The thumb's CMC appears deformed. An X-ray shows a fracture.

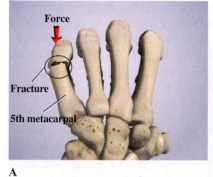 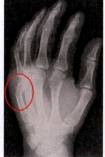

**A**                                        **B**

FIGURE 24–39  **(A)** A boxer's fracture occurs in the fifth metacarpal. **(B)** X-ray view.

(b) Courtesy Jordan B. Renner, MD, Departments of Radiology and Allied Health Sciences, University of North Carolina

An automobile assembly line worker sustains an axial force to the thumb, producing a Bennett's fracture.

**?** What symptoms and signs should the athletic trainer expect in such an injury?

*Management* This condition is structurally unstable and must be referred to an orthopedic surgeon.

## Distal Phalangeal Fracture

*Etiology* The primary cause of distal phalangeal fracture is a crushing force.[14]

*Symptoms and signs* There is a complaint of pain and swelling of the distal phalanx. A subungual hematoma is often seen in this condition.

*Management* Initially, POLICE and analgesics are given. A protective splint is applied as a means for relief of pain. The subungual hematoma is drained.

## Middle Phalangeal Fracture

*Etiology* A middle phalangeal fracture occurs from a direct trauma or twist.[14]

*Symptoms and signs* There is pain and swelling with tenderness over the middle phalanx. There may be deformity. X-rays show bone displacement.

*Management* POLICE and analgesics are given as needed. Depending on the fracture site and if there is no deformity, a buddy tape may be used with a thermoplastic splint for sports activity. If there is deformity, immobilization is applied for 3 to 4 weeks and a protective splint for an additional 9 to 10 weeks.[45]

## Proximal Phalangeal Fracture

*Etiology* Fractures of the proximal phalanges may be spiral and angular.

*Symptoms and signs* The patient complains of pain, swelling, and deformity. Inspection reveals varying degrees of deformity.

*Management* POLICE and analgesics are given as needed. Fracture stability is maintained by immobilization of the wrist in slight extension, MCP in 70 degrees of flexion, and buddy taping.

## PIP Fracture and Dislocation

*Etiology* The cause of this combination of fracture and dislocation is an axial load on a partially flexed finger.

*Symptoms and signs* This condition causes pain and swelling in the region of the PIP joint. There is localized tenderness over the PIP joint.

*Management* POLICE and analgesics are given initially, followed by reduction of the fracture. If there is a small fragment, buddy taping is used. If there is a large fragment, a splint of 30 to 60 degrees of flexion is applied.

**Fingernail Deformities** Changes in the normal appearance of the fingernails can indicate a number of diseases.[52]

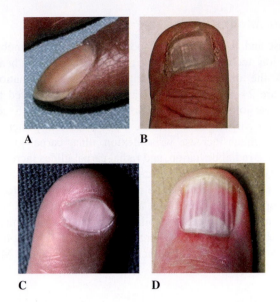

FIGURE 24–40   Fingernail deformities. **(A)** Clubbed nail. **(B)** Scaling or ridging nail. **(C)** Spooning or depression nail. **(D)** Vertical ridges nail.

(a, c) Courtesy Dean Morrell, MD, Department of Dermatology, University of North Carolina; (b, d) © William E. Prentice

Some of the more common changes in the fingernails and their causes are as follows (Figure 24–40).[52]

- Clubbing and cyanosis—congenital heart disorders or chronic respiratory disease
- Scaling or ridging (onycholysis)—psoriasis
- Spooning or depression (koilonychia)—thyroid problems, iron-deficiency anemia
- Ridging (vertical) and poor development—nutritional deficiencies

# REHABILITATION OF INJURIES TO THE FOREARM, WRIST, HAND, AND FINGERS

Reconditioning of the hand, wrist, and forearm must commence as early as possible.[54] Immobilization of the forearm or wrist requires that the muscles be exercised almost immediately after an injury occurs if atrophy and contracture are to be prevented.[49]

## General Body Conditioning

Patients who sustain forearm, wrist, or hand injuries must maintain their preinjury level of conditioning. This conditioning includes cardiorespiratory endurance, strength, flexibility, and neuromuscular control.[42] Patients have many exercise options, such as walking, running, stair climbing, aerobics, cycling, and a variety of resistance and flexibility activities. Modified sports activities can be adapted to the individual injury.[42]

## Joint Mobilization

Wrist and hand injuries respond to traction and mobilization techniques.[43] Distal glides of the radial head with the ulna stabilized can help increase pronation (Figure 24–41). Radiocarpal joint glides can be used to increase joint accessory motions. If the radius is fixed, anterior carpal glides increase wrist extension, posterior carpal glides increase wrist flexion, ulnar carpal glides increase radial deviation, and radial carpal glides increase ulnar deviation. Carpometacarpal joint anterior/posterior glides can help increase the mobility of the hand. Metacarpophalangeal (MP) joint anterior glides in which the proximal metacarpal is stabilized and the distal segment is mobilized are used to increase flexion of the MP joint, whereas posterior glides increase extension of the MP joint.[43]

## Flexibility

A full, pain-free ROM is a primary goal of rehabilitation following injury to the forearm, wrist, hand, and fingers. The flexibility program should include active assisted and active pain-free stretching exercises to increase wrist flexion, extension, ulnar deviation, and radial deviation (Figure 24–42). These exercises should be done with the elbow in full extension to get the greatest stretch.[49] Wrist extension can be improved by progressing from wall, to table, to floor push-up positions (Figure 24–43). If there are neural signs, such as tingling, numbness, or pain, stretching to relieve neural tension in the median and radial nerves reduces those symptoms (Figure 24–44). Regaining thumb ROM is critical to normal hand function. ROM exercises should include opposition, flexion, and abduction exercises (Figure 24–45).

## Strength

Strengthening exercises for the wrist, hand, and fingers present some special challenges for the injured patient and for the athletic trainer supervising the rehabilitation program. Resistive exercises using a weighted device should include flexion, extension, ulnar deviation, radial deviation, pronation, and supination (Figure 24–46). Restoring grip strength is essential for regaining normal hand function. It can be regained by gripping a number of different devices (Figure 24–47).[49] Resistive rubber band exercises can be used to strengthen the fingers (Figure 24–48). A handheld dynamometer can be used to objectively measure grip strength (Figure 24–49).

## Neuromuscular Control

Regaining normal function of the hand requires reestablishing not only gross motor function but also fine motor function and control. Hand and finger rehabilitation requires a restoration of dexterity, which includes pinching and other fine motor activities, such as buttoning buttons, tying shoes, and picking up small

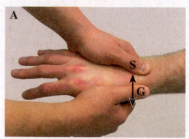
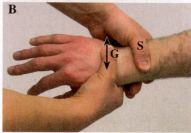
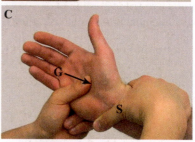
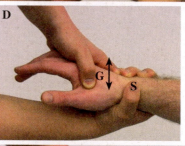
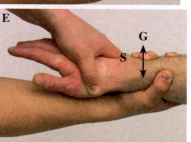
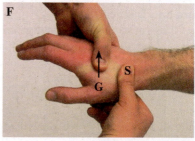

FIGURE 24–41 **(A)** Distal anterior/posterior radial glides. **(B)** Radiocarpal joint anterior glides. **(C)** Radiocarpal joint posterior glides. **(D)** Carpometacarpal joint anterior/posterior glides. **(E)** Radiocarpal joint ulnar glides. **(F)** Carpometacarpal joint anterior posterior glides. (S = stabilize, G = glide)

© William E. Prentice

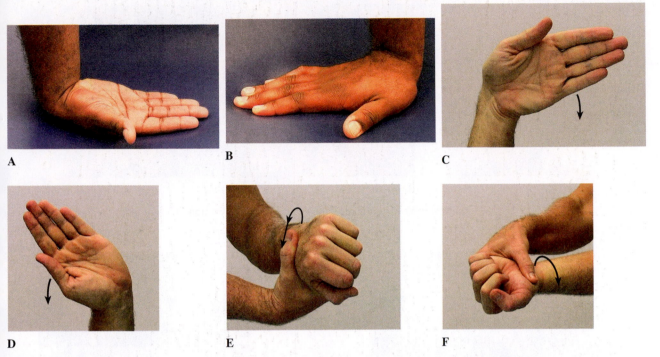

FIGURE 24–42   Static wrist stretching. **(A)** Wrist extensors. **(B)** Wrist flexors. **(C)** Wrist radial deviators. **(D)** Wrist ulnar deviators. **(E)** Wrist pronation. **(F)** Wrist supination.
© William E. Prentice

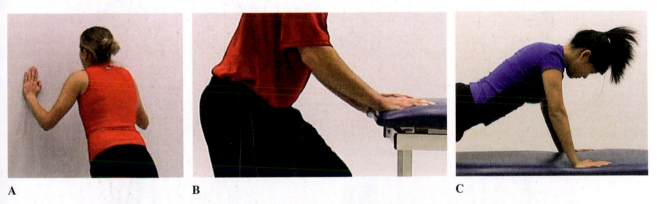

FIGURE 24–43   Wrist extension range of motion progression from **(A)** wall to **(B)** table to **(C)** floor push-ups.
© William E. Prentice

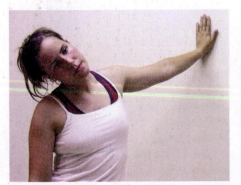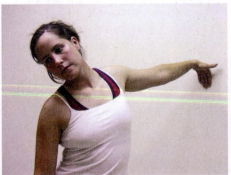

FIGURE 24–44   Neural tension stretches. **(A)** Median nerve. **(B)** Radial nerve.
© William E. Prentice

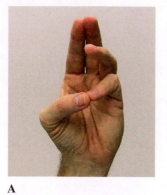
A

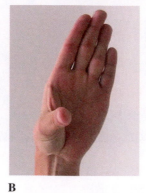
B

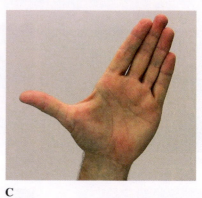
C

FIGURE 24–45   Regaining thumb range of motion. **(A)** Opposition. **(B)** Flexion. **(C)** Abduction.
© William E. Prentice

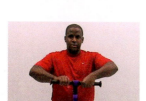
A

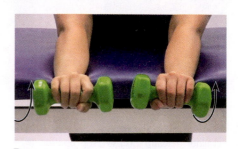
B

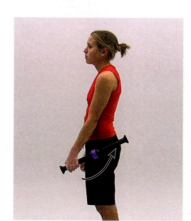
C

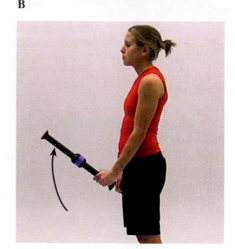
D

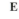
E

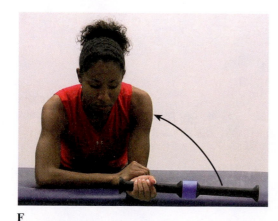
F

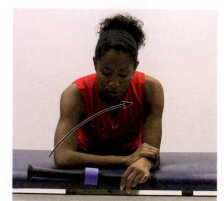
G

FIGURE 24–46   Wrist strengthening. **(A)** Flexion. **(B)** Extension. **(C)** Wrist rolls (flexion or extension). **(D)** Ulnar deviation. **(E)** Radial deviation. **(F)** Pronation. **(G)** Supination.
© William E. Prentice

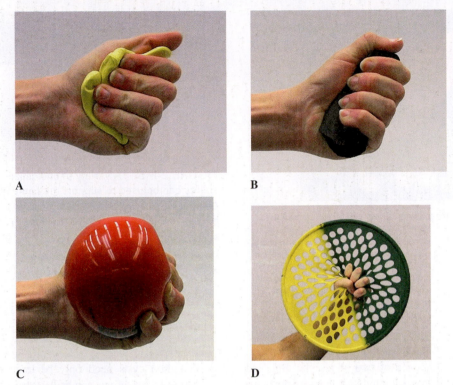

FIGURE 24–47   A variety of resistance devices are available for restoring hand grip function. **(A)** Putty. **(B)** Foam. **(C)** Rubber ball. **(D)** Power web.
© William E. Prentice

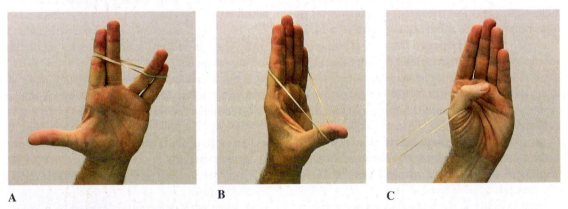

FIGURE 24–48   Finger strengthening using rubber bands. **(A)** Finger abduction exercise. **(B)** Thumb abduction exercise. **(C)** Thumb opposition exercise.
© William E. Prentice

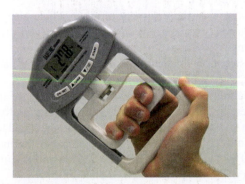

FIGURE 24–49   Increases in grip strength can be measured using a digital handheld dynamometer.
© William E. Prentice

objects (Figure 24–50).[23] It is important to design and incorporate functional activities that allow the patient to perform the normal activities of daily living that generally require fine motor control of hand and finger function.

## Return to Activity

The criteria for the return to activity after wrist or hand injury are grip strength equal to the unaffected limb, full range of motion, and full dexterity. A variety of customized bracing splints and taping techniques are available to protect the injured wrist and hand (Figure 24–51).

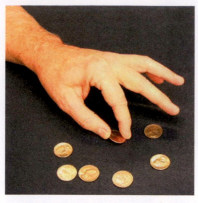

FIGURE 24–50   Restoring finger dexterity by picking up coins.
© William E. Prentice

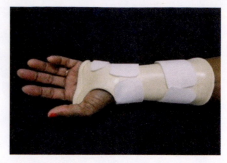

FIGURE 24–51   A variety of customized braces and splints can be used to support the hand and/or wrist.
Barbosa, Rafael Inácio et al. "Effectiveness of Low-Level Laser Therapy for Patients with Carpal Tunnel Syndrome: Design of a Randomized Single-Blinded Controlled Trial." BMC Musculoskeletal Disorders 13: 248 (2012). PMC. © 2012 by Barbosa, Rafael Inácio et al. All rights reserved. Used with permission.

## SUMMARY

- The forearm is composed of two bones, the ulna and the radius, as well as associated soft tissue. Sports injuries to the region commonly consist of contusions, chronic forearm splints, acute strains, and fractures.
- Forearm splints are like shinsplints and involve pain in the forearm muscles upon exertion.
- A Colles' fracture of the distal radius and/or ulna is the most common forearm fracture.
- Injuries to the wrist usually occur as a result of a fall on an outstretched hand or repeated movements involving flexion, extension, and/or rotation. Common injuries are sprains, lunate dislocation, scaphoid fracture, and hamate fracture.
- Wrist sprains are a diagnosis of exclusion. All other pathology must be ruled out prior to return to activity.
- TFCC injuries can result in permanent disability if not properly managed.
- Carpal tunnel syndrome is a tenosynovitis occurring in the anterior wrist.
- Nerve compression or palsy can result in benediction deformity, bishop's deformity, claw hand, drop wrist, or ape hand deformity.
- deQuervain's syndrome should be immobilized for 2 to 3 weeks with gentle, pain-free range of motion exercises performed daily to maintain mobility.
- Lunate dislocations are serious injuries that require lengthy rehabilitation.
- Scaphoid fractures may not be seen on an initial X-ray. If a fracture is suspected but the X-ray is negative, the patient should be treated as if a fracture were present, with X-rays repeated in 2 weeks to confirm the diagnosis. Early, proper immobilization is important to the long-term outcome.
- Hamate hook fractures usually occur through contact with a sports implement, such as a bat or golf club.

- Ganglion cysts need only be treated if symptomatic. Multiple aspirations can be performed during the season with excision postseason, if necessary.
- Injuries to the hand occur frequently. Common injuries include those caused by contusions and chronic pressure; by tendons receiving sustained irritation, which leads to tenosynovitis; and by tendon avulsions. Sprains, dislocations, and fractures of the fingers are also common.
- Both a mallet finger and a boutonniere deformity involve injury to the extensor expansion and must be splinted in full extension uninterrupted for 5 to 8 weeks.
- Jersey finger is a rupture of the flexor digitorum profundus tendon.
- Dupuytren's contracture eventually results in a flexion contracture.
- A swan neck deformity is caused by a volar plate injury at the PIP joint.
- Flexor tendon injuries are very labor-intensive, significant injuries.
- The goal in the treatment of ulnar collateral ligament injuries (gamekeeper's thumb) is stability of the MCP joint.
- Dislocations of the MCP joints are very rare and are often complicated. Dorsal PIP dislocations without fracture are common and need early range of motion exercise and edema control. Splinting for comfort during competition is acceptable but does not need to continue off the field unless the dislocation is unstable. DIP dislocations are frequently open and require surgery. They are treated like a mallet finger.
- Boxer's fractures tend to heal without incident, with full return of motion in 4 to 6 weeks. Splint immobilization should leave the PIP joint and wrist free to move.

American Occupational Therapy Association:
www.aota.org
American Orthopaedic Society for Sports Medicine:
www.sportsmed.org
American Society for Surgery of the Hand:
www.assh.org

Medline Plus: www.nlm.nih.gov/medlineplus
/handinjuriesanddisorders.html
Wheeless' Textbook of Orthopaedics:
www.wheelessonline.com

## SOLUTIONS TO CLINICAL APPLICATION EXERCISES

24-1   This condition is commonly called forearm splints. Its mechanism is from static contractions of the extensor forearm muscles. As a result, minute tears are produced in the interosseous membrane.

24-2   This is a Colles' fracture, which is caused by the fracture displacement of the distal radius. The athletic trainer should apply an ice compress, a splint, and a sling and should refer the waitress to a physician for an X-ray and definitive treatment.

24-3   The patient's hand is cold to the touch. Pinching a fingernail makes it blanch, and when released, it does not return to a pink color. Allen's test is carried out last, verifying a problem with hand circulation.

24-4   It is likely that the patient has injured the triangular fibrocartilage complex (TFCC) between the radioulnar joint and the proximal row of carpal bones. TFCC injury is often associated with sprain of the ulnar collateral ligament. The athletic trainer should refer the instructor with TFCC injury to a physician for treatment.

24-5   The patient's repeated wrist flexions against a resistance, while using a keyboard, have caused an inflammation of the tendons and synovial sheaths within the carpal tunnel, resulting in carpal tunnel syndrome. This inflammation in turn has caused a compression of the median nerve and the subsequent symptoms experienced by the student-athlete.

24-6   The compression force is likely to cause a scaphoid fracture, which is often mistaken for a sprained wrist.

24-7   It is likely that the golfer has sustained a fracture to the hook of the hamate. A cast needs to be applied to the wrist.

24-8   POLICE should be applied immediately. An X-ray should be done to rule out a fracture of the distal phalanx. The distal interphylangeal joint should be splinted in extension.

24-9   This injury is most likely gamekeeper's thumb, which is a sprain of the ulnar collateral ligament of the metacarpophalangeal joint. A valgus stress test can be used to evaluate the stability of the collateral ligament.

24-10   The suspected injuries from such a mechanism could be a complete tear of the collateral ligament, a volar plate tear, or a central extensor expansion tear.

24-11   The athletic trainer should suspect a fracture of the fifth metacarpal bone. The injury may appear as an angular or rotational deformity. POLICE and analgesics should be given along with an X-ray examination. The injury should be splinted for about 4 weeks, and the student should engage in early ROM exercises.

24-12   With such a fracture, the patient would complain of pain and swelling at the base of the thumb.

## REVIEW QUESTIONS AND CLASS ACTIVITIES

1.  Compare forearm splints and shinsplints. How does each occur?
2.  Describe the Colles' fracture of the forearm—its cause, appearance, and care.
3.  Demonstrate the major tests for hand and wrist conditions.
4.  Describe the mechanism, symptoms, and signs of a wrist sprain.
5.  Distinguish between the symptoms and signs of a wrist strain and those of a sprain.
6.  What healing problems occur with navicular carpal fractures? Why?
7.  How can a subungual hematoma be released?
8.  What causes stenosing tenosynovitis in the hand?
9.  Describe the circumstances that can produce a mallet finger and a boutonniere deformity in baseball players. What care should each condition receive?
10.  A sprained thumb is common. How does it occur, and what care should it receive?
11.  Should a dislocated finger be reduced by the athletic trainer? Explain your answer.

## REFERENCES

1.   Abraham M: The emergent evaluation and treatment of hand and wrist injuries, *Emergency Medicine Clinics of North America* 28(4):789–809, 2010.

2.   Backstrom K: Mobilization with movement as an adjunct intervention in a patient with complicated deQuervain's tenosynovitis: A case report, *J Orthop Sports Phys Ther* 32(3):86, 2002.

3.   Bickley L: *Bates guide to physical examination and history taking,* Philadelphia, PA, 1999, Lippincott.

4.   Bindra R: Management of proximal interphylangeal joint dislocations in athletes, *Hand Clinics* 25(3):423–35, 2009.

5.   Birkbeck D: Overview of common hand and wrist injuries in athletics, *Athletic Therapy Today* 6(2):6, 2001.

6.   Brooks T: Madelung deformity in a collegiate gymnast: A case report, *J Athl Train* 36(2):170, 2001.

7.   Brukner P: Wrist and hand pain. In Brukner P, ed: *Bruckner and Kahn's clinical sports medicine,* Sydney, 2011, McGraw-Hill.

8.   Carlsen B: Thumb trauma: Bennett fractures, Rolando fractures, and ulnar collateral ligament injuries, *Journal of Hand Surgery* 34(5):945–52, 2009.

9.   Chinchalkar S: Swan neck deformities after distal interphylangeal joint flexion contractures: A biomechanical analysis, *Journal of Hand Therapy* 23(4):420–25, 2010.

10.   Coel R: Hand injuries in young athletes, *Athletic Therapy Today* 15(4):52, 2010.

11.   Combs JA: It's not "just a finger," *J Athl Train* 35(2):168, 2000.

12.   Dang A: Unusual compression neuropathies of the forearm, *Journal of Hand Surgery* 34(10):1915–20, 2009.

13.   David T: Symptomatic, partial union of the hook of the hamate fracture in athletes, *Am J Sports Med* 31(1):106, 2003.

14.   Dean B: Fractures of the metacarpals and phalanges, *Orthopedics and Trauma* 25(1):43–56, 2011.

15.   Dias J: Kienböck's disease, *Journal of Hand Surgery* 35(7):533, 2010.

16.   Edwards S: Hand and wrist injuries in athletes, *Current Orthopedic Practice* 20(4):388, 2009.

17.   Finkbone P: *Wrist injuries,* New York, 2011, Springer.

18.   Haisman J: Acute fractures of the scaphoid, *J Bone Joint Sur* 88(12):275, 2006.

19. Hanker G: Radius fractures in the athlete, *Clin Sports Med* 20(1):189, 2001.
20. Haugstvedt J: Finger injuries. In Bahr R, ed: *Clinical guide to sports injuries,* Champaign, IL, 2004, Human Kinetics.
21. Haugstvedt J: Hand and wrist injuries. In Bahr R, ed: *Clinical guide to sports injuries,* Champaign, IL, 2004, Human Kinetics.
22. Hecht S: Why wrist pain is common in gymnasts, *Athletic Therapy Today* 11(6):62, 2006.
23. Hemsley K: Rehabilitation of athletic hand injuries: Five case studies, *Athletic Therapy Today* 6(2):19, 2001.
24. Katz J: Carpal tunnel syndrome diagnostic utility of history and physical examination findings, *Ann Int Med* 112:321–27, 1990.
25. Kawamura K: Treatment of scaphoid fractures and nonunions, *Journal of Hand Surgery* 33(6):988–97, 2008.
26. Kijima Y: Wrist anatomy and biomechanics, *Journal of Hand Surgery* 34(8):1555–63, 2009.
27. Leggit J: Acute finger injuries: Part II. Fractures. Dislocations and thumb injuries, *American Family Physician* 73(5):828–34, 2006.
28. Leinberry C: Mallet finger injuries, *Journal of Hand Surgery* 34(9):1715–17, 2009.
29. Lillegard W: Hand and wrist injuries. In Birrer R, ed: *Sports medicine for the primary care physician,* ed 2, Boca Raton, FL, 1994, CRC Press.
30. Lord J: Forearm injuries. In Birrer R: *Sports medicine for the primary care physician,* ed 3, Boca Raton, FL, 2004, CRC Press.
31. Marchessault J: Carpal fractures in athletes excluding scaphoid, *Hand Clinics* 25(3):371–88, 2009.
32. Magee D: *Orthopedic physical assessment,* Philadelphia, PA, 2013, Saunders.
33. Martin A: Reliability of Allen's test in selection of patients for radial artery harvest: The society of thoracic surgeons. *Ann Thorac Surg* 70:1362–65, 2000.
34. Metz J: Managing golf injuries: Technique and equipment changes that aid treatment, *Physician Sportsmed* 27(7):41, 1999.
35. Michlovitz S: Conservative interventions for carpal tunnel syndrome, *J Orthop Sports Phys Ther* 34(10):589, 2004.
36. Nagle D: Triangular fibrocartilage complex tears in the athlete, *Clin Sports Med* 20(1):155, 2001.
37. Newmann D: Clinical commentary—the carpometacarpal joint of the thumb: Stability, deformity, and therapeutic intervention, *J Orthop Sports Phys Ther* 33(6):386, 2003.
38. Papadonikolakis A: Trans-scaphoid volar lunate dislocation, *J Bone Joint Surg* 85(9):1805, 2003.
39. Peterson L: Forearm, wrist and hand. In Peterson L, ed.: *Sports injuries: Their prevention and treatment,* Champaign, IL, 2001, Human Kinetics.
40. Petrizzi M: Making an ulnar gutter splint for a boxer's fracture, *Physician Sportsmed* 27(1):111, 1999.
41. Poirier M: Complication from triangular fibrocartilage-complex degenerative tear, *Athletic Therapy Today* 7(1):30, 2002.
42. Prentice W: Maintenance of cardiorespiratory endurance. In Prentice W: *Rehabilitation techniques in sports medicine and athletic training,* Thorofare, NJ, 2015, Slack.
43. Prentice W: Mobilization and traction techniques. In Prentice W: *Rehabilitation techniques in sports medicine and athletic training,* Thorofare, NJ, 2015, Slack.
44. Prosser R: Provocative wrist test and MRI are of limited diagnostic value for suspected wrist ligament injuries: A cross-sectional study, *Journal of Physiotherapy* 57(4):247–53, 2011.
45. Rettig A: Athletic injuries of the wrist and hand, Part I: Traumatic injuries of the wrist, *Am J Sports Med* 31(6):1038, 2003.
46. Rettig A: Athletic injuries of the wrist and hand, Part II: Overuse injuries of the wrist and traumatic injuries to the hand, *Am J Sports Med* 32:262, 2004.
47. Rettig A: Ulnar collateral ligament injury of the thumb MP joint, *Clinical Journal of Sports Medicine* 20(2):106–12, 2010.
48. Rettig A: Wrist and hand overuse syndromes, *Clin Sports Med* 20(3):591, 2001.
49. Schneider AM: Injuries to the hand and wrist. In Prentice, ed.: *Rehabilitation techniques in sports medicine and athletic training,* Thorofare, NJ, 2015, Slack.
50. Stanbury S: Dupuyten contracture, *Journal of Hand Surgery* 36(12):2038–40, 2011.
51. Steinberg B: Acute wrist injuries in the athlete, *Orthopedic Clinics of North America* 33(3):535, 2002.
52. *Taber's cyclopedic medical dictionary,* Philadelphia, PA, 2013, F.A. Davis.
53. Wainner R: Development of a clinical prediction rule for the diagnosis of carpal tunnel syndrome, *Arch Phys Med Rehabil* 86(4):609–18, 2005.
54. Walsh K: Rehabilitation of postsurgical hand and finger injuries in the athlete, *Athletic Therapy Today* 6(2):13, 2001.
55. Waugh A: Perilunate dislocation in a collegiate football player, *Athletic Therapy Today* 14(1):5, 2009.
56. Werner S: Biomechanics of wrist injuries in sports, *Clin Sports Med* 17(3):407, 1998.
57. Williams M: Quick splint for acute boutonniere injuries, *Physician Sportsmed* 29(8):69, 2001.
58. Youngman J: What exactly is wrist tendinitis in athletes, and what are the most effective ways to treat it? *Sports Injury Bulletin* 30:1, 2003.

## ANNOTATED BIBLIOGRAPHY

Burke S, Higgins J, Saunders R: *Hand and upper extremity rehabilitation: A practical guide,* London, 2015, Churchill-Livingstone.

*Blends the technical and clinical skills and knowledge of hand therapy for the treatment of common medical conditions affecting the upper extremity. Also features expanded coverage of the wrist, elbow, and shoulder. Both conservative and postoperative rehabilitation are reviewed, and potential postoperative complications are addressed.*

Falkenstein N, Weiss-Lessard S: *Hand rehabilitation: A quick reference guide and review,* New York, 2013, Elsevier Health Science.

*A wealth of information relating to the hand and upper-extremity rehabilitation, surgery, and anatomy. An excellent resource for health professionals who treat hand and upper-extremity injuries.*

Jacoby S: *Musculoskeletal Examination of the Elbow, Wrist, and Hand: Making the Complex Simple,* Thorofare, NJ, 2012, Slack.

*Provides a thorough review of the most common pathologic elbow, wrist, and hand conditions, techniques for diagnosis, as well as the appropriate treatment for each condition.*

Jebson P, Kasdan M: *Hand secrets,* Philadelphia, PA, 2006, Elsevier Science.

*A complete reference on the evaluation, diagnosis, and medical and surgical management of disorders and diseases of the hand.*

Skirven T: *Rehabilitation of the hand and upper extremity,* Philadelphia, PA, 2011, Elsevier Science.

*Directed at all health professionals involved with the care of hand and upper-extremity conditions.*

Weiland A, Rohde R: *Acute management of hand injuries,* Thorofare, NJ, 2008, Slack.

*Provides excellent material for diagnosing hand injuries in the acute setting.*

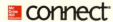

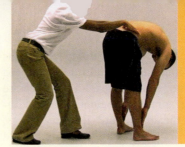
© William E. Prentice

# 25

# The Spine

## Connect Highlights   connect

*Visit connect.mcgraw-hill.com for further exercises to apply your knowledge:*

- Clinical application scenarios covering assessment and recognition of cervical, thoracic, and lumbar spine and nerve root injuries; etiology, symptoms and signs, and management of cervical, thoracic, and lumbar spine and nerve root injuries; and rehabilitation for the cervical, thoracic, and lumbar spine
- Click-and-drag questions covering structural anatomy of the cervical, thoracic, and lumbar spine and nerve roots; assessment of cervical, thoracic, and lumbar spine and nerve root injuries; and rehabilitation plan of the cervical, thoracic, and lumbar spine
- Multiple-choice questions covering anatomy, assessment, etiology, management and rehabilitation of cervical, thoracic, and lumbar spine and nerve root injuries
- Selection questions covering rehabilitation plan for various injuries to the cervical, thoracic, and lumbar spine and nerve roots
- Video identification of special tests for the cervical, thoracic, and lumbar spine and nerve root injuries; and rehabilitation techniques for the cervical, thoracic, and lumbar spine
- Picture identification of major anatomical components of the cervical, thoracic, and lumbar spine and nerve roots; rehabilitation techniques of the cervical, thoracic, and lumbar spine; and therapeutic modalities for management

The spine is one of the most complex regions of the body.[50] It contains a multitude of bones, joints, ligaments, and muscles, all of which are collectively involved in spinal movement. The proximity and relationship of the spinal cord, the nerve roots, and the peripheral nerves to the vertebral column add to the complexity of this region. Low back pain is one of the most common ailments known to humans. *Injury to the cervical spine has potentially life-threatening implications* (see Chapter 12 for emergency management). Thus, the athletic trainer requires an in-depth understanding of the anatomy of the spine, the techniques to assess the spine, the various injuries that can occur to different regions of the spine, and rehabilitative techniques.

# ANATOMY OF THE SPINE

## Bones of the Vertebral Column

The spine, or vertebral column, is composed of 33 individual bones called vertebrae. Twenty-four are classified as movable, or true, and nine are classified as immovable, or false. The false vertebrae, which are fixed by fusion, form the sacrum and the coccyx. The design of the spine allows a high degree of forward and lateral flexibility and limited backward mobility. Rotation around a central axis in the areas of the neck and the low back is also permitted.

| Regions of the spinal column: |
| --- |
| • Cervical |
| • Thoracic |
| • Lumbar |
| • Sacrum |
| • Coccyx |

The movable vertebrae are separated into three divisions, according to location and function. The first division comprises the 7 cervical vertebrae; the second, the 12 thoracic vertebrae; and the third, the 5 lumbar vertebrae. As the spinal segments progress downward from the cervical region, they grow increasingly larger to accommodate the upright posture of the body and to contribute in weight bearing. The shape of the vertebrae is irregular, but the vertebrae possess certain characteristics that are common to all. Each vertebra consists of a neural arch, through which the spinal cord passes, and several projecting processes that serve as attachments for muscles and ligaments. Each neural arch has two laminae and two pedicles. The latter are bony processes that project backward from the body of the vertebrae and connect with the laminae. The laminae are flat, bony processes occurring on either side of the neural arch; they project backward and inward from the pedicles. With the exception of the first and second cervical vertebrae, each vertebra has a spinous and transverse process for muscular and ligamentous attachment, and all vertebrae have an articular process.

**The Cervical Spine** The cervical spine consists of seven vertebrae, with the first two differing from the other true vertebrae (Figure 25–1A). These first two are called the atlas and the axis, respectively, and they function together to support the head on the spinal column and to permit cervical rotation. The atlas, named for its function of supporting the head, displays no body or spinous processes and is composed of lateral masses that are connected to the anterior and posterior arches. The upper surfaces articulate with the occipital condyles of the skull and allow flexion and extension along with some lateral movement. The arches of the atlas form a bony ring sufficiently large to accommodate the odontoid process and the medulla of the spinal cord. The axis, or epistropheus, is the second cervical vertebra and is designed to allow the skull and atlas to rotate on it. Its primary difference from a typical vertebra is the presence of a toothlike projection from the vertebral body that fits into the ring of the atlas. This projection is called the dens (odontoid process). The great mobility of the cervical spine is attributed to the flattened, oblique facing of the spine's articular facets and to the horizontal positioning of the spinous processes (Figure 25–1B).

**The Thoracic Spine** The thoracic spine consists of 12 vertebrae. Thoracic vertebrae have long transverse processes and prominent but thin spinous processes (Figure 25–1C). Thoracic vertebrae 1 through 10 have articular facets on each transverse process with which the ribs articulate. The head of the rib articulates between two vertebrae and thus shares half of an articular facet.

**The Lumbar Spine** The lumbar spine is composed of five vertebrae. These vertebrae are the major support of the low back and are the largest and thickest of the vertebrae, with large spinous and transverse processes (Figure 25–1D). The superior articular processes face medially, while the inferior processes face laterally. The articular processes of the superior vertebrae articulate with the articular processes of the inferior vertebrae. Movement occurs in all the lumbar vertebrae; however, there is much less extension than flexion.

While assessing complaints of back pain in a warehouse stockman, the athletic trainer notes that on lateral observation the low back appears to be excessively curved and the thoracic spine seems to have a curved, rounded appearance.

**?** When assessing posture laterally, the athletic trainer will normally see curves in various regions of the spine. What are the normal curves and their shape within the spine?

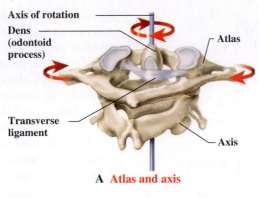

Axis of rotation
Dens (odontoid process)
Atlas
Transverse ligament
Axis

**A  Atlas and axis**

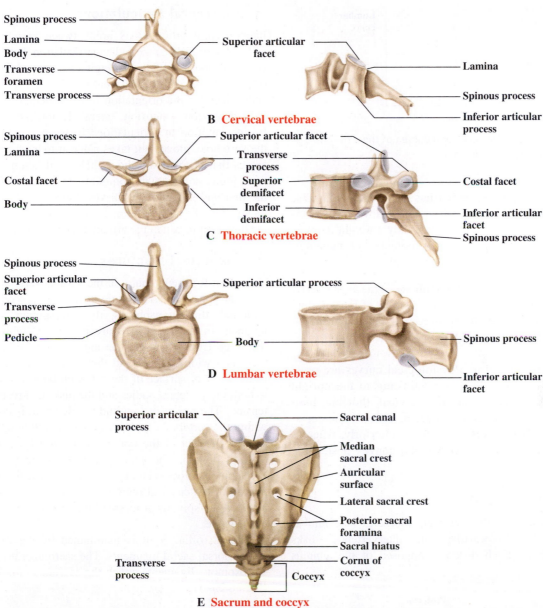

Spinous process
Lamina
Body
Transverse foramen
Transverse process
Superior articular facet
Lamina
Spinous process
Inferior articular process

**B  Cervical vertebrae**

Spinous process
Lamina
Costal facet
Body
Superior articular facet
Transverse process
Superior demifacet
Inferior demifacet
Costal facet
Inferior articular facet
Spinous process

**C  Thoracic vertebrae**

Spinous process
Superior articular facet
Transverse process
Pedicle
Superior articular process
Body
Spinous process
Inferior articular facet

**D  Lumbar vertebrae**

Superior articular process
Sacral canal
Median sacral crest
Auricular surface
Lateral sacral crest
Posterior sacral foramina
Sacral hiatus
Cornu of coccyx
Transverse process
Coccyx
Coccyx

**E  Sacrum and coccyx**

FIGURE 25–1   Bones of the vertebral column. (**A**) Atlas and axis. (**B**) Cervical vertebrae. (**C**) Thoracic vertebrae. (**D**) Lumbar vertebrae. (**E**) Sacrum and coccyx.

**The Sacrum**  The sacrum is formed in the adult by the fusion of five vertebrae (Figure 25–1E) and, with the two hip bones, comprises the pelvis. The roots of the lumbar and sacral nerves, which form the lower portion of the cauda equina, pass through four foramina lateral to the five fused vertebrae.

The sacrum articulates with the ilia to form two sacroiliac joints posteriorly. The ilia meet anteriorly to form

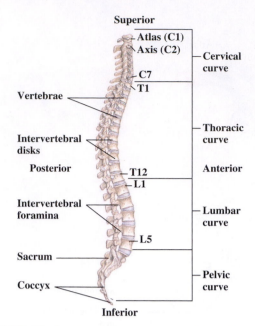

FIGURE 25–2  Vertebrae and curves of the different regions of the spinal column.

the pubis symphysis, which has an interarticular disc with a synovium and is lubricated by synovial fluid. During both sitting and standing, the body's weight is transmitted through these joints. A complex of numerous ligaments makes these joints very stable.[30]

**The Coccyx**  The coccyx, or tailbone, is the most inferior part of the vertebral column and consists of four or more fused vertebrae. The gluteus maximus muscle attaches to the coccyx posteriorly (Figure 25–1E).

**Curves of the Spine**  Physiological curves are present in the spinal column for adjusting to the upright stresses. These curves are the cervical, thoracic, lumbar, and pelvic, or sacrococcygeal, curves. The cervical and lumbar curves are convex anteriorly, whereas the thoracic and pelvic curves are convex posteriorly (Figure 25–2).

## Intervertebral Disks

Between each of the cervical, thoracic, and lumbar vertebrae lie fibrocartilaginous intervertebral disks (Figure 25–3). Each disk is composed of the annulus

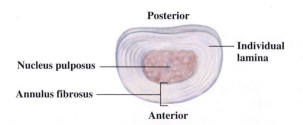

FIGURE 25–3  Intervertebral disk.

fibrosus and the nucleus pulposus. The annulus fibrosus forms the periphery of the intervertebral disk and is composed of strong, fibrous tissue, with its fibers running in several different directions for strength. The disks act as important shock absorbers for the spine.

During the first decade of life, the nucleus of the disk loses much of its vital blood supply, and without sufficient nutrients from blood, cells of the disk begin to die, and the disk (especially the nucleus) becomes depleted of water. The drop in water content is one of the classic signs of disk aging.

## Intervertebral Articulations

Intervertebral articulations are between vertebral bodies and vertebral arches. The articulation between the vertebral bodies is a cartilaginous joint. Movements of the vertebrae in the different regions of the spine are determined by the orientation of the articular facets and include flexion, extension, lateral flexion, and rotation. Besides motion at articulations between the bodies of the vertebrae, movement takes place at four articular processes that derive from the pedicles and laminae. These facet joints are synovial joints except for those between the first and second cervical vertebrae. The direction of movement of each vertebra is somewhat dependent on the direction in which the articular facets face.

## Ligamentous Structures

The major ligaments that join the various vertebral structures are the anterior longitudinal, the posterior longitudinal, the supraspinous, the interspinous, and the ligamentum flavum, which are important stabilizers of the spine (Figure 25–4). The anterior longitudinal ligament is a wide, strong band that extends the full length of the anterior surface of the vertebral bodies. It attaches to both the vertebral bodies and the disks and restricts extension. The posterior longitudinal ligament is contained within the vertebral canal; it extends the full length of the posterior aspect of the bodies of the vertebrae and acts to limit flexion. The supraspinous ligament attaches to each spinous process and is referred to as the ligamentum nuchae in the cervical region. The interspinous ligament between the spinous processes limits rotation and flexion of the spine.

The sacroiliac joint is maintained by the extremely strong dorsal sacral ligaments. The sacrotuberous and the sacrospinous ligaments attach the sacrum to the ischium (Figure 25–5).

## Muscles of the Spine

The muscles that extend the spine and rotate the vertebral column can be classified as either superficial or deep (Figure 25–6). The superficial muscles extend from the vertebrae to ribs. The erector spinae make up the superficial muscles. The erector spinae are a group of paired muscles that consist of three columns, or bands:

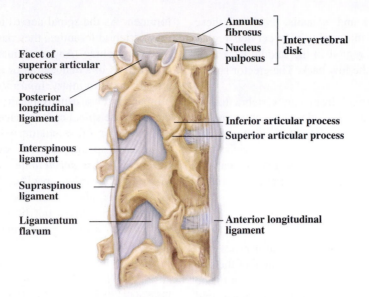

Facet of superior articular process

Posterior longitudinal ligament

Interspinous ligament

Supraspinous ligament

Ligamentum flavum

Annulus fibrosus
Nucleus pulposus
] Intervertebral disk

Inferior articular process
Superior articular process

Anterior longitudinal ligament

FIGURE 25–4   Ligaments of the vertebral column (posterior view).

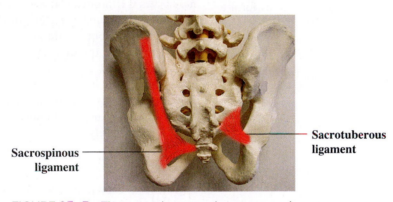

Sacrospinous ligament

Sacrotuberous ligament

FIGURE 25–5   The sacrotuberous and sacrospinous ligaments maintain the position of the sacrum relative to the pelvis.

© William E. Prentice

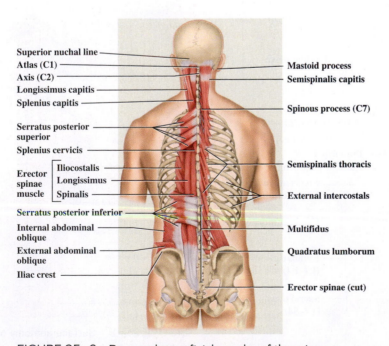

Superior nuchal line
Atlas (C1)
Axis (C2)
Longissimus capitis
Splenius capitis

Serratus posterior superior

Splenius cervicis

Erector spinae muscle
  Iliocostalis
  Longissimus
  Spinalis

Serratus posterior inferior

Internal abdominal oblique

External abdominal oblique

Iliac crest

Mastoid process
Semispinalis capitis

Spinous process (C7)

Semispinalis thoracis

External intercostals

Multifidus

Quadratus lumborum

Erector spinae (cut)

FIGURE 25–6   Deep and superficial muscles of the spine.

iliocostalis, longissimus, and spinalis. Each of these groups is further divided into regions: the cervicis region in the neck, the thoracis region in the middle back, and the lumborum region in the low back. The erector spinae muscles extend the spine.

The deep muscles extend from one vertebra to another. The deep muscles include the interspinales, multifidus, rotatores, semispinalis, and splenius. The semispinalis is divided into the capitus, cervicis, and thoracis regions (the splenius is divided into the capitus and cervicis regions) (Table 25–1). These muscles collectively extend and rotate the spine.

## Spinal Cord

The spinal cord is the portion of the central nervous system that is contained within the vertebral canal of the spinal column. It extends from the foramen magnum of the cranium to the filum terminale, which is the lower end of the cord, in the vicinity of the first or second lumbar vertebra. The lumbar roots and the sacral nerves form a horselike tail called the cauda equina (Figure 25–7).

## Spinal Nerves and Peripheral Branches

Thirty-one pairs of spinal nerves extend from the sides of the spinal cord: 8 cervical, 12 thoracic, 5 lumbar, 5 sacral, and 1 coccygeal (Figure 25–7). Each of these nerves has an anterior root (motor root) and a posterior root (sensory root). The two roots in each case join together and form a single spinal nerve, which passes downward and outward through the intervertebral foramen. As the spinal nerves are conducted through the intervertebral foramina, they pass near the articular facets of the vertebrae. Any abnormal movement of these facets, such as in a dislocation or a fracture, may expose the spinal nerves to injury. Injuries that occur below the third lumbar vertebra usually result in nerve root damage but do not cause spinal cord damage.

Each pair of spinal nerves, with the exception of C1, has a specific area of cutaneous sensory distribution called a *dermatome* (see Figure 25–46). Loss of sensation in a specific dermatome can provide information about the location of nerve damage. Dermatomes should not be confused with myotomes, which are muscles innervated by a single, specific spinal nerve.

The spinal nerve roots combine to form a network of nerves, or a plexus. There are five nerve plexuses: *cervical, brachial, lumbar, sacral,* and *coccygeal* (Figure 25–7). The cervical plexus originates from spinal nerves C1 through C4; the brachial plexus, from C5 through T1; the lumbar plexus, from L1 through L4; the sacral plexus, from L4 through S4; and the coccygeal plexus, from S4 through S5 and the coccygeal nerve. Tables 25–2 and 25–3 indicate each nerve, its nerve roots, the muscle it innervates and that muscle's accompanying action, as well as the cutaneous innervation for the brachial plexus, the lumbar plexus, and the sacral plexus, respectively.

## Surface Anatomy

Figure 25–8 shows the pertinent surface anatomy landmarks for the entire spine.

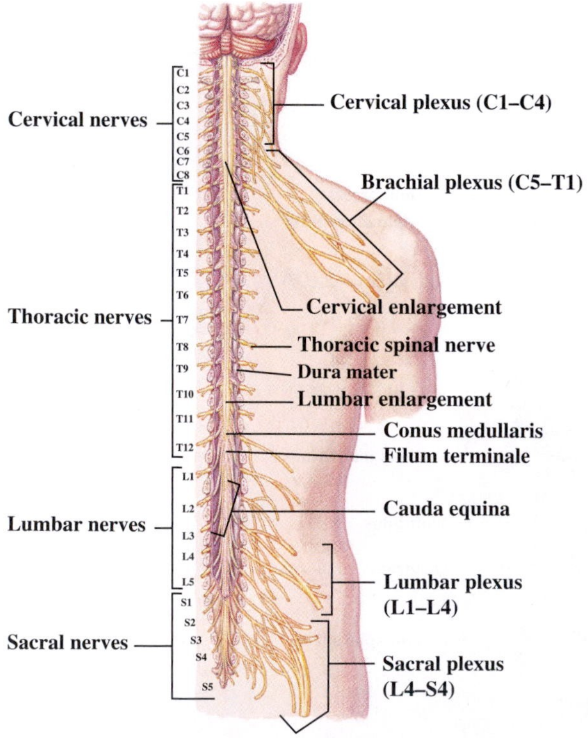

Cervical nerves

C1
C2
C3
C4
C5
C6
C7
C8
T1

Cervical plexus (C1–C4)

Brachial plexus (C5–T1)

Thoracic nerves

T2
T3
T4
T5
T6
T7
T8
T9
T10
T11
T12

Cervical enlargement
Thoracic spinal nerve
Dura mater
Lumbar enlargement
Conus medullaris
Filum terminale

Lumbar nerves

L1
L2
L3
L4
L5

Cauda equina

Lumbar plexus (L1–L4)

Sacral nerves

S1
S2
S3
S4
S5

Sacral plexus (L4–S4)

FIGURE 25–7   The spinal cord, nerve roots, and plexuses.

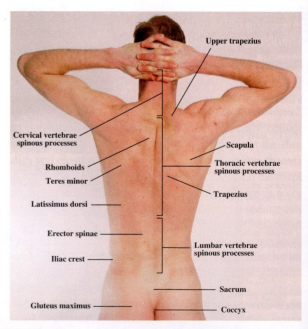

FIGURE 25–8   Surface anatomy of the spine.
© JW Ramsey/McGraw-Hill Education

## TABLE 25–1  Muscles That Move the Vertebral Column*

| Muscle | Origin | Insertion | Action | Innervation/ Nerve Root |
|---|---|---|---|---|
| *Erector spinae* | | | | |
| **Iliocostalis lumborum thoracis cervicis** | Crest of the sacrum; spinous processes of the lumbar and lower thoracic vertebrae; iliac crests; angles of the ribs | Angles of the ribs; transverse processes of the cervical vertebrae | Extends the vertebral column and bends it to one side | Branches of the spinal nerves (dorsal primary divisions) |
| **Longissimus thoracis cervicis capitis** | Transverse processes of the lumbar, thoracic, and lower cervical vertebrae | Transverse processes of the vertebra above the vertebra of origin, and the mastoid process of the temporal bone (capitis) | Extends the vertebral column and head; rotates the head toward the same side | Branches of the spinal nerves (dorsal primary divisions) |
| **Spinalis thoracis cervicis** | Spinous process of the upper lumbar, lower thoracic, and seventh cervical vertebrae | Spinous processes of the upper thoracic and the cervical vertebrae | Extends the vertebral column | Branches of the spinal nerves (C4–C8) |
| **Multifidus** | Posterior surface of the sacrum and the ilium, and the transverse processes of the lumbar, thoracic, and lower cervical vertebrae | Spinous processes of the lumbar, thoracic, and cervical vertebrae | Extends the vertebral column; rotates it toward the opposite side | Branches of the spinal nerves (dorsal primary divisions) |
| **Rotatores˙** | Transverse processes of all the vertebrae | Base of the spinous process of the vertebra above the vertebra of origin | Extends the vertebral column; rotates it toward the opposite side | Branches of the spinal nerves (dorsal primary divisions) |
| **Interspinales˙** | Superior surface of all the spinous processes | Inferior surface of the spinous process of the vertebra above the vertebra of origin | Extends the vertebral column | Branches of the spinal nerves (dorsal primary divisions) |
| **Semispinalis thoracis cervicis capitis** | Transverse processes of the thoracic and the seventh cervical vertebrae | Spinous processes of the second cervical through the fourth thoracic vertebrae, and the occipital bone | Extends the vertebral column and the head (capitis); rotates them to the opposite side | Branches of the spinal nerves (dorsal primary divisions) |
| **Splenius capitis cervicis** | Spinous processes of the upper thoracic and the seventh cervical vertebrae, and from the ligamentum nuchae | Occipital bone, the mastoid process of the temporal bone, and the transverse processes of the upper three cervical vertebrae | Acting together, they extend the head and the neck; acting singly, they abduct and rotate the head toward the same side | Branches of the spinal nerves (dorsal primary divisions) |

Joint Movements of the Spine and Neck**

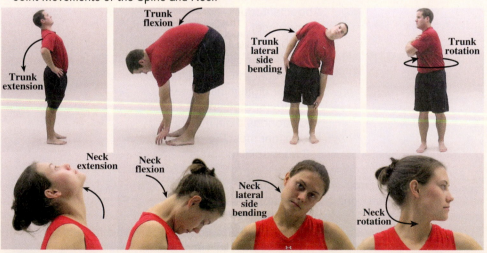

© William E. Prentice

* Manual muscle tests and goniometric measurements of range of motion for the spine and neck can be found in Appendix F and Appendix G at the end of the text.
** Too small to see on Figure 25–6.

TABLE 25–2    Brachial Plexus (Figure 25–7)

| Nerve | Origin | Function, Muscle Innervated | Cutaneous Innervation |
|---|---|---|---|
| **Axillary** | Posterior cord, C5, C6 | Abducts arm<br>    Deltoid<br>Laterally rotates arm<br>    Teres minor | Inferior lateral shoulder |
| **Radial** | Posterior cord, C5–T1 | Extends forearm<br>    Triceps brachii<br>    Anconeus<br>Flexes forearm<br>    Brachialis (part)<br>    Brachioradialis<br>Supinates forearm<br>    Supinator<br>Extends wrist<br>    Extensor carpi radialis longus<br>      (also abducts wrist)<br>    Extensor carpi radialis brevis<br>      (also abducts wrist)<br>    Extensor carpi ulnaris<br>      (also adducts wrist)<br>Extends fingers<br>    Extensor digitorum<br>    Extensor digiti minimi<br>    Extensor indicis<br>Thumb muscles<br>    Abductor pollicis longus<br>    Extensor pollicis longus<br>    Extensor pollicis brevis | Posterior surface of arm and forearm, lateral two-thirds of dorsum of hand |
| **Musculocutaneous** | Lateral cord, C5–C7 | Flexes arm<br>    Coracobrachialis<br>Flexes forearm<br>    Biceps brachii (also supinates)<br>    Brachialis (also small amount of<br>      innervation from radial) | Lateral surface of forearm |
| **Ulnar** | Medial cord, C8–T1 | Flexes wrist<br>    Flexor carpi ulnaris (also adducts wrist)<br>Flexes fingers<br>    Part of flexor digitorum profundus (distal<br>      phalanges of little and ring finger)<br>Abducts/adducts fingers<br>    Interossei<br>Thumb muscle<br>    Adductor pollicis<br>Hypothenar muscles<br>    Flexor digiti minimi brevis<br>    Abductor digiti minimi<br>    Opponens digiti minimi<br>Midpalmar muscles<br>    Two medial lumbricals<br>    Interossei | Medial one-third of hand, little finger, and medial one-half of ring finger |
| **Median** | Medial and lateral cord, C8–T1 | Pronates forearm<br>    Pronator teres<br>    Pronator quadratus | Lateral two-thirds of palm of hand, including lateral half of ring finger |

*Continued*

| TABLE 25-2 | Brachial Plexus (Figure 25-7)—continued |

| Nerve | Origin | Function, Muscle Innervated | Cutaneous Innervation |
|---|---|---|---|
| **Median (cont.)** | | Flexes wrist | |
| | |    Flexor carpi radialis (also abducts wrist) | |
| | |    Palmaris longus | |
| | | Flexes fingers | |
| | |    Part of flexor digitorum profundus | |
| | |      (distal phalanges of middle | |
| | |      and index finger) | |
| | |    Flexor digitorum superficialis | |
| | | Thumb muscle | |
| | |    Flexor pollicis longus | |
| | | Thenar muscles | |
| | |    Abductor pollicis brevis | |
| | |    Opponens pollicis | |
| | |    Flexor pollicis brevis | |
| | | Midpalmar | |
| | |    Two lateral lumbricals | |

# FUNCTIONAL ANATOMY

## Movements of the Vertebral Column

The movements of the vertebral column are flexion and extension, right and left lateral flexion (side bending), and rotation to the left and right. The degree of these movements differs in the various regions of the vertebral column.

> **Movements of the vertebral column:**
> - Flexion
> - Extension
> - Lateral flexion
> - Rotation

- Cervical—facets angled superior and medial, permits flexion, extension, lateral extension, rotation
- Thoracic—facets in coronal plane, permits little or no flexion or extension, rotation, and little lateral flexion
- Lumbar—facets in sagittal plane, permits flexion, extension, limited lateral flexion, limited rotation

Flexion of the cervical region is produced primarily by the sternocleidomastoid muscles and the scalene muscle group on the anterior aspect of the throat. The scalenes flex the head and stabilize the cervical spine as the sternocleidomastoids flex the neck. The upper trapezius, semispinalis capitis, splenius capitis, and splenius cervicis muscles extend the neck. Lateral flexion of the neck is accomplished by all the muscles on one side of the vertebral column contracting unilaterally. Rotation is produced when the sternocleidomastoid, the scalenes, the semispinalis cervicis, and the upper trapezius on the side opposite the direction of rotation contract in addition to a contraction of the splenius capitus, splenius cervicis, and longissimus capitus on the same side as the direction of rotation.

Flexion of the trunk involves the lengthening of the deep and superficial back muscles and the contraction of the abdominal muscles (rectus abdominus, internal oblique, external oblique) and hip flexors (rectus femoris, iliopsoas, tensor fasciae latae, sartorius). Although the thoracic vertebrae have minimal movement, their combined movement between the first and twelfth thoracic vertebrae can account for 20 to 30 degrees of flexion and extension.[16] Seventy-five percent of flexion occurs at the lumbosacral junction (L5–S1), whereas 15 to 20 percent occurs between L4 and L5. The rest of the lumbar vertebrae execute 5 to 10 percent of flexion.[62] Extension involves the lengthening of the abdominal muscles and the contraction of the erector spinae and the gluteus maximus, which extends the hip. Trunk rotation is produced by the external obliques and the internal obliques. Lateral flexion is produced by the quadratus lumborum muscle along with the obliques, latissimus dorsi, iliopsoas, and rectus abdominus on the side of the direction of movement.

> **25-2 Clinical Application Exercise**
>
> A patient has normal neck flexion and extension and lateral flexion but is having difficulty rotating his head toward his left shoulder. The athletic trainer suspects a strain of one of the muscles that rotate the head.
>
> **?** Which muscles rotate the head to the left?

**TABLE 25–3**   Lumbar and Sacral Plexuses (Figure 25–7)

| Nerve | Origin | Function, Muscle Innervated | Cutaneous Innervation |
|---|---|---|---|
| **Obturator** | L2–L4 | Adducts hip<br>    Adductor magnus<br>    Adductor longus<br>    Adductor brevis<br>    Gracilis (also flexes hip)<br>Rotates thigh laterally<br>    Obturator externus | Superior medial side of thigh |
| **Femoral** | L2–L4 | Flexes hip<br>    Iliacus<br>    Psoas major<br>    Pectineus<br>    Sartorius (also flexes knee)<br>Extends knee<br>    Rectus femoris (also flexes hip)<br>    Vastus lateralis<br>    Vastus medialis<br>    Vastus intermedius | Anterior and lateral branches supply the thigh; the saphenous branch supplies the medial leg and foot |
| **Tibial** | L4–S3 | Extends hip, flexes knee<br>    Biceps femoris (long head)<br>    Semitendinosus<br>    Semimembranosus<br>    Adductor magnus<br>Flexes knee<br>    Popliteus<br>Plantar flexes foot<br>    Gastrocnemius<br>    Soleus<br>    Plantaris<br>    Tibialis posterior<br>Flexes toes<br>    Flexor hallucis longus<br>    Flexor digitorum longus | None |
| **Medial and lateral plantar** | Tibial | Plantar muscles of foot | Medial and lateral sole of foot |
| **Sural** | Tibial | None | Lateral and posterior one-third of leg and lateral side of foot |
| **Common peroneal** | L4–S2 | Extends hip, flexes knee<br>    Bicep femoris (short head) | Lateral surface of knee |
| **Deep peroneal** | Common peroneal | Dorsiflexes foot<br>    Tibialis anterior<br>    Peroneus tertius<br>Extends toes<br>    Extensor hallucis longus<br>    Extensor digitorum longus | Skin over great and second toe |
| **Superficial peroneal** | Common peroneal | Plantar flexes and everts foot<br>    Peroneus longus<br>    Peroneus brevis<br>Extends toes<br>    Extensor digitorum brevis | Distal anterior third of leg and dorsum of foot |

# PREVENTION OF INJURIES TO THE SPINE

## Cervical Spine

Acute traumatic injuries to the spine can be life threatening, particularly if the cervical region of the spinal cord is involved. Thus, the athletic trainer must do everything possible to minimize potential injury.

**Muscle Strengthening** Strengthening of the musculature of the neck is critical. The neck muscles can protect the cervical spine by resisting excessive hyperflexion, hyperextension, or rotational forces. During participation, the athlete should constantly be in a state of readiness and, when making contact with an opponent, should "bull" the neck by elevating both shoulders and isometrically co-contracting the muscles surrounding the neck. Protective cervical collars can also help limit movement of the cervical spine. Athletes with long, weak necks are especially at risk. Tackle football players and wrestlers must have highly stable necks.

Specific strengthening exercises are essential for the development of stability. A variety of exercises that incorporate isotonic, isometric, or isokinetic contractions can be used.[95] One of the best methods is manual resistance by a partner who selectively uses isometric and isokinetic resistance exercises.

**Range of Motion** In addition to strong muscles, the neck should have a full range of motion. Ideally, the individual should be able to place his or her chin on the chest and to extend the head back until the face is parallel with the ceiling. There should be at least 40 to 45 degrees of lateral flexion and enough rotation to allow the chin to reach a level even with the tip of the shoulder. Flexibility is increased through stretching exercises and strengthening exercises that are in full range of motion. Where flexibility is restricted, various stretching techniques can be beneficial.

**Using Correct Techniques** Athletes involved in collision sports—in particular, American football and rugby, which involve tackling an opponent—must be taught and required to use techniques that reduce the likelihood of cervical injury. The head, especially one in a helmet, should not be used as a weapon. Football helmets do not protect players against neck injury. In the illegal spearing maneuver, the athlete uses the helmet as a weapon by striking the opponent with its top. Most serious cervical injuries in football result from axial loading while spearing.[96] The NATA has developed a position statement, "Head-down contact and spearing in tackle football," which appears at www.nata.org/sites/default/files/headdowncontactandspearingintacklefb.pdf.

In other sports, such as diving, wrestling, and bouncing on a trampoline, the athlete's neck can be flexed at the time of contact. Energy of the forward-moving body mass cannot be fully absorbed, and fracture or dislocation or both can occur. Diving into shallow water causes many catastrophic neck injuries.[33] Most accidents happen when the diver dives into water that is less than 5 feet (1½ m) deep and fails to keep the arms extended in front of the face. The head strikes the bottom, which produces a cervical fracture at the C5 or C6 level. Many of the same forces are applied in wrestling. In such trauma, paraplegia, quadriplegia, or death can result. Coaches cannot stress enough to the athlete the importance of using appropriate tackling techniques.

## Lumbar Spine

Low back pain is one of the most common and disabling ailments known to humans. Most cases of low back pain do not involve serious or long-lasting pathology.

**Avoiding Stress** Low back pain can be prevented by avoiding unnecessary stresses and strains that are associated with activities of daily living.[81] The back is subjected to these stresses and strains when standing, sitting, lying, working, or exercising. Care should be taken to avoid postures and positions that can cause injuries (see *Focus Box 25–1:* "Recommended postures to prevent low back pain").

**Correction of Biomechanical Abnormalities** The athletic trainer should be aware of any biomechanical anomalies the patients may possess. This knowledge helps the athletic trainer establish individual corrective programs. Basic conditioning should include an emphasis on trunk strengthening.[60] If you do not have the muscle strength to control the flexibility the chances of injury are increased. Strength through a full range of motion should be developed in the spinal extensors (erector spinae).[47] Abdominal wall strength is very important in spinal health as well as in the quadratus lumborum to ensure proper postural alignment.[74] Intensive training programs addressing global muscle strengthening should emphasize maintaining a neutral spine while stressing mobility from the hips and knees.[75]

**Using Correct Lifting Techniques** Weight lifters can minimize their chance of injury to the lumbar spine by using proper lifting techniques.[15] They can help stabilize the spine by incorporating appropriate breathing techniques that involve inhaling and exhaling deeply during lifting. Weight belts can also help stabilize the lumbar spine. Spotters can greatly enhance safety by helping lift and lower the weight. Proper lifting technique was discussed in detail in Chapter 4.

**Core Stabilization** Core stabilization, dynamic abdominal bracing, and maintenance of a neutral position are all aspects of a technique that can be used to increase the stability of the spine and the lumbo-pelvic-hip complex. This increased stability helps maintain the spine and pelvis in

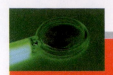

a comfortable and acceptable mechanical position that will control the effects of repetitive microtrauma and protect the structures in the back from further damage.[35] Abdominal muscle control also gives the patient the ability to stabilize the trunk and control posture.[50]

As discussed previously, improving core stability can enhance optimal function of the extremities.

## ASSESSMENT OF THE SPINE

Assessment of injuries to the spine is somewhat more complex than assessment of injuries to the joints of the extremities because of the number of articulations involved in spinal movement.[46] It is also true that injury to the spine—in particular, the spinal cord—may have life-threatening or life-altering implications. Thus, the athletic trainer must perform systematic and detailed evaluations.

### History

The most critical part of the evaluation is to rule out the possibility of spinal cord injury. Questions that address this possibility should first establish the mechanism of injury:

- What do you think happened?

- Did you hit someone with, or land directly on, the top of your head?
- Were you knocked out or unconscious? (Anytime an impact is sufficient to cause unconsciousness, the potential for injury to the spine exists.)
- Do you have any pain in your neck?
- Do you have tingling, numbness, or burning in your shoulders, arms, or hands?
- Do you have equal muscle strength in both hands? (Any sensory or motor change bilaterally may indicate a spinal cord injury.)
- Are you unable to move your ankles and toes?

A positive response to any of these questions necessitates extreme caution when the patient is moved. The athletic trainer who is handling a suspected cervical spine injury should err only in being overly cautious. *Emergency care of the patient with suspected cervical spine injury was discussed in detail in* Chapter 12.

Once cervical spine injury has been ruled out, other general questions may provide some indication as to the nature of the problem:

- Where is the pain located?
- What kind of pain do you have?

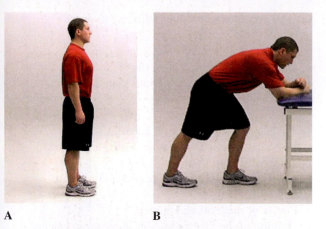

A                          B

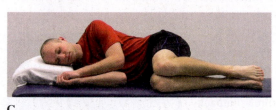

C

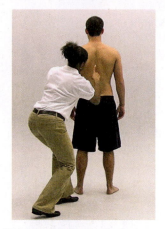

FIGURE 25–10   Observing spinal alignment.
© William E. Prentice

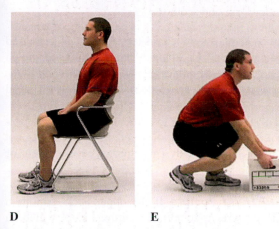

D                          E

FIGURE 25–9   Examples of safe postures.
**(A)** Ideal standing posture. **(B)** Correct leaning posture.
**(C)** Correct sleeping position. **(D)** Ideal sitting position.
**(E)** Correct lifting position.

© William E. Prentice

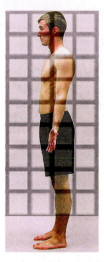

FIGURE 25–11   Using a grid can produce more accurate results during posture screening.
© William E. Prentice

- What were you doing when the pain began?
- Were you standing, sitting, bending, or twisting?
- Did the pain begin immediately?
- How long have you had this pain?
- Do certain movements or positions cause more pain?
- Can you assume a position that gets rid of the pain?
- Is there any tingling or numbness in the arms or legs?
- Is there any pain in the buttocks or the back of the legs?
- Have you ever had any back pain before?
- What position do you usually sleep in? How do you prefer to sit?

It is important to remember that pain in the back may be caused by many different conditions. The source may be musculoskeletal or visceral, or it may be referred.

## Observation

Observing the posture and movement capabilities of the patient during the evaluation can help clarify the nature and extent of the injury.

**Posture Evaluation** It is important to observe the patient's total static posture, paying special attention to the low back, pelvis, and hips.[65] The athletic trainer also should make some decision about somatotype (i.e., ectomorph, mesomorph, or endomorph). When observing the patient's standing static posture, the athletic trainer must accept the fact that postural alignment varies considerably among individuals; therefore, only obvious asymmetries should be considered.[64] The entire body should be observed from all angles—lateral, anterior, and posterior (Figure 25–10). To ensure accuracy of observation, a plumb line or posture screen may be of use (Figure 25–11). A trained observer with a good background in postural observation may not require any special devices. Figure 25–12 shows typical vertical alignment landmarks in the frontal plane from a lateral view. In the anterior and posterior assessment, the

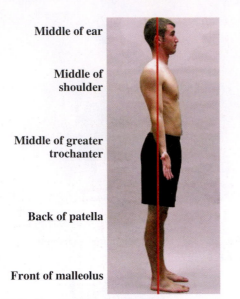

**Middle of ear**

**Middle of shoulder**

**Middle of greater trochanter**

**Back of patella**

**Front of malleolus**

FIGURE 25–12    Typical vertical frontal plane alignment landmarks.
© William E. Prentice

athletic trainer should look for asymmetries or differences in height between anatomical landmarks on each side in the sagittal plane (Figure 25–13).[62]

General observations relative to posture include the following:

- Head is tilted to one side.
- Shoulder is lower on one side.
- One shoulder is carried forward.
- One scapula is lower and more prominent than the other.
- Trunk is habitually bent to one side (hips look shifted to one side).
- Space between the body and arm is greater on one side.
- One hip is more prominent than the other.

- Hips are tilted to one side (iliac crests are not same height).
- Ribs are more pronounced on one side.
- One arm hangs longer than the other.
- One arm hangs farther forward than the other.
- One patella is lower than the other (level of popliteal creases is different).
- Trochanters are of unequal height.
- Posterior superior iliac spine (PSIS) levels are different.
- Anterior superior iliac spine (ASIS) levels are different.
- Levels of malleoli are different.
- Position of the feet (pronation. supination, calcaneal position, tibial position)

Classic postural deviations include kyphosis, forward head posture, flatback posture, swayback posture, lordosis, and scoliosis.

> **Classic postural deviations include kyphosis, forward head posture, flatback posture, swayback posture, lordosis, and scoliosis.**

**Kyphosis**    Kyphosis is characterized by an increased thoracic curve and by scapulae that are protracted, which produces a rounded shoulder appearance (Figure 25–14A). Kyphosis is usually associated with a forward head posture.

*Scheuermann's disease* is a disease of unknown etiology that usually affects adolescent males, which is not only painful but also may cause progressive thoracic or lumbar kyphosis.

**Forward Head Posture**    If the upper back exhibits a kyphotic posture in standing or sitting, there will be a compensatory change in the position of the head and neck.

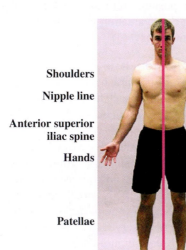
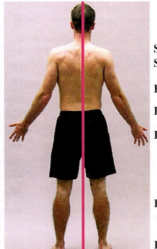

**Shoulders**

**Nipple line**

**Anterior superior iliac spine**

**Hands**

**Patellae**

**Feet Position**

**Shoulders**
**Scapulae**

**Elbows**

**Posterior dimples**

**Hands**

**Popliteal fossae**

**Feet Position**

FIGURE 25–13    Typical sagittal plane alignment landmarks.
© William E. Prentice

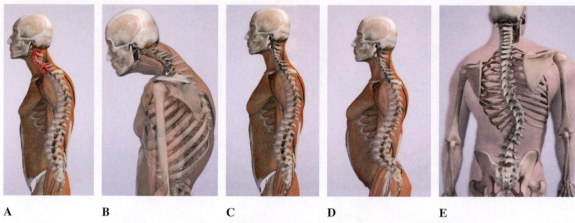

FIGURE 25–14    Postural malalignments. **(A)** Kyphosis. **(B)** Forward head. **(C)** Swayback. **(D)** Lordosis. **(E)** Scoliosis.

To keep the eyes level in spite of a slumped or rounded shoulder posture, the patient must extend the cervical spine, which tends to produce short but strong neck extensors and weak, long neck flexors. Thus, the head will be held in a forward position (Figure 25–14B).

***Swayback Posture*** A swayback posture involves an anterior shifting of the entire pelvis that results in hip extension. The thoracic segment shifts posteriorly, causing flexion of the thorax on the lumbar spine. Thus, there is a decrease in lordosis in the lumbar spine and an increase in kyphosis in the thoracic spine (Figure 25–14C).

***Lordosis*** Lordotic posture is characterized by an increased curve in the lumbar spine and an increase both in anterior tilt of the pelvis and in hip flexion (Figure 25–14D). Lordosis combined with kyphosis and a forward head posture is referred to as a kypho-lordotic posture. Lordosis can result from obesity, osteoporosis, or spondylolisthesis.

***Scoliosis*** Scoliosis is a lateral curvature of the spine (Figure 25–14E). The patient with scoliosis exhibits a recognizable abnormal curve in one direction and a compensatory secondary curve in the opposite direction. Scoliosis can be functional or structural. A functional scoliosis can be caused by some nonspinal defect, such as unequal leg length, muscle imbalance, or nutritional deficiency. Structural scoliosis is caused by some defect in the bony structure of the spine. When the patient bends forward, the spine with a functional scoliosis may straighten, whereas the spine with a structural scoliosis remains twisted. With the patient in this position, one side of the spine may be more prominent than the other.

***Flatback Posture*** Flatback posture is caused by a decreased lumbar curve and an increase in posterior pelvic tilt and in hip flexion. When this happens the patient appears to be stooped forward and has difficulty standing up straight. This can occur as a result of degenerative arthritis or from a spinal fusion.

**Cervical Spine Observation** When evaluating a case of cervical injury, the athletic trainer should look at the position of the head and neck. Are the shoulders level and symmetrical? Is the patient willing to move the head and neck freely? The athletic trainer should check passive, active, and resisted range of motion in the neck, including flexion, extension, rotation, and lateral bending (Figure 25–15).[70]

**Thoracic Spine Observation** The patient is first asked to flex, extend, laterally flex, and rotate the neck. Pain accompanying the movement in the upper back region could be referred from a lesion of the cervical disk. Additionally, pain in the scapular area could stem from an irritation of a myofascial trigger point or from irritation of the long thoracic or suprascapular nerves, which requires evaluation of the shoulder complex (see Chapter 22). The patient should also be asked to flex forward laterally and to extend and rotate the trunk. Pain felt during movement may indicate nerve root irritation to the lower thoracic region.

The most common cause of thoracic pain is dysfunction of one or more joint articulations and usually involves the facet joints. Increased pain upon placing the chin on the chest or upon deep inspiration is often indicative of a facet joint problem.

**Lumbar Spine and Sacroiliac Joint Observation** Normal functional movement in the low back region depends on coordinated motion of the lumbar vertebrae, the sacrum, and the pelvis.[100] The pelvis and shoulders should be level. Both the soft tissue and bony structures on both sides of the midline should be symmetrical. Any unusual curve in the lumbar area that is observed when the patient is standing or walking could be due to muscular, capsular, or ligamentous injuries, disk-related problems, or some idiopathic or structural problem.[100]

The patient should be observed in standing, sitting, supine, side-lying, and prone positions, and special tests should be done in each of those positions to determine the nature of the problem.[79]

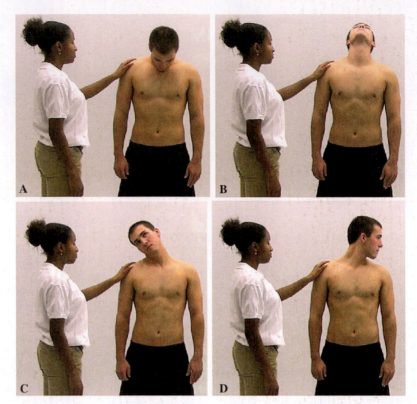

FIGURE 25–15 Checking neck range of motion. **(A)** Flexion.
**(B)** Extension. **(C)** Lateral flexion. **(D)** Rotation.
© William E. Prentice

## Palpation

Palpation should be performed with the patient lying
prone and the spine as straight as possible. The head and
neck should be slightly flexed. In cases of low back pain,
a pillow placed under the hips might make the patient
more comfortable. Palpation should progress from proximal to distal as the athletic trainer attempts to identify
points of tenderness, muscle spasm or guarding, and defects in bone or soft tissue.

The musculature on each side of the spine should be
palpated for tenderness or guarding. Referred pain can
produce tender areas. At some point in the evaluation of
the lumbar spine, the abdominal musculature should also
be palpated; the patient should perform a partial sit-up to
determine symmetry and tone.

The spinous processes are the easiest landmark to locate. Pressure and release should be applied to the spinous process of each vertebra in an anterior direction
to determine whether pain is increased either centrally
or laterally. The gaps between the spinous processes
should be palpated. Tenderness may indicate a ligamentous or disk-related problem. Each spinous process
should be in a direct line with the one directly above
and directly below (Figure 25–16). Misalignment usually occurs in the cervical or lumbar areas, indicating
some rotation of an individual vertebral segment. The
transverse processes on both sides of each vertebra can
also be palpated. Pressure on one side only produces

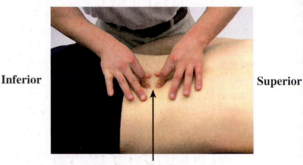

Inferior                                    Superior

**Space between
lumbar spinous processes**

FIGURE 25–16 Each spinous process should be in a
direct line with the one above and below.
© William E. Prentice

rotation of that segment, which can increase pain. The
facet joints and laminae are difficult to palpate because
of the paraspinal muscles.

The sacroiliac joints should be palpated bilaterally
for tenderness. Posterior pressure on the sacrum may increase pain if the sacroiliac joint is involved.

## Special Tests for the Cervical Spine

Special tests for the cervical spine should not be done
until trauma to either the vertebrae or the spinal cord has
been ruled out.

### Brachial Plexus Test[59]

Lateral flexion or bending of the cervical spine by the application of pressure on both the head and the shoulder duplicates the mechanism of injury to the brachial plexus (Figure 25–17). If the cervical spine is flexed to the right and pain radiates to the right shoulder and arm, a compression injury exists. Conversely, if the pain radiates to the left shoulder and arm, a traction or stretch injury has occurred. Sn. 0.83 | Sp. 0.69 | +LR 4.06 | -LR 0.37

**Cervical Compression and Spurling's Tests[38]** Axial compression of the cervical spine by the application of a downward force compresses cervical facet joints and the cervical spinal nerve roots (Figure 25–18). The level of the associated pain will determine specifically which nerve root has been injured. Spurling's test also uses cervical compression but with lateral bending and slight extension, which produces pain in the shoulder and arm on the side of flexion (Figure 25–19).[99] Pain is caused by impingement of the nerve root. Sn. 0.50 | Sp. 0.88 | +LR 0.58 | -LR 3.5

**Vertebral Artery Test[29]** This test is done with the patient supine. The athletic trainer extends, then laterally bends and rotates the cervical spine in the same direction (Figure 25–20). Dizziness or abnormal movement of the eyes (nystagmus) indicates that the cervical vertebral artery is being partially occluded because of some abnormal compression. The patient should be immediately referred

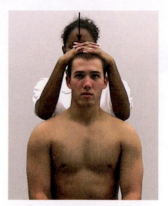

FIGURE 25–18   Cervical compression test.
© William E. Prentice

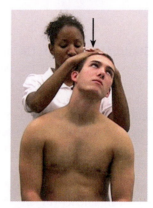

FIGURE 25–19   Spurling's test.
© William E. Prentice

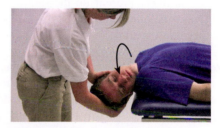

FIGURE 25–20   Vertebral artery test.
© William E. Prentice

to a physician for additional testing and diagnosis.[107] Sn. 0.0 | Sp. 0.83 | +LR 0.54 | -LR 1.21

**Shoulder Abduction Test (Bakody's Sign)[31]** The patient abducts the shoulder by placing the hand on top of the head (Figure 25–21). A decrease in radicular symptoms may indicate the presence of a nerve root compression, possibly due to a herniated disk. Sn. 0.46 | Sp. 0.90 | +LR* 0.05 | -LR* 0.60

### Special Tests for the Lumbar Spine and Sacroiliac Joint

Special tests for the lumbar spine should be performed in standing, sitting, supine, side-lying, and prone positions.[50]

*Calculated from sensitivity and specificity.

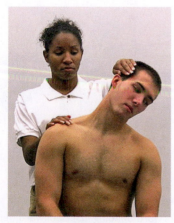

FIGURE 25–17   Brachial plexus test.
© William E. Prentice

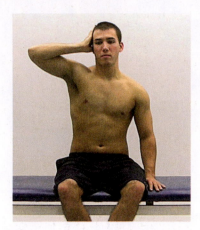

FIGURE 25–21  Shoulder abduction test.
© William E. Prentice

**Tests Done in Standing Position** The athletic trainer should observe the patient's gait. Is the patient's trunk bent, or are the hips shifted to one side? Is there a limp or any difficulty in walking? The athletic trainer should check the alignment and symmetry of the malleoli, popliteal crease, trochanters, anterior and posterior superior iliac spines (ASIS and PSIS), and iliac crests.

**Forward Bending** Forward bending involves stretching of the posterior spinal ligaments (Figure 25–22A). With forward bending or flexion, the PSISs on each side should move together. If one moves farther than the other, a motion restriction is likely present on the side that moves most. If they move at different times, the side that moves first usually has a restriction.

**Backward Bending** Backward bending places the spine in a hyperextended position and stretches the anterior ligaments of the spine (Figure 25–22B). Restrictions and pain present in backward bending are usually

associated with a disk problem. However, the pain may also be related to spondylolysis or spondylolisthesis (to be discussed later in this chapter).

**Side Bending** For the patient with a lumbar lesion or with sacroiliac dysfunction, side bending toward the painful side will increase the pain (see Figure 25–22C). In the case of a herniated disk, the patient will usually side bend toward the side of the herniation to relieve the nerve from external compression by the disk.

**Rotation** With the arms folded across the chest, the athletic trainer should rotate the trunk to the left, then to the right, checking the movement of the lumbar spine for symmetry. This test may be done while standing. However, since the pelvis should not move during the rotation it is best tested in a sitting position.

**Stork Test**[54] The patient is standing on one leg and leans backward with the support of the clinician. If extension done in the one-leg standing position (stork position) produces pain in the lumbar or sacral regions of the spine, it may indicate a lesion in the pars interarticularis on the side opposite the raised leg (Figure 25–23). This is referred to as a spondylolysis. Sn. 0.96 | Sp. 0.88 | +LR 2.80 | -LR 0.18

**Gillet Test**[36] In the Gillet test the patient is standing. The clinician palpates the posterior superior iliac spine

> A recreational weight lifter complains of a centrally located back pain that radiates down her left leg. She describes a sudden onset after a workout that becomes more severe as she tries to rest it. Forward bending and sitting postures increase pain. Backward bending is restricted. Side bending toward the affected side increases pain.
>
> ? Based on the athletic trainer's assessment, what is likely causing this pain?

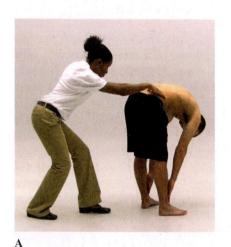
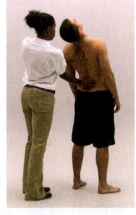
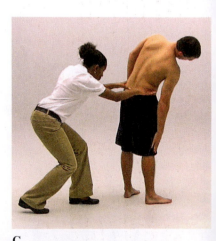

A                                    B                                    C

FIGURE 25–22  Checking lumbar range of motion in standing position. **(A)** Forward bending. **(B)** Backward bending. **(C)** Side bending.
© William E. Prentice

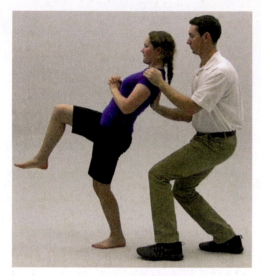

FIGURE 25–23    Stork test—single-leg stance extension.
© William E. Prentice

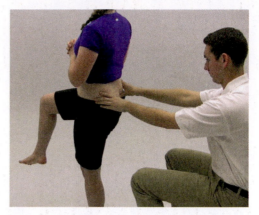

FIGURE 25–24    Gillet test for sacroiliac joint hypomobility.
© William E. Prentice

with one thumb and the sacrum with the other thumb at a parallel level. The patient lifts the leg on the side being palpated to at least 90 degrees (Figure 25–24). A positive test is if the PSIS does not move inferiorly indicating sacroiliac joint hypomobility. The test is repeated on the opposite side and the results are compared.
Sn. 0.43 | Sp. 0.69 | +LR 1.34 | -LR 0.84

### Tests Done in Sitting Position

*Forward Bending*    In seated forward bending or flexion, as in standing forward bending, the PSISs should move together. If one moves farther than the other, a motion restriction is likely present on the side that moves most.

*Rotation*    The patient sits with arms folded across the chest and rotates the trunk to the left and then to the right while the athletic trainer checks the movement of the lumbar spine for symmetry and provides overpressure to see whether pain increases (Figure 25–25A).

*Hip Rotation*    With the patient in the sitting position, the hip should be rotated internally and externally (Figure 25–25B&C). Internal rotation that produces pain is likely a piriformis irritation (discussed later in this chapter), and pain is produced as the muscle is stretched.

*Slump Test*[57]    The slump test begins with the patient sitting with knees flexed and feet on the ground (Figure 25–26). The thoracic and lumbar spines are flexed with overpressure. Pain is assessed first in this starting position. From this starting position, the following series of positional changes occurs, with pain being assessed in each position: (1) The cervical spine is flexed, (2) one knee is extended, (3) the ankle is dorsiflexed, (4) neck flexion is released, (5) both legs are extended simultaneously, and (6) steps 1 through 4 are repeated with the other leg.[40] This test is done to detect an increase in nerve root tension that has been labeled *neural tension,* which may be caused by lateral disk herniation, nerve root adhesions, or vertebral impingement.[42,61]
Sn. 0.84 | Sp. 0.83 | +LR NA | -LR NA

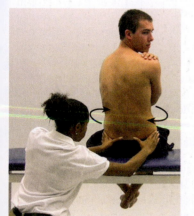
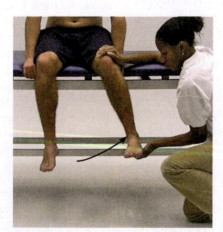
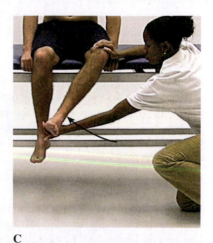

A                                B                                C

FIGURE 25–25    Checking lumbar range of motion in sitting position. **(A)** Rotation. **(B)** Internal hip rotation. **(C)** External hip rotation.
© William E. Prentice

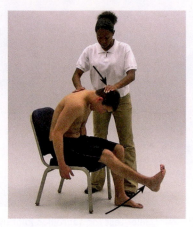

FIGURE 25–26    Slump test.
© William E. Prentice

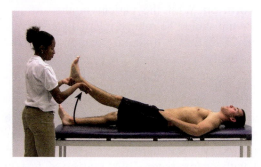

FIGURE 25–27    Straight-leg raising test.
© William E. Prentice

**Tests Done in Supine Position** The athletic trainer should first note the leg position. If there is asymmetrical and exaggerated external rotation on one side, there may be a piriformis contracture on that side. The iliopsoas, adductors, pubic tubercles, and symphysis pubis should be palpated for symmetry and tenderness in the supine position prior to performing the following tests.

***Straight-Leg Raises (Lasegue's Test)*[34]** The *straight-leg raising* test applies pressure to the sacroiliac joint and may indicate a problem in the sciatic nerve, the sacroiliac joint, or the lumbar spine (Figure 25–27). Pain at 30 degrees of straight-leg raising indicates either a hip problem or an inflamed nerve. Pain from 30 to 60 degrees indicates some sciatic nerve involvement. If dorsiflexing the ankle at maximum straight-leg raising increases the pain, the problem is likely due to some nerve root (L3–L4, S1–S3) or sciatic nerve irritation (Laseague's sign). Pain between 70 and 90 degrees is indicative of a sacroiliac joint problem. Sn. 0.91 | Sp. 0.26 | +LR 0.35 | -LR 1.2

***Kernig's Test*[94]** In Kernig's test, the patient is supine with the knee and hip flexed to 90 degrees (Figure 25–28). The test is performed by passively extending the knee and eliciting pain in the hamstrings. Back pain may be a sign of nerve root irritation or a sign of meningitis. Sn. 0.05 | Sp. 0.95 | +LR 0.97 | -LR 1.0

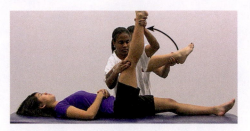

FIGURE 25–28    Kernig's test.
© William E. Prentice

***Brudzinski's Test*[94]** Brudzinski's test is done with the patient in a supine position. Flexing the neck causes a reflex flexion of one or both knees and increase in pain. This may indicate either a lumbar disk or some nerve root irritation, or a sign of meningitis (Figure 25–29). Sn. 0.05 | Sp. 0.95 | +LR 0.97 | -LR 1.0

***Crossed Straight-Leg Raising Test (Well Test)*[101]** The crossed straight-leg raising test (Well test), done on the unaffected side, may also produce pain in the low back on the affected side, as well as radiating along the sciatic nerve. This test provides additional proof of nerve root inflammation or a disk herniation (Figure 25–30). Sn. 0.32 | Sp. 0.98 | +LR 16.0 | -LR 0.69

***Milgram Test*** An inability to hold both legs off the treatment table for 30 seconds on the Milgram straight-leg raising test indicates some problem with the lumbar spine. This test increases intrathecal pressure that causes a disk to put pressure on a lumbar nerve root (Figure 25–31).

***Hoover Test*** The patient is supine and the athletic trainer cups the calcaneous in each hand (Figure 25–32). The patient is instructed to lift the leg on the involved side. A positive test occurs when the patient makes no attempt to lift the involved side and the athletic trainer does not sense any pressure from the uninvolved side pressing down into the hand. A positive test may indicate that the patient is malingering.

***Bowstring Test*[67]** The bowstring test is another way to determine sciatic nerve irritation. The leg on the affected side is lifted until pain is felt. The knee is then flexed until the pain is relieved, at which time pressure is applied to the popliteal fossa. The test result is positive if pain is felt during palpation along the sciatic nerve (Figure 25–33). A positive test indicates a radiculopathy. To confirm that the pain stems from a nerve root involvement and

A volleyball player comes to the athletic trainer, complaining of recurring low back pain. She has been seen by a therapist in her hometown, who has told her that she has a positive straight-leg raising test, but the patient still does not understand what is causing her pain.

**?** How should the athletic trainer explain what having a positive straight-leg raising test means?

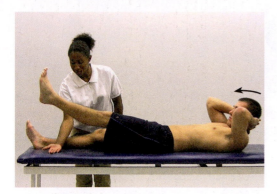

FIGURE 25-29   Brudzinski's test.
© William E. Prentice

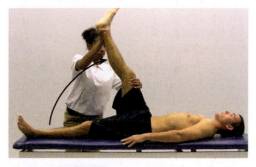

FIGURE 25-30   Crossed straight-leg raising test (Well Test).
© William E. Prentice

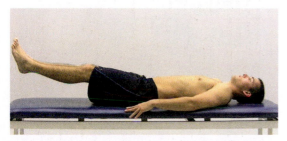

FIGURE 25-31   Milgram straight-leg raising test. The patient cannot hold the legs up for 30 seconds.
© William E. Prentice

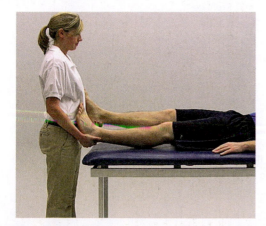

FIGURE 25-32   Hoover test. The athletic trainer holds the patient's calcaneous in each hand. The patient does not attempt to lift the leg on the involved side.
© William E. Prentice

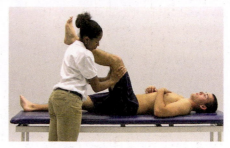

FIGURE 25-33   Bowstring test for sciatic nerve irritation.
© William E. Prentice

not from hamstring tightness, the leg is lowered to a point at which pain ceases. In this position, the foot is dorsiflexed and the neck flexed. If pain returns, it is a verification of a pathological condition of the nerve root. **Sn. 0.71 | Sp. NA | +LR NA | -LR NA**

***FABER Test*[89]** A flexion, abduction, and external rotation (FABER) test, also known as the *Patrick test,* is done with the patient supine and the involved leg in the figure 4 position (see Figure 21–18). With the leg in this position, there may be pain in the inguinal region anterior to the hip, indicating hip pathology. When overpressure to the knee produces pain, some SI joint pathology is indicated. **Sn. 0.57 | Sp. 0.71 | +LR 1.19 | -LR 0.61**

***FADDIR Test*[75]** A flexion, adduction, and internal rotation (FADDIR) test is done with the patient supine and the involved side hip and knee flexed (see Figure 21–17). The athletic trainer adducts and internally rotates the hip. The test is positive if the patient indicates an increase in low back pain. A positive test indicates lumbar pathology. **Sn. 0.94 | Sp. 0.08 | +LR 1.02 | -LR 0.48**

***Gaenslen's Test*[54]** In a supine position, with the affected side on the edge of the table, the unaffected thigh is flexed toward the abdomen. Pressure is applied to the knee on the affected side, moving the sacroiliac joint into extension. The test is positive if hyperextension on the affected side increases pain (Figure 25–34). **Sn. 0.53 | Sp. 0.77 | +LR 2.2 | -LR 0.65**

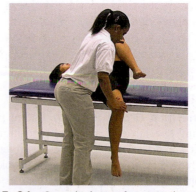

FIGURE 25-34   Gaenslen's test for sacroiliac joint pain.
© William E. Prentice

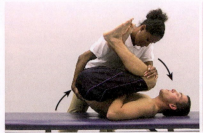 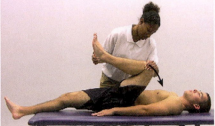 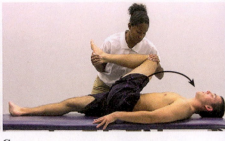

**A**            **B**            **C**

FIGURE 25–35   **(A)** Bilateral knees to chest. **(B)** Single knee to chest. **(C)** Knee to opposite shoulder.
© William E. Prentice

***Knees to ChestTests*** Pulling the knees to the chest bilaterally will increase symptoms in the lumbar spine (Figure 25–35A). If pulling a single knee to the chest causes pain in the posterolateral thigh, there may be some irritation to the sacrotuberous ligament (Figure 25–35B). If pain is reported in the area of the PSIS when pulling a single knee to the opposite shoulder, there may be sacroiliac ligament irritation (Figure 25–35C).

***SI Compression Tests***[54] The sacroiliac compression test is used to stress the posterior sacroiliac ligaments. Standing behind the patient, the clinician exerts a downward force at the iliac crest. Pain on compression is a positive sign and is indicative of sacral joint irritation or sprain (Figure 25–36A). Sn. 0.69 | Sp. 0.69 | +LR 2.20 | -LR 0.46

***SI Distraction Test***[54] The sacroiliac distraction test is also referred to as the "gapping" test and is used to test the anterior sacroiliac ligaments. If the patient reports posterior gluteal or leg pain, the test is positive, which may indicate sacral joint irritation or sprain (Figure 25–36B). Sn. 0.60 | Sp. 0.81 | +LR 3.2 | -LR 0.5

***Pelvic Tilt Tests*** Anterior and posterior pelvic tilts that increase the pain on the side being stressed indicate irritation of the sacroiliac joint (Figure 25–37). Occasionally, this test may be done on an athlete in a side-lying position.

***Thigh Thrust Test***[54] With the patient supine, the clinician stands on the side opposite the side being tested, places one hand under the sacrum, and the other on the flexed knee. A downward force is applied through the femur (Figure 25–38). An increase in pain in the sacroiliac joint may indicate SI joint dysfunction. Sn. 0.88 | Sp. 0.69 | +LR 2.80 | -LR 0.18

**Tests Done in a Prone Position** Before performing the following special tests in a prone position, the athletic trainer should palpate a number of structures, feeling for increased tension, attempting to provoke a tender pain response, and checking for landmark asymmetries. The structures that are easily palpated in a prone position include the lumbar spinous processes, iliac crests, PSIS,

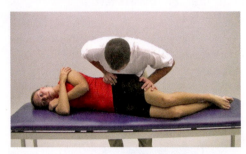

**A**

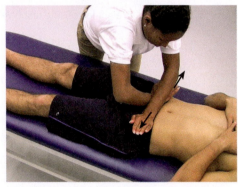

**B**

FIGURE 25–36   **(A)** Sacral compression. **(B)** Sacral distraction.
© William E. Prentice

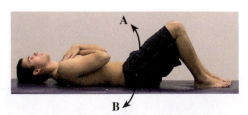

FIGURE 25–37   **(A)** Anterior pelvic tilt. **(B)** Posterior pelvic tilt.
© William E. Prentice

sacrum, trochanters, sacral sulcus, sacrotuberous ligament, sacrospinous ligament, sciatic nerve region, quadratus lumborum, erector spinae, gluteus maximus, gluteus medius, and piriformis.

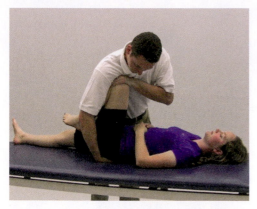

FIGURE 25–38   Thigh thrust test for sacroiliac joint dysfunction.
© William E. Prentice

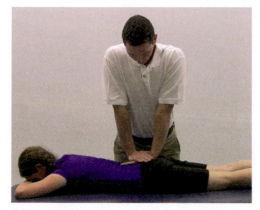

FIGURE 25–39   Sacral thrust for sacroliliac dysfunction
© William E. Prentice

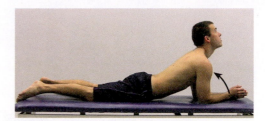

FIGURE 25–40   Press-ups.
© William E. Prentice

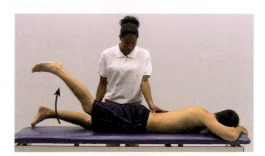

FIGURE 25–41   Prone hip extension.
© William E. Prentice

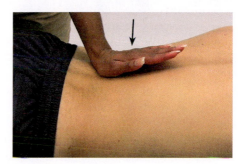

FIGURE 25–42   Spring test.
© William E. Prentice

***Sacral Thrust***[54] With the patient lying prone, the clinician's hands are placed over the sacrum one on top of the other. Pressure is applied downward through the sacrum (Figure 25–39). The test is positive if pain is increased in the sacroiliac joint. Sn. 0.63 | Sp. 0.75 | +LR 2.50 | -LR 0.50

***Press-Ups***   Press-ups, which extend the spine, are done to see whether pain radiates into the buttocks or thigh, which may indicate a herniated disk. If pain localizes in this position, conservative care is recommended. If pain is more generalized, surgical care may be required (Figure 25–40).

***Prone Hip Extension Test***[11] In a prone hip extension test, the patient lies prone and lifts the affected leg. If pain occurs in the low back, an L2–L4 nerve root irritation may be present (Figure 25–41). Sn. 0.27 | Sp. 0.78 | +LR* 1.23 | -LR* 0.94

***Spring Test***[36] In the spring test, a downward pressure is applied through the spinous process of each vertebra to assess anterior/posterior motion. The spring test can also be done on the transverse process to assess rotational movement. This test can determine either hypermobility

*Calculated from sensitivity and specificity.

or hypomobility of a specific vertebral segment (Figure 25–42). Sn. 0.75 | Sp. 0.35 | +LR* 1.15 | -LR* 0.71

***Prone Knee Flexion Test***   A comparison of apparent leg lengths is made with the patient prone with knees extended and prone with knees flexed to 90 degrees. The leg lengths are compared by inspecting the heels; if there is a short side, that side is indicative of a posterior rotated SI joint. If, on flexing the knees, the apparent length of the legs equalizes, this indicates a posteriorly rotated SI joint on that side (Figure 25–43).

***Prone Instability Test***[48] The patient is positioned prone with legs off the table while toes touch the floor (Figure 25–44). The clinician, positioned on either side of the table, places the hands at the suspected lumbar segment. The patient is asked to lift his or her feet off of the floor 2 to 3 inches and extend the hips toward the ceiling while the clinician applies direct downward force to the segment. The test is positive if the pain decreases during the procedure. Sn. 0.72 | Sp. 0.58 | +LR 1.7 | -LR 0.48

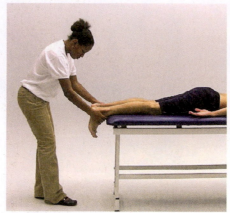
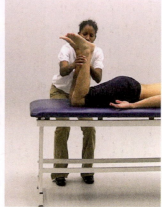

A             B

FIGURE 25–43   Prone knee flexion test. **(A)** Knees extended.
**(B)** Knees flexed.

© William E. Prentice

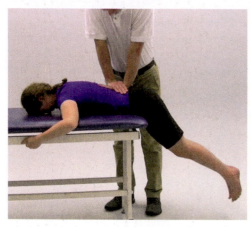

FIGURE 25–44   Prone instability test for lumbar segment
instability.

© William E. Prentice

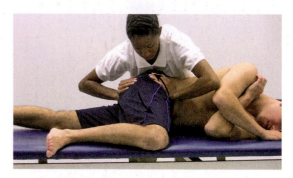

FIGURE 25–45   Posterior rotation stress test.

© William E. Prentice

### Tests Done in a Side-Lying Position

***Posterior Rotation Stress Test*** Pain on movement located near the PSIS indicates irritation in the sacroiliac
joint. This does not indicate the direction of the dysfunctional movement, but the pain localizes the problem to a
specific side (Figure 25–45).

***Iliotibial Band Stretch Test*** Long-standing SI joint
problems sometimes lead to shortness of the iliotibial
band and a perpetuation or recurrence of the SI problem.
This test will often provoke pain in the contralateral PSIS
area, indicating an SI problem (Figure 25–46).

***Quadratus Lumborum Stretch Test*** A pillow roll
placed under the patient's waist will side bend the lumbar spine and open the upper quadratus to easy palpation. Dropping the leg off the side of the table while
maintaining this position will provide some stretch to
the muscle, provoking pain or demonstrating tightness
(Figure 25–47).

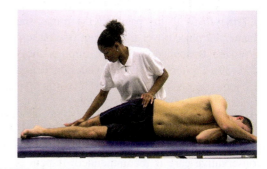

FIGURE 25–46   Iliotibial band stretch test.

© William E. Prentice

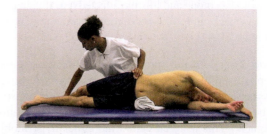

FIGURE 25–47   Quadratus lumborum stretch test.

© William E. Prentice

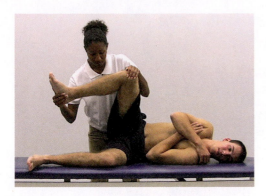

FIGURE 25–48   Piriformis muscle test.
© William E. Prentice

***Piriformis Muscle Test***[37]   A piriformis lesion can be identified by flexing the hips to 90 degrees with the patient side-lying and resisting hip abduction in the top leg (Figure 25–48). A positive test indicates tightness or myofascial pain in that muscle. This test can also be done seated, with the hip and knee at 90 degrees. Resisting hip external rotation can also elicit pain if there is a problem with the piriformis muscle (see Figure 25–25C). Sn. 0.88 | Sp. 0.83 | +LR 5.2 | -LR 0.14

***Femoral Nerve Traction Test***[88]   The femoral nerve traction test is done with the hip extended and the knee flexed to 90 degrees. As the hip is extended, pain occurs in the anterior thigh, which indicates nerve root impingement in the lumbar area. This test may also be done in a prone position (Figure 25–49). Sn. 0.50 | Sp. 1.0 | +LR >10 | -LR 0.5

***Clinical Prediction Rules***   The following clinical prediction rules are currently used for the spine and neck:

- Cervical Manipulation for Neck Pain[72]—identifies patients with mechanical neck pain who will demonstrate favorable outcomes following cervical manipulation.
- Canadian Cervical Spine Rules[85]—developed to determine the need for radiographs after acute head/neck injury secondary to the risk of fracture.
- Cervical Myelopathy[26]—diagnoses patients with cervical myelopathy so that patients can be treated with the appropriate interventions and/or referred for further radiological/surgical procedures.

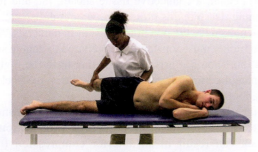

FIGURE 25–49   Femoral nerve traction test.
© William E. Prentice

- Cervical Radiculopathy[103]—diagnoses patients with cervical radiculopathy so that patients can be treated with the appropriate interventions.
- Cervical Closed Fracture[25]—identifies historical findings indicative of a closed cervical spine fracture.
- Vertebral Compression Fracture[77]—identifies patients likely to present with a vertebral compression fracture.
- Lumbar Spinal Stenosis[27]—identifies signs and symptoms indicative of lumbar spinal stenosis.
- Manipulation for Low Back Pain[19]—identifies patients with low back pain who likely will improve with spinal manipulation.
- Mechanical Traction for Low Back Pain[13]—identifies patients with low back pain who likely will respond favorably to mechanical lumbar traction.
- Mechanical Traction for Neck Pain[73]—identifies patients with neck pain likely to improve with cervical traction and exercise.
- Stabilization for Low Back Pain[48]—identifies patients presenting with low back pain who will likely respond favorably to a stabilization exercise program.
- Thoracic Manipulation for Neck Pain[23]—identifies patients with neck pain who are likely to experience early success from thoracic spine thrust manipulation, exercise, and patient education.
- Sacroiliac Joint Pain[54]—diagnoses patients with sacroiliac joint pain so that patients can be treated with the appropriate interventions.
- Fear Avoidance Belief Questionnaire (FABQ)[48]—determines how a patient's fear-avoidance beliefs about physical activity and work may contribute to their low back pain.

## Neurological Exam

The neurological exam was discussed in detail in Chapter 13. In cases in which the spinal cord and associated nerve roots are potentially injured, sensation testing and reflex testing should be a routine aspect of the assessment process.

***Sensation Testing***   When there is a nerve root involvement, sensation can be partially or completely disrupted in dermatomal patterns. Figure 25–50A&B indicates the locations of general disruption or loss of sensation as a result of cervical and lumbosacral nerve root involvement.

***Reflex Testing***   Deep tendon reflexes were discussed in Chapter 13. Three reflexes in the upper extremity are the biceps, brachioradialis, and triceps reflexes. In the biceps reflex, the C5 and C6 nerve roots are being tested. The brachioradialis reflex assesses the C6 nerve root. C7 nerve root dysfunction is indicated by the triceps reflex.

Two reflexes in the lower extremity are the patellar and the Achilles tendon reflexes. A diminished or absent patellar reflex is an indication of an L4 nerve root problem. The Achilles tendon reflex can determine the presence or absence of an S1 nerve root problem.

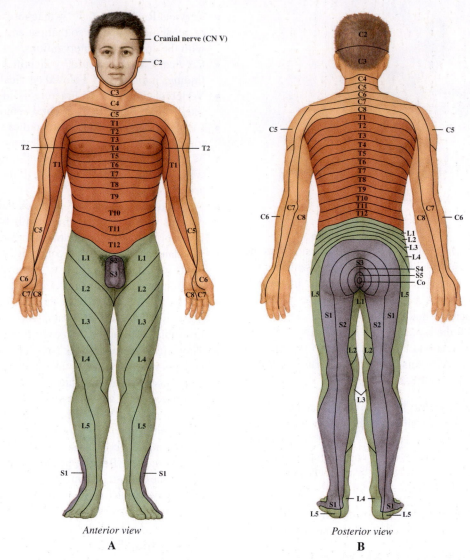

FIGURE 25–50   Dermatomal patterns of sensation. **(A)** Anterior. **(B)** Posterior.

Table 25–4 summarizes the special tests for the spine.

# RECOGNITION AND MANAGEMENT OF SPECIFIC INJURIES AND CONDITIONS

## Cervical Spine Conditions

Because the neck is so mobile, it is extremely vulnerable to a wide range of injuries.[3] Severe injury to the neck, although relatively uncommon, can produce catastrophic impairment of the spinal cord.[8] The neck can be seriously injured by the following traumatic events (Figure 25–51): an axial load force to the top of the head, a flexion force, a hyperextension force, a rotation and flexion force, a rotation and hyperextension force, and a lateral flexion force. The neck is also prone to

subtle injuries stemming from stress, tension, and postural malalignments.

### Cervical Fractures

*Etiology*   Fortunately, neck fracture is relatively uncommon. The spinal cord is well protected by a bony vertebral canal, a connective tissue sheath, fat, and fluid cushioning. Despite this protection, vertebral dislocations and fractures have the potential to result in paralysis.[5] The athletic trainer must constantly be prepared to handle such a situation, should it arise.[90] Sports that have the highest incidence of cervical fracture are gymnastics, ice hockey, diving, football, and rugby.[22]

Axial loading of the cervical vertebra from a force to the top of the head combined with flexion of the neck can result in an anterior compression fracture or a dislocation.[91] Fractures are most common in the fourth, fifth, or sixth cervical vertebra. If the head

| TABLE 25–4 | Summary of Special Tests for the Spine |
|---|---|
| **Test** | **A Positive Test Indicates** |
| *Cervical spine* | |
| Brachial plexus test | Brachial plexus injury |
| Cervical compression test | Nerve root impingement |
| Spurling's test | Nerve root impingement |
| Vertebral artery test | Occluded cervical vertebral artery |
| Shoulder abduction test | Nerve root impingement |
| *Lumbar spine and Sacroiliac Joint* | |
| **Standing Position** | |
| Forward bending | Restriction in PSIS |
| Backward bending | Disk problem; spondylolysis |
| Side bending | Herniated disk; SI dysfunction |
| Stork test | Spondylolysis |
| Gillet test | SI hypomobility |
| **Sitting Position** | |
| Forward bending | Restriction in PSIS |
| Rotation | Asymmetry in lumbar spine |
| Internal hip rotation | Piriformis injury |
| Slump test | Increased neural tension |
| **Supine Position** | |
| Straight-leg raising 30° | Hip problem; nerve root impingement |
| Straight-leg raising 30–60° | Sciatic nerve; nerve root impingement |
| Straight-leg raising 70–90° | SI joint dysfunction |
| Kernig's test | Nerve root irritation |
| Brudzinski's test | Lumbar disk; nerve root irritation |
| Crossed straight-leg raising (Well test) | Nerve root irritation |
| Milgram straight-leg raising | Lumbar disk |
| Hoover test | Identifies malingerers |
| Bowstring test | Sciatic nerve irritation |
| FABER/Patrick test | SI joint dysfunction |
| FADDIR test | Lumbar strain |
| Gaenslen's test | SI joint dysfunction |
| Bilateral knees to chest | Lumbar sprain |
| Single knee to chest | Sacrotuberous ligament sprain |
| Single knee to opposite shoulder | Sacroiliac ligament sprain |
| SI joint compression | SI joint dysfunction |
| SI joint distraction | SI joint dysfunction |
| Pelvic tilt | SI joint irritation |
| Thigh thrust | SI joint dysfunction |
| **Prone Position** | |
| Sacral thrust | SI joint pain |
| Press-ups | Herniated disk |
| Prone hip extension | L4 nerve root irritation |
| Spring test | Vertebral hypermobility/hypomobility |
| Prone knee flexion test | Posteriorly rotated SI joint |
| Prone instability test | Lumbopelvic instability |
| **Side-Lying Position** | |
| Posterior rotation stress test | SI joint irritation |
| Iliotibial band stretch test | SI joint irritation |
| Quadratus lumborum stretch test | Quadratus lumborum tightness |
| Piriformis muscle stretch test | Piriformis muscle tightness |
| Femoral nerve traction test | Nerve root irritation |

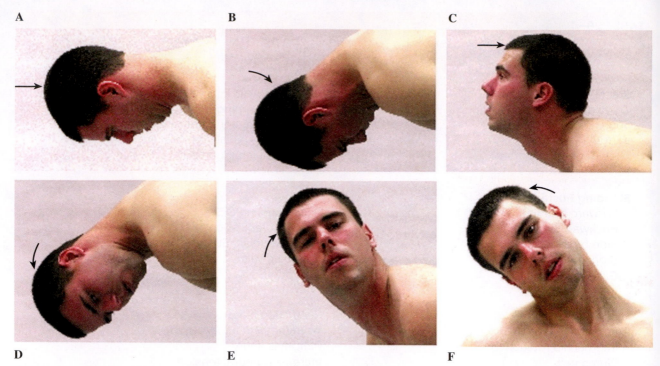

**A**      **B**      **C**

**D**      **E**      **F**

FIGURE 25–51   Mechanisms of cervical neck injury. **(A)** Axial load. **(B)** Flexion. **(C)** Hyperextension. **(D)** Rotation and flexion. **(E)** Rotation and hyperextension. **(F)** Lateral flexion.
© William E. Prentice

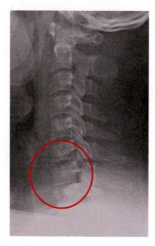

FIGURE 25–52   Fracture of C7.
Courtesy Jordan B. Renner, MD, Departments of Radiology and Allied Health Sciences, University of North Carolina

is also rotated when contact is made, a dislocation may occur along with the fracture. Fractures can also occur during a sudden forced hyperextension of the neck (Figure 25–52).

***Symptoms and signs*** The patient may have one or more of the following signs of cervical fracture: neck point tenderness and restricted movement, cervical muscle spasm, cervical pain and pain in the chest and extremities, numbness in the trunk and/or limbs, weakness

or paralysis in the limbs and/or trunk, and loss of bladder and/or bowel control.

***Management*** Patients with suspected cervical spine fractures should be stabilized, collared, and spine boarded regardless of whether they are conscious or unconscious.[90] An unconscious patient should be treated as if a serious neck injury were present until this possibility is ruled out by the physician.[3] Extreme caution must be used in moving the patient.[8] The athletic trainer must always be aware that a patient can sustain a catastrophic spinal injury from improper handling and transportation[32] (see Chapter 12 for *detailed* emergency care of spinal injuries).

### Cervical Dislocations

***Etiology*** Cervical dislocations are not common, but they do occur much more frequently than fractures (Figure 25–53).[5] Cervical dislocations usually result from violent flexion and rotation of the head. Most injuries of this type happen in pool diving accidents. The cervical vertebrae are more easily dislocated than are the vertebrae in other spinal regions, principally because of their horizontally arranged articular facets. The superior articular facet moves beyond its normal range of motion and either completely passes the inferior facet (luxation) or catches on its edge (subluxation).[5] The latter is far more common and, as in the case of the complete luxation, most often affects the fourth, fifth, or sixth vertebra.

***Symptoms and signs*** For the most part, a cervical dislocation produces many of the same signs as a

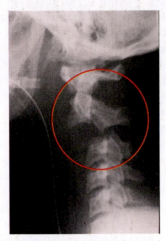

FIGURE 25–53    Complete cervical vertebra (C2–C3) dislocation.

Courtesy Jordan B. Renner, MD, Departments of Radiology and Allied Health Sciences, University of North Carolina

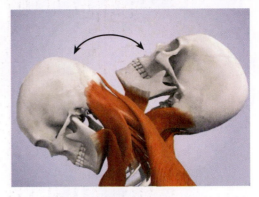

FIGURE 25–54    Whiplash injury involves a sudden forward or backward acceleration of the head relative to the spine.

fracture. Both can result in considerable pain, numbness, and muscle weakness or paralysis. The most easily discernible difference is the position of the neck in a dislocation: A unilateral dislocation causes the neck to be tilted toward the dislocated side, with extreme muscle tightness on the elongated side and a relaxed muscle state on the tilted side.[69]

***Management***    Because a dislocation of a cervical vertebra has a greater likelihood of causing injury to the spinal cord, even greater care must be exercised when moving the patient.[90] Again, the procedures described in Chapter 12 should be applied to cervical dislocations.

## Acute Strains of the Neck and Upper Back

***Etiology***    In a strain of the neck or upper back, the patient has usually turned the head suddenly or has forced flexion, extension, or rotation.[10] The muscles involved are typically the upper trapezius, the sternocleidomastoid, the scalenes, and the splenius capitis and cervicis.[10]

***Symptoms and signs***    Localized pain, point tenderness, and restricted motion are present. Muscle guarding resulting from pain is common, and the patient is reluctant to move the neck in any direction.

***Management***    Care usually includes the use of POLICE immediately after the strain occurs and the application of a cervical collar. Follow-up management may include ROM exercises, followed by isometric exercises and progressing to full-range isotonic strengthening exercises, cryotherapy or superficial heat, and analgesic medications as prescribed by the physician.

## Cervical Sprain (Whiplash)

***Etiology***    A cervical sprain can occur from the same mechanism as the strain but usually results from a more violent motion. More commonly, cervical sprain occurs

from a sudden snap of the head (Figure 25–54). Frequently, muscle strains occur with ligament sprains. A sprain of the neck produces tears in the major supporting tissue of the anterior or posterior longitudinal ligaments, the interspinous ligament, and the supraspinous ligament.[45]

***Symptoms and signs***    The sprain displays all the signs of the strained neck, but the symptoms persist longer. There may also be tenderness over the transverse and spinous processes that serve as sites of attachment for the ligaments.

Pain may not be experienced initially but always appears the day after the trauma. Pain stems from the inflammation of injured tissue and a protective muscle spasm that restricts motion.

***Management***    As soon as possible, the patient should have a physician evaluation to rule out the possibility of fracture, dislocation, or disk injury.[45] Neurological examination is performed by the physician to ascertain spinal cord or nerve root injury. A soft cervical collar may be applied to reduce muscle spasm. POLICE is used for 48 to 72 hours while the injury is in the acute stage of healing. For a patient with a severe injury, the physician may prescribe 2 to 3 days of bed rest along with analgesics and anti-inflammation agents. Therapy might include cryotherapy or heat and massage. Mechanical traction may also be prescribed to relieve pain and muscle spasm.[42] Manual therapy has been shown to be effective in treating whiplash injuries.

## Acute Torticollis (Wryneck)

***Etiology***    Acute torticollis, a very common condition, is more frequently called wryneck, stiff neck, or acute cervical joint lock. The patient usually complains of pain on one side of the neck on awakening. Wryneck usually occurs when a small piece of synovial membrane lining the joint capsule is impinged or trapped within a facet joint in the cervical vertebra. This problem also can follow exposure to a cold draft of air or holding of the head in an unusual position over a period of time.[79]

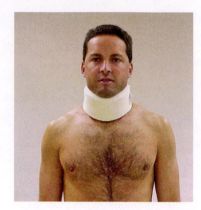

FIGURE 25–55   A soft collar can make the neck feel more comfortable.
© William E. Prentice

**Symptoms and signs**   During inspection, there is palpable point tenderness and muscle spasm. Head movement is restricted to the side opposite the irritation, with marked muscle guarding. X-ray examination will rule out a more serious injury.

**Management**   Various therapeutic modalities may be used to modulate pain in an attempt to break a pain-spasm-pain cycle. Muscle guarding can be reduced through joint mobilizations that involve gentle traction, rotation, and lateral bending, first in the pain-free direction, then in the direction of pain. The patient may find it helpful to wear a soft cervical collar for comfort (Figure 25–55). This muscle guarding will generally last for 2 to 3 days while the athlete progressively regains motion.

### Cervical Cord and Nerve Root Injuries

**Etiology**   The spinal cord and nerve roots may be injured via five basic mechanisms: laceration by bony fragments, hemorrhage, contusion, cervical cord neuropraxia, and shock.[16] These mechanisms may be combined into a single trauma or may act as separate conditions.

> The spinal cord and nerve roots may be injured via five basic mechanisms: laceration by bony fragments, hemorrhage, contusion, cervical cord neuropraxia, and shock.

**Laceration**   Laceration of the cord is usually produced by the combined dislocation and fracture of a cervical vertebra. The jagged edges of the fragmented vertebral body cut and tear nerve roots or the spinal cord and cause varying degrees of paralysis below the point of injury.

**Hemorrhage**   Hemorrhage develops from all vertebral fractures and from most dislocations as well as from sprains and strains. It seldom causes harmful effects in the musculature extradurally or even within the arachnoid space, where it dissipates faster than it can accumulate. However, hemorrhage within the cord itself causes irreparable damage.

**Contusion**   Contusion in the cord or nerve roots can arise from any force that is applied to the neck violently but does not cause a cervical dislocation or fracture. Such an injury may result from sudden displacement of a vertebra that compresses the cord and then returns to its normal position. This compression causes edematous swelling within the cord, resulting in various degrees of temporary and/or permanent damage.

**Cervical cord neuropraxia**   Occasionally, a patient, after receiving a severe twist of the neck, presents all the signs of a spinal cord injury. The patient is unable to move certain parts of the body and complains of numbness and a tingling sensation in the arms. After a short while, all these signs leave. The patient is then able to move the limbs quite freely and has no symptoms other than a sore neck. This condition is considered a cervical cord neuropraxia and is caused by cervical spine stenosis. In such cases, the patient should be cared for in the same manner used for any severe neck injury.

**Spinal cord shock**   Spinal cord shock is usually seen with severe trauma to the spinal cord, most often a cord transaction, in which there is immediate loss of function below the level of the lesion. The limbs are flaccid, in contrast to the later development of spasticity. Also, there is a total loss of deep tendon reflexes, in contrast to the later development of hyperreflexia.

**Symptoms and signs**   Each of these situations can result in various types of paralysis that affect the motor and/or sensory systems.[16] The level of the injury obviously determines the extent of the functional deficits. Spinal cord lesions may be either complete or incomplete. A complete lesion is one in which the spinal cord has been totally severed and there is a complete loss of all motor function and sensation below the level of the injury. Recovery of significant function below the level of the injury is unlikely, although some nerve root function may eventually recover one to two levels below the injury. Complete cord lesions at or above C3 impair respiration and result in death. Lesions at spinal segment levels below C4 allow for return of some nerve root function as follows:

- C4–C5—return of deltoid function
- C5–C6—return of elbow flexion and wrist extension
- C6–C7—return of elbow and finger extension and wrist flexion
- C7–T1—return of grip function

Incomplete lesions can result in central cord syndrome, Brown-Sequard syndrome, anterior cord syndrome, or posterior cord syndrome (Figure 25–56).[97] *Central cord syndrome* is caused by hemorrhage or ischemia in the central portion of the cord and results in complete quadriplegia with nonspecific sensory loss and in sexual as well as bowel-bladder dysfunction. *Brown-Sequard syndrome* is caused by an injury to one side of the spinal cord that results in loss of motor function, touch, vibration, and position sense on one side of the body and loss of pain and temperature

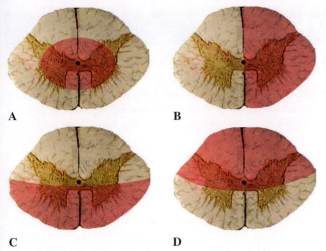

**A**              **B**

**C**              **D**

FIGURE 25–56   Incomplete cervical cord lessions.
**(A)** Central cord syndrome. **(B)** Brown-Sequard syndrome.
**(C)** Anterior cord syndrome. **(D)** Posterior cord syndrome.
© William E. Prentice

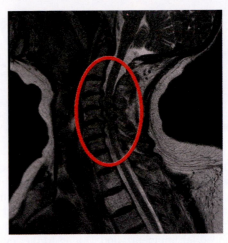

FIGURE 25–57   MRI showing cervical stenosis of the spinal canal with impingement on the spinal cord.
Courtesy Jordan B. Renner, MD, Departments of Radiology and Allied Health Sciences, University of North Carolina

sensation on the other side. *Anterior cord syndrome* is caused by an injury to the anterior two-thirds of the cord that results in loss of motor function and pain and temperature sensation. However, sexual and bowel-bladder function are present. *Posterior cord syndrome,* although rare, is caused by injury to the posterior cord. This type of injury may leave the person with good muscle power and pain and temperature sensation; however, he or she may experience difficulty in coordinating movement of the limbs.

*Management*   Like suspected cervical fractures and dislocations, suspected injuries to the spinal cord must be handled with extreme caution.[90] Care must be taken to minimize potential damage to the spinal cord. In cases in which evidence of spinal cord damage accompanied by varying degrees of paralysis exists immediately with injury, management efforts must attempt to minimize additional trauma to the cord.[8] Chapter 12 presents a detailed discussion of the recommended procedures for managing athletes with suspected spinal cord injury.

### Cervical Spine Stenosis

*Etiology*   Cervical spine stenosis is a syndrome characterized by a narrowing of the spinal canal in the cervical region that can impinge the spinal cord (Figure 25–57).[53] This stenosis occurs either as a congenital variation or from some change in the vertebrae, including the development of bone spurs, osteophytes, or disk bulges.[55] There are two methods of determining cervical spinal stenosis: the Torg ratio and the space available for the cord (SAC).[96] The Torg ratio is determined by dividing the sagittal spinal-canal diameter by the corresponding sagittal vertebral-body diameter. The SAC is determined by subtracting the sagittal spinal-cord diameter from the corresponding sagittal spinal-canal diameter.[22] The Torg

ratio and SAC are measured in millimeters. The SAC measure relies more on the spinal canal compared with the Torg ratio and therefore may be a more effective indicator of spinal stenosis. This is relevant clinically because neurological injury related to stenosis is a function of the spinal canal and the spinal cord, not the vertebral body.[96] A ratio of the sagittal canal diameter relative to anteroposterior width of the same vertebra at its midpoint of less than 0.80 suggests cervical stenosis.[22]

*Symptoms and signs*   Transient quadriplegia may occur from axial loading, hyperextension, or hyperflexion. Neck pain may be absent initially. The symptoms may be purely sensory with burning or tingling, or the athlete may have some associated motor weakness in the arms, the legs, or all four extremities.[105] Complete recovery normally occurs within 10 to 15 minutes but may be delayed. Following neurological recovery, full neck ROM is possible.

*Management*   Cervical spine stenosis may be present without any symptoms and signs. The presence of transient quadriplegia necessitates extreme caution initially. The athlete must have diagnostic tests, including X-rays or an MRI, to determine the extent of the problem.[6] Athletes, particularly those in contact sports who have been identified as

**25–6 Clinical Application Exercise**

A football linebacker is making a tackle and makes initial contact with the ball carrier with his head, forcing the neck into hyperflexion. The athlete immediately has transient quadriplegia with burning and tingling and associated motor weakness in the arms and legs. Neck pain is absent initially. Within 15 minutes, the athlete recovers completely and has full range of motion.

**?** What type of injury should the athletic trainer suspect with this athlete, and how should this condition be managed?

# MANAGEMENT PLAN

## Cervical Sprain (Whiplash)

**Injury Situation** A male patient was rear-ended in an automobile accident. Because he was not properly set for the force, his head was snapped vigorously backward into extension and forward into flexion. In this process, the patient experienced a sudden, sharp pain and a tearing sensation at the base of the posterior neck region.

**Symptoms and Signs** The patient complained to the athletic trainer that immediately after the accident there was a dull ache, stiffness, and weakness in the neck region.

Palpation revealed severe muscle spasm and point tenderness of the erector spinae muscles and the lateral aspect of the neck and upper shoulder. A neurological exam did not reveal any changes in motor or sensory abilities. X-ray examination ruled out fracture, dislocation, and spinal cord injury. Gentle passive movement produced some pain. A soft neck collar was applied for immobilization. During further evaluation, there was pain during both gentle active and resistive movement. The condition was considered to be a second-degree neck sprain with muscle involvement produced by a whiplash mechanism.

**Management Plan** The nature of a neck sprain dictates that management should follow a conservative course. A soft cervical collar was to be worn 24 hours a day for comfort until the patient was symptom free. Wearing this collar could be followed by wearing the brace just during the waking hours for 1 or 2 additional weeks.

---

*Phase* **1** *Acute Injury*   **GOALS:** To control initial hemorrhage, swelling, spasm, and pain.
**ESTIMATED LENGTH OF TIME (ELT):** 2 to 3 days.

- **Therapy** Ice pack (20 min) intermittently 6 to 8 times daily. Transcutaneous electrical nerve stimulation (TENS) can be used successfully to reduce spasm and pain in the early stages of injury.
- **Exercise rehabilitation** Patient should wear soft cervical collar. Patient should be taught to hold head in good alignment in relation to shoulder and spine; this alignment should be practiced every waking hour. Begin gentle grade 1 and 2 cervical mobilizations as tolerated.

---

*Phase* **2** *Repair*   **GOALS:** To restore 90% neck range of motion and 50% strength.
**ELT:** 7 to 10 days.

- **Therapy** Ice pack (5 to 15 min) or ice massage (7 min) 3 or 4 times; precedes active motion.
- **Exercise rehabilitation** Active stretching 2 or 3 times daily, including neck flexion with depressed shoulders, lateral neck flexion, and right and left head rotation; each position should be held 5 to 10 seconds and repeated 5 times or within pain-free limits. Gentle passive static stretching within pain-free limits (2 or 3 times each direction) once daily; each stretch should be held for 20 to 30 seconds. Manual isotonic resistive exercise to the neck should be performed once daily by the patient or athletic trainer (5 repetitions). Progress to grade 3 and 4 cervical mobilizations as tolerated.

---

*Phase* **3** *Remodeling*   **GOALS:** To restore full range of motion and full strength. To return to competition and full neck muscle bulk.
**ELT:** 4 to 7 days.

- **Therapy** Ice pack (5 to 15 min) or ice massage (7 min) once daily preceding exercise.
- **Exercise rehabilitation** Continue manual resistive exercise once daily; add resistance devices, such as weighted helmet and/or machine neck strengthener (3 sets of 10 repetitions) concept, 3 times a week. Begin practice once daily with a neck roll protective brace during first few weeks of return. Work on maximum neck resistance 3 or 4 times daily.

*Criteria for Return to Full Activity*

1. The patient is completely symptom free.
2. The patient's head has full range of motion.
3. The patient's neck has full strength and bulk.

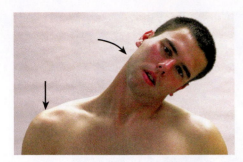

**FIGURE 25–58** Mechanism of injury for brachial plexus neuropraxia.
© William E. Prentice

having some degree of cervical stenosis, should be advised of the potential risks of continued participation in that sport. There is a growing consensus among physicians that continued participation should be discouraged.[55]

### Brachial Plexus Neuropraxia (Burner)

***Etiology*** Transient neuropraxia, resulting from stretching or compression of the brachial plexus, is the most common of all cervical neurological injuries.[80] Neuropraxia involves a disruption in normal function of a peripheral nerve, without any degenerative changes.[104] Other terms commonly used to indicate this condition are *stinger, burner,* and *pinched nerve.*[80] The primary mechanism of injury is stretching of the brachial plexus when the neck is forced laterally to the opposite side while the shoulder is depressed, as would occur with a shoulder block in football. A second mechanism compresses the brachial plexus when the neck is extended, compressed, and rotated toward the affected side (Figure 25–58).

An injury mimicking the stretch palsy is the direct injury to the upper brachial plexus from the edge of the shoulder pads impacting this area. The tip-off here is that there is usually exquisite tenderness over the trapezius, and the rhomboid muscles are spared, if there is associated weakness.[102] Injury can result in a partial rupture of the nerve without complete rupture (axontomesis), in which the myelin sheath is damaged. In this case, the nerve will eventually heal itself. In some instances, a nerve can be completely torn or avulsed. In these situations, there is no potential for recovery unless surgical reconnection is made in a timely manner.

***Symptoms and signs*** With the common burner or stinger, the patient usually complains of pain and numbness, radiating into all fingers of the hand. This implies involvement of, at least, cervical roots 6, 7, and 8. However, if there is associated weakness (most of the time there isn't), it is limited to the deltoid and biceps/brachialis muscles (especially the deltoid), implicating the C5 root. Therefore, if there is no weakness of the deltoid on on-field testing, the athlete can return to play when asymptomatic.

The patient complains of a burning sensation, numbness and tingling, and pain extending from the shoulder down to the hand, with some loss of function of the arm and hand that lasts for several minutes.[104] Rarely, symptoms persist for several days. Neck range of motion is usually normal. Repeated brachial plexus nerve stretch injuries may result in neuritis, muscular atrophy, and permanent damage.[53]

***Management*** Once the symptoms have completely resolved and there are no associated neurological symptoms, the athlete may return to full activity. Thereafter the patient should begin strengthening and stretching exercises for the neck musculature.[15] The patient should have a negative Spurling's test, full cervical and shoulder ROM, and strength to be able to return to play, as there can be associated shoulder weakness due to the nerve irritation. A football player should be fitted with shoulder pads and a cervical neck roll to limit neck range of motion during impact.[55]

### Cervical Disk Injuries

***Etiology*** Herniation of a cervical disk is relatively common. A herniation usually develops from an extruded posterolateral disk fragment or from degeneration of the disk (Figure 25–59).[22] The primary mechanism involves sustained, repetitive cervical loading during contact sports.

***Symptoms and signs*** The symptoms and signs include neck pain with some restriction in neck motion. There is radicular pain (nerve root) in the upper extremity, with associated motor weakness or sensory changes.[22]

***Management*** Initial treatment involves rest and immobilization of the neck to decrease discomfort. Neck mobilizations may help the athlete regain some range of motion. Cervical traction may also help reduce symptoms. The patient should be instructed on the importance of maintaining a neutral spine and demonstrating correct posture to facilitate stable, safe, and pain-free cervical posture during strenuous activity. If conservative treatment is not helpful or if the neurological deficits increase, surgery may be necessary.

## Thoracic Spine Conditions

Injuries to the thoracic region of the spine have a much lower incidence than do injuries to the cervical or lumbar region. This lower rate of injury is due to the articulation of the thoracic vertebrae with the ribs, which stabilizes and limits the motion of the vertebrae and thus minimizes the likelihood of injury to this area. Thoracic fractures, therefore, are relatively rare and occur in high-impact

During a preparticipation exam, a high-school wrestler describes a history of stingers.

**?** What is a stinger, and what are the symptoms of this injury?

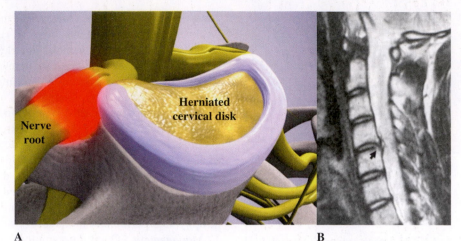

**FIGURE 25–59** **(A)** Herniated cervical disk compressing nerve root. **(B)** MRI view.

(b) Abe, Toshiki et al. "Symptomatic Cervical Disc Herniation in Teenagers: Two Case Reports." *Journal of Medical Case Reports* 7:42 (2013). PMC. © 2013 by Abe, Toshiki et al. All rights reserved. Used with permission.

sports, such as skiing, tobogganing, skydiving, and automobile racing.

### Scheuermann's Disease (Dorsolumbar Kyphosis)

*Etiology*   Scheuermann's disease is characterized by kyphosis that results from wedge fractures of 5 degrees or greater in three or more consecutive vertebral bodies, with associated disk space abnormalities and irregularity of the epiphyseal endplates. This degeneration allows the disk's nucleus pulposus to prolapse into a vertebral body. Characteristically, there is an accentuation of the kyphotic curve and backache in the young patient. Adolescents engaging in sports such as gymnastics and swimming—the butterfly stroke, particularly—are prone to this condition. The cause of Scheuermann's disease is unknown, but the occurrence of multiple minor injuries to the vertebral epiphyses seems to be an etiological factor. These injuries apparently disrupt circulation to the epiphyseal endplate, causing avascular necrosis.

*Symptoms and signs*   In the initial stages, the young patient has kyphosis of the thoracic spine and lumbar lordosis without back pain. In later stages, there is point tenderness over the spinous processes, and the young patient may complain of backache at the end of a very physically active day. Hamstring muscles are characteristically very tight.

*Management*   The major goal of management is to prevent progressive kyphosis. In the early stages of the disease, extension exercises and postural education are beneficial. Bracing, rest, and antiinflammatory medication may also be helpful. The patient may stay active but should avoid aggravating movements.

## Lumbar Spine Conditions

**Mechanisms of Low Back Pain**   Pain in the low back is second only to foot problems in order of incidence in humans throughout their life span.[68] Back problems are relatively common and are most often the result of either congenital (present at birth) or idiopathic (mechanical or traumatic) causes.[41] Many authorities think that the human back is still undergoing structural changes as a result of its upright position,

> Low back problems are most often either congenital or idiopathic.

and therefore humans are prone to slight spinal defects at birth that may cause pain later in life. The usual cause of back pain among athletes is overuse that produces strains and/or sprains of paravertebral muscles and ligaments.[21]

*Congenital anomalies*   Anomalies of bony development are the underlying cause of many back problems. Such conditions would have remained undiscovered, had it not been for some abnormal stress or injury in the area of the anomaly. The most common causes of these anomalies are excessive length of the transverse process of the fifth lumbar vertebra, incomplete closure of the neural arch (spina bifida occulta), nonconformities of the spinous processes, atypical lumbosacral angles or articular facets, and incomplete closures of the vertebral laminae.[21] All these anomalies may produce mechanical weaknesses that make the back prone to injury when it is subjected to excessive postural strains.

An example of a congenital defect that may develop into a more serious condition when aggravated by a blow or a sudden twist is spondylolisthesis. Spondylolisthesis is a forward subluxation of the body of a vertebra, usually the fifth lumbar.

***Mechanical Defects of the Spine***   Mechanical back defects are caused mainly by faulty posture, obesity, and faulty body mechanics—all of which may affect the patient's activity.[50] Traumatic forces produced either directly or indirectly can result in contusions, sprains, strains, and/or fractures. Sometimes even minor injuries can develop into chronic and recurrent conditions, which may have serious complications for the patient. To fully understand a back complaint, the athletic trainer should make a logical investigation into the history and the site of any injury, the type of pain produced, and the extent of impairment of normal function.[12]

Maintaining proper segmental alignment of the body during standing, sitting, lying, running, jumping, and throwing is of utmost importance for keeping the body in good condition. Habitual violations of the principles of good body mechanics occur in many sports and produce anatomical deficiencies that subject the body to constant abnormal muscular and ligamentous strain. In all cases of postural deformity, the athletic trainer should determine the cause and attempt to rectify the condition through proper strength and mobilization exercises.[4]

### Recurrent and Chronic Low Back Pain
Following an episode of low back pain it is likely that a patient will have further recurrent episodes of pain.[83] Repeated strains or sprains in the low back can cause the supporting tissues to lose their ability to stabilize the spine and thus produce tissue laxity. After repeated episodes, the patient may develop what is referred to as chronic low back pain.[60] Recurrent or chronic low back pain can have many causes, including malalignment of the vertebral facets, discogenic disease, and nerve root compression, all of which can result in pain. Gradually, this problem could lead to muscular weakness and impairment of sensation and reflex responses. The incidence of this condition at the secondary-school level is relatively low but becomes progressively greater with increasing age. Adolescents have a 70 to 80 percent incidence of back pain before the age of 20.[51] The older the patient, the more prone he or she is to developing chronic low back pain.[78] Females are more likely to have low back pain than males. An acute back condition is the culmination of a long, progressive degeneration aggravated or accentuated by sudden flexion, extension, or rotation.[71]

### Lumbar Vertebrae Fracture and Dislocation

*Etiology* Fractures of the vertebral column, in terms of bone injury, are not serious in themselves, but they pose dangers when related to spinal cord damage. Vertebral fractures of the greatest concern are compression fractures and fractures of the transverse and spinous processes.[76]

The compression fracture may occur as a result of hyperflexion of the trunk (Figure 25–60). Falling from a height and landing on the feet or buttocks may also produce a compression fracture. The vertebrae that are most often compressed are those in the dorsolumbar curves. The vertebrae usually are crushed anteriorly by the traumatic force of the body

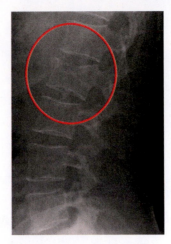

FIGURE 25–60   Lumbar compression fracture.
Courtesy  Jordan B. Renner, MD, Departments of Radiology and Allied Health Sciences, University of North Carolina

above the site of injury. The crushed vertebral body may spread out fragments and protrude into the spinal canal, compressing and possibly even cutting the cord.[21]

Fractures of the transverse and spinous processes result most often from kicks or another direct impact to the back. Because these processes are surrounded by large muscles, fracture produces extensive soft-tissue injury. The fractures themselves present little danger and usually permit the patient considerable activity within the range of pain tolerance. Most care and treatment will be oriented toward therapy of the soft-tissue pathology.[21]

Dislocations of the lumbar vertebrae are rare and occur only with an associated fracture. This infrequency is due to the orientation of the facet joints in the lumbar vertebrae.

*Symptoms and signs* Recognition of the compression fracture is difficult without an X-ray examination. A basic evaluation may be made through knowledge of the history and through point tenderness over the affected vertebrae. Fractures of the transverse and spinous processes may be directly palpable. There is point tenderness with some localized swelling, along with muscle guarding to protect the area.

*Management* If the symptoms and signs associated with a fracture are present, the injured athlete should be X-rayed. Transporting and moving the patient should be done on a spine board, as described in Chapter 12, in an effort to minimize movement of the fractured segment.

### Low Back Muscle Strains

*Etiology* There are two mechanisms of the typical low back strain.[21] The first is a sudden extension contraction on an overloaded, unprepared, or underdeveloped spine, usually in combination with trunk rotation. The second is

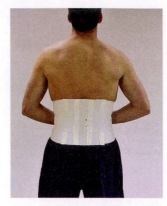

**FIGURE 25–61** An abdominal brace helps support the lumbar area.
© William E. Prentice

the chronic strain, commonly associated with faulty posture, that involves excessive lumbar lordosis.[50] However, other postures, such as flatback posture or scoliosis, can also predispose a patient to strain.

***Symptoms and signs*** Evaluation should be performed immediately after injury to rule out the possibility of fracture. Discomfort in the low back may be diffused or localized in one area. In the case of muscle strain, pain is present on active extension and with passive flexion. There is no radiating pain farther than the buttocks or thigh and no neurological involvement that causes muscle weakness, sensation impairment, or reflex impairments.

***Management*** In the acute phase of this injury, it is essential that cold packs and/or ice massage be used intermittently throughout the day to decrease muscle spasm. An elastic wrap or corset-type brace will help compress the area. A graduated program of stretching and strengthening begins slowly during the acute stage. Progressive strengthening exercises should include stabilization exercises (e.g., planks) using abdominal bracing and modified activity to activate the muscles that are shutting down (e.g., multifidus). Postural control is important. The physician may prescribe oral analgesic medication. Cryotherapy, ultrasound, and an abdominal support (Figure 25–61) are often beneficial following the acute phase. Exercise must not cause pain.

### Myofascial Pain Syndrome

***Etiology*** Myofascial pain syndrome is defined as a regional pain with referred pain to a specific area that occurs with pressure or palpation of tender spots or trigger points within a specific muscle.[49] A trigger point is an area of tenderness in a tight band of muscle. Palpation of the trigger point produces pain in a predictable distribution of referred pain.[58] There may also be some restricted range of motion because of pain. Pressure on the trigger point produces a twitch or jump response from the pain.

Pain can be increased by passive or active stretching of the involved muscle. Painful or active trigger points most often develop because of some mechanical stress to the muscle. This stress could involve either an acute muscle strain or static postural positions that produce constant tension in the muscle.[49] Trigger points occur most typically in the neck, upper back, and low back. In the low back, there are two muscles in which trigger points commonly occur: the piriformis and the quadratus lumborum.

The piriformis muscle was discussed in Chapter 21. It is an external rotator of the thigh and is located posterior to the hip joint in the sciatic notch. The piriformis muscle is important because of its proximity to the sciatic nerve. The sciatic nerve either pierces the piriformis or courses directly above or below it.

The quadratus lumborum originates on the 12th rib and the transverse processes of L1 through L4. It inserts on the iliac crest. The quadratus elevates the pelvis.

***Symptoms and signs*** Palpation of or pressure on a trigger point in the piriformis muscle in the sciatic notch refers pain to the posterior sacroiliac region, to the buttocks, and occasionally down to the posterior or posterolateral thigh. Pain is a deep ache that increases with exercise or with prolonged sitting while the hip is adducted, flexed, and medially rotated. Isometric abduction and passive internal rotation increase pain. Sciatic pain may also occur, with diminished sensation in the leg.[49]

A trigger point in the quadratus lumborum produces a sharp, aching pain in the lateral low back or flank. Pain may be referred to the upper buttocks and posterior sacroiliac region and sometimes to the abdominal wall. Pain increases when the patient stands for long periods, moves from sitting to standing, or coughs or sneezes. There will be muscle spasm with pain that is localized to one side. Pain increases when the patient side bends toward the side of the trigger point.

***Management*** Rehabilitation exercises should include both stretching and strengthening of the involved muscle. The key in treating myofascial pain is to stretch the muscle back to a normal resting length and thus relieve the irritation that created the trigger point.[1] The patient should be placed in a comfortable position that also stretches the involved muscle. Active stretching should be mild and progressive. The use of electrical stimulation in combination with ultrasound is helpful in relieving the pain associated with a trigger point. A spray and stretch technique has also been used successfully (see Chapter 15). Progressive strengthening exercises should also be included.

### Lumbar Sprains

***Etiology*** Sprains may occur in any of the ligaments in the lumbar spine. The most common sprain involves lumbar facet joints. Facet joint sprain typically occurs when the patient bends forward and twists while lifting or moving some object.[50] A traumatic force overextends the spinal joints and causes a sudden onset of a deep, sharp pain. It can occur with a single episode or with chronic, repetitive stress that causes a gradual onset that becomes progressively worse with activity.

*Symptoms and signs*   The pain is localized and is located just lateral to the spinous process. Pain becomes sharper with certain movements or postures, and the athlete will limit movement in painful ranges. Passive anteroposterior or rotational movement of the vertebrae will increase pain. Pain can be reproduced with certain movements.

*Management*   Like sprains to other joints in the body, the lumbar sprain requires some time to heal. Initial treatment should include POLICE to reduce pain. Joint mobilizations that use anteroposterior and rotational glides can be used to help decrease pain. Strengthening exercises for abdominals and back extensors as well as stretches in all directions should be limited to a pain-free range. The patient should be instructed in trunk stabilization exercises.[50] A brace or support should be worn to limit movement during early return to activity. It is important to guard against the development of postural changes that may occur in response to pain.

## Back Contusions

*Etiology*   Back contusions rank third to strains and sprains in incidence. Because of its surface area, the back is quite vulnerable to contusion. A history that includes a significant impact to the back could indicate an extremely serious condition. Contusion of the back must be distinguished from a vertebral fracture.[50] In some instances, this distinction is possible only through an X-ray examination.

*Symptoms and signs*   The bruise causes local pain, muscle spasm, and point tenderness. A swollen, discolored area may be visible.

*Management*   Cold and pressure should be applied immediately for approximately 72 hours or longer, along with rest. Ice massage combined with gradual stretching benefits soft-tissue contusion in the region of the low back. Recovery usually ranges from 2 days to 2 weeks. Ultrasound is effective in treating the deep muscles.

## Sciatica

*Etiology*   Sciatica is an inflammatory condition of the sciatic nerve that can accompany recurrent or chronic low back pain. The term *sciatica* has been incorrectly used as a general term to describe all low back pain without reference to exact causes. Sciatica is commonly associated with peripheral nerve root compression from intervertebral disk protrusion, structural irregularities within the intervertebral foramina, or tightness of the piriformis muscle. The sciatic nerve is particularly vulnerable to torsion or direct blows that tend to impose abnormal stretching and pressure on it as it emerges from the spine, thus effecting a traumatic condition.[60]

*Symptoms and signs*   Sciatica may begin either abruptly or gradually. It produces a sharp, shooting pain that follows the nerve pathway along the posterior and medial thigh. There may also be some tingling and numbness along its path. The nerve may be extremely sensitive to palpation. Straight-leg raising usually intensifies the pain.

*Management*   In the acute stage, rest is essential. The cause of the inflammation must be identified and treated. If there is a disk protrusion, lumbar traction may be appropriate. Stretching of a tight piriformis muscle may also decrease symptoms. Because recovery from sciatica usually occurs within 2 to 3 weeks, surgery should be delayed to see whether symptoms resolve. Oral antiinflammatory medication may help reduce inflammation.[50]

## Herniated Lumbar Disk

*Etiology*   The lumbar disks are subject to constant abnormal stresses that stem from faulty body mechanics, trauma, or both, which, over a period of time, can cause degeneration, tears, and cracks in the annulus fibrosus.[63] The disk most often injured lies between the L4–L5 vertebrae. The L5–S1 disk is the second most commonly affected.

The mechanism of a disk injury is the same as for the lumbosacral sprain—forward bending and twisting that places abnormal strain on the lumbar region. The movement that produces herniation, or bulging, of the nucleus pulposus may be minimal, and associated pain may be significant.[44] Besides injuring soft tissues, such a stress may herniate an already degenerated disk by causing the nucleus pulposus to protrude into or through the annulus fibrosis (Figure 25–62).

> A herniated lumbar disk can be prolapsed, extruded, or sequestered.

---

A swimmer complains of an area of tenderness in a tight band of muscle in the middle of her upper back. Palpation of the trigger point refers pain around the chest wall. Pain is increased by both passive and active stretching of the involved muscle. Pain is usually increased following a long training workout in the pool.

**?** What type of muscular problem frequently develops in the middle or low back of athletes who engage in repetitive motions that fatigue a muscle? How is this problem best managed?

# MANAGEMENT PLAN

## Lumbosacral Strain

**Injury Situation** A patient who works for a moving company is seen by an athletic trainer working in a hospital-based clinic. The patient complains of a very sore back. He indicates that he woke up with the problem and was not sure how it occurred.

**Symptoms and Signs** The patient complains of a constant, dull ache and an inability to flex, extend, or rotate the trunk without increasing the pain. Inspection of the injury indicates the following:

1. The patient has a pronounced lumbar lordosis.
2. There is an obvious muscle contraction of the right erector spinae.
3. There is severe point tenderness in the right lumbar region.
4. The right pelvis is elevated.
5. Passive movement does not cause pain; however, active and resistive movements produce severe pain.
6. Range of motion in all directions is restricted.
7. All tests for nerve root, hip joint, and sacroiliac joint are negative.
8. Leg length was measured, and the patient has a functional shortening but no apparent structural shortening.
9. Both the left and right hamstring muscle groups and iliopsoas muscles are abnormally tight.
10. X-ray examination showed no pathological conditions of the lumbar vertebrae.

Based on the examination, it was concluded that the patient has sustained a grade 1 to grade 2 strain of the lumbar muscles, primarily in the right erector spinae region.

---

*Phase* **1** *Acute Injury*  **GOALS:** To relieve muscle spasm and pain.
**ESTIMATED LENGTH OF TIME (ELT):** 2 or 3 days.

- **Therapy** Ice pack (20 min) followed by exercise and then TENS (15 to 20 min) 3 or 4 times daily.
- **Exercise rehabilitation** Following cold application, gentle passive stretch of low back region and hamstring and iliopsoas muscles—all within pain tolerance levels—3 or 4 times daily, along with grade 1 and 2 mobilizations of affected segments.

---

*Phase* **2** *Repair*  **GOALS:** To increase low back, hamstring, and iliopsoas ROM to at least begin postural correction and 50% normal extensibility of the low back, hamstring, and iliopsoas muscles. Appropriate abdominal strength.
**ELT:** 4 to 12 days.

- **Therapy** Ice massage followed by exercise 2 or 3 times daily. If there still is pain, TENS therapy should be used. Ultrasound 1 to 1.5 watts/cm² once daily.
- **Exercise rehabilitation** Repeat Phase 1 exercise and begin PNF to hip and low back regions 2 or 3 times daily; or static low back, hamstring, and iliopsoas stretching (2 or 3 repetitions) and lower abdominal strengthening 2 or 3 times daily. Continue grade 1 and 2 mobilizations, progressing to grades 3 and 4 as tolerated. Practice realigning pelvis. General body maintenance exercises should be conducted (as long as they do not aggravate the injury) 3 times a week.

---

*Phase* **3** *Remodeling*  **GOALS:** To restore 90% of ROM, strength, and proper back alignment.
**ELT:** 13 days to 3 weeks.

- **Exercise rehabilitation** Patient should be instructed about proper back alignment when lifting. Patient should wear a back brace or belt while working. Patient should begin a spinal stabilization program.

*Criteria for Return to Work*

1. The patient's back must be pain free and spasm free.
2. The patient must be near normal in hamstring, low back, and iliopsoas extensibility.
3. The patient must be making good progress toward correcting lumbar lordosis.
4. The patient must be able to perform lifting activities with the spine and pelvis in good alignment.

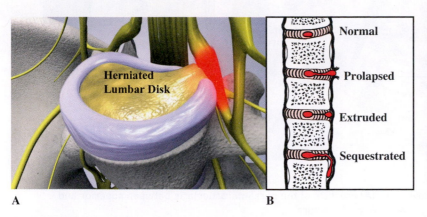
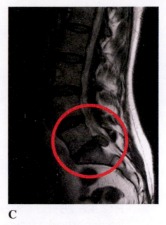

A                                    B                                    C

FIGURE 25–62 **(A)** A herniated lumbar disk compressing a nerve root. **(B)** Further degeneration can lead to a prolapsed disk, an extruded disk, or a sequestrated disk. **(C)** MRI image of a herniated lumbar disk.

(c) Courtesy Jordan B. Renner, MD, Departments of Radiology and Allied Health Sciences, University of North Carolina

A disk that progressively degenerates may develop into a *prolapsed disk,* in which the nucleus moves completely through the annulus. If the nucleus moves into the spinal canal and comes in contact with a nerve root, the result is an *extruded disk.* This protrusion of the nucleus pulposus may place pressure on the cord of spinal nerves and thus cause radiating pains similar to those of sciatica. A *sequestrated disk* occurs when the material of the nucleus separates from the disk and begins to migrate.[44]

Pressure within the intervertebral disks changes with various positions or postures. Studies that used intervertebral pressure in the standing position as a constant found that pressure was decreased by 75 percent when the spine was in the supine position and by 25 percent when the spine was in the side-lying position. Pressure was increased by 33 percent while the patient was sitting, by 33 percent while the patient was standing slightly bent forward, by 45 percent while the patient was sitting slightly bent forward, by 52 percent while the patient was standing bent far forward, and by 63 percent while the patient was sitting bent well forward.

***Symptoms and signs*** There is usually a sharp, centrally located pain that radiates unilaterally in a dermatomal pattern to the buttocks and down the back of the leg, or pain that spreads across the back.[50] The patient may describe weakness in the lower limb. Symptoms are worse in the morning with axial loading, such as when the patient gets out of bed. Onset may be sudden or gradual, and pain may increase after the patient sits and then tries to resume activity. Forward bending and sitting increase pain. Backward bending reduces pain. The patient's posture will exhibit a slight forward bend with side bending away from the side of pain. Side bending toward the side of pain is limited and increases pain. There is tenderness around the painful area. Straight-leg raising to 30 degrees increases

pain. Tendon reflexes may be diminished. Muscle testing may reveal weakness with bilateral differences. A Valsalva maneuver increases the pain (e.g., coughing, sneezing). The athlete has difficulty putting on shoes and socks.[50]

***Management*** Initial treatment should involve pain-reducing modalities, such as ice or electrical stimulation. Manual traction combined with passive backward bending or extension makes the athlete more comfortable. The goal is to reduce the protrusion and restore normal posture. Thus, the patient should be taught appropriate posture self-correction exercises. As pain and posture return to normal, back extensor and abdominal strengthening should be used.[63]

If the disk is extruded or sequestrated, all the athletic trainer can do is to modulate pain with electrical stimulation. Doing flexion exercises and lying supine in a flexed position may help with comfort. Sometimes the symptoms resolve with time. However, if there are signs of nerve damage, surgery may be required to eliminate pain and dysfunction.[108]

### Spondylolysis and Spondylolisthesis

***Etiology*** Spondylolysis is a degeneration of the vertebrae and, more commonly, a defect in the pars interarticularis, which is the region between the superior and inferior articulating facets of a vertebra (Figure 25–63).[52] The condition is often attributed to a congenital weakness, and the defect occurs as a stress fracture.[52] It is more common among boys.[93] Spondylolysis may produce no symptoms unless a disk herniation occurs or there is sudden trauma, such as hyperextension.[82] Movements that characteristically hyperextend the spine, such as the back arch in gymnastics, the lifting of weights, the football block, the tennis serve, the volleyball spike, and the butterfly stroke in swimming,[67] are most likely to cause this condition.

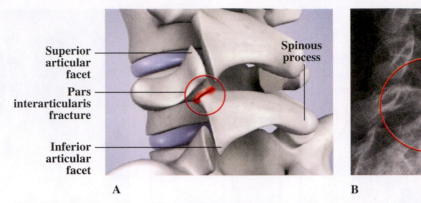

Superior
articular
facet

Spinous
process

Pars
interarticularis
fracture

Inferior
articular
facet

**A**                    **B**

FIGURE 25–63   Spondylolysis. **(A)** Fracture of the pars interarticularis between superior and inferior articular facets. **(B)** X-ray view of fracture.

(b) Courtesy Jordan B. Renner, MD, Departments of Radiology and Allied Health Sciences, University of North Carolina

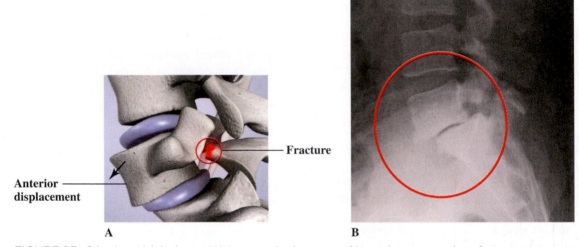

Fracture

Anterior
displacement

**A**                    **B**

FIGURE 25–64   Spondylolisthesis. **(A)** Anterior displacement of L5 with pars articularis fracture. **(B)** X-ray view.

(b) Courtesy Jordan B. Renner, MD, Departments of Radiology and Allied Health Sciences, University of North Carolina

Commonly, spondylolysis begins unilaterally. If it extends bilaterally, however, there may be some slipping of one vertebra on the one below it. This condition, called a spondylolisthesis, is considered to be a complication of spondylolysis that often results in hypermobility of a vertebral segment.[82] Spondylolisthesis's highest incidence is with L5 slipping on S1, which is referred to as a *step deformity* (Figure 25–64).[39] Although pars interarticularis defects are more common among boys, the incidence of slippage is higher in girls. Spondylolisthesis may be asymptomatic.[50] The patient with this condition usually has a lumbar hyperlordosis postural impairment. A direct blow, a sudden twist, or chronic low back strain may cause the defective vertebra to displace itself forward on the sacrum. A spondylolisthesis is easily detectable on X-ray.

> Spondylolisthesis is considered to be a complication of spondylolysis.

***Symptoms and signs***
The patient complains of persistent mild to moderate aching pain across the low back or a stiffness in the low back, with increased pain after, but not usually during, physical activity.[92] There is usually a complaint that the low back area feels tired and fatigues easily. The patient feels the need to change positions frequently or to self-manipulate the low back to reduce the pain. Movements of the trunk are full range

A gymnast constantly hyperextends her low back. She complains of stiffness and persistent, aching pain across the low back, with increased pain after, but not usually during, practice. The athlete feels that she needs to change positions frequently or self-manipulate her low back to reduce the pain. She is beginning to develop pain in her buttock and some muscle weakness in her leg.

**?** What type of injury should the athletic trainer suspect the gymnast has, and what can be done about it?

and painless, with some hesitation in forward bending. At extreme ranges held for 30 seconds, an aching pain develops. The patient feels weak when straightening from forward bending. There may be tenderness localized to one segment. When applying posteroanterior pressure to the spinous process during palpation, the athletic trainer may note some segmental hypermobility. If displacement is great enough, there may be some neurological signs.[92]

***Management*** Bracing and, occasionally, bed rest for 1 to 3 days will help reduce pain. The major focus in rehabilitation should be directed toward exercises that control or stabilize the hypermobile segment. Progressive trunk strengthening exercises, especially through the midrange, should be incorporated. Dynamic core stabilization exercises that concentrate on abdominal muscles should also be used. Braces are most helpful during high-level activities. Hypermobility of a lumbar vertebra may make the patient more susceptible to lumbar muscle strains and ligament sprains. Thus, it may be necessary for the athlete to avoid vigorous activity.[50]

## Sacroiliac Joint Dysfunction

The sacroiliac is the junction formed by the ilium and the sacrum, and it is fortified by strong ligaments that allow little motion to take place. Because the sacroiliac joint is a synovial joint, disorders can include sprain, inflammation, hypermobility, and hypomobility.

### Sacroiliac Sprain

***Etiology*** A sprain of the sacroiliac joint may result when the patient twists with both feet on the ground, stumbles forward, falls backward, steps too far down and lands heavily on one leg, or bends forward with the knees locked during lifting.[71] It may also occur from downhill running or repetitive unilateral activities, such as overrotating a golf swing, dancing, punting, high jumping, hurdling, or performing gymnastics. Any of these mechanisms can produce irritation and stretching of the sacrotuberous or sacrospinous ligaments. These mechanisms may also cause either an anterior or a posterior rotation of one side of the pelvis relative to the other. With rotation of the pelvis, there is hypomobility.[50] As healing occurs, the joint on the injured side may become hypermobile, allowing that joint to sublux in either an anteriorly or a posteriorly rotated position.[14] Stress fracture, although uncommon, can also occur in the sacrum with repetitive unilateral activities.[7]

***Symptoms and signs*** With a sprain of the sacroiliac joint, there may be palpable pain and tenderness directly over the joint just inferior and medial to the PSIS, with some associated muscle guarding. Occasionally, pain radiates to the posterior, lateral, or anterior thigh, and there may be a vaguely located groin pain without associated tenderness. Pain is increased or

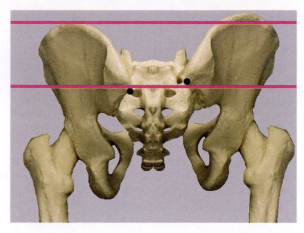

**FIGURE 25–65** The black dots identify the PSIS on each side. The right PSIS appears higher than the left. In this case, there is an anterior rotation of the right innominate.
© William E. Prentice

generated with unilateral stance on that leg and walking, with increased pain uphill or downhill. Rolling over will often precipitate or increase the pain. Sitting is usually comfortable, but movement from sitting to standing creates pain. The athletic trainer may observe that the ASIS and/or PSIS may be asymmetrical when compared with the opposite side, which is caused by either anterior or posterior rotation of one side of the pelvis relative to the other (Figure 25–65). There may also be a measurable leg-length difference. Forward bending reveals a block to normal movement, and the PSIS on the injured side moves sooner than the one on the normal side. Straight-leg raising increases pain after 45 degrees. Side bending toward the painful side increases pain.[50]

***Management*** Modalities can be used to reduce pain. A supportive brace is also helpful in an acute sprain. Manual therapy techniques such as muscle energy or mobilizations can be used to correct asymmetries. If one side of the pelvis is posteriorly rotated, it should be mobilized in an anterior direction.[71] Strengthening exercises should be incorporated to improve stability to a hypermobile joint.

## Coccygeal Injuries

***Etiology*** Coccygeal injuries are prevalent and occur primarily from direct impact, which may result from forcibly sitting down, falling, or being kicked by an opponent. Injuries to the coccyx include sprains, subluxations, and fractures. With healing, the sacrococcygeal joint may become hypermobile and thus restrict passive motion.

***Symptoms and signs*** Patients with persistent coccyalgia, or pain in the coccyx, should be referred to a physician for X-rays and rectal examinations. Pain in the coccygeal region is often-prolonged and at times chronic.

Such conditions are identified by the term *coccygodynia* and occur as a result of an irritation to the coccygeal plexus.

***Management*** Treatment consists of analgesics and a ring seat to relieve the pressure on the coccyx while sitting. Pain from a fractured coccyx may last for many months. Once a coccygeal injury has healed, the patient should be protected against reinjury by appropriately applied padding.

# REHABILITATION TECHNIQUES FOR THE NECK

## Joint Mobilizations

Mobilization techniques for the cervical spine are extensively used in rehabilitating the injured neck. Mobilization can decrease pain, restore mobility, and increase range of motion.[28] The most common joint mobilization techniques for the cervical spine are the following (Figure 25–66):

1. Cervical flexion mobilizations, which increase forward bending and flexion
2. Cervical extension mobilizations, which increase backward bending and extension
3. Cervical rotation mobilizations, which treat pain or stiffness when there is some resistance in the same direction as the rotation

4. Cervical side bending mobilizations, which treat pain and stiffness when there is some resistance to side bending of the neck
5. Cervical traction, which is used to relieve discogenic pain or increase range of motion

## Flexibility Exercises

The first consideration in neck rehabilitation should be restoration of the neck's normal range of motion. The patient who had a prior restricted range of motion should work on increasing it to a more normal range. A second goal is to strengthen the neck as much as possible. All mobility exercises should be performed pain free. Stretching exercises include passive and active movement.[50]

The patient sits in a straight-backed chair while the athletic trainer applies a gentle passive stretch through a pain-free range. Extension, flexion, lateral flexion, and rotation in each direction is sustained for a count of six and repeated three times. Passive stretching should be conducted daily.

The patient is also instructed to actively stretch the neck two or three times daily. Each exercise is performed for 8 to 10 repetitions, with each endpoint held for a count of six. All exercises are performed without force. Figure 25–67 shows forward flexion, extension, lateral flexion, and rotation.

Stretching can progress gradually to a more vigorous procedure, such as the *Billig procedure*. In this exercise,

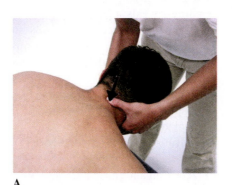

A

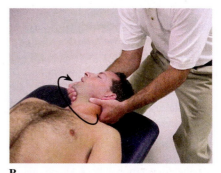

B

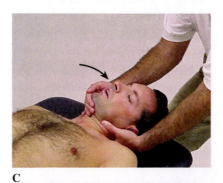

C

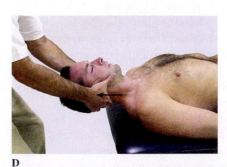

D

FIGURE 25–66 Cervical mobilizations. **(A)** Cervical facet anterior-posterior glides. **(B)** Cervical rotation. **(C)** Cervical side bending. **(D)** Cervical traction.
© William E. Prentice

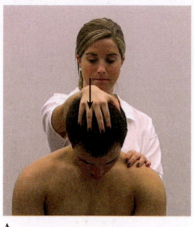
A

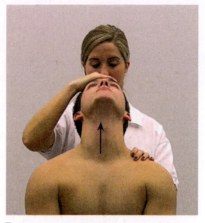
B

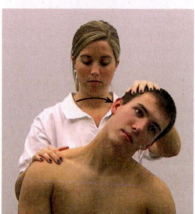
C

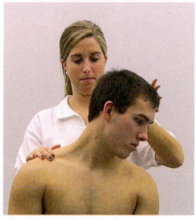
D

FIGURE 25–67   Neck stretching is important in increasing neck mobility after injury. **(A)** Forward flexion. **(B)** Extension. **(C)** Lateral flexion. **(D)** Rotation.
© William E. Prentice

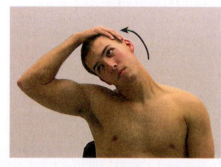

FIGURE 25–68   Stretching the lateral neck flexors by the Billig procedure.
© William E. Prentice

the patient sits on a chair, with one hand firmly grasping the seat of the chair. The other hand, over the top of the head, is placed above the ear on the side of the support hand. Keeping that hand in place, the patient gently pulls the opposite side of the neck. The stretch should be held for 6 seconds (Figure 25–68). The patient can apply a rotary stretch in each direction in the same manner.

## Strengthening Exercises

When the patient has gained near-normal range of motion, a strength program should be instituted. All exercises should be conducted pain free. In the beginning, each exercise is performed with the head in an upright position facing straight forward. Exercises are performed isometrically; each resistance is held for a count of six. The patient should start with 5 repetitions and progress to 10 repetitions (Figure 25–69).

1. Flexion—press forehead against palm of hand.
2. Extension—lace fingers behind head and press head back against hands.
3. Lateral flexion—place palm on side of head and press head into palm.
4. Rotation—put one palm on side of forehead and the other at back of the head. Push with each hand, attempting to rotate head. Change hands and reverse direction.

Strengthening progresses to isotonic exercises through a full range of motion, using manual resistance, special equipment (such as a towel), or weighted devices (Figure 25–70). Each exercise is performed

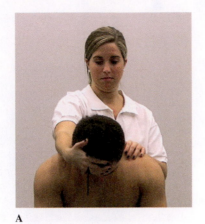

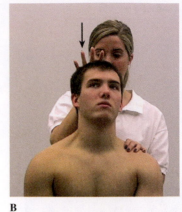

**A**

**B**

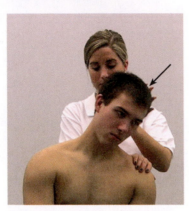

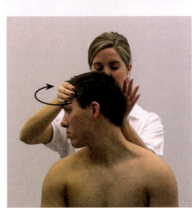

**C**

**D**

FIGURE 25–69    Manual neck-strengthening exercises. **(A)** Flexion. **(B)** Extension. **(C)** Lateral flexion. **(D)** Rotation.

© William E. Prentice

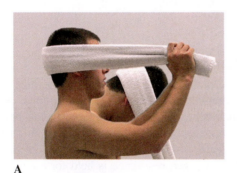

**A**

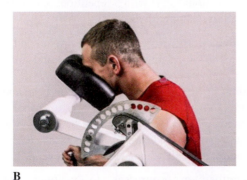

**B**

FIGURE 25–70    Neck strengthening using resistive devices. **(A)** Towel. **(B)** Exercise machine.

(a) © William E. Prentice; (b) Courtesy Rogers Athletic Company

for 10 repetitions and two or three sets. NOTE: The patient must be cautioned against overstressing the neck and must be encouraged to increase resistance gradually.

## REHABILITATION TECHNIQUES FOR THE LOW BACK

Over the years, many techniques for the treatment and rehabilitation of low back pain have been recommended. Individuals such as Williams, McKenzie, Cyriax, Maitland, Paris, Saal, and McGill have proposed effective and specific philosophical approaches for managing individuals with low back pain.[35] In some instances, the approach used the same exercises for all low back pain patients, regardless of the existing etiology. Today the techniques for treating low back pain incorporate a more eclectic approach and use a combination of the most applicable and useful aspects of each of the philosophical approaches.[50]

Factors to consider in a rehabilitation program are fitness level, training goals, previous lumbar injury, workplace environment, sport, and psychosocial issues. Other issues are proper breathing, lumbar and lower extremity flexibility, low back and pelvis muscle strength, low back and pelvis muscle endurance, cardiovascular fitness, order and amount of exercise, and time of day to exercise.[60]

The initial treatment for low back pain should focus on modulating pain.[56] Following acute injury, ice should be used along with electrical stimulating currents for analgesia. Rest is also helpful in allowing the injured structures to begin the healing process. It is essential that the athletic trainer avoid movements or positions that increase pain, while positioning the patient in a posture that minimizes pain and discomfort.

Analgesics and oral antiinflammatory agents are commonly given to inhibit pain and reduce inflammation in the patient with a low back problem.[56] If muscle spasm or guarding is severe, muscle relaxants may be prescribed.

Progressive relaxation techniques can also be useful in treating low back pain. With constant pain come anxiety and increased muscular tension that compounds the low back problem. By systematically contracting and completely "letting go" of the body's major muscles, the patient learns to recognize abnormal tension and to relax the muscles consciously. Various relaxation techniques are discussed in Chapter 11.

## General Body Conditioning

The low back pain that patients most often encounter is an acute, painful experience that rarely lasts longer than 3 weeks. In the initial stages of acute injury, however, there can be a great deal of pain and disability. In some of the conditions described in this chapter, any movement at all can produce incapacitating low back pain. Thus, patients with certain conditions may find it difficult to maintain general body conditioning, particularly during the acute stage of healing. It may be necessary to eliminate any type of conditioning during the first several days. The patient should resume conditioning activities as soon as the condition has resolved to the point that discomfort can be tolerated.[98] The patient may find it helpful to use aquatic exercise as a method for maintaining cardiorespiratory endurance, because the pain that often occurs with weight bearing may be minimized.

## Joint Mobilizations

Joint mobilization of the lumbar spine may be used to improve joint mobility or to decrease joint pain by restoring to the joint accessory movements that will help the patient achieve a nonrestricted, pain-free range of motion.[18,24] Vertebral joints in the lumbar region are capable of both anterior and posterior gliding or rotation, or some combination of the two; mobilization techniques should address all restricted joint motions. Grade 1 and 2 mobilizations may be incorporated early in the rehabilitation program for managing pain. Mobilization may progress to grades 3 and 4 once pain

and muscle guarding are decreased. For best results, mobilization should be combined with manual traction techniques.

Joint mobilization techniques for the low back are indicated when:

- Pain is centralized at a specific joint and increases with activity and decreases with rest.
- Active and passive range of motion are decreased.
- There is muscle tightness.
- Forward and backward bending deviates from the midline.
- Rotation and side bending produce asymmetrical movements.
- Accessory motion at individual spinal segments is decreased.

Specific mobilization techniques for the low back are the following (Figure 25–71):

A. Anterior/posterior lumbar vertebrae mobilizations to decrease pain and increase the mobility of individual vertebrae
B. Lumbar lateral distraction to reduce pain associated with some compression of a spinal nerve
C. Lumbar vertebral rotation mobilizations to decrease pain and increase the mobility of individual vertebrae
D. Anterior sacral mobilizations to reduce pain and muscle guarding around the sacroiliac joint
E. Anterior rotation mobilizations to correct a unilateral posterior rotation
F. Posterior rotation mobilizations to correct a unilateral anterior rotation
G. SI posterior rotation mobilization to correct a posterior rotation
H. SI lateral rotation mobilization to correct a postural asymmetry
I. Thoracic rib facet joint mobilization to correct rib alignment

A clinical prediction rule has been developed to help the clinician decide when a spinal manipulation is appropriate. The criteria include:[19]

- Duration of the current episode is less than 16 days.
- No symptoms distal to the knee.
- One hypermobile segment exists in the lumbar spine.
- Hip internal rotation is greater than 35 degrees.

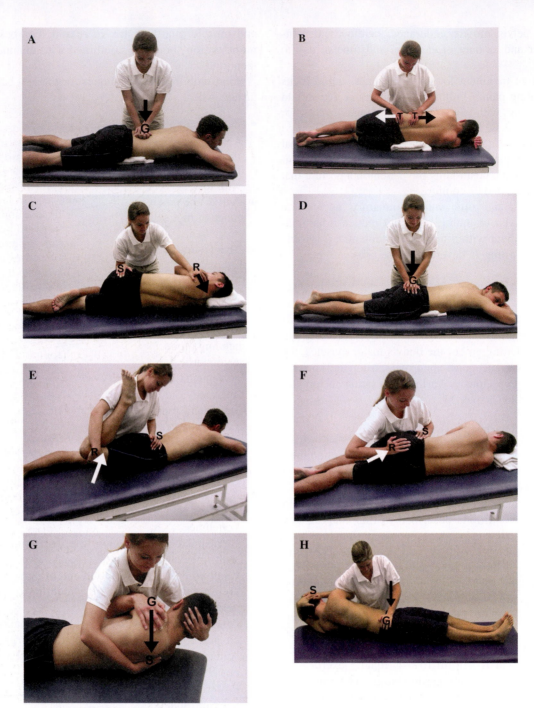

FIGURE 25–71   Low back and thoracic mobilizations. **(A)** Anterior lumbar vertebrae mobilization. **(B)** Lumbar lateral distraction. **(C)** Lumbar vertebral rotation. **(D)** Anterior sacral mobilization. **(E)** Anterior inominate rotation mobilization. **(F)** Posterior innominate rotation mobilization. **(G)** Thoracic facet joint mobilization **(H)** SI posterior rotation mobilization.
(S = stabilize, G = glide R = rotate)
© William E. Prentice

**Traction** Traction is the treatment of choice when there is a small protrusion of the nucleus pulposus. Through traction, the lumbar vertebrae are distracted; a subatmospheric pressure is created, which tends to pull the protrusion to its original position; and there is tightening of the longitudinal ligament, which tends to push the protrusion toward its original position within the disk.[50] Traction may be done manually or with a traction machine. Sustained traction for at least 30 minutes with a force commensurate with body weight is preferred. An 80-pound (35-kilogram) force would be the minimum for a small woman, and a 180-pound (80-kilogram) force would be the minimum for a large man.[50] Traction is usually applied daily (five times per week) for 2 weeks.

## Flexibility Exercises

Back pain may be caused by tightness or a lack of flexibility in a number of different muscle groups related to movement of the low back.[2] An assessment of the flexibility of the muscle groups will indicate which ones are tight and need to be stretched. The following muscle groups may need to be stretched (Figure 25–72):

A. Low back extensors
B. Lumbar rotators and hip abductors
C. Lumbar lateral flexors
D. Hip adductors
E. Hip rotators
F. Hip flexors
G. Hamstrings
H. Thoracic spine flexibility (mobility)

## Strengthening Exercises

Strengthening exercises should routinely be incorporated into the rehabilitation program to encourage the patient to remain active and to regain lumbar motion.[50] Strengthening exercises that reinforce pain-reducing movements and postures should be used. Any exercise

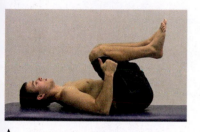

A

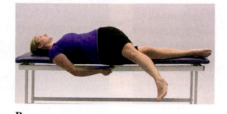

B

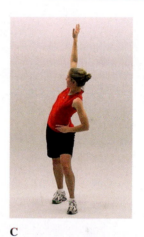

C

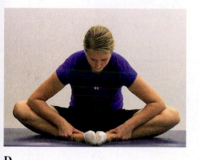

D

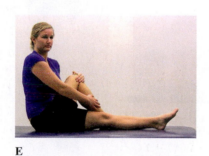

E

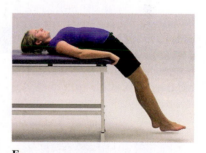

F

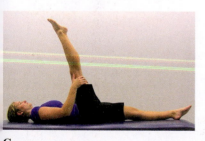

G

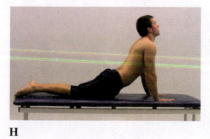

H

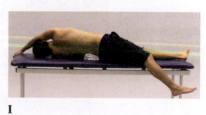

I

FIGURE 25–72   Low back stretching exercises. **(A)** Low back extensors. **(B)** Lumbar rotators and hip abductors. **(C)** Lumbar lateral flexors. **(D)** Hip adductors. **(E)** Hip rotators. **(F)** Hip flexors. **(G)** Hamstrings. **(H)** Prone extension stretch on hands. **(I)** Quadratus lumborum stretch.
© William E. Prentice

or movement that causes pain to spread over a larger area should be avoided. Thus, selecting the correct strengthening exercises should centralize or diminish pain.[2]

**Flexion versus Extension Exercises** Generally, strengthening exercises can involve either extension or flexion exercises.[59] Extension exercises are used to strengthen the back extensors, to stretch the abdominals, and to reduce the pressure on the

> Extension exercises are used to strengthen the back extensors, to stretch the abdominals, and to reduce the pressure on the intervertebral disks.

intervertebral disks (Figure 25–73).[9,105] Patients should engage in extension exercises when

- Back pain diminishes when the patient is lying down and increases when the patient is sitting.
- Backward bending is limited, yet the movement diminishes pain.
- Forward bending is extremely limited and increases pain.
- Straight-leg raising is limited and painful.

Flexion exercises are used to strengthen the abdominal muscles, to stretch the back extensors, and to take pressure off a nerve root by separating the lumbar facet joints and opening the intervertebral foramina

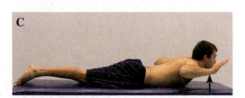
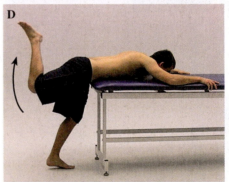
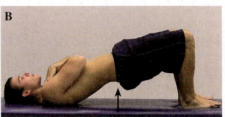
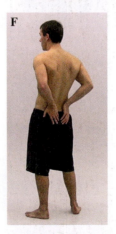
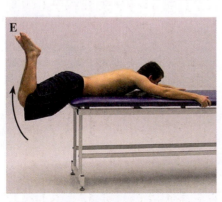
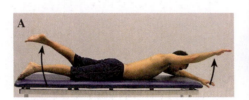

FIGURE 25–73   Extension strengthening exercises. **(A)** Alternating leg extension. **(B)** Supine hip extension. **(C)** Trunk extension. **(D)** Prone single hip extension. **(E)** Prone double-leg hip extension. **(F)** Standing extension.

© William E. Prentice

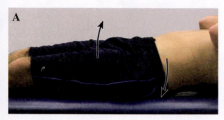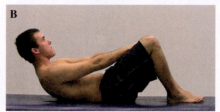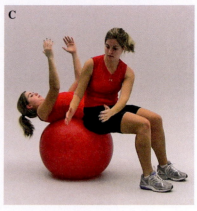

FIGURE 25–74   Flexion strengthening exercises. **(A)** Posterior pelvic tilt. **(B)** Partial sit-up. **(C)** Partial sit-up with rotation on a stability ball.

© William E. Prentice

(Figure 25–74). Patients should engage in flexion exercises when

- Back pain diminishes when the patient is sitting and increases when the patient is lying down or standing.
- Forward bending decreases the pain.
- The lordotic curve in the lumbar area does not reverse itself in forward bending.
- Backward bending is painful, especially at the end range.
- There is poor abdominal muscle strength.

**PNF Exercises** PNF upper-trunk chopping and lifting patterns may be used to strengthen the trunk musculature. Besides increasing strength, PNF exercises can help establish neuromuscular control and proprioception. Rhythmic stabilization, using isometric exercise, can facilitate the cocontraction of antagonistic muscle groups (see Chapter 16).

## Neuromuscular Control (Core Stabilization)

Despite the fact that the patient may have adequate strength and flexibility, he or she may have difficulty controlling the spine if the patient does not learn to contract the appropriate muscles in a desired sequence.[43] Stabilization, especially during complex functional movements, relies heavily on the patient's learned response to control the movement.[50] Stabilization exercises for the trunk and spine may help minimize the cumulative effects of repetitive microtrauma to the spine. Spinal stabilization does not mean that the patient maintains a static position. *Dynamic,* or *core, stabilization* involves maintaining a controlled range of motion that varies with the position and the activity

being performed.[20] Core stabilization is achieved by conscious repetitive training that, over time, becomes an unconscious, natural response.[106] Core stabilization techniques are widely used in rehabilitation programs for the low back.[50]

The first step in core stabilization is for the patient to learn to control the pelvis in a neutral position.[50] An ab-

> Dynamic stabilization involves maintaining a controlled range of motion that varies with the position and the activity being performed.

dominal brace or "drawing in" maneuver similar to a posterior tilt of the pelvis, which flattens the lumbar curve, as if someone is going to punch you in the stomach, is caused by a simultaneous cocontraction of the transversus abdominus and multifidus muscles to maintain a "corset" control of the lumbar spine.[50] Once the patient has learned to simultaneously contract these muscles, then progressively more advanced activities should be incorporated that involve movements of both the spine and the extremities while the abdominal brace is maintained in a neutral position (Figure 25–75).[17] (See Figures 4–11, 16–2 and 21–42 for more examples of core stabilization exercises.) Core stabilization exercises may also be incorporated into aquatic therapy.[64]

A clinical prediction rule has been developed to determine which patients with low back pain will respond to a stabilization exercise program based on the following criteria:[48]

- Positive prone instability test
- No aberrant movement
- FABQ physical activity < 9
- No hypermobility with lumbar spring testing.

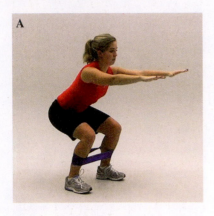

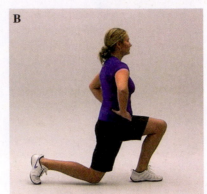

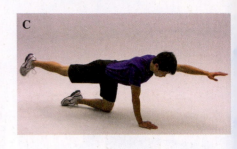

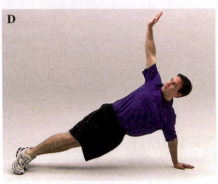

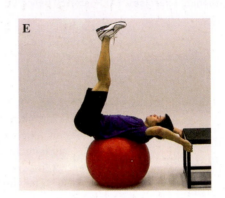

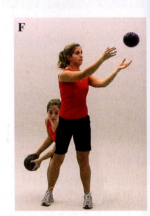

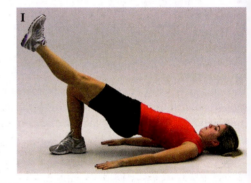

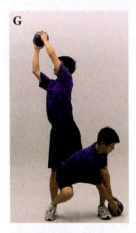

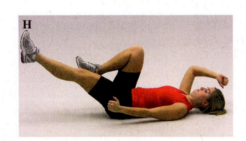

FIGURE 25-75    Core Stabilization Exercises **(A)** Squats with Theraband. **(B)** Lunges. **(C)** Alternating arm-leg extension. **(D)** Rolling plank. **(E)** Straight-leg raises on stability ball. **(F)** Weighted ball double-arm rotation toss. **(G)** Weighted ball D2 PNF pattern. **(H)** Dying bug. **(I)** Bridge with single-leg extension.
© William E. Prentice

## Functional Progressions

The progression of stabilization exercises should be from supine activities, to prone activities, to kneeling activities, and eventually to weight-bearing activities,[43] all performed while the patient actively stabilizes the trunk. The patient should be taught to perform a stabilization contraction before starting any movement.[86] As the movement begins, he or she will become less aware of the stabilization contraction. The patient may begin by incorporating stabilization into every movement performed in the strengthening exercises.[84] Stabilization contractions can also be used in aerobic conditioning activities. The exercises should include activities that replicate the demands of a specific sport. The various components of an activity should be broken down into separate activities or skills that allow

A college student has been told by his family physician that he has an unstable back. The physician referred him to a therapist, who recommended that the patient perform dynamic stabilization exercises. Unfortunately, the student had to leave home and return to college before he had a chance to learn the exercises.

**?** The patient asks the athletic trainer to show him the appropriate dynamic stabilization exercises. What progression should the athletic trainer recommend?

the patient to consciously practice the stabilization technique with each drill. Each patient will differ in degree of control and in the speed at which the skills of dynamic core stabilization are acquired.[50]

## Return to Activity

Most acute muscular strains or ligament sprains in the low back take as long to heal as acute strains and sprains in the extremities do. However, if the injury becomes recurrent or the problem becomes chronic, achieving full return to activity may be frustrating to both the patient and the athletic trainer. Injuries to the low back can be incapacitating for anyone, but the physical demands of activity increase the likelihood of recurrent injury.[76] Thus, the athletic trainer must take whatever time is required to fully rehabilitate the patient with a low back problem and must educate the patient about the skills and techniques that can minimize additional injury.

## SUMMARY

- The spine, or vertebral column, is composed of 33 individual vertebrae. The design of the spine allows for flexion, extension, lateral flexion, and rotation. The movable vertebrae are separated by intervertebral disks, and their position is maintained by a series of muscular and ligamentous supports. The spine can be divided into three regions: cervical, thoracic, and lumbar. The sacrum and coccyx are fused vertebrae within the vertebral column.

- The spinal cord is the portion of the central nervous system that is contained within the vertebral canal of the spinal column. Thirty-one pairs of spinal nerves extend from the sides of the spinal cord. The spinal nerve roots combine to form the peripheral nerves, which provide motor and sensory innervation. Each pair of spinal nerves has a specific area of cutaneous sensory distribution called a dermatome.

- Acute traumatic injuries to the spine can be life threatening, particularly if the cervical region of the spinal cord is involved. Thus, the patient must do everything possible to minimize the possibility of injury. Strengthening the musculature of the neck is critical. In addition to strong muscles, the neck should have a full range of motion. Individuals involved in collision sports must be taught and required to use techniques that reduce the likelihood of cervical injury.

- Low back pain is one of the most common and disabling ailments known to humans. Back pain can be prevented by avoiding unnecessary stresses and strains that are associated with standing, sitting, lying, working, and exercising. The individual should take care to avoid postures and positions that can cause injuries.

- The most critical part of evaluating spine injuries is to rule out the possibility of spinal cord injury. Observing the posture and movement capabilities of the patient during the evaluation can help clarify the nature and extent of the injury. Classic postural deviations include kyphosis, forward head posture, lordosis, flatback posture, swayback posture, and scoliosis. Special tests may be performed with the patient in standing, sitting, supine, side-lying, and prone positions.

- Because the cervical and lumbar regions of the spine are so mobile, they are extremely vulnerable to a wide range of injuries, including fractures, dislocations, strains, sprains, contusions, lesions of the intervertebral disks, injuries to spinal nerves, and degenerative conditions. Although relatively uncommon, severe injury to the neck can produce catastrophic impairment of the spinal cord.

- The first consideration in neck rehabilitation should be restoration of the neck's normal range of motion.

When the patient has gained near-normal range of motion, a strength program should be instituted. Mobilization techniques for the cervical spine are extensively used in rehabilitating the injured neck.

- Rehabilitation of low back pain focuses on teaching the patient dynamic stabilization techniques that involve exercises for the trunk and spine to minimize the cumulative effects of repetitive microtrauma to the spine. Exercises are designed to strengthen or stretch specific muscles of spinal movement and are divided into extension and flexion exercises.

## WEB SITES

### NATA Position, Official, and Consensus Statements
*Head-Down Contact and Spearing in Tackle Football (2004):*
www.nata.org/sites/default/files
/headdowncontactandspearingintacklefb.pdf

AAFP—Diagnosis and Management of Acute Low Back Pain: www.aafp.org/afp/20000315/1779.html
*This site provides information on managing low back pain from the American Academy of Family Practice.*

Back Pain: www.orthopedics.about.com/cs/backpain
*This site discusses the many causes of low back pain.*

MEDLINEplus: Back Pain:
www.nlm.nih.gov/medlineplus/backpain.html
*This site has information on back pain from the Mayo Foundation for Medical Education and Research.*

Spine-Health: www.spine-health.com
*Written and updated by a multispecialty team of medical professionals, this site provides a comprehensive overview of causes and treatments for low back pain and a variety of services and in-depth features.*

Cleveland Clinic Foundation: Spinal Cord Trauma:
http://my.clevelandclinic.org/disorders/spinal_cord_injury/hic_the_spinal_cord_and_injury.aspx

## SOLUTIONS TO CLINICAL APPLICATION EXERCISES

25-1 The normal curves are the cervical, thoracic, lumbar, and sacrococcygeal. The cervical and lumbar curves are convex anteriorly, whereas the thoracic and sacrococcygeal curves are convex posteriorly. Lordotic posture is characterized by an increased curve in the lumbar spine, with an increase in both anterior tilt of the pelvis and hip flexion. When combined with kyphosis and a forward head posture, this condition is referred to as a kypholordotic posture.

25-2 Left rotation is produced when the sternocleidomastoid, scalenes, semispinalis cervicis, and upper trapezius on the right side contract in addition to contractions of the left splenius capitus, splenius cervicis, and longissimus capitus.

25-3 The athletic trainer should look for symmetry of the ASIS, PSIS, and iliac crests. Sacroiliac compression and distraction tests and a positive Patrick, or FABER, test are all useful in determining a problem in the sacroiliac joint. In forward bending or flexion, the PSISs on each side should move together. If one moves farther than the other, a motion restriction is likely present in the sacroiliac joint on the side that moves most. Usually, if they move at different times, the side that moves first has a restriction.

25-4 Pain present in forward bending and restriction in backward bending with radiating pain are usually associated with a disk problem. However, such pain may also be related to spondylolysis or spondylolisthesis.

25-5 Straight-leg raising applies pressure to the sacroiliac joint and may indicate a problem in the sciatic nerve, sacroiliac joint, or lumbar spine. Pain at 30 degrees of straight-leg raising indicates either a hip problem or an inflamed nerve. Pain from 30 to 60 degrees indicates some sciatic nerve involvement. Pain between 70 and 90 degrees is indicative of a sacroiliac joint problem. Pain on bilateral straight-leg raising indicates some problem with the lumbar spine.

25-6 The patient may have cervical spine stenosis, which involves a narrowing of the spinal canal in the cervical region that can impinge on the spinal cord. The presence of cervical stenosis is determined by an X-ray that measures the canal diameter and divides that by the anteroposterior width of the same vertebral body. The patient should be advised of the potential risks of continued participation in football.

25-7 A stinger is an injury to the brachial plexus, resulting in transient neuropraxia. Common symptoms of a brachial plexus injury are burning, numbness and tingling, possible loss of function, and pain from the shoulder to the hand.

25-8 The patient has most likely developed a myofascial trigger point. The key in treating myofascial pain is to stretch the muscle back to a normal resting length and thus relieve the irritation that created the trigger point. Active stretching should be mild and progressive. The use of electrical stimulation in combination with ultrasound is helpful in relieving the pain associated with a trigger point. Progressive strengthening exercises should also be included.

25-9 The patient likely has a spondylolisthesis that has resulted in hypermobility of a vertebral segment. Initially, rest will help reduce pain. Rehabilitation should consist of exercises that control or stabilize the hypermobile segment and progressive trunk-strengthening exercises, especially to the abdominal muscles through the midrange. A brace can be helpful during practice.

25-10 Given this set of conditions, the athletic trainer should have the patient engage in extension exercises to strengthen the back extensors, to stretch the abdominals, and to reduce the pressure on the intervertebral disks.

25-11 It is likely that some pressure on the nerve root is causing this pain. The athletic trainer should recommend using flexion exercises to strengthen the abdominal muscles, to stretch the back extensors, and to take pressure off a nerve root by separating the lumbar facet joints and opening the intervertebral foramina.

25-12 The first step in core stabilization is for the patient to learn to control the lumbo-pelvic-hip complex in a neutral position. Once the patient has learned the "drawing in" maneuver, the athletic trainer should incorporate progressively more advanced activities that involve movements of both the spine and the extremities while the pelvis is maintained in a neutral position. Abdominal muscle control is another key to stabilization of the low back. Stabilization exercises include weight shifting in kneeling, standing lunges, bridging on a ball, wall slides, and alternating arm and leg extensions.

25-13 It could be that the patient should not be stretching for his back problem except during a warm-up before playing. Perhaps a better way to manage his back pain is to engage in a core stabilization training program to make his back more stable. It might also help to suggest that, before hitting a golf shot, he perform the "drawing in" maneuver to stabilize the lumbo-pelvic-hip complex.

# REVIEW QUESTIONS AND CLASS ACTIVITIES

1. Identify the regions of the spine.
2. Describe the mechanisms of a catastrophic neck injury.
3. What is the relationship among the spinal cord, the nerve roots, and the peripheral nerves?
4. Describe the various postural abnormalities.
5. Describe the special tests used in evaluating the lumbar and sacroiliac portions of the spine.
6. Discuss the various considerations in the prevention of cervical injuries.
7. What are the mechanisms of injury to the spinal cord?
8. What can be done to minimize the incidence of low back pain?
9. Describe the types of herniated disks.
10. How does a spondylolysis become a spondylolisthesis?
11. What is the usual mechanism for injury to the sacroiliac joint?
12. Explain when flexion exercises should be used and when extension exercises should be used in treating conditions of the low back.
13. Explain the rationale for using dynamic stabilization to rehabilitate low back pain.

# REFERENCES

1. Annaswamy T: Emerging concepts in the treatment of myofascial pain: A review of medications, modalities, and needle-based interventions, *Physical Medicine and Rehabilitation* 3(10):940–61, 2011.
2. Ashmen K: Strength and flexibility characteristics of athletes with chronic low-back pain, *J Sport Rehabil* 5(4):275, 1996.
3. Bailes J: Management of cervical spine injuries in athletes, *J Athl Train* 42(1):126–34, 2007.
4. Barry D: Managing low back pain with exercise interventions, *Athletic Therapy Today* 10(5):31, 2005.
5. Boden B: Catastrophic cervical spine injuries in high school and college football players, *Am J Sports Med* 34(8):1223, 2006.
6. Bogner E: Imaging of the cervical spine in athletes, *Sports Health: A Multidisciplinary Approach* 1(5):384–91, 2009.
7. Boissonnault W: Differential diagnosis of a sacral stress fracture, *J Orthop Sports Phys Ther* 32(12):613, 2002.
8. Broglio S: Emergency management of head and cervical-spine injuries, *Athletic Therapy Today* 10(2):24, 2005.
9. Browder D: Effectiveness of an extension oriented treatment approach in a subgroup of subjects with low back pain: A randomized clinical trial, *Physical Therapy* 87(12):1608–18, 2007.
10. Brox J: Acute neck and back injuries. In Bahr R: *Clinical Guide to Sports Injuries, Champaign,* IL, 2003, Human Kinetics.
11. Bruno P: Inter-rater agreement, sensitivity, and specificity of the prone hip extension test and active straight leg raise test, *Chiropractic Manipulative Therapy* 22:23, 2014.
12. Burns R: Low back pain in a female varsity ice-hockey player, *Athletic Therapy Today* 11(3):34, 2006.
13. Cai C: A clinical prediction rule for classifying patients with low back pain who demonstrate short-term improvement with mechanical lumbar traction, *Eur Spine J* 18(4): 554–61, 2009.
14. Cappaert T: The sacroiliac joint as a factor in low back pain: A review, *J Sport Rehabil* 9(2):169, 2000.
15. Carpenter D: Low back strengthening for the prevention and treatment of low back pain, *Med Sci Sports Exerc* 31(1):18, 1999.
16. Chao S: The pathomechanics, pathophysiology and prevention of cervical spinal cord and brachial plexus injuries in athletics, *Sports Medicine* 40(1):59–75, 2010.
17. Chen L: Endurance times for trunk-stabilization exercises in healthy women: Comparing three kinds of trunk flexor exercises, *J Sport Rehabil* 12(3):199, 2003.
18. Childs J: Clinical decision making in the identification of patients likely to benefit from spinal manipulation: A traditional versus an evidence-based approach, *J Orthop Sports Phys Ther* 33(5):259, 2003.
19. Childs J: A clinical prediction rule to identify patients with LBP most likely to benefit from spinal manipulation: A validation study, *Ann Int Med* 141:920–28, 2004.
20. Cholewicki J: Neuromuscular function in athletes following recovery from a recent acute low back injury, *J Orthop Sports Phys Ther* 32(11):568, 2002.
21. Chou R: Diagnosis and treatment of low back pain: A joint clinical practice guideline from the American College of Physicians and the American Pain Society, *Annals of Internal Medicine* 147(7):478–91, 2007.
22. Clark A: Cervical spinal stenosis and sports-related cervical cord neuropraxia, *Neurological Focus* 31(5):7, 2011.
23. Cleland J: Examination of a clinical prediction rule to identify patients with neck pain likely to benefit from thoracic spine thrust manipulation and a general cervical range of motion exercise: Multi-center randomized clinical trial, *Phys Ther* 90(9): 1239–50, 2010.
24. Cleland J: The use of a lumbar spine manipulation technique by physical therapists in patients who satisfy a clinical prediction rule: A case series, *J Orthop Sports Phys Ther* 36(4):209–14, 2006.
25. Cook C: Clinical identifiers for detecting underlying closed cervical fractures, *Pain Practice* 14(2):109–16, 2014.
26. Cook C: Clustered clinical findings for diagnosis of cervical spine myelopathy, *J Man Manip Ther* 18(4):175–80, 2010.
27. Cook C: The clinical value of a cluster of patient history and observational findings as a diagnostic support tool for lumbar spine stenosis, *Physiother Res Int* 16(3): 170–78, 2011.
28. Coppieters M: The immediate effects of a cervical lateral glide treatment technique in patients with neurogenic cervicobrachial pain, *J Orthop Sports Phys Ther* 33(6):369, 2003.
29. Côté P: The validity of the extension-rotation test as a clinical screening procedure before neck manipulation: A secondary analysis, *J Manipulative Physiol Ther* 19(3):159–64[A2], 1996.
30. Cuppett M: The anatomy and pathomechanics of the sacroiliac joint, *Athletic Therapy Today* 6(4):6, 2001.
31. Davidson R: The shoulder abduction test in the diagnosis of radicular pain in cervical extra-dural compressive mono radiculopathies, *Spine* 6:441–46, 1981.
32. Del Rossi G: Management of cervical spine injuries, *Athletic Therapy Today* 7(2):46, 2002.
33. Demetrios S: Diving injuries of the cervical spine in amateur divers, *The Spine Journal* 6(1):44–49, 2006.
34. Deville W: The test of Lasegue. Systematic review of the accuracy in diagnosing herniated discs, *Spine* 25: 1140–47, 2000.
35. Drezner J: Exercises in the treatment of low-back pain, *Physician Sportsmed* 29(8): 67, 2001.
36. Dreyfuss P: The value of medical history and physical examination in diagnosing sacroiliac joint pain, *Spine* 21(22):2594–602, 1996.
37. Fishman L: Piriformis syndrome: Diagnosis, treatment and outcome—a 10 year study, *Arch Phys Med Rehabil* 83:295–301, 2002.
38. Flynn T: *Users' Guide to the Musculoskeletal Examination.* Louisville, KY, 2008, Evidence in Motion.
39. Fras C: MRI imaging in diagnosing lumbar spondylolisthesis, *Spine Journal* 10(9):22s, 2010.
40. George S: Characteristics of patients with lower extremity symptoms treated with slump stretching: A case series, *J Orthop Sports Phys Ther* 32(8):391, 2002.
41. Geraci J: Low back pain in adolescent athletes: Diagnosis, rehabilitation, and prevention, *Athletic Therapy Today* 10(5):6, 2005.
42. Grant R: Physical therapy of the cervical and thoracic spine, New York, 2002, Churchill-Livingstone.
43. Hammann L: Functional back rehabilitation, *Athletic Therapy Today* 5(2):22, 2000.
44. Hangai M: Lumbar intervertebral disk degeneration in athletes, *Am J Sports Med* 37(1): 149–55, 2009.
45. Haperin J: Whiplash, *Physician Sportsmed* 81(11):856, 2002.
46. Heck J: A classification system for the assessment of lumbar pain in athletes, *J Athl Train* 35(2):204, 2000.
47. Henchoz Y: Exercise and non-specific low back pain: A literature review, *Joint Bone Spine* 75(5):533–39, 2008.
48. Hicks G: Preliminary development of a clinical prediction rule for determining which patients with low back pain will respond to a stabilization exercise program, *Arch of Phys Med Rehabil* 86:1753–62, 2005.
49. Hong C: Treatment of myofascial pain syndrome, *Current Pain and Headache Reports* 10(5)345–49, 2006.
50. Hooker D: Back rehabilitation. In Prentice W: *Rehabilitation techniques in sports medicine and athletic training,* Thorofare, NJ, 2015, Slack.

51. Jones G: Epidemiology of low back pain in children and adolescents, *Archives Dis Child* 90:312–16, 2005.

52. Kalichman L: Spondylolysis and spondylolisthesis: Prevalence and association with low back pain in the adult community–based population, *Spine* 34(2):199–205, 2009.

53. Kelly J, Aliquo D, Sitler M: Association of burners with cervical canal and foraminal stenosis, *Am J Sports Med* 28(2):214, 2000.

54. Laslett M: Diagnosis of sacroiliac joint pain: Validity of individual provocation tests and composites of tests, *Man Ther* 10:207–18, 2005.

55. Lee M: Prevalence of cervical spine stenosis, *J Bone Joint Surg* 89(2):376, 2007.

56. Liebenson C: *Rehabilitation of spine: A practitioner's manual,* Philadelphia, PA, 2005, Lippincott, Williams and Wilkins.

57. Majlesi J: The sensitivity and specificity of the slump and the straight leg raising tests in patients with lumbar disc herniation, *Journal of Clinical Rheumatology* 14(2):87–92, 2008.

58. Malanga G: Myofascial low back pain: A review, *Physical Medicine and Rehabilitation Clinics of North America* 21(4):711–24, 2010.

59. McGee D: *Orthopedic Physical Assessment,* Philadelphia, PA, 2014, Saunders.

60. McGill S, ed: *Low back disorders: Evidence-based prevention and rehabilitation,* Champaign, IL, 2015, Human Kinetics.

61. McHugh M: The role of neural tension in hamstring flexibility, *Scandinavian Journal of Medicine and Science in Sports* 22:164–69, 2012.

62. McKenzie R: *The lumbar spine: Mechanical diagnosis and therapy,* ed 2, Wellington, New Zealand, 2003, Spinal Publications.

63. Mooney V: Nonoperative management of low back pain and lumbar disc degeneration, *J Bone Joint Surg* 87(5):1165, 2005.

64. Moss C: Aquatic core strengthening for preventing low back manifestations, *Athletic Therapy Today* 7(4):26, 2002.

65. Moss R: Posture and pathology, *Athletic Therapy Today* 6(5):38, 2001.

66. Nourbakhsh M: Relationship between mechanical factors and incidence of low back pain, *J Orthop Sports Phys Ther* 32(9):447, 2002.

67. Nyska M: Spondylolysis as a cause of low back pain in swimmers, *Int J Sports Med* 21(5):375, 2000.

68. Oldridge N: Low back pain syndrome. In American College of Sports Medicine: *ACSM's exercise management for persons with chronic disease and disabilities,* Champaign, IL, 2009, Human Kinetics.

69. Olson K: Diagnosis and treatment of cervical spine clinical instability, *J Orthop Sports Phys Ther* 31(4):194, 2001.

70. Olson S: Tender point sensitivity, range of motion, and perceived disability in subjects with neck pain, *J Orthop Sports Phys Ther* 30(1):13, 2000.

71. Prather H: Sacroiliac joint pain: Practical management, *Cl J Sports Med* 13(4):252, 2003.

72. Puentedura E: Development of a clinical prediction rule to identify patients with neck pain likely to benefit from thrust joint manipulation to the cervical spine, *J Orthop Sports Phys Ther* 42(7):577–92, 2012.

73. Raney N: Development of a clinical prediction rule to identify patients with neck pain likely to benefit from cervical traction and exercise, *Eur Spine J* 18(3):382–91, 2009.

74. Reed J: Lower back pain in golf: A review, *Current Sports Medicine Reports* 9(1):57–59, 2010.

75. Reiman M: Trunk stabilization training: An evidence basis for the current state of affairs, *Journal of Back and Musculoskeletal Rehabilitation* 22(1):131–42, 2009.

76. Resnik L: Guide to outcomes measurement for patients with low back pain syndromes, *J Orthop Sports Phys Ther* 33(6):307, 2003.

77. Roman, M: The development of a clinical decision making algorithm for detection of osteoporotic vertebral compression fracture or wedge deformity, *Journal of Manual and Manipulative Therapy* 18(1): 44–49, 2010.

78. Ross M: Treating low back pain in a middle-age recreational athlete, *Athletic Therapy Today* 4(2):22, 1999.

79. Saunders-Ryan R: *Evaluation, treatment and prevention of musculoskeletal disorders: The spine,* Atlanta, GA, 2004, Saunders Group.

80. Shannon B: Cervical burners in the athlete, *Clin Sports Med* 21(1):29, 2002.

81. Speicher T: Managing low back pain through activities-of-daily-living education, *Athletic Therapy Today* 1(6):74, 2006.

82. Standaert C: Spondylolysis: A critical review, *British Journal of Sports Medicine* 34(6):415, 2000.

83. Stanton T: How do we define the condition "recurrent low back pain"? A systematic review, *European Spine Journal* 19(4):533–39, 2009.

84. Stevans J: Motor skill acquisition strategies for rehabilitation of low back pain, *J Orthop Sports Phys Ther* 28(3):165, 1998.

85. Stiell I: Implementation of the Canadian C-spine rule: Prospective 12 centre cluster randomised trial, *British Medical Journal* 339:b4146, 2009.

86. Stone J: Back stabilization exercises, *Athletic Therapy Today* 4(3):23, 1999.

87. Supik L: Sciatic tension signs and lumbar disk Herniation, *Spine* 19:1066–69, 1994.

88. Suri P: The accuracy of the physical examination for the diagnosis of mid lumbar and lower lumbar nerve root impingement, *Spine* 36(1):63–73, 2011.

89. Sutlive T: Development of a clinical prediction rule for diagnosing hip osteoarthritis in individuals with unilateral hip pain, *J Orthop Sport Phys Ther* 38: 542–50, 2008.

90. Swartz E: NATA Position Statement: Acute management of the cervical spine-injured athlete, *J Athl Train* 44(3):306–31, 2009.

91. Swartz E: Cervical spine functional anatomy and the biomechanics of injury due to compressive loading, *J Athl Train* 40(3):155, 2003.

92. Tallarico R: Spondylolysis and spondylolisthesis in the athlete, *Sports Medicine and Arthroscopy Review* 16(1):32–38, 2008.

93. Thein-Nissenbaum J: Differential diagnosis of spondylolysis in a patient with chronic low back pain, *J Orthop Sports Phys Ther* 35(5):319, 2005.

94. Thomas K: The diagnostic accuracy of Kernig's sign and Brudzinski's sign and nuchal rigidity in adults with suspected meningitis, *Clinical Infectious Diseases* 35(1):46–52, 2002.

95. Tierney RT: Measuring isometric strength in the cervical spine, *Athletic Therapy Today* 8(3):56, 2003.

96. Tierney R: Cervical spine stenosis measures in normal subjects, *J Athl Train* 37(2):190, 2002.

97. Timm K: An algorithm for assessing lumbar spine injuries, *Athletic Therapy Today* 3(2):18, 1998.

98. Timm K: Therapeutic exercise guidelines for rehabilitating lumbar spine injuries in athletes, *Athletic Therapy Today* 4(2):17, 1998.

99. Tong H: The Spurling test and cervical radiculopathy, *Spine* 27(2):156–59, 2002.

100. Udermann B: Quantitative assessment of lumbar paraspinal muscle endurance, *J Athl Train* 38(3):259–62, 2003.

101. Vroomen P: Diagnostic value of history and physical examination in patients suspected of sciatica due to disc herniation: A systematic review, *J Neurol* 246:899–906, 1999.

102. Wainner R: Diagnosis and nonoperative management of cervical radiculopathy, *J Orthop Sports Phys Ther* 30(12):728, 2000.

103. Waldrop M: Diagnosis and treatment of cervical radiculopathy using a clinical prediction rule and a multimodal intervention approach: A case series, *J Orthop Sports Phys Ther* 36(3):152–59, 2006.

104. Weinberg J: Etiology, treatment, and prevention of athletic "stingers," *Clin Sports Med* 22(3):493, 2003.

105. Whalen R: EMG analysis of patients with unilateral neck pain, *J Sport Rehabil* 8(1):32, 1999.

106. Wisbey-Roth T: Dysfunctional muscle recruitment patterns affecting core stability: The theory of synergistic stabilizer retraining. Abstract from Australian Conference of Science and Medicine in Sport, National Convention Centre, Canberra, October 1996.

107. Wrisley D: Cervicogenic dizziness: A review of diagnosis and treatment, *J Orthop Sports Phys Ther* 30(12):755, 2000.

108. Young J: The disk at risk in athletes: Perspectives on operative and nonoperative care, *Med Sci Sports Exerc* 29(7 suppl):S222, 1997.

## ANNOTATED BIBLIOGRAPHY

Grant R: *Physical therapy of the cervical and thoracic spine,* ed 3, New York, 2002, Churchill-Livingstone.
*Provides guidance for the evaluation and treatment of cervical and thoracic problems. An overview is presented in three sections: anatomy, biomechanics, and innervation; examination and assessment; and clinical management.*

Key J: *Back pain—A movement problem: A clinical approach incorporating relevant research and practice,* Philadelphia, PA, 2010, Churchill-Livingston.
*Examines aspects of motor control and functional movement in the spine and the development of the spine, and explores probable reasons why the spine is altered in people with back pain,*

Liebenson C: *Rehabilitation of the spine: a practitioner's manual,* Philadelphia, PA, 2006, Lippincott, Williams and Wilkins.

*Presents the most current and significant spinal rehab information, showing how to apply simple and inexpensive rehabilitation in the office.*

McGill S, editor: *Low back disorders: evidence-based prevention and rehabilitation,* Champaign, IL, 2007, Human Kinetics.

*Presents approaches to help professionals make clinical decisions for building prevention and rehabilitation programs.*

McKenzie R: *The cervical and thoracic spine: Mechanical diagnosis and therapy,* Minneapolis, MN, 2006, Orthopedic Physical Therapy Products.

*Provides evidence-based and clinically relevant information explores, in-depth, literature relating to mechanical syndromes, and neck/trunk pain.*

Morris C: *Low back syndromes: Integrated clinical management,* New York, 2005, McGraw-Hill.

*The most thorough examination of the principles and practices of conservative care of the lower back. Covers nonsurgical and nonmedicinal methods of treating low back pain and other common disorders and dysfunction.*

Richardson C, Hides J, Hodges P: *Therapeutic exercise for lumbopelvic stabilization: A motor control approach for the treatment and prevention of low back pain,* New York, 2004, Elsevier Health Sciences.

*Presents the latest information and research on the prevention and management of musculoskeletal pain and dysfunction. It introduces the reader to an approach to clinical management and prevention based on that research.*

Saunders-Ryan R: *Evaluation, treatment, and prevention of musculoskeletal disorders,* Chaska, MN, 2004, The Saunders Group.

*A manual therapy approach to treating and rehabilitating musculoskeletal injuries in general and injuries to the spine in particular.*

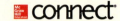

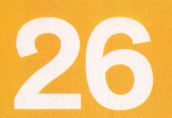

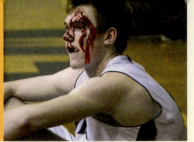

Courtesy Phil Stapleton

# 26

# The Head, Face, Eyes, Ears, Nose, and Throat

## ■ Objectives

*When you finish this chapter you should be able to*

- Propose a plan for helping prevent or at least minimize the frequency of injuries to the head.
- Review the related anatomy of the head.
- Establish a systematic process for evaluating concussions and mild head injuries.
- Make an informed decision regarding the sideline and follow-up management of sport-related concussions based on a comprehensive presentation of the available options.

- Recognize the seriousness of a variety of injuries to the head and be aware of the length of time potentially needed for recovery.
- Discuss the value of neurocognitive tests in determining the state of recovery following concussion.
- Be able to correctly identify the various injuries that can occur to the face, eyes, ears, nose, and throat.

## ■ Outline

## ■ Key Terms

coup injury                contrecoup injury                epistaxis                diplopia

## ■ Connect Highlights    connect

*Visit connect.mcgraw-hill.com for further exercises to apply your knowledge:*

- Clinical application scenarios covering evaluation of concussions, neuropsychological tests, and injuries to the face, eyes, ears, nose and throat.
- Click-and-drag questions covering facial anatomy, concussions, and various head injuries
- Multiple-choice questions covering prevention of head injuries, sport-related concussions, neuropsychological testing, and injuries to the face, eyes, ears, nose and throat.
- Selection questions covering injuries to the nose

Injuries to the region of the head, face, eyes, ears, nose, and throat are common. The severity of injuries to this region can vary from something as benign as a nosebleed to severe concussions of the cortex.

# PREVENTION OF INJURIES TO THE HEAD, FACE, EYES, EARS, NOSE, AND THROAT

Although injuries to the head and face are more prevalent in collision and contact sports, the potential for head injuries exists in all sports (Table 26–1).[34] The use of helmets or other protective headgear and, in some instances, face masks in sports such as football, ice hockey, lacrosse, wrestling, and baseball has dramatically reduced the incidence of injuries to the head, face, eyes, ears, and nose. Some have argued that if the face mask were eliminated in a sport such as football, the number of cervical spine and head injuries would be reduced because the athlete would be less likely to use the head when making contact. It is certain, however, that the incidence of injuries to the face, eyes, ears, and nose would significantly increase. A helmet can do only so much in preventing injury to the brain. Manufacturers of protective headgear for soccer have made unsubstantiated claims about its ability to minimize concussions.[9] All football helmets have written warnings that discourage the use of the head

as a weapon (see Chapter 7). The athletic trainer should take responsibility for educating coaches, athletes, and parents about the limitations of protective equipment for concussion prevention, and should ensure that everyone reads all warning labels associated with protective equipment.[10] SoR:C The athletic trainer has a responsibility to make certain that coaches are teaching and athletes are using correct and safe techniques.[3]

The single most important consideration in reducing injuries to this region involves educating the athlete in (1) proper techniques for initiating contact and (2) the danger of concussive brain injury and second-impact syndrome discussed later in this chapter.

# THE HEAD

## Anatomy of the Head

**Bones** The skull is composed of 22 bones. With the single exception of the mandible, all the bones of the skull are joined together in immovable joints called sutures. The cranial vault, which houses the brain, is enclosed by the cranium, or skull, and is made up of the frontal, the ethmoid, the sphenoid, two parietal, two temporal, and the occipital bones. The skull's thickness varies in different locations; it is thinner over the temporal regions (Figure 26–1).

**Scalp** The scalp is the covering of the skull. It has five layers of soft tissue. The skin, connective tissue, and aponeurosis epicranius are the three outermost tissue layers. They are fused and move as a single layer. The aponeurosis epicranius is a thick connective tissue sheet that acts as an attachment for the occipitalis and frontalis muscles. Between the first three tissue layers and the periosteum lies a loose connective tissue layer.

**Brain** The *brain*, or encephalon, is the part of the central nervous system that is contained within the bony cavity of the cranium (Figure 26–2). It is divided into four sections. The *cerebrum* is the largest part of the brain and is divided into two hemispheres separated by a deep longitudinal

| TABLE 26–1 | Sports with a High Risk of Head Injury[34] | |
|---|---|---|
| Boxing | Rugby | Gymnastics |
| Football | Wrestling | Motorcycle |
| Ice hockey | Soccer | racing |
| Lacrosse | Auto racing | Diving |
| (see Chapter 7) | Equestrian | Bicycling |
| Martial arts | events | Snow skiing |

Jordan B: Head injuries in sports. In Jordan B, Tsairis P, Warren R, editors: Sports neurology, Philadelphia, 1998, Lippincott, Williams and Wilkins.

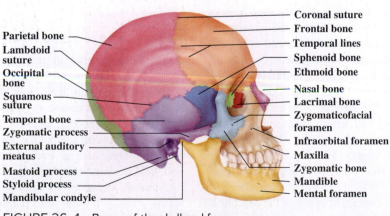

Parietal bone
Lambdoid suture
Occipital bone
Squamous suture
Temporal bone
Zygomatic process
External auditory meatus
Mastoid process
Styloid process
Mandibular condyle

Coronal suture
Frontal bone
Temporal lines
Sphenoid bone
Ethmoid bone
Nasal bone
Lacrimal bone
Zygomaticofacial foramen
Infraorbital foramen
Maxilla
Zygomatic bone
Mandible
Mental foramen

FIGURE 26–1 Bones of the skull and face.

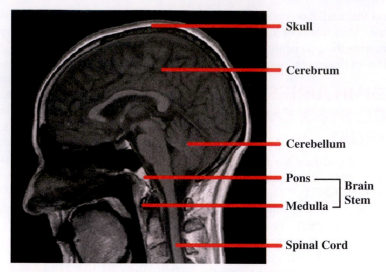

FIGURE 26–2    MRI showing major areas of the brain (sagittal cross-sectional view).

Courtesy Jordan B. Renner, MD, Departments of Radiology and Allied Health Sciences, University of North Carolina

fissure. The cerebrum, also referred to as the *cortex*, coordinates all voluntary muscle activities and interprets sensory impulses in addition to controlling higher mental functions, including memory, reasoning, intelligence, learning, judgment, and emotions. The *cerebellum* controls synergistic movements of skeletal muscle and plays a critical role in the coordination of voluntary muscular movements. The *pons* controls sleep, posture, respiration, swallowing, and the bladder. The *medulla oblongata* is the lowest part of the brain stem and regulates heart rate, breathing, and blood pressure as well as coughing, sneezing, and vomiting.[82]

**Meninges**  Investing the spinal cord and the brain are the *meninges,* which are the three membranes that protect the brain and the spinal cord. Outermost is the dura mater, consisting of a dense, fibrous, and inelastic sheath that encloses the brain and cord. In some places, it is attached directly to the vertebral canal, but, for the most part, a layer of fat that contains the vital arteries separates this membrane from the bony wall and forms the epidural space. The arachnoid, an extremely delicate sheath, lines the dura mater and is attached directly to the spinal cord by many silklike tissue strands. The dura and arachnoid are separated by the *subdural space,* which contains the veins. The space between the arachnoid and the pia mater, the membrane that helps contain the spinal fluid, is called the *subarachnoid space.* The subarachnoid cavity projects upward and, running the full length of the spinal cord, connects with the ventricles of the brain. The pia mater is a thin, delicate, and highly vascularized membrane that adheres closely to the spinal cord and to the brain (Figure 26–3).[82]

*Cerebrospinal fluid* is contained between the arachnoid and the pia mater membrane and completely surrounds

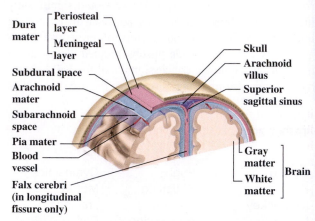

FIGURE 26–3    The meningeal membranes covering the brain.

and suspends the brain. Its main function is to buoy the brain, helping diminish the transmission of shocking forces.

## Assessment of Head Injuries

Head trauma results in more fatalities than any other sports injury. The morbidity and mortality associated with traumatic brain injury have been labeled a silent epidemic. Brain injury is common in collision or contact sports, such as football, soccer, lacrosse, boxing, ice hockey, and wrestling. But head trauma has also been reported in noncontact sports, such as track, baseball, gymnastics, softball, field hockey, volleyball, and cheerleading.

Athletes engaging in high-risk contact or collision sports should, before the competitive season, undergo annual baseline examinations, consisting of a clinical history (including any symptoms), physical and neurologic evaluations, measures of motor control, and neurocognitive function.[10] SoR:B

An individual who receives either a direct blow to the head or body contact that causes the head to snap forward, backward, or rotate to the side must be carefully evaluated for injury to the brain.[7] These injuries are best defined as a *brain injury,* and they represent the most common type of head trauma.[51] It is important for the athletic trainer to use, and educate others in using, the proper terminology of concussion and traumatic brain injury and to discourage the use of colloquial terms such as "ding" and "bell ringer."[10] SoR:B *Concussions* are a type of traumatic brain injury. Concussion may result in disorientation or amnesia; motor, coordination, or balance deficits; cognitive deficits; and, rarely, unconsciousness. The majority of concussions sustained by athletes do not involve loss of consciousness. Nevertheless, the athletic trainer must be prepared to manage those injuries in which there is a loss of consciousness.

On-the-field management of the unconscious patient was discussed in detail in Chapter 12. The athletic trainer must be adept at recognizing and interpreting the signs that an unconscious patient presents. Priority first aid for any head injury must always deal with any life-threatening condition, but in particular with loss of breathing. When assessing an unconscious patient, the athletic trainer must always suspect a cervical neck injury and manage the situation accordingly, as described in Chapter 12.[1] A patient who has been unconscious should be removed from the field on a spine board.

> The majority of concussions do not involve loss of consciousness; they present with dizziness, headaches, blurred vision, and concentration problems.

If no life-threatening condition exists, the athletic trainer should note the length of time that the patient is unconscious and should not move the patient until he or she regains consciousness. Once the patient regains consciousness, or if the patient never lost consciousness, the athletic trainer should obtain a history from the patient.

> An ice skater falls and hits the back of her head on the ice, incurring a possible cerebral concussion.
>
> **?** Initially, what observational signs may indicate a cerebral injury?

**History** The primary purpose of the history is to establish whether the patient has, in fact, sustained a concussion. However, current guidelines recommend not grading a concussion, as initial presentation does not always predict recovery.[10,51] Concussion may be caused by a direct blow to the head, face, neck, or elsewhere on the body, with a force transmitted to the head. There is usually a rapid onset of short-lived impairment of neurologic function that resolves spontaneously. With a concussion, there may be neuropathological changes; however, the acute clinical symptoms largely reflect a functional disturbance rather than a structural injury.[51] A patient who has sustained a concussion may or may not be able to respond to questions about exactly what happened to cause the concussion. Nevertheless, the following questions should be asked:

- Can you tell me what happened to you?
- Can you remember the score or whom we played last week? (This question will determine whether there is retrograde amnesia.)
- Can you remember walking off the field? (This question will determine whether there is anterograde amnesia.)
- Does your head hurt?
- Do you have any pain in your neck?
- Can you move your hands and feet?
- Have you experienced tinnitus (ringing in the ears)?

**Observation** The athletic trainer who is usually around an individual both on and off the field has the advantage of knowing the individual's normal affect and behavior. The following observations should be made:

- Is the patient disoriented and unable to tell where he or she is, what time it is, what date it is, and who the opponent is?
- Does the patient have a blank or vacant stare? Does he or she have difficulty keeping his or her eyes open?
- Does the patient have slurred or incoherent speech?
- Does the patient have delayed verbal and motor responses (slow to answer questions or follow instructions)?
- Does the patient have a gross coordination disturbance (e.g., stumbling, inability to walk a straight line, can't touch finger to nose)?
- Is the patient unable to focus attention, and is he or she easily distracted?
- Does the patient appear to have a memory deficit exhibited by repeatedly asking the same questions or no knowledge of what happened?
- Does the patient have normal cognitive function (serial sevens, assignment on a particular play, three-word recall)?
- Does the patient elicit a normal emotional response?
- How long was the patient's affect abnormal?

> A football player sustains a cerebral concussion while making a tackle during a game.
>
> **?** How should the athletic trainer determine the athlete's level of orientation and memory?

- Is the patient's scalp swollen or bleeding?
- Does the patient have a clear or straw-colored fluid in the ear canal (cerebrospinal fluid leakage that would occur with skull fracture)?

**Palpation**  Palpation of both the neck and the skull should be performed in a systematic manner to identify areas of point tenderness or deformity. Deformity of either structure may indicate the presence of a fracture and requires immediate and advanced medical care.

### Special Tests

***Neurological Exam***  In all cases of head injury, the athletic trainer should administer an on-the-field neurological exam. The neurological exam was discussed in detail in Chapter 13. It consists of six major areas: cerebral testing, which assesses cognitive function; cranial nerve testing; cerebellar testing, which assesses coordination and motor function; sensory testing; reflex testing; and motor testing (see Chapter 13).

***Eye Function Tests***  Abnormal eye function is often related to head injury. The following conditions should be tested:

1. Pupils are equal and reactive to light (PEARL).
    a. Dilated or irregular pupils. Checking for equal pupil sizes may be particularly difficult at night and under artificial lights. Some individuals normally have pupils that differ in size.[38]

> Checking eye signs can yield crucial information about possible brain injury or a deteriorating neurological condition.

    b. Inability of the pupils to accommodate rapidly to light variance. The athletic trainer can test eye accommodation by covering one of the patient's eyes with a hand. The covered eye normally will dilate, whereas the uncovered pupil will remain the same. When the hand is removed, the previously covered pupil normally accommodates readily to the light. A slowly accommodating pupil may indicate cerebral injury.[38]
2. Eyes track smoothly. The patient is asked to hold the head in a neutral position with both eyes looking straight ahead. The patient is then asked to follow the top of a pen or pencil, first up as far as possible, then down as far as possible. The eyes are observed for smooth movement and any signs of pain. Next, the tip of the pen or pencil is slowly moved from left to right to determine whether the eyes follow the tip smoothly across the midline of the face or whether they make involuntary movements. A constant involuntary back and forth, up and down, or rotary movement of the eyeball is called *nystagmus* and indicates possible lesion in the posterior fossa of the brain, often involving the brain stem or cerebellum.[13] Recently, a screening tool has been developed to identify concussed athletes

by assessing eye movements.[54] Called the Vestibular/Ocular Motor Screening (VOMS) assessment, it includes five domains: (1) smooth pursuit, (2) horizontal and vertical saccades, (3) near point of convergence (NPC) distance, (4) horizontal vestibular ocular reflex (VOR), and (5) visual motion sensitivity (VMS).

3. Vision is blurred. The athletic trainer can test for blurred vision by determining whether the patient has difficulty reading or is unable to read a game program or the scoreboard.

### Balance Tests

***Romberg Test***  In the past, if the patient was capable of standing following head injury, a Romberg test was used to assess static balance. Originally, the test was to have the patient shut the eyes and stand erect with the hands at the sides. Normally, a person can stand motionless in this position, but the tendency to sway or fall to one side is considered a positive Romberg sign indicating a loss of proprioception. A positive sign is one in which the patient begins to sway, cannot keep the eyes closed, or obviously loses balance. Over the years, there have been several variations and modifications to the original Romberg test, most involving changes in foot positions during static stance to alter the base of support. The most commonly used variations have involved a single-leg stance and a tandem (heel to toe) stance. Evidence suggests that the best on-the-field balance test uses a tandem stance performed on a foam surface or a single-limb (nondominant) stance on a foam surface (Figure 26–4).[67] The standard Romberg test has, however, been criticized for its lack of sensitivity and objectivity. It is considered to be a rather qualitative assessment of static balance because a considerable amount of stress is required to make the subject sway enough for an observer to characterize the sway.

***Balance Error Scoring System***  The use of a quantifiable clinical test battery called the *Balance Error Scoring System (BESS)* is recommended over the standard Romberg

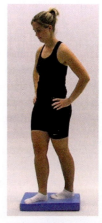

**FIGURE 26–4**  A tandem Romberg test on an unstable foam surface (Airex Pad).

© William E. Prentice

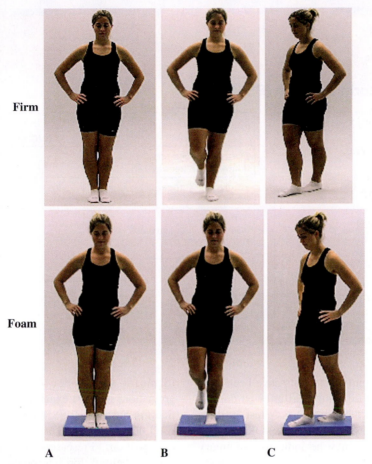

**FIGURE 26–5** Balance Error Scoring System (BESS) performed with three different stances on two different surfaces (firm, foam). **(A)** Double-leg. **(B)** Single-leg. **(C)** Tandem.

© William E. Prentice

test.[23,60,67] Three different stances (double, single, and tandem) are completed twice, once while on a firm surface and once while on a 10 cm thick piece of medium-density foam (Airex, Inc.) for a total of six trials (Figure 26–5). Patients are asked to assume the required stance by placing their hands on the iliac crests and then to close their eyes for 20 seconds. During the single-leg stance, patients are asked to maintain the contralateral limb in 20 to 30 degrees of hip flexion and 40 to 50 degrees of knee flexion. The patient is also asked to stand quietly and as motionless as possible in the stance position, keeping the hands on the iliac crest and eyes closed. The single-leg stance tests are performed on the nondominant foot. The same foot is placed toward the rear in the tandem stance. Subjects are told that, on losing their balance, they are to make any necessary adjustments and return to the testing position as quickly as possible. Performance is scored by adding one error point for each error committed (see *Focus Box 26–1: "Balance Error Scoring System [BESS]"*). Trials are considered to be incomplete if the patient cannot sustain the stance position for longer than 5 seconds during the entire 20-second testing period.

These trials are assigned a standard maximum error score of 10. Balance test results during injury recovery are best compared with baseline measurements, and athletic trainers working with patients on a regular basis should try to attain baseline measurements when possible. The focus box provides a sheet for scoring the BESS. The results from this test have been shown to correlate strongly with the results from more sophisticated tests conducted on highly sensitive computerized force plate systems.[8] There does appear to be a slight practice effect with repeated administration of the BESS.[81] It also appears that fatigue decreases performance on the BESS.[86] More sensitive testing can be done off the field with sophisticated balance systems, such as those manufactured by NeuroCom, Biodex, Chattex, and Breg.

Recently, mobile applications for smartphones, tablets, and other devices have also been developed to assess balance in an efficient manner. These mechanisms are not as well studied, but clinicians should be aware of their utility and existence.[2] Additionally, measures of more dynamic balance, such as tandem gait tasks, have been discussed.[51]

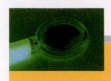

# FOCUS 26–1 Focus on Examination, Assessment, and Diagnosis

## Balance Error Scoring System (BESS)

| Balance Error Scoring System– Types of Errors |
|---|
| 1. Hands lifted off iliac crest |
| 2. Opening eyes |
| 3. Step, stumble, or fall |
| 4. Moving hip into > 30 degrees abduction |
| 5. Lifting forefoot or heel |
| 6. Remaining out of testing position > 5 seconds |

The BESS is calculated by adding one error point for each error during the six 20-second tests.

| SCORE CARD (# errors): | FIRM Surface | FOAM Surface |
|---|---|---|
| Double-Leg Stance (narrow stance–feet together) | | |
| Single-Leg Stance (nondominant foot) | | |
| Tandem Stance (nondominant foot in back) | | |
| Total Scores: | | |
| Total Score: | | |

**Coordination Tests** A number of tests have been used to determine whether a head injury has affected coordination. These tests include the finger-to-nose test, heel-to-toe walking, and the standing heel-to-knee test. Inability to perform any of these tests may be indicative of injury to the cerebellum.

**Cognitive Tests** The purpose of cognitive testing is to establish the effects of head trauma on various cognitive functions and to obtain an objective measure to assess the patient's status and improvement.[17,34] Cognitive tests may be performed as part of the on-the-field neurological exam. Among the more traditional commonly used on-the-field cognitive tests are serial sevens, in which the patient counts backward from 100 by 7; spelling a word backward; and naming the months in reverse order. Tests of recent memory (the game score, who won last week, what was eaten at breakfast, three-word recall) have also been used as brief memory tests.

Currently, the most widely used on-the-field test for assessing concussion-related signs and symptoms, cognition, balance, and coordination is the Sport Concussion Assessment Tool 3 (SCAT3) and the child SCAT3.[51] The SCAT3 test can be used with children ages 10 and older. For children younger than 10, a child version of SCAT3 is available, but validation of this tool has not been fully completed.[51] This tool was developed by a group of concussion experts at the Fourth International Conference on Concussion in Sport in Zurich in 2012.[51] It represents a standardized method of evaluating injured athletes for concussion by medical and health professionals. It can be used for athletes ages 10 years and older. The SCAT3 consists of eight sections: the Glasgow Coma Scale (GCS); Maddocks scale; a symptom evaluation; a cognitive assessment (Standard Assessment of Concussion [SAC]); neck examination; balance examination (modified Balance Error Scoring System [BESS]); coordination examination; and a SAC delayed recall. The SCAT3 has a separate score for each section.[51] Preseason baseline testing with the SCAT3 can be helpful for interpreting post-injury test scores. Focus Box 26–2 shows the entire SCAT3 evaluation tool.

The *Standardized Assessment of Concussion (SAC)* is a brief mental status test that was designed to provide athletic trainers and other medical personnel with immediate, objective data concerning the presence and severity of neurocognitive impairment associated with concussion.[48] The test has been designed to be used either on or off the field and includes measures of orientation, immediate memory recall, concentration, and delayed recall. Although the SAC is most often used as a stand-alone tool, it is included as part of the SCAT3 and can be found on pages 831–834.

*Neuropsychological assessments* have been developed for use in both on- and off-the-field evaluation.[19,66] A number of additional neuropsychological assessments focus on short-term memory, working memory, attention, concentration, visual spatial capacity, verbal learning, information processing speed, and/or reaction time. Paper-and-pencil tests have been available for several years and include the *Hopkins Verbal Learning Test, Trail-Making Test Parts A and B, Symbol Digit Modalities Test, Wechsler Digit Span Test—Forward and Backward, Stroop Color Word Test,* and *Controlled Oral Word Association Test.* These traditional tests are valid and reliable assessment tools but are not practical when instituting a baseline assessment program.[19] They take a significant amount of time and resources to administer.

Computerized neurocognitive tests, adapted from traditional neuropsychological tests, programs, which are

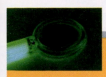

# SCAT3™

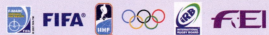

## Sport Concussion Assessment Tool – 3rd Edition*

For use by medical professionals only

---

Name _____    Date/Time of Injury: _____    Examiner: _____
                              Date of Assessment: _____

## What is the SCAT3?[1]

The SCAT3 is a standardized tool for evaluating injured athletes for concussion and can be used in athletes aged from 13 years and older. It supersedes the original SCAT and the SCAT2 published in 2005 and 2009, respectively[2]. For younger persons, ages 12 and under, please use the Child SCAT3. The SCAT3 is designed for use by medical professionals. If you are not qualified, please use the Sport Concussion Recognition Tool[1]. Preseason baseline testing with the SCAT3 can be helpful for interpreting post-injury test scores.

Specific instructions for use of the SCAT3 are provided on page 3. If you are not familiar with the SCAT3, please read through these instructions carefully. This tool may be freely copied in its current form for distribution to individuals, teams, groups and organizations. Any revision or any reproduction in a digital form requires approval by the Concussion in Sport Group.
**NOTE:** The diagnosis of a concussion is a clinical judgment, ideally made by a medical professional. The SCAT3 should not be used solely to make, or exclude, the diagnosis of concussion in the absence of clinical judgement. An athlete may have a concussion even if their SCAT3 is "normal".

## What is a concussion?

A concussion is a disturbance in brain function caused by a direct or indirect force to the head. It results in a variety of non-specific signs and/or symptoms (some examples listed below) and most often does not involve loss of consciousness. Concussion should be suspected in the presence of **any one or more** of the following:

- Symptoms (e.g., headache), or
- Physical signs (e.g., unsteadiness), or
- Impaired brain function (e.g. confusion) or
- Abnormal behaviour (e.g., change in personality).

# SIDELINE ASSESSMENT

## Indications for Emergency Management

**NOTE:** A hit to the head can sometimes be associated with a more serious brain injury. Any of the following warrants consideration of activating emergency procedures and urgent transportation to the nearest hospital:

- Glasgow Coma score less than 15
- Deteriorating mental status
- Potential spinal injury
- Progressive, worsening symptoms or new neurologic signs

## Potential signs of concussion?

If any of the following signs are observed after a direct or indirect blow to the head, the athlete should stop participation, be evaluated by a medical professional and **should not be permitted to return to sport the same day** if a concussion is suspected.

| | | |
|---|---|---|
| Any loss of consciousness? | Y | N |
| "If so, how long?" _____ | | |
| Balance or motor incoordination (stumbles, slow/laboured movements, etc.)? | Y | N |
| Disorientation or confusion (inability to respond appropriately to questions)? | Y | N |
| Loss of memory: | Y | N |
| "If so, how long?" _____ | | |
| "Before or after the injury?" _____ | | |
| Blank or vacant look: | Y | N |
| Visible facial injury in combination with any of the above: | Y | N |

---

## 1  Glasgow coma scale (GCS)

**Best eye response (E)**

| | |
|---|---|
| No eye opening | 1 |
| Eye opening in response to pain | 2 |
| Eye opening to speech | 3 |
| Eyes opening spontaneously | 4 |

**Best verbal response (V)**

| | |
|---|---|
| No verbal response | 1 |
| Incomprehensible sounds | 2 |
| Inappropriate words | 3 |
| Confused | 4 |
| Oriented | 5 |

**Best motor response (M)**

| | |
|---|---|
| No motor response | 1 |
| Extension to pain | 2 |
| Abnormal flexion to pain | 3 |
| Flexion/Withdrawal to pain | 4 |
| Localizes to pain | 5 |
| Obeys commands | 6 |

| | |
|---|---|
| **Glasgow Coma score (E + V + M)** | of 15 |

GCS should be recorded for all athletes in case of subsequent deterioration.

## 2  Maddocks Score[3]

*"I am going to ask you a few questions, please listen carefully and give your best effort."*
Modified Maddocks questions (1 point for each correct answer)

| | | |
|---|---|---|
| What venue are we at today? | 0 | 1 |
| Which half is it now? | 0 | 1 |
| Who scored last in this match? | 0 | 1 |
| What team did you play last week/game? | 0 | 1 |
| Did your team win the last game? | 0 | 1 |
| **Maddocks score** | | of 5 |

Maddocks score is validated for sideline diagnosis of concussion only and is not used for serial testing.

**Notes:** Mechanism of Injury ("tell me what happened"?):

_____
_____
_____
_____

**Any athlete with a suspected concussion should be REMOVED FROM PLAY, medically assessed, monitored for deterioration (i.e., should not be left alone) and should not drive a motor vehicle until cleared to do so by a medical professional. No athlete diagnosed with concussion should be returned to sports participation on the day of injury.**

---

*The SCAT3 form in this focus box will become obsolete at some point in early 2017 and will be replaced by a new modified version. However, at the time this book was published, the form shown here was the most current version available.

*(continued)*

## BACKGROUND

Name: _____ Date: _____

Examiner: _____

Sport/team/school: _____ Date/time of injury: _____

Age: _____ Gender: ☐ M ☐ F

Years of education completed: _____

Dominant hand: ☐ right ☐ left ☐ neither

How many concussions do you think you have had in the past? _____

When was the most recent concussion? _____

How long was your recovery from the most recent concussion? _____

Have you ever been hospitalized or had medical imaging done for a head injury? ☐ Y ☐ N

Have you ever been diagnosed with headaches or migraines? ☐ Y ☐ N

Do you have a learning disability, dyslexia, ADD/ADHD? ☐ Y ☐ N

Have you ever been diagnosed with depression, anxiety or other psychiatric disorder? ☐ Y ☐ N

Has anyone in your family ever been diagnosed with any of these problems? ☐ Y ☐ N

Are you on any medications? If yes, please list: ☐ Y ☐ N

_____

**SCAT3 to be done in resting state. Best done 10 or more minutes post excercise.**

## SYMPTOM EVALUATION

### 3 How do you feel?

*"You should score yourself on the following symptoms, based on how you feel now".*

| | none | mild | | moderate | | severe | |
|---|---|---|---|---|---|---|---|
| Headache | 0 | 1 | 2 | 3 | 4 | 5 | 6 |
| "Pressure in head" | 0 | 1 | 2 | 3 | 4 | 5 | 6 |
| Neck Pain | 0 | 1 | 2 | 3 | 4 | 5 | 6 |
| Nausea or vomiting | 0 | 1 | 2 | 3 | 4 | 5 | 6 |
| Dizziness | 0 | 1 | 2 | 3 | 4 | 5 | 6 |
| Blurred vision | 0 | 1 | 2 | 3 | 4 | 5 | 6 |
| Balance problems | 0 | 1 | 2 | 3 | 4 | 5 | 6 |
| Sensitivity to light | 0 | 1 | 2 | 3 | 4 | 5 | 6 |
| Sensitivity to noise | 0 | 1 | 2 | 3 | 4 | 5 | 6 |
| Feeling slowed down | 0 | 1 | 2 | 3 | 4 | 5 | 6 |
| Feeling like "in a fog" | 0 | 1 | 2 | 3 | 4 | 5 | 6 |
| "Don't feel right" | 0 | 1 | 2 | 3 | 4 | 5 | 6 |
| Difficulty concentrating | 0 | 1 | 2 | 3 | 4 | 5 | 6 |
| Difficulty remembering | 0 | 1 | 2 | 3 | 4 | 5 | 6 |
| Fatigue or low energy | 0 | 1 | 2 | 3 | 4 | 5 | 6 |
| Confusion | 0 | 1 | 2 | 3 | 4 | 5 | 6 |
| Drowsiness | 0 | 1 | 2 | 3 | 4 | 5 | 6 |
| Trouble falling asleep | 0 | 1 | 2 | 3 | 4 | 5 | 6 |
| More emotional | 0 | 1 | 2 | 3 | 4 | 5 | 6 |
| Irritability | 0 | 1 | 2 | 3 | 4 | 5 | 6 |
| Sadness | 0 | 1 | 2 | 3 | 4 | 5 | 6 |
| Nervous or Anxious | 0 | 1 | 2 | 3 | 4 | 5 | 6 |

**Total number of symptoms** (Maximum possible 22) ☐

**Symptom severity score** (Maximum possible 132) ☐

Do the symptoms get worse with physical activity? ☐ Y ☐ N

Do the symptoms get worse with mental activity? ☐ Y ☐ N

☐ self rated ☐ self rated and clinician monitored

☐ clinician interview ☐ self rated with parent input

**Overall rating:** If you know the athlete well prior to the injury, how different is the athlete acting compared to his/her usual self?

Please circle one response:

☐ no different ☐ very different ☐ unsure ☐ N/A

**Scoring on the SCAT3 should not be used as a stand-alone method to diagnose concussion, measure recovery or make decisions about an athlete's readiness to return to competition after concussion. Since signs and symptoms may evolve over time, it is important to consider repeat evaluation in the acute assessment of concussion.**

## COGNITIVE & PHYSICAL EVALUATION

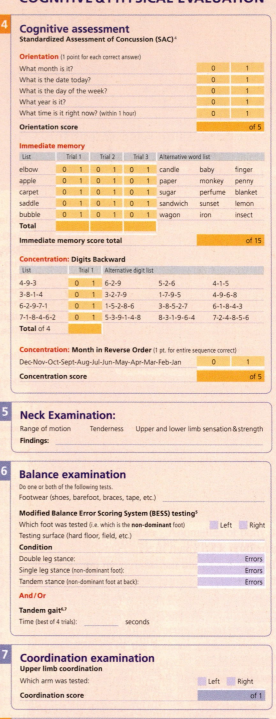

### 4 Cognitive assessment
**Standardized Assessment of Concussion (SAC)[4]**

**Orientation** (1 point for each correct answer)

| | | |
|---|---|---|
| What month is it? | 0 | 1 |
| What is the date today? | 0 | 1 |
| What is the day of the week? | 0 | 1 |
| What year is it? | 0 | 1 |
| What time is it right now? (within 1 hour) | 0 | 1 |
| **Orientation score** | | of 5 |

**Immediate memory**

| List | Trial 1 | | Trial 2 | | Trial 3 | | Alternative word list | | |
|---|---|---|---|---|---|---|---|---|---|
| elbow | 0 | 1 | 0 | 1 | 0 | 1 | candle | baby | finger |
| apple | 0 | 1 | 0 | 1 | 0 | 1 | paper | monkey | penny |
| carpet | 0 | 1 | 0 | 1 | 0 | 1 | sugar | perfume | blanket |
| saddle | 0 | 1 | 0 | 1 | 0 | 1 | sandwich | sunset | lemon |
| bubble | 0 | 1 | 0 | 1 | 0 | 1 | wagon | iron | insect |
| Total | | | | | | | | | |

**Immediate memory score total** — of 15

**Concentration: Digits Backward**

| List | Trial 1 | | Alternative digit list | | |
|---|---|---|---|---|---|
| 4-9-3 | 0 | 1 | 6-2-9 | 5-2-6 | 4-1-5 |
| 3-8-1-4 | 0 | 1 | 3-2-7-9 | 1-7-9-5 | 4-9-6-8 |
| 6-2-9-7-1 | 0 | 1 | 1-5-2-8-6 | 3-8-5-2-7 | 6-1-8-4-3 |
| 7-1-8-4-6-2 | 0 | 1 | 5-3-9-1-4-8 | 8-3-1-9-6-4 | 7-2-4-8-5-6 |
| **Total** of 4 | | | | | |

**Concentration: Month in Reverse Order** (1 pt. for entire sequence correct)

| | | |
|---|---|---|
| Dec-Nov-Oct-Sept-Aug-Jul-Jun-May-Apr-Mar-Feb-Jan | 0 | 1 |
| **Concentration score** | | of 5 |

### 5 Neck Examination:
Range of motion    Tenderness    Upper and lower limb sensation & strength

**Findings:** _____

### 6 Balance examination
Do one or both of the following tests.

Footwear (shoes, barefoot, braces, tape, etc.)

**Modified Balance Error Scoring System (BESS) testing[5]**

Which foot was tested (i.e. which is the **non-dominant** foot) ☐ Left ☐ Right

Testing surface (hard floor, field, etc.) _____

**Condition**

| | |
|---|---|
| Double leg stance: | Errors |
| Single leg stance (non-dominant foot): | Errors |
| Tandem stance (non-dominant foot at back): | Errors |

**And/Or**

**Tandem gait[6,7]**

Time (best of 4 trials): _____ seconds

### 7 Coordination examination
**Upper limb coordination**

Which arm was tested: ☐ Left ☐ Right

**Coordination score** — of 1

### 8 SAC Delayed Recall[4]

**Delayed recall score** — of 5

# INSTRUCTIONS

Words in *Italics* throughout the SCAT3 are the instructions given to the athlete by the tester.

## Symptom Scale

*"You should score yourself on the following symptoms, based on how you feel now".*

To be completed by the athlete. In situations where the symptom scale is being completed after exercise, it should still be done in a resting state, at least 10 minutes post exercise.
For total number of symptoms, maximum possible is 22.
For Symptom severity score, add all scores in table, maximum possible is 22 x 6 = 132.

## SAC[4]

### Immediate Memory

*"I am going to test your memory. I will read you a list of words and when I am done, repeat back as many words as you can remember, in any order."*

### Trials 2 & 3:

*"I am going to repeat the same list again. Repeat back as many words as you can remember in any order, even if you said the word before."*

Complete all 3 trials regardless of score on trial 1 & 2. Read the words at a rate of one per second. **Score 1 pt. for each correct response.** Total score equals sum across all 3 trials. Do not inform the athlete that delayed recall will be tested.

### Concentration
### Digits backward

*"I am going to read you a string of numbers and when I am done, you repeat them back to me backwards, in reverse order of how I read them to you. For example, if I say 7-1-9, you would say 9-1-7."*

If correct, go to next string length. If incorrect, read trial 2. **One point possible for each string length.** Stop after incorrect on both trials. The digits should be read at the rate of one per second.

### Months in reverse order

*"Now tell me the months of the year in reverse order. Start with the last month and go backward. So you'll say December, November … Go ahead"*

**1 pt. for entire sequence correct**

### Delayed Recall

The delayed recall should be performed after completion of the Balance and Coordination Examination.

*"Do you remember that list of words I read a few times earlier? Tell me as many words from the list as you can remember in any order."*

**Score 1 pt. for each correct response**

## Balance Examination

### Modified Balance Error Scoring System (BESS) testing[5]

This balance testing is based on a modified version of the Balance Error Scoring System (BESS)[5]. A stopwatch or watch with a second hand is required for this testing.

*"I am now going to test your balance. Please take your shoes off, roll up your pant legs above ankle (if applicable), and remove any ankle taping (if applicable). This test will consist of three twenty second tests with different stances."*

### (a) Double leg stance:

*"The first stance is standing with your feet together with your hands on your hips and with your eyes closed. You should try to maintain stability in that position for 20 seconds. I will be counting the number of times you move out of this position. I will start timing when you are set and have closed your eyes."*

### (b) Single leg stance:

*"If you were to kick a ball, which foot would you use? [This will be the dominant foot] Now stand on your non-dominant foot. The dominant leg should be held in approximately 30 degrees of hip flexion and 45 degrees of knee flexion. Again, you should try to maintain stability for 20 seconds with your hands on your hips and your eyes closed. I will be counting the number of times you move out of this position. If you stumble out of this position, open your eyes and return to the start position and continue balancing. I will start timing when you are set and have closed your eyes."*

### (c) Tandem stance:

*"Now stand heel-to-toe with your non-dominant foot in back. Your weight should be evenly distributed across both feet. Again, you should try to maintain stability for 20 seconds with your hands on your hips and your eyes closed. I will be counting the number of times you move out of this position. If you stumble out of this position, open your eyes and return to the start position and continue balancing. I will start timing when you are set and have closed your eyes."*

### Balance testing – types of errors
1. Hands lifted off iliac crest
2. Opening eyes
3. Step, stumble, or fall
4. Moving hip into > 30 degrees abduction
5. Lifting forefoot or heel
6. Remaining out of test position > 5 sec

Each of the 20-second trials is scored by counting the errors, or deviations from the proper stance, accumulated by the athlete. The examiner will begin counting errors only after the individual has assumed the proper start position. **The modified BESS is calculated by adding one error point for each error during the three 20-second tests. The maximum total number of errors for any single condition is 10.** If a athlete commits multiple errors simultaneously, only one error is recorded but the athlete should quickly return to the testing position, and counting should resume once subject is set. Subjects that are unable to maintain the testing procedure for a minimum of **five seconds** at the start are assigned the highest possible score, ten, for that testing condition.

**OPTION:** For further assessment, the same 3 stances can be performed on a surface of medium density foam (e.g., approximately 50 cm x 40 cm x 6 cm).

### Tandem Gait[6,7]

*Participants are instructed to stand with their feet together behind a starting line (the test is best done with footwear removed). Then, they walk in a forward direction as quickly and as accurately as possible along a 38mm wide (sports tape), 3 meter line with an alternate foot heel-to-toe gait ensuring that they approximate their heel and toe on each step. Once they cross the end of the 3m line, they turn 180 degrees and return to the starting point using the same gait. A total of 4 trials are done and the best time is retained. Athletes should complete the test in 14 seconds. Athletes fail the test if they step off the line, have a separation between their heel and toe, or if they touch or grab the examiner or an object. In this case, the time is not recorded and the trial repeated, if appropriate.*

## Coordination Examination

### Upper limb coordination
Finger-to-nose (FTN) task:

*"I am going to test your coordination now. Please sit comfortably on the chair with your eyes open and your arm (either right or left) outstretched (shoulder flexed to 90 degrees and elbow and fingers extended), pointing in front of you. When I give a start signal, I would like you to perform five successive finger to nose repetitions using your index finger to touch the tip of the nose, and then return to the starting position, as quickly and as accurately as possible."*

**Scoring: 5 correct repetitions in < 4 seconds = 1**
**Note for testers:** Athletes fail the test if they do not touch their nose, do not fully extend their elbow or do not perform five repetitions. **Failure should be scored as 0.**

## References & Footnotes

1. McCrory P. Meeuwisse W, Aubry M, Cantu RC, Dvorak J, Echemendia R, Engebretsen L, Johnston K, Ktcher J, Raftery M, Sills A, Benson B, Davis G, Ellenbogen R, Guskeiwicz K, Herring SA, Iverson G, Jordan B, Kissick J, McCrea M, McIntosh A, Maddocks D, Makdissi M, Purcell L, Putukian M, Schneider K, Tator C, Turner M. Consense Statement on Concussion in Sport – The 4th International Conference on Concussion in Sport Held In Zurich, November 2012. BR J Sports Med 2013; 47: 250–258.

2. McCrory P et al., Consensus Statement on Concussion in Sport – the 3rd International Conference on Concussion in Sport held in Zurich, November 2008. British Journal of Sports Medicine 2009; 43: i76-89.

3. Maddocks, DL; Dicker, GD; Saling, MM. The assessment of orientation following concussion in athletes. Clinical Journal of Sport Medicine. 1995; 5(1): 32–3.

4. McCrea M. Standardized mental status testing of acute concussion. Clinical Journal of Sport Medicine. 2001; 11: 176–181.

5. Guskiewicz KM. Assessment of postural stability following sport-related concussion. Current Sports Medicine Reports. 2003; 2: 24–30.

6. Schneiders, A.G., Sullivan, S.J., Gray, A., Hammond-Tooke, G. & McCrory, P. Normative values for 16-37 year old subjects for three clinical measures of motor performance used in the assessment of sports concussions. Journal of Science and Medicine in Sport. 2010; 13(2): 196–201.

7. Schneiders, A.G., Sullivan, S.J., Kvarnstrom. J.K., Olsson, M., Yden. T. & Marshall, S.W. The effect of footwear and sports-surface on dynamic neurological screening in sport-related concussion. Journal of Science and Medicine in Sport. 2010; 13(4): 382–386

*(continued)*

## ATHLETE INFORMATION

**Any athlete suspected of having a concussion should be removed from play, and then seek medical evaluation.**

### Signs to watch for

Problems could arise over the first 24–48 hours. The athlete should not be left alone and must go to a hospital at once if they:

- Have a headache that gets worse
- Are very drowsy or can't be awakened
- Can't recognize people or places
- Have repeated vomiting
- Behave unusually or seem confused; are very irritable
- Have seizures (arms and legs jerk uncontrollably)
- Have weak or numb arms or legs
- Are unsteady on their feet; have slurred speech

**Remember, it is better to be safe.**
**Consult your doctor after a suspected concussion.**

### Return to play

Athletes should not be returned to play the same day of injury.
When returning athletes to play, they should be **medically cleared and then follow a stepwise supervised program,** with stages of progression.

**For example:**

| Rehabilitation stage | Functional exercise at each stage of rehabilitation | Objective of each stage |
|---|---|---|
| No activity | Physical and cognitive rest | Recovery |
| Light aerobic exercise | Walking, swimming or stationary cycling keeping intensity, 70 % maximum predicted heart rate. No resistance training | Increase heart rate |
| Sport-specific exercise | Skating drills in ice hockey, running drills in soccer. No head impact activities | Add movement |
| Non-contact training drills | Progression to more complex training drills, eg passing drills in football and ice hockey. May start progressive resistance training | Exercise, coordination, and cognitive load |
| Full contact practice | Following medical clearance participate in normal training activities | Restore confidence and assess functional skills by coaching staff |
| Return to play | Normal game play | |

There should be at least 24 hours (or longer) for each stage and if symptoms recur the athlete should rest until they resolve once again and then resume the program at the previous asymptomatic stage. Resistance training should only be added in the later stages.

If the athlete is symptomatic for more than 10 days, then consultation by a medical practitioner who is expert in the management of concussion, is recommended.

**Medical clearance should be given before return to play.**

## CONCUSSION INJURY ADVICE

(To be given to the **person monitoring** the concussed athlete)

This patient has received an injury to the head. A careful medical examination has been carried out and no sign of any serious complications has been found. Recovery time is variable across individuals and the patient will need monitoring for a further period by a responsible adult. Your treating physician will provide guidance as to this timeframe.

**If you notice any change in behaviour, vomiting, dizziness, worsening head-ache, double vision or excessive drowsiness, please contact your doctor or the nearest hospital emergency department immediately.**

**Other important points:**

- Rest (physically and mentally), including training or playing sports until symptoms resolve and you are medically cleared
- No alcohol
- No prescription or non-prescription drugs without medical supervision. Specifically:
  · No sleeping tablets
  · Do not use aspirin, anti-inflammatory medication or sedating pain killers
- Do not drive until medically cleared
- Do not train or play sport until medically cleared

**Clinic phone number**

### Scoring Summary:

| Test Domain | Score | | |
|---|---|---|---|
| | Date: | Date: | Date: |
| Number of Symptoms of 22 | | | |
| Symptom Severity Score of 132 | | | |
| Orientation of 5 | | | |
| Immediate Memory of 15 | | | |
| Concentration of 5 | | | |
| Delayed Recall of 5 | | | |
| **SAC Total** | | | |
| BESS (total errors) | | | |
| Tandem Gait (seconds) | | | |
| Coordination of 1 | | | |

### Notes:

Patient's name _____

Date/time of injury _____

Date/time of medical review _____

Treating physician _____

Contact details or stamp

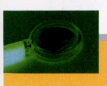

## FOCUS 26–3 Focus on Examination, Assessment, and Diagnosis

### Commonly used neurocognitive tests for sport concussion

| *Paper-and-pencil tests* | *Cognitive domain assessed* |
|---|---|
| 1. Hopkins Verbal Learning Test | Verbal learning, immediate and delayed memory |
| 2. Wechsler Digit Span (WMS-R) Test | Attention, concentration |
| 3. Trail-Making Test | Visual scanning, attention, information processing speed, psychomotor speed |
| 4. Stroop Color Word Test | Attention, information processing speed |
| 5. Controlled Oral Word Association Test | Verbal fluency |
| 6. Symbol Digit Modalities Test | Psychomotor speed, attention, concentration |

| *Computerized tests* | |
|---|---|
| 7. Automated Neuropsychological Assessment Matrix (ANAM) | Simple reaction metrics, Sternberg memory, math processing, continuous performance, matching to sample, spatial processing, code substitution |
| 8. AxonSport | Simple reaction time, complex reaction time, one-back, continuous learning |
| 9. Concussion Resolution Index (CRI) | Reaction time, cued reaction time, visual recognition 1, visual recognition 2, animal decoding, symbol scanning |
| 10. ImPACT | Verbal memory, visual memory, information processing speed, reaction time, impulse control |
| 11. CNS Vital Signs | Verbal memory, visual memory, processing speed, executive function, psychomotor speed, reaction time, complex attention, cognitive flexibility, and reasoning |

more practical for athletic trainers, have gained popularity in recent years. The *Automated Neuropsychological Assessment Metrics (ANAM)*, the AxonSport, *Headminder's Concussion Resolution Index (CRI)*, the *Immediate Postconcussion Assessment and Cognitive Test (ImPACT)*, and *CNS Vital Signs* are the most commonly used tests. These software packages eliminate some of the logistical challenges of baseline testing hundreds of athletes in a timely fashion. Computerized neurocognitive testing can provide useful information in the management of concussion. However, there are limitations to the testing, and athletic trainers should be cautioned against trying to interpret the results of neuropsychological tests without the assistance of a licensed neuropsychologist. Neuropsychological assessment scores can be used as part of the decision for return to play following head injury but should be viewed as only one piece of the concussion puzzle.[19,20] See *Focus Box 26–3:* "Commonly used neurocognitive tests for sport concussion."

## Recognition and Management of Specific Head Injuries

### Skull Fractures

***Etiology*** Skull fractures occur most often from a blunt trauma, such as a baseball to the head, a shot put to the head, or a fall from a height.

***Symptoms and signs*** The patient complains of severe headache and nausea. The patient may also be unconscious. Palpation may infrequently reveal a defect, such as a skull indentation. There may be blood in the middle ear, blood in the ear canal, bleeding through the nose, ecchymosis around the eyes (raccoon eyes), or ecchymosis behind the ear (Battle's sign). Cerebrospinal fluid (straw-colored fluid) may appear in the ear canal and nose.[43]

***Management*** It is not the skull fracture itself that causes the most serious problem but complications that stem from intracranial bleeding, bone fragments embedded in the brain, and infection.[43] Such an injury requires immediate hospitalization and referral to a neurosurgeon.

### Cerebral Concussions (a Form of Traumatic Brain Injury)
Concussion has become a widely publicized public health concern, and deciding when a patient can safely return to participation following a concussion is perhaps the most challenging task for any sports medicine clinician.[10,25,79] An estimated 1.6 to 3.8 million cases of MTBI occur in sports and recreation each year in the United States, including nearly 63,000 concussions annually in high-school sports.[15,29,40,64] The athletic trainer should gain an understanding of prevention, mechanisms of injury, recognition and referral, appropriate return to participation, physical and cognitive restrictions for concussed athletes, and ramifications of improper concussion

management, and use that knowledge to educate athletes, parents, and administrators.[10] **SoR:B**

***Etiology*** Direct blows usually occur when the athlete is struck in the head by some object (e.g., a ball, a baseball bat, a lacrosse stick, or another player). A direct blow may also occur when the athlete's moving head strikes some fixed object (e.g., the floor, a goalpost), which results in impact deceleration of the brain. A blow to the head can produce an injury to the brain either at the point of contact, a **coup injury,** or on the opposite side of the head, a **contrecoup injury.** Acceleration/deceleration forces, and particularly rotational forces, produce shaking of the brain within the skull, which results in shearing forces that disrupt diffuse axonal connections running between the cortex and midbrain.[44] These injuries are not visible lesions.[40]

***Symptoms and signs*** The most current thinking relative to diagnosing an acute concussion is that assessment should involve a variety of symptoms and signs, including these:[51]

- Clinical symptoms
  - somatic (e.g. headache),
  - cognitive (e.g. feeling like in a fog)
  - emotional (e.g. liability)
- Physical signs (e.g. loss of consciousness, amnesia)
- Behavioral changes (e.g. irritability)
- Cognitive impairment (e.g. slowed reaction times)
- Sleep disturbance (e.g. drowsiness)

If any one or more of these components is present, a concussion should be suspected and the appropriate management strategy instituted.

For many years, the medical community in general, and sports medicine practitioners particularly, have attempted to classify concussions into various grades by looking primarily at the physical symptoms, which included the level of consciousness and posttraumatic amnesia that can be either anterograde amnesia (no memory for things that occurred after the injury) or retrograde amnesia (no memory for things that occurred before the injury).[14] The medical community uses the Glasgow Coma Scale to determine level of consciousness and the severity of the injury after head injury. (The Glasgow Coma Scale is part of the SCAT3 and can be found on page 831.) More recently, considerable debate has raged over a variety of classification systems that have been proposed for determining severity of concussion.[12,21,30,31,33,34,35,55,59,69]

> The Glasgow Coma Scale is rarely used by athletic trainers on the sidelines.

**26–3 Clinical Application Exercise**

An ice hockey player is checked hard into the boards head first and sustains a concussion. It is his second concussion this season.

**?** What guidelines should be followed regarding his return to play?

In most of these classification systems, the grades of concussion have been based primarily on the length of time that the patient is unconscious or experiences posttraumatic amnesia. However, it has been demonstrated that loss of consciousness occurs in less than 10 percent of all concussions and that unconsciousness lasts longer than one minute in less than 1 percent of all concussions.[31] Additionally, amnesia is found in less than 30 percent of all concussions. Thus, several of the more recent classification systems take into account other parameters such as concentration deficits, attention span difficulties, and balance and coordination problems rather than focusing on loss of consciousness and posttraumatic amnesia.

It now seems that there may have been too much emphasis placed on these grading scales.[26] **It appears that the most logical approach is to determine the severity of the concussion based on the presence and overall duration of symptoms only after all concussion signs and symptoms have resolved, if the injury is graded.**[10,24,51] This approach places less emphasis on loss of consciousness as a potential predictor of subsequent impairment and additional weight on overall symptom duration.[24] Additionally, attention should be focused on the patient's recovery via symptoms, neurocognitive tests, and postural stability tests, and not by using a grading scale at all.[4] In this approach, the focus is on whether the patient is symptomatic or asymptomatic. The Graded Symptoms Checklist that lists the most common signs and symptoms that occur with concussion can be found in the SCAT3.

***Management*** Returning a patient to competition following concussion has always created a difficult dilemma for both athletic trainers and physicians.[25] A poor decision to return a patient to competition too early can be very costly, one that can lead to death.[8]

When a patient loses consciousness for any reason, the athletic trainer has only one choice, and that is to remove the patient from further activity immediately. If the patient has sustained a head injury that causes unconsciousness, the athletic trainer must always suspect that the patient also has a cervical neck injury and must remove the patient from the field using a spine board.[57,58] Since May 2009, all 50 states have passed some concussion legislation that includes some version of the following requirements: (1) any athlete suspected of having suffered a concussion must be immediately taken out of the game or

A 40-year-old former professional football player with a history of numerous concussions begins to complain of memory difficulty, difficulty in concentrating, and, on occasion, some irritability and problems in visual focusing.

**?** What problem does this patient have? How should his condition be managed?

## TABLE 26–2  On-Field or Sideline Evaluation of Acute Concussion

When an athlete shows *any* signs of a concussion:

1. The athlete should be medically evaluated on-site using standard emergency management principles, and particular attention should be given to excluding a cervical spine injury.
2. The appropriate disposition of the athlete must be determined by the treating health care provider in a timely manner. If no health care provider is available, the athlete should be safely removed from practice or play and urgent referral to a physician arranged.
3. Once the first-aid issues are addressed, then an assessment of the concussive injury should be made using the SCAT3 or other similar tool.
4. The athlete should not be left alone following the injury, and serial monitoring for deterioration is essential over the initial few hours following injury.
5. An athlete with diagnosed concussion should not be allowed to return to play on the day of injury.

Modified from: Consensus statement on concussion in sport: The 4th International Conference on Concussion in Sport, Zurich, November 2012 *Clinical J Sports Med* 23:89–117, 2013.

practice; (2) the athlete is not allowed to return to play on the day of injury, and (3) the athtlete can return to play or practice only after receiving written medical clearance from a physician.[51] Table 26–2 details the procedures that should be followed on the sideline with an athlete who has sustained a concussion. The athletic trainer should be cognizant of the potential for the patient's condition to deteriorate, either immediately (within minutes to hours) or over several days after the injury. Serial assessments and physician follow-up are essential in managing a concussion.[74]

The decision on when to allow a patient with a concussion to return to play is more difficult and to date has been based primarily on the subjective judgment of the athletic trainer or physician. For a number of years, subjective tests for determining when a patient may return to play following concussion (e.g., the Romberg test, among others) have been criticized for their lack of sensitivity and objectivity.[20] The newer, more objective tests, such as the SCAT3, the BESS and the SAC, discussed previously, enable the athletic trainer to make better decisions regarding return to play.[80] The recommendations that have been used in the past for long-term management of concussions over several weeks have changed dramatically. Recent studies have indicated that the recovery period following even a mild head injury may be longer than has been thought in the past.[63] When cognition is tested over a period of several days following concussion, using various neurocognitive assessments, and when balance and postural sway are tested with more sensitive devices[76,85] (e.g., NeuroCom or other force plate systems), it appears that even those patients with mild head injury do not return to normal baseline measures until approximately 3 to 5 days following injury.[23] Patients who have sustained a concussion should not be permitted to return to any type of physical activity until it is either self-reported or

> After a cerebral injury, an athlete must be free of symptoms and signs before returning to competition.

directly observed that *all* postconcussive symptoms have resolved.[53,65]

Following a thorough examination of a patient with a concussion, a decision must be made as to whether the patient can return home or should be admitted to the hospital for overnight observation. If the patient is allowed to return home, the athletic trainer should identify a teammate, friend, or parent who can closely monitor the patient. A concussion instruction sheet such as the one in *Focus Box 26–4* "Home instructions for concussion" can be given to the patient or the person responsible for monitoring the patient.[10]

Once the patient is free of postconcussive symptoms, the patient should not be placed back into practice or competition immediately. Instead, the patient should be gradually progressed through physical activities that have specific criteria for progression from one step to the next (Table 26–3).[51]

Even after postconcussive symptoms have disappeared and the patient has returned to play, there is still a danger of recurrent concussions that can produce cumulative traumatic injury to the brain.[27] Permitting a patient, particularly one in a contact sport, to return before postconcussive symptoms resolve may place the patient at risk of postconcussion syndrome or second-impact syndrome.[28,49]

For many years, clinicians and researchers agreed that cognitive and physical rest was the best rehabilitation for concussed patients. However, recent evidence suggests that strict rest may not be beneficial following a concussion.[78] More recently, researchers have begun investigating the efficacy of *dual task rehabilitation strategies* (combined postural stability and cognitive tasks) for treating patients with lingering postconcussion symptoms.[68] Although there is little research on this rehabilitation strategy, there is promise for its use in the sports medicine community. These techniques involve a divided-attention task, in which the patient is asked to perform a balance task and a neurocognitive task simultaneously. For example, the patient might be asked to perform the BESS while conducting serial sevens or reciting the months of the year

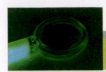

## Home instructions for concussion

*Home Care Plan*

I believe that _____ sustained a concussion on_____.

To make sure he or she recovers, please follow the following important recommendations:

1. _____ must report to the athletic training facility on _____ at _____ for a follow-up evaluation.

2. If any of the problems below develop before the follow-up visit, please call _____ at _____ or contact the local emergency medical system or your family physician.

- Decreasing level of consciousness
- Increasing confusion
- Increasing irritability
- Loss of or fluctuating level of consciousness
- Numbness in the arms or legs
- Pupils becoming unequal in size

- Repeated vomiting
- Seizures
- Slurred speech or inability to speak
- Inability to recognize people or places
- Worsening headache

Otherwise, you can follow the instructions outlined below.

**It is OK to**
- Use acetaminophen (Tylenol) for headaches
- Use ice pack on head and neck as needed for comfort
- Eat a carbohydrate-rich diet
- Go to sleep
- Rest (no strenuous activity or sports)

**There is No need to**
- Check eyes with flashlight
- Wake up frequently (unless otherwise instructed)
- Test reflexes
- Stay in bed

**Do NOT**
- Drink alcohol
- Drive a car or operate machinery
- Engage in physical activity (eg, excerise, weight lifting, physical education, sport participation) that makes symptoms worse
- Engage in mental activity (eg, school, job, homework, computer games) that makes symptoms worse

Other recommendations:

Recommendations provided to: _____

Please feel free to contact me if you have any questions. I can be reached at _____.

Please follow up in the athletic training facility on _____ (date).

Recommendations provided by: _____

Signature: _____ Date: _____

Broglio, S, et al.: National Athletic Trainers' Association position statement: Management of Sport Concussion, Journal of Athletic Training 49(2):245–265, 2014. Reprinted with permission from the National Athletic Trainers' Association.

| TABLE 26–3 | Graduated Return-to-Play Protocol | |
|---|---|---|
| **Rehabilitation Stage*** | **Functional Exercise at Each Stage of Rehabilitation** | **Objective of Each stage** |
| 1. No activity | Complete physical and cognitive rest | Recovery |
| 2. Light aerobic exercise | Walking, swimming or stationary cycling, keeping intensity < 70% MPHR | Increase HR |
| 3. Sport-specific | Skating drills in ice hockey, exercise running drills in soccer. No head impact activities. | Add movement |
| 4. Noncontact | Progression to more training drills and complex training drills, e.g., passing drills in football and ice hockey | Exercise, cognitive load |
| 5. Full contact | Following medical clearance, participate in normal training activities | Restore confidence and assess functional skills by coaching staff |
| 6. Return to play | Normal game play | |

\* With this stepwise progression, the athlete should continue to proceed to the next level if asymptomatic at the current level. Generally, each step should take 24 hours, so that an athlete would take approximately 1 week to proceed through the full rehabilitation protocol once asymptomatic at rest and with provocative exercise.[51]

Modified from Consensus statement on concussion in sport: The 4th International Conference on Concussion in Sport, Zurich, November 2012 *Clinical J Sports Med* 23:89–117, 2013.

in reverse order. More research is necessary to help determine the efficacy of concussion rehabilitation. The first question that must be answered is, Which patients are the best candidates for rehabilitation, and how soon after the injury should these techniques be introduced?

It has been clearly shown that following a concussion, cognitive function may be reduced. It has also been demonstrated that with repeated concussions the severity and duration of functional impairment may be greater and that these changes may be cumulative.[16,18] Once a patient has sustained an initial cerebral concussion, his or her chances of incurring a second one are three to six times greater than for a patient who has never sustained a concussion.[16] Therefore, if a patient sustains more than one concussion, the team physician must decide whether to allow the patient to continue to compete.[28]

In cases of repetitive concussion or brain injury, some evidence suggests it is possible that the patient can develop *chronic traumatic encephalopathy (CTE)*. CTE is a progressive degenerative disease of brain tissue that also involves an accumulation of tau protein within the tissue.[52] CTE has been most recently discovered posthumously in athletes involved in contact sports and in military personnel with a history of multiple concussions and other forms of head injury. Patients who are developing chronic traumatic encephalopathy may show signs of dementia that can include depression, confusion, memory loss, or aggression, however, an accurate clinical description is not widely accepted. These can begin to appear within months following repeated injury but may not appear for decades following injury.[52]

In 2014, the NATA released a position statement management of sport concussion (www.nata.org/sites/default/files/Concussion_Management_Position_Statement.pdf).[10]

## Postconcussion Syndrome

***Etiology*** Postconcussion syndrome is a poorly understood condition that occurs following concussion. It may occur in cases of mild head injury that do not involve loss of consciousness or in cases of severe concussions.[46]

***Symptoms and signs*** The patient complains of a range of postconcussion problems, including persistent headache, impaired memory, lack of concentration, anxiety and irritability, giddiness, fatigue, depression, and visual disturbances (see Table 26–3).[46] These symptoms can begin immediately or within several days following the initial trauma and may last for weeks or even months before resolving.

***Management*** There is no clear-cut treatment for postconcussion syndrome. The patient should not be allowed to return to play until all the symptoms of this condition have resolved.

## Second-Impact Syndrome

***Etiology*** Second-impact syndrome occurs because of rapid swelling and herniation of the brain after a second head injury that occurs before the symptoms of a previous head injury have resolved.[50] This second impact may be relatively minor and, in some cases, may not even involve a blow to the head. A blow to the chest or back may

**26–5 Clinical Application Exercise**

A high-school lacrosse player experienced a concussion with a brief loss of consciousness. One week later, the patient is symptom free except for a headache.

**?** Should the athletic trainer allow the patient to resume normal contact activity at this point?

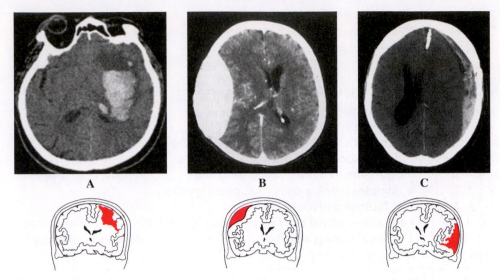

FIGURE 26–6 CT scans showing intracranial hematomas. **(A)** Intracerebral hematoma.
**(B)** Epidural hematoma. **(C)** Subdural hematoma.

create enough force to snap the patient's head and send acceleration/deceleration forces to an already compromised brain. The resulting symptoms occur because a disruption of the brain's blood autoregulatory system leads to swelling of the brain, which significantly increases intracranial pressure, and to herniation. Second-impact syndrome is most likely to occur in individuals less than 20 years of age.

***Symptoms and signs*** Often, the patient does not even lose consciousness and may look stunned. The patient may remain standing and be able to leave the playing field under his or her own power. However, within 15 seconds to several minutes, the patient's condition worsens rapidly, with dilated pupils, loss of eye movement, loss of consciousness leading to coma, and respiratory failure.[50] Second-impact syndrome is a life-threatening situation that has a mortality rate of approximately 50 percent.

***Management*** Second impact syndrome is a life-threatening emergency that must be addressed within approximately 5 minutes by dramatic life-saving measures performed in an emergency care facility.[50] From the athletic trainer's perspective, the best way to manage second-impact syndrome is to prevent it from occurring. Thus, the decision to allow a patient to return to play following an initial head injury must be carefully made based on the absence of postconcussive symptoms.

### Cerebral Contusion

***Etiology*** A contusion of the cerebrum is a focal injury to the brain that involves small hemorrhages, or

*intracerebral bleeding,* within the cortex, the brain stem, or the cerebellum (Figure 26–6A).[21] Brain contusions usually result from an impact injury in which the head strikes a stationary, immovable object, such as the floor.

***Symptoms and signs*** Depending on the extent of trauma and the injury site, symptoms and signs may vary significantly. In most instances, the patient experiences a loss of consciousness but subsequently becomes very alert and talkative. A neurological exam will be normal; however, symptoms such as headaches, dizziness, and nausea persist.

***Management*** Hospitalization and CT or MRI tests are standard for a cerebral contusion. Treatment varies according to the clinical status of the patient.[21] A decision to return to play can be made only when the patient is asymptomatic and a CT scan is normal.

> **The three major types of intracranial hematoma:**
>
> - Intracerebral
> - Epidural
> - Subdural

### Malignant Brain Edema Syndrome

***Etiology*** This condition occurs in the young population. In adults, this syndrome occurs due to an intracranial clot. However, in children there is diffuse brain swelling resulting from hyperemia or vascular engorgement with little or no injury to the brain. The serious or perhaps life-threatening consequences of this condition are due to raised intracranial pressure with herniation.[72]

***Symptoms and signs*** There is rapid neurological deterioration from a normal alert state that progresses to coma and occasionally death within minutes to several hours following head trauma.

***Management*** This condition is a life-threatening situation that requires immediate recognition and subsequent rapid treatment in an emergency care facility.

## Epidural Hematoma

***Etiology*** A blow to the head or a skull fracture can cause a tear of the meningeal arteries, which are embedded in bony grooves in the skull (Figure 26–6B). Because of arterial blood pressure, blood accumulation and the creation of a hematoma occur extremely quickly—usually within minutes to a few hours.[11]

***Symptoms and signs*** In most cases, initially, there is a loss of consciousness. In some cases, once the patient regains consciousness, he or she may be lucid and show few or none of the symptoms of serious head injury. Gradually, symptoms begin to worsen, and the patient experiences severe head pains; dizziness; nausea; dilation of one pupil, usually on the same side as the injury; or sleepiness (see *Focus Box 26–5:* "Conditions indicating the possibility of increasing intracranial pressure"). Later stages of an epidural hematoma are characterized by deteriorating consciousness, neck rigidity, depression of pulse and respiration, and convulsions.[4] An epidural hematoma is a life-threatening situation that necessitates urgent neurosurgical care.[11]

***Management*** A CT scan is necessary to diagnose an epidural hematoma. The pressure of an epidural hematoma must be surgically relieved as soon as possible to avoid the possibility of death or permanent disability.

## Subdural Hematoma

***Etiology*** Acute subdural hematomas occur much more frequently than do epidural hematomas and are the most common cause of death in athletes.[46] Subdural hematomas result from acceleration/deceleration forces that tear vessels that bridge the dura mater and the brain (Figure 26–6C).[46]

A professional firefighter falls from a ladder, striking his head on the pavement, and develops a subdural hematoma.

**?** How can an athletic trainer distinguish the symptoms of a subdural hematoma from the symptoms of an epidural hematoma?

There are three kinds of subdural hematoma. One is an acute subdural hematoma, which progresses rapidly and acts as an epidural hematoma. It occurs due to arterial bleeding. The second is the subdural hematoma seen in association with other brain (contusions) and skull injuries. The third is a chronic subdural hematoma, which occurs due to venous bleeding. If the bridging veins are

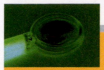

## FOCUS 26–5 Focus on Examination, Assessment, and Diagnosis

### Conditions indicating the possibility of increasing intracranial pressure

- Worsening headache
- Nausea and vomiting
- Unequal pupils
- Disorientation
- Progressive or sudden impairment in consciousness
- Gradual increase in blood pressure
- Decrease in pulse rate

Adapted from Vegso, JJ and Lehman, RC: Field evaluation and management of head and neck injuries. In Torg, JS (ed.): Head and neck injuries, *Clinics in Sports Medicine*, vol. 6, no. 1, Philadelphia: WB Saunders, 1987.

torn, low-pressure venous bleeding occurs into the subdural space, but because of the low pressure, the rising intracranial pressure tamponades the bleeding before serious intracranial pressure occurs. Most subdural hematomas that occur are the acute rapidly progressing form. The acute subdural hematoma is also a common cause of death in boxers.

***Symptoms and signs*** With a simple subdural hematoma, the patient is not likely to be unconscious; the patient with a complicated subdural hematoma almost always is unconscious and exhibits dilation of one pupil, usually on the same side as the injury. Both types show signs of headache, dizziness, nausea, or sleepiness.

***Management*** An acute subdural hematoma is a life-threatening situation that calls for immediate medical attention. A diagnostic CT scan or MRI is necessary to determine the extent and location of the hemorrhage.

## Migraine Headaches

***Etiology*** A migraine is a type of headache that usually happens in episodes or attacks that last anywhere from 4 hours to 72 hours. A migraine is a distinct neurological disorder and is more common in women than men. The exact cause of migraines is unknown; however, they are thought to be an inherited problem. Many factors may trigger a migraine. Triggers include certain foods, medications, sensory stimuli (flickering/bright lights, bright sunlight, odors), or lifestyle changes (sleep patterns, eating habits, stress). Falling estrogen levels that occur just before menstruation can precipitate a migraine headache in many women.[82]

***Symptoms and signs*** The pain of a migraine headache is generally moderate to severe and can disrupt normal activities. It may feel like it is throbbing or pulsating and may be located on one side of the head. It is not uncommon for the pain and other symptoms to be so severe

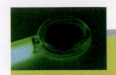

## FOCUS 26-6 Focus on Therapeutic Intervention

### Care of scalp lacerations

*Materials needed*

Antiseptic soap, water, antiseptic, 4-inch (10 cm) gauze pads, sterile cotton, and hair clippers

*Position of the patient*

The patient lies on the table with the wound upward.

*Procedure*

1. The entire area of bleeding is thoroughly cleansed with antiseptic soap and water. Washing the wound to remove dirt and debris is best done in lengthwise movements.
2. After the injury site is cleansed and dried, it is exposed and, if necessary, the hair is cut away. Enough scalp should be exposed so that a bandage and tape may be applied.
3. Firm pressure or an astringent can be used to reduce bleeding if necessary.
4. Wounds that are more than ½ inch (1.25 cm) in length and ⅛ inch (0.3 cm) in depth should be referred to a physician for treatment. In less severe wounds, the bleeding should be controlled and an antiseptic applied, followed by the application of a protective coating, such as collodion and a sterile gauze pad. A tape adherent is then painted over the skin area to ensure that the tape sticks to the skin.

that the person only wants to lie down in a dark room and go to sleep. The pain may be accompanied by nausea; vomiting; sensitivity to sound, smell, or light (photophobia). Some people experience an aura 10 to 30 minutes before they have a migraine headache, which can include visual changes such as bright, flashing lights or colored, zigzag lines; blind spots; or loss of vision on one side. An aura also can include a tingling sensation or numbness in the arms or legs and dizziness. The cause of this aura is still unknown.[82]

*Management* The best management of migraines is prevention. Prophylactic medications, such as promethazine, can help reduce the recurrence of migraines. For severe attacks, the administration of a prescription drug, such as ergotamine tartrate or sumatriptan succinate (Imitrex), has a high success rate.

**Scalp Injuries** The scalp can receive lacerations, abrasions, contusions, and hematomas.

*Etiology* The cause of scalp injury is usually blunt or penetrating trauma. A scalp laceration can exist in conjunction with a serious skull or cerebral injury.

*Symptoms and signs* The patient complains of being hit in the head. Bleeding is often extensive, making it difficult to pinpoint the exact site. Matted hair and dirt can also disguise the actual point of injury.

*Management* The treatment of a scalp laceration poses a special problem because of its general inaccessibility. (See *Focus Box 26–6:* "Care of scalp lacerations.")

BIOHAZARD

# THE FACE

## Anatomy of the Face

The facial skin covers subcutaneous bone that has very little protective muscle, fascia, or fat. The supraorbital ridges house the frontal sinuses. In general, the facial skeleton is composed of dense, bony buttresses combined with thin sheets of bone. The middle third of the face consists of the maxillary bone, which supports the nose and nasal passages. The lower aspect of the face consists of the lower jaw, or mandible. Besides supporting teeth, the mandible also supports the larynx, trachea, upper airway, and upper digestive tract (see Figure 26–1).

**Temporomandibular Joint** The temporomandibular joint (TMJ) is the articulation between the mandibular condyle and the mandibular fossa of the temporal bone.[83] It moves in a hingelike manner when the mouth is opened and closed and glides forward, backward, and side to side when biting or chewing. The TMJ is surrounded by a joint capsule. Within the joint capsule lies a fibrocartilaginous meniscus that separates and cushions the bones and provides for a better fit between the articulating surfaces. The joint capsule is supported by sphenomandibular, temporomandibular, and stylomandibular ligaments (Figure 26–7).

## Recognition and Management of Specific Facial Injuries

With any type of injury to the face, the athletic trainer should always suspect the possibility of an associated head injury.[73]

### Mandible Fracture

*Etiology* Fractures of the lower jaw, or mandible (Figure 26–8), occur most often in collision sports. They are the second most common type of all facial fractures. Because it has relatively little padding and sharp contours, the lower jaw is prone to injury from a direct blow. The most frequently fractured area is near the jaw's frontal angle.

*Symptoms and signs* The main indications of a fractured mandible are deformity, loss of normal occlusion of the teeth, pain when biting down, trismus (guarding of the jaw muscles causing the mouth to be tightly closed), bleeding around the teeth, and lower lip anesthesia.[72]

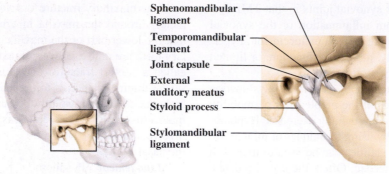

Sphenomandibular ligament
Temporomandibular ligament
Joint capsule
External auditory meatus
Styloid process
Stylomandibular ligament

FIGURE 26–7   Temporomandibular joint (TMJ).

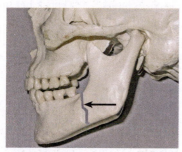

A

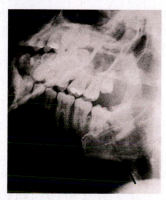

B

FIGURE 26–8   **(A)** Mandibular fracture. **(B)** X-ray view.
© William E. Prentice

**Management**   Fracture of the mandible requires temporary immobilization with an elastic bandage followed by reduction and fixation of the jaw by a physician. After fixation, mild repetitive activities can be carried out, such as lightweight lifting, swimming, or cycling. Recovery time is from 4 to 6 weeks. Full activity is resumed in 2 to 3 months.[74]

## Mandibular Luxation

*Etiology*   A dislocation of the jaw, or *mandibular luxation,* involves the temporomandibular joint (see Figure 26–7). Because of its wide range of motion and the inequity of size between the mandibular condyle and the temporal fossa, the jaw is somewhat prone to dislocation. The mechanism of injury in dislocations is usually a side blow to the open mouth of the patient, which forces the mandibular condyle forward out of the temporal fossa. This injury may occur as either a luxation (complete dislocation) or a subluxation (partial dislocation).

*Symptoms and signs*   The major signs of the luxated jaw are a locked-open position, with jaw movement being almost impossible, and an overriding malocclusion of the teeth.

*Management*   Initially, cold is applied along with elastic bandage immobilization and reduction. Follow-up care includes a soft diet, NSAIDs, and analgesics when needed for 1 to 2 weeks. A gradual return to activity can begin 7 to 10 days after the acute period.[72] Complications of jaw luxation are recurrent dislocation, malocclusion, and TMJ dysfunction.

### Temporomandibular Joint Dysfunction

*Etiology*   The TMJ is important for both communication and mastication, and it has a high degree of mobility. Because of this extreme mobility, the stability of the joint is compromised. The bony configuration of the joint does not limit its mobility, so the muscles and ligaments provide the primary stability.

The most common cause of TMJ dysfunction is a disk-condyle derangement in which the disk is positioned anteriorly with respect to the condyle when the jaw is closed. As the jaw opens and the condyle translates forward, the disk relocates over the condyle, producing an audible click. A second click may occur when the jaw is closed. This chronic derangement eventually leads to deterioration of the posterior stabilizing structures and, ultimately, anterior dislocation of the disk. This chronic derangement is most typically treated through the use of a custom-designed removable mouthpiece that repositions the condyles anteriorly.[83]

A dislocation of the TMJ occurs when one or occasionally both condyles are dislocated forward and prevent the jaw from closing.

*Symptoms and signs*   TMJ dysfunction has been identified as a cause of various signs and symptoms within the head and neck, including headache, earache, vertigo, inflammation, and neck pain associated with trigger points and muscle guarding. Problems in and about the TMJ are similar to those of other synovial joints in that TMJ dysfunction may result from inflammation of the synovial capsule, internal disk derangement, malocclusion, hypermobility or hypomobility, muscle dysfunction, or limited mandibular joint range of motion.[83]

**Management** Management of TMJ dysfunction should address the causes of the problem. Hypermobility can be corrected using strengthening exercises. Hypomobility may be corrected by using techniques of joint mobilization. Therapeutic modalities can be used to treat pain and to provide heat as needed. Often, the use of a dental appliance is recommended. A custom-fitted mouth guard or even a manufactured mouth guard can be used to correct occlusion problems. If these corrective measures fail, the patient should be referred to a dentist for treatment.

### Zygomatic Complex (Cheekbone) Fracture

**Etiology** A fracture of the zygoma represents the third most common facial fracture.[75] The mechanism of injury is a direct blow to the cheekbone (the common name for the zygoma). The zygoma is a very thick facial bone, and is attached to three adjacent facial bones; the maxilla medially and inferiorly, the frontal bone superiorly, and the temporal bone posteriorly (Figure 26–7). Because of its thickness, when the zygoma is hit, it usually fractures at one or more of the suture lines that attach it to the three other facial bones. If only one or two suture lines are affected, the fracture would be nondisplaced, as the remaining attachment would keep the zygoma in place. However, if all three suture lines are involved, this is called a "tripod fracture," and the zygoma will be displaced.

**Symptoms and signs** If the zygoma fracture is nondisplaced, symptoms would be primarily pain and swelling in the region of the fracture. Depending on the location of the fracture(s), symptoms could also include trismus and/or numbness of the face. If all three suture lines are involved, the zygoma is usually rotated downward, leading to loss of prominence of the cheekbone on the involved side as well as a lowering of the infraorbital rim.

**Management** If an obvious facial deformity is present, referral to a hospital is recommended to both evaluate the extent of the zygoma fracture as well as to rule out other facial fractures. For nondisplaced fractures, ice and anti-inflammatories for 24 hours and referral to a physician the next day is sufficient.

### Maxillary Fracture

**Etiology** A severe blow to the upper jaw, such as from a hockey puck or stick, can fracture the maxilla. This injury ranks as the fourth most common type of facial fracture.

**Symptoms and signs** Usually, only the front wall of the maxilla is fractured, as it is quite thin. In this case, symptoms may be minimal and would include swelling of the front of the face between the eye and the mouth, as well as possible numbness of this same area if the fracture involves the infraorbital foramen and nerve. Rarely, there may be some epistaxis, as blood from the torn maxillary sinus mucosa makes its way into the nose.

If the maxillary fracture is severe, it may extend completely around the maxilla in a horizontal direction, so that the lower part of the maxilla and the attached maxillary teeth are now totally separated from the skull. This is called a "Lefort fracture" and is usually only seen when severe trauma is applied to the maxilla, as in a motor vehicle accident. This would obviously result in significant malocclusion as well as epistaxis, as the fracture would involve the lateral wall of the nasal cavity.

**Management** If there is no malocclusion or significant epistaxis, ice and ibuprofen for 24 hours followed by referral to a physician is appropriate. If facial numbness is present, the referral should be expedited so that a CT of the facial bones can be performed to determine the extent of the injury.

A field hockey player sustains a severe blow to her cheek by a stick. The blow fractures her maxilla but does not knock her unconscious.

**?** How should the patient be transported to the hospital and why?

### Facial Lacerations

**Etiology** Facial lacerations are common in contact and collision sports. Lacerations about the face are caused by a direct impact to the face with a sharp object or by an indirect compressive force.

**Symptoms and signs** The patient feels pain, and there is substantial bleeding and obvious tearing of the epidermis, the dermis, and often the subcutaneous layer of skin (Figure 26–9).

**Management** The procedures for facial lacerations are presented in the section on wound care in Chapter 28. The patient should be referred to a physician for definitive care, such as suturing. Athletic trainers should note that, with *eyebrow lacerations,* they should not shave the eyebrow because it may not regrow or, if it does, it may do so in an irregular pattern.[82] Lip, oral, ear, cheek, and nasal

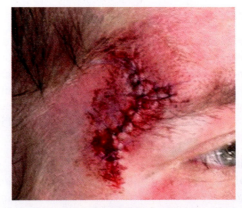

FIGURE 26–9 Facial lacerations usually require either Steri-strips or sutures to close the wound and reduce the chance of having a significant scar.
© William E. Prentice

lacerations, like all facial lacerations, are grossly contaminated and must be carefully cleaned before suturing to avoid infection. Systemic antibiotics and tetanus prophylaxis may be necessary.[82]

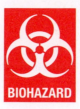

# DENTAL INJURIES

## Anatomy of the Teeth

The tooth is a composite of mineral salts, of which calcium and phosphorus are the most abundant. The portion protruding from the gum, called the *crown,* is covered by the hardest substance within the body, the enamel. The portion that extends into the alveolar bone of the mouth is called the *root* and is covered by a thin, bony substance known as *cementum.* Underneath the enamel and cementum lies the bulk of the tooth, a hard material known as *dentin.* Within the dentin is a central canal and chamber containing the *pulp,* which is composed of nerves, lymphatics, and blood vessels that supply the entire tooth (Figure 26–10). With the use of face guards and properly fitting mouth guards, most dental injuries can be prevented (see Chapter 7).

## Preventing Dental Injuries

There is universal agreement within the dental community that all athletes, but particularly those in contact/collision sports, should routinely wear mouth guards to prevent injuries to the teeth.[7,52] Chapter 7 includes a discussion of the different types of mouth guards available and the relative advantages and disadvantages of each. Without question, the mandatory use of mouth guards by both high-school and collegiate football players has significantly reduced the incidence of oral injuries in those sports.[7] However, there is still a high incidence of dental injuries in the sports that do not require mouth guards to be worn.[36]

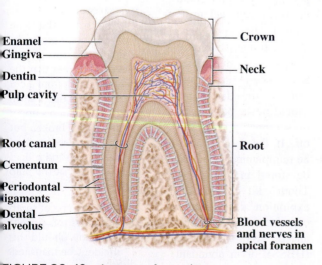

FIGURE 26–10   Anatomy of a tooth.

Labels: Enamel, Gingiva, Dentin, Pulp cavity, Root canal, Cementum, Periodontal ligaments, Dental alveolus, Crown, Neck, Root, Blood vessels and nerves in apical foramen

Individuals should practice good dental hygiene that includes regular brushing, rinsing, and flossing. Everyone should have dental screenings at least once each year to prevent the development of dental caries (cavities), which is a gradual decay and degeneration of soft or bony tissue of a tooth. If this decay progresses, the tissue surrounding the tooth can become inflamed, and an *abscess* forms from a bacterial infection of the tooth. Poor dental hygiene can also lead to *gingivitis,* which is an inflammation of the gums that causes swelling, redness, tenderness, and a tendency to bleed easily. Chronic gingivitis can lead to *periodontitis,* in which there is an inflammation and/or a degeneration of the dental periosteum, the surrounding bone, and the cementum; loosening of the teeth; recession of the gingiva; and infection.[82]

## Recognition and Management of Specific Dental Injuries

### Tooth Fractures

*Etiology*   Any impact to the upper or lower jaw or direct trauma can fracture the teeth.[69] Three types of fractures can occur to the teeth: an *uncomplicated crown fracture,* a *complicated crown fracture,* and a *root fracture* (Figure 26–11).

*Symptoms and signs*   In an *uncomplicated crown fracture,* a small portion of the tooth is broken, but there is no bleeding from the fracture and the pulp chamber is not exposed. In a *complicated crown fracture,* a portion of the tooth is broken, and there is bleeding from the fracture. The pulp chamber is exposed, and there is a great deal of pain (Figure 26–12). A *root fracture* occurs below the gum line; therefore, diagnosis is difficult and may require an X-ray. Root fractures account for only 10 to 15 percent of all dental fractures. The tooth may appear to be in the normal position, but there is bleeding from the gum around the tooth, and the crown of the tooth may be pushed back or loose.

Any impact great enough to cause a fracture of a tooth could also produce a fracture of the mandible or even a concussion.[69]

*Management*   Neither uncomplicated nor complicated crown fractures require immediate treatment by a dentist.[32] The fractured piece of tooth can simply be placed in a plastic bag, and if the fractured tooth is not extremely sensitive to air or cold, the athlete can continue to play and can see the dentist within 24 to 48 hours after the game. If there is bleeding, a piece of gauze can be placed over the fracture. For the sake of appearance, the fractured piece of tooth can be bonded in place or the tooth can be capped with a synthetic composite or gold material by a dentist.

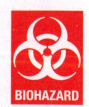

In the case of a root fracture, the patient may continue to play if there is no excessive bleeding or tooth mobility but should see a dentist as soon as possible after the game. A tooth that is pushed back should not be forced forward because doing so is likely to make the fracture worse. The

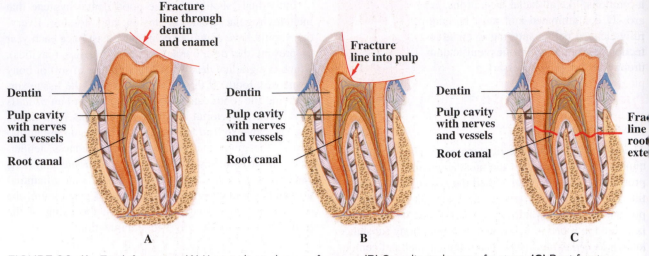

FIGURE 26-11   Tooth fractures. **(A)** Uncomplicated crown fracture. **(B)** Complicated crown fracture. **(C)** Root fracture.

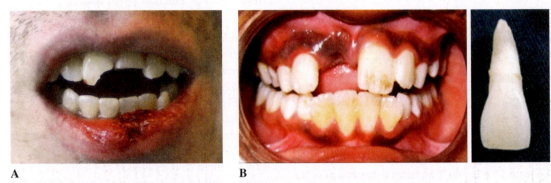

FIGURE 26-12   Tooth injuries. **(A)** A fractured tooth. **(B)** Avulsed tooth.

dentist will reposition the tooth and apply a brace to be worn for 3 to 4 months. The patient must wear a mouth guard while competing.

### Tooth Subluxation, Luxation, Avulsion

*Etiology*   The same mechanisms that can cause a tooth fracture can also cause loosening or dislocation of the tooth.[69] Loosening of the tooth can result in concussion or subluxation, luxation, or avulsion.

*Symptoms and signs*   A tooth may be slightly loosened or totally dislodged. In the case of a concussion or subluxation, the tooth is still in its normal place and is only slightly loose. The patient feels little or no pain but indicates that the tooth just feels different or is sensitive to tapping (percussing) or biting. In a luxation, the tooth is not fractured but is very loose and has moved either outward to an extruded position or inward to an intruded position. In an avulsion, the tooth is knocked completely out of the mouth.

*Management*   For a concussion or subluxation, no immediate treatment is required, and the patient should be referred to a dentist within 48 hours for evaluation only. In a luxation, the tooth should be moved back into its normal position only if it is easy to move. The patient should be referred to a dentist immediately, especially if the tooth could not be moved back to its normal position. The athletic trainer should try to reimplant an avulsed tooth. The avulsed tooth can be rinsed off but should never be scraped or scrubbed to get dirt off. If the tooth cannot be reimplanted, it should be stored in a "Save a Tooth" kit (check the expiration date), which contains Hank's Balanced Salt Solution (HBSS), or in abundant saliva from the athlete in

A basketball player is elbowed in the mouth while fighting for a rebound. He goes to the sidelines with blood in his mouth, saying that he thinks he has chipped a tooth. On examination, the athletic trainer determines that the blood is coming from a cut in the lip and that a small portion of one of his upper front teeth is broken but there is no bleeding from the fracture and it does not appear that the pulp chamber has been exposed.

**?**  What type of tooth fracture does this patient have, and how should this incident be managed?

a plastic bag, milk, or saline.[69] If the patient is conscious and a Save a Tooth kit is not available, the tooth can be placed between the cheek and gum while the patient is transported to a dentist. The patient should be referred to the dentist immediately. The sooner the tooth can be reimplanted, the better the prognosis.[6]

# NASAL INJURIES

## Anatomy of the Nose

The nose cleans, warms, and humidifies inhaled air. The external portion of the nose is formed by a combination of bone in the superior portion and fibrocartilage inferiorly that spreads laterally to form the ala. The nasal cavity extends from the nostrils posteriorly to the choanae, which are openings into the pharynx. The hard palate is a plate that covers the floor of the nasal cavity and separates the nasal cavity from the oral cavity. A nasal septum divides the nasal cavity into right and left chambers (Figure 26–13).

## Recognition and Management of Specific Nose Injuries

### Nasal Fractures

*Etiology* A fracture of the nose is the most common fracture of the face (Figure 26–14 ). The force of the

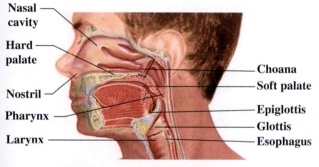

**Nasal cavity**
**Hard palate**
**Nostril**
**Pharynx**
**Larynx**
**Choana**
**Soft palate**
**Epiglottis**
**Glottis**
**Esophagus**

FIGURE 26–13 Anatomy of the nasopharynx.

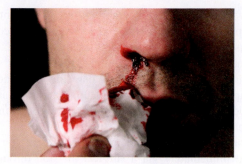

FIGURE 26–14 A nasal fracture will usually cause bleeding, swelling and deformity.
© powerofforever/Getty Images

blow to the nose may come either from the side or from a straight frontal force. A lateral force causes greater deformity than a straight-on blow does.

*Symptoms and signs* With nasal fractures, hemorrhage is common but may or may not be present depending on whether the nasal mucosa was torn or not because of the fracture. Swelling is immediate. Deformity is usually present if the nose has received a lateral blow, but may not be present if the blow was straight on.

*Management* The athletic trainer should control the bleeding and then refer the patient to a physician for X-ray examination and reduction of the fracture. Simple and uncomplicated fractures of the nose will not hinder the patient or be unsafe, and he or she will be able to return to competition within a few days. Fracture deformity reduction must be performed by a trained person.[71] Adequate protection can be provided through splinting (see *Focus Box 26–7:* "Nose splinting").

### Deviated Septum

*Etiology* A nasal hematoma is due to a fracture of the cartilaginous portion of the nasal septum. It is usually the result of a forceful blow directly to the nasal tip.

*Symptoms and signs* A septal hematoma will not show up for at least 24 to 48 hours after the nasal injury.

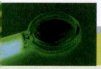

# FOCUS 26–7 Focus on Therapeutic Intervention

## Nose splinting

The following procedure is used for nose splinting.

### Materials needed

Two pieces of gauze, each 2 inches (5 cm) long and rolled to the size of a pencil; three strips of 1½-inch (3.8 cm) tape cut approximately 4 inches (10 cm) long; and clear tape adherent.

*Position of the patient*

The patient lies supine on the training table.

*Procedure*

1. The rolled pieces of gauze are placed on either side of the patient's nose.
2. Gently but firmly, 4-inch (10 cm) lengths of tape are laid over the gauze rolls.

The two most common symptoms are persistent low-grade pain in the septal area and persistent nasal congestion, usually more on one side than the other. Exam of the nasal passages using a penlight or other light source will show obstruction of usually one side of the nose by what appears to be a deviated septum, but which, in fact, is blood underneath the septal mucosa, bulging it into the nasal passage.

***Management*** When a hematoma is present, it must be drained immediately via a surgical incision through the nasal septal mucosa. After surgical drainage, a small wick is inserted for continued drainage, and the nose is firmly packed to prevent the hematoma from reforming. If a hematoma is neglected, an abscess will form, causing bone and cartilage loss and, ultimately, a difficult-to-correct deformity.

### Epistaxis (Nosebleed)

***Etiology*** Nosebleeds are usually the result of direct blows that cause varying degrees of contusion to the septum. Epistaxis can be classified as either anterior or posterior. Anterior epistaxis originates from the nasal septum, and posterior epistaxis from the lateral wall. Anterior epistaxis is more common by far and may result from a direct blow, a sinus infection, high humidity, allergies, a foreign body lodged in the nose, or some other serious facial or head injury.[84] nasal dryness, or from inflamed capillaries secondary to a viral or allergic rhinitis.

***Symptoms and signs*** Hemorrhages arise most often from the highly vascular anterior aspect of the nasal septum. In most situations, the nosebleed presents only a minor problem and stops spontaneously after a short period of time. However, there are persistent types that require medical attention and possibly cauterization. As always when blood is present, universal precautions must be used.

***Management*** The patient should sit upright with his or her head held forward and tilted slightly up, in what is called the "sniffing position" (as when you sniff a flower). This keeps the blood from going down the back of the throat. Ice can be applied over the bridge of the nose using a plastic bag. Pressure against the septum should be applied by pressing the nostril(s) closed using the patient's thumb and forefinger. Ideally, before applying digital pressure, a topical nasal decongestant such as oxymetazoline (Afrin) should be either sprayed directly into the nose or used to soak a piece of cotton gauze that is then placed in the nose and pressure is applied. Pressure should be held for 5 minutes, and may be repeated once if bleeding persists. After bleeding has ceased, the patient may resume activity but should be reminded not to blow the nose under any circumstances for at least 2 hours after the initial insult.

A wrestler is hit in the nose, which injures the lateral nasal wall and causes epistaxis.

**?** How should this nosebleed be managed?

# EAR INJURIES

## Anatomy of the Ear

The ear (Figure 26–15) is responsible for the sense of hearing and for equilibrium. It is composed of three parts: the external ear; the middle ear (tympanic membrane), lying just inside the skull; and the internal ear (labyrinth), which is formed in part by the temporal bone

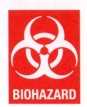
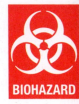
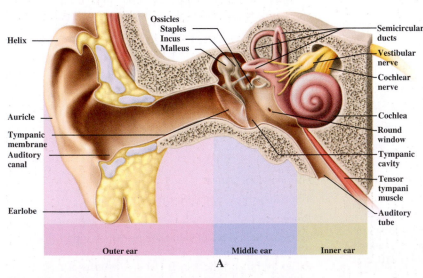
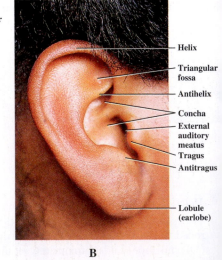

FIGURE 26–15  Anatomy of the ear. **(A)** Internal. **(B)** Auricular.

© Joe DeGrandis/McGraw-Hill Education

of the skull. The middle ear and internal ear are structured to transport auditory impulses to the brain. Aiding the organs of hearing and equalizing pressure between the middle and the internal ear is the eustachian tube, a canal that joins the nose and the middle ear.[70]

Injuries to the ear occur most often to the external portion. The external ear is separated into the auricle (pinna) and the external auditory canal (meatus). The auricle, which is shaped like a shell, collects and directs sound waves into the auditory canal. It is composed primarily of flexible cartilage and is covered by a closely adhering, thin layer of skin. Most of the blood vessels and nerves of the auricle are in the skin and also the perichondrium, which overlays the cartilage itself.

## Recognition and Management of Specific Ear Injuries

### Auricular (Pinna) Hematoma (Cauliflower Ear)

*Etiology*  Hematomas of the ear are common in boxing, rugby, and wrestling. They are most common in individuals who do not wear protective headgear. This condition usually occurs either from compression or from a shearing injury (single or repeated) to the auricle that causes bleeding from blood vessels in the perichondrium, which then fills the space between the perichondrium and the ear cartilage.

*Symptoms and signs*  Trauma may tear the overlying tissue away from the cartilaginous plate, resulting in hemorrhage and fluid accumulation. A hematoma usually forms before the limited circulation can absorb the fluid. If the hematoma goes unattended, a sequence of coagulation, organization, and fibrosis results in a keloid that appears elevated, rounded, white, nodular, and firm, resembling a cauliflower (Figure 26–16). Often, the neocartilage forms

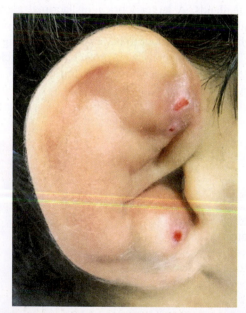

FIGURE 26–16  Hematoma of the auricle, also called cauliflower ear.
© William E. Prentice

in the region of the helix fossa or concha; once developed, the keloid can be removed only through surgery.[39]

*Management*  To prevent this disfiguring condition from arising, some friction-reducing agent, such as petroleum jelly, should be applied to the ears of athletes susceptible to this condition. These athletes should also routinely wear ear guards in practice and in competition.

If an ear becomes "hot" because of excessive rubbing or twisting, the immediate application of a cold pack to the affected spot will alleviate hemorrhage. Once swelling is present in the ear, special care should be taken to prevent the fluid from solidifying; a cold pack should be placed immediately over the ear and held tightly by an elastic bandage for at least 20 minutes. If the swelling is still present at the end of this time, aspiration by a physician is required.[41] After drainage, pressure is applied to the area to prevent the return of the hematoma. The physician may suture dental rolls into position to ensure uniform pressure.[41]

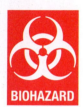

### Rupture of the Tympanic Membrane

*Etiology*  Rupture of the tympanic membrane is commonly seen in contact and collision sports as well as in water polo and diving.[42] A fall or slap to the unprotected ear or sudden underwater variation can rupture the tympanic membrane. It can also be a problem for an individual who is traveling on an airplane who has an existing ear infection or inflammation. When the pressure changes abruptly in the cabin, the tympanic membrane can be ruptured.

*Symptoms and signs*  The patient complains of a loud pop followed by pain in the ear, nausea, vomiting, and dizziness.[42] The patient demonstrates hearing loss and visible rupture of the tympanic membrane. Tympanic membrane ruptures can be seen through an otoscope, an instrument used to visually examine the ear canal and the tympanic membrane (Figure 26–17).

*Management*  Small to moderate perforations of the tympanic membrane usually heal spontaneously in 1 to 2 weeks. Infection can occur and must be continually monitored.

### Otitis Externa (Swimmer's Ear)

*Etiology*  A common condition in individuals engaged in water activities is otitis externa, or *swimmer's ear*. Swimmer's ear is an infection of the ear canal caused by *Pseudomonas aeruginosa,* a type of gram-negative bacillus. Contrary to current thought among swimming coaches, swimmer's ear is not usually associated with a fungal infection. Water can become trapped in the ear canal as a result of obstructions created by cysts, bone growths, plugs of earwax, or swelling caused by allergies.[39]

*Symptoms and signs*  The patient complains of pain and dizziness and may complain of itching, discharge, or even a partial hearing loss.

*Management*  Individuals can best prevent ear infection by drying the ears thoroughly with a soft towel, using

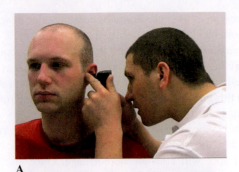

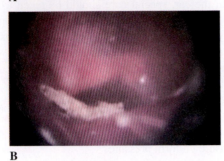

FIGURE 26–17 Examining the ear with an otoscope. **(A)** The position of the examiner. **(B)** A realistic view of what is seen in a normal ear canal by the examiner through an otoscope.

© William E. Prentice

ear drops containing a mild acid (3% boric acid) and alcohol solution before and after each swim, and avoiding situations that can cause ear infections, such as overexposure to cold wind or sticking foreign objects into the ear.

When a swimmer displays symptoms of otitis external, he or she should be referred immediately to a physician. Tympanic membrane rupture should be ruled out. Treatment may include acidification through drops into the ear to make an inhospitable environment for the gram-negative bacteria. Antibiotics may be used in patients with a mild ear infection.[39] In the event of a ruptured tympanic membrane, custom-made earplugs must be used.

### Otitis Media (Middle Ear Infection)

*Etiology* Otitis media is an accumulation of fluid in the middle ear caused by local and systemic inflammation and infection.[70]

*Symptoms and signs* There is usually intense pain in the ear, fluid draining from the ear canal, and a transient loss of hearing. In addition, the systemic infection may also cause fever, headache, irritability, loss of appetite, and nausea.[70] If examined through an otoscope, the tympanic membrane will appear to be bulging and possibly bleeding (Figure 26–17C).

*Management* A physician may choose to draw a small amount of fluid from the middle ear to determine the most appropriate antibiotic therapy. Analgesics can be used to help reduce pain. The problem generally begins to resolve within 24 hours, although pain may last for 72 hours.

### Impacted Cerumen

*Etiology* Cerumen, or earwax, is secreted by glands in the outer portion of the ear canal. Occasionally, an excessive amount of earwax accumulates, clogging the ear canal.

*Symptoms and signs* Impacted cerumen causes some degree of muffled hearing or hearing loss. However, there is generally little or no pain because no infection is involved.[82]

*Management* Initially, an attempt can be made to remove excess cerumen by irrigation of the ear canal with warm water. The athlete should not attempt to remove the cerumen with a cotton tip applicator because that may increase the degree of impaction. If irrigation fails, the impacted cerumen must be physically removed by a physician.

## EYE INJURIES

Eye injuries account for approximately 2 percent of all sports injuries.[5] In the United States, basketball, baseball, boxing, soccer, swimming, and racquet sports have a high incidence of eye injuries (Table 26–4).[22]

### Anatomy of the Eye

The eye has many protective anatomical features.[61] It is firmly retained within an oval socket formed by the bones of the head. A cushion of soft, fatty tissue surrounds it, and a thin skin flap (the eyelid), which functions by reflex action, covers the eye for protection. Foreign particles are prevented from entering the eye by the lashes and eyebrows, which act as a filtering system. A soft mucous lining that covers the inner conjunctiva transports and spreads tears, which are secreted by many accessory lacrimal glands. A larger lubricating lacrimal gland, located above the eyeball, secretes large quantities of tears through the lacrimal duct to help wash away foreign particles. The eye proper is well protected by the sclera, a tough, white, outer layer possessing a transparent center portion called the *cornea*.

| TABLE 26–4 | Percentage of Sports Eye Injuries in the United States |
|---|---|
| **Sport** | **Percent (%)** |
| Baseball | 27 |
| Racquet sports | 20 |
| Basketball | 20 |
| Football and soccer | 7 |
| Ice hockey | 4 |
| Ball hockey | 1 |

Adapted from Pashby, RC and Pashby, TJ: Ocular injuries in sport. In Welsh, PR and Shepard, RJ (eds.): *Current therapy in sports medicine*, 1985–1986, Philadelphia: BC Decker, 1985.

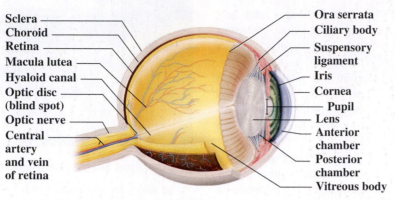

FIGURE 26–18 Anatomy of the eye.

Sclera
Choroid
Retina
Macula lutea
Hyaloid canal
Optic disc (blind spot)
Optic nerve
Central artery and vein of retina

Ora serrata
Ciliary body
Suspensory ligament
Iris
Cornea
Pupil
Lens
Anterior chamber
Posterior chamber
Vitreous body

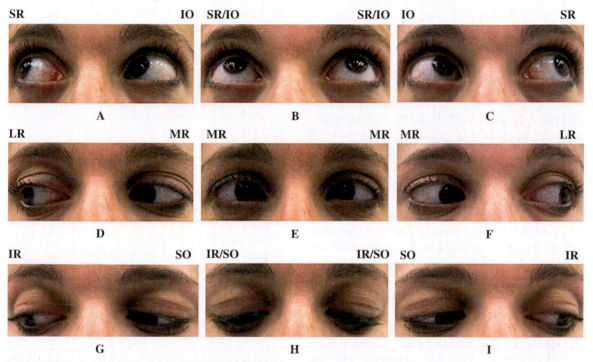

FIGURE 26–19 Nine cardinal planes of gaze. The prime mover for each eye is identified for each of the nine cardinal gazes. (A) Up and right. (B) Up. (C) Up and left. (D) Right. (E) Convergence. (F) Left. (G) Down and right. (H) Down. (I) Down and left.

SR = superior rectus          SO = superior oblique          LR = lateral rectus
MR = medial rectus            IR = inferior rectus           IO = inferior oblique

© William E. Prentice

The cornea covers the pupil, which is the central opening of the eye. Light passes through the cornea, then through the anterior chamber and pupil past the iris and the lens, and finally through the vitreous body, all of which function collectively to focus an image on the retina, where the image is relayed to the brain by the optic nerve (Figure 26–18).

The muscles that move the eye are innervated by cranial nerves III (occulomotor), IV (trochlear), and VI (abducens). There are six muscles that move each eye: medial rectus (III), lateral rectus (VI), inferior rectus (III), superior rectus (III), superior oblique (IV), and inferior oblique (III).

Injury to any one of the muscles, or injury to any of the three cranial nerves, affects the eye's ability to move in one or more of the nine cardinal planes of gaze: up and left, up and right, up, left, right, down, down and left, down and right, and in convergence (Figure 26–19).

## Preventing Eye Injuries

The eye can be injured in a number of ways. Shattered eyeglass or goggle lenses can lacerate; ski pole tips can penetrate; and fingers, racquetball balls, and larger projectiles can seriously compress and injure the eye. High-energy sports, such as ice hockey, football, and lacrosse,

**26–10 Clinical Application Exercise**

A 30-year-old male is accidently poked in the left eye while playing basketball with a few friends in his driveway.

❓ What symptoms indicate that this may be a serious eye injury?

require full-face and helmet protection, whereas low-energy sports, such as racquetball and tennis, require eye guards that rest on the face.[22] Protective devices must provide protection from front and lateral blows.

Sport goggles can be made with highly impact-resistant polycarbonate lenses for refraction. The major problem with sport goggles is that they distort peripheral vision and tend to become fogged under certain weather conditions (see Chapter 7).

## Assessment of the Eye

It has been said that "evaluating and managing eye injuries is no place for amateurs." Thus, the athletic trainer must use extreme caution in evaluating eye injuries. If any of the following conditions are evident, the patient should be immediately referred to an ophthalmologist:[62] retinal detachment, perforation of the globe, a foreign object embedded in the cornea, blood in the anterior chamber, decreased vision, loss of the visual field, poor pupillary response, double vision, laceration, or impaired lid function. An object impaled in the globe should be stabilized and left in place pending transport to the hospital ER.

Ideally, the patient with a serious eye injury should be transported to the hospital by ambulance in a recumbent position. Because the eyes move together, both eyes must be covered during transport; otherwise, moving the unaffected eye will cause the injured eye to move as well. At no time should pressure be applied to the eye. In case of surrounding soft-tissue injury, a cold compress can be applied for 30 to 60 minutes to control hemorrhage. See *Focus Box 26–8:* "Supplies for managing eye injuries."

> **Extreme care must be taken with any eye injury: Transport the athlete in a recumbent position; cover both eyes, but do not put pressure on the eye.**

The athletic trainer's first concerns are to understand the mechanism of injury and to determine whether there is also a condition related to the head, face, or neck.[22] The evaluation process should include the following steps.

### History
- What was the mechanism of injury (sharp and penetrating or blunt)?
- Was loss of vision gradual or immediate?
- What was the visual status before injury?
- Was there loss of consciousness?

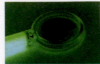

### Observation
- Inspect the external ocular structures for swelling and discoloration, penetrating objects, deformities, and movement of the lid.
- Inspect the globe of the eye for lacerations, foreign bodies, hyphema, and deformities.
- Inspect the conjunctiva and sclera for foreign bodies, hemorrhage, and deformities.
- Check eye movements through the nine cardinal planes of gaze.

**Palpation** Palpate the orbital rim for point tenderness and bony deformity.

### Special Tests
***Pupillary Response*** Tests to determine pupillary response were described in the section on the assessment of head injuries; they include pupil dilation and accommodation by covering the eye and then exposing it to light.

***Visual Acuity*** The evaluator determines visual acuity by asking the patient to report what is seen when he or she looks at some object with the unaffected eye covered. A Snellen eyechart can be used to determine the extent of impairment (Figure 26–20). There may be blurring of vision, diplopia, floating black specks, or flashes of light, all of which indicate serious eye involvement.

***Ophthalmoscope*** An ophthalmoscope is an instrument for observing the interior of the eye, especially the retina (Figure 26–21). An athletic trainer may use an ophthalmoscope to look into the eye. Obviously, special training is

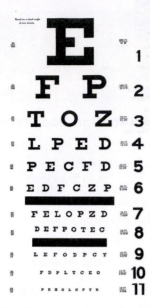

FIGURE 26–20 When using the Snellen eyechart to check visual acuity, one eye is covered at a time. The vision of each eye, as well as both eyes together, is recorded separately. In the Snellen fraction 20/20, the top number is related to the test distance, and the bottom number is related to the size of the letter seen. For reporting visual acuity, record the test used, the distance tested, and the lowest line correctly seen.
© William E. Prentice

necessary to recognize the presence of specific conditions or injuries.

## Recognition and Management of Specific Eye Injuries

### Orbital Hematoma (Black Eye)

*Etiology* Although well protected, the eye may be bruised by direct contact. The severity of eye injuries varies from a mild bruise to an extremely serious condition affecting vision to the fracturing of the orbital cavity. Fortunately, most eye injuries sustained in sports are mild. A blow to the eye may initially injure the surrounding tissue and produce capillary bleeding into the tissue spaces. If the hemorrhage goes unchecked, the result may be a classic black eye (Figure 26–22).[22]

*Symptoms and signs* The signs of a more serious contusion may be displayed as a subconjunctival hemorrhage or as reduced vision.

*Management* Care of an eye contusion requires cold application for at least half an hour, plus a 24-hour rest period if the patient has distorted vision. A patient should avoid blowing the nose after an acute eye injury. To do so might increase hemorrhaging.

### Orbital Fractures

*Etiology* A fracture of the bony framework of the orbit surrounding the eye can occur when a blow to the eyeball forces it posteriorly, compressing the orbital fat until a blowout or rupture occurs to the floor of the orbit. Both fat and the inferior extraocular muscles can herniate through this fracture.[5] This is occasionally referred to as a *trap door injury.*

*Symptoms and signs* The patient with a fracture of the orbit often exhibits diplopia, restricted movement of the eye, a downward displacement of the eye, and pain accompanied by soft-tissue swelling and hemorrhage. There may be numbness associated with injury to the infraorbital nerve on the floor of the orbit. An X-ray or CT scan must be taken to confirm the fracture.

*Management* A physician should administer antibiotics prophylactically to decrease the likelihood of infection. A fracture in the orbital floor allows communication with the maxillary sinus, which may contain infectious bacteria. Most orbital fractures are treated surgically, although

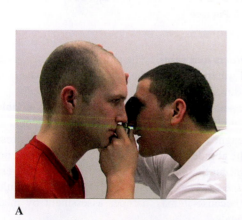

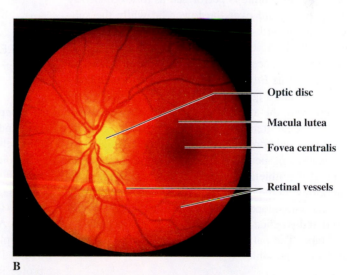

Optic disc

Macula lutea

Fovea centralis

Retinal vessels

**A**                         **B**

FIGURE 26–21 Examining the eye with an ophthalmoscope. (A) Position of the examiner. (B) View of the normal eye through the ophthalmoscope. (*Note:* the handheld ophthalmoscope field of view is about six times smaller than the photographic image in B.)

(a) © William E. Prentice; (b) © Steve Allen/Getty Images

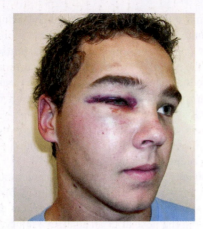

**FIGURE 26–22** Orbital hematoma (black eye).
© William E. Prentice

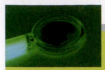

**Removing a foreign body from the eye**

*Materials needed*

Sterile cotton-tipped swab, eyecup, and eyewash (solution of sterile saline or artificial tears).

*Position of the patient*

The patient lies supine on a table.

*Procedure*

1. Gently pull the eyelid up or down, depending on location of foreign body (FB).
2. Have the patient look up or down; then grasp the lashes.
3. Holding the lid open with one hand, use the sterile cotton swab to lift out the FB.
4. Rinse with sterile saline or artificial tears.

some physicians prefer to wait and see whether the symptoms resolve on their own.

### Foreign Bodies in the Eye

*Etiology*　Foreign bodies in the eye are a frequent occurrence in sports and are potentially dangerous.

*Symptoms and signs*　A foreign object produces considerable pain and disability. No attempt should be made to remove the body by rubbing or to remove it with the fingers.

*Management*　The athletic trainer should instruct the patient to close the eye until the initial pain has subsided and then attempt to determine whether the object is in the vicinity of the upper or lower lid. Foreign bodies in the lower lid are relatively easy to remove by depressing the tissue and then wiping it with a sterile cotton applicator. Foreign bodies in the area of the upper lid are usually much more difficult to localize. Two methods may be used. The first technique is performed as follows: Gently pull the upper eyelid over the lower lid while the subject looks downward. This causes tears to be produced, which may flush the object down onto the lower lid. If this method is unsuccessful, the second technique should be used (see *Focus Box 26–9:* "Removing a foreign body from the eye" and Figure 26–23). After the foreign particle is removed, the affected eye should be washed with a saline solution. Often, after removal of the foreign body there is a residual soreness, which may be alleviated by the application of petroleum jelly or some other mild ointment. If the athletic trainer encounters extreme difficulty in removing the foreign body, or if the foreign body has become embedded in the eye itself, the eye should be closed and patched with a gauze pad held in place by strips of tape. The patient should be referred to a physician as soon as possible.[5]

### Corneal Abrasions and Lacerations

*Etiology*　A patient who gets a foreign object in his or her eye usually tries to rub it away. In doing so, the cornea can become abraded or perhaps sustain a small laceration.

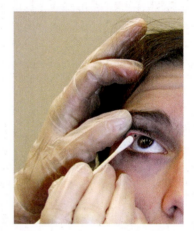

**FIGURE 26–23** Removing a foreign body from the eye.
© William E. Prentice

*Symptoms and signs*　The patient complains of severe pain and watering of the eye, photophobia, and spasm of the eyelid muscles.

*Management*　The eye should be patched, and the patient should be sent to an eye care provider. Corneal abrasion is diagnosed through the application of a fluorescein strip to the abraded area, which stains the abrasion a bright green. Antibiotic ointment is applied with a semipressure patch placed over the closed eyelid. Dilation should be avoided because it may hamper assessment by medical professionals.

### Hyphema

*Etiology*　A blunt blow to the anterior aspect of the eye can produce a hyphema, which is a collection of blood

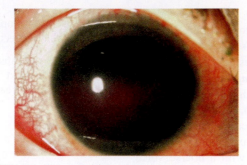

FIGURE 26–24 Hyphema. Blood accumulates in the anterior chamber of the eye.

within the anterior chamber.[77] This injury is often caused when an individual is struck in the eye with a racquetball ball or squash ball when not wearing the appropriate protective eyewear.[77]

*Symptoms and signs* Initially, there is a visible reddish tinge in the anterior chamber and, within the first 2 hours, the blood settles inferiorly or may fill the entire chamber (Figure 26–24). The blood may turn to a pea green color. Vision may be partially or completely blocked. The athletic trainer must be aware that a hyphema is a major eye injury that may be associated with serious problems of the lens, choroid, or retina.

*Management* A patient with a hyphema should be immediately referred to an eye care professional. Historical treatment included hospitalization and bed rest with the head elevated 30 to 40 degrees, patching of both eyes, sedation, and medication. Current therapy is usually more conservative. While awaiting treatment, the athletic trainer should recommend limited activity and avoiding aspirin products, which may act as a blood thinner and cause rebleeds. If not managed properly, irreversible vision damage can occur.[77]

### Rupture of the Globe

*Etiology* A blow to the eye by an object smaller than the eye orbit produces extreme pressure that can rupture the globe. A golf ball or racquetball fits this category. Larger objects, such as a tennis ball or a fist, often fracture the bony orbit before the eye is overly compressed. Even if it does not cause rupture of the globe, such a force can cause internal injury that may ultimately lead to blindness.[5]

*Symptoms and signs* The patient complains of severe pain, decreased visual acuity, and diplopia.

A racquetball player who is not wearing protective goggles is hit in his eye with a ball and develops a collection of blood in the anterior chamber.

❓ What type of eye injury is this, and what complications may follow?

Inspection reveals irregular pupils, increased intraocular pressure, and orbital leakage.

*Management* Immediate referral to an ophthalmologist must be made. Treatment depends on the clinical signs and may involve exploratory surgery.

### Retinal Detachment

*Etiology* A blow to the eye can partially or completely separate the retina from its attachment in the back of the eye. Retinal detachment is more common among athletes who have myopia (nearsightedness).[22]

*Symptoms and signs* Detachment is painless; however, early signs include specks floating before the eye, flashes of light, or blurred vision. As the detachment progresses, the patient complains of a "curtain" falling over the field of vision.

*Management* The patient with a suspected detachment should immediately be referred to an ophthalmologist to determine if surgery is required. Small retinal tears or detachments can sometimes be treated with laser. Large retinal detachments require major surgery.

### Acute Conjunctivitis (Pink Eye)

*Etiology* The conjunctiva is the tissue that lines the back of the eyelid, moves into the space between the eyelid and eye globe, and spreads up over the sclera to the cornea.[82] Acute conjunctivitis is usually caused by various bacteria or allergens. It may begin with conjunctival irritation from wind, dust, smoke, or air pollution. It may also be associated with the common cold or other upper respiratory conditions. Conjunctivitis is not always highly contagious but should be treated as such until a final diagnosis is made by a physician.

*Symptoms and signs* The patient complains of redness, discomfort, and eyelid swelling, sometimes with a purulent discharge (Figure 26–25). Itching is associated with allergy. Eyes may burn or itch.

*Management* Acute conjunctivitis can be highly infectious. Athletes with signs or symptoms of pink eye should avoid contact with other people, discontinue contact lens wear, and isolate their materials, such as washcloths and towels. Treatment typically includes antibiotic eye drops prescribed by an eye care practitioner.

### Stye and Blepharitis

*Etiology* Stye is the common name for a clogged or infected oil gland located in the eyelid. Blepharitis is a

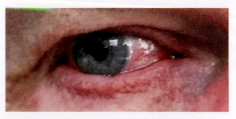

FIGURE 26–25 Conjuctivitis in the right eye.
© William E. Prentice

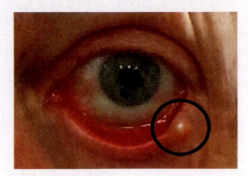

FIGURE 26–26    Stye on the lower eyelid.
© William E. Prentice

low-grade infection of the eyelid margins near the base of the lashes. Staphylococcal bacteria common in the environment is often the cause.

***Symptoms and signs***    The condition starts as erythema of the eye. It localizes into a painful pustule within a few days (Figure 26–26).

***Management***    Most sties will resolve on their own in less than 4 weeks. Treatment consists of the application of hot, moist compresses. Antibiotics and ointments are not necessary unless the entire lid becomes inflamed or infected. Recurrent sties require the attention of an ophthalmologist vider. Treatment with staph-sensitive oral and topical antibiotics can be useful.

## THROAT INJURIES

### Contusions

***Etiology***    Blows to the throat do not occur frequently in sports, but occasionally an athlete receives a kick or blow to the throat. One type of trauma is known as clotheslining, in which the patient is struck in the throat region by another player's outstretched arm. Such a force could injure the carotid artery, causing a clot to form that occludes the blood flow to the brain. The same clot could become dislodged and migrate to the brain. In either case, serious brain injury may result.

***Symptoms and signs***    Immediately after throat trauma, the patient may experience severe pain and spasmodic coughing, speak with a hoarse voice, and complain of difficulty in swallowing. The patient may also have difficulty breathing, particularly if the vocal cords have been traumatized.[56]

Fracture of throat cartilages of the larynx is rare, but it is possible and may be indicated by an inability to breathe and by expectoration of frothy blood. Cyanosis may be present. Throat contusions are extremely uncomfortable and are often frightening to the athlete.

***Management***    The most immediate concern is the integrity of the airway. The patient who is experiencing difficulty breathing should be sent to an emergency care facility immediately. In most situations, cold should be applied intermittently to control superficial hemorrhage and swelling, and, after a 24-hour rest period, moist hot packs may be applied. For the most severe neck contusions, stabilization with a well-padded collar is beneficial.

> A patient develops an eyelash follicle infection.
>
> **?** What is the cause of this condition, and how should it be treated?

> While carrying the ball, a football back is clotheslined and seriously injures his throat.
>
> **?** What should the athletic trainer be concerned with in such an injury?

## SUMMARY

- The skull is lined with the meninges, which collectively protect the underlying cortex and midbrain from trauma.
- An individual who receives either a direct blow to the head or body contact that causes the head to snap forward, backward, or rotate to the side must be carefully evaluated for injury to the brain. Injuries to the brain may or may not result in unconsciousness; disorientation or amnesia; motor coordination or balance deficits; and cognitive deficits.
- It is important to realize that the majority of concussions do not involve loss of consciousness.

- Concussions usually occur as a result of a direct impact or through a combination of rotational and acceleration/deceleration forces.
- A variety of classification systems have been proposed for determining the severity of concussion. To date, none of these classification systems have been universally endorsed, and thus debate continues.
- Returning an athlete to competition following concussion often creates a difficult dilemma for the athletic trainer. There must be ongoing concern for postconcussion syndrome, second-impact syndrome, and epidural and subdural hematomas.

- Injuries to the face could involve fractures of the mandible, maxilla, or zygoma; dislocations of the mandible; temporomandibular dysfunction; and facial lacerations.
- Impact to the upper or lower jaw or direct trauma to the teeth can result in one or more of three types of fracture to the teeth: an uncomplicated crown fracture, a complicated crown fracture, and a root fracture. A tooth may also be subluxated, luxated, or avulsed. The athletic trainer should know when to refer a patient for dental care.
- Most injuries to the ear involve the auricle, with cauliflower ear being the most common injury. Rupture of the tympanic membrane, swimmer's ear, and middle ear infections are common.
- Injuries to the eye should be treated by physicians who are specifically trained. Even injuries as simple as a black eye, a stye, or a corneal abrasion have the potential to cause some irreversible damage to vision if not properly managed. An orbital fracture, a foreign body in the eye, a hyphema, a rupture of the globe, and a retinal detachment are all considered serious injuries to the eye.
- The most serious consequence of a throat contusion is airway interference.

## WEB SITES

### NATA Position, Official, and Consensus Statements
*Management of Sport Concussion (2014):*
www.nata.org/sites/default/files/Concussion_Management_Position_Statement.pdf
American Academy of Neurology: www.aan.com

American Academy of Ophthalmology:
www.aao.org
American Academy of Otolaryngology—Head and Neck Surgery: www.entnet.org
American Dental Association: www.ada.org

## SOLUTIONS TO CLINICAL APPLICATION EXERCISES

26-1  The patient's face color is pale, her skin moist, her pulse is rapid with shallow breathing, and her pupils may become dilated.

26-2  The athletic trainer should ask the patient questions that are related to recently acquired information, such as the current date, the name of last week's opponent, who won that game, and who scored this game's last goal.

26-3  The patient should be held out of all activity until he is completely asymptomatic and can perform at baseline levels on neuropsychological tests and balance tests, no matter how long this takes. The physician may consider terminating the patient for the rest of the season.

26-4  This patient is experiencing a postconcussion syndrome. The patient cannot return completely to play until cleared by a thorough neurological examination.

26-5  In a patient of this age, there should always be some concern about the possibility of second-impact syndrome. From the athletic trainer's perspective, the decision to allow a patient to return to play after an initial head injury must be carefully made based on the absence of postconcussive symptoms and clearance by a physician.

26-6  A subdural hematoma is due to venous bleeding, and the symptoms appear gradually over hours or even days. However, an epidural hematoma results from arterial bleeding, and therefore the symptoms appear rapidly.

26-7  The conscious patient with a fractured maxilla is transported to the hospital in a forward-leaning position. This position allows external drainage of saliva and blood.

26-8  This appears to be an uncomplicated crown fracture, which does not require immediate treatment by a dentist. The fractured piece of tooth, if found, can be placed in a plastic bag. The patient can finish the game and then should be seen by a dentist within 24 to 48 hours.

26-9  The patient should sit up with a cold compress placed over the nose and ipsilateral carotid artery. Digital pressure should also be applied to the affected nostril for 5 minutes.

26-10  The symptoms that the athletic trainer should look for are blurred vision, a loss in the visual field, major pain, and double vision.

26-11  Blood in the anterior eye chamber is known as a hyphema, which could lead to major lens, choroid, or retinal problems.

26-12  This stye is caused by a staphylococcal organism that is commonly spread by rubbing or by dust particle contamination. The condition should be managed with hot, moist compresses and a 1 percent yellow oxide or mercury ointment.

26-13  The compressive force of clotheslining could produce a blood clot in the carotid artery. A large enough force could fracture the larynx and cause a breathing crisis.

## REVIEW QUESTIONS AND CLASS ACTIVITIES

1. What is the difference between the terms *concussion* and *mild traumatic brain injury?*
2. What are the different classification systems for determining grades of concussion?
3. How are postconcussion syndrome and second-impact syndrome related to concussion?
4. Demonstrate the following procedures in evaluating a concussion: testing eye signs, testing balance, testing coordination, testing cognition.
5. What immediate care procedures should be performed for patients with facial lacerations?
6. Describe the immediate care procedures that should be performed when a tooth is fractured and when it is dislocated.
7. Describe the procedures that should be performed for a patient with a nosebleed.
8. How can cauliflower ear be prevented?
9. How can eye injuries be prevented?

# REFERENCES

1. Almquist J: Assessment of mild head injuries, *Athletic Therapy Today* 6(1):13, 2001.
2. Alberts J, et al.: Quantification of the balance error scoring system with mobile technology, *Medicine and Science in Sport and Exercise* 47(10):2233–40, 2015.
3. Aubry M: Summary and agreement statement: Recommendations for the improvement of safety and health of athletes who may suffer concussive injuries, *British Journal of Sports Medicine* 15:509–11, 2009.
4. Bailes J: Sports-related concussion: What do we know in 2009: A neurosurgeon's perspective, *Journal of the International Neuropsychological Society* 15:509–11, 2009.
5. Barr A: Ocular sports injuries: The current picture, *British Journal of Sports Medicine* 34(6):456, 2000.
6. Beachy G: Dental injuries in intermediate and high school athletes: A 15-year study at Punahou School, *J Athl Train* 39(4):310, 2004.
7. Berry D: Athletic mouth guards and their role in injury prevention, *Athletic Therapy Today* 6(5):52, 2001.
8. Broglio S: Generalizability theory analysis of balance error scoring system reliability in healthy young adults, *J Athl Train* 44(5):497–502, 2009.
9. Broglio S: Soccer heading: Are there risks involved? *Athletic Therapy Today* 6(1):28, 2001.
10. Broglio S, et al.: National Athletic Trainers' Association position statement: Management of sport concussion, *Journal of Athletic Training* 49(2):245–65, 2014.
11. Bruzzone E: Intracranial delayed epidural hematoma in a soccer player: A case report, *Am J Sports Med* 28(6):901, 2000.
12. Cameron K: A standardization protocol for the initial evaluation and documentation of mild brain injury, *J Athl Train* 34(1):34, 1999.
13. Cantu R: Posttraumatic retrograde and anterograde amnesia: Pathophysiology and implications in grading and safe return to play, *J Athl Train* 36(3):244, 2001.
14. Cass S: Ocular injuries in sports, *Current Sports Medicine Reports* 11(1):11–15, 2012.
15. Cooper E: Definitional problems in mild head injury epidemiology, *Athletic Therapy Today* 6(1):6, 2001.
16. Covassin T: Immediate post-concussion assessment and cognitive testing (ImPACT) practices of sports medicine professionals, *J Athl Train* 44(6):639–44, 2009.
17. Covassin T: Sex differences and the incidence of concussions among collegiate athletes, *J Athl Train* 38(3):238, 2003.
18. Covassin T: Investigating baseline neurocognitive performance between male and female athletes with a history of multiple concussion, *Journal of Neurology*, 81:597–601, 2010.
19. Erlanger D: Monitoring resolution of post concussion symptoms in athletes: Preliminary results of a web-based neuropsychological test protocol, *J Athl Train* 36(3):280, 2001.
20. Ferrara M: A survey of practice patterns in concussion assessment and management, *J Athl Train* 36(2):145, 2001.
21. Gennarelli T: Closed head injuries. In Torg JS, Shephard RJ, editors: *Current therapy in sports medicine*, St. Louis, MO, 1995, Mosby.
22. Gunter G: Eye injuries in sports, *Athletic Therapy Today* 15(5):14–18, 2010.

23. Guskiewicz K: Balance assessment in the management of sport-related concussions, *Clinics in Sports Medicine* 30(1):89–102, 2011.
24. Guskiewicz K: Concussion in sport: The grading system dilemma, *Athletic Therapy Today* 6(1):18, 2001.
25. Guskiewicz K, et al.: National Athletic Trainers' Association position statement: Management of sport-related concussion, *J Athl Train* 39(3):280, 2004.
26. Guskiewicz K: The concussion puzzle: Evaluation of sport-related concussion, *Am J Sports Med* 6:13, 2004.
27. Guskiewicz K: Cumulative effects of recurrent concussion in collegiate football players, *JAMA* 290:2549, 2003.
28. Guskiewicz K: Recurrent concussion in a collegiate football player equipped with the head impact telemetry system (abstract), *J Athl Train* 40(2 Suppl):S-81, 2005.
29. Guskiewicz K: Epidemiology of mild head injury in high school and college football players, *Am J Sports Med* 28(5):643–50, 2000.
30. Guskiewicz K: Alternative approaches to the assessment of mild head injury in athletes, *Med Sci Sports Exerc* 29(7):S213, 1997.
31. Guskiewicz K: Postural stability and neuropsychological deficits after concussion in collegiate athletes, *J Athl Train* 36(3):263, 2001.
32. Honsik K: Steps to take for dental injuries, *Physician Sportsmed* 32(9):35, 2004.
33. Hugenholtz H: Return to athletic competition following concussion, *Canadian Medical Assoc J* 127:827, 1982.
34. Jordan B: Head injuries in sports. In Jordan B, ed: *Sports neurology*, Philadelphia, PA, 1998, Lippincott, Williams and Wilkins.
35. Kelly J: Loss of consciousness: pathophysiology and implications in grading and safe return to play, *J Athl Train* 36(3):249, 2001.
36. Knapik J: Mouthguards in sport activities, *Sports Med* 37(2):117, 2007.
37. Kelly J: Traumatic brain injury and concussion in sports, *JAMA* 282:989, 1999.
38. Laio J: Eye injuries in sports, *Athletic Therapy Today* 4(5):36, 1999.
39. Landry G: Eye, ear, and maxillofacial pathologies. In Landry G: *Essentials of primary care sports medicine*, Champaign, IL, 2003, Human Kinetics.
40. Langlois J: The epidemiology and impact of traumatic brain injury: A brief overview, *Journal of Head Trauma Rehabilitation* 21:375, 2006.
41. Lavasani L: Management of acute soft tissue injury to the auricle, *Facial Plastic Surgery*, 26(6):445–50, 2010.
42. Lenker C: Traumatic tympanic membrane perforation in a collegiate football player, *Athletic Therapy Today* 5(1):43, 2000.
43. Liu R: Skull fracture and brain contusion in a baseball player, *Athletic Therapy Today* 14(1):7, 2009.
44. Livingston S: The neurophysiology behind concussion signs and symptoms, *Athletic Therapy and Training* 16(5):5–9, 2011.
45. Logan K: Recognition and management of postconcussion syndrome, *Athletic Therapy Today* 15(3):62, 2010.
46. Logan S: Acute subdural hematoma in a high school football player after two unreported episodes of head trauma: A case report, *J Athl Train* 36(4):433, 2001.

47. Maddocks D: The assessment of orientation following concussion in athletes, *Clinical Journal Sports Med* 5(1):32, 1995.
48. McCrea M: An integrated review of recovery after mild traumatic brain injury (MTBI): Implications for clinical management, *The Clinical Neuropsychologist* 23(8):1368–90, 2009.
49. McCrea M: Standardized mental status testing on the sideline after sport-related concussion, *J Athl Train* 36(3):274, 2001.
50. McCrory P: Second impact syndrome or cerebral swelling after sporting head injury, *Current Sports Medicine Reports*, 11(1):21–23, 2012.
51. McCrory P, et al.: Consensus statement on concussion in sport: The 4th International Conference on Concussion in Sport, Zurich, November 2012, *Journal of Athletic Training* 48(4):554–75, 2013.
52. McKee A, et al.: Chronic traumatic encephalopathy in athletes: Progressive tauopathy following repetitive head injury, *Journal of Neuropathologic Experimental Neurology* 68(7):709–35, 2009.
53. Moss R: Preventing postconcussion sequelae, *Athletic Therapy Today* 6(2):28, 2001.
54. Mucha A, et al.: A brief Vestibular/Ocular Motor Screening (VOMS) assessment to evaluate concussions, *American Journal of Sports Medicine* 42(10):2479–86, 2014.
55. Nelson W: Minor head injury in sports: A new system of classification and management, *Physician Sportsmed* 12:103, 1984.
56. Newsham K: Paradoxical vocal cord dysfunction: Management in athletes, *J Athl Train* 37(3):325, 2002.
57. Okonkwo D: Basic science of closed head injuries and spinal cord injuries, *Clin Sports Med* 22(3):467, 2003.
58. Oliaro S: Management of cerebral concussion in sports: The athletic trainer's perspective, *J Athl Train* 36(3):257, 2001.
59. Ommaya A: A spectrum of mild head injuries in sport. In National Athletic Trainers' Association: *Proceedings of mildbrain injury in sports summit*, Dallas, TX, 1994, NATA.
60. Onate J: A comparison of sideline versus clinical cognitive test performance in collegiate athletes, *J Athl Train* 35(2):155, 2000.
61. Parver D: Anatomy of the eye, *Athletic Therapy Today* 4(5):13, 1999.
62. Parver D: Recognizing diseases and disorders of the eye, *Athletic Therapy Today* 4(5):22, 1999.
63. Piland S: Investigation of baseline self-report concussion symptom scores, *J Athl Train* 45(3):273–78, 2010.
64. Piland S: Evidence for the factorial and construct validity of a self report concussion symptoms scale, *J Athl Train* 38(2):104, 2003.
65. Powell J: Traumatic brain injury in high school athletes, *JAMA* 282:958, 1999.
66. Randolph C: Implementation of neuropsychological testing models for the high school, collegiate, and professional sport settings, *J Athl Train* 36(3):280, 2001.
67. Reimann B: Relationship between clinical and forceplate measures of postural stability, *J Sport Rehab* 8(2):71–82, 1999.
68. Resch J: Balance performance with a cognitive task: A continuation of the dual task testing paradigm, *J Athl Train* 46(2): 170–75, 2011.
69. Roberts W: Field care of the injured tooth, *Physician Sportsmed* 28(1):101, 2000.

70. Robinson T: Ear injuries. In Birrer R, ed: *Sports medicine for the primary care physician*, ed 2, Boca Raton, FL, 1994, CRC Press.

71. Robinson T: Nasal injuries. In Birrer R, ed: *Sports medicine for the primary care physician*, ed 2, Boca Raton, FL, 1994, CRC Press.

72. Robinson T: Head injuries. In Birrer R, ed: *Sports medicine for the primary care physician*, ed 2, Boca Raton, FL, 1994, CRC Press.

73. Romeo S: Facial injuries in sports: A team physician's guide to diagnosis and treatment, *Physician Sportsmed* 33(4):45, 2005.

74. Shrier I: Concussion risk factors and return-to-play variables, *Physician Sportsmed* 33(9):6, 2005.

75. Snouse S: Zygomatic arch fracture in women's ice hockey, *Athletic Therapy Today* 3(6):13, 1998.

76. Sosnoff J: Previous mild traumatic brain injury and postural-control dynamics, *J Athl Train* 46(1): 85–91, 2011.

77. Stilger V: Traumatic hyphema in an intercollegiate baseball player: A case report, *J Athl Train* 34(1):25, 1999.

78. Thomas D, et al.: Benefits of strict rest after acute concussion: A randomized controlled trial, *Pediatrics* 135(2):213–23, 2015.

79. Tommasone B, Valovich-McLeod T: Contact sport concussion incidence, *J Athl Train* 41(4):470, 2006.

80. Valovich T: Repeat administration elicits a practice effect with the balance error scoring system but not with the standardized assessment of concussion in high school athletes, *J Athl Train* 38(1):51, 2003.

81. Valovich-McLeod, T: The value of various assessment techniques in detecting the effects of concussion on cognition, symptoms, and postural control, *J Athl Train* 44(6):663–65, 2009.

82. Venes D: *Tabor's cyclopedic medical dictionary*, Philadelphia, PA, 2013, F.A. Davis.

83. Weiler R: Prevalence of signs and symptoms of temporomandibular dysfunction in male adolescent athletes and non-athletes, *International Journal of Pediatric Otorhinolaryngology* 74(9):896–900, 2010.

84. Weir J: Effective management of epistaxis in athletes, *J Athl Train* 32(3):254, 1997.

85. Whitney S: Vestibular disorders in mild head injury, *Athletic Therapy Today* 6(1):33, 2001.

86. Wilkins J: Performance on the balance error scoring system decreases after fatigue, *J Athl Train* 39(2):156, 2004.

## ANNOTATED BIBLIOGRAPHY

Cantu R: *Concussions and our kids: America's leading expert on how to protect young athletes and keep sports safe,* Orlando, FL, 2013, Mariner Books.

*This book is not geared to the professional caregiver or scientist, but directly to parents and people who work with kids in athletics, both formally organized or not.*

Currie D, Ritchie E, Scott S: *The management of head injuries,* London, 2000, Oxford University Press.

*Chapters cover initial assessment, resuscitation, neurological deterioration, scalp and skull injuries, cervical spine injuries, children's injuries, and more.*

Magnus W: *Concussions in sports: Protecting the players*, Hauppauge, NY, 2011, Nova Science Publishers Inc.

*This book examines efforts to protect football players from concussions and explores the legal issues relating to football head injuries and the impact of concussions on high-school athletes.*

Meehan W: Concussion in sports, an issue of *Clinics in Sports Medicine*, Philadelphia, PA, 2010, Saunders.

*This issue of* Clinics in Sports Medicine *explores all aspects of sports-related concussion, such as the biomechanics and epidemiology of concussions, and includes articles on return-to-play and retiring decisions after sports-related concussions.*

McCrea M: *Mild traumatic brain injury and post-concussion syndrome: The new evidence base for diagnosis and treatment*, New York, 2007, Oxford University Press.

*This text provides a welcome evidence base for all clinicians involved in the clinical diagnosis and treatment of MTBI.*

Roush K: *Sports concussion and neck trauma: Preventing injury for future generations,* Bloomington, IN, 2012, Authorhouse.

*This book educates coaches, athletes, parents, and physicians on the danger of an athlete continuing to play with a probable head/neck injury, and how to do their part to prevent further injury.*

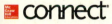

# 27

© William E. Prentice

# The Thorax and Abdomen

## ■ Connect Highlights   Mc Graw Hill Education **connect**

*Visit connect.mcgraw-hill.com for further exercises to apply your knowledge:*

- Clinical application scenarios covering assessment and recognition of thoracic and abdominal injuries; etiology, symptoms and signs, and management of thoracic and abdominal and internal organ injuries; and rehabilitation for the thorax and abdomen
- Click-and-drag questions covering structural anatomy of the thorax, abdomen, and internal organs; assessment of thorax, abdomen, and internal organ injuries; and rehabilitation plan of the thorax and abdomen
- Multiple-choice questions covering anatomy, assessment, etiology, management, and rehabilitation of thorax, abdomen, and internal organ injuries

- Selection questions covering rehabilitation plan for various injuries to the thorax and abdomen
- Video identification of special tests for the thorax, abdomen, and internal organ injuries, and rehabilitation techniques for the thorax and abdomen
- Picture identification of major anatomical components of the cervical, thoracic, and lumbar spine and nerve roots; thorax; abdomen; and internal organs; and rehabilitation techniques of the thorax and abdomen; and therapeutic modalities for management

This chapter deals with sports injuries to the thorax and abdomen. In an athletic environment, injuries to the thorax and abdomen have a lower incidence than do injuries to the extremities. However, unlike the musculoskeletal injuries to the extremities discussed to this point, injuries to the heart, lungs, and abdominal viscera can be serious and even life threatening if not recognized and managed appropriately. It is imperative for the athletic trainer to be familiar with the anatomy of and more common injuries seen in the abdomen and thorax (Figure 27–1).

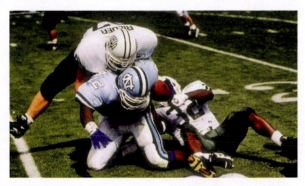

FIGURE 27–1 Collision sports can produce serious thoracic and abdominal injuries.

© William E. Prentice

## ANATOMY OF THE THORAX

The thoracic cavity is the portion of the body commonly known as the chest, which lies between the base of the neck and the diaphragm. It consists of the thoracic vertebrae, the 12 pairs of ribs with their associated costal cartilages, and the sternum (Figure 27–2). Its main functions are to protect the vital respiratory and circulatory organs and to assist the lungs in inspiration and expiration during the breathing process. Within the thoracic cage lie the lungs, the heart, and the thymus.

> The thoracic cage protects the heart and lungs.

### Ribs, Costal Cartilage, and Sternum

The ribs are flat bones that are attached to the thoracic vertebrae in the back and to the sternum in the front. The upper seven ribs are called sternal, or true, ribs, and each rib is joined to the sternum by a separate costal cartilage. The 8th, 9th, and 10th ribs (false ribs) have a common cartilage that joins the 7th rib before attaching to the sternum. The 11th and 12th ribs (floating ribs) remain unattached to the sternum but do have muscle attachments. The individual rib articulation produces a slight gliding action.

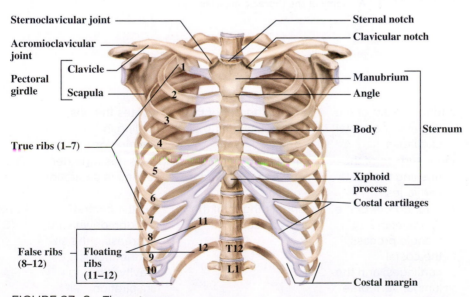

FIGURE 27–2 Thoracic cage.

The inside of the thoracic cage is lined with the pleura, a thin, double-layer membrane filled with pleural fluid, that permits the lungs to slide along the thoracic cage.

## Thoracic Muscles

There are 11 pairs of both external intercostal muscles and internal intercostal muscles between the ribs (Figure 27–3). They attach on the inferior border of the rib above and the superior border of the rib below. The external intercostals elevate the diaphragm during inspiration, whereas the internal intercostals depress the rib cage to assist with expiration. The intercostal muscles are innervated by the intercostal nerves (Table 27–1).

The pectoralis minor, trapezius, serratus anterior, serratus posterior, levator scapula, and rhomboids are muscles that originate on the thorax and were discussed in Chapter 22. Their primary function is controlling movement of the scapula.

## Lungs

The trachea, or windpipe, branches into right and left primary bronchi, which branch into smaller divisions called bronchioles that control air resistance, and ultimately terminate in clusters of air sacs called alveoli within the lungs (Figure 27–4). Alveoli facilitate the exchange of oxygen and carbon dioxide with the capillaries. The lungs are elastic and expand and constrict in response to contraction of the diaphragm muscle.

**Respiratory Muscles** The diaphragm is a large, dome-shaped muscle that separates the thoracic cavity from the abdominal cavity. When the diaphragm contracts, the dome flattens, which increases the volume of the thorax and results in inspiration of air. Expiration occurs when the diaphragm relaxes and the elastic components of the lungs and thoracic cage passively decrease thoracic volume.

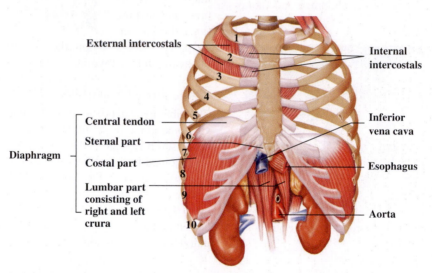

FIGURE 27–3   Anatomy of the thoracic muscles.

| TABLE 27–1 | Muscles of the Thorax | | | |
|---|---|---|---|---|
| **Muscle** | **Origin** | **Insertion** | **Muscle Action** | **Innervation (Nerve Root)** |
| **External intercostals** | Inferior border of the ribs and the costal cartilages | Superior border of the rib below the rib of origin | Elevates the ribs, aiding in inspiration | T1–T11 |
| **Internal intercostals** | Inner surface of the ribs and the costal cartilages | Superior border of the rib below the rib of origin | Draws ribs together, aiding in expiration | T1–T11 |
| **Diaphragm** | Inferior border of the rib cage; the xiphoid process; the costal cartilages; and the lumbar vertebrae | Central tendon of the diaphragm | Pulls the central tendon downward, increasing the size of the thoracic cavity, causing inspiration | Phrenic (C3–C5) |

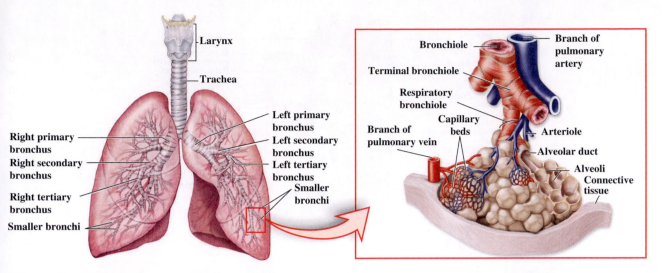

FIGURE 27–4    The lungs and the respiratory apparatus.

**Blood Supply** Blood flows to the lungs through the pulmonary arteries to the alveoli, where it is oxygenated and returns to the heart through the pulmonary veins to supply the entire arterial system.

The bronchi are supplied with oxygenated blood through the bronchial arteries that branch from the aorta. Deoxygenated blood returns to the heart from the bronchi via both the bronchial and pulmonary veins.

## Heart

The heart is the main pumping mechanism; it circulates oxygenated blood throughout the body to the working tissues. The transport of oxygen involves the coordinated function of the heart, the blood vessels, the blood, and the lungs.

The adult heart lies under the sternum, slightly to the left, between the lungs and in front of the vertebral column (Figure 27–5). It is about the size of a clenched fist. It extends from the first rib to the space between the fifth and sixth ribs.

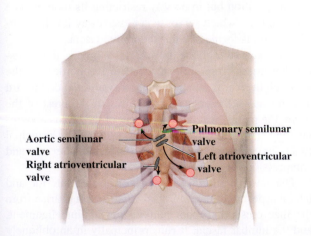

FIGURE 27–5    Location of the heart and valves in the thorax. (The colored dots indicate the points where valve sounds are best heard.)

The heart consists of four chambers: the right and left atria and the right and left ventricles (Figure 27–6). Deoxygenated blood returns from all parts of the body through the venous system to the right atrium and passes through the tricuspid valve to the right ventricle. The right ventricle pumps the blood through the pulmonary valve to the pulmonary artery and into the lungs, where it is oxygenated. Blood returns from the lungs via the pulmonary vein to the left atrium and passes through the mitral valve into the left ventricle. Blood is ejected past the aortic valve into the aorta, which supplies the entire body through the arterial system.

A single heartbeat consists of a contraction of both atria followed quickly by a contraction of both ventricles. There must be some time between contraction of the atria and contraction of the ventricles to allow for the ventricle to fill with blood. Contraction of the chambers is referred to as systole, relaxation as diastole.[57]

**Blood Supply** The heart is supplied by right and left coronary arteries branching from the aorta. Cardiac veins drain into the right atrium.

## Thymus

The thymus is located in the thorax just anterior to and above the heart. The function of the thymus is to mature lymphocytes into T cells, which migrate to other lymphatic tissues to respond to foreign substances. The thymus is relatively large in the infant and after puberty gradually decreases in size (Figure 27–7).[61]

## ANATOMY OF THE ABDOMEN

The abdominopelvic cavity lies between the diaphragm and the bones of the pelvis and is bounded by the margin of the lower ribs, the abdominal muscles, and the vertebral column. In the abdominopelvic cavity, there is no physical separation between the abdominal and pelvic

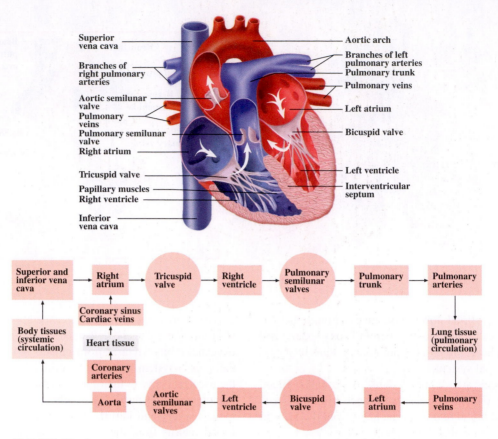

FIGURE 27–6    Blood flow through the heart.

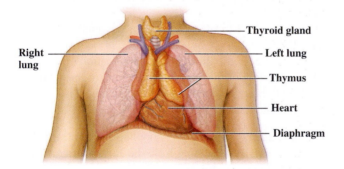

FIGURE 27–7    The thymus is just anterior and superior to the heart.

cavities. The *parietal peritoneum* is a moist serous membrane that lines the surface of the body wall in the abdominopelvic cavity. The portion of the peritoneum that reflects and covers the surface of internal organs is called the *visceral peritoneum.* Between these two layers is the *peritoneal cavity,* a potential space where the peritoneal layers face each other and secrete a lubricating serous fluid that reduces any friction resulting from the movement, allowing the abdominal organs to move freely.[57]

## Abdominal Muscles

The abdominal muscles are the rectus abdominis, the external oblique, the internal oblique, and the transversus abdominis (Figure 27–8). They are invested with both superficial and deep fasciae (Table 27–2).

The rectus abdominis muscle, a trunk flexor, is attached to the rib cage above and to the pubis below. It is divided into three segments by transverse tendinous inscriptions; longitudinally it is divided by the linea alba. It functions in trunk flexion, rotation, and lateral flexion and in compression of the abdominal cavity. A heavy fascial sheath encloses the rectus abdominis muscle, holding it in its position but in no way restricting its motion. The inguinal ring, which serves as a passageway for the spermatic cord, is formed by the abdominal fascia.

The external oblique muscle is a broad, thin muscle that arises from slips attached to the borders of the lower eight ribs. It runs obliquely forward and downward and inserts on the anterior two-thirds of the crest of the ilium, the pubic crest, and the fascia of the rectus abdominis and the linea alba at their lower front. Its principal functions are trunk flexion, rotation, lateral flexion, and compression.

The internal oblique muscle forms the anterior and lateral aspects of the abdominal wall. Its fibers arise from the iliac crest, the upper half of the inguinal ligament, and the lumbar fascia. It runs principally in an obliquely upward direction to the cartilages of the 10th, 11th, and 12th ribs on each side. The main functions of the internal oblique are trunk flexion, lateral flexion, and rotation.

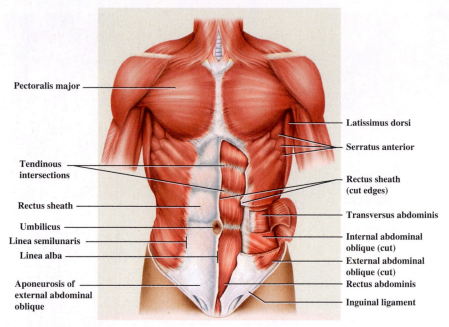

Pectoralis major

Latissimus dorsi

Serratus anterior

Tendinous intersections

Rectus sheath (cut edges)

Transversus abdominis

Rectus sheath

Umbilicus

Linea semilunaris

Linea alba

Internal abdominal oblique (cut)

External abdominal oblique (cut)

Rectus abdominis

Aponeurosis of external abdominal oblique

Inguinal ligament

FIGURE 27–8   Abdominal muscles.

## TABLE 27–2   Muscles of the Abdominal Wall

| Muscle | Origin | Insertion | Muscle Action | Innervation |
|---|---|---|---|---|
| **External abdominal oblique** | External surface of the lower eight ribs | Linea alba and the anterior half of the iliac crest | Compresses the abdominopelvic cavity; assists in flexing and rotating the vertebral column | 8–12 intercostals, iliohypogastric, and ilioinguinal |
| **Internal abdominal oblique** | Inguinal ligament, the iliac crest, and the lumbodorsal fascia | Linea alba, the pubic crest, and the lower four ribs | Compresses the abdominopelvic cavity; assists in flexing and rotating the vertebral column | 8–12 intercostals, iliohypogastric, and ilioinguinal |
| **Transversus abdominis** | Inguinal ligament, the iliac crest, the lumbodorsal fascia, and the costal cartilages of the last six ribs | Linea alba and the pubic crest | Compresses the abdominopelvic cavity | 7–12 intercostals, iliohypogastric, and ilioinguinal |
| **Rectus abdominis** | Pubic crest | Xiphoid process and the costal cartilages of the fifth through the seventh ribs | Compresses the abdominopelvic cavity; flexes the vertebral column | 7–12 intercostals |
| **Quadratus lumborum** | Iliac crest and the iliolumbar ligament | Lower border of the twelfth rib; the transverse processes of the upper lumbar vertebrae | Pulls the thoracic cage toward the pelvis; abducts the vertebral column toward the side that is being contracted | 12th thoracic and first lumbar |

**Joint Movements of the Trunk and Abdomen**

Trunk extension

Trunk flexion

Trunk lateral side bending

Trunk rotation

*Manual muscle tests and goniometric measurements of range of motion for the trunk and abdomen can be found in Appendix F and Appendix G of this text.

© William E. Prentice

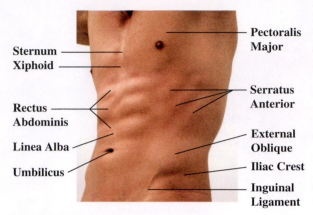

FIGURE 27–9  Surface anatomy of the thorax and abdomen.
© William E. Prentice

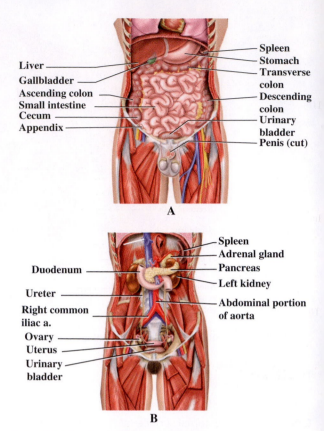

FIGURE 27–10  **(A)** Anterior abdominal viscera.
**(B)** Posterior abdominal viscera.

The transversus abdominis is the deepest of the abdominal muscles. Its fibers run transversely across the abdominal cavity, arising from the outer third of the inguinal ligament, the iliac crest, the lumbar fascia of the back, and the lower six ribs. It inserts into the linea alba and the front half of the iliac crest. The main functions of the transversus abdominis are to hold the abdominal contents in place and to aid in forced expiration. All the abdominal muscles work together in performing defecation, urination, and forced expiration.

## Surface Anatomy

Figure 27–9 shows the pertinent surface anatomy landmarks on the thorax and abdomen from an anterior view.

## Abdominal Viscera

The abdominal viscera are composed of both hollow and solid organs. The solid organs are the kidneys, spleen, liver, pancreas, and adrenal glands. The hollow organs include vessels, tubes, and receptacles, such as the stomach, intestines, gallbladder, and urinary bladder (Figure 27–10). Organs in the abdominal cavity may be classified as being part of the urinary system, the digestive system, the reproductive system, or the lymphatic system.

> Abdominal viscera are part of the urinary, digestive, reproductive, and lymphatic systems.

**Urinary System Organs**  The kidneys, the ureters, and the urinary bladder are the urinary system organs (Figure 27–11).

*Kidneys*  The kidneys are situated on each side of the spine, approximately in the center of the back. They are bean-shaped, approximately 4½ inches (11.25 cm) long, 2 inches (5 cm) wide, and 1 inch (2.5 cm) thick. The right kidney is usually slightly lower than the left because of the pressure of the liver. The uppermost surfaces

of the kidneys are connected to the diaphragm by strong, ligamentous fibers. As breathing occurs, the kidneys move up and down as much as ½ inch (1.25 cm). The inferior aspect is positioned 1 to 2 inches (2.5 to 5 cm) above the iliac crest. Resting anterior to the left kidney are the stomach, spleen, pancreas, and small and large intestines. The organs that are situated anterior to the right kidney are the liver and the intestines. The kidneys lie posterior to the abdominal cavity. Their primary function is to filter metabolic wastes, ions, and drugs from the blood and expel them from the body via urination.[61]

*Adrenal glands*  Although part of the endocrine system rather than the urinary system, the adrenal glands, also called the suprarenal glands, are located on top of each kidney. They secrete the hormones epinephrine, norepinephrine, cortisol, estrogen, aldosterone, and androgen, which have a variety of physiological functions throughout the body.[67]

A soccer player is kicked in the abdomen above the umbilicus. Initially, she had the wind knocked out of her. Now she is complaining of pain and her abdomen is tight on palpation.

**?** What should the athletic trainer be most concerned about, and what organs may be involved?

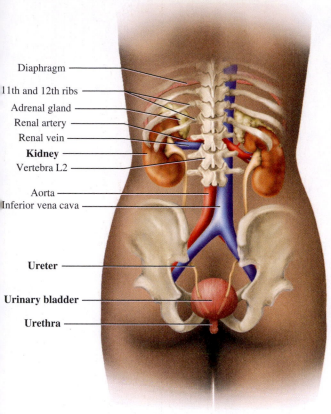

Diaphragm
11th and 12th ribs
Adrenal gland
Renal artery
Renal vein
**Kidney**
Vertebra L2

Aorta
Inferior vena cava

**Ureter**

**Urinary bladder**

**Urethra**

FIGURE 27–11   Organs of the urinary system.

**Ureters and Urinary Bladder** The ureters are small tubes that extend inferiorly from the kidneys to the urinary bladder, which stores urine. The bladder is a hollow container that lies posterior to the symphysis pubis. In the male, the bladder is anterior to the rectum; in the female, it is anterior to the vagina and inferior to the uterus.

**Digestive System Organs** The liver, gallbladder, pancreas, stomach, small intestine, and large intestine are digestive system organs (Figure 27–12).

**Liver** The liver is the largest internal organ of the body. It lies in the right upper quadrant of the body against the inferior surface of the diaphragm and weighs about 3 pounds (~1.4 kg). It consists of two major lobes, right and left. The liver performs digestive and excretory functions, absorbs and stores excess glucose, processes nutrients, and detoxifies harmful chemicals. It secretes bile, which is essential in neutralizing and diluting stomach acid and for digesting fat in the small intestine during the digestive process.

**Gallbladder** The gallbladder is a pear-shaped, saclike structure located on the inferior surface of the liver. It serves as a storage reservoir for bile secreted from the liver. Shortly after a meal, the gallbladder secretes the stored bile into the small intestine.

**Pancreas** The pancreas is located between the small intestine and the spleen. It secretes pancreatic juice, which

is critical in the digestion of fats, carbohydrates, and proteins. It also produces insulin and glucagon, which are hormones that control the amount of glucose and amino acids in the blood.

**Stomach** The stomach is found primarily in the left upper quadrant between the esophagus and the small intestine. It functions mainly as a storage and mixing chamber for food that has been ingested, although some digestion and absorption occur there. Gastric secretions assist in the partial digestion of protein and the absorption of alcohol and caffeine. Ingested food is mixed with secretions from the stomach glands to form a semifluid material called chyme, which passes from the stomach into the small intestine.[66]

**Small Intestine** The small intestine is connected to the stomach via a series of tubelike folds. The small intestine has three portions: the duodenum, the jejunum, and the ileum. In total, it is approximately 20 feet (6 m) long. Secretions from the liver and pancreas mix with secretions from the small intestine, which are essential to the process of digestion. Mucus is secreted in large amounts to lubricate and protect the wall of the intestine. It is a mixture of chyme and the digestive enzymes propelled through the small intestine by a series of peristaltic contractions. Chyme moves through the small intestine over a period of 3 to 5 hours. Most of the digestion and absorption of food occurs in the small intestine.[57]

**Large Intestine** The large intestine extends from the small intestine to the anus and is approximately 6½ feet (2 m) long. It has three divisions: the cecum, the colon, and the rectum. The vermiform appendix extends from the cecum. The colon also has three divisions: the ascending, transverse, and descending colon. In the colon, chyme is converted to feces through the absorption of water, the secretion of mucus, and the activity of microorganisms. Feces remain in the colon and rectum until the time of defecation.

**Lymphatic System Organs** The spleen and the thymus, which is discussed in the section on the thoracic cavity, are organs of the lymphatic system.[66]

**Spleen** The spleen is the largest lymphatic organ in the body. It weighs approximately 6 ounces (170 grams) and is approximately 5 inches (12.5 cm) long. It lies under the diaphragm on the left side and behind the 9th, 10th, and 11th ribs. It is surrounded by a fibrous capsule that is firmly invested by the peritoneum. The spleen's main functions are to serve as a reservoir of red blood cells, to regulate the number of red blood cells in the general circulation, to destroy ineffective red cells, to produce antibodies for immunological function, and to produce lymphocytes.[67]

**Reproductive System Organs** Unlike the other organ systems discussed to this point, the reproductive system differs considerably between males and females. The

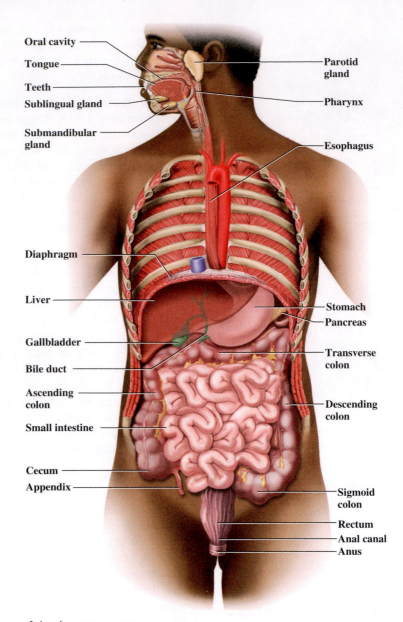

FIGURE 27–12    Organs of the digestive system.

female reproductive organs include the ovaries, uterus, uterine tubes (fallopian tubes), and vagina. The male reproductive organs include the seminal vesicles, prostate gland, testes, vas deferens, epididymis, urethra, and penis.

***Female Reproductive Organs*** The reproductive organs in the female are between the urinary bladder and the rectum; the uterus and vagina are in the midline, and the uterine tubes and ovaries extend to each side (Figure 27–13). Their position is maintained by a group of ligaments, the primary one being the broad ligament. The vagina is a receptacle for sperm, which swim upward into the uterus to fertilize the egg.

The ovaries produce and store the female eggs (ova), which are released one at a time each month into the uterine tubes. The uterine tubes transport each ovum to the uterus, where a fertilized ovum attaches to the uterine wall and becomes a developing embryo. If the ovum is not fertilized, the process of menstruation begins.

The reproductive organs in the female are well protected by the pelvis. Thus, traumatic injury to these structures is rare.

***Male Reproductive Organs*** The reproductive organs in the male are found both inside and outside the abdominal cavity (Figure 27–14). The prostate is dorsal to the symphysis pubis and inferior to the bladder. The urethra and the ejaculatory ducts pass through the prostate. The prostate is made of both glandular and muscular tissue and is similar in size to a walnut. The prostate secretes a milky fluid that is discharged by 20 to 30 ducts into the prostatic portion of the urethra as a component of semen. The seminal vesicles are also glandular structures found posterior and superior to the prostate gland under the bladder. The

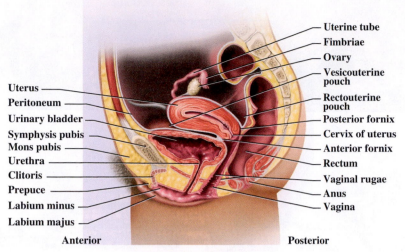

FIGURE 27–13   Female reproductive organs.

Labels (clockwise from top right):
Uterine tube
Fimbriae
Ovary
Vesicouterine pouch
Rectouterine pouch
Posterior fornix
Cervix of uterus
Anterior fornix
Rectum
Vaginal rugae
Anus
Vagina

Labels (left side):
Uterus
Peritoneum
Urinary bladder
Symphysis pubis
Mons pubis
Urethra
Clitoris
Prepuce
Labium minus
Labium majus

Anterior                                Posterior

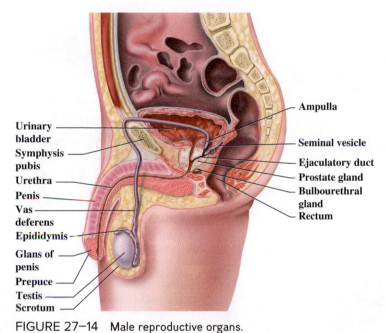

FIGURE 27–14   Male reproductive organs.

Labels (left side):
Urinary bladder
Symphysis pubis
Urethra
Penis
Vas deferens
Epididymis
Glans of penis
Prepuce
Testis
Scrotum

Labels (right side):
Ampulla
Seminal vesicle
Ejaculatory duct
Prostate gland
Bulbourethral gland
Rectum

seminal vesicles contribute the majority of the fluid to the semen through the ejaculatory ducts.

The remainder of the male reproductive organs are exposed outside the abdominal cavity and are more susceptible to injury. The testes are the primary male sex organs. They are located within the scrotum and produce spermatozoa and testosterone. The epididymis is a comma-shaped structure connected to the posterior surface of the testis in which the sperm are stored until mature. The vas deferens is a duct running from the epididymis to the ejaculatory duct. The urethra runs from the bladder to the tip of the penis and serves as a pathway through which both urine and semen are ejected through the penis. The penis consists of three layers of erectile tissue, which, when engorged with blood, cause an erection.

# PREVENTION OF INJURIES TO THE THORAX AND ABDOMEN

Injuries to the thorax may be prevented by appropriate protective equipment, particularly in collision sport activities. In football, for example, shoulder pads are usually designed to extend to at least below the level of the sternum. Rib protectors may be worn to cover the entire thoracic cage if necessary.

The muscles of the abdomen should be strengthened to provide protection to the underlying viscera (Figure 27–15). A consistent regimen of core stabilization exercises done in various positions can markedly increase the strength and size of the abdominal musculature (see Figures 4–11, 21–47, and 25–75).

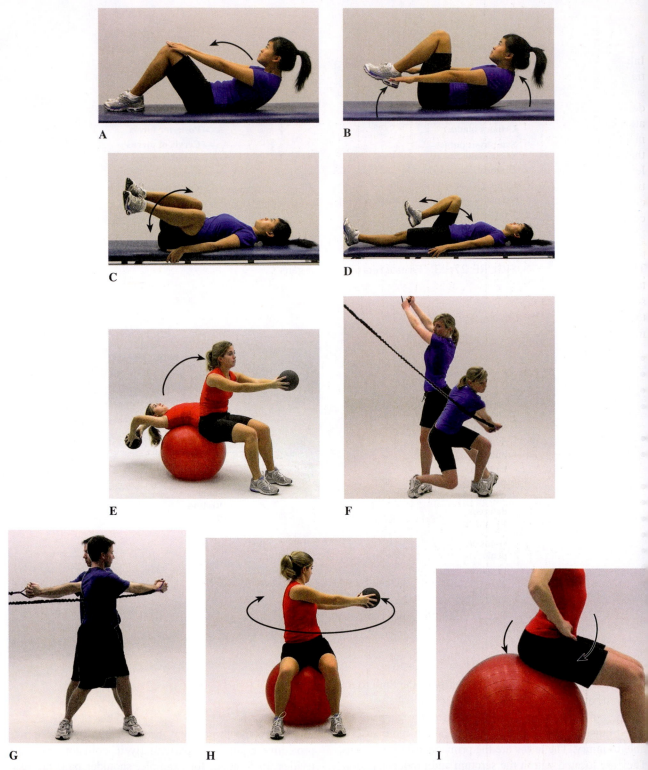

FIGURE 27–15  Abdominal strengthening exercises. **(A)** Crunches. **(B)** Lying tucks. **(C)** Trunk rotation with bent knee. **(D)** Bicycles. **(E)** Stability ball pullover crunch with weighted ball. **(F)** Chopping using cable or tubing. **(G)** Standing trunk rotations using cable or tubing. **(H)** Stability ball trunk rotations with weighted ball. **(I)** Pelvic tilts on stability ball.
© William E. Prentice

Making sure that the hollow organs—in particular, the stomach and bladder—are emptied prior to activity can reduce the chance of injury to those structures. Meals should be eaten at least 3 to 4 hours before activity to allow foods to clear the stomach. Urination immediately before stepping onto the field or court will protect the bladder from injury.

# ASSESSMENT OF THE THORAX AND ABDOMEN

Injuries to the thorax and abdomen can produce potentially life-threatening situations.[55] An injury that may seem to be relatively insignificant at first may rapidly develop into one that requires immediate and appropriate medical attention.[6] Thus, the athletic trainer's primary survey should focus on the signs and symptoms that indicate some life-threatening condition. The athletic trainer should continually monitor the injured patient to identify any disruption of normal breathing or circulation or any indication of internal hemorrhage that could precipitate shock.

## History

The questions that the athletic trainer should ask to determine a history for thoracic and abdominal injuries are somewhat different than the questions that are pertinent to musculoskeletal injuries of the extremities.[61] The primary mechanism of injury should be determined first:

- What happened to cause this injury?
- Was there direct contact or a direct blow?
- What position were you in?
- What type of pain is there (sharp, dull, localized, etc.)?
- Was the pain immediate or gradual?
- Do you feel any pain other than in the area where the injury occurred?
- Have you had any difficulty breathing?
- Are certain positions more comfortable than others?
- Do you feel faint, light-headed, or nauseated?
- Do you feel any pain in your chest?
- Did you hear or feel a pop or crack in your chest?
- Have you had any muscle spasms?
- Have you noticed any blood in your urine?
- Have you had any difficulty or pain in urinating?
- Was the bladder full or empty?
- How long has it been since you have eaten?
- Is there a personal or family history of any heart problems, any abdominal problems, or any other diseases involving the thorax and abdomen?

## Observation

The athletic trainer should observe the patient immediately following injury to check for normal breathing and respiratory patterns:

- Most importantly, is the patient breathing at all?
- Is the patient having difficulty breathing deeply, or is he or she catching the breath?
- Does breathing cause pain?
- Is the patient holding the chest wall?
- Is there symmetry in movement of the chest during breathing?
- If the patient's wind was knocked out, is normal breathing returning rapidly or is there prolonged difficulty? Prolonged difficulty may indicate a more severe injury.

The patient's body position should be observed. A patient who has sustained some type of thoracic injury often leans toward the side that is injured, holding or splinting the area with the opposite hand (Figure 27–16A). In the case of an abdominal injury, the patient typically lies on his or her side, with the knees pulled up toward the chest (Figure 27–16B).[67] The male who has sustained an injury to the external genitalia lies on his side, holding the scrotum (Figure 27–16C).

The athletic trainer should check for areas of discoloration, swelling, or deformities that may produce asymmetries. Discoloration or ecchymosis around the umbilicus is indicative of intraabdominal bleeding, whereas ecchymosis on the flanks may indicate swelling outside the abdomen.

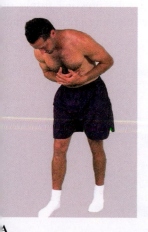
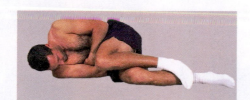
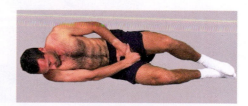

A     B     C

FIGURE 27–16   Typical body position after injury. **(A)** Thoracic injury. **(B)** Abdominal injury. **(C)** External genitalia injury.
© William E. Prentice

- Is there protrusion or swelling of any portion of the abdomen? Such swelling may indicate internal bleeding.
- Does the thorax appear to be symmetrical? Rib fractures can cause one side to appear different.
- Are the abdominal muscles tight and guarding?
- Is the patient holding or splinting a specific part of the abdomen?

Other observable signs and symptoms may indicate the nature of a thoracic or abdominal injury. Bright red blood being coughed up indicates some injury to the lungs. Bright red, frothy blood being vomited may indicate injury to the esophagus or stomach, although the blood may also be swallowed from the mouth or nose and then vomited. Cyanosis generally indicates some respiratory difficulty, whereas pale, cool, clammy skin indicates lowered blood pressure.

It is important to monitor vital signs, including pulse, respirations, and blood pressure (see Chapter 12). A rapid, weak pulse and/or a significant drop in blood pressure is an indication of a potentially serious internal injury, which very often involves loss of blood.

### Palpation

**Thorax** The athletic trainer should first place his or her hands on each side of the chest wall to check for symmetry in chest wall movement during deep inspiration and expiration and to begin to isolate areas of tenderness (Figure 27–17).[33] Once a tender area is identified, the athletic trainer should palpate along the ribs in the intercostal

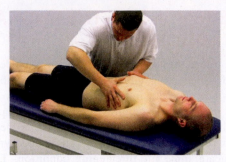

FIGURE 27–17 Checking asymmetry of the chest wall during breathing.
© William E. Prentice

space between the ribs and at the costochondral junction to locate a specific point of tenderness. Applying anteroposterior compression to the thoracic cage is done to identify potential rib fractures (Figure 27–18A). Transverse compression applied laterally identifies costochondral injuries (Figure 27–18B). If the patient is having difficulty breathing, it may be helpful to use a semireclining position for these tests.

**Abdomen** For abdominal palpation, the patient should be supine with the arms at the side and with the hips and knees flexed to relax the abdominal muscles. Palpation should occur in a systematic manner using the four abdominopelvic quadrants, which were discussed in Chapter 13 (see Figure 13–1). Palpation should begin in the right upper quadrant and move clockwise to the left upper quadrant, the left lower quadrant, and finally the right lower quadrant (appendix). The athletic trainer should begin palpating uninjured areas first, using the tips of the fingers to feel for any tightness or rigidity (Figure 27–19).[53] A patient with an abdominal injury will voluntarily contract the abdominal muscles to guard or protect the tender area. If there is bleeding or irritation inside the abdominal cavity, the abdomen exhibits boardlike rigidity and cannot be voluntarily relaxed. **Rebound tenderness** may also accompany intraabdominal bleeding. The athletic trainer can produce rebound tenderness by pressing firmly on the abdomen and then quickly releasing pressure, which

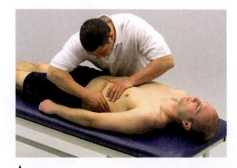

A

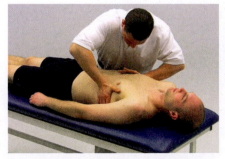

B

FIGURE 27–18 **(A)** Checking for rib fractures. **(B)** Checking for costochondral injuries.
© William E. Prentice

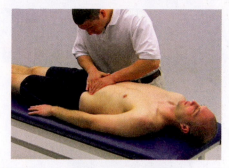

FIGURE 27–19 Palpating the abdomen for guarding or rigidity.
© William E. Prentice

causes intense pain. If the patient is exhibiting only voluntary guarding, the athletic trainer can palpate over the liver, gallbladder, spleen, stomach, small intestine, large intestine, vermiform appendix, and bladder while searching for tenderness, swelling, or enlargement. The kidneys should be palpated, with the patient in a prone position.

Pressure on the abdominal organs may elicit referred pain in predictable patterns away from the source.[55] Figure 27–20 identifies patterns of referred pain.

## Special Tests

**Auscultation** Auscultation involves listening to body sounds through a stethoscope.[38] It has been suggested that auscultation should be done prior to obtaining a history, as described on page 855. When the athletic trainer chooses to perform auscultation in the assessment sequence is a matter of personal preference. If the patient is experiencing respiratory difficulties and for whatever reason is not capable of providing a history, then logic dictates that auscultation should be done immediately to try and identify what is causing the problem. Auscultation is often used to listen to heart sounds, breathing sounds, and bowel sounds (Figure 27–21A).[3]

**Heart Sounds** A normal cardiac cycle includes two sounds, often called "lubb-dupp," which are caused by the turbulence of the blood as the valves close. In children, it is not unusual to hear a third sound.[57] Figure 27–21A shows the positions for auscultation of the heart with a stethoscope. When auscultating the heart, the clinician should stand on the right side of the patient, who is in either a seated or semi-reclined position and breathing normally. To listen to the heart, the stethoscope should be placed over four general areas: over the mitral region in the fifth left intercostal space, 1 cm medial to the midclavicular line; over the tricuspid region in the fourth intercostal space, at lower-left sternal border; over the aortic region in the second right intercostal space; and over the pulmonary region in the second left intercostal space. Most stethoscopes have two surfaces, a diaphragm and a bell. The bell of the stethoscope is better for detecting lower-frequency sounds, whereas the diaphragm is better for higher frequencies. The bell is usually used to listen to the mitral valve, the diaphragm at all other sites.

**Breath Sounds** The rate of breathing patterns should be even and consistent. Abnormal breathing patterns include *Cheyne-Stokes* breathing, in which the rate speeds up and then slows down over a 1- to 3-minute period; *Biot's* breathing, in which a series of breaths at the normal rate are followed by complete cessation of breathing; *apneustic* breathing, in which there are pauses in the

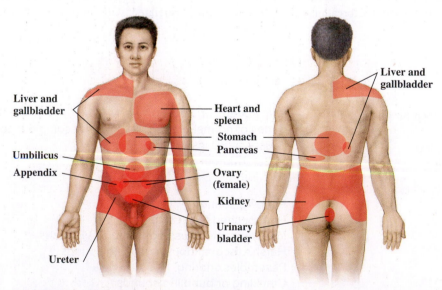

Liver and gallbladder

Heart and spleen

Stomach

Pancreas

Umbilicus

Appendix

Ovary (female)

Kidney

Urinary bladder

Ureter

Liver and gallbladder

FIGURE 27–20 Patterns of referred pain.

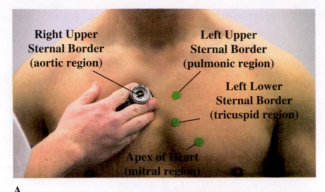

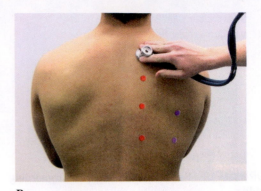

**A**

**B**

Right Upper
Sternal Border
(aortic region)

Left Upper
Sternal Border
(pulmonic region)

Left Lower
Sternal Border
(tricuspid region)

Apex of Heart
(mitral region)

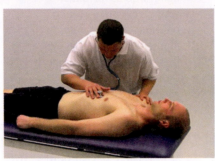

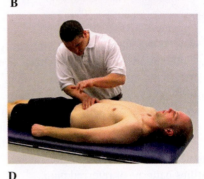

**C**

**D**

FIGURE 27–21 Points of auscultation. **(A)** Heart sounds. **(B)** Breath sounds. **(C)** Bowel sounds (anywhere in lower abdomen). **(D)** Percussion.
© William E. Prentice

respiratory cycle at full inspiration; and *thoracic* breathing, which occurs without diaphragmatic breathing. Abnormal breathing sounds are often superimposed on normal breathing sounds. Adventitious breath sounds are those that are not normally heard and may be continuous, musiclike sounds with a high pitch, called *wheezes;* popping sounds called *crackles;* continuous wheezes called *stridor;* harsh, crackling sounds called *stertor*; snoringlike sounds called *ronchi;* and crackling or bubbling sounds called *rales.* Figure 27–21B shows the points of auscultation on the back for breath sounds. Both sides of the back should be examined. Table 27–3 summarizes the breathing patterns and

sounds. Positions for auscultation should be over the apex, centrally, and at the base of each lung, both anteriorly and posteriorly.[61]

**Bowel Sounds** Normal bowel sounds are liquidlike, gurgling sounds created by normal peristaltic actions that propel intestinal contents through the lower gastrointestinal tract. Following abdominal injury, bowel signs may be absent or diminished, which may indicate paralytic ilieus (pseudo-obstruction) or peritonitis (inflammation of the peritoneum). High-pitched tinkling sounds are associated with intestinal obstruction.[67] Certainly,

| **TABLE 27–3** | **Summary of Breathing Patterns and Sounds** |
|---|---|
| **Breathing patterns** | |
| Cheyne-Stokes breathing | Rate speeds up and slows down over 1 to 3 minutes |
| Biot's breathing | Series of normal breaths followed by complete cessation |
| Apneustic breathing | Pauses at full inspiration |
| Thoracic breathing | Occurs without diaphragmatic breathing |
| **Adventitious (abnormal) sounds** | |
| Crackles | Popping sounds |
| Wheezes | High-pitched musical tones |
| Stridor | Intense, continuous, monophonic wheezes |
| Stertor | Harsh, discontinuous, crackling sounds |
| Ronchi | Resembles snoring |
| Rales | Crackling or bubbling sounds |

auscultation may provide valuable diagnostic information. The stethoscope can be placed in multiple positions anywhere over the lower abdomen (Figure 27–20C).[61] If there are no bowel sounds over a 30-second period, the patient should be referred to a physician.

**Percussion**  The athletic trainer performs percussion by placing a finger of one hand over an organ and then using one or two fingers from the other hand to strike that finger (Figure 27–21D). The resulting sound may provide some indication as to the status of the organ being percussed. A solid organ, such as the liver, produces a dull sound, whereas a hollow organ, such as a lung, produces a tympanic or resonant sound.

Some special training is required to know exactly what to listen for in auscultation and percussion. The athletic trainer should know what sounds are normal and be able to determine when something sounds abnormal. The physician is certainly better qualified to make diagnostic decisions based on auscultation and percussion.

# RECOGNITION AND MANAGEMENT OF SPECIFIC INJURIES AND CONDITIONS OF THE THORACIC REGION

The thorax is vulnerable to a variety of injuries to the ribs, the costochondral junction, and the muscles. Injuries to the lungs and heart are more serious and require special attention.

## Rib Contusions

***Etiology***  A blow to the rib cage can contuse intercostal muscles or, if severe enough, produce a fracture. Because the intercostal muscles are essential for the breathing mechanism, both expiration and inspiration become very painful when they are bruised.

***Symptoms and signs***  Characteristically, the pain is sharp during breathing, there is point tenderness, and pain is elicited when the rib cage is compressed. X-ray examination should be routine in such an injury.

***Management***  POLICE and antiinflammatory agents are commonly used. Like most rib injuries, contusions to the thorax are self-limiting; they respond best to rest and to the cessation of strenuous activities.

## Rib Fractures

***Etiology***  Rib fractures (Figure 27–22) are not uncommon and have their highest incidence in collision sports, particularly wrestling and football. Fractures can be caused by either direct or indirect traumas and can, infrequently, be the result of violent muscular contractions.[40] A direct injury is caused by a kick or a well-placed block, with the fracture developing at the site of force application. An indirect fracture is produced as a result of general compression of the rib cage, as may occur in football or wrestling.

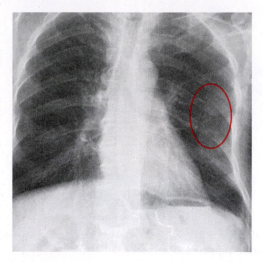

**FIGURE 27–22**  Rib fractures.

Ribs have also been known to fracture from forces caused by coughing and sneezing. Ribs 5 through 9 are the most commonly fractured. Multiple rib fractures can be severe. A *flail chest* involves a fracture of three or more consecutive ribs on the same side.

The structural and functional disruption sustained in a rib fracture varies according to the type of injury that has been received.[12] The *direct fracture* causes the most serious damage, because the external force fractures and displaces the ribs inwardly. Such a mechanism may completely displace the bone and cause an overriding of fragments. The jagged edges of the fragments may cut, tear, or perforate the tissue of the pleurae, causing hemothorax, or they may collapse one lung (pneumothorax). Contrary to the direct injury, the indirect fracture usually causes the rib to spring and fracture outward, producing an oblique or transverse fissure. Stress fracture of the first rib is becoming more prevalent. It can result from repeated arm movements, such as those used in pitching or in rowing. Stress fractures to other ribs have resulted from repeated coughing or laughing. Injury to the pectoral muscles may mask signs of a rib fracture.[11]

***Symptoms and signs***  The rib fracture is usually detected quite easily. The history informs the athletic trainer of the type and degree of force to which the rib cage has been subjected. After trauma, the patient complains of severe pain during inspiration and has point tenderness. A fracture of the rib is readily evidenced by a severe, sharp pain and possibly crepitus during palpation.

> A rib fracture may be indicated by a severe, sharp pain during breathing.

***Management***  The patient should be referred to a physician for X-ray examination if there is any indication of fracture.

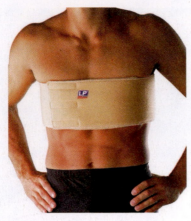

FIGURE 27–23   A commercial rib brace can provide moderate support to the thorax.

Courtesy La Pointique Int'l Ltd./Oppo Medical Inc.

An uncomplicated rib fracture is often difficult to identify on an X ray. Therefore, the physician plans the treatment according to the symptoms presented. The rib fracture is usually managed with support and rest. Simple transverse or oblique fractures heal within 3 to 4 weeks. A rib brace can offer the patient some rib cage stabilization and comfort (Figure 27–23). However, rib supports may predispose the patient to develop hypostatic pneumonia, which has the potential to occur whenever an individual does not take full inspirations because of pain and some mechanical restriction.[12,67]

### Costochondral Separation and Dislocation

*Etiology*   A costochondral separation or dislocation has a higher incidence than do fractures (Figure 27–24). This injury can occur from a direct blow to the anterolateral aspect of the thorax or indirectly from a sudden twist or a fall on some object that compresses the rib cage. The costochondral injury displays many signs that are similar to the rib fracture, with the exception that pain is localized in the junction of the rib cartilage and rib.

*Symptoms  and  signs*   The patient complains of sharp pain during sudden movement of the trunk and has

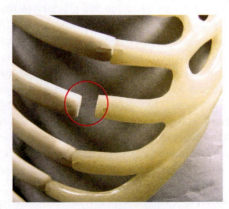

FIGURE 27–24   Costochondral separation.

© William E. Prentice

difficulty breathing deeply. There is point tenderness with swelling. In some cases, there is a rib deformity and a complaint that the rib makes a crepitus noise as it moves in and out of place.

*Management*   Like a rib fracture, the costochondral separation is managed by rest and immobilization by rib brace. Healing takes from 1 to 2 months and precludes any strenuous activity until the patient is symptom free.

### Rib Tip Syndrome

*Etiology*   Rib tip syndrome involves ribs 8, 9, and 10. Because these ribs are attached to each other by fibrous tissue and not by costal cartilage, if these connections are damaged or even ruptured as a result of trauma, the ribs can slip and impinge on the intercostal nerve, producing pain. It is most common in contact sports.

*Symptoms  and  signs*   Pain is localized in the upper abdomen or inferior costal area and is described as sharp or stabbing. It occurs when the patient laterally flexes and hyperextends toward the opposite side. It is not uncommon for the patient to report a popping sensation or a slipping movement of the ribs. Symptoms can be reproduced by hooking the fingers under the inferior rib and pulling anteriorly. A positive test produces a click.

*Management*   Using a compression wrap or an abdominal brace will make the patient comfortable; it may be worn until fibrous adhesions have had a chance to develop. Mobilization and/or manipulation of the rib to reposition it may also be effective. A physician may choose injection of a local anesthetic and corticosteroid.

### Sternum Fracture

*Etiology*   Fracture of the sternum results from a high-impact blow to the chest. Sternum fractures are more likely to occur in automobile accidents than in athletics.[12] Injuries to the ribs or the costochondral junction are much more likely in the athlete. An impact severe enough to cause fracture of the sternum may also cause contusion to the underlying cardiac muscle.

*Symptoms  and  signs*   There may be point tenderness over the sternum at the site of the fracture that is exacerbated by deep inspiration or forceful expiration. Signs of shock or a weak, rapid pulse may indicate more severe internal injury.

*Management*   The patient should be sent for X-rays and should be closely monitored for signs of trauma to the heart.

### Muscle Injuries

*Etiology*   The muscles of the thorax are all subject to contusions and strains in sports. The intercostals are especially vulnerable. Traumatic injuries occur most often from direct blows or sudden torsion of the athlete's trunk.

*Symptoms  and  signs*   Pain occurs on active motion. Injuries to muscles in this region, however, are particularly painful during inspiration and expiration, laughing, coughing, or sneezing.

***Management*** The care of thoracic muscle injuries requires immediate pressure and applications of cold for approximately 1 hour. After hemorrhaging has been controlled, immobilization should be used to make the patient more comfortable.

### Breast Injury

***Etiology*** Many active individuals, but particularly females, can have breast problems. Violent up-and-down and lateral movements of the breasts, as are encountered in running and jumping, can bruise and strain the breast, especially in large-breasted women. Constant, uncontrolled movement of the breast over a period of time can stretch the Cooper's ligament, which supports the breast at the chest wall, and lead to premature ptosis of the breasts (see Figure 7–17).[58]

Another condition that occurs to the breasts in both males and females is runner's nipples, in which the shirt rubs the nipples and causes an abrasion. Runner's nipples can be prevented by placing an adhesive bandage over each nipple before participation. Bicyclist's nipples occur as a result of a combination of cold and the evaporation of sweat, which causes the nipples to become painful. Wearing a windbreaker can prevent this problem.[58]

***Management*** Female athletes should wear a well-designed bra that has minimum elasticity and allows little vertical or horizontal breast movement (see Figure 7–18).[58] Breast injuries usually occur during physical contact with either an opponent or equipment. In sports such as fencing and field hockey, female athletes should protect themselves by wearing plastic cup-type brassieres.

### Breast Cancer

***Etiology*** Breast cancer is the most common type of cancer in women and is the second leading cause of death by cancer in women, following only lung cancer.[57] Although breast cancer is primarily a disease of women, about 1 percent of breast cancers occur in men. Many women who develop breast cancer have no risk factors other than age and gender. Breast cancer may occur at any age, though the risk of breast cancer increases with age. Family history has long been known to be a risk factor for breast cancer. The risk is highest if the affected relative developed breast cancer at a young age, had cancer in both breasts, or is a close relative. Hormonal influences play a role in the development of breast cancer. Women who start their periods at 11 years of age or younger and those who experience menopause later than 55 years of age have a higher risk of developing breast cancer. Breast cancer occurs more frequently in women with high dietary intake of fat.[57] Metastatic cancers spread from the place where they started into other tissues. The most common place for breast cancer to metastasize is into the lymph nodes under the arm or to the brain, the bones, and the liver.

***Symptoms and signs*** In the early stages, breast cancer usually has no symptoms and is not painful. Quite often, breast cancer is discovered before symptoms are present, either by feeling a lump on the breast or in the armpit or by finding an abnormality on mammography. Other possible symptoms are breast discharge, nipple inversion (in instead of out), and redness and/or puckering in the skin overlying the breast.

***Management*** Breast self-exams should be done frequently. *Focus Box 27–1:* "Five steps of a breast self-exam" describes this process. Not all lumps are malignant, but all should be evaluated by a physician, who may use mammography, MRI, ultrasound, or a biopsy. If a malignancy is found, surgery is the primary treatment for breast cancer. Breast-sparing surgery is often possible. Additional treatments may include radiation therapy, chemotherapy, and hormonal therapy. The decision about which additional treatments are needed is based on the stage and type of cancer and the patient's health and preferences.[67]

### Injuries to the Lungs

***Etiology*** Fortunately, injuries to the lungs resulting from sports trauma are rare.[35] However, because of the seriousness of these injuries, the athletic trainer should be able to recognize the basic signs.[9] The most serious of the conditions are pneumothorax, tension pneumothorax, hemothorax (hemorrhaging into the lungs), and traumatic asphyxia.[68]

> Lung injuries include pneumothorax, tension pneumothorax, hemothorax, and traumatic asphyxia.

***Symptoms and signs***

***Pneumothorax*** Pneumothorax is a condition in which the pleural cavity becomes filled with air that has entered through an opening in the chest (Figure 27–25A).[27] As the negatively pressured pleural cavity fills with air, the lung on that side collapses. The loss of one lung may produce pain, difficulty in breathing, and anoxia.[27,60]

***Tension pneumothorax*** A tension pneumothorax occurs when the pleural sac on one side fills with air and displaces the lung and the heart toward the opposite side, which compresses the opposite lung (Figure 27–25B).[68] There is shortness of breath and chest pain on the side of the injury. There may be absence of breath sounds, cyanosis, and distention of neck veins. The trachea may deviate away from the side of injury. A total collapse of the opposite lung is possible; therefore, medical attention is required immediately.[27]

***Hemothorax*** Hemothorax is the presence of blood within the pleural cavity (Figure 27–25C). It results from the tearing or puncturing of the lung or pleural tissue, which involves the

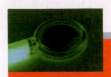

# FOCUS 27-1 Focus on Injury/Illness Prevention and Wellness Promotion

## Five steps of a breast self-exam

**Step 1:** Begin by looking at the breasts in the mirror, with the shoulders straight and the arms on the hips. Look for
- Breasts that are their usual size, shape, and color
- Breasts that are evenly shaped without visible distortion or swelling
- Dimpling, puckering, or bulging of the skin (bring any of these to your doctor's attention)
- A nipple that has changed position or an inverted nipple (pushed inward instead of sticking out)
- Redness, soreness, rash, or swelling

**Step 2:** Now, raise the arms and look for the same changes.

**Step 3:** While at the mirror, gently squeeze each nipple between the finger and thumb and check for nipple discharge (this could be a milky or yellow fluid or blood).

**Step 4:** Next, feel the breasts while lying down, using the right hand to feel the left breast and then the left hand to feel the right breast. Use a firm, smooth touch with the first few fingers of the hand, keeping the fingers flat and together.

Cover the entire breast from top to bottom, side to side—from the clavicle to the top of the abdomen, and from the armpit to the cleavage. Follow a pattern to be sure to cover the whole breast. Begin at the nipple, moving in larger and larger circles until reaching the outer edge of the breast. Also move the fingers up and down vertically, in rows, as if mowing a lawn. Be sure to feel all the breast tissue: just beneath the skin with a soft touch and down deeper with a firmer touch. Begin examining each area with a very soft touch, and then increase pressure to feel the deeper tissue, down to the ribcage.

**Step 5:** Finally, feel the breasts while standing or sitting. Many women find that the easiest way to feel their breasts is when their skin is wet and slippery, so they like to do this step in the shower. Cover the entire breast, using the same hand movements described in Step 4.

From: Breastcancer.org.www.breastcancer.org/symptoms/testing/types/self_exam/bse_steps

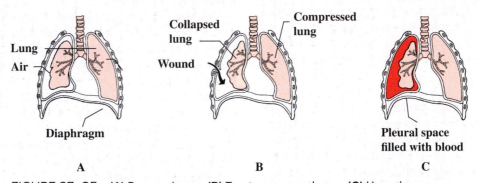

FIGURE 27-25   **(A)** Pneumothorax. **(B)** Tension pneumothorax. **(C)** Hemothorax.

**27–5 Clinical Application Exercise**

A lacrosse player is hit in the thorax with an opponent's stick. He has immediate, localized pain over his ribs and within minutes begins to develop some respiratory difficulty. The athletic trainer suspects that the player has likely fractured a rib and is extremely concerned that the fracture has damaged the lungs.

**?** What lung injuries are possible, and how should this injury be managed?

blood vessels in the area. Like pneumothorax, hemothorax produces pain, difficulty in breathing, and cyanosis.

A violent blow or compression of the chest without an accompanying rib fracture may cause a lung hemorrhage. This condition results in severe pain during breathing, dyspnea (difficult breathing), coughing up of frothy blood, and signs of shock. If these signs are observed, the athlete should be treated for shock and immediately referred to a physician.

**Traumatic asphyxia** Traumatic asphyxia occurs as a result of a violent blow to or a compression of the rib cage that causes a cessation of breathing.[35] Signs include purple discoloration of the upper trunk and head, and the conjunctivas of the eyes display a bright red color. A condition of this type demands immediate mouth-to-mouth resuscitation and medical attention.

**Management** Each of these conditions is a medical emergency that requires immediate physician attention.[4,7] The patient must be transported to a hospital emergency room as quickly as possible.

## Hyperventilation

*Etiology* A patient who has an excessively rapid rate of ventilation, usually due to anxiety-induced stress or asthma, gradually develops a decreased amount of carbon dioxide in the blood (hypocapnia).[63]

***Symptoms and signs*** The patient appears to be having great difficulty in getting air and seems to be struggling to breathe. He or she is in somewhat of a panic state. There may also be some gasping and wheezing. Although it appears that the patient is not getting enough oxygen, the problem is that the levels of carbon dioxide are too low relative to the amount of oxygen.

***Management*** The immediate treatment consists of decreasing the rate of carbon dioxide loss. This is accomplished by first having the patient slow the rate of respiration and concentrate on breathing in through the nose and exhaling through the mouth. A second technique is to have the patient inhale and exhale through one nostril, with the other pinched closed and the mouth closed. A third technique, which has been recommended in the past but is no longer used very often, involves having the patient breathe slowly into a paper or plastic bag. All of these techniques should help rapidly increase the level of carbon dioxide. Typically within 1 or 2 minutes, the patient has returned to a normal respiratory pattern. After the acute phase of hyperventilation has been treated, it is necessary to determine the underlying cause and take appropriate treatment measures.

## Sudden Cardiac Death (SCD) Syndrome in Athletes

***Etiology*** It is catastrophic when a young individual dies suddenly for no apparent reason. It is estimated that 1 in 280,000 men under age 30 experience sudden death each year.[41] More than 20 causes have been identified.[29] In individuals 35 years and younger, the most common cause of exercise-induced sudden cardiac death is a congenital cardiovascular abnormality.[65] The three most prevalent conditions are hypertrophic cardiomyopathy, anomalous origin of the coronary artery, and Marfan's syndrome.[18]

*Hypertrophic cardiomyopathy (HCM)* is a condition in which there is thickened cardiac muscle, with a decrease in the size of the chamber and extensive myocardial scarring. With this condition, there is an increased frequency of ventricular arrhythmia.[24] In an *anomalous origin of the coronary artery,* one of the two coronary vessels originates in a different site than normal, which compromises or obstructs that artery because of its unusual course. People with *Marfan's syndrome* have an abnormality of the connective tissue that results in a weakening of the structure of the aorta and cardiac valves, which can lead to a rupture of either a valve or the aorta itself.[65] Mitral valve prolapse has been associated with both HCM and Marfan's syndrome.[65]

Other potential causes of sudden cardiac death include *coronary artery disease (CAD),* which results from atherosclerosis, in which there is a narrowing of the coronary arteries that is usually due to hypercholesterolemia in the young patient; *peripheral artery disease (PAD),* which involves the dislodgement of relatively large portions of plaques (containing red blood cells, fibrin aggregates, and cholesterol) from arteries in the extremities, which then migrate as an embolus of sufficient size to occlude a major coronary artery; *right ventricular dysplasia,* in which enlargement of the right ventricle causes a potentially lethal disturbance in heartbeat; *cardiac conduction system abnormalities,* which can result from abnormalities of the sinus or atrioventricular nodes; aortic stenosis, which is usually associated with a heart murmur and can cause a fall in blood pressure and cardiac collapse during exercise; *Wolff-Parkinson-White syndrome,* in which an abnormality in cardiac rhythm manifests itself as ventricular tachycardia; and *myocarditis,* an inflammation of the heart associated with a viral condition.[8,13,16,18,34,41,42,47]

Sudden death also has several noncardiac causes, including the use of certain drugs, such as alcohol, cocaine, amphetamines, and erythropoietin (stimulates red blood cell production). A vascular event—bleeding in the brain caused by a cerebral aneurysm, for example, or head trauma that causes intracranial bleeding—may also result in sudden death. Obstructive respiratory diseases, such as asthma, can result in sudden death because of drug toxicity or undertreatment.[41]

***Symptoms and signs*** Most afflicted patients have no symptoms before death.[29] Common symptoms and signs associated with sudden cardiac death include chest pain or discomfort during exertion, heart palpitations or flutters,

---

A football player is running 60-yard sprints during a conditioning workout with the rest of the team. Even before beginning the first practice, the athlete knew that he was not very fit and was worried about how he would do. On the fifth sprint, he called for the athletic trainer and said that he felt as if he could not breathe. He appeared to be gasping for air.

**?** What might the athletic trainer suspect is wrong with this patient, and what is the immediate treatment?

---

The most common causes of sudden cardiac death syndrome are hypertrophic cardiomyopathy, anomalous origin of the coronary artery, and Marfan's syndrome.

---

A basketball player collapses during a practice session when running sprints. The player is conscious and complains of chest pain, heart palpitations or flutters, syncope, nausea, profuse sweating, shortness of breath, and general malaise. The athletic trainer suspects a cardiac-related problem, yet the player has no history of such a condition.

**?** What can cause these symptoms, and how can the athletic trainer provide the most appropriate and immediate care for this patient?

---

syncope, nausea, profuse sweating, heart murmurs, shortness of breath, general malaise, and fever.[5,49]

*Management* It has been suggested that a major number of deaths could be avoided by counseling, screening, and early identification of preventable causes of sudden death.[36,48] The use of diagnostic tests to screen for cardiovascular abnormalities has proven to be ineffective.[44] It appears that currently a history and physical exam in accordance with American Heart Association guidelines are the most effective methods of preparticipation screening.[29] Initial screening should include the following questions:

- Has a physician ever told you that you have a heart murmur?
- Have you had chest pain during exercise?
- Have you fainted during exercise?
- Has anyone in your family under age 35 died suddenly?
- Has anyone in your family been diagnosed with a thickened heart?
- Does anyone in your family have Marfan's syndrome?

If the answer to any of these questions is yes, a more in-depth medical examination should be performed. Resting and exercise electrocardiograms and echocardiograms may be necessary to determine existing pathology.[8]

### Heart Murmur

*Etiology* An abnormal periodic sound that occurs in auscultation of the heart is called a *murmur*. A murmur does not necessarily mean that a pathogenic condition exists in the heart. There are two types of heart murmurs: functional and abnormal. A murmur that exists in the absence of any organic disease in the heart is called *a functional murmur*.[67] Most heart murmurs are functional and are caused by blood flowing through healthy valves in a healthy heart and no treatment is necessary. Functional murmurs arc common in athletes because high cardic output in trained athletes creates high flow velocity and thus a turbulent flow, which results in the presence of murmurs during the ejection phase of the cardiac cycle.

Abnormal heart murmurs can be caused by blood flowing through a damaged heart valve. A heart valve defect may be present congenitally, at birth, or heart valve disease may result from infection, disease, or aging. There are several types of heart valve disease. In mitral valve prolapse, the mitral valve does not close completely when the left ventricle contracts, allowing blood to flow back into the left atrium. This causes a clicking sound as the heart beats. Often, this common condition is not serious; however, it may lead to infective endocarditis or mitral and/or aortic regurgitation (backward blood flow through the valve), both of which can be serious. In mitral valve or aortic stenosis, the mitral and/or aortic valves can become narrowed by scarring from infections, such as rheumatic fever, or may be narrow at birth, forcing the heart to work harder to pump enough blood to satisfy oxygen needs. If untreated, stenosis can lead to

heart failure. In aortic sclerosis, there is scarring, thickening, or stiffening of the aortic valve, which is usually seen in older people with atherosclerosis, or hardening of the arteries. This condition is generally not dangerous; the valve can function for years after the murmur is detected.

*Symptoms and signs* A heart murmur creates an abnormal heart sound described as a clicking, whooshing, or swishing noise heard through auscultation using a stethoscope. In an innocent heart murmur, there are usually no other symptoms or signs of heart problems. People who have abnormal murmurs may have symptoms or signs of other heart problems.

*Treatment* Treatments for a heart murmur vary depending on the cause. Innocent heart murmurs and mitral valve prolapse usually do not indicate disease and require no treatment. Other types of heart valve disease may require different medications to reduce the risk of heart infection, to prevent blood clots, to control irregular heartbeat, to control rapid heartbeat or heart fluttering, or to relax and dilate blood vessels. In some cases, surgery is required either to correct congenital heart defects or to correct certain types of heart valve disease.

### Athletic Heart Syndrome

*Etiology* Athletic heart syndrome involves both structural and functional changes that occur in the hearts of individuals who train for greater than 1 hour on most days.[52] These changes include an increase in the mass of the left ventricle due to increases in left ventricle diastolic cavity dimension, wall thickness, or both. Maximal stroke volume and cardiac output increase, contributing to a lower resting heart rate and longer diastolic filling time. These changes in cardiac morphology are demonstrated using echocardiography (ECG). Despite these changes, systolic and diastolic function remains normal. Differences between athlete and nonathlete populations are generally small, but athletic heart syndrome typically occurs less often in women than in men.

*Symptoms and signs* Athletic heart syndrome is essentially asymptomatic. Signs include bradycardia (decreased heart rate), a systolic murmur, and extra heart sounds. ECG abnormalities are common. The syndrome is significant because it must be distinguished from disorders that cause similar findings but are life threatening (such as hypertrophic cardiomyopathy).[52]

*Management* Once a definitive diagnosis has been made and other, more serious cardiac abnormalities have been ruled out, essentially no treatment is necessary.

### Commotio Cordis

*Etiology* **Commotio cordis** is a syndrome that occurs from a traumatic blunt impact to the chest, resulting in cardiac arrest.[32] It occurs in healthy, young individuals and is primarily a result of the unfortunate timing of a blow during a narrow window within the repolarization phase of the cardiac cycle, 15 to 30 msec prior to the peak of the T wave (see Figure 13–15).[39] Young athletes are especially at risk because of the pliability of their chest walls. Since 1998, 130 cases have been documented in baseball, lacrosse, hockey, softball, football, basketball, cricket, martial arts, and boxing. The true number of deaths is unknown because of underreporting and misclassification.[37]

*Symptoms and signs* Ventricular fibrillation is the most common associated arrhythmia. In most cases, the blow occurs to the precordial area (the chest wall in front of the heart), but cases of left lateral chest trauma have also been reported. Immediate death occurs in about half of the cases, while in others there is a brief period of consciousness before collapse.

*Management* Resuscitation of the victims of commotio cordis is seldom successful. Time is a critical factor after the onset of the event. Early cardiopulmonary resuscitation, and especially early defibrillation with an AED, is essential.[28] A link to the NATA official statement on "Commotio cordis," can be found at www.nata.org/sites/default/files/CommotioCordis.pdf.

### Heart Contusion

*Etiology* A heart contusion may occur when the heart is compressed between the sternum and the spine by a strong outside force. For example, it can occur if an individual is hit by a pitched ball or if an athlete bounces a barbell off the chest in a bench press. The right ventricle is most often injured. The most severe consequence of a violent impact to the heart is a rupture of the aorta, which is immediately life threatening.[43]

*Symptoms and signs* This injury produces severe shock and heart pain. The heart may exhibit certain arrhythmias that cause a decrease in cardiac output, which is followed by death if medical attention is not administered immediately.[37]

*Management* The patient should be taken immediately to a hospital emergency room. The athletic trainer should be prepared to administer CPR and treat the athlete for shock (see Chapter 12).

# RECOGNITION AND MANAGEMENT OF SPECIFIC INJURIES AND CONDITIONS OF THE ABDOMEN

Although abdominal injuries constitute only about 10 percent of sports injuries, they can require long recovery periods and can be life threatening.[1,23] The abdominal area is particularly vulnerable to injury in all contact sports. A blow can produce superficial or even deep internal injuries, depending on its location and intensity.[2] In internal injuries of the abdomen that occur in sports, the solid organs are most often affected. Strong abdominal muscles give good protection when they are tensed, but, when relaxed, they are easily damaged.[10] It is very important to protect the trunk region properly against the traumatic forces of collision sports. Good conditioning is essential, as are the use of proper protective equipment and the application of safety rules.

## Injuries and Conditions Related to the Urinary System

### Kidney Contusion

*Etiology* The kidneys are seemingly well protected within the abdominal cavity. However, on occasion, contusions and even ruptures of these organs occur. The

> Kidney and bladder contusions can cause hematuria.

kidneys may be susceptible to injury because of their normal distention by blood. An external force, usually one applied to the patient's back, causes abnormal extension of an engorged kidney, resulting in injury. The degree of renal injury depends on the extent of the distention and the angle and force of the blow.[20]

*Symptoms and signs* A patient who has received a contusion of the kidney may display signs of shock, nausea, vomiting, rigidity of the back muscles, and hematuria (blood in the urine).[50] Like injuries to other internal organs, kidney injuries may cause referred pain to the outside of the body. Pain may be felt high in the costovertebral angle posteriorly and may radiate forward around the trunk into the lower abdominal region.[62] Any patient who reports having received a severe blow to the abdomen or back region should be instructed to urinate two or three times and to look for the appearance of blood in the urine. If there is any sign of hematuria, the athlete must be referred to a physician immediately.[67]

*Management* Medical care of the contused kidney usually consists of 24-hour hospital observation and a gradual increase of fluid intake. If the hemorrhage fails to stop, surgery may be indicated. Controllable contusions usually require 2 weeks of bed rest and close surveillance after activity is resumed. In questionable cases, complete withdrawal from one active playing season may be required.

### Kidney Stones

*Etiology* Kidney stones are small crystals that form in the kidneys, although the precise cause is not known. They can be as small as a grain of sand or as large as a

27–8 Clinical Application Exercise

A football receiver jumps to catch a high pass thrown over the middle. A defensive back hits the receiver in the low back. The athlete does not seem to have a specific injury. After the game, the patient notices blood in the urine and gets really worried.

**?** Is blood in the urine a cause for concern? What should the athletic trainer do to manage this condition?

marble. They can be smooth, although most are jagged, which makes them harder to pass. A stone may stay in the kidney, causing blockage and pressure in the renal (kidney) system, or it may break loose and travel down the urinary tract, which is very painful.[15] The most common type (75 percent) is a calcium stone, formed when too much calcium in the urine combines with other waste products.[61]

***Symptoms and signs***   The onset of pain is sudden, severe, and sharp and later the pain becomes intermittent as the stone moves. Pain is referred to the low back or in the flank on one side and shoots toward the groin on the same side.[6] It is difficult to find any position of comfort, but pacing seems to help. There may be nausea and vomiting. The skin is cool, clammy, pale, and sweaty. There may be burning with frequent urination and blood in the urine.[61]

***Management***   The patient should drink plenty of fluids, especially water. Urine should be watched for blood or stones. Over-the-counter medications may help with the pain, particularly anti-inflammatory medications. In 80 to 85 percent of cases, smaller stones move through the ureter, drop into the bladder, and come out in the urine. Larger stones, particularly those that are irregularly shaped, may need to be broken up or surgically removed.[61]

## Contusion of the Ureters, Bladder, and Urethra

***Etiology***   On rare occasions, a blunt force to the lower abdominal region avulses a ureter or contuses or ruptures the urinary bladder. Injury to the urinary bladder usually occurs only if it is distended by urine. Hematuria is often associated with contusion of the bladder during running and has been referred to as a *runner's bladder.*[22] Abnormal concentrations of protein in urine is referred to as proteinuria. Injury to the urethra is more common in men because the male's urethra is longer and more exposed than is the female's. Injury may produce severe perineal pain and swelling.

***Symptoms and signs***   After a severe blow to the pelvic region, the patient may display the following recognizable signs: pain and discomfort in the lower abdomen; abdominal rigidity; nausea, vomiting, and signs of shock; blood coming from the urethra; and the passing of a great quantity of bloody urine, which indicates possible injury to the kidney. With a bladder contusion, the patient is able to urinate. With a bladder rupture, the patient is unable to urinate. Bladder injury commonly causes referred pain to the lower trunk, including the upper thigh anteriorly and suprapubically.

***Prevention***   With any impact to the abdominal region, the possibility of internal damage must be considered; after such trauma, the patient should be instructed to check periodically for blood in the urine. To lessen the possibility of rupture, the patient must always empty the bladder before practice or game time. The bladder can also be irritated by intraabdominal pressures during long-distance running. In this situation, repeated impacts to the bladder's base are produced by the jarring of the abdominal contents, resulting in hemorrhage and blood in the urine.

## Cystitis and Urinary Tract Infections

***Etiology***   *Cystitis* is an inflammation or infection of the urinary bladder. When caused by bacteria, it is called a *urinary tract infection (UTI).*[61] Bacterial cystitis, the most common type, is commonly caused by *coliform bacteria* transferred from the bowel through the urethra into the bladder. In females, it most often occurs from wiping incorrectly from back to front after a bowel movement. It can also occur due to frequent or rough sexual intercourse or other activities that push bacteria into the bladder. Females are much more prone to cystitis than males. Cystitis occurs most often in sexually active females ages 20 to 50. It also may occur in women or teenagers who are not sexually active, or in young girls. Cystitis rarely occurs in men with normal urinary tracts. In men, an enlarged prostate gland can cause bladder infections.[22]

***Symptoms and signs***   Patients with bladder infections may develop any or all of the following: a strong, persistent urge to urinate; a burning sensation when urinating; frequent, small amounts of urine; blood in the urine (hematuria); cloudy or strong-smelling urine; a feeling of pressure in the lower abdomen; or a low-grade fever.

***Management***   Oral antibiotics are used to treat cystitis. Symptoms usually disappear within a few days, and further tests probably will be unnecessary. It is essential to drink plenty of liquids, especially water. Cranberry juice has been recommended to change the pH of urine to make it a hostile environment for the infective bacteria. Practicing sanitary bowel and bladder habits, washing the genitals before intercourse, emptying the bladder after intercourse, and immediately removing contraceptive diaphragms after intercourse can help reduce urinary tract infections, which can lead to cystitis.[22]

## Urethritis

***Etiology***   Urethritis is an inflammation of the urethra, most often caused by gonorrhea, chlamydia, the herpes virus, or bacterial infections transmitted during sexual activity.[61] Chemical irritation caused by soaps or lotions, spermicide in condoms, and contraceptive jelly, cream, or foam can also cause inflammation.

***Symptoms and signs***   Burning and pain when urinating are classic symptoms of urethritis. There is an urge to urinate more often. There may also be itching, tenderness, or swelling in the penis, pain with sexual intercourse, ulcers on the genitals, discharge from the penis, or blood in urine or semen. If the infection spreads to other organs, there may be back or abdominal pain, fever, nausea, or swollen joints.[61]

***Management***   Antibiotics are required to treat infections due to bacteria or sexually transmitted diseases. The patient should drink fluids to dilute the urine, thus lessening the pain when urinating. Nonsteroidal antiinflammatory medications and acetaminophen can be used for pain control.

# INJURIES AND CONDITIONS RELATED TO THE DIGESTIVE SYSTEM

A patient may develop various complaints of digestive system disorders resulting from poor eating habits or stress. The athletic trainer should recognize the more severe conditions and cases so that early referrals to a physician can be made.

## Gastrointestinal Bleeding

*Etiology*   Gastrointestinal bleeding that is reflected in bloody stools occurs in a variety of individuals. Distance runners often have blood in their stools during and following a race. The causes of gastrointestinal bleeding can vary. Possible reasons are gastritis, iron-deficiency anemia, ingestion of aspirin or other antiinflammatory agents, stress, bowel irritation, and colitis. Colitis is an inflammation of the colon, usually caused by an ulceration of the mucosal lining of the colon.

*Symptoms and signs*   Signs of colitis include abdominal pain with colic, watery stools that contain pus; dehydration; intermittent fever; and possible hemorrhage and perforation.

*Management*   Patients displaying gastrointestinal bleeding must be referred immediately to a physician.[14]

## Liver Contusion

*Etiology*   Compared with other organ injuries from blunt trauma, injuries to the liver are the second most common.[46] However, liver injury is relatively infrequent. A hard blow to the right side of the rib cage can tear or seriously contuse the liver, especially if it has been enlarged as a result of some disease, such as hepatitis. Hepatitis is an inflammation of the liver caused by viral infection or alcohol consumption. If it is not corrected, the cells in the liver may die and be replaced by scar tissue, which can lead to cirrhosis or impaired liver function.[66] Cirrhosis is a progressive disease of the liver that results in diffuse scarring, fibrosis, and disruption of hepatic blood flow, which can eventually result in liver failure. Cirrhosis has many causes, but it is most often associated with chronic alcoholism.[67]

*Symptoms and signs*   Liver injury can cause hemorrhage and shock, requiring immediate surgical intervention. Liver injury commonly produces a referred

> Hepatitis can cause enlargement of the liver.

pain that is just below the right scapula, right shoulder, and substernal area and, on occasion, a referred pain located in the anterior left side of the chest.[46]

*Management*   A liver contusion requires immediate referral to a physician for diagnosis and treatment.

## Gallbladder Conditions

*Etiology*   The gallbladder stores bile produced by the liver. Before eating a meal, the gallbladder may be filled with bile. After meals, the bile is emptied into the small intestine and the gallbladder is flat, like a deflated balloon. Injury to the gallbladder via direct trauma is most likely when it is filled with bile.

Inflammation of the gallbladder is known as cholecystitis. Cholesterol, which is secreted by the liver, may cause the gallbladder to produce a gallstone, which can block the release of bile. A gallstone that blocks the pancreatic duct may lead to pancreatitis. There is also risk of bacterial infection.

*Symptoms and signs*   *Cholecystitis* is likely to cause pain and fever, as well as tenderness in the upper right quadrant of the abdomen. If gallstones develop, they can be harmless and asymptomatic, but they can also cause jaundice, nausea, and severe pain in the upper right quadrant.

*Management*   Cholecystitis is treated with rest and antibiotics. Diagnostic ultrasound can be used to check for gallstones. Gallstones are initially managed by waiting for them to be passed naturally. In patients who have recurrent gallstones, surgery to remove the gallbladder may be considered.[67] The gallbladder is not essential, and removing it causes no difficulties with digestion or a patient's health.

## Pancreatitis

*Etiology*   Inflammation of the pancreas may be either acute or chronic and is often related to obstruction of the pancreatic duct. An acute inflammation leads to necrosis, suppuration, gangrene, and hemorrhage. Chronic inflammation results in the formation of scar tissue that causes malfunction of the pancreas; inflammation may occur gradually from chronic alcoholism.[67]

*Symptoms and signs*   Acute epigastric pain causes vomiting, belching, constipation, and potentially shock. There may also be tenderness and rigidity on palpation. Chronic pancreatitis causes jaundice, diarrhea, and mild to moderate pain that radiates to the back.

*Management*   Acute pancreatitis requires rehydration, pain reduction, treatment of shock, reduction of pancreatic secretions using medication, and prevention of secondary infection. Surgery would be indicated only if the pancreatic duct were blocked. Treatment of chronic pancreatitis is difficult and requires large doses of analgesics, the administration of pancreatic enzymes, and a low-fat diet.

## Indigestion (Dyspepsia)

*Etiology*   Some patients have food idiosyncrasies that cause them considerable distress after eating. Others develop reactions when eating before competition. The term given to digestive upset is *indigestion* (dyspepsia). Indigestion can be caused by any number of conditions. The most common are emotional stress, esophageal and stomach spa-

> Indigestion, vomiting, diarrhea, and constipation are common problems among athletes.

sms, and inflammation of the mucous lining of the esophagus and stomach.[14]

**Symptoms and signs**   Dyspepsia causes an increased secretion of hydrochloric acid (sour stomach), nausea, and flatulence (gas).

**Management**   Care of acute dyspepsia involves eliminating irritating foods from the diet, developing regular eating habits, and avoiding anxieties that may lead to gastric distress.

Constant irritation of the stomach may lead to more chronic and serious disorders, such as gastritis, an inflammation of the stomach wall, or ulcerations of the gastrointestinal mucosa. Patients who appear nervous and high-strung and suffer from dyspepsia should be examined by a physician.

### Vomiting

**Etiology**   Vomiting results from some type of irritation, most often in the stomach. This irritation stimulates the vomiting center in the brain to cause a series of forceful contractions of the diaphragm and abdominal muscles, thus compressing the stomach and forcefully expelling the contents.[66]

**Management**   Antinausea medications should be administered (see Chapter 17). Fluids to prevent dehydration should be administered by mouth if possible. If vomiting persists, fluids and electrolytes must be administered intravenously.

### Food Poisoning (Gastroenteritis)

**Etiology**   Food poisoning, which ranges from mild to severe, results from infectious organisms (bacteria of the salmonella group, certain staphylococci, streptococci, or dysentery bacilli) that enter the body in either food or drink. Foods become contaminated, especially during warm weather, when improper food refrigeration permits the organisms to multiply rapidly. Contamination can also occur if the food is handled by an infected food handler.[61]

**Symptoms and signs**   Infection results in nausea, vomiting, cramps, diarrhea, and anorexia. The symptoms of staphylococcal infections usually subside in 3 to 6 hours. Salmonella infection symptoms may last from 24 to 48 hours or more.

**Management**   Management requires the rapid replacement of lost fluids and electrolytes, which, in severe cases, may need to be replaced intravenously. Bed rest is desirable in all but mild cases; as long as the nausea and vomiting continue, nothing should be given by mouth. If tolerated, light fluids or foods—such as clear broth, bouillon with a small amount of added salt, soft-cooked eggs, or bland cereals—may be given.

### Peptic Ulcer

**Etiology**   A peptic ulcer is a condition in which the acids secreted in the stomach destroy the mucous lining either in the stomach or in the small intestine. Peptic ulcers occur most often in people who experience severe anxiety for long periods of time.[66] *H. pylori* is a type of bacteria thought to be responsible for the majority of peptic ulcers.

*H. pylori* weakens the mucous lining of the stomach and small intestine, allowing acid to penetrate the wall, irritating the lining and causing a sore or ulcer.

**Symptoms and signs**   A gnawing pain, localized in the epigastric region, usually appears between 1 and 3 hours following a meal. Other symptoms include dyspepsia, heartburn, nausea, and vomiting. Pain usually lasts for minutes rather than hours.[67]

**Management**   Occasionally, symptoms disappear without the aid of medication. Antacids may be helpful in neutralizing gastric secretions. Altering the diet has not proven to be effective in managing the peptic ulcer. If the cause is bacterial, antibiotics should be prescribed. If hemorrhaging or perforation occur, surgery may be necessary.

### Gastroesophageal Reflux Disease (GERD)

**Etiology**   This condition occurs when there is a reflux, or backward flow, of the acidic gastric contents into the esophagus, usually due to a malfunction of the lower esophageal sphincter. It can also occur as a result of a hiatal hernia. The incidence is increased with exercise. If this occurs repeatedly, the lower esophagus can become inflamed, and this condition is referred to as *esophagitis*.[66]

**Symptoms and signs**   There is heartburnlike retrosternal pain that can progress to a gripping chest pain similar to angina pectoris. There is a burning feeling with a sour liquid taste in the throat. The athlete also may have difficulty swallowing.

**Management**   Usually, this regurgitation can be controlled by medication. However, if the medication does not stop the reflux, surgery may be needed.

### Diarrhea

**Etiology**   Diarrhea is abnormal stool looseness or passage of a fluid, unformed stool and is categorized as acute or chronic, according to the type present. Diarrhea can be caused by problems in the diet, inflammation of the intestinal lining, gastrointestinal infection, the ingestion of certain drugs, and psychogenic factors. *"Travelers'" diarrhea* is the most common illness, affecting as many as half of travelers to high-risk international destinations. It most often occurs during the first week of travel but may occur even after returning home. It is most likely to affect young adults, immunosuppressed persons, individuals with inflammatory-bowel disease or diabetes, and people taking antacids.[67]

**Symptoms and signs**   Diarrhea is characterized by abdominal cramps, nausea, and possibly vomiting, coupled with frequent elimination of stools, ranging from 3 to 20 a day. The infected person often has a loss of appetite and a light brown or gray, foul-smelling stool. Extreme weakness caused by fluid dehydration is usually present.

**Management**   The cause of diarrhea is often difficult to establish. The loose stool may be caused by any irritant, including an infestation of parasitic organisms or an emotional upset. Management of diarrhea requires a knowledge of its cause. The athletic trainer can care for less severe cases by having the athlete omit foods that cause irritation, drink boiled milk, eat bland food until symptoms have ceased, and use pectins two or three times daily for the absorption of excess fluid.[14]

## Constipation

**Etiology**  Some individuals are subject to constipation, which is the failure of the bowels to evacuate feces.[14] There are numerous causes of constipation, the most common of which are lack of peristalsis; insufficient moisture in the feces, causing it to be hard and dry; lack of a sufficient proportion of roughage and bulk in the diet to stimulate peristalsis; poor bowel habits; nervousness and anxiety; and overuse of laxatives and enemas.[67]

**Symptoms and signs**  Constipation results in a feeling of fullness, with occasional cramping and pain in the lower abdomen. When an individual strains hard to defecate, some vessels may be ruptured in the rectum and bleeding from the anus may occur.

**Management**  The best means of overcoming constipation is to regulate eating patterns to include foods that will encourage normal defecation. Cereals, fruits, vegetables, and fats stimulate bowel movement, whereas sugars and carbohydrates tend to inhibit it. Some persons become constipated as a result of psychological factors. In such cases, the athletic trainer may try to determine the causes of stress and, if needed, refer the athlete to a physician or school psychologist for counseling. Above all, laxatives and enemas should be avoided unless their use has been prescribed by a physician.

## Irritable Bowel Syndrome

**Etiology**  Irritable bowel syndrome (IBS) is a group of disorders related to the gastrointestinal tract that present themselves differently, depending on the individual.[67] IBS is thought to occur in 10 to 20 percent of the adult population and is slightly more common in women than men. No psychological factors have been identified as a cause of IBS, but psychological factors often determine how the individual experiences and handles the condition.

**Symptoms and signs**  The individual with IBS experiences abdominal pain that is relieved with defecation. There is an irregular pattern of defecation at least 25 percent of the time. In addition, there may be some alteration in stool frequency, stool form, stool passage, the passage of mucus, and abdominal bloating and distention.

**Management**  The patient should be referred for long-term physician management. Initially, treatment should include modifying the diet to eliminate foods that seem to cause a problem.[61] Most often, dairy foods and gas-forming foods are the cause. Antidiarrheal or antispasmodic medications may help reduce the symptoms. Some psychological counseling intervention may also prove helpful. The long-term prognosis for this condition is positive.

## Appendicitis

**Etiology**  Inflammation of the vermiform appendix can be chronic or acute. It is caused by a variety of conditions, such as a fecal obstruction, lymph swelling, or even a carcinoid tumor. Its highest incidence is in males between the ages of 15 and 25. Appendicitis can be mistaken for a common gastric complaint.[67] In early stages, the appendix becomes red and swollen; in later stages, it may become gangrenous, rupturing into the bowels or peritoneal cavity and causing peritonitis.[67] Bacterial infection is a complication of rupture of the inflamed appendix.

**Symptoms and signs**  The patient may complain of a mild-to-severe pain in the lower abdomen, associated with nausea, vomiting, and a low-grade fever ranging from 99°F to 100°F (37°C to 38°C). Later, the cramps may localize into a pain in the right side, and palpation may reveal abdominal rigidity and tenderness at a point (McBurney's point) between the anterior superior spine of the ilium and the umbilicus, about 1 to 2 inches (2.5 to 5 cm) above the latter.[67]

A strain of the psoas muscle or an abcess in the sheath of the psoas is sometimes mistaken for appendicitis.

**Management**  Surgical removal of the appendix is often necessary. Appendicitis is at least an urgent situation.[21] An obstructed bowel with an acute rupture is a life-threatening condition.

## Hemorrhoids (Piles)

**Etiology**  Hemorrhoids are varicosities of the hemorrhoidal venous plexus of the anus. There are both internal and external anal veins. Chronic constipation or straining at the stool may stretch the anal veins, resulting in either a protrusion (prolapse) and bleeding of the internal or external veins or a thrombus in the external veins.[67]

**Symptoms and signs**  Hemorrhoids are painful, nodular swellings near the sphincter of the anus. They may cause slight bleeding and itching. The majority of hemorrhoids are self-limiting and heal spontaneously within 3 weeks.

**Management**  The management of hemorrhoids is mostly palliative to eliminate discomfort until healing takes place. The following measures can be suggested: using

> Appendicitis is often mistaken for a common gastric problem.

**27–9 Clinical Application Exercise**

Immediately after finishing a meal, a patient begins to complain of a mild-to-severe pain in the lower abdomen. She has nausea, vomiting, and a low-grade fever. The athletic trainer suspects that she has indigestion; in about an hour, however, the cramps begin to localize into a pain in the right side, and palpation reveals abdominal rigidity and tenderness at McBurney's point.

**?** What should the athletic trainer suspect is wrong with this patient, and how should this illness be managed?

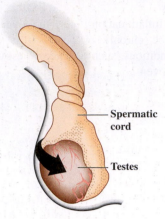

FIGURE 27–26   Spermatic cord torsion.

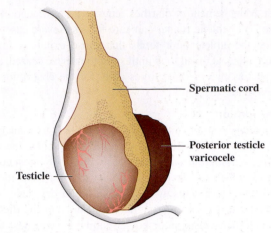

FIGURE 27–27   Hydrocele of the tunica vaginalis.

proper bowel habits, ingesting 1 tablespoon of mineral oil daily to assist in lubricating dry stool, applying an astringent suppository (tannic acid), and applying a local anesthetic to control pain and itching (dibucaine). If palliative measures are unsuccessful, surgery may be required.[67]

## Injuries and Conditions Related to the Reproductive Organs

Injuries to the reproductive organs are much more likely to occur in the male because the genitalia are more exposed.

### Scrotal Contusion

*Etiology*   As a result of its considerable sensitivity and particular vulnerability, the scrotum may sustain a contusion that causes a very painful, nauseating, and disabling condition.

*Symptoms and signs*   Like any other contusion, the scrotal contusion causes hemorrhage, fluid effusion, and muscle spasm, the degree of which depends on the intensity of the impact to the tissue.

*Management*   Immediately following a scrotal contusion, the patient must be put at ease and testicular spasms must be reduced. Several techniques have been proposed to help reduce testicular pain following contusion. The first of these techniques is to place the patient in a kneeling position and have him bounce up and down. The second technique is to place the patient supine with knees and hips flexed to 90 degrees and have him perform a Valsalva maneuver. These maneuvers aid in reducing discomfort and relaxing the muscle spasm. After the pain has diminished, a cold pack is applied to the scrotum. Increasing or unresolved pain after 15 to 20 minutes requires prompt referral to a physician for evaluation.

### Testicular Torsion

*Etiology*   Testicular torsion occurs when the spermatic cord twists in the scrotum, impairing the blood supply to the testicle. Men who get testicular torsion tend to have an inherited trait that allows the testicle to freely move and

rotate within the scrotum. It usually occurs several hours following vigorous activity (Figure 27–26).

*Symptoms and signs*   Cord torsion produces acute testicular pain (in the lower abdomen and groin), swelling of the scrotum, the testicle positioned higher than normal, nausea, vomiting, with tenderness and redness in the area.

*Management*   In this case, the patient must receive immediate medical attention to prevent irreparable complications. Twisting of the spermatic cord may present the appearance of a cluster of swollen veins and may cause a dull pain combined with a heavy, dragging feeling in the scrotum. This condition may eventually lead to atrophy of the testicle. A physician should be consulted within no more than 6 hours when this condition is suspected.[59] Surgery may be necessary to correct this problem.

### Traumatic Hydrocele of the Tunica Vaginalis

*Etiology*   Traumatic hydrocele of the tunica vaginalis is an excess fluid accumulation caused by a severe blow to the testicular region. The venous plexus on the posterior aspect of the testicle can become engorged, creating a varicocele (Figure 27–27). A rupture of this plexus results in a rapid accumulation of blood in the scrotum, called a hematocele.

*Symptoms and signs*   After trauma, the patient complains of pain. Swelling in the scrotum can significantly increase the size of the sac.

*Management*   Cold packs should be applied to the scrotum, and the athlete should be referred to a physician. Irreversible damage can occur to the testicle if medical treatment is delayed.

A male soccer player receives a blow to the genitalia. Shortly after the hit, the patient is in significant pain and begins vomiting.

**?** How should this injury be managed?

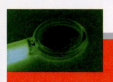

## Testicular Cancer

***Etiology*** Testicular cancer is the most common cancer in American males between the ages of 15 and 34 and accounts for 1 percent of all cancers in men.[67] Although the exact cause of testicular cancer is unknown, several factors seem to increase risk, including a medical history of undescended testicle(s), abnormal testicular development, low levels of male hormones, sterility, previous testicular cancer, and family history of testicular cancer. Cancer usually affects only one testicle.

***Symptoms and signs*** Testicular cancer can result in pain or discomfort in a testicle or the scrotum, a lump or an enlargement in either testicle, swelling or a sudden collection of fluid in the scrotum, a feeling of heaviness in the scrotum, a dull ache in the abdomen or groin, unexplained fatigue, and enlargement or tenderness of the breasts.[57]

***Management*** Testicular cancer is highly treatable when diagnosed early. Depending on the type and stage of testicular cancer, a patient may receive one of several treatments, including surgical removal of the testicle, chemotherapy, radiation therapy, or a combination. Regular testicular self-examinations can help identify dangerous growths early, when the chance for successful treatment of testicular cancer is highest. *Focus Box 27–2:* "Self-examination of the testes" discusses proper technique.

## Vaginitis

***Etiology*** Vaginitis is an inflammation of the vagina caused by a variety of microorganisms, many of which are associated with sexually transmitted diseases (STDs)[56] (discussed in Chapter 29). Other non-STD causes exist, however, including bacterial infection, strong chemicals from douching, irritation from a tampon, and poor hygiene habits.[69]

***Symptoms and signs*** There will be purulent (filled with pus) and, occasionally, bloody vaginal discharge. There may also be a strong odor with vaginal itching. Urination is frequent and painful. The vagina is red and painful to touch.

***Management*** For vaginitis caused by an STD, appropriate antibiotic or antifungal medications should be given. The patient should also be instructed in correct bowel and bladder hygiene and cleanliness and should be counseled regarding sexual behavior.

### Contusion of the Female Genitalia

***Etiology*** The female reproductive organs have a low incidence of injury. By far, the most common gynecological injury in the female patient involves a contusion to the external genitalia, or vulva, which includes the labia, clitoris, and vestibule of the vagina.

***Symptoms and signs*** A hematoma results from the contusion, which most often occurs with a direct impact to this area. A contusion of this area may also injure the symphysis pubis, producing osteitis pubis (discussed in Chapter 21).

***Management*** As long as the skin is intact, the contusion can be treated with ice to minimize swelling. If pain persists over several days, the patient should be evaluated by a physician to rule out fracture and osteitis pubis.

## Injury to Lymphatic Organs

### Injury of the Spleen

***Etiology*** Injuries to the spleen are relatively uncommon. If injury does occur, it is most often due

A baseball player is hit with a pitch in the left upper quadrant. Initially, he appears to be all right, but, toward the end of the game, he becomes nauseated and starts to vomit. He complains of pain in the left upper quadrant and pain in his left shoulder, extending down his arm. The athletic trainer palpates the abdomen and detects rigidity. Within a matter of minutes, the player begins to develop shocklike symptoms.

**?** What should the athletic trainer suspect has happened to this patient, and how should the injury be treated?

27–11 Clinical Application Exercise

to a fall or a direct blow to the left upper quadrant of the abdomen (see Figure 13–1) when an existing medical condition has caused splenomegaly (enlargement of the spleen).[64] Infectious mononucleosis is the most likely cause of spleen enlargement. Athletes with mononucleosis should not engage in any activity for 3 weeks because approximately 50 percent of sufferers exhibit splenomegaly, which is difficult to diagnose clinically (see Chapter 29).

***Symptoms and signs*** The gross indications of a ruptured spleen must be recognized, so that an immediate

medical referral can be made. Indications include a history of a severe blow to the abdomen and possibly signs of shock, abdominal rigidity, nausea, and vomiting. There may be a reflex pain occurring approximately 30 minutes after injury, called Kehr's sign, which radiates to the left shoulder and one-third of the way down the left arm.[19]

The great danger with a ruptured spleen lies in its ability to splint itself and then produce a delayed hemorrhage. Splinting of the spleen is effected by a loose hematoma formation and the constitution of the supporting and surrounding structures. Any slight strain may disrupt the splinting effect and allow the spleen to hemorrhage profusely into the abdominal cavity, causing the patient to die of internal bleeding days or weeks after the injury.[17]

***Management*** Conservative, nonoperative treatment is recommended initially with a week of hospitalization. At 3 weeks, the patient can engage in light conditioning activities, and, at 4 weeks, the patient can return to full activity as long as no symptoms appear. If surgical repair is necessary, the patient will require 3 months to recover, whereas removal of the spleen will require 6 months before the patient can return to activity.[64]

## Injuries to the Abdominal Wall

A number of other abdominal pain sites can be disabling. The athletic trainer should be able to discern the pain sites that are potentially more serious and refer the patient accordingly.[45]

### Abdominal Muscle Strains

***Etiology*** An abdominal muscle strain, also called a pulled abdominal muscle, is an injury to one of the muscles of the abdominal wall, most commonly involving the rectus abdominis.[54] Other abdominal muscles that are subject to strain are the internal and external obliques and the transversus abdominis. Strains most often occur when the muscle is stretched, usually in combination with a twisting motion, or when the muscle is maximally contracted in a shortened position and is then stretched.

***Symptoms and signs*** Abdominal muscle strains usually cause immediate pain in the area of the injured muscle. It can be hard to flex the muscle because of this pain. The other common symptom is muscle spasm of the injured muscle. Less commonly, swelling and bruising result from the muscle injury.

***Management*** Treatment of abdominal muscle injuries is difficult—there is no way to completely splint the abdomen, although an elastic wrap can help provide support and make the patient more comfortable. It is important to rest the muscle by avoiding exercise to allow the injured muscle to heal. Activities that cause pain or spasm of the abdominal muscles should be avoided. Gentle stretching is helpful, but it should not be painful.

### Contusions of the Abdominal Wall

***Etiology*** Compressive forces that injure the abdominal wall are not common in sports. When they do happen, they are more likely to occur in collision sports, such as football or ice hockey; however, any sports implements or high-velocity projectiles can injure. Hockey goalies and baseball catchers would be very vulnerable to injury without their protective torso pads. Contusion may occur superficially to the abdominal skin or subcutaneous tissue or much deeper to the musculature. The extent and type of injury vary, depending on whether the force is blunt or penetrating.[54]

***Symptoms and signs*** A contusion of the rectus abdominis muscle can be very disabling. A severe blow may cause a hematoma that develops under the fascial tissue surrounding this muscle. The pressure that results from hemorrhage causes pain and tightness in the region of the injury.

***Management*** A cold pack and a compression elastic wrap should be applied immediately after injury. The athletic trainer must look for signs of possible internal injury.

### Hernia

***Etiology*** The term *hernia* refers to the protrusion of abdominal viscera through a portion of the abdominal wall. Hernias may be congenital or acquired.[26] A congenital hernial sac is developed before birth, and an acquired hernia develops after birth. Structurally, a hernia has a mouth, a neck, and a body. The mouth, or hernial ring, is the opening from the abdominal cavity into the hernial protusion; the neck is the portion of the sac that joins the hernial ring and the body. The body is

the sac that protrudes outside the abdominal cavity and contains portions of the abdominal organs.[25]

Hernias most often occur in the groin area. Inguinal hernias (Figure 27–28A), which occur in men (more than 75 percent), and femoral hernias (Figure 27–28B), most often occurring in women, are the most prevalent types. Externally, the inguinal and femoral hernias appear similar because of the groin protrusion, but a considerable difference is indicated internally. The inguinal hernia results from an abnormal enlargement of the opening of the

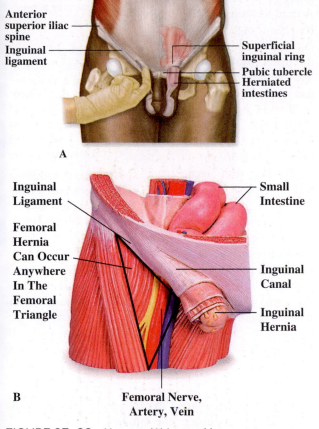

**Anterior superior iliac spine**

**Inguinal ligament**

**Superficial inguinal ring**

**Pubic tubercle**

**Herniated intestines**

**A**

**Inguinal Ligament**

**Small Intestine**

**Femoral Hernia Can Occur Anywhere In The Femoral Triangle**

**Inguinal Canal**

**Inguinal Hernia**

**B**

**Femoral Nerve, Artery, Vein**

FIGURE 27–28 Hernias. (A) Inguinal hernias appear in the inguinal canal and (B) femoral hernias can occur anywhere in the femoral triangle.

(b) © William E. Prentice

inguinal canal, through which the vessels and nerves of the male reproductive system pass. In contrast, the femoral hernia arises in the canal that transports the vessels and nerves that go to the thigh and lower limb.[25]

Under normal circumstances, the inguinal and femoral canals are protected by muscle control against abnormal opening. When intraabdominal tension affects these areas, muscles produce contractions around these canal openings. If the muscles fail to react or if they prove inadequate in their shutter action, intestinal loops may be pushed through the opening. Repeated protrusions stretch the size of the opening. Some physicians think that any patient who has a hernia should be prohibited from engaging in hard physical activity until surgical repair has been made.

One danger of a hernia is that it may become irritated by falls or blows. Besides the hernial aggravations caused by trauma, another concern that athletic trainers need to be aware of is the development of a *strangulated hernia*, in which the inguinal ring constricts the protruding sac and occludes normal blood circulation. A strangulated hernia produces intense pain and marked tenderness. Because the intestine is obstructed, there is gross abdominal pain and vomiting. If the strangulated hernia is not surgically repaired immediately, gangrene and death may ensue.

*Symptoms and signs* The acquired hernia occurs when a natural weakness is further aggravated by either a strain or a direct blow. An acquired hernia may be recognized by the following signs: history of a blow or strain to the groin area that produced pain and prolonged discomfort, superficial protrusion in the groin area that is increased by coughing, and a reported feeling of weakness and pulling sensation in the groin area.

*Management* The treatment preferred by most physicians is surgery.[31] Mechanical devices, which prevent hernial protrusion, are for the most part unsuitable because of the friction and irritation they produce. Exercise has been thought by many to be beneficial to a mild hernia, but such is not the case. Exercise will not positively affect the stretched inguinal or femoral canals.

### Blow to the Solar Plexus

*Etiology* A blow to the sympathetic celiac plexus (solar plexus) produces a transitory paralysis of the diaphragm ("wind knocked out"). There may also be a loss of residual volume in the lungs due to the blow, forcing a large amount of air from the lungs.

*Symptoms and signs* Paralysis of the diaphragm stops respiration and leads to anoxia. When the athlete is unable to inhale, hysteria because of fear may result. These symptoms are usually transitory. It is necessary to allay such fears and instill confidence in the athlete.

*Management* In dealing with a patient who has had the wind knocked out of him or her, the athletic trainer should adhere to the following procedures: help the patient overcome apprehension by talking in a confident manner, loosen the patient's belt and the clothing around the abdomen, have the patient bend the knees, and encourage the athlete to relax by initiating short inspirations and long expirations. Panting helps restore the normal amount of residual volume air, and symptoms subside.

> A blow to the solar plexus can lead to transitory paralysis of the diaphragm and unconsciousness.

Because of the fear of not being able to breathe, the patient may hyperventilate. Hyperventilation is rapid breathing that results in a lowered carbon dioxide level. It causes a variety of physical reactions, such as dizziness, a lump in the throat, a pounding heart, and fainting.

The athletic trainer should always be concerned that a blow hard enough to knock out the wind could also cause internal organ injury.

## Stitch in the Side

***Etiology*** A "stitch in the side" is the name given to an idiopathic condition that occurs in some patients. The cause is obscure, although several hypotheses have been advanced. Among the possible causes are constipation, intestinal gas, overeating, diaphragmatic spasm as a result of poor conditioning, lack of visceral support because of weak abdominal muscles, distended spleen, breathing techniques that lead to a lack of oxygen in the diaphragm, ischemia of either the diaphragm or the intercostal muscles, and a fluid-engorged gut that tugs on visceral ligaments.

***Signs and symptoms*** A stitch in the side is a cramplike pain that develops on either the left or right costal angle during hard physical activity. Sports that involve running apparently produce this condition.

***Management*** Immediate care of a stitch in the side demands relaxation of the spasm, for which three methods have proved beneficial. First, the patient is instructed to stretch the arm on the affected side as high as possible. If this method is inadequate, flexing the trunk forward on the thighs while tightening the abdominal muscles may prove of some benefit.[51] A third technique, which has been suggested but not confirmed, is to have the patient walk and exhale while stepping on the opposite foot—that is, if there is a stitch in the left side, the patient exhales while stepping on the right foot.

Patients with recurrent abdominal spasms may need special study. The identification of poor eating habits, poor elimination habits, or an inadequate conditioning program may explain the patient's problem.[30] A stitch in the side, although not considered serious, may require further evaluation by a physician if abdominal pains persist.

> A cross-country runner complains of a recurring stitch in the side. She has a cramplike pain that develops on the left costal angle during a hard run. She indicates that, when she stops running, the cramp disappears, but it comes back when she starts to run again.
>
> **?** What can the athletic trainer recommend that might help this runner alleviate her problem?

## SUMMARY

- Injuries to the heart, lungs, and abdominal viscera can be serious and even life threatening if not recognized and managed appropriately.
- The thorax is the portion of the body commonly known as the chest, which lies between the base of the neck and the diaphragm. Its main functions are to protect the vital respiratory and circulatory organs and to assist the lungs in inspiration and expiration during the breathing process. Within the thoracic cage lie the lungs, the heart, and the thymus.
- The abdominal cavity lies between the diaphragm and the bones of the pelvis and is bounded by the margin of the lower ribs, the abdominal muscles, and the vertebral column. The abdominal viscera are composed of both hollow and solid organs. Organs in the abdominal cavity may be classified as being part of the urinary system, the digestive system, the reproductive system, or the lymphatic system.
- The primary survey by the athletic trainer who is evaluating an injury to the abdomen or thorax should focus on the signs and symptoms that indicate some life-threatening condition. Asking pertinent questions, observing body positioning, and palpating the injured structures are critical in assessing the nature of the injury.
- Rib fractures and contusions, costochondral junction separations, sternum fractures, muscle strains, and breast injuries are all common injuries to the chest wall.
- Injuries involving the lungs include pneumothorax, tension pneumothorax, hemothorax, and traumatic asphyxia.
- The most common cause of sudden cardiac death is some congenital cardiovascular abnormality. The three most prevalent conditions are hypertrophic cardiomyopathy, anomalous origin of the coronary artery, and Marfan's syndrome.
- With any injury to the abdominal region, internal injury to the abdominal viscera must be considered. Injuries to the liver, spleen, and kidneys are among the more common injuries to the abdominal viscera.
- A number of conditions of the digestive system, such as diarrhea, constipation, and gastroenteritis, are common.
- Injuries to the reproductive organs are much more likely to occur in the male because the genitalia are more exposed.
- Injuries to the abdominal wall include muscle strains, getting the wind knocked out, and developing an inguinal or femoral hernia.

## WEB SITES

**NATA Position, Official, and Consensus Statements**
*Commotio Cordis (2007):*
www.nata.org/sites/default/files/CommotioCordis.pdf
Acute Appendicitis: www.emedicine.com/emerg/topic41.htm

American Society of Abdominal Surgeons:
www.abdominalsurg.org

American Thoracic Society—about ATS:
www.thoracic.org

## SOLUTIONS TO CLINICAL APPLICATION EXERCISES

27-1 The athletic trainer should be concerned about the possibility of injury to an organ that can lead to internal blood loss and eventually result in shock. It is possible that the spleen, liver, stomach, small intestine, pancreas, and gallbladder are all injured. It is also possible that there is a contusion to the muscles of the abdominal wall that is causing muscle guarding.

27-2 For palpation of the abdominal structures, the patient should be supine with the hips and knees flexed. A patient with an abdominal injury voluntarily contracts the abdominal muscles to guard, or protect, the tender area. If there is bleeding or irritation inside the abdominal cavity, the abdomen exhibits boardlike rigidity and cannot be relaxed voluntarily. The athletic trainer can produce rebound tenderness by pressing firmly on the abdomen and then quickly releasing pressure, which causes intense pain.

27-3 The athletic trainer should know what sounds are normal and be able to identify abnormal sounds. Abnormal breathing sounds are often superimposed on normal breathing sounds. Adventitious breath sounds are not normally heard and may be either continuous, musiclike sounds with a high pitch, called wheezes or rhonchi, or crackling or bubbling sounds, called rales.

27-4 The athletic trainer should palpate along the rib, in the intercostal space between the ribs, and at the costochondral junction to locate a specific point of tenderness. The athletic trainer should also apply anteroposterior compression to the thoracic cage to identify potential rib fractures. If the patient complains of increased pain or tenderness on transverse compression applied laterally to the rib cage, a costochondral injury is more likely.

27-5 Injuries severe enough to cause a rib fracture might also result in pneumothorax, tension pneumothorax, hemothorax, or traumatic asphyxia. All of these conditions should be considered life threatening, and the athletic trainer should access the rescue squad immediately. The athletic trainer should also be prepared to initiate CPR if indicated.

27-6 It is most likely that the athlete is hyperventilating. This was likely caused by the anxiety that existed over having to do these sprints. The athletic trainer needs to increase the level of carbon dioxide in the lung and can do this by having the patient either breathe slowly through one nostril or breathe into a paper bag.

27-7 Potential causes include myocardial infarction, hypertrophic cardiomyopathy, Marfan's syndrome, coronary artery disease resulting from atherosclerosis, right ventricular dysplagia, cardiac conduction system abnormalities, aortic stenosis, and myocarditis. All these causes have been attributed to sudden cardiac death syndrome. The athletic trainer is dealing with a life-threatening situation and must seek emergency medical care as soon as possible.

27-8 Anytime blood appears in the urine, there is cause for concern. In this case, it is likely that the kidneys have been contused, and the blood that appears in the urine will disappear over the next couple of days. Nevertheless, the patient should be referred to a physician for diagnosis.

27-9 It is possible that the patient has an inflamed vermiform appendix. Most often, surgical removal of the appendix is necessary. Occasionally, an inflamed appendix results from an obstructed bowel. A rupture of the appendix because of bowel obstruction is a life-threatening emergency.

27-10 This patient may have spermatic cord torsion and needs to be evaluated by a physician immediately to avoid permanent damage.

27-11 The patient is exhibiting the symptoms and signs of a ruptured spleen. The spleen has the ability to splint itself and stop hemorrhage. However, because of the potential of shock, the athletic trainer should treat this injury as life threatening. Usually, treatment is conservative and involves brief hospitalization, but surgical management is necessary when the spleen has ruptured and is hemorrhaging.

27-12 Most often, the patient has a history of a blow or strain to the groin area that produced pain and prolonged discomfort. There may be a superficial protrusion in the groin area that is increased when the patient coughs, or the patient may experience a feeling of weakness and a pulling sensation in the groin area. An inguinal hernia results from an abnormal enlargement of the opening of the inguinal canal through which the abdominal contents may be pushed.

27-13 The athletic trainer should try to modify the patient's eating habits, which might produce constipation or gas. Cramps can be caused by improper breathing techniques, which may cause a lack of oxygen in the diaphragm and ischemia of either the diaphragm or the intercostal muscles. Cramps may also be caused by diaphragmatic spasm that results from poor conditioning or by a lack of visceral support because of weak abdominal muscles. Patients with recurrent abdominal spasms should have further evaluation by a physician if abdominal pains persist.

## REVIEW QUESTIONS AND CLASS ACTIVITIES

1. Describe the anatomy of the thorax.
2. Differentiate among rib contusions, rib fractures, and costochondral separations.
3. Compare the signs of pneumothorax, tension pneumothorax, hemothorax, and traumatic asphyxia.
4. Identify the possible causes of sudden cardiac death syndrome.
5. List the abdominal viscera and other structures associated with the urinary system, the digestive system, the lymphatic system, and the reproductive system.
6. What muscles protect the abdominal viscera?
7. What conditions of the abdominal viscera produce pain in the abdominal region?
8. Contrast the signs of a ruptured spleen with the signs of a severely contused kidney.
9. What are the most common sports injuries and conditions related to the digestive system?
10. How should a patient who has had his or her wind knocked out be managed?
11. Distinguish an inguinal hernia or a femoral hernia from a groin strain.
12. Describe the signs of a stitch in the side.

# REFERENCES

1. Aitkins J: Acute and overuse injuries of the abdomen and groin in athletes, *Current Sports Medicine Reports* 9(2):115–20, 2010.
2. Aune A: Abdominal injuries. In Bahr R, ed: *Clinical guide to sports injuries,* Champaign, IL, 2004, Human Kinetics.
3. Barrett M: Cardiac auscultation in sports medicine: Strategies to improve clinical care, *Curr Sports Med Reports* 11(2):78–84, 2012.
4. Brims F: Respiratory chest pain: Diagnosis and treatment, *Medical Clinics of North America* 94:217–32, 2010.
5. Brukner P: Thoracic and chest pain. In Brukner P, ed: *Bruckner and Kahn's clinical sports medicine,* Sydney, 2011, McGraw-Hill.
6. Cartwright S: Evaluation of acute abdominal pain in adults, *American Family Physician* 77(7):971–78, 2008.
7. Ciocca M: Pneumothorax in a weight lifter: The importance of vigilance, *Physician Sportsmed* 28(4):97, 2000.
8. Corrado D: Preparticipation screening of young competitive athletes for prevention of sudden cardiac death, *Journal of the American College of Cardiology* 52(24):1981–89, 2008.
9. Curtin S: Pneumothorax in sports: Issues in recognition and follow-up care, *Physician Sportsmed* 28(8):23, 2000.
10. Dennis R: Abdominal wall injuries occurring after blunt trauma: Incidence and grading system, *American Journal of Surgery* 193(3):413–17, 2009.
11. Dodds S: Injuries to the pectoralis major, *Sports Med* 32(14):945, 2002.
12. Du Preez G: Fractured ribs may result in serious complications, *Nursing Times* 99(20):37, 2003.
13. Durakovic Z: Sudden cardiac death due to physical exercise in male competitive athletes. A report of six cases, *J Sports Med Phys Fitness* 45(4):532, 2005.
14. Eichner E: Gut reactions: Athletes' gastrointestinal problems, *Sports Med Digest* 21(10):111, 1999.
15. Eichner E: Throw no stones: How to prevent kidney stones, *Sports Med Digest* 24(2):22, 2002.
16. Evans C: Sudden cardiac death in athletes: What sport-rehabilitation specialists need to know, *J Sport Rehabil* 12(3):259, 2003.
17. Fait P: Third-degree spleen laceration in a male varsity athlete, *Athletic Therapy Today* 8(3):32, 2003.
18. Favalle S: Sudden death due to atrial fibrillation in hypertrophic cardiomyopathy, *Pacing and Clinical Electrophysiology* 26(2):637, 2003.
19. Gannon E: Splenic injuries in athletes: A review, *Current Sports Medicine Reports* 9(2):111–14, 2010.
20. Gazzillo-Diaz L: A severed kidney as a result of blunt trauma in a high school football player (poster session), *J Athl Train* 39(2 Suppl):S-81, 2004.
21. Hardin D: Acute appendicitis: Review and update, *Am Fam Phys* 60(7):2027–34, 1999.
22. Harrahill M: Bladder trauma: A review, *Journal of Emergency Nursing* 30(3):287, 2004.
23. Haycock C: Abdominal injuries. In Fu F, ed: *Sports injuries: Mechanisms, prevention, and treatment,* Philadelphia, PA, 2001, Lippincott, Williams and Wilkins.
24. Hipp A: Hypertrophic cardiomyopathy—sports-related aspects of diagnosis, therapy, and sports eligibility, *Int J Sports Med* 25(1):20, 2004.
25. Johnson J: Primary care of the sports hernia, *Physician Sportsmed* 33(2):35, 2005.
26. Kemp S: The "sports hernia": A common cause of groin pain, *Physician Sportsmed* 26(1):3, 1998.
27. Kersey R: Primary spontaneous pneumothorax in a collegiate soccer player, *Athletic Therapy Today* 5(2):48, 2000.
28. Kim J: Commotio cordis in the athlete, *Athletic Therapy Today* 15(4):67, 2010.
29. Koester M: A review of sudden cardiac death in young athletes and strategies for preparticipation cardiovascular screening, *J Athl Train* 36(2):197, 2001.
30. Konrad P: Neuromuscular evaluation of trunk-training exercises, *J Athl Train* 36(2):109, 2001.
31. Lacroix V: A complete approach to groin pain, *Physician Sportsmed* 28(1):66, 2000.
32. Lateef F: Commotio cordis: An underappreciated cause of sudden death in athletes, *Sports Med* 30(4):301, 2000.
33. Leaver-Dunn D: Assessment of respiratory conditions in athletes, *Athletic Therapy Today* 5(6):14, 2000.
34. Link M: Sudden cardiac death in athletes, *Progress in Cardiovascular Diseases* 51(1): 44–57, 2008.
35. Lively M: Pulmonary contusion in football players, *Cl J Sports Med* 16(2):177, 2006.
36. Maron B: Hypertrophic cardiomyopathy: Practical steps for preventing sudden death, *Physician Sportsmed* 30(1):19, 2002.
37. Maron B: Commotio cordis, *N Engl J Med* 362(6):917–27, 2010.
38. McChesney J: Auscultation of the chest and abdomen by athletic trainers, *J Athl Train* 36(2):190, 2001.
39. McCrory P: Commotio cordis: Instantaneous cardiac arrest caused by a blow to the chest depends on the timing of the blow relative to the cardiac cycle, *Brit J Sports Med* 36(4):236, 2002.
40. McGown A: Blunt abdominal and chest trauma, *Athletic Therapy Today* 9(1):40, 2004.
41. McGrew C: Sudden cardiac death in competitive athletes, *J Orthop Sports Phys Ther* 33(10):589, 2003.
42. McKnight J: Chest pain in the athlete: Differential diagnosis, evaluation, and treatment, In Lawless C, ed: *Sports cardiology essentials: Evaluation, management and case studies,* New York, 2010, Springer.
43. Meghoo C: Complete occlusion after blunt injury to the abdominal aorta (includes abstract), *Journal of Trauma* 55(4):795, 2003.
44. Merrick M: Cardiovascular pathologies: To screen or not to screen? *Athletic Therapy Today* 6(4):28, 2001.
45. Meyers W: Management of severe lower abdominal or inguinal pain in high-performance athletes, *Am J Sports Med* 28(1):2, 2000.
46. Mileski W: Injuries to the liver. In Flint L: *Trauma: Contemporary principles and therapy,* Philadelphia, PA, 2007, Lippincott, Williams and Wilkins.
47. Norris R: Assessment of cardiovascular conditions in the athlete, *Athletic Therapy Today* 5(6):11, 2000.
48. Paterick T: Medical and legal issues in the cardiovascular evaluation of competitive athletes, *Journal of the American Medical Association* 294(23):3011–18, 2005.
49. Perron A: Chest pain in athletes, *Clin Sports Med* 22(1):37, 2003.
50. Piccininni J: Kidney laceration in a university football player, *Athletic Therapy Today* 7(5):42, 2002.
51. Plunkett B: Investigation of the side pain "stitch" induced by running after fluid ingestion, *Med Sci Sports Exerc* 31(8):1169, 1999.
52. Puffer J: The athletic heart syndrome: Ruling out cardiac pathologies, *Physician Sportsmed* 30(7):41, 2002.
53. Putukian M: Assessment of abdominal conditions in athletes, *Athletic Therapy Today* 5(6):20, 2000.
54. Rifat S: Chest and abdominal wall. In McKeag D, ed: *ACSM's primary care sports medicine,* Philadelphia, PA, 2007, Lippincott, Williams and Wilkins.
55. Ryan J: Abdominal injuries and sport, *British Journal of Sports Medicine* 33(3):155, 1999.
56. Ryan S: Managing urinary tract and vaginal infections, *Physician Sportsmed* 24(7):101, 1996.
57. Saladin K: *Anatomy and physiology: The unity of form and function,* New York, 2014, McGraw-Hill.
58. Scurr J: The effect of breast support on the kinematics of the breast during the running gait cycle, *Journal of Sport Sciences* 28(10):1103–09, 2010.
59. Sharp V: Testicular torsion: Diagnosis, evaluation and management, *Am Fam Phys* 88(12):835–40, 2013.
60. Smith D: Chest injuries, what the sports physical therapist should know, *Int J Sports Phys Ther* 6(4):357–60, 2011.
61. *Stedman's concise medical dictionary for the health professions,* Baltimore, MD, 2014, Lippincott, Williams and Wilkins.
62. Stopka CB: Referred visceral pain: What every sports medicine professional needs to know, *Athletic Therapy Today* 4(1):29, 1999.
63. Suman O: Airway obstruction during exercise and isocapnic hyperventilation in asthmatic subjects, *J App Physiol* 87(3):1107, 1999.
64. Terrell T: Management of splenic rupture and return-to-play decisions in a college football player, *Clin Sports Med* 12(6):400, 2002.
65. Turk E: Natural and traumatic sports-related fatalities: A 10-year retrospective study, *Brit J Sports Med* 42:604–08, 2008.
66. VanPutte C: *Seeley's anatomy and physiology,* New York, 2010, McGraw-Hill.
67. Venes D: *Taber's cyclopedic medical dictionary,* Philadelphia, PA, 2013, F.A. Davis.
68. Weder M: Pulmonary disorders in athletes, *Clinics in Sports Medicine* 30(3):525–36, 2011.
69. Wegenlehner F: An update on uncomplicated urinary tract infections in women, *Current Opinion in Urology* 19(4):368–74, 2009.

## ANNOTATED BIBLIOGRAPHY

VanPutte C, Seeley R, Stephens T, Tate P: *Seely's anatomy and physiology,* ed 5, New York, 2010, McGraw-Hill.

*Helps clarify the anatomy of the various systems of the abdomen and thorax and provides clinical correlations for specific injuries and illnesses.*

Venes D: *Taber's cyclopedic medical dictionary,* Philadelphia, PA, 2011, F.A. Davis.

*Despite the dictionary format, an excellent guide for the athletic trainer who is searching for clear, concise descriptions of various injuries and illnesses accompanied by brief recommendations for management and treatment.*

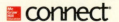

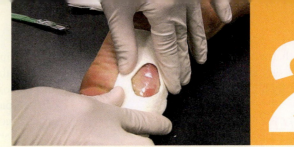

© William E. Prentice

# Skin Disorders

## ■ Objectives

*When you finish this chapter you should be able to*

- Explain the structure and function of the skin and identify the lesions that result from skin abnormalities.
- Describe in detail how skin trauma occurs, how it may be prevented, and how it may be managed.
- Identify bacterial skin infections that are potentially contagious.

- Describe the correct hygiene practices to use to avoid fungal infections.
- Identify potentially threatening viral infections.
- Contrast allergic, thermal, and chemical reactions of the skin.
- Identify infestations and insect bites and contrast them with other skin infections.

## ■ Outline

## ■ Key Terms

sebaceous cyst
cellulitis
hyperkeratosis

macerated skin
staphylococcus
streptococcus

bacillus
tetanus (lockjaw)
tinea (ringworm)

## ■ Connect Highlights  connect

*Visit connect.mcgraw-hill.com for further exercises to apply your knowledge:*

- Clinical application scenarios covering identification and management of skin disorders
- Click-and-drag questions covering identification, classification, and signs and symptoms of skin disorders and infections
- Multiple-choice questions covering skin trauma, skin reactions, bacterial and fungal infections, and skin infestations

It is essential that athletic trainers understand conditions that adversely affect the skin and mucous membranes, especially highly contagious conditions.[24,86]

# SKIN ANATOMY AND FUNCTION

The skin is the largest organ of the human body. The average adult skin varies in total weight from 6 to 7½ pounds (2.7 to 3.4 kg) and is from ⅟₃₂ to ⅛ inch (0.031 to 0.125 cm) thick. It is composed of three layers: the epidermis, dermis, and subcutis (Figure 28–1 and Table 28–1).[38]

## Epidermis

The epidermis acts as a barrier against invading microorganisms, foreign particles from dirt and debris, chemicals, and ultraviolet rays, and it helps contain the body's water and electrolytes.[85] The epidermis is the outermost layer of the skin and itself is composed of several layers identified as the stratum corneum, stratum granulosum, stratum spinosum, and stratum basale. The stratified nature of the epidermal cell layers results from the migration of keratinocytes, the epidermal epithelial cells, from the basal layer outward to the stratum corneum. During this migration process, the cells undergo a well-described change in shape from round basal cells to flat, elongated cells. In the final stage of differentiation, the flattened keratinocytes secrete a variety of substances into the extracellular space and then lose their nuclei to form the horny layer known as the stratum corneum. The stratum corneum acts as a permeability barrier, allowing only small molecules to diffuse into the lower regions of the epidermis, and thus it protects against environmental irritants, toxins, and pathogens. Other cells, including melanocytes and Langerhans cells, are also found in the epidermis. Melanocytes synthesize and transfer to

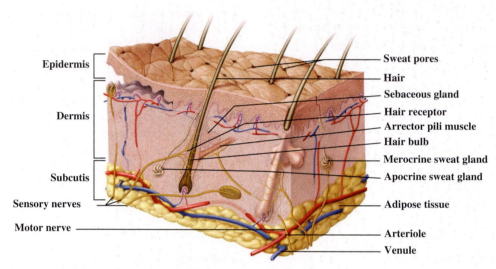

FIGURE 28–1  Cross section of the skin.

| TABLE 28–1 | The Skin's Structure and Function | |
|---|---|---|
| **Layer** | **Subregion** | **Function** |
| Epidermis | Stratum corneum | Prevents intrusion of microorganisms, debris, chemicals, and ultraviolet radiation |
| | | Prevents loss of water and electrolytes |
| | | Performs heat regulation for conduction, radiation, and convection |
| | Melanin (pigmentation) | Prevents intrusion of ultraviolet radiation |
| Dermis | | Protects against physical trauma |
| | | Contains sensory nerve endings |
| | | Holds water and electrolytes |
| | Appendages | Contains eccrine and apocrine sweat glands, hair, nails, and sebaceous glands |
| Subcutis | | Stores fat and regulates heat |

keratinocytes the pigment melanin, which blocks harmful solar radiation. Langerhans cells aid in immunological surveillance by collecting and presenting to lymphocytes foreign substances, such as bacterial proteins.

## Dermis

The dermis, beneath the epidermis, is composed of connective tissue. The dermis provides mechanical support to the epidermis and contains blood vessels, nerves, sweat glands, hair follicles, and sebaceous glands. The dermis forms a series of fingerlike projections, the dermal papilla, that reach into the epidermis. This creates an interlocking arrangement that increases the surface area of dermal-epidermal contact and thereby prevents the epidermis from slipping off the dermis.

**Adnexal Structures: Hair, Sebaceous Glands, and Eccrine Glands** Hair grows from hair follicles in the skin. It extends into the dermis, where it is nourished by the blood capillaries. Small muscles called arrectores pilorum connect to the hair and, when contracted by stimuli (such as cold or fear), pull the hair into a vertical position, creating a "standing-on-end" effect, or goose bumps. This increases the hair's insulating effect, protecting the body from cold.

The sebaceous glands, which surround the hair, secrete sebum, an oily substance, which is extruded into the hair follicles. Sebaceous glands can become enlarged, a condition known as sebaceous hyperplasia. This is a benign condition; however, the appearance of the enlarged glands can sometimes be confused with basal cell carcinoma, a form of skin cancer. The term **sebaceous cyst** is a misnomer, because it is not derived from the sebaceous glands, but is an epithelial-lined space originating from the upper portion of the hair follicle. Enlargement of this cyst results from the accumulation of keratin, the major skin protein, into the cavity of the cyst. The more correct term, *epithelial inclusion cyst,* should be used to describe this common and benign skin lesion.

**Sweat Glands** Sweat glands are necessary for cooling the surface of the body and the internal organs. Patients with anhidrotic ectodermal dysplasia, a rare inherited disease, do not make functional sweat glands and are susceptible to significant overheating with physical exertion. There are two main types of glands: eccrine glands, which are present at birth and are generally present throughout the skin, and apocrine glands, which are much larger than eccrine glands and mature during adolescence in conjunction with the axillary and pubic hair. Sweat gland secretions contain antibacterial agents that aid in controlling infection.

**Nails** The nails are horny cell structures that come from the phalanges. The nail matrix, located beneath the proximal nail fold and visible as a white, semicircular structure beneath the proximal nail plate, synthesizes the hard, keratinaceous nail plate. The nails grow approximately ½ inch

(1.3 cm) in 4 months. Abnormalities of the fingernails were discussed in Chapter 24.

**Sensory Nerve Endings** Besides its many other functions, the dermis contains sensory nerve endings. These peripheral nerves provide tactile sensation and detect temperature changes and pain.

## Subcutis

The subcutis contains fat. Subcutaneous fat has a role in temperature regulation/insulation and energy storage, and it increases the mobility of the skin over the underlying tissues.

## SKIN LESIONS DEFINED

Skin that is healthy has a smooth, soft appearance. Different amounts of the skin pigment melanin are responsible for ethnic variations in skin color. Areas of increased melanin can result in pale brown areas of skin and are referred to as *café au lait spots* or macules (Figure 28–2). These are common in infancy and disappear with age. Café au lait spots are harmless but sometimes are a sign of *neurofibromatosis,* a genetic disorder of the nervous system that primarily affects the development and growth of nerve cell tissues. The presence of six or more café au lait spots of 1.5 centimeters or more in diameter is diagnostic of neurofibromatosis.[38]

Additional and sometimes transient changes in skin color are due to anatomical, physiological, or pathophysiological changes in skin blood flow. Increased blood flow to the skin capillaries results in a red-colored skin, whereas decreased blood flow to the skin causes pallor.[1]

The normal appearance of the skin can be altered by external and internal factors. Some changes may be signs of other involvements. The different intensities of paleness or redness of the skin, which is related to the extent

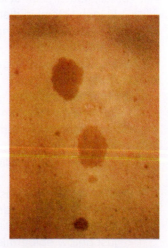

**FIGURE 28–2** Café au lait spot on low back.
Courtesy Dean Morrell, MD, Department of Dermatology, University of North Carolina

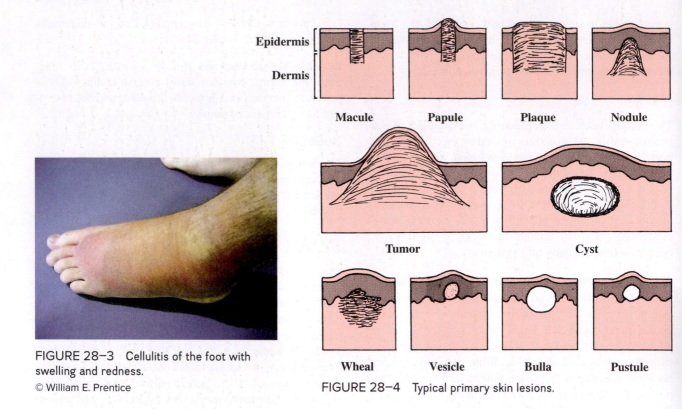

Epidermis

Dermis

Macule     Papule     Plaque     Nodule

Tumor                Cyst

Wheal     Vesicle     Bulla     Pustule

FIGURE 28–3   Cellulitis of the foot with swelling and redness.
© William E. Prentice

FIGURE 28–4   Typical primary skin lesions.

of superficial circulation, may be hereditary. Pigment variation may result from an increase of sun exposure or from organic disease; a yellowish discoloration, for example, may be indicative of jaundice. **Cellulitis,** the infectious inflammation of deep skin structures, is characterized by a reddening of the skin called erythema and by increased warmth (Figure 28–3).

Skin abnormalities may be divided into primary and secondary lesions. Primary lesions include macules, papules, plaques, nodules, tumors, cysts, wheals, vesicles, bullae, and pustules (Figure 28–4 and Table 28–2). Secondary lesions, such as excoriations, result from primary lesions that have been manipulated (Figure 28–5 and Table 28–3).

| TABLE 28–2 | Primary Skin Lesions | |
|---|---|---|
| **Type** | **Description** | **Example** |
| Macule | Small, flat, circular discoloration smaller than ½ inch (<1cm) in diameter | Freckle or flat nevus café au lait macule (spot) |
| Papule | Solid elevation less than ½ inch (<1cm) in diameter | Wart |
| Plaque or patch | Macule or papule larger than ½ inch (<1cm) in diameter | Vitiligo patch (patch of depigmentation) |
| Nodule | Solid mass less than ½ inch (<1cm), deeper into the dermis than a papule | Dermatofibroma fibrosis |
| Tumor | Solid mass larger than ½ inch (<1cm) | Cavernous hemangioma (tumor filled with blood vessels) |
| Cyst | Encapsulated, fluid-filled lesion in the dermis or subcutis | Epidermoid cyst |
| Wheal | Papule or plaque caused by serum collection into the dermis, allergic reactions | Urticaria (hives) |
| Vesicle | Fluid-filled elevation less than ½ inch (<1cm), just below epidermis | Smallpox, chickenpox |
| Bulla | Like a vesicle but larger | Second-degree burn, friction blister |
| Pustule | Like a vesicle or bulla but contains pus | Acne |

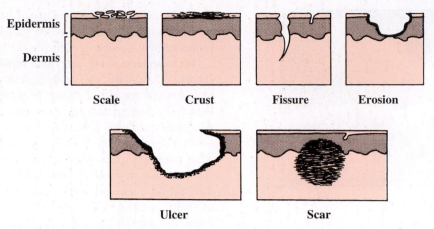

Epidermis

Dermis

Scale    Crust    Fissure    Erosion

Ulcer    Scar

FIGURE 28–5    Typical secondary skin lesions.

| TABLE 28–3 | Secondary Skin Lesions | |
|---|---|---|
| **Type** | **Description** | **Example** |
| Scales | Flakes of skin | Psoriasis |
| Crust | Dried fluid or exudates on the skin | Impetigo |
| Fissure | Skin crack | Chapping |
| Excoriation | Superficial scrape | Abrasion |
| Erosion | Loss of the superficial epidermis | Scratch (superficial) |
| Ulcer | Destruction of the entire epidermis | Pressure sore |
| Scar | Healing of the dermis | Vaccination, laceration |

# SKIN TRAUMA

Physical activity can place a great deal of mechanical force on the skin. These forces can include friction, compression, shearing, stretching, scraping, tearing, avulsing, and puncturing, all of which can lead to painful and serious injuries.[71]

## Friction and Pressure Problems

Excessive rubbing back and forth over the skin, along with abnormal pressure, can cause thickening of the stratum corneum, or horny layer, of the epidermis, especially on the soles of the feet and the palms of the hands. This causes **hyperkeratosis,** which is characteristic of callus formation.[37] Pressure, shearing, and frictional forces can also produce corns and blisters.

### Hyperkeratosis of the Feet and Hands

*Etiology*    Skin, typically the epidermal skin layer, increases in thickness when constant friction and pressure are applied externally. Excessive callus accumulation may occur over bony protuberances.

Foot calluses may become excessive on a patient who wears shoes that are too narrow or short.[32] As with the foot, hand calluses can become painful when the subcutaneous fatty layer loses its elasticity, which is an important cushioning effect. The callus moves as a mass when pressure and a shearing force are applied. Hyperkeratotic skin is less pliable, and mechanical stress on hyperkeratotic skin, as occurs with movement, can result in epidermal tears or cracks that are painful and that facilitate the entry of infectious organisms into the body.[7]

*Symptoms and signs*    The callus appears as a circumscribed thickening and hypertrophy of the horny layer of the skin. It may be ovular, elongated, brownish, and/or slightly elevated. Calluses may not be painful when pressure is applied.

*Management*    Because callus formation is a protective response to frictional and shearing forces applied to the skin, exposure to such forces should be minimized.[7] The use of emery files or pumice stones should be discouraged because their use results in frictional forces that stimulate the skin to produce additional calluses. Patients who are prone to excess calluses should be encouraged to use moisturizers and keratolytic agents. Massaging small amounts of lanolin into calluses twice a day may help maintain some tissue elasticity. A keratolytic agent, such as 25 percent urea (Ultramide), lactic acid (Lachydrin), or salicylic acid (3 percent salicylic acid in petrolatum), may be applied. Additional formulations of salicylic acid, such

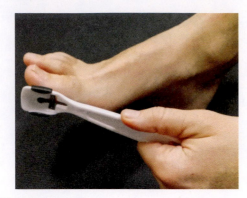

**FIGURE 28–6** Callus trimmer.
© William E. Prentice

as 5 to 10 percent in a flexible collodion, can be applied at night and peeled off in the morning. Before applying a keratolytic ointment, the athletic trainer might manually decrease the thickness of a callus by carefully paring it with a callus trimmer (Figure 28–6). Great care should be taken not to remove the callus totally and the protection it affords a pressure point.[37] A doughnut pad may be cut to size and placed on a pressure point to prevent pain.

Patients whose shoes are properly fitted but who still develop heavy calluses commonly have foot mechanics problems that may require orthotics.

Cushioning devices, such as wedges, doughnuts, and arch supports, may help distribute the weight on the feet more evenly and thus reduce skin stress. Excessive callus accumulation can be prevented by wearing two pairs of socks, a thin cotton or nylon pair next to the skin and a heavy pair over the cotton pair, or a single doubleknit sock; wearing shoes that are the correct size and are in good condition; routinely applying materials, such as lubricants, to reduce friction; and shaving the callus with a callus trimmer. Hand calluses also can be controlled by using a special glove for direct protection, as is used in batting, or by applying elastic tape or moleskin. In sports such as gymnastics, athletic trainers and athletes go to great lengths to protect the athlete's hands against tearing calluses. Gymnastic grips are routinely used to protect the hands and prevent tearing of hand calluses.

### Blisters

*Etiology*  Like calluses, blisters are often a major problem in all forms of repetitive physical activity. Shearing forces produce a raised area that contains a collection of fluid below or within the epidermis.

Blisters are particularly associated with rowing, pole vaulting, basketball, football, and weight events in track and field, such as the shot put and discus. Such activities commonly cause the skin to be subjected to horizontal shearing, which produces a friction blister.[21]

*Symptoms and signs*  The patient normally feels a hot spot—a sharp, burning sensation as the blister is formed. The area of sensation should be examined immediately. The blister may be superficial, containing clear liquid. On

the other hand, a blood blister may form, in which deeper tissue is disrupted, causing blood vessels to rupture. Pain is caused by the pressure of the fluid.[43]

*Management*  Soft feet and hands, coupled with shearing skin stress, can produce severe blisters. A dusting of talcum powder or a dab of petroleum jelly can protect the skin against abnormal friction. Wearing tubular socks or two pairs of socks is also desirable, particularly for patients who have sensitive feet. Individuals who have feet that perspire excessively should wear moisture wicking socks. These use moisture-wicking fibers throughout the sock, particularly along the sole portion and instep to wick away the moisture from the surface of the skin of the foot and transfer it through the sock to the upper of the shoe and insole. Wearing the correct-size shoe is essential. If, however, a friction area ("hot spot") does arise, the patient has several options. The patient can cover the irritated skin with a friction-reducing material, such as "second skin," Another method that has proved effective against blisters is applying ice over skin areas that have developed abnormal friction. Once developed, blisters can be a serious problem for the patient, as well as for the athletic trainer. *Focus Box 28–1:* "Managing blisters" presents general rules for dealing with them (OSHA standards must be followed; see Chapter 14).

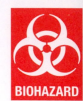

### Soft Corns and Hard Corns

*Etiology*  Soft corns and hard corns are hyperkeratoses caused by abnormal skin pressure and friction.[37]

A hard corn (clavus durus) is the most serious type. It is caused by the pressure of improperly fitting shoes and other anatomical abnormalities—the same mechanisms that cause calluses.[32] Hammertoes are usually associated with the hard corns that form on the tops of deformed toes (Figure 28–8). Symptoms are local pain and disability, with inflammation and thickening of soft tissue. Because of the chronic nature of this condition, it requires a physician's care.[37]

A soft corn (clavus mollis) is a result of wearing narrow shoes and having excessive foot perspiration. It is also associated with an exostosis. Because of the pressure of the shoe coupled with the exudation of moisture, the corn usually forms between the fourth and fifth toes (Figure 28–9).[32] A circular area of thickened, white, **macerated skin** appears between the toes at the base of

An inexperienced runner wearing new shoes during a 3K charity race sustains a completely denuded blister on the back of the heel.

**?** How should this condition be managed after the race?

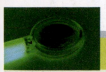
## Managing blisters

### A closed blister

1. If the blister is not affecting activity, leave the blister intact. Apply the "second-skin" dressing by Spenco (Spenco Medical Corporation, Waco, Texas) over the blister to reduce friction. A doughnut pad can also be used to protect the blister and lessen irritation.
2. If the blister is affecting activity or contains cloudy fluid, clean the blister roof and periwound tissues by scrubbing with sterile gauze soaked in an antiseptic.
3. With a sterile, sharp instrument, cut a small incision in the roof and allow the blister to drain. NOTE: In some states, this procedure is considered a surgical technique and this would be a violation of certain practice acts.
4. Using conservative sharp debridement, remove the roof with sterile instruments. Cut along the border between the nonviable (roof) and viable tissue. NOTE: Check appropriate state practice acts prior using to this technique.
5. Clean the wound bed with normal saline or tap water irrigation using a syringe.
6. Pat the periwound tissues dry with sterile gauze, avoiding contact with the wound bed.
7. Dress the wound with a film, foam, hydrogel, or hydrocolloid or nonocclusive dressing based on wound depth and amount of exudate.

8. For active patients, apply adhesive gauze over the dressing to further secure the dressing to the periwound tissues. A doughnut pad and/or "second-skin" can be used over the dressing to further protect the wound.
9. Monitor the patient and blister area daily for clinical features of adverse reactions and infection.

### An open (torn) blister (Figure 28–7)

1. Debride the roof of the blister by conservative sharp debridement with sterile instruments.
2. Clean the wound with normal saline or tap water irrigation.
3. Clean periwound tissues with saline or tap water irrigation or scrubbing with sterile gauze soaked with saline, tap water, or antiseptic.
4. Dry the periwound tissues with sterile gauze. Do not touch the wound bed.
5. Apply an occlusive (i.e., film, foam, hydrogel, or hydrocolloid) or nonocclusive dressing based on wound depth and amount of exudate.
6. If needed, apply adhesive gauze to secure the dressing. A doughnut pad and/or "second-skin" can be used to protect the wound and reduce friction.
7. Monitor the patient and wound area daily for adverse reactions and infection.

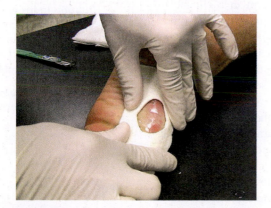

FIGURE 28–7   Managing an open blister.
© William E. Prentice

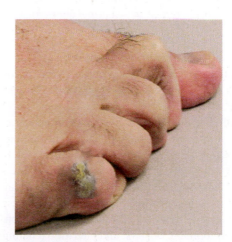

FIGURE 28–8    Hard corn (clavus durus) on second toe.
© William E. Prentice

the proximal head of the phalanges. Both pain and inflammation are likely to be present.[3]

**Symptoms and signs**   With a soft corn, the patient complains of pain laterally on the fifth toe. During inspection, the soft corn appears as a circular piece of thickened, white, macerated skin on the lateral side of the fifth toe at the base of the proximal head of the phalanges. In contrast,

hard corns are on the tops of hammertoes. The bony prominence of the toe is forced up, and it presses on the inner top of the shoe, causing the corn to form. It appears hard and dry, with a callus that is sharply demarcated.

**Management**   The corn is difficult to manage. If pain and inflammation are major, referral to a podiatrist for surgical removal may be advisable. The athletic trainer

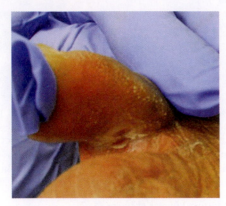

**FIGURE 28–9** Soft corn (clavus mollis).
Courtesy Dr. Howard Kashefsky, Podiatry, University of North Carolina

may ameliorate the condition by having the athlete wear properly fitting shoes and socks and may alleviate further irritation of the corn by protecting it with a small felt pad or sponge pad, which can act as a buffer between the shoe and the toe. In caring for a soft corn, the best procedure is to have the athlete wear properly fitting shoes, keep the skin between the toes clean and dry, decrease pressure by keeping the toes separated with cotton or lamb's wool, and apply a keratolytic agent, such as 25 percent urea (Ultramide) or 40 percent salicylic acid in liquid or plasters.

The primary way to prevent a soft or hard corn is to wear properly fitted shoes.[37] Soft corns can be avoided by wearing shoes that are wide enough. Conversely, hard corns can be avoided by wearing shoes that are long enough.

### Excessive Perspiration (Hyperhidrosis)

*Etiology* Excessive perspiration (hyperhidrosis) occurs in a small segment of the population. Emotional excitement often makes the situation worse. Hyperhidrotic perspiration from palms is syruplike in appearance and extremely high in sodium chloride. This problem also increases the possibility of skin irritations and often makes the adherence of bandages difficult, especially where adhesive tape is necessary. The condition makes callus development, blisters, and intertrigo (chafing) much more likely to occur.[22]

> Excessive perspiration can be a cause of serious skin irritation.

*Management* Treatment of excessive perspiration should include using an astringent, such as alcohol, or an absorbent powder[22] (see *Focus Box 28–2:* "Foot hygiene for excessive perspiration and odor"). Aluminum chloride (Drysol) applied topically or electrical current (iontophoresis) is also used to control hyperhidrosis.

### Chafing of the Skin

*Etiology* Chafing of the skin stems from friction. It occurs particularly in individuals who are obese or

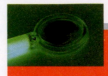
heavy-limbed. It results from the combined friction and maceration of the skin in a climate of heat and moisture.[7]

*Symptoms and signs* Repeated skin rubbing, as in the groin and axilla, can separate the keratin from the granular layer of the epidermis. This separation causes oozing wounds, which develop into crusting and cracking lesions.

*Management* The chafed area should be cleansed once daily with mild soap and lukewarm water. Treatment of a chafed area includes wet packs, using a medicated solution, such as Burrows, for 15 to 20 minutes, three times daily. This is followed by applying a 1 percent hydrocortisone cream.

To prevent chafing, keep the skin dry, clean, and friction free. For groin conditions, the patient should wear loose, soft, cotton underwear. A male athlete should wear his supporter over a pair of loose cotton boxer shorts.

> An overweight construction worker complains of a skin irritation in his groin region. The area appears red and macerated. Some of the tissue is cracked, and there are oozing sores.
>
> **?** How could this chafing have been prevented?

### Xerotic (Dry) Skin

*Etiology* Dry skin is a condition that patients commonly experience during the winter months.[64] Individuals who are exposed to weather and bathe commonly develop dry or chapped skin. The drying cold of winter tends to dehydrate the stratum corneum. Some patients naturally may have fewer skin lipids, which increases its tendency to lose water.[64] Lower humidity and cold winds cause the skin to lose water.

***Symptoms and signs*** The skin appears dry with variable redness and scaling. It occurs first on the shins, forearms, backs of the hands, and face. There may be itching. The skin may crack and develop fissures.

***Management*** The major goals in treatment are to prevent water loss and to replace lost water.[54] The following treatment procedures should be followed:

- Bathe in tepid water and shower one time per day.
- Use moisturizing soaps. Avoid soaping dry areas. Restrict washing to genitalia, underarms, hands, feet, and face.
- Use emollient lotions, which hydrate the skin. Apply them after each washing.
- When the condition is more severe, the patient should be referred to a physician for antipruritics, alpha-hydroxy acids, and perhaps topical corticosteroids.[54]

### Ingrown Toenails

***Etiology*** An ingrown toenail is a common condition. The great toe is the most often affected. The nail grows into the lateral nail fold and penetrates the skin.[34] In general, the ingrown nail results from the lateral pressure of poorly fitting shoes, improper toenail trimming, or trauma, such as repeated pressure from sliding to the front of the shoe (Figure 28–10).

***Symptoms and signs*** The first indications of an ingrown toenail are pain and swelling. If not treated early,

the penetrated skin becomes severely inflamed and purulent. The lateral nail fold becomes swollen and irritated.[43]

***Management*** There are a number of ways to manage the ingrown toenail. If it is in the first stages of inflammation, a more conservative approach can be taken:[43]

- Soak the inflamed toe in warm water (105°F to 110°F) and Betadine for approximately 20 minutes.
- After soaking, the nail will be soft and pliable and may be pried out of the skin. Using sterile forceps or scissors, lift the nail from the soft tissue and insert a piece of cotton to keep the nail out of the skin. This also relieves the pain. Perform this procedure daily until the corner of the nail has grown past the irritated tissue.

If the condition becomes chronically irritated, a more aggressive approach should to be taken by a physician:

- After applying an anesthetic (e.g., 1 or 2 percent lidocaine), slip the nail-splitting scissor under the ingrown nail.[34]
- With the scissor inserted to the point of resistance, cut away and remove the wedge-shaped nail. Keep a moist antiseptic compress in place until the inflammation has subsided.

Because of the disabling nature of this condition, prevention of ingrown toenails is much preferred over management. Properly fitted shoes and socks are essential. The toenails should be trimmed weekly by cutting straight across, avoiding rounding, so that the margins do not penetrate the tissue on the sides (Figure 28–11). The nail should be left sufficiently long so that it is clear of the underlying skin, but it should be cut short enough so as to not irritate the skin by pushing against shoes or socks.[43]

Individuals with recurrent ingrown nails may require the use of phenol for permanent destruction of the lateral portion of the nail.

## Wounds

Traumatic skin lesions, commonly called wounds, are extremely prevalent in sports; abrasions, punctures, lacerations, incisions, avulsions, and bruises are daily occurrences (Figure 28–12).

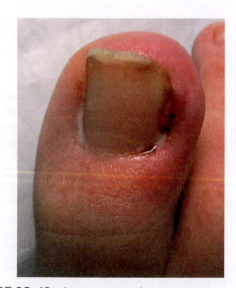

FIGURE 28–10 Ingrown toenail.
Courtesy Dr. Howard Kashefsky, Podiatry, University of North Carolina

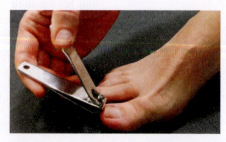

FIGURE 28–11 Preventing an ingrown toenail requires proper trimming with the nail cut straight across.
© William E. Prentice

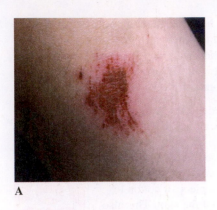

A

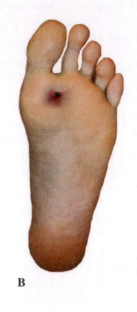

B

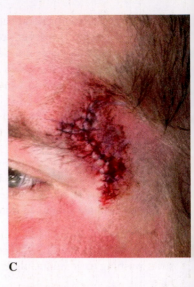

C

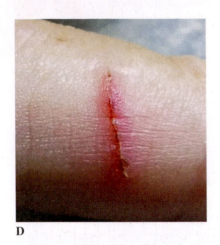

D

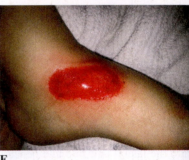

E

FIGURE 28–12   Wounds. **(A)** Abrasion on forearm. **(B)** Puncture on sole of foot. **(C)** Laceration on eyebrow. **(D)** Incision on finger. **(E)** Avulsion on foot.

(a, e) Courtesy Dean Morrell, MD, Department of Dermatology, University of North Carolina; (b, c, d) © William E. Prentice

**Abrasions** Abrasions are common and occur when the skin is scraped against a rough surface. The top layer of skin is worn away, thus exposing numerous blood capillaries. This general exposure, with dirt and foreign materials scraping and penetrating the skin, increases the probability of infection unless the wound is properly debrided and cleansed (Figure 28–12A).

**Punctures** Puncture wounds can easily occur during physical activities and have a high potential for infection. Direct penetration of tissues by a pointed object, such as a track shoe spike, can introduce the tetanus bacillus into the bloodstream. All puncture wounds and severe lacerations should be referred immediately to a physician (Figure 28–12B).

**Lacerations** Lacerations are also common; they occur when a sharp or pointed object tears the tissues, giving the wound the appearance of a jagged-edged cavity.[35] Also, blunt trauma over a sharp bone can cause a wound that is similar in appearance to a laceration. As with abrasions, lacerations present an environment conducive to severe infection (Figure 28–12C).[35]

**Incisions** Incisions are similar to lacerations, but the cut is smooth, as would occur with a knife or piece of glass.[2] Incision wounds often occur where a blow has been delivered over a sharp bone or over a bone that is poorly padded (Figure 28–12D).

**Avulsions** Avulsions occur when skin is torn from the body; they are often associated with major bleeding.[2] The avulsed tissue should be wrapped in saline-soaked gauze and placed in a watertight bag. The bag is immersed in ice water or placed on top of an ice bag. The tissue and bag are sent to the physician for further evaluation and possible reattachment (Figure 28–12E).

**Bruises** The consequence of a sudden compressive, blunt force to the skin is a bruise. The skin is not broken, but the soft tissue is traumatized. A bruise (ecchymosis) results from the disruption of superficial blood vessels and results in black and blue discoloration. A great force affects the underlying structures, producing a bone or muscle contusion. Rest, ice, compression, and elevation (POLICE) are the treatment of choice to control the hemorrhage that may occur.

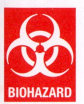 **Wound Management*** All open wounds should be cared for immediately (Table 28–4). Traumatic skin lesions initially must be considered contaminated and receive appropriate cleansing, debridement, and dressing as soon as possible. Although most traumatic skin lesions heal without consequence, appropriate management can lessen the risk of adverse reactions and infection and create an environment conducive to healing (i.e., moist, clean, warm).

***Wound Cleansing*** Wound cleansing is the delivery of a nontoxic solution to the wound bed to remove exudate, foreign bodies/debris, dressing residue, and bacteria.[4] Common cleansing techniques include irrigation, showering, scrubbing and swabbing, and whirlpool baths and soaks. Irrigation, the controlled flow of a solution across the wound bed and periwound tissues, is the preferred cleansing technique for open traumatic wounds. This technique has been shown to be effective in the removal of foreign bodies/debris and bacteria while preserving the healing tissues.[29,30] Showering can be used for larger traumatic wounds and postoperative incisions, although control of the water pressure is difficult.[30] Scrubbing and swabbing involves direct contact of a soft brush or gauze with tissues to remove debris and bacteria. The brush or gauze is moistened with a cleansing solution and wiped across the tissues. Scrubbing and swabbing is not recommended for cleaning the wound bed because it can damage granulation tissues and is ineffective in lowering bacterial counts.[81] Scrubbing and swabbing can be used to safely clean noninjured periwound tissues. Whirlpool baths and soaks are the immersion of the body part and wound into a tub or container of a cleansing solution to hydrate and loosen contaminants and necrotic tissue from the wound bed. While this technique is commonly used, whirlpool baths and soaks increase the risk of cross-contamination and maceration of the tissues.

Cleansing solutions for traumatic skin lesions should be chosen based on their effectiveness and cytotoxicity to the tissues. Normal saline is the most appropriate cleansing solution for all traumatic wounds.[30] Tap water can also be used for traumatic wounds, except those that have bone or tendon exposed. Evidence-based reviews and clinical studies have demonstrated that normal

* Provided by Joel Beam, PhD, ATC, University of North Florida.

saline and tap water are effective as cleansing solutions and do not increase rates of infection.[29,30] Antiseptics such as povidone-iodine and hydrogen peroxide are used to kill or reduce the number of bacteria on tissue and their use has been an area of controversy for many years. Some researchers have revealed that antiseptics are cytotoxic to tissues and ineffective in reducing bacterial counts.[49,56,66] Others found diluted concentrations of antiseptics effective against bacteria and not harmful to human fibroblasts.[29,66] As a result, antiseptics should be used with caution as cleansing solutions on the wound bed, but can safely be used on periwound tissues. The cleansing solution should be delivered to the wound bed between 98.6° and 107.6°F (37° and 42°C).[58] A decrease in wound temperature after cleansing can delay cellular and chemical activities for up to 3 hours, which may delay the healing process.[58]

**Wound Debridement** Debridement is the removal of necrotic tissue, foreign bodies/debris, and bacteria from the wound bed.[63] Debridement should be performed as soon as possible to lessen the risk of infection and create a suitable environment for healing to progress. Debridement techniques for athletic trainers include irrigation, wet-to-moist, scrubbing, conservative sharp, and autolytic. Irrigation can be used as an extension of cleaning to remove loose superficial debris and necrotic tissue.[5] Wet-to-moist is the placement of woven gauze that is premoistened with normal saline or tap water directly on the wound bed. The gauze is left in place for minutes to hours and removed prior to complete drying. This technique can remove debris, necrotic tissue, and eschar from the wound bed in a rapid fashion. Scrubbing can be used to scour a wound that contains large quantities of small debris.[62] However, this technique can damage healthy tissue and increase levels of pain from the mechanical pressure of the brush or gauze. Conservative sharp is the removal of loosely adhering devitalized tissue that lies superficial to the wound bed. Sterile scissors and tweezers or forceps are used to cut along the border between viable and nonviable tissue. Note: Athletic trainers should review applicable state practice acts prior to performing this technique. Autolytic is the softening and digesting of necrotic tissue by the body's mechanisms in a moist wound environment created under occlusive dressings. This technique is painless and occurs over several days, but should not be used with infected wounds.[5,62]

**Wound Dressing** Dressing is the application of materials over the wound bed to produce an environment conducive to healing, prevent cross-contamination and infection, and provide protection. All traumatic skin lesions should be covered with a dressing rather than left uncovered and exposed to the external environment.[12,13] Dressings used with traumatic skin lesions can be categorized into two groups, nonocclusive and occlusive. Nonocclusive dressings possess high permeability, allow desiccation of the

TABLE 28-4 Care of Open Wounds

| Type of Wound | Action of Athletic Trainer | Initial Care | Follow-Up Care |
|---|---|---|---|
| Abrasion | Cleanse, debride, and dress wound. | Cleanse and debride wound bed with normal saline or tap water irrigation. Cleanse periwound tissues with saline or tap water irrigation or scrubbing with sterile gauze soaked with saline, tap water, or antiseptic. Dry the periwound tissues. Dress the wound with a nonocclusive or occlusive dressing based on wound depth and amount of exudate. Apply secondary dressing if needed. | Change dressing based on type; visually inspect daily for adverse reactions and infection. |
| Laceration/ Incision | Change dressing based on type; visually inspect daily for adverse reactions and infection. | Cleanse and debride wound with saline or tap water irrigation. Avoid using tap water if bone or tendon is exposed. Clean periwound tissues with irrigation or scrubbing. Dry the periwound tissues. Tissue approximation and closure will depend on wound length, width, depth, and location. With tissue approximation of superficial- to partial-thickness wounds, dress the wound with a nonocclusive or occlusive dressing based on amount of exudate. With successful tissue approximation of full-thickness wounds in areas of low skin tension, close the wound with dermal adhesives or wound closure strips. With unsuccessful tissue approximation of full-thickness wounds or in areas of high skin tension, cover the wound with saline-soaked gauze and immediately refer to a physician for further cleansing and wound closure. | Change dressing based on type; visually inspect daily for adverse reactions and infection. |
| Puncture | Clean around wound; avoid Visually inspect wound and possible embedded object; clean, debride, and dress wound; refer to physician if necessary. | Leave large or broken-off embedded objects in wound. Apply sterile gauze around object and immobilize the object and/or joint. Refer to a physician. Remove small and visible objects with sterile instruments. Avoid pushing the object deeper into the cavity. Allow bleeding to occur to self-cleanse the wound. Control venous or arterial bleeding. Clean the wound and periwound tissues with saline or tap water irrigation. Use gentle irrigation to prevent pushing debris and bacteria into the cavity. Dress wound with a nonocclusive or occlusive dressing based on wound depth and amount of exudate. | Closely monitor patient and wound area daily for adverse reactions and infection; change dressing based on type; check tetanus immunization. |
| Avulsion | Clean, debride, and dress wound; refer to physician if necessary. | Clean and debride wound with saline or tap water irrigation. Avoid using tap water if exposed bone or tendon is present. Apply saline-soaked gauze over the wound and cover with additional gauze. Gently irrigate completely avulsed tissue with saline. Wrap the avulsed tissue in saline-soaked gauze and place in a watertight bag. Place the bag in ice water or on top of an ice bag. Avoid direct contact of the tissue with the ice. | Closely monitor patient and wound area daily for adverse reactions and infection; change dressing based on type; check tetanus immunization. |

wound bed, and lack barrier properties to microorganisms. Occlusive dressings are semipermeable or impermeable, create a moist wound environment, and provide a barrier to microorganisms. Nonocclusive and occlusive dressings can be used as primary dressings, placed directly on the wound bed, and as secondary dressings, used in combination with primary dressings to provide additional absorption, protection, or occlusion. Evidence-based reviews and clinical investigations have examined the effects of nonocclusive and occlusive dressings on rates of healing, infection, and pain among various traumatic skin lesions. Compared with nonocclusive dressings, occlusive dressings were associated with increased rates of healing, decreased rates of infection, and decreased levels of pain.[8,9,16,17,45,83] Topical antimicrobials are commonly used with dressings and have been found to be effective in reducing rates of infection.[82] However, topical antimicrobials should only be used for a short period of time to prevent the emergence of resistant bacterial strains and adverse effects on healing.[44]

Nonocclusive dressings are commonly used by athletic trainers and include woven, nonwoven, and impregnated sterile gauze, nonadherent pads, adhesive strips and patches, and wound closure strips. As primary dressings, woven and nonwoven gauze can be used with infected wounds and may be more cost-effective than other dressings based on the frequent dressing changes that are required.[62] Woven, nonwoven, and impregnated gauze are indicated for puncture wounds with cavities to eliminate dead space and promote healing from the base upward.[61] Wound closure strips have been shown to be effective for the closure of superficial, linear lacerations and postoperative incisions in areas of minimal static and dynamic tension such as the face and neck.[25,28] Gauze, nonadherent pads, and adhesive strips and patches premoistened with normal saline or tap water are effective as temporary dressings to allow patients an immediate return to practices and competitions. In these cases, appropriate follow-up in the athletic training facility must be conducted. As secondary dressings, woven and nonwoven gauze can be used over primary dressings to absorb excess exudate. Adhesive strips and patches can assist in securing primary dressings to the periwound tissues. Woven, nonwoven, and impregnated sterile gauze, nonadherent pads, and adhesive strips and patches require daily changes to prevent adherence to the wound bed and desiccation and maceration of tissues.[61,62] Wound closure tapes are designed to remain on the wound edges for 5 to 10 days or until they separate from the periwound tissues.

Occlusive dressings are designed to interact with the wound and include alginates, films, foams, hydrogels, hydrocolloids, and dermal adhesives. As primary dressings, films and hydrogels are indicated for wounds that produce minimal levels of exudate such as superficial-thickness abrasions. Films trap moisture underneath the dressing and are nonabsorbent.[20] Hydrogels are constructed with a high water content and can donate moisture to the wound. Partial-thickness wounds with moderate exudate amounts can be managed with hydrogels and hydrocolloids. Hydrocolloids interact with exudate to produce a gel that conforms to the wound contours. Alginates and foams are designed for partial- to full-thickness wounds with heavy exudate. The high absorbency of alginates and foams allows the dressings to control large exudate amounts. Dermal adhesives are used with lacerations and traumatic and postoperative incisions in areas of low skin tension (i.e., the face) that require tissue approximation.[22,23] Films can be used as secondary dressings to secure other occlusive dressings to the periwound tissues, provide occlusion, and prevent leakage of excess exudate. Occlusive dressings can remain on the wound bed for longer periods of time compared with nonocclusive dressings.

Athletic trainers should monitor the patient, wound area, and periwound tissues until healing is complete. Daily visual inspections are conducted to identify signs and symptoms of adverse reactions and infection. Adverse reactions can develop from the use of some cleansing solutions, dressings, and topical antimicrobials. Signs and symptoms include erythematous rash, eczematous reaction, vesicles, maceration, tenderness, and pruritus.[50] Signs and symptoms of infection include pain, edema, erythema, and warmth around the wound, fever, wound dehiscence, and delayed wound healing.[6] If these signs and symptoms are recognized, the patient should immediately be referred to a physician. *Focus Box 28–3:* "Wound Care" suggests procedures to use in the athletic training clinic to cut down the possibility of wound infections.

> **Signs of wound infection, which appear 2 to 7 days after injury:**
> - Red, swollen, hot, and tender tissue
> - Swollen and painful lymph glands near the area of infection (groin, axilla, or neck)
> - Mild fever and headache

**Are Sutures Necessary?** Deeper lacerations, incisions, or puncture wounds may require manual closure using sutures.[35] If a patient has a wound that appears to be severe, the patient should be sent to the physician, who will decide whether sutures are needed to close the wound. Wounds are generally sutured if underlying tissues, such as fat, tendons, bone, or vessels, are exposed. Wounds of this type tend to have significant bleeding. Sutures should be put in as soon as possible but certainly within

> A patient has sustained a laceration just above the eyebrow and there is a good deal of bleeding. On close inspection, the athletic trainer realizes that, despite the large amount of bleeding, the laceration is not very long, but it is fairly deep.
>
> **?** Should this laceration be closed with steri-strips or a butterfly band-aid or should it be sutured by a physician?
>
> **28–4 Clinical Application Exercise**

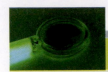
### Wound care

1. Follow all OSHA standards when managing traumatic skin lesions.
2. Cleanse the wound bed and periwound tissues as soon as possible with normal saline or tap water irrigation.
3. Use antiseptics (i.e., povidone-iodine, hydrogen peroxide) with caution.
4. If necessary, debride the wound using irrigation, wet-to-moist, and conservative sharp debridement.
5. Cover the wound with a nonocclusive or occlusive dressing based on the type and depth of the wound and amount of exudate.
6. Nonocclusive dressings can delay normal healing, increase the risk of infection, and should be used with caution.
7. Occlusive dressings and a moist wound environment increase rates of healing and decrease rates of infection.
8. Visually inspect the patient, wound bed, and periwound tissues daily for signs and symptoms of the development of adverse reactions and infection.

12 hours following injury. In relatively simple wounds, the edges may be brought in close approximation by the use of sutures to minimize scar formation. Before closing a wound with a suture, the physician usually anesthetizes the local area with a short-acting anesthetic. Fine suture material and minimal tightening limit any additional tissue damage, inflammation, and scarring. Wounds in areas that heal more slowly (areas that are less vascularized) and wounds in high-stress areas require larger suture material and the stitches must be left in longer.[26] Sometimes sutures are removed after only a few days to minimize scarring. Most sutures are eventually dissolved without having to be removed. Sutures coated with antimicrobial drugs can be used to reduce the chances of wound infection.

The physician may decide that the wound does not require sutures and that the torn tissues may be approximated using steri-strips or butterfly bandages. The most recent alternative is to use a topical skin adhesive or glue (sometimes called "liquid stitches") that forms a strong bond across apposed wound edges, allowing normal healing to occur beneath.[10] It may not be appropriate for all wounds or skin surfaces, such as eyes and mouth, or for patients with certain skin sensitivities. It is used to replace small sutures for small, superficial incisions and lacerations. It protects the wound by sealing out the most common infection-causing bacteria. This adhesive is relatively easy to use following appropriate wound preparation. It has been shown to save time during wound repair by forming a strong, flexible bond; to provide a water-resistant protective coating; and to eliminate the need for suture removal.[10,26] The long-term cosmetic outcome is comparable to that of traditional methods of repair. Patients, especially children, readily accept the idea of being "glued" over traditional methods of repair. Generally, lacerations, incisions, and puncture wounds require an innoculation with tetanus toxoid if a booster has not been given within 10 years.

## BACTERIAL INFECTIONS

Bacteria are single-celled microorganisms that can be seen only with a microscope after they are stained with specific dyes. They are of three major shapes: spherical (cocci), which occur in clumps; doublets, or chains, and rods (bacilli); and spirochetes, which are corkscrew-shaped.

*Staphylococcus* is a genus of gram-positive bacteria that commonly appear in clumps on the skin and in the upper respiratory tract. It is a common cause of skin infection.[80]

*Streptococcus* is also a genus of gram-positive bacteria, but unlike staphylococci, it appears in long chains. Most species are harmless, but some are among the most dangerous bacteria affecting humans. They can be associated with serious systemic diseases such as scarlet fever and, along with staphylococci, are common causes of skin infections.[80]

*Bacillus* is a genus of bacteria belonging to the family Bacillaceae. They are spore forming, aerobic, and gram-positive, and some are mobile. Most bacilli are not pathological; those that are can cause major systemic damage.[69,80] Diagnosis of bacterial infections is most often based on the history and characteristic appearance of the lesions and if necessary culture of any questionable lesion.[86] **SoR:B**

### Methicillin-Resistant *Staphylococcus aureus* (MRSA)

*Etiology* In recent years, some strains of *Staphylococcus* bacteria have become resistant to some antibiotics. *Methicillin-resistant Staphylococcus aureus* (MRSA) strains are resistant not only to the antibiotic called methicillin but also to many other types of antibiotics.[74] Originally, MRSA was most commonly seen in people who were already in the hospital, who were ill, or who had wounds or open sores, such as bed-sores or burns. The wounds or sores may become infected with MRSA, which is difficult to treat. MRSA can also cause infections in people outside a hospital.[70] More recently MRSA has become a rapidly emerging, problematic infection in the community. Community-acquired MRSA (CA-MRSA) can be easily transmitted via superficial abrasions and minor skin trauma.[72] MRSA has become a significant cause of skin and soft tissue infections in athletes who engage in sports such as wrestling and football, in which there is a lot of direct skin-to-skin contact, sharing of equipment and uniforms, and potential improper use of disinfectants.[67]

*Symptoms and signs* MRSA infections can cause a broad range of symptoms, depending on the part of the body that is infected. Infection often results in redness, swelling, and tenderness at the site of infection (Figure 28–13).[57] Sometimes, people carry MRSA without having any symptoms.

*Management* Recognition and referral of athletes with suspicious lesions are critical and those with suspicious lesions must be isolated from other team members.[86] SoR:B Antibiotics are not completely powerless against MRSA, but those infected with this bacteria may require a much higher dose over a much longer period or the use of an alternative antibiotic.[57] Treatment with antibiotics must be guided by local susceptibility data and be determined on a case-by-case basis.[86] SoR:A Many MRSA infections can only be treated with antibiotics that need to be given directly into a vein. The course of treatment is often required for several weeks.[47] Athletes may return to play if there are no new lesions for 48 hours, if there has been 72 hours of antibiotic treatment, and there is no drainage from the wound. Active infections cannot be covered for competition.[86] SoR:B A link to the NATA official statement "Community acquired MRSA infections" can be found at www.nata.org/sites/default/files/MRSA.pdf.

## Impetigo Contagiosa

*Etiology* *Impetigo contagiosa* is an extremely common skin disease, primarily observed in children, with the greatest number of cases occurring in late summer and early fall.[18] Impetigo contagiosa is caused by group A beta-hemolytic streptococci, *S. aureus,* or a combination of these two bacteria. It is spread rapidly when infected patients are in close contact with one another. Wrestling presents a particular risk of spreading this disease.[52]

*Symptoms and signs* *Impetigo contagiosa* is first characterized by mild itching and soreness, which are followed by the eruption of small vesicles and/or pustules that rupture to form honey-colored crusts (Figure 28–14).[18] Up to 20 percent of people carry *Staphylococcus aureus* in and about their nostrils. In general, impetigo develops in body folds that are subject to friction.[14]

*Management* Impetigo usually responds rapidly to proper treatment: thorough cleansing of the crusted area, followed by the application of a topical antibacterial agent, such as Bactroban, Fucidin H or Altabax.[86] SoR:B

An athlete may return to play if there are no skin lesions for 48 hours, there has been 72 hours of antibiotic therapy, and there is no existing drainage from the wound.[86] SoR:B (see *Focus Box 28–4:* "Management of impetigo"). Systemic antibiotics are also used.

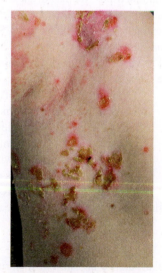

FIGURE 28–14 Impetigo contagiosa.
Courtesy Dean Morrell, MD, Department of Dermatology, University of North Carolina

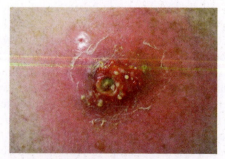

FIGURE 28–13 Methicillin-resistant *Staphylococcus aureus* (MRSA) on the leg.
CDC/Gregory Moran, M.D.

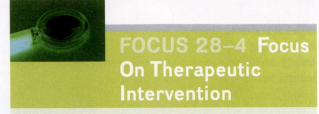

## FOCUS 28–4 Focus On Therapeutic Intervention

### Management of impetigo

1. Wash vigorously four or five times daily, using a medicated cleansing agent and hot water to remove all the crustations.
2. After cleansing, dry the area by patting gently.
3. When completely dried, apply an antibiotic or prescribed medicated ointment.
4. Every precaution should be taken to make sure that the patient uses isolated clothing and towels to prevent the spread of the disease.

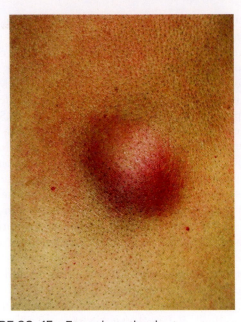

FIGURE 28–15   Furuncle on the chest.
Courtesy Dean Morrell, MD, Department of Dermatology, University of North Carolina

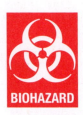

### Furuncles (Boils)

*Etiology*   Furuncles (boils) are infections of the hair follicle that usually result in pustule formation.[14] Staphylococci are usually the responsible organisms.

*Symptoms and signs*   The areas of the body most affected are the back of the neck, the face, and the buttocks. The pustule becomes enlarged, reddened, and hard from internal pressure. As pressure increases, extreme pain and tenderness develop (Figure 28–15). Most furuncles mature and rupture spontaneously, emitting the contained pus. NOTE: Furuncles should not be squeezed, because squeezing forces the infection into adjacent tissue or extends it to other skin areas.[32] Furuncles on the face can be dangerous, particularly if they drain into veins that lead to venous sinuses of the brain. Such conditions should be referred immediately to a physician.

> Individuals with bacterial infections associated with pus may pass the infection on to other people through direct contact.

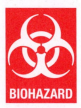

*Management*   Care of the furuncle involves protecting it from additional irritation, referring the patient to a physician for antibiotic treatment, and keeping the patient from contact with other team members while the boil is draining. The common practice of hot dressings or special drawing salves is not beneficial to the maturation of the boil.

### Carbuncles

*Etiology*   Carbuncles are similar to furuncles in their early stages, having also developed from staphylococci.[14]

*Symptoms and signs*   The principle difference between a carbuncle and a furuncle is that the carbuncle is larger and deeper and usually has several openings in the skin. It may produce fever and elevation of the white cell count. A carbuncle starts as a painful node covered by tight, reddish skin that later becomes very thin.[14] The site of greatest occurrence is the back of the neck, where it appears early as a dark red, hard area and then in a few days emerges into a lesion that discharges yellowish-red pus from a number of places.

One must be aware of the dangers inherent in carbuncles—they may result in the patient's developing an internal infection or they may spread to adjacent tissue or to other patients.[14]

*Management*   The most common treatment is surgical drainage combined with the administration of antibiotics. A warm compress is applied to promote circulation to the area.[39]

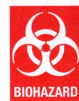

### Folliculitis

*Etiology*   Folliculitis is an inflammatory condition of the hair follicle. It is common in the hair follicles of the beard, scalp, groin, and buttocks (Figure 28–16); however, it can occur anywhere that hair exists on the body.

Folliculitis can be caused by either noninfectious or infectious agents. Occlusive folliculitis is a common form of noninfectious folliculitis in athletes. Moist, warm environments and mechanical occlusion contribute to create a primary irritant folliculitis. This is often seen in bicyclists who wear tight biking shorts. *Pseudofolliculitis barbae* (PFB) is common in African Americans and is due to penetration of the epidermis by curved hair; this creates a foreign body reaction in the skin that can mimic the appearance of folliculitis. PFB occurs most often in

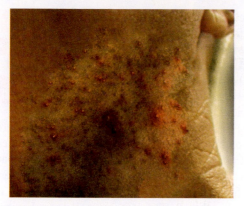

FIGURE 28–16   Folliculitis on the neck.
© William E. Prentice

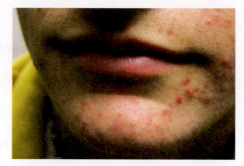

FIGURE 28–17   Acne vulgaris on the chin.
Courtesy Dean Morrell, MD, Department of Dermatology,
University of North Carolina

areas in which hair is shaved or rubs against clothing, such as the neck, face, buttocks, and thigh.[55] Infectious folliculitis can be due to bacteria (*Staphylococcus* or *Pseudomonas*), yeast (*Pityrosporum*), or mites (*Demodex follicularum*).

**Symptoms and signs**   Folliculitis starts with redness around the hair follicle and is followed by the development of a papule or pustule at the hair follicle opening. This may be followed by the development of a crust that can later slough off along with the hair. A deeper infection may cause scarring and permanent baldness (alopecia) in that area. The most common microorganism associated with this condition is *Staphylococcus.*

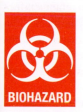

**Management**   The management of acute folliculitis is similar to that of impetigo. Moist heat is applied intermittently to increase local circulation. Antibiotic medication may be applied locally, as well as systemically, depending on the scope of the condition and can be effective in controlling local cellulitis.[86] SoR:B.

### Hidradenitis Suppurativa

**Etiology**   *Hidradenitis suppurativa* is a chronic inflammatory condition of the apocrine glands, or large sweat glands, commonly found in the axilla, scrotum, labia majora, and nipples. The exact cause of this condition is unclear. Some authorities have suggested that a primary inflammatory event in the hair follicle results in secondary blockage and inflammation of the apocrine gland. The role of bacteria is not known.

**Symptoms and signs**   The condition begins as a small papule and grows to the size of a small tumor, which is filled with purulent material. Deep dermal inflammation can occur, resulting in large abscesses that result in bands of scar tissue.[65]

**Management**   Treatment of this problem includes avoiding the use of antiperspirants, deodorants, and shaving creams; using medicated soaps, such as those containing chlorhexidine or povidone-iodine (Betadine); and applying a prescribed antibiotic lotion. Systemic antibiotics, such as tetracycline and mincocyline, are used for their antiinflammatory effects. In severe cases, surgical excision of skin containing the involved aprocrine glands can be curative.

### Acne Vulgaris

**Etiology**   *Acne vulgaris* is an inflammatory disease that involves the hair follicles and the sebaceous glands. It occurs near puberty and usually is less active after adolescence. Acne is characterized by closed comedones (whiteheads), open comedones (blackheads), papules, pustules, and cysts.[65]

Although most adolescents experience some form of acne, only a few develop an extremely disfiguring case (Figure 28–17). Its cause is not known, but it has been suggested that sex hormones may contribute to the development of the acne. The hair follicles of acne patients have increased numbers of the anaerobic bacterium *Propionobacterium acnes*. *P. acnes* breaks down sebaceous gland triglycerides into free fatty acids, which contributes to the inflammatory reaction by attracting inflammatory cells to the follicle.

**Symptoms and signs**   Acne can present with different types of lesions, including whiteheads, blackheads, flesh- or red-colored papules, pustules, or cysts. Commonly affected areas are the face, neck, and back. The superficial lesions usually heal spontaneously, whereas the deeper ones may become chronic and form disfiguring scars.[65]

The patient with a serious case of acne vulgaris has a scarring disease and may have serious emotional problems because of it. The individual may become nervous, shy, and even antisocial, with feelings of inferiority in interpersonal relations with peer groups. The athletic trainer's major responsibility in aiding patients with acne is to help them follow the physician's directions and to give constructive guidance and counseling.[65]

**Management**   A variety of topical and systemic agents are used to treat acne. Over-the-counter preparations containing benzoyl peroxide formulated as washes

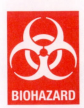

or creams are helpful in mild cases. Topical antibiotics—such as clindamycin (Cleocin) or erythromycin in combination with a topical retinoid, such as Retin-A—are useful for moderate acne. Treatment of more severe or inflammatory acne involves the use of the systemic antibiotics tetracycline, doxycycline, or mincocycline, which are used for their antiinflammatory effect. Severe, cystic acne is treated with the systemic retinoid Accutane. Accutane can cause profound birth defects, and its use is absolutely contraindicated in pregnant women. Women using Accutane are strongly advised to employ methods of birth control. Other therapeutic modalities include the manipulation of endogenous hormone levels with the use of certain formulations of oral contraceptives. Acne is not a result of having dirty skin, and excessive washing or the use of drying agents, such as ethanol or isopropanol, should be avoided, as these irritate the skin and cause excessive redness. Mild soaps and cleansers are recommended. Acne sufferers wishing to use cosmetics are advised to look for products labeled "noncomedogenic"; noncomedogenic products have been formulated to lessen the likelihood that they will block the hair follicles.

### Paronychia and Onychia

***Etiology*** Fingernails and toenails are continually subject to injury and infection. A common infection is *paronychia,* a purulent infection of the proximal and/or lateral nail folds (the skin surrounding the nail) (Figure 28–18). An *onychia* is an infection of the nail bed itself.

Paronychia and onychia develop from staphylococci, streptococci, and fungal organisms that accompany the contamination of open wounds or hangnails.[78] Loss of or damage to the cuticle, which forms a water-tight seal between the nail folds and the nail plate, is a risk factor for the development of paronychial infections.

***Symptoms and signs*** Acute paronychia has a rapid onset, with painful, bright red swelling of the proximal and lateral nail fold. An accumulation of purulent material occurs within the nail fold.[71] The infection may spread

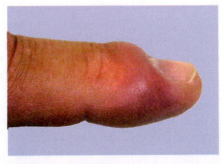

FIGURE 28–18   Paronychia.
© William E. Prentice

and cause onychia and inflammation of the nail bed.

***Management*** The athletic trainer should recognize paronychia early and have the patient soak the affected finger or toe in a hot solution of Betadine or boric acid three times daily. Topical antibiotics are often used between soakings. Severe bacterial paronychia may require systemic antibiotics. The yeast *Candida albicans,* a common cause of nonbacterial paronychia in individuals whose hands are immersed in water for prolonged periods, can be treated with topical thymol in ethanol. The infected nail must be protected while the individual is competing. Uncontrollable paronychia may require medical intervention, consisting of pus removal through a skin incision or the removal of a portion of the infected nail.

### Tetanus Infection

***Etiology*** Tetanus (lockjaw) is an acute infection of the muscles and central nervous system caused by the tetanus bacillus often found in soil, saliva, or feces. The bacteria usually enter the blood through a deep laceration or puncture wound, such as those caused by stepping on a nail on which the tetanus bacteria can be found.

***Symptoms and signs*** The first sign of a tetanus infection is stiffness of the jaw and muscles of the neck. The muscles of facial expression produce contortion and become painful. The muscles of the back and extremities become tetanic. Fever becomes markedly elevated. Tetanus can be fatal.

***Management*** The patient with an acute tetanus infection should be treated in an intensive care unit. Initial childhood immunization by tetanus toxoid is usually completed by the time a child reaches 6 years of age. Boosters should be given every 5 to 10 years. An individual who has not been immunized should receive an injection of tetanus immune globulin (Hyper-Tet) immediately after injury.

## FUNGAL INFECTIONS

Fungi are a group of organisms that include yeasts and molds. Fungal infections of the skin, hair, and nails are relatively common. Athlete's foot and jock itch are fungal infections of the foot and groin, respectively, that are so named because of their prevalence in athletes.[84]

Infection with superficial fungi takes place within the superficial keratinized tissue found in the hair, the nails, and the stratum corneum of the epidermis. These organisms are given the common name of ringworm (tinea) and are classified according to the area of the body infected. The contagious spores of these fungi may be spread by direct contact, contaminated clothing, or dirty locker rooms and showers.[65] Diagnosis of a fungal infection can be made by microscopic examination of skin scrapings.

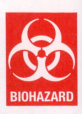

## Dermatophytes (Ringworm Fungi)

Dermatophytes, also known as ringworm fungi, are the cause of most skin, nail, and hair fungal infections. They belong to three genera: *Microsporum, Trichophyton,* and *Epidermophyton.*[48]

### Tinea of the Scalp (Tinea Capitis)

***Symptoms and signs*** Tinea (**ringworm**) of the scalp *(capitis),* beginning as a small papule of the scalp and spreading peripherally, is most common among children. The lesions appear as small, grayish scales, resulting in scattered bald patches. The primary sources of tinea capitis infection are contaminated animals, barber clippers, hairbrushes, and combs. This infection is easily spread among individuals with close physical contact. A culture of lesion scrapings is the most definitive test.[86] **SoR:B**

***Management*** Most patients have cases that are difficult to eradicate. Tinea capitis should be treated with systemic antifungal drugs, such as terbinafine, fluconazole, itraconazole, or ketoconazole for 2 weeks before returning to competition. Additionally, washing the scalp with selenium sulfide shampoo is also recommended.[86] **SoR:B**

### Tinea of the Body (Tinea Corporis)

***Symptoms of signs*** Tinea of the body *(tinea corporis)* commonly involves the extremities and trunk and presents as an itchy, red-brown, scaling, annular (ring-shaped) plaque that expands peripherally and clears centrally (Figure 28–19). Excessive perspiration and friction increase susceptibility to the condition.[41]

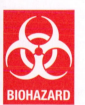

***Management*** Treatment usually consists of a topical antifungal cream, such as terbinafine, naftifine, ciclopirox, or oxiconazole (or more than one of these), twice a day, for at least 72 hours in cases of localized lesions. More diffuse inflammatory conditions should be treated with systemic antifungal medication.[38,86] **SoR:B**

### Tinea of the Nail (Tinea Unguium/Onychomycosis)

***Symptoms and signs*** Tinea of the nail *(tinea unguium* or *onychomycosis)* is a fungal infection of the toenails and/or fingernails. It is often seen among individuals who are involved in water sports or who have chronic athlete's foot. Trauma predisposes the individual to infection.[79] Many different organisms, including the dermatophyte species *Trichophyton* and *Epidermophyton,* the molds *Scopulariopsis* and *Aspergillus,* and the yeast *Candida,* can infect the nail plate. Culture of the infected nail plate is helpful in identifying the causative agent. When infected, the nail becomes thickened, brittle, and separated from its bed (see Figure 24–40).

***Management*** The treatment of tinea unguium can be difficult. In general, topical creams and lotions do not penetrate the nail; however, a topical antifungal (Penlac) has been shown to clear infections in 12 percent of patients. The systemic medications itraconazole (Sporanox) and terbinafine (Lamisil) are the most effective drugs for onychomycosis, but they must be used for at least 3 months to clear up the infection. Surgical removal of the nail may have to be performed on the athlete with extremely infected nails.[79]

### Tinea of the Groin (Tinea Cruris)

***Symptoms and signs*** Tinea of the groin *(tinea cruris),* more commonly called jock itch, appears as a bilateral and often symmetrical red-brown scaling plaque with a serpiginous (snakelike) border.[38] Tinea cruris may resemble the outline of a butterfly in the groin area. Erythrasma, a bacterial infection, can mimic the appearance of tinea cruris, but it is characterized by the absence of scale. The patient complains of mild to moderate itching, resulting in scratching and the possibility of a secondary bacterial infection (Figure 28–20).

***Management*** The athletic trainer must be able to identify lesions of tinea cruris and handle them accordingly.

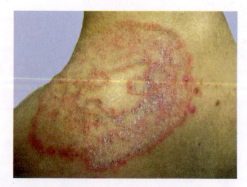

FIGURE 28–19    Tinea of the body (tinea corporis).
Courtesy Dean Morrell, MD, Department of Dermatology, University of North Carolina

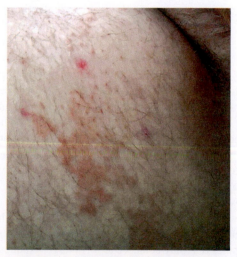

FIGURE 28–20    Tinea of the groin (tinea cruris).
© William E. Prentice

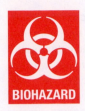

Conditions of this type must be treated until cured. Most ringworm infections will respond to many of the nonprescription medications that are available as aerosol sprays, liquids, powders, or ointments. Ointments are perhaps the most commonly used medication. Medications that are irritating or tend to mask the symptoms of a groin infection, such as the topical corticosterone hydrocortisone, should be avoided. The failure to respond to normal management may suggest a nonfungal skin problem, such as the bacterial infection erythrasma or a primary inflammatory dermatosis, and the athlete should be referred to a physician.[38]

Atypical or complicated groin infections must receive medical attention. Secondary bacterial infections are not an uncommon problem and will not respond to topical antifungals. Superficial fungal infections in immunocompromised individuals may not respond to topical over-the-counter medications. Additional topical and oral prescription medications are available and effective in treating these patients.

### Athlete's Foot (Tinea Pedis)

***Etiology*** The dermatophyte infection of the foot *tinea pedis* is the most common form of superficial fungal infection.[31] *Tricophyton* species, particularly *T. rubrum,* are the most common cause of athlete's foot. *T. rubrum* causes a moccasin-style tinea pedis characterized by an itchy, dry, scaling infection of the sole of the foot. Web space infections between the toes are often caused by *T. mentagrophytes.* Toe webs that become macerated and infected may result from a mixed infection with the yeast *Candida* and gram-negative rods, in addition to or replacing the original dermatophyte.[31] The athlete wearing shoes that are enclosed will perspire, encouraging fungal growth. However, contagion is based mainly on the patient's individual susceptibility. There are other conditions that may also be thought to be athlete's foot, such as allergic contact or eczematous dermatitis (Figure 28–21).

***Symptoms and signs*** Athlete's foot can present in many ways but appears most often as an extreme itching on the soles of the feet and between and on top of the toes. It appears as a dry, scaling patch or inflammatory, scaling red papules that may coalesce to form larger plaques. More inflammatory, blistering variants of athlete's foot are due to zoophilic dermatophytes, fungi such as *Microsporum*

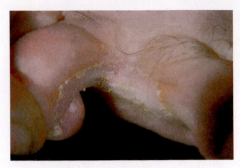

**FIGURE 28–21** Tinea pedis (athlete's foot).
CDC/Dr. Lucille K. Georg

*canis* that normally infect animals. Scratching can cause the tissue to become inflamed and secondarily infected with bacteria.[31]

***Management*** Topical antifungals, as discussed previously for tinea corporis, are effective in the treatment of tinea pedis. Of major importance is good foot hygiene (see *Focus Box 28–5:* "Basic care of athlete's foot").[54]

### Candidiasis

***Etiology*** *Candidiasis* is a skin, mucous membrane, or internal infection caused by the yeastlike fungus *Candida albicans* and some other species. It will attack the skin, as well as other structures, if the environment is right. Weather that is hot and humid, tight clothing that rubs, and poor hygiene provide the ideal environment for fungal growth.[39]

***Symptoms and signs*** Candidiasis commonly causes candidal intertrigo, a skin infection of body folds, such as the axilla and groin. Noninfectious intertrigo, a dermatitis of the same body folds, that may be precipitated by occlusion, heat, and moisture, can predispose an individual to develop secondary candidal intertrigo. Both candidal and noninfectious intertrigo present as beefy red patches, but *candidal intertrigo* can be distinguished from noncandidal variants by the additional presence of satellite pustules.[32] In cases in which it occurs where the skin is folded, a white, macerated border may surround the red area. Later, deep, painful fissures may develop where the skin creases (Figure 28–22).

***Management*** The first concern in treatment is to maintain a dry area. Antifungal creams containing miconazole, ketoconazole, or econazole applied twice daily will clear the infection. (NOTE: Genital candidiasis is discussed in Chapter 29 in the section on sexually transmitted diseases.)

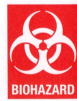

### Tinea Versicolor

***Etiology*** *Tinea versicolor* is a common fungal infection of young adults. Tinea versicolor is caused by the yeast *Malassezia furfur* (synonyms *Pityrosporum ovale, P. orbiculare,* and *M. ovalis*). *M. furfur* is a normal part of

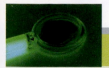

## FOCUS 28–5 Focus on Therapeutic Intervention

### Basic care of athlete's foot

- Keep the feet as dry as possible through frequent use of talcum powder.
- Wear clean white socks to avoid reinfection, and change them daily.
- Use a standard fungicide for specific medication. Over-the-counter medications, such as Desenex and Tinactin, are useful in the early stages of the infection. For stubborn cases, see the team physician; a dermatologist may need to make a culture from foot scrapings to determine the best combatant to be used.

The best cure for the problem of athlete's foot is prevention. To keep the condition from spreading to other individuals, the following steps should be faithfully followed by individuals in the sports program:

- All individuals should powder their feet daily.
- All individuals should dry their feet thoroughly, especially between and under the toes, after every shower.
- All individuals should keep sports shoes and street shoes dry by dusting them with powder daily.
- All individuals should wear clean sports socks and street socks daily.
- The shower and dressing rooms should be cleaned and disinfected daily.

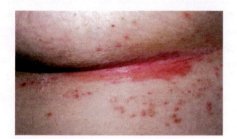

FIGURE 28–22 Candidiasis on the neck.
Courtesy Dean Morrell, MD, Department of Dermatology, University of North Carolina

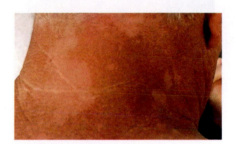

FIGURE 28–23 Tinea versicolor.
© William E. Prentice

the skin's flora, appearing commonly in areas in which sebaceous glands actively secrete body oils (Figure 28–23).[39]

***Symptoms and signs*** The fungus characteristically produces multiple, small, circular macules that are pink, brown, or white. They commonly occur on the abdomen, neck, and chest. The lesions do not tan when exposed to the sun and are usually asymptomatic.

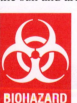
BIOHAZARD

***Management*** Treatment of tinea versicolor is straightforward; however, recurrences are common. Treatment options include selenium sulfide (Selsun shampoo) applied topically for 10 minutes each day for 1 to 2 weeks, topical econazole nitrate or ketoconazole, and systemic ketoconazole. Once the microorganism has been eradicated, repigmentation of the affected areas will occur but may take up to several months.

## VIRAL INFECTIONS

Viruses are ultramicroscopic organisms that require host cells to complete their life cycle. Entering a tissue cell, the virus exists as nucleic acid. Inside, the virus may stimulate the cell chemically to produce more virus until the host cell dies or the virus is ejected to infect additional cells. Instead of killing the cell, a budlike growth may occur, with harm to the cell, or the virus may remain within a cell without ever causing an infection.[19] A number of skin infections are caused by viruses.

### Herpes Simplex Labialis and Gladiatorum and Herpes Zoster

***Etiology*** Herpes *simplex* is a strain of virus that is associated with skin and mucous membrane infection. Types 1 and 2 cause cutaneous lesions and are

**Common viruses that attack the skin:**

- Herpes simplex
- Herpes zoster
- Verruca
- Molluscum contagiosum

A patient goes into a hospital sports medicine clinic concerned about multiple, small, white, circular macules on the abdomen, neck, and chest.

**?** What infection could cause these symptoms?

28–7 Clinical Application Exercise

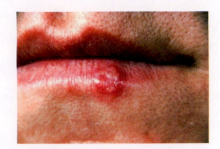

**FIGURE 28–24** Herpes simplex labialis (type 1).
Centers for Disease Control

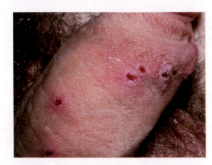

**FIGURE 28–25** Genital herpes simplex (type 2).
Courtesy Dean Morrell, MD, Department of Dermatology,
University of North Carolina

indistinguishable from one another (Figures 28–24 and 28–25); however, type 1 is found, for the most part, extragenitally and type 2 genitally. However, both can be found anywhere on the skin or mucous membrane.[19]

Herpes simplex is highly contagious and is usually transmitted directly through a lesion in the skin or mucous membrane.[15] After the initial outbreak, it is thought to move down a sensory nerve's neurilemmal sheath to reside in a resting state in a local ganglion. Recurrent attacks can be triggered by sunlight, emotional disturbances, illness, fatigue, infection, or other situations that may stress the organism.[19] However, sunlight does not adversely affect the reactivation rate if a sunscreen of sun protection factor (SPF) 15 is used.

***Symptoms and signs*** Not all individuals infected with the virus develop overt symptoms.[19] An early indication that a herpes infection is about to erupt is a tingling or hypersensitivity in the infected area 24 hours before the appearance of lesions. Local swelling occurs, followed by the appearance of vesicles. The patient may feel generally ill with a headache and sore throat, lymph gland swelling, and pain in the area of lesions. The vesicles generally rupture in 1 to 3 days, spilling out a serous material that will form into a yellowish crust. The lesions will normally heal in 10 to 14 days.[53]

Genital herpes is discussed in Chapter 29. *Herpes labialis* (cold sore) is usually less symptomatic than *herpes simplex gladiatorum,* which occurs quite often in

wrestlers, with lesions commonly on the side of the face, neck, or shoulders.[3,53] Herpes simplex infection is so highly contagious that it may run rampant through an entire team in a short time. Wrestlers having any signs of a herpes infection should be disqualified from body contact until these lesions have crusted and dried.[46] *Herpes zoster,* also called *shingles,* appears in a specific pattern on the body in an area that is innervated by a specific nerve root. It may appear on the face or anywhere on the trunk. It is the chickenpox virus that has remained present in the body but asymptomatic for many years (Figure 28–26).

***Management*** Herpes simplex lesions are self-limiting. Therapy usually is directed toward reducing pain and promoting early healing.[3] New active lesions may be treated with oral antiviral drugs, such as valacyclovir, are used to shorten the course and reduce the recurrence of herpes outbreaks and to reduce the chance of transmission. Antiviral medication is useless in those lesions which are crusty.[17,86] **SoR:B** Quite often, valacyclovir is administered prophylactically.

Herpes simplex, if not carefully managed, can lead to secondary infection. A major problem is keratoconjunctivitis, an inflammation of the cornea and conjunctiva, which can lead to loss of vision and must be considered a medical emergency. Athletes may be allowed to return to play following a bout with herpes if no symptoms such as fever or malaise persist; there are no new blisters developed for 72 hours; lesions have crusted over; there has been 5 days of systemic antiviral treatment; and, lesions are covered.[86] **SoR:B**

> A patient experiences a tingling and sometimes painful sensation in the upper lip region. Twenty-four hours later, swelling occurs, followed by the formation of vesicles. The patient also experiences a mild headache, sore throat, and lymph gland swelling.
>
> **?** What condition does this scenario describe, and how could the later symptoms have been prevented?

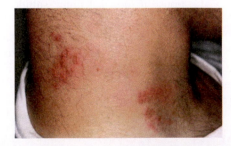

**FIGURE 28–26** Herpes zoster (shingles) on neck.
Courtesy Dean Morrell, MD, Department of Dermatology,
University of North Carolina

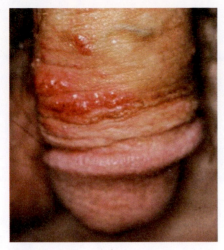

FIGURE 28–27   Genital warts.
CDC/Dr. M.F. Rein

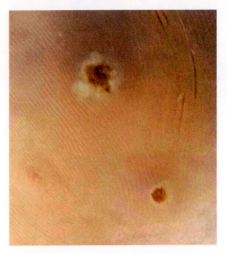

FIGURE 28–29   Plantar warts on the ball of the foot.
© William E. Prentice

## Verruca

Numerous forms of verruca exist, including the *verruca plana* (flat wart), *verruca plantaris* (plantar wart), and *condyloma acuminatum* (venereal wart) (Figure 28–27). Various isotypes of human papillomavirus have been identified. The human papillomavirus uses the skin's epidermal layer for reproduction and growth. The verruca virus enters the skin through a lesion that has been exposed to contaminated fields, floors, or clothing. Contamination can also occur from exposure to other warts.

### Common Wart

*Etiology*   Verruca plana are prevalent on the hands of children (Figure 28–28).

*Symptoms and signs*   This wart appears as a small, round, elevated lesion with rough, dry surfaces. It may be painful if pressure is applied. These warts are subject to secondary bacterial infection, particularly if they are located on the hands or feet, where they may be constantly irritated.[19]

*Management*   Vulnerable warts must be protected until they can be treated by a physician. The application of a topical salicylic acid preparation or liquid nitrogen and electrocautery are the most common ways of managing this condition.

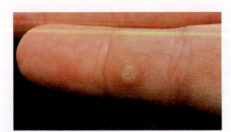

FIGURE 28–28   Common warts on a finger.
© William E. Prentice

### Verruca Plantaris (Plantar Wart)

*Etiology*   Plantar warts are found on the sole of the foot, on or adjacent to areas of abnormal weight bearing. The papillomavirus can be spread to the hands and other body parts.[76]

*Symptoms and signs*   Plantar warts are seen as areas with excessive epidermal thickening and cornification (Figure 28–29). They produce general discomfort and point tenderness in the areas of excessive callus formation. Commonly, the athlete complains that the condition feels as though he or she has stepped on broken glass. A major characteristic of the plantar wart is hemorrhagic puncta, which look like clusters of small, black seeds.

*Management*   There are many approaches to the treatment of warts. In general, a conservative approach is taken. Concern is to protect the wart against infection and to keep the growth of the warts under control. A common approach to controlling plantar warts is the careful paring away of accumulated callous tissue and the application of a keratolytic, such as 40 percent salicylic acid plaster. When the competitive season is over, the physician may decide to remove the wart by freezing it with liquid nitrogen or by electrodessication. Until its removal, a wart should be protected by a doughnut pad. A plantar wart may also be treated using salicylate iontophoresis.[76]

> **28–9 Clinical Application Exercise**
>
> A tennis player complains to the athletic trainer that she has a sharp pain in the ball of her right foot. She says that it feels as though she has stepped on a piece of glass. On inspection, the athletic trainer observes excessive callus formation on the ball of the foot that is dotted with a cluster of black specks.
>
> **?** What is this condition, and how should it be managed?

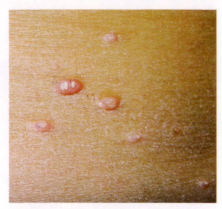

FIGURE 28–30   Molloscum contagiosum.
Courtesy Dean Morrell, MD, Department of Dermatology,
University of North Carolina

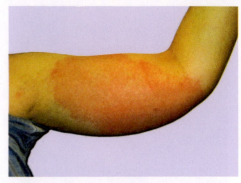

FIGURE 28–31   Cold reaction on the upper arm.
© William E. Prentice

## Molluscum Contagiosum

*Etiology*   *Molluscum contagiosum* is a poxvirus infection. It is more contagious than warts, particularly during direct body contact activities, such as wrestling (Figure 28–30).[73]

*Symptoms and signs*   Molluscum contagiosum appear as small, red or flesh-colored, smooth-domed papules with a central umbilication. When this condition is identified, the patient must be referred immediately to a physician.[73]

*Management*   Treatment often consists of cleansing thoroughly and using a procedure to destroy the lesion, such as the use of a powerful counterirritant (e.g., mupirocin, fusidic acid, or retapamulin), surgical removal of the lesion, or cryosurgery using liquid nitrogen.[61,86] **SoR:B**

# ALLERGIC, THERMAL, AND CHEMICAL SKIN REACTIONS

The skin can react adversely to a variety of nonpathogenic influences. Among the most common affecting athletes are allergies, temperature extremes, and chemical irritants.[13]

| Skin reactions to allergy: |
| :--- |
| • Reddening |
| • Elevated patches |
| • Eczema |

### Allergic Reactions

The skin displays allergic reactions in various ways (Figures 28–31 and 28–32). An allergy is an immunologically mediated reaction to molecules (allergens) against which the body's immune system has been sensitized. Allergens may be foods, drugs, clothing, dusts, pollens, plants, animals, heat, cold, or light. The skin may reflect an allergy in several ways, one of which is reddening and swelling of the tissue, which may occur either locally or generally from an increased dilation of blood capillaries. Different clinical patterns of allergy are reflective of the causative immunological mechanism. For example,

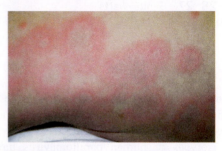

FIGURE 28–32   Hives.
Courtesy Dean Morrell, MD, Department of Dermatology,
University of North Carolina

immediate hypersensitivity reactions manifest as *urticaria,* or *hives,* which appear as red, edematous elevations (wheal, papule, or plaque) of the skin, characterized by a burning or an itching sensation. Delayed-type hypersensitivity reactions can manifest as acute dermatitis, which appears as intensely pruritic (itchy) erythematous papules, plaques, and vesicles. *Eczema* is a term commonly used to describe an acute inflammatory dermatosis characterized by redness, edema, papules, and/or vesicles or a chronic inflammatory dermatosis characterized by erythema, lichenification (thickening of the skin that exaggerates the skin lines), and scale.

The athletic trainer should be able to recognize gross signs of allergic reactions and should then refer the patient to the physician[12] Treatment usually includes avoidance of the sensitizing agents and the use of a topical or systemic antipruritic agent (such as calamine lotion and antihistamines, respectively) and/or topical or systemic corticosteroids.

### Contact Dermatitis (Allergic and Irritant)

*Etiology*   People can be allergic to many substances that will cause a skin reaction (contact dermatitis). Allergic contact dermatitis is an immunologically mediated reaction to a foreign substance, whereas irritant contact dermatitis is a nonimmunological reaction to a chemical irritant.[47]

The most common plants that cause allergic contact dermatitis are poison ivy, poison oak, sumac, ragweed, and primrose.[33] Over time, an individual may become allergic to topical medications, such as antibiotics, antihistamines, anesthetics, or antiseptics. Chemicals such as fragrances and preservatives commonly found in soaps, detergents, and deodorants can create an allergic reaction; detergents and soaps themselves are more likely to cause an irritant contact dermatitis, which is not a hypersensitivity reaction, but rather represents a primary chemical irritant.[47] Some individuals are allergic to materials in the adhesive used in athletic tape. Also, the countless chemicals used in the manufacture of shoes, clothing, and other materials have been known to produce allergic contact dermatitis.

*Symptoms and signs* The period of onset from the time of initial exposure may range from 1 day to 1 week.[11] The skin reacts with redness, swelling, and the formation of vesicles that ooze fluid and form a crust. A constant itch develops that is increased with heat and made worse by rubbing. Secondary infection is a common result of scratching (Figure 28–33). Over time, the morphology may change from the redness and blistering of acute contact dermatitis to the erythematous, scaling,[33] lichenified papules and plaques characteristic of chronic contact dermatitis.

> A patient is seen in a clinic for a knee injury after a ski trip. The athletic trainer notices that her face is sunburned and peeling.
>
> **?** What should this patient be told about protecting the skin from exposure to sunlight?

*Management* The most obvious treatment approach is to determine the allergic contactant or irritant and avoid it. This may not be simple and may require extensive testing. In the acute phase, tap water compresses or soaks soothe and dry the vesicles. Topical corticosteroids may be beneficial.[11]

### Miliaria (Prickly Heat)

*Etiology* Prickly heat is common and occurs most often during the hot season of the year in those individuals who perspire profusely and who wear heavy clothing.

Continued exposure to heat and moisture causes retention of perspiration by the sweat glands and subsequent miliaria.

*Symptoms and signs* Miliaria results in redness and itching and burning vesicles and pustules.[39] It occurs most often on the arms, trunk, and bending areas of the body (Figure 28–34).

*Management* The care of prickly heat requires the avoidance of overheating, frequent bathing with a nonirritating soap, loose-fitting clothing, and the use of antipruritic lotions.

### Chilblains (Pernio)

*Etiology* Chilblains is a common type of dermatitis caused by excessive exposure to cold.

*Symptoms and signs* The tissue does not freeze but reacts with edema, reddening, possibly blistering, and a sensation of burning and itching after exposure to cold. The parts of the body most often affected are the ears, face, hands, and feet.

*Management* Treatment consists of exercise and a gradual warming of the part. Massage and the application of heat are contraindicated in cases of chilblains. The systemic drug nifedipine can be used for more severe cases. (See Chapter 6 for more information about reactions to cold.)

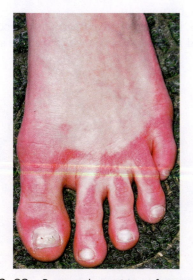

FIGURE 28–33  Contact dermatitis on foot to shoes.
Courtesy Dean Morrell, MD, Department of Dermatology, University of North Carolina

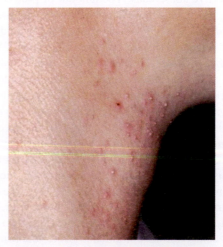

FIGURE 28–34  Miliaria (prickly heat) on the neck.
Courtesy Dean Morrell, MD, Department of Dermatology, University of North Carolina

## Burns

Burns can result from excessive exposure to thermal, chemical, electrical, or radiation sources. In a sports environment, the athlete is certainly most susceptible to radiation burns from exposure to sunlight.

### Sunburn

*Etiology*  Serious skin damage can occur from overexposure to the sun's rays. Sunburn represents an inflammatory response to ultraviolet radiation–induced skin damage—that is caused by ultraviolet solar radiation that varies in intensity from a mild erythema (pink color) to a severe blistering reaction.[20] Every protection should be given to individuals who have thin, white skin. Their skin tends to absorb a greater amount of ultraviolet radiation than more pigmented individuals. Individuals who are taking photosensitizing drugs, such as thiazide diuretics, some tetracyclines, and phenothiazine, are also sensitive. The chemical psoralen in the oil of limes, parsnips, and celery, as well as other foods, can produce a severe adverse reaction in some individuals who expose themselves to sunlight.

*Symptoms and signs*  If a large area of the skin is sunburned, the patient may display all the symptoms of severe inflammation accompanied by shock.[2] A sunburn can cause malfunctioning of the organs within the skin, which in turn may result in the infection of structures such as hair follicles and sweat glands.

Sunburn appears 2 to 8 hours after exposure. The symptoms become most extreme in approximately 12 hours and dissipate in 72 to 96 hours. After once receiving a severe sunburn, the skin is more susceptible to burning.[16] The skin remains injured for months after a severe sunburn has been sustained. Prevention of sunburn should be accomplished by the judicial use of sunscreens and/or moisturizers with sunscreens that filter ultraviolet light. Products containing chemical blocks, such as parsol 1789, or physical blocks, such as titanium dioxide, are very effective sunscreens. The amount of protection provided by sunscreens is determined by the *sun protection factor (SPF)*.[59] An SPF of 15 means that it would require 15 times longer to sustain the same amount of UV radiation with the sunscreen than without. Water-resistant or waterproof sunscreens are recommended for athletics because nonwaterproof sunscreens are easily washed away by perspiration. Constant overexposure to the sun can lead to chronic skin thickening, damage, and skin cancers.[59]

*Management*  A sunburn is treated according to the degree of inflammation present. Mild burns are best treated using cool water in a shower or bath. Aloe-based compounds have also proved beneficial. Over-the-counter antiinflammatory medications may help reduce pain. Moderate and severe burns can be relieved by a cool-water tub bath using colloidal ointment. Severe sunburn may be treated by a physician with corticosteroids and other antiinflammatory drugs. Moisturizers can help reduce dryness and peeling in mild sunburns.

Ultraviolet radiation is damaging—it can prematurely age the skin and can increase the risk of skin cancer. Basal cell and squamous cell carcinomas are the most common cancers.[59,75]

## INFESTATION AND BITES

Certain parasites cause dermatoses, or skin irritations, when they suck blood, inject venom, and even lay their eggs under the skin. Individuals who come in contact with these organisms may develop various symptoms, such as itching, allergic skin reactions, and secondary infections from insult or scratching. The more common parasitic infestations and bites are caused by mites, lice, fleas, ticks, mosquitoes, and stinging insects, such as bees, wasps, hornets, and yellow jackets.[60]

> Depending on the part of the country in which an individual resides, parasites such as mites, lice, fleas, ticks, mosquitoes, and stinging insects can cause serious discomfort and infection.

### Mites (Scabies)

*Etiology*  Scabies is a skin disease caused by the mite *Sarcoptes scabiei*, which produces extreme nocturnal itching (Figure 28–35). The parasitic itch mite is small, with the female causing the greatest irritation. The mite burrows a tunnel approximately ¼ to ½ inch (0.6 to 1.25 cm) long into the skin to deposit its eggs.[39]

*Symptoms and signs*  The mite's burrows appear as dark lines between the fingers, toes, body flexures, nipples, and genitalia. Excoriations, pustules, and papules

> A cross-country runner complains to the athletic trainer of extreme nocturnal itching. Observation of the athlete's skin reveals dark lines in the area of the fingers and toes.
>
> **?** What insect infestation does this scenario describe?

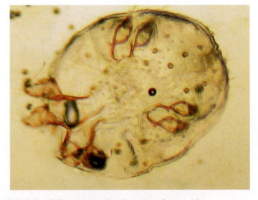

FIGURE 28–35   Magnified view of a scabie.
Courtesy Dean Morrell, MD, Department of Dermatology, University of North Carolina

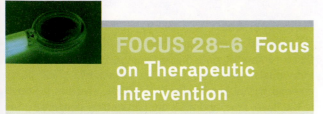

## FOCUS 28-6 Focus on Therapeutic Intervention

### Treatment of scabies

- The entire body should be thoroughly cleansed, with attention to skin lesions.
- Bedding and clothing should be disinfected.
- A coating of Permethrin should be applied to the lesions overnight.
- All individuals who have come in contact with the infected individual should be examined by the physician.
- Locker and game equipment must be disinfected.

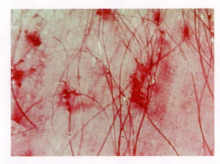

FIGURE 28-36   Lice.
CDC/Joe Miller

caused by the resulting scratching frequently hide the true nature of the disease. The young mite matures in a few days and returns to the skin surface to repeat the cycle. The skin often develops a hypersensitivity to the mite, which produces extreme itching.[39]

***Management*** Permethrin 5 percent cream (Elimite) is the treatment of choice for individuals over 2 months of age. It should be applied topically from the neck down overnight. Affected family members should be similarly treated, and bedding and clothing should be thoroughly washed in hot, soapy water. Gamma benzene hexachloride (Lindane) is no longer the treatment of choice because it is absorbed systemically through the skin and causes central nervous system toxicity. Resistant cases can be treated with the systemic agent Ivermectin. Because of the patient's itching and scratching, secondary infections are common and must also be treated (see *Focus Box 28–6:* "Treatment of Scabies"). After treatment with a scabecide, itching can be controlled with a topical corticosteroid cream.

### Lice (Pediculosis)

***Etiology*** Pediculosis is an infestation by the louse, of which three types are parasitic to humans. The *Pediculus humanus capitis* (head louse) infests the head, where its eggs (nits) attach to the base of the hair shaft (Figure 28–36). The *Phthirus pubis* (crab louse) lives in the hair of the pubic region and lays its eggs at the hair base. The *Pediculus humanus corporis* (body louse) lives and lays its eggs in the seams of clothing.[39]

***Symptoms and signs*** The louse is a carrier of many diseases; its bite causes an itching dermatitis, which, through subsequent scratching, provokes pustules and excoriations.

***Management*** Cure is rapid with the use of any of a number of agents. NIX is an over-the-counter synthetic pyrethroid permethrin that is very effective in treating head and pubic lice. NIX shampoo should be lathered

into the affected area, allowed to sit for 10 minutes, and then rinsed away. The area should be retreated after 7 to 10 days. Body lice can be treated by overnight application of 5 percent permethrin cream. To prevent reinfestation, all clothing and bedding should be washed in hot, soapy water or discarded.

### Fleas

***Etiology*** Fleas are small, wingless insects that suck blood. Singly, their bites cause only minor discomfort to the recipient. Certain species of fleas can transmit the systemic diseases bubonic plague and endemic typhus.[39]

***Symptoms and signs*** When there are a large number of biting fleas, a great deal of discomfort can occur. After attaching themselves to a moving object, such as a dog or a human, most fleas bite in patterns of three. Fleas seem to concentrate their bites on the ankle and lower leg.

***Management*** Once the flea bite has been incurred, the main concern is to prevent itching with an antipruritic lotion, such as calamine or a topical corticosteroid. Scratching the bite should be avoided to prevent a secondary infection. Areas in which fleas abound can be sprayed with selected insecticides containing malathion or some other effective insecticide.

### Ticks

***Etiology*** Ticks are parasitic insects that have an affinity for the blood of many animals, including humans. They are carriers of a variety of microorganisms that can cause Rocky Mountain spotted fever or Lyme disease.[27] Because ticks are commonly found on grass and bushes, they can easily become attached to the athlete who brushes against them.

***Symptoms and signs*** Rocky Mountain spotted

> **28-12 Clinical Application Exercise**
>
> After mountain biking on a trail in the woods, a patient finds a tick on his leg.
>
> **?** What signs and symptoms should the patient look for as a warning sign of a disease transmission?

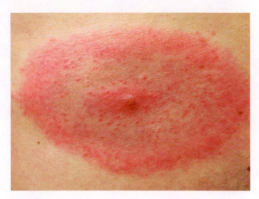

FIGURE 28–37   Lyme disease rash on the inside of the forearm.

Courtesy Dean Morrell, MD, Department of Dermatology, University of North Carolina

fever (RMSF) and Lyme disease are characterized by constitutional symptoms, including headache, fever, malaise, myalgia, and rash.[27] Petechiae and purpura (small, dark spots that retain their color when pressure is applied) localized to the distal arms, legs, hands, and feet characterize the skin manifestations of RMSF. Erythema chronicum migrans, an enlarging annular red ring with or without a central red papule, is the typical rash of Lyme disease (Figure 28–37).

***Management***   To remove a tick, mineral oil or fingernail polish is applied to its body, at which time it will withdraw its head.[2] Grasping or pulling the tick by its head is an acceptable method for removal. RMSF and Lyme disease are serious illnesses with significant morbidity and mortality rates that require systemic antibiotic treatment by a physician.

## Mosquitos

***Etiology***   Mosquitos are blood suckers that produce bites that can be irritating, itchy, and painful. Mosquitos are known to pass blood-borne illnesses from one victim to another. In parts of the world where mosquito-transmitted diseases are common, they are a major health hazard and are responsible for the transmission of yellow fever, malaria, encephalitis, and many other serious diseases.[60] In North America, the West Nile virus (WNV) is carried by mosquitos and occurs as a serious seasonal epidemic that flares up in the summer and continues into the fall. Approximately 80 percent of people who are infected with WNV will not show any symptoms at all. Twenty percent will develop flulike symptoms that may last for 2 weeks. In the United States, it is the bite itself that presents the greatest difficulty.[68]

***Symptoms and signs***   The mosquito bite produces a small, reddish papule. Multiple bites may lead to a great deal of itching.

***Management***   Itching is most often relieved by the application of a topical medication, such as calamine lotion or topical corticosteroids. In climates where mosquitos are prevalent, repellents should be used directly on the skin.

## Stinging Insects

***Etiology***   Bees, wasps, hornets, and yellow jackets inflict a venomous sting that is temporarily painful for most individuals; however, some hypersensitive individuals respond with a potentially fatal allergic reaction.[68] Stings to the head, face, and neck are particularly dangerous. Individuals with a history of allergic reactions from stings must be carefully monitored after a sting for an anaphylactic reaction.[60] The symptoms of an anaphylactic reaction include hives, a sensation of warmth, asthma symptoms, swelling of the mouth and throat area, difficulty breathing, vomiting, diarrhea, cramping, a drop in blood pressure, and loss of consciousness. These symptoms may begin in as little as 5 to 15 minutes to up to 2 hours after a sting, but life-threatening reactions may progress over hours.

***Symptoms and signs***   The allergic patient may respond with an increase in heart rate, fast breathing, chest tightness, dizziness, sweating, and even loss of consciousness.[60]

***Management***   In uncomplicated sting cases, the stinging apparatus must be carefully removed with tweezers, followed by the application of a soothing medication. Detergent soap applied directly on the sting often produces an immediate lessening of symptoms. In severe reactions to a sting, the patient must be treated for anaphylactic shock and referred immediately to a physician.[60] To avoid stings, the individual should not wear scented lotions or shampoos, brightly colored clothes, jewelry, suede, or leather and should not go barefoot. Individuals predisposed to anaphylactic reactions from stings should be provided with and instructed in the use of an EpiPen (see Chapter 17).

> A patient who has had previous allergic reactions is stung by a bee.
>
> **?** What physical reactions might the patient be expected to have?

## Spider Bite

***Etiology***   Most spiders are not dangerous to humans, although all spiders have some amount of venom with varying degrees of potency. Bite marks from most spiders are usually too small to be seen easily. Frequently, the patient will not recall being bitten. Spiders rarely bite more than once. The two spiders most likely to cause significant problems are the black widow and the brown recluse. The black widow spider is a shiny black spider with red to orange markings, usually in the shape of an hourglass on the underside of the belly. The brown recluse has a violin-shaped marking on its back and long legs.[68]

***Symptoms and signs***   Most spider bites result in pain, small puncture wounds, redness, itching, and swelling that lasts a couple of days (Figure 28–38). The wound

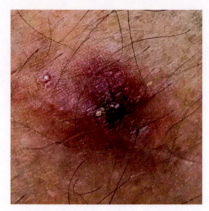

FIGURE 28–38  Spider bite.
© William E. Prentice

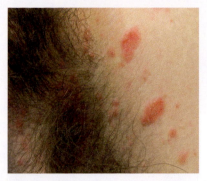

FIGURE 28–39  Pityriasis rosea on the lower chest, showing "herald patch."
Courtesy Dean Morrell, MD, Department of Dermatology, University of North Carolina

has a center blister surrounded by a red ring and then a white ring. The blister breaks open, leaving an ulcer that scabs over. A bite from a black widow or a brown recluse may result in severe muscle pain and cramps in the back, shoulders, abdomen, and thighs within the first 2 hours. Other symptoms include weakness, sweating, headache, anxiety, itching, nausea, vomiting, difficult breathing, and increased blood pressure.

*Management*  Treatment consists of washing the wound and applying an antibiotic ointment. The victim should seek medical attention if there are signs of an infection; an ulcer that does not heal; or a bite accompanied by nausea, vomiting, fever, or a rash. If muscle cramps develop, the victim should be taken to the nearest emergency facility.

## OTHER SKIN CONDITIONS

### Pityriasis Rosea

*Etiology*  This is an acute inflammatory skin rash of unknown origin that occurs most commonly in people between the ages of 10 and 35, but it may occur at any age. It can occur anytime of year, but it is most common in the spring and fall. It is not a sign of any internal disease, nor is it caused by fungi, bacteria, or an allergy. There is recent evidence suggesting that it may be caused by a virus, since the rash resembles certain viral illnesses, and occasionally a person feels slightly ill for a short while just before the rash appears.[77] However, this has not been proven. It does not seem to spread from person to person and it usually occurs only once in a lifetime.

*Symptoms and signs*  Pityriasis rosea is characterized initially by a single, pinkish-red patch called a "herald patch" that appears somewhere on the chest or back and over several days enlarges to a few centimeters. Within 2 days to 3 weeks, a secondary macular eruption occurs on the trunk over the ribs and on the upper extremities. The lesions are red and scaly with a clearing in the center (Figure 28–39). They appear in a symmetrical distribution over the trunk and extremities. Usually, there are no

permanent marks as a result of this condition, although some darker-skinned persons may develop long-lasting flat, brown spots that eventually fade.[77]

*Management*  Most cases usually do not need treatment, and fortunately, even the most severe cases eventually go away. The rash gradually disappears over a 2- to 10-week period. Local application of antipruretics may help relieve itching. Occasionally, antiinflammatory medications, such as a corticosteroid, are necessary to stop the itching or make the rash go away.

### Psoriasis

*Etiology*  This is a relatively common chronic disease of the skin that causes itching. The exact cause of psoriasis is not known, but there is some genetic factor present. Certain conditions, such as infection, smoking, some drugs, climate, and maybe hormonal factors, may cause an outbreak.[36]

*Symptoms and signs*  The lesions begin as reddish papules that collectively form plaques with distinctive borders. As the condition progresses, the lesions develop a yellowish-white, scaly appearance (Figure 28–40). The lesions may occur anywhere but are most likely to appear on the elbows, knees, scalp, genitalia, and trunk, particularly around the umbilicus. Trauma causes new lesions to appear.[36]

*Management*  Treatment involves teaching the patient how to self-manage this condition. Topical glucocorticoids in combination with a kerolytic agent to remove the scales are used, thus enhancing penetration of the glucocorticoids. Calciportriene ointment is used to inhibit the proliferation of keratinocytes. In severe cases that are resistant to treatment, long-term oral medications may be warranted. Counseling may be required to help the individual deal with the psychological aspects of managing these lesions.

### Skin Cancer

*Etiology*  Exposure to ultraviolet light from the sun can ultimately lead to the development of skin cancer.[42] Skin cancer is a malignant tumor that grows in the skin

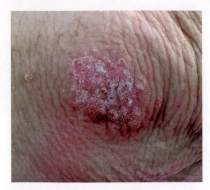

FIGURE 28–40   Psoriasis on the elbow.
© William E. Prentice

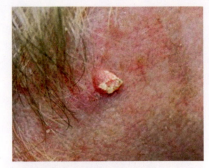

FIGURE 28–42   Squamous cell carcinoma.
National Cancer Institute

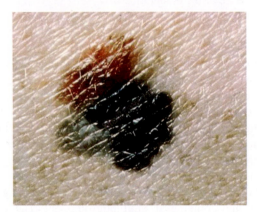

FIGURE 28–43   Malignant melanoma.
National Cancer Institute

cells and accounts for 50 percent of all cancers.[23] The three most common types are basal cell carcinoma, squamous cell carcinoma, and malignant melanoma. *Basal cell carcinoma* accounts for approximately 75 percent of all skin cancers. It starts in the basal cell layer of the epidermis (the top layer of skin) and grows very slowly. *Squamous cell carcinoma* accounts for about 20 percent of all skin cancer cases. It starts in the middle, or squamous, cell layer of skin.[39]

*Malignant melanoma* accounts for 4 percent of all skin cancers. Malignant melanoma starts in the melanocytes—cells that produce pigment in the skin.[69] Unlike basal and squamous cell carcinomas, which are highly treatable, malignant melanoma has a high mortality rate, because this cancer tends to metastasize (spread) to other parts of the body.[59]

**Symptoms and signs**   Basal cell carcinoma usually appears in areas exposed to the sun, such as the head, neck, arms, hands, and face. It begins as a small, shiny bump or nodule on the skin (Figure 28–41). It commonly occurs among persons with light-colored eyes, hair, and complexion. Squamous cell carcinoma may appear as nodules or red, scaly patches of skin and may be found on the face, ears, lips, and mouth (Figure 28–42). However, squamous cell carcinoma can spread to other parts of the body. This type of skin cancer is usually found in fair-skinned people.

Malignant melanomas usually begin as a mole, which turns cancerous and spreads quickly. Certain moles are at higher risk of changing into malignant melanoma. Moles that are present at birth and atypical moles have a greater chance of becoming malignant.[69] Melanomas vary greatly in appearance. Melanomas may show the following *ABCD* characteristics (Figure 28–43).[39]

- Asymmetry—one-half of the mole does not match the other half
- Border—the edges are irregular, or ragged
- Color—the color varies throughout the mole
- Diameter—the mole is larger than a pencil eraser

Some may show all four characteristics, whereas others may show only changes in one or two characteristics. Malignant melanoma most often appears on fair-skinned men and women, but persons with all skin types can be affected.[69]

**Management**   If an athletic trainer suspects that a patient has skin cancer, that patient should be immediately referred to a physician for a medical diagnosis. Surgery is a common treatment for skin cancer, which is used in about 90 percent of treated cases.[23] Some types of skin cancer growths can be removed very easily and require only very minor surgery, whereas others may require a more extensive surgical procedure. Surgery may include cryosurgery (using liquid nitrogen to freeze and destroy

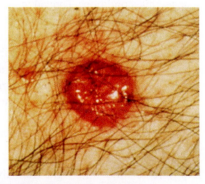

FIGURE 28–41   Basal cell carcinoma.
National Cancer Institute

the tissue); excision (using a scalpel to excise and remove the growth); or Mohs' microscopically controlled surgery (excising a lesion, layer by layer, until no tumor cells are seen under a microscope). Skin cancers may also be treated nonsurgically with laser, radiation, and chemotherapy. It is important to examine the skin on a regular basis and become familiar with moles and other skin conditions, in order to better identify changes. Recognizing changes in moles is crucial in detecting malignant melanoma at its earliest stage.

## SUMMARY

- The skin is the largest organ of the human body. It is composed of three layers: the epidermis, the dermis, and the subcutis. The outermost layer, the epidermis, acts as protection against infections from a variety of sources. The dermis contains sweat glands, sebaceous glands, and hair follicles. The subcutis layer is the major area for fat storage and temperature regulation.
- Primary skin lesions include macules, papules, plaques, nodules, tumors, cysts, wheals, vesicles, bullae, and pustules. Secondary skin lesions include scales, crusts, fissures, erosions, ulcers, and scars.
- Microorganisms, trauma, allergies, temperature variations, chemicals, infestations, and insect bites can cause skin lesions.
- Participation in any physical activity can place a great deal of mechanical force on the skin, which can lead to many different problems. Abnormal friction causes hyperkeratosis, blisters, and intertrigo. Hyperhidrosis adds to the problems of skin friction and infections. A tearing force can lacerate or avulse skin. Compression can bruise, scraping abrades, and a pointed object can puncture.
- Providing immediate proper care is essential to avoid skin infections. Streptococcal and staphylococcal bacteria are associated with wound contamination, and MRSA has become a serious problem in the athletic population.

- Impetigo contagiosa is a highly infectious disease and is associated with both the staphylococcal and streptococcal bacteria. Furuncles, carbuncles, and folliculitis are staphylococcal-caused afflictions and can be spread by direct contact.
- The sports environment, which is often one of excessive moisture, warmth, and darkness, is conducive to fungal growth. An extremely common fungus, ringworm, falls under the general heading of dermatophytes. Under the right conditions, these fungi can attack a wide variety of body tissues.
- Herpes simplex is a virus associated with herpes labialis and herpes gladiatorum. Human papillomavirus causes a variety of warts, such as the plantar wart verruca plantaris and the common wart verruca vulgaris. The poxvirus causes molluscum contagiosum, a highly contagious wart spread by direct contact.
- Individuals are also subject to many other causes of skin conditions, including allergies, extremes of heat or cold, and chemical irritations.
- One major problem that produces an insidious destruction of the skin is prolonged overexposure to sunlight.
- Different parts of the country have problems with insect infestations and bites. Two of these problems are scabies (caused by mites) and pediculosis (from lice), and there are others, produced by fleas, ticks, mosquitos, and stinging insects.

## WEB SITES

**NATA Position, Official, and Consensus Statements**
*Community Acquired MRSA Infections (2005):*
   www.nata.org/sites/default/files/MRSA.pdf
American Academy of Dermatology: www.aad.org
American Society for Dermatologic Surgery:
   www.asds.net

American Society of Dermatology: www.asd.org
Canadian Dermatology Association:
   www.dermatology.ca
Dermatology Foundation:
   www.dermatologyfoundation.org

## SOLUTIONS TO CLINICAL APPLICATION EXERCISES

28–1   Initially, the skin flap should be completely removed. The area should be cleaned with soap and water, and the antiseptic liquid benzalkonium should be applied along with an occlusive dressing, such as second-skin.

28–2   To prevent intertrigo, the skin should be kept dry, clean, and friction free. The patient who is prone to this problem should wear loose cotton underwear. Males should wear a supporter over underwear.

28–3   A major concern for this abrasion is contamination from the gravel and possible development of infection. The wound should be cleaned and debrided with normal saline or tap water irrigation. Continue until all visible debris is removed from the wound bed and periwound tissues. Cover the wound with a dressing to promote a moist wound environment.

28–4   Because this laceration is on the face, the best advice is to have this wound sutured by a qualified physician as soon as possible.

28–5 This skin condition is the highly contagious disease impetigo contagiosa. The patient must not have physical contact with other athletes until the disease is resolved. It is managed with daily thorough cleansing of crusted material followed by an application of an antibiotic salve or oral medication.

28–6 With tinea pedis, there is severe itching on the top of and between the toes and on the soles of the feet. A rash occurs, with blisters that secrete a yellow serum. Scratching can cause an infection. A red, white, or grayish scaling may also be present.

28–7 It is likely that the patient has tinea versicolor. Treatment of this condition is difficult and recurrences are common. Perhaps the most effective treatment is to use selenium sulfide. Pigment changes occur slowly even after the microorganism has been eradicated.

28–8 This condition is a herpes simplex viral infection. Once the herpes virus is contracted, it is impossible to get rid of it. When symptoms begin to appear, the patient should be referred immediately to a physician for a prescription drug called valacyclovir, which can minimize symptoms.

28–9 The black specks are plantar warts. The accumulated callus should be pared down and a 40 percent salicylic acid plaster should be applied. A doughnut pad should be used to protect the area.

28–10 Individuals should be cautioned to use sunscreen routinely, even in cold weather, to prevent the damaging effects of overexposure to sunlight.

28–11 This scenario describes infestation by the mite *Sarcoptes scabiei*. Another name for this condition is scabies. The mite burrows a tunnel under the skin to deposit its eggs. The eggs hatch, and the young mites return to the skin surface to repeat the cycle. A hypersensitivity develops that causes extreme itching at night.

28–12 Headache, fever, malaise, myalgia, and a rash are symptoms of both Rocky Mountain spotted fever and Lyme disease. Any small, dark spots or an enlarging red ring also indicate that the athlete has contracted a disease from the tick.

28–13 The patient may experience an anaphylactic reaction, with an increase in heart rate, fast breathing, chest tightness, dizziness, sweating, and possibly a loss of consciousness. This condition is a medical emergency.

## REVIEW QUESTIONS AND CLASS ACTIVITIES

1. Describe the skin's anatomy and functions. Describe lesions that are indicative of infection.
2. Contrast the microorganisms that are related to skin infections.
3. Relate the mechanical forces of friction, compression, shearing, stretching, scraping, tearing, avulsing, and puncturing to specific skin injuries.
4. List the steps to take in managing major skin traumas.
5. How should wounds be managed to avoid serious infections?
6. Characterize the viruses that are associated with common skin infections.
7. What bacterial skin infections are commonly seen?
8. Tinea (ringworm) is a fungus that can be present on different parts of the body. Name the body parts.
9. How may skin infections related to microorganisms be avoided?
10. Why is candidiasis considered one of the most serious fungal infections?
11. What allergic, thermal, and chemical skin reactions could an individual sustain in the typical sports environment?
12. Different parts of the United States have their own problems with insects that infect the skin of humans. Identify the insects in your area that can cause problems. How may they be avoided?

## REFERENCES

1. Adams B: Skin infections in athletes, *Expert Review of Dermatology* 5(5):567–77, 2010.
2. American Red Cross: *First-aid—Responding to emergencies,* Samford, CT, 2007, Staywell.
3. Anderson B: Managing herpes gladiatorum outbreaks in competitive wrestling: The 2007 Minnesota experience, *Current Sports Medicine Reports* 7(6):323–27, 2008.
4. Atiyeh B: Wound cleansing, topical antiseptics and wound healing, *Int Wound J* 6(6):420–30, 2009.
5. Ayello E: Skip the knife: Debriding wounds without surgery, *Nursing* 32(9):58–63, 2002.
6. Bailey E: Cellulitis: diagnosis and management, *Dermatol Ther* 24(2):229–39, 2011.
7. Basler R: Athletic skin injuries: Combating pressure and friction, *Physician Sportsmed* 32(5):33, 2005.
8. Beam J: Effects of occlusive dressings on healing of partial-thickness abrasions, *Athletic Training and Sports Health Care* 4(2):58–66, 2012.
9. Beam J: Occlusive dressings and the healing of standardized abrasions, *J Athl Train*, 43(6):600–07, 2008.
10. Beam J: Tissue adhesive for simple traumatic lacerations, *J Athl Train* 43(2):222–24, 2008.
11. Berger T: Dermatologic disorders. In McPhee S, ed: *Current medical diagnosis and treatment*, New York, 2012, McGraw-Hill.
12. Bobo L: Photoallergic contact dermatitis (PACD) caused by sunscreen lotion, *Athletic Therapy Today* 14(6):15, 2009.

13. Brooks C: Cutaneous allergic reactions induced by sporting activities, *Sports Med* 33(9):699, 2003.
14. Canadian Medical Association: Sports dermatology, Part 1: Common dermatoses, *Canadian Medical Assoc J* 171(8):85, 2004.
15. Cernik C: The treatment of herpes simplex infections: An evidence-based review, *Archives of Internal Medicine* 168(11):137–44, 2008.
16. Chaby G: Dressings for acute and chronic wounds: A systematic review, *Arch Dermatol* 143(10):1297–1304, 2007.
17. Claus E: Comparison of the effects of selected dressings on the healing of standardized abrasions, *J Athl Train*, 33(2):145–49, 1998.
18. Cole C: Diagnosis and treatment of impetigo, *American Family Physician* 75(6):859–64, 2007.
19. Cyr P: Viral skin infections, *Physician Sportsmed* 32(7):33, 2004.
20. Davis J: Sun and active patients: Preventing acute and cumulative skin damage, *Physician Sportsmed* 28(7):79, 2000.
21. Dawson C: Treatment of friction blisters in professional baseball players, *Athletic Therapy Today* 9(3):62, 2004.
22. DeCampos J: Treatment options for primary hyperhidrosis, *American Journal of Clinical Dermatology* 13(2):139, 2012.
23. Dewald L: The ABCDs of skin cancer: A primer for athletic trainers and therapists, *Athletic Therapy Today* 7(3):29, 2002.

24. Dougherty T: Sports dermatology: What certified athletic trainers and therapists need to know, *Athletic Therapy Today* 8(3):46, 2003.
25. Dumville J: Tissue adhesives for closure of surgical incisions, *Cochrane Database Syst Rev*, 11:CD004287, 2014.
26. Ediger M: Closure options for skin lacerations, *Athletic Therapy Today* 15(2):7, 2010.
27. Elston D: Tick bites and skin rashes, *Current Opinions in Infectious Diseases* 23(2):132–38, 2010.
28. Farion K: Tissue adhesives for traumatic lacerations in children and adults, *Cochrane Database Syst Rev* (3): CD003326, 2002.
29. Fernandez R: Effectiveness of solutions, techniques and pressure in wound cleansing, *JBI Reports* 2(7):231–70, 2004.
30. Fernandez R: Water for wound cleansing, *Cochrane Database Syst Rev,* 2:CD003861, 2012.
31. Field L: Tinea pedis in athletes, *International Journal of Dermatology* 47(5):485–92, 2008.
32. Freeman D: Corns and calluses resulting from mechanical hyperkeratosis, *American Family Physician* 65(11):2277–80, 2002.
33. Garner L: Poison ivy, oak, and sumac dermatitis: Identification, treatment, and prevention, *Physician Sportsmed* 27(5):33, 1999.
34. Glasser R: Simple ingrown toenail relief, *Physician Sportsmed* 33(7):17, 2005.
35. Glazer JL: Laceration care, *Physician Sportsmed* 30(7):50, 2002.

36. Griffiths C: Pathogenesis and clinical features of psoriasis, *The Lancet*, 370(9583):21–27, 2007.

37. Grouios G: Corns, calluses in athletes' feet: A cause for concern, *The Foot* 14(4):175–84, 2004.

38. Gupta A: Tinea corporis, tinea cruris, tinea nigra and piedra, *Dermatology Clinics* 21:395–400, 2003.

39. Habif T: *Clinical dermatology*, Philadelphia, PA, 2009, Elsevier Science.

40. Habif T: Skin disease: Diagnosis and treatment, Philadelphia, PA, 2005, Elsevier.

41. Hand J: Prevention of tinea corporis in collegiate wrestlers, *J Athl Train* 34(4):350, 1999.

42. Harrison S: Ultraviolet light and skin cancer in athletes, *Sports Health: A Multidisciplinary Approach* 1(4):335–40, 2009.

43. Heidelbaugh J: Management of the ingrown toenail, *American Family Physician* 79(4):303–308, 2009.

44. Hood R: A prospective, randomized pilot evaluation of topical triple antibiotic versus mupirocin for the prevention of uncomplicated soft tissue wound infection, *Am J Emerg Med* 22(1):1–3, 2004.

45. Hutchinson J: Occlusive dressings: A microbiologic and clinical review, *Am J Infect Control* 18(4):257–68, 1990.

46. Johnson R: Herpes gladiatorum and other skin diseases, *Clinics Sports Med* 23(3):473, 2004.

47. Kahanov L: Certified athletic trainers' knowledge of methicillin-resistant staphylococcus aureus and common disinfectants, *J Athl Train* 46(4):415–23, 2011.

48. Kockentiet B: Contact dermatitis in athletes, *Journal of the American Academy of Dermatology* 56(6):1048–55, 2007.

49. Kohl T: Berks County Scholastic Athletic Trainers' Association: Wrestling mats: Are they a source of ringworm infections? *J Athl Train* 35(4):427, 2000.

50. Kramer S. Effect of providone-iodine on wound healing: A review, *J Vasc Nurs* 17(1):17–23, 1999.

51. Krautheim A: Chlorhexidine anaphylaxis: Case report and review of the literature, *Contact Dermatitis* 50(3):113–16, 2004.

52. Landry G: Dermatological pathologies. In Landry G. ed: *Essentials of primary care sports medicine*, Champaign, IL, 2003, Human Kinetics.

53. Landry G: Herpes and tinea in wrestling, *Physician Sportsmed* 32(10):34, 2004.

54. Leski M: Common dermatological conditions in sports: A review of environmental, traumatic, and infectious causes, *Athletic Therapy Today* 7(3):8, 2002.

55. Likness L: Common dermatologic infections in athletes and return to play guidelines, *Journal of the American Osteopathic Association* 111(6):373–79, 2011.

56. Lineaweaver W: Topical antimicrobial toxicity, *Arch Surg* 120(3):267–70, 1985.

57. List P: MRSA skin infections: What athletic trainers need to know, *Athletic Therapy Today* 10(4):51, 2005.

58. Lock P: The effects of temperature on mitotic activity at the edge of experimental wounds, *Symposia on Wound Healing: Plastic Surgical and Dermatological Aspects*, 1980.

59. Marshall S: Sunscreen use and malignant melanoma risk: The jury's still out, *Am J Public Health* 93(1):11, 2003.

60. Moffit J: Allergic reactions to insect stings and bites, *Southern Medical Journal* 96(11):1073–79, 2003.

61. Myer A: Dressings. In Kloth L, ed: *Wound healing alternatives in management*, Philadelphia, PA, 2002, F.A. Davis Company.

62. Myers B: *Wound management: Principles and practice*, Upper Saddle River, NJ, 2008, Pearson Prentice Hall.

63. National Institute for Health and Clinical Excellence: *Surgical site infection: Prevention and treatment of surgical site infection*, www.nice.org.uk /guidance/cg74/resources/surgical-site-infections-prevention-and-treatment-975628422853, 2008.

64. Pecci M: Skin conditions in the athlete, *Am J Sports Med* 37(2):406–18, 2009.

65. Pleacher M: Cutaneous fungal and viral infections in athletes, *Clinics in Sports Medicine* 26(3):397–411, 2007.

66. Rabenberg V: The bactericidal and cytotoxic effects of antimicrobial wound cleansers, *J Athl Train* 37(1):51–54, 2002.

67. Redziniak D: Methicillin-resistant staphylococus aureus (MRSA) in the athlete, *International Journal of Sports Medicine* 30(8):557–62, 2009.

68. Rhoads J: Managing bites and stings, *The Nurse Practitioner* 34(8):37–43, 2009.

69. Robinson J: Prevention of melanoma with regular sunscreen use, *JAMA* 306(3): 302–03, 2011.

70. Romano R: Outbreak of community-acquired methicillin-resistant staphylococcus aureus skin infections among a collegiate football team, *J Athl Train* 41(2):141, 2006.

71. Rush S: Sports dermatology, *ACSM's Health & Fitness Journal* 6(4):24, 2002.

72. Saben B: MRSA in athletes: What athletic trainers and therapists need to know, *Athletic Therapy Today* 14(6):28, 2009.

73. Scheinfeld N: Molluscum contagiosum, *SKINmed: Dermatology for the Clinician* 7(2):89–92, 2008.

74. Schnirring L: MRSA infections, *Physician Sportsmed* 32(10):12, 2004.

75. Simandl G: Alterations in skin function and integrity. In Porth C, ed: *Pathophysiology: Concepts of altered health states*, Philadelphia, PA, 2004, Lippincott, Williams and Wilkins.

76. Soroko Y: Treatment of plantar verrucae using 2% sodium salicylate iontophoresis, *Phys Ther* 82:1184, 2002.

77. Stulberg D: Pityriasis rosea, *Amercian Family Physician* 69(1):87–91, 2004.

78. Sutton A: *Dermatological disorders sourcebook*, Detroit, MI, 2005, Omnigraphics.

79. Tanzi E: Managing common nail disorders in active patients and athletes, *Physician Sportsmed* 27(9):35, 1999.

80. Thibodeau G: *Anatomy and physiology*, Philadelphia, PA, 2006, Elsevier Science.

81. Towler J: Cleansing traumatic wounds with swabs, water or saline. *J Wound Care*;10(6):231–34, 2001.

82. Waterbrook A: Do topical antibiotics help prevent infection in minor traumatic uncomplicated soft tissue wounds? *Ann Emerg Med* 61(1):86–88, 2013.

83. Wiechula R: The use of moist wound-healing dressings in the management of split-thickness skin graft donor sites: A systematic review, *Int J Nurs Pract* 9(2):S9–S17, 2003.

84. Winokur R: Fungal infections and parasitic infestations in sports, *Physician Sportsmed* 32(10):23, 2004.

85. Wolff K: Fitzpatrick's color atlas and synopsis of clinical dermatology, New York, 2009, McGraw-Hill.

86. Zinder S: National Athletic Trainers' Association position statement: Skin diseases, *J Athl Train* 45(4):411–28, 2010.

# ANNOTATED BIBLIOGRAPHY

Bolognia J, Jorizzo J, Rapini R: *Dermatology,* Philadelphia, PA, 2012, Elsevier Science.

*Features over 3,000 full-color photographs and line drawings; focuses on the clinical aspects of dermatology and includes only "need-to-know" basic science.*

DuViver A: *Atlas of clinical dermatology,* Philadelphia, PA, 2012, Elsevier Health Science.

*Covers the clinical aspects of skin disease, with an emphasis on how diagnosis can be made. Illustrated with more than 2,000 color photographs.*

Habif T: *Clinical dermatology: A color guide to diagnosis and therapy,* Philadelphia, PA, 2009, Elsevier Science.

*An illustrated guide to the diagnosis and treatment of skin abnormalities and diseases, covering various topical therapies as well as specific skin diseases, such as dermatitis, warts, and tumors.*

James W, Berger T: *Andrew's diseases of the skin: Clinical dermatology,* Philadelphia, PA, 2011, Elsevier Health Sciences.

*Covers clinical presentation and therapy for a full range of common and rare skin diseases.*

Kloth L, McCulloch JM: *Wound healing: Alternatives in management,* ed 3, Philadelphia, PA, 2002, F.A. Davis.

*Originally intended for physical therapists; appropriate for any health professional involved in the management of wounds.*

Wolff K: *Fitzpatrick's color atlas and synopsis of clinical dermatology,* New York, 2009, McGraw-Hill.

*Presents an outstanding and varied array of skin conditions, from the most common to those that are life threatening.*

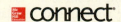

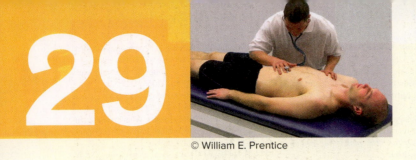

© William E. Prentice

# 29

# Additional General Medical Conditions

## ■ Objectives

*When you finish this chapter you should be able to*

- Analyze the role of the immune system in preventing disease.
- Differentiate different viral infections that may affect the patient.
- Identify symptoms and signs of respiratory infections.
- Categorize disorders of the muscular system.
- Examine disorders associated with the nervous system.
- Recognize disorders of the vascular and lymphatic systems.
- Explain diabetes mellitus, and contrast diabetic coma and insulin shock.

- Indicate the causes of epilepsy and explain how to perform the appropriate action when a seizure occurs.
- Explain what causes hypertension and how it may be controlled.
- Describe the classic symptoms and signs of cancer.
- Compare and contrast the symptoms and signs of the most common sexually transmitted diseases.
- Explain menstrual irregularities and their effect.
- Review female reproduction and pregnancy.

## ■ Outline

## ■ Key Terms

malaise
coryza
photophobia
hemolysis

thrombi
embolus
bacteremia
epilepsy

benign
malignant
amenorrhea

## ■ Connect Highlights   connect

*Visit connect.mcgraw-hill.com for further exercises to apply your knowledge:*

- Clinical application scenarios covering identification and management of viral infections, respiratory infections; muscular, nervous, and vascular and lymphatic system disorders; and the female triad
- Click-and-drag questions covering identification, classification, and signs and symptoms of viral infections; respiratory infections; muscular, nervous, and vascular and lymphatic system disorders
- Multiple-choice questions covering role of the immune system; viral and respiratory infections; disorders to the muscular, nervous, and vascular and lymphatic systems; diabetes; cancer; sexually transmitted diseases; and the female triad

In addition to the many injuries that have been discussed in previous chapters, a variety of additional medical conditions can affect a patient. When illnesses occur, it is the athletic trainer's responsibility to recognize these conditions and to follow up with appropriate care. Appropriate care for the illnesses and conditions discussed in this chapter often means referring the patient to a physician to provide medical care that is beyond the scope of the athletic trainer. The information provided in this chapter serves as a reference for the athletic trainer in making appropriate decisions regarding care of the sick patient.

## THE ROLE OF THE IMMUNE SYSTEM

The immune system is not an organ system but is instead a collection of disease-fighting cells populating the lymphatic and other organ systems that recognize the presence of foreign substances in the body and act to neutralize or destroy them.[62] Illness results when the immune system fails to neutralize or destroy the invading offender. Immunity means being protected from a disease by having been previously exposed to an invading agent, called an *antigen.* Immunity may be acquired *actively,* as a result of a natural infection or invasion of antigens, or *passively* from inoculation.[69]

An immune response disposes of the antigen and thus prevents damage. The immune response may be *cell-mediated,* in which lymphocytes (T cells) are produced by the thymus in response to the antigen exposure. There may also be a *humoral immune response,* in which plasma lymphocytes (B cells) are produced, with the subsequent formation of *antibodies.* An innate, or *nonspecific, immune response*—inflammation—is the reaction of the tissues to injury from trauma, chemicals, or ischemia that always occurs, regardless of the cause. These are all positive responses that collectively destroy or neutralize an antigen.[38]

However, an autoimmune response directed against an individual's own tissues causes damage. Autoimmune diseases include diabetes mellitus, rheumatoid arthritis, multiple sclerosis, hemolytic anemia, myasthenia gravis, and HIV.[33]

## VIRAL INFECTIONS

Everyone is susceptible to viral infections. Among the more common viral infections are rhinovirus (common cold), influenza (flu), infectious mononucleosis, rubella (German measles), rubeola (measles), parotitis (mumps), and varicella (chicken pox).

### Rhinovirus (Common Cold)

*Etiology* More than 100 different rhinoviruses cause colds. The common cold is the most prevalent of all communicable diseases. It is as an upper respiratory infection transmitted by either direct or indirect contact. One method of infection is by touching a contaminated article and then rubbing the eyes.[45]

*Symptoms and signs* Frequently, the cold begins with a scratchy or sore throat, watery discharge or stopped-up nose, and sneezing. Not all colds follow the same pattern. In some instances, a secondary bacterial infection occurs, which produces a thickened, yellowish nasal discharge; watering eyes; mild fever; sore throat; headache; **malaise;** myalgia; and dry cough. In addition to the secondary infection can be laryngitis (hoarseness), tracheitis (irritation of the trachea), acute bronchitis, sinusitis, and even an inflammation of the middle ear (otitis media).[45]

*Management* Treatment of the common cold is symptomatic. Most colds last for 5 to 10 days regardless of treatment. Nonprescription cold medications may help ease some symptoms. To avoid colds, athletes should stay out of crowds, wash their hands frequently, avoid sharing personal items, eat a balanced diet, and drink at least eight 8-ounce glasses of water per day. Emotional stress and extreme fatigue should be avoided as much as possible.[73] Late in 2001, medical researchers developed the first medicine proven to reduce the length and severity of the common cold. The drug called *pleconaril* seems to cause the symptoms to clear up sooner than normal. It is thought that the medication attacks the rhinovirus.

The use of Breathe Right nasal strips has been recommended as a drug-free alternative for managing nasal congestion due to colds and allergies. When adhered to the nose, the nasal strips have two springlike pieces that pull upward, mechanically "lifting" open the nasal passages.[48] Many athletes routinely use these nasal strips to facilitate breathing (Figure 29–1).

### Influenza (Flu)

*Etiology* Influenza, commonly known as the flu, is one of the most persistent and debilitating diseases. It usually occurs in various forms as an annual epidemic that causes severe illness among the population.[43]

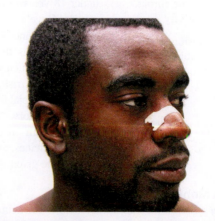

**FIGURE 29–1** Nasal strips mechanically lift open the nasal passages.
© William E. Prentice

Influenza is caused by myoviruses classified as types A, B, and C. Type A influenza is the most common and causes serious and widespread epidemics. The most recent epidemics were caused by type A/H1N1 virus (swine flu) in 2009 and type A/N5H1 virus (avian flu) in 2004. The virus controls the cell through its genetic material. The virus has to enter the cell through the membrane and later enters the nucleus. The virus multiplies and is released from the cell by a budding process, to be spread throughout the body. Not all athletes need influenza vaccines; however, athletes engaging in winter sports, basketball, wrestling, and swimming may require them.[47]

*Symptoms and signs* The patient with the flu has the following symptoms: fever, cough, headache, malaise, and inflamed respiratory mucous membranes with **coryza**.[46] Certain viruses can increase the body's core temperature. Flu generally has an incubation period of 48 hours and comes on suddenly, accompanied by chills and a fever of 102°F to 103°F (39°C to 39.5°C), which develops over a 24-hour period. The patient complains of a headache and general aches and pains—mainly in the back and legs. The headache increases in intensity, and the patient may develop **photophobia** and an aching at the back of the skull. There is often sore throat, burning in the chest, and in the beginning a nonproductive cough, which later may develop into bronchitis. The skin is flushed, and the eyes are inflamed and watery. The acute stage of the disease usually lasts up to 5 days. Weakness, sweating, and fatigue may persist for many days. Flu prevention includes avoiding infected persons and maintaining good resistance through healthy living. Vaccines, including those to cover prevalent strains, are often recommended to individuals to decrease the incidence or severity of illness.[45]

*Management* If the flu is uncomplicated, its management consists of bed rest and supportive care. During the acute stage, the temperature often returns to normal. Symptomatic care is the preferential treatment. But aspirin should be avoided in febrile illnesses for all individuals under 18 years of age because of Reye's syndrome. Amantadine and Relenza are medications that may be used for influenza A for individuals at risk. They are also beneficial for fever and respiratory symptoms.[59] Steam inhalation, cough medicines, and gargles may be given.

### Infectious Mononucleosis

*Etiology* Infectious mononucleosis is an acute viral disease that affects mainly young adults and children. Infectious mononucleosis, commonly called mono, is caused by the Epstein-Barr virus (EBV), a member of the herpes group.[32] It can produce severe fatigue and raise the risk of splenic rupture.[60] Incubation is 4 to 6 weeks. The EBV is carried in the throat and transmitted to another person through saliva. It has been called the kissing disease.[26]

*Symptoms and signs* The EBV syndrome usually starts with a 3- to 5-day prodrome of headache, fatigue, loss of appetite, and myalgia. From days 5 to 15, there is fever, swollen lymph glands, and a sore throat.[4] By the second week, 50 to 70 percent of those infected with EBV have an enlarged spleen, 10 to 15 percent have jaundice, and 5 to 15 percent have a skin rash, a pinkish flush to the cheeks, and puffy eyelids.[69] A blood test reveals an elevated white blood cell count. Complications include ruptured spleen, meningitis, encephalitis, hepatitis, and anemia.[26]

*Management* Treatment is supportive and symptomatic. Acetaminophen is often given for headache, fever, and malaise. Patients may resume easy training in 3 weeks after the onset of illness if (1) the spleen is not markedly enlarged or painful, (2) they are afebrile, (3) liver function tests are normal, and (4) pharyngitis and any complications have resolved.[60] A CT scan or ultrasound may be used to determine whether the spleen is enlarged.

### Rubella (German Measles)

*Etiology* Rubella is a highly contagious viral disease that usually occurs during childhood. Infection occurs between 13 and 24 days following exposure. If the disease occurs in the pregnant female, defects may occur in the developing fetus.[69]

*Symptoms and signs* Slight temperature elevation, sore throat, drowsiness, swollen lymph glands, and the appearance of red spots on the palate all occur for about 1 to 5 days prior to the appearance of a rash that occurs about 50 percent of the time. The rash begins on the face and forehead, spreads down the trunk and extremities, and lasts for about 3 days.[65]

*Management* Rubella is a viral infection and thus cannot be treated with antibiotics. To relieve minor discomfort, the patient can be given acetaminophen or ibuprofen. Aspirin should be avoided because its use in such cases has been associated with the development of Reye's syndrome. If body temperature rises above 102°F (39°C), a physician should be consulted. Otherwise, unless there are complications, rubella resolves on its own. Any pregnant female who has been exposed to rubella should contact her obstetrician immediately. Rubella may be prevented by early childhood immunization with a combination vaccine that prevents measles and mumps in addition to rubella (MMR).[65]

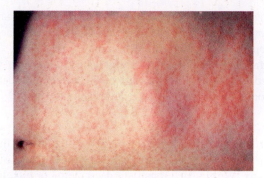

FIGURE 29–2  Measles.
CDC/Dr. Heinz F. Eichenwald

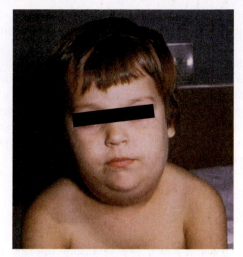

FIGURE 29–3  Mumps.
CDC/Public Health Image Library

### Rubeola (Measles)

*Etiology*  Like rubella, rubeola (measles) is a highly contagious disease that often occurs during childhood. An individual who once has this disease becomes immune to further exposure. The incubation period is approximately 10 days following exposure.[69]

*Symptoms and signs*  The onset of measles causes sneezing, nasal congestion, coughing, malaise, photophobia, spots in the mouth, conjunctivitis, and fever that may elevate to 104°F (39°C) at about 4 days. When the fever reaches that level, a rash appears, usually first on the face, as small, red spots that rapidly increase in size and spread to the trunk and extremities. The rash causes an uncomfortable itching. The rash lasts for about 5 days, after which the temperature returns to normal (Figure 29–2).[69]

*Management*  Any child who has not had measles should be inoculated with the MMR vaccine at 12 to 15 months and at 4 to 6 years. If measles do occur, bed rest, isolation in a darkened room, and the use of anti-pyretic and anti-itching medication can provide some relief while the disease runs its course.[65]

### Parotitis (Mumps)

*Etiology*  Mumps is a contagious viral disease that results in the inflammation of the parotid and other salivary glands. Mumps usually appears within 25 days following exposure.[65]

*Symptoms and signs*  Symptoms begin with malaise, headache, chills, and a moderate fever. There is pain in the neck below and in front of the ear, which progresses to marked swelling on one or both sides (Figure 29–3). Swelling may last for as long as 7 days. It is painful to move the jaw, and swallowing may be difficult. Saliva production may be either increased or decreased.[59] Adults who contract mumps often have significant symptoms.

*Management*  Immunization with MMR should be done in children older than 1 year to prevent the disease. If mumps does occur, the patient should be isolated while contagious, confined to bed rest, and given a soft diet. Analgesics may be used along with cold applications to control swelling; later, heat applications should be used.[59]

### Varicella (Chicken Pox)

*Etiology*  This highly contagious viral disease is caused by the varicella-zoster virus, which also causes herpes zoster, or shingles (discussed in Chapter 28). Children are vaccinated for varicella-zoster between 12 and 18 months, which significantly lowers the chances of getting chicken pox, although a patient may develop shingles later in life. Chicken pox may occur at any age but is much more likely to occur in children under the age of 15 years. The average incubation time is 13 to 17 days following exposure. An individual who has chicken pox is contagious for approximately 11 days, beginning 5 days before the first signs of a rash appear.[65]

*Symptoms and signs*  Chicken pox begins with a slight elevation in temperature for 24 hours, followed by an eruption of a rash. The rash first appears as individual red crops or spots, each of which progressively evolves through stages of macules, papules, vesicles, and crusts over a period of 2 to 3 days (Figure 29–4). The rash begins on the back and chest; relatively few lesions appear on the extremities.

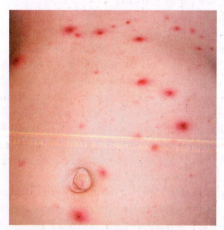

FIGURE 29–4  Chicken pox on torso.
Courtesy Dean Morrell, MD, Department of
Dermatology, University of North Carolina

Occasionally, infection occurs from scratching and rupturing the vesicles. A few scars nearly always remain. The disease may last for 2 to 3 weeks.[69]

***Management*** The administration of varicella-zoster immune globulin (VZIg) within 96 hours of exposure prevents clinical symptoms in normal, healthy children. Acyclovir medication should be administered to adolescents and adults within 24 hours following the appearance of symptoms. Anti-itch medication should be used to prevent scratching.[65]

# RESPIRATORY CONDITIONS

Individuals may be prone to conditions that affect the upper respiratory tract, which includes the nose, sinuses, throat, larynx, trachea, and bronchi.[24] Specific conditions discussed here include upper respiratory infections (URIs), sinusitis, pharyngitis (sore throat), tonsillitis, seasonal atopic rhinitis (hay fever), acute bronchitis, pneumonia, bronchial asthma, and cystic fibrosis.

> Respiratory tract infections can be highly communicable among sports team members.

## Sinusitis

***Etiology*** Sinusitis is an inflammation of the paranasal sinuses. It can stem from an upper respiratory infection caused by a variety of bacteria. As a result, nasal mucous membranes swell and block the ostium of the paranasal sinus. A pressure, occurring from an accumulation of mucus, produces pain.[28]

***Symptoms and signs*** The skin area over the sinuses may be swollen and painful to the touch. A headache and malaise may be present. A purulent nasal discharge may also occur.

***Management*** If the infection is purulent, antibiotics may be warranted. Steam inhalation and other nasal topical sprays containing oxymetazalone (e.g., Afrin) can produce vasoconstriction and drainage.

## Pharyngitis (Sore Throat)

***Etiology*** Acute inflammation of the throat, or pharyngitis, can be related to the common cold, influenza, or a more serious condition, such as mononucleosis.

Pharyngitis can be caused by a virus such as the Epstein-Barr virus of mononucleosis or by the *Streptococcus* bacterium, as in scarlet fever or tonsillitis.[59] Approximately 95 percent of all bacterial pharyngitis is caused by a streptococcal infection.[15] Transmission is often by direct contact with an actively infected person or one who is a carrier. The ingestion of contaminated food can lead to a streptococcal sore throat.[15]

***Symptoms and signs*** Pharyngitis is characterized by pain on swallowing, fever, inflamed and swollen lymph glands (called *lymphadenitis*), swollen tonsils, malaise, and weakness. The mucous membranes of the throat may be severely inflamed with a covering of purulent matter.[59] Laryngitis may develop due to an inflammation of the laryngeal mucosa, which causes hoarseness and occasionally pain. A throat culture for determining the presence of a streptococcal bacterial infection may be necessary.

***Management*** Topical gargles and rest may be warranted. Antibiotic therapy is given for a streptococcal infection to prevent scarlet fever and rheumatic fever.[69]

## Tonsillitis

***Etiology*** The tonsils are pieces of lymphatic tissue covered by epithelium that are found at the entrance of the pharynx. Within each tonsil are deep clefts, or pits, lined by lymphatic nodules. Ingested or inhaled pathogens collect in the pits and penetrate the epithelium, where they come in contact with lymphocytes and cause an acute inflammation and bacterial infection.[62] Complications include sinusitis, middle ear infections (otitis media), and tonsillar abcesses.

***Symptoms and signs*** The tonsils appear inflamed, red, and swollen, with yellowish exudate in the pits. The patient has difficulty swallowing and may have a relatively high fever with chills. Headache and pain in the neck and back may also be present.[69]

***Management*** The throat should be cultured to look for streptoccocal bacteria; if the culture is positive, antibiotics should be used for 10 days. Gargling with warm saline solution, a liquid diet, and antipyretic medication should all be recommended. Frequent bouts of tonsillitis may eventually necessitate surgical removal of the tonsils.[69]

## Seasonal Atopic (Allergic) Pollinosis (Hay Fever)

***Etiology*** Hay fever, or pollinosis, is an acute seasonal allergic condition that results from airborne pollens, dust, dander, or mold. These allergens can be found either outdoors or indoors.

Hay fever can occur during the spring as a reaction to pollens from trees, such as oak, elm, maple, alder, birch, and cottonwood. During the summer, grass and weed pollens can be the culprits. In the fall, ragweed pollen is the prevalent cause. Airborne fungal spores also have been known to cause hay fever. These substances act as allergens. The body's immune system produces allergic antibodies that release the chemical histamine, which produces the symptoms of hay fever.[15]

***Symptoms and signs*** In the early stages, the patient's eyes, throat, mouth, and nose begin to itch; these symptoms are followed by watering of the eyes, sneezing, and a clear, watery nasal discharge. The patient may complain of a sinus-type headache, emotional irritability, difficulty sleeping, red and swollen eyes and nasal mucous membranes, and a wheezing cough.[29] Other adverse allergic conditions are asthma, anaphylaxis, urticaria, angioedema, and rhinitis.[67]

***Management*** Most patients obtain relief from hay fever through oral antihistamines. However, antihistamines may cause a sedating effect that the patient must be aware of. The use of decongestants can cause a stimulating effect.

## Acute Bronchitis

*Etiology*   An inflammation of the mucous membranes of the bronchial tubes is called bronchitis. It occurs in both acute and chronic forms. If it occurs in a physically active individual, bronchitis is more likely to be in the acute form.[65]

Acute bronchitis usually occurs as an infectious winter disease that follows a common cold or other viral infection of the nasopharynx, throat, or tracheobronchial tree. Secondary to this inflammation is a bacterial infection that may follow overexposure to air pollution. Fatigue, malnutrition, or becoming chilled could be predisposing factors.

*Symptoms and signs*   The symptoms of a patient with acute bronchitis usually start with an upper respiratory infection, nasal inflammation and profuse discharge, slight fever, sore throat, and back and muscle pains.[39] A cough signals the beginning of bronchitis. In the beginning, the cough is dry, but in a few hours or days a clear mucous secretion begins, which becomes yellowish, indicating an infection. In most cases, the fever lasts 3 to 5 days, and the cough lasts 2 to 3 weeks or longer. The patient may wheeze, and rales may be present when auscultation of the chest is performed. Pneumonia can complicate bronchitis. To avoid bronchitis, a patient should not sleep in an area that is extremely cold or exercise in extremely cold air without wearing a face mask to warm inhaled air.[62]

*Management*   Management of acute bronchitis requires that the patient rest until fever subsides, drink 3 to 4 quarts (3 to 4 liters) of water per day, and ingest an antipyretic analgesic, a cough suppressant, and an antibiotic (when severe lung infection is present) on a daily basis.

## Pneumonia

*Etiology*   Pneumonia is an infection of the alveoli and bronchioles that may be caused by viral, bacterial, or fungal microorganisms. It may also be caused by irritation from chemicals, aspiration of vomitus, or other agents.[47] The alveolar spaces become filled with exudate, inflammatory cells, and fibrin.

*Symptoms and signs*   If the cause of pneumonia is bacterial, there is a rapid onset. High fever with chills, pain on inspiration, decreased breath sounds and rhonchi on auscultation, and the coughing up of purulent, yellowish sputum are all associated with bacterial pneumonia. Although most patients with bacterial pneumonia get sick very quickly, the symptoms of viral pneumonia usually go on for several days to a few weeks.[24] The patient experiences a low-grade fever (less than 102°F [39°C]), muscle aches, and fatigue and coughs up small amounts of mucus. Certain types of fungus can also cause pneumonia. When the fungus is inhaled, some individuals develop symptoms of acute pneumonia and others develop a form that lasts for months, although most patients experience few, if any, symptoms.

*Management*   Bacterial pneumonia must be treated with antibiotics. Deep breathing exercises and removal of sputum through a productive cough are helpful. Analgesics and antipyretics may also be useful for controlling pain and fever.[24] With viral pneumonia, the patient should be encouraged to rest and stay well hydrated.

## Asthma

*Etiology*   Asthma is one of the most common respiratory diseases. The exact cause of asthma is not clear. Metabolic acidosis, postexertional hypocapnia, stimulation of tracheal irritant receptors, adrenergic abnormalities (such as a defective catecholamine metabolism), and psychological factors have been suggested as possible causes. Asthma can be triggered by a number of stressors, such as a viral respiratory tract infection, emotional upset, changes in barometric pressure or temperature, inhalation of a noxious odor, exposure to a specific allergen, or exercise.[50] Asthma that is triggered by exercise is known as *exercise-induced asthma (EIA)*.[72] It is also referred to as *exercise-induced bronchospasm (EIB)*. An exercise-induced asthmatic attack can be stimulated by exercise in some individuals; in others, the attack may be provoked, only on rare occasions, during moderate exercise. Loss of heat and water causes the greatest loss of airway reactivity. Sinusitis can also trigger an attack in an individual with chronic asthma. EIA may be the only asthma condition the patient has.[37] A link to the NATA consensus statement "Management of asthma in the athlete" can be found at www.nata.org/sites/default/files/MgmtOfAsthmaInAthletes.pdf.

*Symptoms and signs*   Asthma is characterized by a spasm of the smooth muscle walls of the bronchioles, causing a narrowing of the airway, edema, and inflammation of the mucous membrane, producing copious amounts of mucus (Figure 29–5).[30] Bronchoconstriction occurs in the bronchioles. Difficulty breathing may cause the patient to hyperventilate, resulting in dizziness. The attack may begin with chest tightness, coughing, wheezing, shortness of breath, and fatigue.[71] The patient may show signs of nausea, hypertension,[71] respiratory stridor (high-pitched noise on respiration), headaches, and redness of the skin. Symptoms may occur within 8 minutes of strenuous activity.[57] Patients who have a chronic inflammatory asthmatic condition (bronchiectasis) characteristically have a constant dilation of the bronchi or bronchioles.

*Management*   A regular exercise program can benefit asthmatics.[51] The patient should engage in gradual warmups and cool-downs.[14] Swimming produces the fewest bronchospasms, which may be a result of the moist, warm environment. A mask or scarf may be beneficial in avoiding cold, dry air. Conditioning reduces bouts of asthma.[57] The duration of exercise should build slowly to 30 to 40 minutes, four or five times a week. Exercise intensity and loading also should be graduated slowly—for example, 10 to 30 seconds of work followed by 30 to 90 seconds of rest. Slow nasal breathing is suggested, and patients should avoid exercising in areas with high levels of air pollution or high pollen counts.[57]

Many patients with chronic or exercise-induced asthma use an inhaled bronchodilator (see Table 17–6). The most commonly prescribed B$_2$ agonist for asthma is

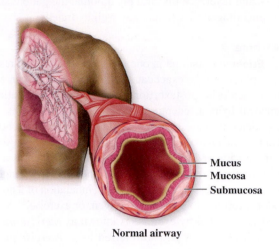

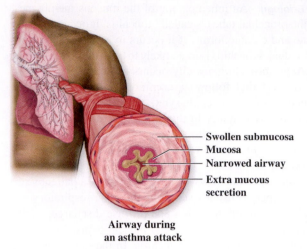

Mucus
Mucosa
Submucosa

Normal airway

Swollen submucosa
Mucosa
Narrowed airway
Extra mucous
secretion

Airway during
an asthma attack

FIGURE 29–5   The airway becomes constricted and narrowed during an asthma attack.

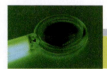

A soccer player has a history of exercise-induced asthma (EIA).

**?** How should the patient avoid incidences of EIA?

albuterol, which acts for about 2 hours. Salmeterol provides a prophylaxis for up to 12 hours. Albuterol should be administered 15 minutes before exercise; salmeterol, 30 to 60 minutes before exercise. Cromolyn sodium should be inhaled 30 minutes before exercise. Metered-dose inhalers are preferred for administration (see Figure 17–1).[71] It has also been found

that prophylactic use of the bronchodilator 15 minutes before exercise delays the symptoms by 2 to 4 hours.[14] Asthmatic athletes who receive medication for their condition should make sure that what they take is legal for competition.[50] *Focus Box 29–1:* "Management of the acute asthmatic attack" provides specific recommendations.

### Cystic Fibrosis

*Etiology*   Cystic fibrosis is a genetic disorder that can affect many different body systems; it can manifest as a type of chronic obstructive pulmonary disease, as pancreatic deficiency, as urogenital dysfunction, and as increased electrolytes in sweat.[74] It usually begins in infancy and is a major cause of severe chronic lung disease in children. Maximum life expectancy is about 30 years.

## FOCUS 29–1  Focus on Therapeutic Intervention

### Management of the acute asthmatic attack

Patients who have a history of asthma usually know how to care for themselves when an attack occurs. However, the athletic trainer must be aware of what to look for and what to do if called on.

*Early symptoms and signs*

- Anxious appearance
- Sweating and paleness
- Flared nostrils
- Breathing with pursed lips
- Fast breathing (hyperventilation)
- Vomiting
- Hunched-over body posture
- Physical fatigue unrelated to activity
- Indentation in the notch below the Adam's apple
- Sinking in of rib spaces as the patient inhales

- Coughing for no apparent reason
- Excessive throat clearing
- Irregular, labored breathing or wheezing
- Tingling and numbness in hands and feet

*Actions to take*

- Attempt to relax and reassure the patient.
- If medication has been cleared by the physician, have the patient use it.
- Encourage the patient to drink water.
- Have the patient perform controlled breathing along with relaxation exercises.
- If an environmental factor triggering the attack is known, remove it or the patient from the area.
- If these procedures do not help, immediate medical attention may be necessary.

**Symptoms and signs**  A number of physical symptoms may exist, including bronchitis, pneumonia, respiratory failure, gallbladder disease, pancreatitis, diabetes, and nutritional deficiencies. There is an abnormally high production of mucous secretions in the lungs and susceptibility to heat illnesses.[52]

**Management**  Drug therapy, including ibuprofen, can help slow the progress of the disease. Antibiotics are used to control pulmonary disease. The patient must undergo consistent postural drainage, using a cupping or hacking massage technique followed by deep breathing and coughing to help mobilize secretions. High fluid intake to thin the secretions and the breathing of humidified air are also recommended.[74]

# MUSCULAR SYSTEM DISORDERS

The muscular system suffers from fewer disorders than other systems do. However, two serious muscular disorders are Duchenne muscular dystrophy and myasthenia gravis.

## Duchenne Muscular Dystrophy

**Etiology**  Duchenne muscular dystrophy is a hereditary disease in which there is degeneration of skeletal muscle with an associated loss in strength.[42] Muscle tissue is gradually replaced by adipose and fibrous connective tissue. This connective tissue impedes circulation, which accelerates the degenerative process. Onset is usually in early childhood, between the ages of 2 and 10 years.[9]

**Symptoms and signs**  The problem begins to appear as the child learns to walk; he or she takes frequent falls and has difficulty standing up. The progressive degeneration first affects the hips, then the legs, and finally the abdominal and spinal musculature. Muscles tend to shorten as they atrophy, which causes scoliosis and other postural abnormalities.[9]

**Management**  Duchenne muscular dystrophy cannot be cured; however, consistent exercise can retard muscle atrophy. Individuals may ambulate with braces for a while before they are confined to a wheelchair. Death usually occurs before the age of 20.[42]

## Myasthenia Gravis

**Etiology**  Myasthenia gravis is an autoimmune disease in which antibodies attack the synaptic junctions between nerves and muscles. A deficiency in aceytlcholine (a neurotransmitter) creates an abnormality that produces early fatigue of skeletal muscle.[12] Myasthenia gravis occurs most often in females between the ages of 20 and 40 years.

**Symptoms and signs**  One of the first signs is a drooping of the upper eyelid and double vision due to weakness in the extraocular muscles. Following the initial symptoms, there may be difficulty in chewing and swallowing, weakness of the extremities, and a general decrease in muscular endurance.[12]

**Management**  The disease may be treated with drugs that inhibit the breakdown of aceytlcholine, enabling it to stimulate the muscle for longer periods. Corticosteroids may also be used to suppress the immune system and thus reduce the production of antibodies that destroy acetylcholine receptors.[12]

# NERVOUS SYSTEM DISORDERS

Disorders that can affect the nervous system include meningitis, multiple sclerosis, amyotrophic lateral sclerosis, and reflex sympathetic dystrophy.

## Meningitis

**Etiology**  Meningitis is an inflammation of the meninges, or membranes, that surround the spinal cord and brain. Viral, or "aseptic," meningitis, which is the most common type, is caused by an infection with one of several types of viruses. About 90 percent of cases are caused by a group of viruses known as enteroviruses.[19] Viral meningitis is serious but rarely fatal. The symptoms last for 7 to 10 days, and the patient usually recovers completely. Bacterial meningitis, on the other hand, can be very serious and result in disability or death if not treated promptly.[19] Meningococcus bacteria enter the central nervous system through the nose or throat, following infections of the ear, throat, or respiratory tract. The bacteria get into the arachnoid or pia mater, and inflammation spreads to the adjacent nervous tissue, causing swelling of the brain, enlargement of the ventricles, and hemorrhage of the brain stem.[19] Meningitis occurs in patients of all ages and recently has infected groups of college-aged students living in clustered dorms or personnel in military barracks. Meningitis is a serious disease in children; it usually occurs between the ages of 3 months and 2 years.

**Symptoms and signs**  Symptoms include a high fever, a stiff neck, an intense headache, and sensitivity to light and sound, and they progress to vomiting, convulsions, and coma. Often, the symptoms of viral and bacterial meningitis are the same.[69]

**Management**  The cerebrospinal fluid (CSF) must be analyzed for bacteria or viruses and the presence of white blood cells. CSF is taken through a puncture in the lumbar area, or spinal tap. If meningococcus bacteria are identified, isolation is necessary for at least 24 hours due to the highly contagious nature of the condition. Intravenous antibiotics must begin immediately.[19] Because of the severity of this condition, the patient should be monitored and treated in an intensive care unit. Individuals who have been in contact with a contagious patient should be given prophylactic antibiotics. No specific treatment for viral meningitis exists at this time. Most patients completely recover on their own. Doctors often recommend bed rest, plenty of fluids, and medicine to relieve the fever and headache.

## Multiple Sclerosis

***Etiology*** Multiple sclerosis (MS) is an autoimmune inflammatory disease of the central nervous system that causes deterioration and permanent damage to the myelin sheath that surrounds each nerve cell axon.[66] Nerve conduction is disrupted, causing diverse symptoms. MS most often affects individuals between the ages of 20 and 40 years. There is currently no cure.[65]

***Symptoms and signs*** Specific signs depend on the part of the nervous system that is affected, and damage may occur in several locations. Blurred vision with blind spots, speech defects, tremors, and muscle weakness and numbness in the extremities are common. Some people experience tremor, spasticity, and unusual behavior that involves mood swings. The disease may progress steadily, or there may be acute attacks followed by partial or complete temporary remission of symptoms.[66]

***Management*** Management involves dealing with the symptoms as they appear and disappear. The individual should avoid overexertion and fatigue, exposure to extreme temperatures, and stressful situations. A regular plan for daily activity and exercise should be established. Several drugs, including interferon, appear to slow the progression of the disease.[69]

## Amyotrophic Lateral Sclerosis

***Etiology*** Amyotrophic lateral sclerosis (ALS), also known as Lou Gehrig's disease, involves a sclerosis of the lateral regions of the spinal cord along with degeneration of motor neurons and significant atrophy of muscles.[27]

***Symptoms and signs*** There is a distinction between upper and lower trunk disease in ALS. Those with upper disease have a much worse prognosis than those with lower. Symptoms include difficulty in speaking, swallowing, and using the hands. However, sensory and intellectual functions remain intact. There is rapid progression of muscle atrophy, usually resulting in paralysis and confinement to a wheelchair.[27]

***Management*** Although there is no cure for this devastating disease, the individual who is totally incapacitated still has normal intellectual function but simply is unable to communicate feelings and ideas.[27] Eighty percent of ALS patient die within 3–5 years of diagnosis.[65]

## Complex Regional Pain Syndrome (CRPS)

***Etiology*** Complex regional pain syndrome, previously called reflex sympathetic dystrophy (RSD) or causalgia, is an abnormal and excessive response of the sympathetic portion of the autonomic nervous system that occurs following injury.[61] Most commonly, it is seen in the hand or the foot, resulting from the immobilization of an injured part due to pain. It has been associated with injuries to bone, soft tissue, nerve, and blood vessels.

***Symptoms and signs*** There is a series of changes, mediated by the sympathetic nervous system, that progressively result in extreme hypersensitivity to touch, redness, sweating, burning/aching pain, swelling with palpable tightness and shining of the skin, and atrophy. Symptoms may persist for months and even as long as a year. With ongoing chronic pain, there is certainly a potential for psychological depression to occur.[61]

***Management*** Early recognition and intervention are essential for a good prognosis. Treatment should be directed at disrupting the abnormal sympathetic response. A sympathetic ganglion nerve block administered by a physician is critical to treatment. Active range of motion exercise through a pain-free range along with the use of various therapeutic modalities for managing pain and reducing swelling also have been recommended. If symptoms persist for months, antidepressant medication may be necessary.[61]

> A gymnast has been casted for a radial styloid fracture from falling off the balance beam. She comes into the sports medicine clinic concerned about her hand, which looks swollen and red and is extremely sensitive to the touch.
>
> **?** What should the athletic trainer be concerned about?

# BLOOD AND LYMPH DISORDERS

Diseases that can affect the vascular and lymphatic systems include anemias, hemophilia, and lymphangitis.

**Iron-Deficiency Anemia** Iron deficiency is the most common cause of true anemia among athletes. Stores of iron are depleted before clinical signs occur. Iron is stored mainly in blood hemoglobin (64 percent) and bone marrow (27 percent).[17] Iron-deficiency anemia is most prevalent among menstruating females, and among males, 11 to 14 years of age.[31]

***Etiology*** Three conditions occur during anemia: erythrocytes (red blood cells) are too small, hemoglobin is decreased, and ferritin concentration is low. Ferritin is an iron-phosphorus-protein complex that normally contains 23 percent iron. There are many ways that individuals can become iron deficient. Gastrointestinal (GI) losses are common in runners because of bowel ischemia. Aspirin or NSAIDs may cause GI blood loss. Runners absorb 16 percent of iron from the GI tract compared with 30 percent in nonathletes who are iron deficient.[17] Menstrual losses account for most iron loss in females. Average menstrual iron loss is 0.6 to 1.5 mg per day. Inadequate dietary intake of iron is the primary cause of iron deficiency. The recommended daily allowance (RDA) is 15 mg per day for females and 10 mg per day for males. The average diet contains 5 to 7 mg of iron per 100 kcal. Because many females eat less than they need, they also fail to consume enough iron. Also, individuals who are vegetarians might lack iron.[31]

***Symptoms and signs*** In the first stages of iron deficiency, performance begins to decline. The patient may complain of burning thighs and nausea from becoming anaerobic. Ice craving is also common. Patients with mild iron-deficiency anemia may display some mild impairment in their maximum performance. Determining serum ferritin is the most accurate test of iron status. Two factors must be checked by the physician: the patient's mean corpuscular volume (MCV), which is the average volume of individual cells in a cubic micron, and the relative sizes of the erythrocytes.

***Management*** Individuals can manage iron deficiency in the following ways: eat a proper diet, including more red meat or dark poultry; avoid coffee and tea, which hamper iron absorption from grains; ingest vitamin C sources, which enhance iron absorption; and take an iron supplement (dosage depends on the degree of anemia).[17]

### Runners' Anemia

***Etiology*** Runners' anemia, or **heelstrike hemolysis,** is the second most prevalent cause of iron deficiency in athletes. The cause of runners' anemia, as its name implies, is the impact of the foot as it strikes the surface. Impact forces destroy normal erythrocytes within the vascular system.[65] Excessive turbulence in the blood is also postulated as a cause of runners' anemia. Swimmer's also get this so it is not only because of the running.

***Symptoms and signs*** Heelstrike hemolysis is characterized by mildly enlarged red cells, an increase in circulatory reticulocytes, and a decrease in the concentration of haptoglobin, which is a glycoprotein bound to hemoglobin and released into the plasma. Even if the patient wears a well-designed and well-constructed running shoe, this condition can occur. Runners' anemia varies according to the amount of running performed.

***Management*** The only way to manage runners' anemia is by reducing running distance.

### Sickle-Cell Anemia

***Etiology*** Sickle-cell anemia is a chronic, hereditary hemolytic anemia. The frequency of the genetic defect responsible for this disorder is highest in the African American, Native American, and Mediterranean populations.[1] In these populations, 8 to 13 percent are not anemic but carry this trait in their genes. If both parents carry the defective gene, the child will still have sickle-cell anemia; if only one parent carries the gene, the child will still have the sickle-cell trait.[1] The person with sickle-cell anemia or the trait can have sickle-shaped red blood cells. The person with the sickle-cell trait may participate in physical activity and never encounter problems until symptoms are brought on by some stress or unusual circumstance.[18]

Individuals with sickle-cell anemia have red cells that are sickle-, or crescent-, shaped.[62] Within the red cells, an abnormal type of hemoglobin exists. It has been speculated that the sickling of the red blood cells results from an adaptation to malaria, which is prevalent in Africa.

The sickle cell has less potential for transporting oxygen and is fragile when compared with normal cells. A sickle cell's life span is 15 to 25 days, compared with the 120 days of a normal red cell; the short life of the sickle cell can produce severe anemia in individuals with acute sickle-cell anemia.[62] The cell's distorted shape inhibits its passage through the small blood vessels and can cause clustering of the cells and, consequently, clogging of the blood vessels and thus ischemia. This clogging produces **thrombi,** which block circulation. For individuals with this condition, death can occur (in the severest cases of sickle-cell anemia) from a stroke, heart disease, or an **embolus** in the lungs. Conversely, persons with the sickle-cell trait may never experience any problems. Four factors of exercise can cause sickling: acidosis; hyperthermia; dehydration of red blood cells, which increases hemoglobin concentration; and severe hypoxemia.[1] A link to the NATA consensus statement "Sickle cell trait and the athlete" can be found at www.nata.org/sites/default/files/SickleCellTraitAndTheAthlete.pdf.

***Symptoms and signs*** A patient may never experience any complications from having the sickle-cell trait. However, a sickle-cell crisis can be brought on by exposure to high altitudes or by overheating of the skin, as is the case with a high fever. Crisis symptoms include fever, severe fatigue, skin pallor, muscle weakness, and severe pain in the limbs and abdomen.[18] Abdominal pain in the upper-left quadrant may indicate a splenic syndrome in which there is an infarction.[1] This syndrome is especially characteristic of a crisis triggered by a decrease in ambient oxygen while the individual is flying at high altitudes. The patient may also experience headache and convulsions.

***Management*** Treatment of a sickle-cell crisis is usually symptomatic. The physician may elect to give anticoagulants and analgesics for pain.[1]

### Hemophilia

***Etiology*** Hemophilia is a hereditary disease characterized by a deficiency in any one of a number of clotting factors in the blood. Consequently, there is prolonged coagulation time, failure of the blood to clot, and abnormal bleeding.[22] Hemophilia occurs predominantly in males.

***Symptoms and signs*** In hemophiliacs, physical exertion can cause bleeding into muscles and joints, which can be extremely painful. Eventually, joints may become immobilized.[17,23]

***Management*** A hemophiliac who begins bleeding should be taken to an emergency medical care facility immediately.[21] Unfortunately, there is no cure for hemophilia, but concentrated clotting factors have been developed that can control the bleeding for several days. Patients may be taught to self-administer these clotting factors, should bleeding occur. The hemophiliac should avoid trauma and should wear a medical alert bracelet to alert care providers to his or her condition.[22,23]

## Lymphangitis

*Etiology*   Lymphangitis is an inflammation of the lymphatic channels; it is most often caused by streptococcal bacteria.[62] A bacterial infection may also occur in the blood, which is referred to as **bacteremia**.

*Symptoms and signs*   Lymphangitis usually occurs in the extremities. There is a deep reddening of the skin, warmth, lymphandentitis, and a raised border over the affected area, particularly in cases of infection. The condition is accompanied by an onset of chills and high fever with moderate pain and swelling. Lymphangitis is sometimes called blood poisoning.[62]

*Management*   The patient should be hospitalized and vital signs should be closely monitored. The affected extremity should be elevated and warm, moist compresses applied. Antibiotics should be administered, and fluid intake is encouraged to restore fluid balance.[69]

# ENDOCRINE SYSTEM DISORDERS

## Diabetes Mellitus

*Etiology*   Diabetes mellitus is a syndrome that results from an interaction of physical and environmental factors. Its etiology is not distinct. There is a complete or partial decrease in the secretion of insulin by the pancreas.[69]

Diabetics engaging in vigorous physical activity should eat before exercising, and if the exercise is protracted, should have hourly glucose supplementation.[34] As a rule, the insulin dosage is not changed, but food intake is increased. The response of diabetics varies among individuals and depends on many variables. Although there are some hazards, with proper medical evaluation and planning by a professional, diabetics can feel free to engage in most physical activities.[7] The most common types of diabetes are type 1, and type 2.[70] Type 1 diabetes is found primarily in individuals under 35 years of age and represents between 5 and 10 percent of all cases. Type 2 diabetes is most commonly associated with obesity and occurs in all age groups. It is becoming increasingly prevalent in younger individuals as childhood obesity increases. It represents 80 percent of all cases.[44]

*Symptoms and signs*   Type 1 may occur suddenly; symptoms include frequent urination, constant thirst; weight loss; constant hunger; tiredness and weakness; itchy, dry skin; and blurred vision. Type 2 is usually associated with being overweight. Diabetes can be diagnosed by measuring blood glucose levels. After fasting for 8 hours, plasma glucose levels in the blood should range between 60 and 109 mg/dl. If it is 126 mg/dl or higher, the patient is considered diabetic. It causes cells to resist the insulin

that is produced and available. Like type 1, type 2 can be a threat to the heart, kidneys, blood vessels, and eyes.[34]

*Management*   It is essential that blood glucose levels be controlled at acceptable levels. This control includes a balanced diet and, when needed, daily doses of insulin. Regular vigorous exercise can be effective in increasing peripheral insulin action to enhance glucose tolerance. Exercise, in general, improves the diabetic person's quality of life. It helps increase type I insulin sensitivity and use and may reduce long-term complications. In persons with type II diabetes, exercise decreases insulin resistance, improves glycemic control, and reduces or eliminates the need for insulin.[34] The athletic trainer should be aware that the diabetic can adversely respond to extreme temperature variations or to an unpredictable level of activity duration or intensity and may require rapid-acting carbohydrates.[7,34] A link to the NATA position statement "Management of the athlete with type 1 diabetes mellitus" can be found at www .nata.org/sites/default/files/mgmtofathletewithtype1diabete-smellitus.pdf.

It is important that athletic trainers who work with patients who have diabetes mellitus be aware of the major symptoms of diabetic coma and insulin shock and the proper actions to take when either one occurs.[44]

**Diabetic Coma**   If diabetes is not treated adequately through proper diet or too little insulin is produced, the diabetic can develop ketoacidosis.[44]

*Etiology*   A loss of sodium, potassium, and ketone bodies through excessive urination produces ketoacidosis, which can lead to coma.

*Symptoms and signs*   Symptoms and signs include labored breathing, fruity-smelling breath caused by acetone, nausea and vomiting, thirst, dry mucous membrane of the mouth, flushed skin, and mental confusion or unconsciousness followed by coma.[70]

> A diabetic field hockey player appears irritable and weak during practice. In the middle of a scrimmage, the player is unable to continue playing and has shallow respirations and a rapid heartbeat.
>
> **?** What is this patient experiencing, and how should it be treated?

*Management*   Because of the life-threatening nature of diabetic coma, early detection of ketoacidosis is essential. This can be accomplished by monitoring blood glucose levels prior to, during, and after activity. Urine can also be monitored for ketones with dipstick testing. The injection of insulin into the patient may in part help prevent coma.

### Insulin Shock

*Etiology*   Unlike diabetic coma, insulin shock occurs when the body has too much insulin and too little blood sugar; hypoglycemia results.[69]

**Symptoms and signs**   The patient complains of tingling in the mouth, hands, or other body parts; physical weakness; headaches; and abdominal pain. It may be observed that the patient has normal or shallow respirations, rapid heartbeat, and tremors, along with irritability and drowsiness.

**Management**   The diabetic patient who engages in intense exercise and metabolizes large amounts of glycogen could inadvertently take too much insulin and thus have a severe reaction.[44] To avoid this problem, the patient must adhere to a carefully planned diet that includes a snack before exercise. The snack should contain a combination of a complex carbohydrate and protein, such as cheese and crackers. Activities that last for more than forty minutes should be accompanied by snacks of simple carbohydrates. Some diabetics carry glucose packets or have candy or orange juice readily available in the event that an insulin reaction seems imminent.[49]

### Thyroid Gland Disorders

**Etiology**   The thyroid gland is located in the base of the neck on both sides of the lower larynx and upper trachea. It produces two hormones, thyroxine and triiodothyronine. Two disorders related to the function of the thyroid gland are *hyperthyroidism* and *hypothyroidism.*[69]

**Symptoms and signs**   Hyperthyroidism involves the overproduction of thyroxine and results in impaired glucose metabolism, increased metabolism, rapid fatigue during exercise, weight loss, and hyperthermia during exercise. *Graves' disease* is a form of hyperthyroidism that, in addition to the symptoms already mentioned, may lead to weakness, tremors, and difficulty swallowing and/or speaking. Hypothyroidism is a condition caused by deficient secretion of thyroid hormone, resulting in lowered metabolism, poor circulation, dry skin, low blood pressure, slow pulse, depressed muscle activity, intolerance to cold, increasing obesity, and potentially the development of a goiter, which is an enlargement of the thyroid gland.[26]

**Management**   A patient who shows signs of hyper- or hypothyroidism should be referred to a physician for diagnosis. The treatment for hyperthyroidism usually involves medication to slow the production of thyroxine or surgery to remove a part of the thyroid gland. The treatment of hypothyroidism most often involves hormone replacement therapy.

## SEIZURE DISORDERS

Berkow defines seizure disorders as "a recurrent paroxysmal disorder of cerebral function characterized by sudden, brief attacks of altered consciousness, motor activity, sensory phenomena, or inappropriate behavior caused by an abnormal excessive discharge of cerebral neurons."[59]

### Epilepsy

**Etiology**   Any recurrent seizure pattern is termed **epilepsy.** Epilepsy is not a disease but is a symptom that can be caused by a large number of underlying disorders.[36]

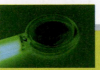

### FOCUS 29–2 Focus on Therapeutic Intervention

#### Management during a seizure

- Be emotionally composed.
- If possible, cushion the patient's fall.
- Keep the patient away from injury-producing objects by clearing the area.
- Loosen restrictive clothing.
- Allow the patient to awaken normally after the seizure.
- Do not restrain the patient during the seizure.

For some types of epilepsy, there is a genetic predisposition and a low threshold to having seizures. In others, altered brain metabolism or a history of injury may be the cause. A seizure can range from extremely brief episodes that last 5 to 15 seconds (petit mal seizures) to major episodes (tonic/clonic or grand mal seizures) that last a few minutes and include unconsciousness and uncontrolled tonic/clonic muscle contractions. There are approximately 1 million epileptics in the United States, most of whom can participate in some form of physical activity.[56] Activity-related injuries are not increased in the epileptic, nor is the sudden cardiac death syndrome linked to strenuous activity by the epileptic.[36]

**Symptoms and signs**   Each person with epilepsy must be considered individually as to whether he or she should engage in competitive sports. If an individual has daily or even weekly major seizures, collision sports should be prohibited. This prohibition is not because a hit on the head will necessarily trigger a seizure, but because a blow during participation that causes unconsciousness could result in a serious injury. If the seizures are properly controlled by medication or occur only during sleep, little, if any, sports restriction should be imposed, except for scuba diving, swimming alone, and participating in activities that occur at a great height.[36,56]

> Individuals who have major daily or weekly seizures should avoid collision sports.

**Management**   The epileptic patient commonly takes an anticonvulsant medication that is specific for the type and degree of seizures that occur. On occasion, the patient may experience some undesirable side effects from drug therapy, such as drowsiness, restlessness, nystagmus, nausea, vomiting, problems with balance, or skin rash.

When a patient with epilepsy becomes aware of an impending seizure, he or she should take measures to avoid injury, such as immediately sitting or lying down. When a seizure occurs without warning, the athletic trainer should follow the steps outlined in *Focus Box 29–2:* "Management during a seizure."

# HYPERTENSION (HIGH BLOOD PRESSURE)

***Etiology*** Excessive pressure applied against arterial walls while blood circulates is known as hypertension, or high blood pressure (HBP). A normal resting blood pressure is 120/80 mm/Hg (systolic/diastolic). Hypertension is classified as either primary (essential) or secondary.[3] Primary hypertension accounts for 90 percent of all cases and has no disease associated with it. Secondary hypertension is related to a specific underlying cause, such as kidney disorder, overactive adrenal glands, hormone-producing tumors, narrowing of the aorta, pregnancy, and medications (oral contraceptives, cold remedies, etc.). The presence of prolonged high blood pressure increases the chances of premature mortality and morbidity due to such causes as coronary artery disease, congestive heart failure, and stroke.[53]

> Hypertension may be a factor that excludes players from sports participation.

***Symptoms and signs*** Primary hypertension is usually asymptomatic until complications occur.[53] High blood pressure may cause dizziness, flushed appearance, headache, fatigue, epistaxis, and nervousness.

***Management*** The upper range of normal blood pressure is a systolic pressure of 120 mm/Hg and a diastolic pressure of 80 mm/Hg. The risk of death from heart disease and stroke begins to rise at blood pressures as low as 115 over 75, and it doubles for each 20 over 10 mm/Hg increase. Blood pressure is classified as follows: normal—less than 120/less than 80 mm/Hg; prehypertension—120–139/80–89 mm/Hg; Stage 1 hypertension—140–159/90–99 mm/Hg; Stage 2 hypertension—at or greater than 160/at or greater than 100 mm/Hg (Table 29–1).[53] Medication is not recommended for those with prehypertension unless it is required by another condition, such as diabetes or chronic kidney disease. However, those with prehypertension should make any needed lifestyle changes, including losing excess weight, becoming physically active, limiting alcoholic beverages, quitting smoking, and following a heart-healthy eating plan. It is recommended that those who have Stage 1 or 2 hypertension be on medication.

# CANCER

***Etiology*** Cancer is the second leading cause of death in adults, behind coronary artery disease. It is estimated that about 30 percent of all Americans will get cancer during their lifetime, and one of five will eventually die from it.[62] Cancer is a condition in which body cells no longer perform their normal functions. In general, cancer cells do not multiply at an increased rate. Instead, whatever causes cancer alters the cell's genetic makeup and changes the way it functions. This abnormal cell then divides, forming additional cancer cells; over a period of time, this tumor, or collection of abnormal cells, tends to invade and ultimately take over normal tissue.

***Tumors*** Tumors are either **benign** or **malignant.** Benign tumors typically pose only a small threat to a tissue and tend to remain confined in a limited space. Malignant tumors, though, grow out of control and spread. Unfortunately, malignancies can invade surrounding tissues and can spread via the blood and lymphatic systems (metastasize) to the entire body, making it difficult to control the cancer.[62]

Malignancies are classified according to the type of tissue in which they occur and according to the rate at which they affect the tissue. Although different types of cancer cells share similar characteristics, each is separate and distinct. Some types are relatively easy to cure, whereas others are difficult to cure and are life threatening. Skin cancer is the most common type and, fortunately, one of the easiest to detect and cure. Males and females have a different incidence of other types of cancers. In males, the type of cancer with the highest incidence is prostate, followed closely by lung, colon/rectal, urinary, and leukemias/lymphomas. In females, the highest incidence is breast, followed by colon/rectal, lung, uterus, and leukemias/lymphomas.

> **Warning signs of cancer:**
> - A change in bowel and bladder habits
> - A sore that does not heal
> - Unusual bleeding or discharge
> - Thickening or a lump in the breast or elsewhere
> - Indigestion or difficulty swallowing
> - Obvious change in a wart or mole
> - A nagging cough or hoarseness

| TABLE 29–1 | Blood Pressure | | |
|---|---|---|---|
| **Blood Pressure Classification** | **Systolic (mm/Hg)** | | **Diastolic (mm/Hg)** |
| Normal | Less than 120 | and | Less than 80 |
| Prehypertension | 120–139 | or | 80–89 |
| High | | | |
|     Stage 1 | 140–159 | or | 90–99 |
|     Stage 2 | 160 or higher | or | 100 or higher |

*Causes of cancer* The precise causes of cancer are not easily identified. Researchers have identified more than 100 types of cancer with genetic origins. The onset of most cancers has also been attributed to certain environmental factors, including viruses; exposure to ultraviolet light, radiation, and certain chemicals, such as tobacco; and alcohol use. A fatty diet has also been linked to cancer. It is likely that a combination of hereditary and environmental factors is responsible for the development of cancer.[62]

*Symptoms and signs* Specific signs of cancer can vary tremendously, depending on the type of cancer. The American Cancer Society has identified the classic warning signs of cancer: a change in bowel and bladder habits, a sore that does not heal, unusual bleeding or discharge, thickening or a lump in the breast or elsewhere, indigestion or difficulty swallowing, obvious change in a wart or mole, and a nagging cough or hoarseness. The presence of any of these signs warrants immediate attention by a physician.

*Management* Unquestionably, early detection and treatment of cancer markedly improves the patient's chances of beating the disease. The most effective forms of treatment involve three traditional techniques: surgery, radiation, and chemotherapy.

# SEXUALLY TRANSMITTED DISEASES (STDs)

The sexually transmitted diseases with the highest incidence are chlamydia, trachomatis, genital herpes, trichomoniasis, genital candidiasis, condyloma acuminata, gonorrhea, and syphilis.[68] HIV and hepatitis B were discussed in Chapter 14.

### Chlamydia Trachomatis

*Etiology* Chlamydia trachomatis is considered by many to be the most common STD in the United States. It is more common than gonorrhea.[59] In females, chlamydia may result in pelvic inflammatory disease and is a major cause of infertility and ectopic pregnancy.

*Symptoms and signs* In males, inflammation occurs, along with a purulent discharge, 7 to 28 days after intercourse.[11] On occasion, painful urination and traces of blood in the urine occur. Most females with this infection are asymptomatic, but some experience a vaginal discharge, painful urination, pelvic pain, and pain and inflammation in other sites.

*Management* A bacteriological examination is given to determine the exact organisms present. Once identified, the infection must be treated promptly to prevent complications. Organism identification and treatment must take place immediately in women who are pregnant. Chlamydia can cause conjunctivitis and pneumonia in the newborn from an infected mother.[11] Uncomplicated cases are usually treated with antibiotics. Approximately 20 percent of the sufferers have one or more relapses.

### Genital Herpes

*Etiology* Genital herpes is a venereal infection that is common. Type 2 herpes simplex virus is associated with genital herpes infection, which is now the most prevalent cause of genital ulcerations. Signs of the disease appear approximately 4 to 7 days after sexual contact. Primary (initial) genital herpes crusts in 14 to 17 days, and secondary (recurrent) cases crust in 10 days.[68]

*Symptoms and signs* The first signs in the male are itching and soreness, but women may be asymptomatic in the vagina and cervix. It is estimated that 50 to 60 percent of individuals who have had one attack of genital herpes will have no further episodes, or if they do, the lesions are few and insignificant. Like the lesions in herpes labialis and gladiatorum, the lesions that develop in genital herpes eventually become ulcerated with a red areola. Ulcerations crust and heal in approximately 10 days, leaving a scar (see Figure 28–25, in Chapter 28). Of major importance to a pregnant woman with a history of genital herpes is whether there is an active infection when she is nearing delivery. Herpes simplex can be fatal to a newborn. There may be some relationship between a higher incidence of cervical cancer and the incidence of genital herpes.[11]

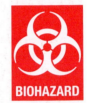

*Management* At this time, there is no cure for genital herpes. Systemic medications—specifically, antiviral medications, such as acyclovir (Zovirax), valaciclovir, and vidarabine (Vira-A)—are being used to lessen the early symptoms of the disease.[68]

### Trichomoniasis

*Etiology* Trichomoniasis is an infection that affects 20 percent of all females during their reproductive years and 5 percent to 10 percent of males.[11] It is caused by the flagellate protozoan *Trichomonas vaginalis.*

> Trichomoniasis affects **20 percent of all females and 5 percent to 10 percent of all males.**

*Symptoms and signs* The female with trichomoniasis typically has a vaginal discharge that is greenish yellow and frothy. The disease causes irritation of the vulva, perineum, and thighs. The female may also experience painful urination. Males are usually asymptomatic, although some may experience a frothy, purulent urethral discharge.

*Management* Two grams of metronidazole in one dose, usually the drug of choice in the treatment of trichomoniasis, cures up to 95 percent of women. Men, in contrast, should be treated with 500 milligrams twice a day for 7 days. The sexual partner should be treated concurrently. Complete cure is required before the individual can again engage in sexual intercourse.

## Genital Candidiasis

***Etiology*** As discussed in Chapter 27, *Candida* (a genus of yeastlike fungi) is commonly part of the normal flora of the mouth, skin, intestinal tract, and vagina.

The *Candida* organism is one of the most common causes of vaginitis in women of reproductive age. The infection may be transmitted sexually, but there can be numerous other causes.[26]

***Symptoms and signs*** The symptoms and signs are similar to those of other, related conditions. The female complains of vulval irritation that begins with redness, severe pain, and a vaginal discharge (scanty). The male is usually asymptomatic but may develop some irritation and soreness of the glans penis, especially after intercourse. Rarely, a slight urethral discharge occurs.

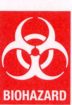

***Management*** Because of the highly infectious nature of this disease, all sexual contact should cease until the completion of treatment. An antifungal cream should be applied to the vagina, labia, perineum, and perianal region for 3 days.

## Condyloma Acuminata (Venereal Warts)

***Etiology*** Another sexually transmitted infection that should be referred to a physician is condyloma acuminata, or venereal warts (see Figure 28–27). They appear on the glans penis, vulva, or anus.

***Symptoms and signs*** This form of wart virus produces nodules that can have a cauliflower-like lesion or can be singular. In their early stage, the nodules are soft, moist, pink or red swellings that rapidly develop a stem with a flower-like head. They may be mistaken for secondary syphilis or carcinoma[11] (see Figure 28–27). The warts become whitish and more visible if swabbed with ¼% acetic acid (vinegar).

***Management*** Moist condylomas are treated with a solution containing 20 to 25 percent podophyllin. Dry warts may be treated with a freezing process, such as liquid nitrogen.

## Gonorrhea

***Etiology*** Gonorrhea is an acute venereal disease that can infect the urethra, cervix, and rectum. The organism of infection is the gonococcal bacteria *Neisseria gonorrhoea*.[11]

***Symptoms and signs*** In men, the incubation period is 2 to 10 days. The onset of the disease is marked by a tingling sensation in the urethra, followed in 2 or 3 hours by a greenish-yellow discharge of pus and painful urination. Sixty percent of infected women are asymptomatic. For those who have symptoms, onset is between 7 and 21 days. In these cases, symptoms are mild, with some vaginal discharge. Gonorrheal infection of the throat and rectum is also possible.[11]

***Management*** Because of embarrassment, some individuals fail to secure proper medical help for the treatment of gonorrhea, and although the initial symptoms will disappear, such an individual is not cured and can still spread the infection. Untreated gonorrhea becomes latent and manifests itself in later years, usually causing sterility or arthritis. Treatment consists of large amounts of penicillin or other antibiotics. Recent experimental evidence suggests an increasing resistance of the gonococci to penicillin. The athletic trainer who sees evidence of any of the symptoms should immediately remand the individual to a physician for testing and treatment. *All sexual contact must be avoided* until it has been medically established that the disease is no longer active. Because of the latent residual effects, including sterility and arthritis, immediate medical treatment is mandatory. Additionally, such treatment alleviates the discomfort that accompanies the initial stages of the disease.[11]

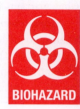

## Syphilis

***Etiology*** A sexually transmitted infection that is on the increase is syphilis. Reasons for this increase are high-risk sexual behavior, drug usage, and lack of knowledge about preventing infection.[26]

*Treponema pallidum,* a spirochete bacteria, is the organism that causes syphilis. It enters the body through mucous membranes or skin lesions.[59]

***Symptoms and signs*** Untreated syphilis may have a course of four stages within the body: primary, secondary, latent, and late, or tertiary. The incubation period of syphilis is normally 3 to 4 weeks but can range from 1 to 13 weeks. A painless chancre, or ulceration, develops and heals within 8 weeks. Syphilis during this primary stage is highly contagious. Ulcerations can occur on the penis, urethra, vagina, cervix, mouth, hand or foot, or around the eye.

The secondary stage of syphilis occurs within 12 weeks after the initial infection. It is characterized by a skin rash, lymph swelling, body aches, and mild flulike symptoms. Hair may fall out in patches.

Latent syphilis follows the secondary stage and is characterized by no or few symptoms. If untreated, approximately one-third of persons with latent syphilis will develop late, or tertiary, syphilis.

The late stage of syphilis is characterized by a deep penetration of spirochetes that damage skin, bone, and the cardiovascular and nervous systems. Tertiary syphilis can develop 3 to 10 years after infection. Neurosyphilis can progress to severe muscle weakness, paralysis, and various types of mental disorders.[26]

***Management*** Penicillin is currently the appropriate antibiotic for all stages of syphilis. Those patients allergic

A male college basketball player confides in the athletic trainer about a greenish-yellow urethral discharge and painful urination.

**?** How should this situation be managed by the athletic trainer?

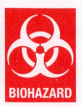

**BIOHAZARD**

to penicillin may be treated with erythromycin. Because *T. pallidum* can exist only in body fluids, air drying and cleaning with soap and water will destroy it. Because of the rise of penicillin resistance, ceftriaxone may be the drug of choice.

# MENSTRUAL IRREGULARITIES AND THE FEMALE REPRODUCTIVE SYSTEM

Females who engage in intense physical activity have special menstrual and reproductive concerns. This section addresses some of the more prevalent issues.

## Physiology of the Menstrual Cycle

Menstruation is the periodic discharge of bloody fluid from the uterus, usually at regular intervals, during the life of a woman from puberty to menopause. Puberty is a period of adolescence in which either sex becomes able to reproduce.

**Menarche** Menarche—the onset of the menses—and puberty normally occur between ages 9 and 17, with the majority of girls entering puberty between ages 13 and 15.

> During the prepubertal period, girls are equal to, and often superior to, boys of the same age in activities that require speed, strength, and endurance.

There is indication that strenuous sports training and competition delay the onset of menarche. The greatest delay is related to the higher-caliber competition. In itself, a delay in the first menses does not appear to pose any significant danger to the young athlete. Delayed menarche, or primary amenorrhea, is defined as menstruation not occurring by age 16 or a failure to develop secondary sex characteristics by age 14.

> The onset of menarche may be delayed by strenuous training and competition.

The late-maturing girl commonly has longer legs, narrower hips, and less adiposity and body weight for her height, all of which are more conducive to sports.

**Menstruation** The effects of sustained and strenuous training and competition on the menstrual cycle and the effects of menstruation on performance still cannot be fully explained with any degree of certainty.

The classic 28-day cycle consists of the follicular and luteal phases, each of which is approximately 14 days long (Figure 29–6). The menses vary from 2 to 10 days, with an average of 4 to 7 days. The majority of women tend to show some variation in the length of their cycles; these differences occur principally because of differences in the duration of the preovulatory phase rather than the premenstrual phase.

With the onset of menarche, a cyclic hormonal pattern commences, which establishes the menstrual cycle (Figure 29–6).[62] These hormonal changes result from complex feedback mechanisms and specifically controlled interactions that occur among the hypothalamus, ovaries, and pituitary gland. Two gonadotropins induce the release of the egg from the mature follicle at midcycle (ovulation): follicle-stimulating hormone (FSH), which stimulates the maturation of an ovarian follicle, and luteinizing hormone (LH), which stimulates the development of the corpus luteum—a small body that develops within a ruptured ovarian follicle after ovulation—and the endocrine structure that secretes progesterone and estrogens. The control and eventual inhibition of the production of FSH when the follicle reaches maturity is brought about by the estrogenic steroids

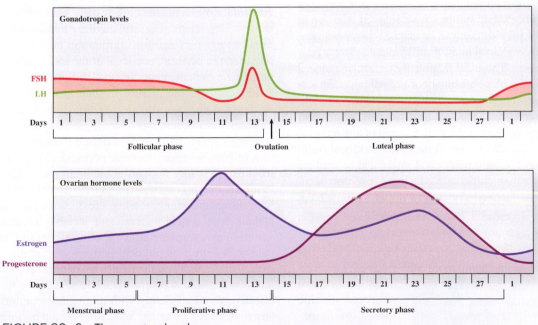

**FIGURE 29–6** The menstrual cycle.

produced by the ovaries. Progesterone, a steroid hormone produced within the corpus luteum, eventually inhibits the production of LH. Estrogen is secreted principally by the luteal cells. Before the onset of a new menstrual period, FSH levels are already rising, probably to initiate the maturation of new follicles to institute the next cycle.[62]

## Menstrual Cycle Irregularities

Highly active females, such as those participating in ballet, gymnastics, and long-distance running, can experience irregularities in the normal menstrual cycle of 25 to 38 days. *Oligomenorrhea* (a reduction in the number of periods and blood flow) refers to fewer than six cycles per year.[62] **Amenorrhea** is the complete cessation of the cycle, with ovulation occurring seldom or not at all because of the low level of circulating estrogen.[62] Approximately 10 to 20 percent of vigorously exercising women have amenorrhea.

### Amenorrhea

*Etiology*   Primary amenorrhea is a condition in which a female has not had any menstrual periods by age 16. Secondary amenorrhea occurs when a female was previously menstruating but then stopped having periods.[25] The cause of secondary amenorrhea, or athlete's amenorrhea, is often a hypothalamic dysfunction. The amount of gonadotropin-releasing hormone (GnRH) produced by the hypothalamus is often deficient.[25] Many factors must be ruled out, by a physical examination, before athlete's amenorrhea is diagnosed. Pregnancy and abnormalities of the reproductive or genital tract must be ruled out, as well as ovarian failure and pituitary tumors.[5,41] See *Focus Box 29–3:* "Suggested factors in secondary amenorrhea."

*Symptoms and signs*   The primary sign of amenorrhea is that there is no menstrual period. In primary amenorrhea, there is no menstrual period by age 16. In secondary amenorrhea, there is no period for 3 to 6 months or longer. Depending on the cause of amenorrhea, a patient might experience other symptoms or signs in addition to the absence of periods, such as headache, vision changes, hair loss or excess facial hair, or milky nipple discharge.

*Management*   The ideal treatment of exercise-induced amenorrhea is the reestablishment of normal hormone levels and the return of the normal menstrual cycle.[41] It is important that a medical evaluation be performed before other intervention procedures are started. Cleared of any physical abnormalities, the athlete should be given nutritional counseling to balance calorie output and intake and to regulate the proper amount of nutrients. Reduction of exercise intensity and counseling to reduce emotional stress can be helpful. Estrogen replacement may be considered.[20]

### Dysmenorrhea

*Etiology*   Dysmenorrhea (painful menstruation) apparently is prevalent among more active women; however,

| Girls who have moderate to severe dysmenorrhea require examination by a physician. |

it is inconclusive whether specific sports participation can alleviate

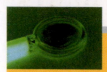

or produce dysmenorrhea.[62] For girls with moderate to severe dysmenorrhea, gynecological consultation is warranted to rule out a pathological condition.[28]

Dysmenorrhea may be caused by ischemia (a lack of normal blood flow to the pelvic organs), a hormonal imbalance, or endometriosis (uterine cells growing outside the uterus).

*Symptoms and signs*   This syndrome, which is identified by cramps, nausea, lower abdominal pain, headache, and occasionally emotional lability, is the most common menstrual disorder.

*Management*   Mild to vigorous exercises that help ameliorate dysmenorrhea are usually prescribed by physicians. Physicians generally advise a continuance of the usual sports participation during the menstrual period, provided the performance level of the individual does not drop below her customary level of ability. Among athletes, swimmers have the highest incidence of dysmenorrhea; it, along with menorrhagia (excessive bleeding during menstruation) occurs most often, probably as a result of strenuous sports participation during the menses. Generally, oligomenorrhea (irregular periods), amenorrhea, and irregular or scanty flow are more common in sports that require strenuous exertion over a long period of time (e.g., long-distance running, rowing, cross-country skiing, basketball, tennis, field hockey, and soccer). Because great variation exists among athletes with respect to menstrual pattern, its effect on physical performance, and the effect of physical activity on the menstrual pattern, each individual must learn to adjust to her cycle so that she functions effectively and efficiently with minimal discomfort or restriction. Evidence to date indicates that top performances are possible in all phases of the cycle.

## Ovarian Cyst

***Etiology*** Each month, the ovaries grow tiny follicular cysts that hold the eggs. When an egg is mature, the follicular cyst breaks open to release the egg so that it can travel through the fallopian tube for fertilization. If a follicular cyst fails to rupture and release the egg, the fluid remains and can form an ovarian cyst within one of the ovaries. Ovarian cysts are small, fluid-filled sacs surrounded by a very thin wall. Most ovarian cysts are benign, meaning they are not cancerous, and many disappear on their own in a matter of weeks without treatment. But some cause problems, such as bleeding and pain, and some can grow quite large. Surgery may be required to remove those cysts. Factors that can lead to the development of an ovarian cyst include early menstruation (11 years or younger), irregular menstrual cycles, increased upper-body fat distribution, hormonal imbalance, ovarian cancer, and cancer that has spread outside the ovary.[65,69]

***Symptoms and signs*** Many women have ovarian cysts without having any symptoms. Among the more common symptoms are a dull ache in the low back and thighs, problems passing urine completely, pressure, breast tenderness, nausea or vomiting, a feeling of fullness or pain in the abdomen, weight gain, painful menstrual periods, and abnormal bleeding and pain during sexual intercourse.[65]

***Management*** Pain relievers, including NSAIDs, can be used. Oral contraceptives may be helpful in regulating the menstrual cycle, thus preventing the formation of follicles that can turn into cysts. Limiting strenuous activity may reduce the risk of cyst rupture or torsion. If the patient develops more serious symptoms, including pain with fever and vomiting, sudden severe abdominal pain, faintness, dizziness, weakness, or rapid breathing, a physician should be consulted immediately. Laparoscopic surgery may be necessary to remove the cyst or correct a torsion.

## Bone Health

The female who has a prolonged decrease of FSH, LH, estrogen, and progesterone shows a profile similar to that of a postmenopausal woman.[8] Osteoporosis is most common in women older than age 50 whose bone mass (bone mineral density) has fallen below a critical threshold. Physically active women who have irregular menses because of endocrine changes are strong candidates for bone loss. Low bone mass leads to bone fragility and increased susceptibility to stress fractures in females with premature osteoporosis, especially females with late menarche.[16] There is evidence that estrogen receptors on bone cells have a direct relation to growth and bone function.[26] Calcium nutrition is also needed; a recommended daily allowance for adolescents through age 24 is 1,200 milligrams daily.[6]

A female experiencing loss of periods with low bone mass should decrease training intensity and volume, increase total calories, and ingest 1,500 milligrams of calcium daily. A program of resistance training designed for both muscle mass and strength may enhance the skeletal profile and protect against muscle injury. Estrogen replacement therapy may be warranted if other means fail.[16] It should be added that estrogen supplementation is used for a variety of reasons, not as a primary treatment for bone health.[12]

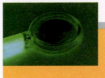

## Female Athlete Triad

***Etiology*** The relationship among three medical disorders—disordered eating, amenorrhea, and osteoporosis—is called the *female athlete triad*.[13,65] A young female, driven to excel in her chosen sport and pressured to fit a specific athletic image to reach her goals, is at risk for the development of disordered patterns of eating, which "may lead to menstrual dysfunction and subsequent premature osteoporosis."[5] This triad has the potential for serious illness and risk of death.[5,6]

***Symptoms and signs*** Disordered eating follows the same patterns of eating characteristics that anorexia nervosa and bulimia do (see Chapter 5).[63] Amenorrhea is discussed earlier in this chapter. Osteoporosis in young women includes premature bone loss and inadequate bone development that result in low bone mass, microarchitectural destruction, increased skeletal fragility, and increased risk of fracture.[63] Physicians and athletic trainers must be aware of the female's potential for risk. Special concern must be directed toward those females who participate in sports that focus on an ideal body type and weight, who exhibit signs of disordered eating, and who experience disruption in menarche or the menstrual cycle[35] (see *Focus Box 29–4:* "Identifying a woman at risk for female athlete triad").

***Management*** Management of this triad lies in prevention. Those concerned with the patient's total health must be

A female patient has been diagnosed as having a serious eating disorder and amenorrhea.

**?** Why may these two medical disorders eventually lead to osteoporosis?

**29–8 Clinical Application Exercise**

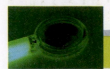

# FOCUS 29–5 Focus on Therapeutic Intervention

## American College of Obstetricians and Gynecologists guidelines for exercise during pregnancy and postpartum[2,5]

1. During pregnancy, women can continue to exercise and derive health benefits, even from a mild to moderate exercise routine. Regular exercise (at least three times per week) is preferable to intermittent activity.

2. Women should avoid exercise in the supine position after the first trimester. Such a position is associated with decreased cardiac output in most pregnant women; because the remaining cardiac output will be preferentially distributed away from splanchnic beds (including the uterus) during vigorous exercise, such regimens are best avoided during pregnancy. Prolonged periods of motionless standing should also be avoided.

3. Women should be aware of the decreased amount of oxygen available for aerobic exercise during pregnancy. They should be encouraged to modify the intensity of their exercise according to maternal symptoms. Pregnant women should stop exercising when fatigued and not exercise to exhaustion. Under some circumstances, weight-bearing exercises may be continued throughout pregnancy at intensities similar to those before pregnancy. Non-weight-bearing exercise, such as cycling or swimming, minimizes

the risk of injury and facilitates the continuation of exercise during pregnancy.

4. Morphological changes in pregnancy should serve as relative contraindications to types of exercise in which loss of balance could be detrimental to maternal or fetal well-being, especially in the third trimester. Any type of exercise involving the potential for even mild abdominal trauma should be avoided.

5. Pregnancy requires an additional 300 kcal per day to maintain metabolic homeostasis. Thus, women who exercise during pregnancy should be particularly careful to ensure an adequate diet.

6. Pregnant women who exercise in the first trimester should augment heat dissipation by ensuring adequate hydration, appropriate clothing, and optimal environmental surroundings during exercise.

7. Many of the physiological and morphological changes of pregnancy persist 4 to 6 weeks postpartum. Thus, the woman's prepregnancy exercise routine should be resumed gradually based on her physical capability.

http://www.ncbi.nlm.nih.gov/pmc/articles/PMC1724598/pdf/v037p00006.pdf

---

educated.[63] A concerted effort must be made to identify and screen athletes who are at risk.

## Contraceptives and Reproduction

Female athletes have been known to take extra oral contraceptive pills to delay menstruation during competition. This practice is not recommended because the pills should be taken for 21 days, followed by a 7-day break. Birth control pills are available that allow the female to reduce the number of periods she has each year. Side effects range from nausea, vomiting, fluid retention, and amenorrhea to the extreme effects of hypertension and double vision. Some oral contraceptives make women hypersensitive to the sun. Any use of oral contraceptives related to physical performance should be under the express direction and control of a physician. However, oral contraceptive use is acceptable for females with no medical problems who have coitus at least twice a week. New low-dose preparations, containing less than 50 mg of estrogen, add negligible risks for the healthy woman.[10]

A number of other contraceptive options are available to female athletes, such as an intrauterine device (IUD) that is inserted into the uterus: one type is made of copper that lasts for 10 to 12 years, and another type releases the hormone progestin that lasts for 3 years. Other types include the NuvaRing, inserted into the vagina for 3 weeks then removed for a week; a birth-control shot

that lasts for 3 months; a birth-control implant that is a match-sized rod inserted into the upper arm and that lasts for 3 years; and the transdermal birth-control patch, which adheres to the skin and must be changed every 7 days.

## Pregnancy

Generally, females can participate in physical activity and even competition well into the third month of pregnancy, unless bleeding or cramps are present, and she can continue such activity until the seventh month if no disabling or physiological complications arise.[58] Such activity may make pregnancy, childbirth, and postparturition less stressful. Many women do not continue beyond the third month because of a drop in their performance. This decline has a number of causes, some related to the pregnancy, others perhaps psychological. It is during the first 3 months that the dangers of disturbing the pregnancy are greatest.[40] After that period, there is less danger to the mother and fetus because the pregnancy is stabilized.[58]

**Exercise and Pregnancy** There is no evidence that mild to moderate exercise during pregnancy is harmful to fetal growth and development or causes reduced fetal mass, increased perinatal or neonatal mortality, or physical or mental retardation.[2,54] It has been found, however, that extreme exercise may lower birth weight (see *Focus Box 29–5:* "American College of Obstetricians and Gynecologists guidelines for exercise during pregnancy and postpartum").[2] Many females compete during pregnancy with no ill effects. Most physicians, although advocating moderate activity during this period, believe that especially vigorous

> In general, childbirth is not adversely affected by a history of hard physical exercise.

performance, particularly in activities with severe body contact, heavy jarring, or falls, should be avoided.[64] Contraindications to exercise include the following:

- Pregnancy-induced hypertension
- Preterm rupture of membranes
- Preterm labor during the prior or current pregnancy or both
- Incompetent cervix or cerclage
- Persistent second- or third-trimester bleeding
- Intrauterine growth retardation

**Ectopic Pregnancy**  In ectopic pregnancy, the fertilized egg is implanted outside the uterine cavity because of inflammation of the fallopian tubes or a mechanical blockage to the normal downward movement of the ovum.[3,62] The symptoms include amenorrhea, tenderness, soreness and pain on the affected side, referred pain in the shoulders, pallor, and signs of shock and hemorrhage. Operative treatment is necessary to terminate the nonviable pregnancy and to control the hemorrhage if a rupture of the tube has occurred.

## SUMMARY

- The immune system is not an organ system, but rather a collection of disease-fighting cells that recognize the presence of foreign substances in the body and act to neutralize or destroy them.
- Among the more common viral infections are rhinovirus (common cold), influenza (flu), infectious mononucleosis, rubella (German measles), rubeola (measles), mumps, and varicella (chicken pox).
- Conditions that affect the respiratory system include sinusitis, pharyngitis, tonsillitis, seasonal rhinitis, acute bronchitis, pneumonia, bronchial asthma, and cystic fibrosis.
- The muscular system suffers from fewer disorders than do other systems. Two serious muscular disorders are Duchenne muscular dystrophy and myasthenia gravis.
- Disorders that affect the nervous system include meningitis, multiple sclerosis, and amyotrophic lateral sclerosis.
- Diseases that affect the vascular and lymphatic systems include anemias, hemophilia, and lymphangitis.
- Diabetes mellitus is a complex hereditary or developmental disease. Diabetics must be extremely cautious about the possibility of going into diabetic coma or insulin shock.
- Some patients have a history of epilepsy that could lead to an alteration of consciousness. Epilepsy is not a disease, and each person with epilepsy must be considered individually.
- The individual with high blood pressure may have to be monitored carefully by a physician. Hypertension may require the avoidance of heavy resistive activities.
- Cancer is a condition in which cellular behavior becomes abnormal. Malignant tumors are cancerous; they grow out of control and spread within a specific tissue. Skin cancer is the most common type. In males, the highest incidence of cancer is in the prostate, followed closely by lung, colon/rectal, urinary, and leukemias/lymphomas. In females, the highest incidence is found in the breast, followed by colon/rectal, lung, uterus, and leukemias/lymphomas.
- The sexually transmitted diseases with the highest incidence are chlamydia, genital herpes, trichomoniasis, genital candidiasis, condyloma acuminata, gonorrhea, and syphilis.
- The highly active female may have menstrual irregularities, including dysmenorrhea, amenorrhea, or ovarian cysts. Menstrual irregularities could lead to a thinning of bone and subsequent fractures.
- Many females compete during pregnancy with no ill effects. There is no indication that mild to moderate exercise during pregnancy is harmful to fetal development.

## WEB SITES

**NATA Position, Official, and Consensus Statements**
*Management of Asthma in the Athlete (2005):*
www.nata.org/sites/default/files
   /MgmtOfAsthmaInAthletes.pdf
*Sickle Cell Trait and the Athlete (2007):*
www.nata.org/sites/default/files
   /SickleCellTraitAndTheAthlete.pdf

*Management of the Athlete with Type 1 Diabetes Mellitus (2007):*
www.nata.org/sites/default/files
   /mgmtofathletewithtype1diabetesmellitus.pdf
American Board of Obstetrics and Gynecology: www
   .abog.org
American Cancer Society: www.cancer.org

*The American Cancer Society is dedicated to eliminating cancer as a major health problem by preventing cancer, saving lives, and diminishing suffering.*

American Diabetes Association: www.diabetes.org
*This site offers the latest information on diabetes and living with the disease.*

American Epilepsy Society: www.aesnet.org
*The American Epilepsy Society promotes research and education for professionals dedicated to the prevention, treatment, and cure of epilepsy.*

American Gastroenterological Association: www.gastro.org
*This site includes information for physicians and the public about digestive disease symptoms, treatments, and research.*

The American Sickle Cell Anemia Association: www.ascaa.org
*The American Sickle Cell Anemia Association (ASCAA) provides quality and comprehensive services through diagnostic testing, evaluation, counseling, and supportive services to individuals and families at risk for Sickle Cell Disease and its variants.*

American Society of Hypertension, Inc.: www.ash-us.org
*This site is dedicated to hypertension and related cardiovascular disease.*

Amyotrophic Lateral Sclerosis Association: www.alsa.org
*This nonprofit health organization is dedicated solely to the fight against Lou Gehrig's disease.*

Asthma and Allergy Foundation of America (AAFA): www.aafa.org
*Asthma and Allergy Foundation of America (AAFA) is dedicated to helping people with asthma and allergic diseases through education and support for research.*

Cystic Fibrosis Foundation: www.cff.org
*The Cystic Fibrosis Foundation seeks the means to cure and control cystic fibrosis and to improve the quality of life for those with the disease.*

eMedicine World Medical Library: emedicine.medscape.com

eMedicine features up-to-date, searchable, peer-reviewed medical journals, online physician reference textbooks, and a full-text article database.

Medline Plus Medical Encyclopedia: www.nlm.nih.gov/medlineplus
*This site reviews the symptoms, causes, incidence, diagnosis, treatment, and prognosis of various acute and chronic conditions and diseases.*

Meningitis Foundation of America: www.meningitisfoundationofamerica.org
*This site provides information about the organization as well as the disease, including FAQs, symptoms, treatment, prevention, course of recovery, and support.*

Multiple Sclerosis Foundation (MSF): www.msfocus.org
*MSF was established as a service-based organization to provide the best information about MS.*

Muscular Dystrophy Association: www.mda.org
*The Muscular Dystrophy Association provides information, research, and recommendations for dealing with muscular dystrophy.*

National Hemophilia Foundation: www.hemophilia.org
*The National Hemophilia Foundation is dedicated to finding better treatments and cures for inheritable bleeding disorders and to preventing the complications of these disorders through education, advocacy and research.*

Reflex Sympathetic Dystrophy (RSD): www.rsdfoundation.org
*The International Research Foundation for RSD/CRPS is dedicated to education and research on Reflex Sympathetic Dystrophy and Complex Regional Pain Syndrome. The primary mission of the Foundation is to establish an international research network which will help educate medical professionals and support research worldwide.*

World Health Organization: www.who.int/influenza
*This site offers information on worldwide surveillance of influenza, recommendations for flu vaccines, pandemic preparedness, and more.*

## SOLUTIONS TO CLINICAL APPLICATION EXERCISES

29–1 This scenario describes flu symptoms. There should be symptomatic care, but aspirin should be avoided.

29–2 It is possible that this patient has infectious mononucleosis. Treatment should be supportive and symptomatic. Acetaminophen is often given for headache, fever, and malaise. The patient may resume activity in about three weeks after the onset of illness if (1) the spleen is not markedly enlarged or painful, (2) he is afebrile, (3) liver function tests are normal, and (4) pharyngitis and any complications have resolved.

29–3 The patient should maintain a high level of conditioning, including running longer distances, and should always warm up and cool down gradually. All exercise intensity and loading should be graduated slowly. A bronchodilator may be employed. A mask or scarf should be used in cold, dry air. The patient should avoid exercising in areas with high levels of air pollution or when there is a high pollen count.

29–4 It is possible that the gymnast has complex regional pain syndrome (CRPS). Her concern is justified because this problem could persist for months. The physician will likely do a sympathetic ganglion nerve block. The athletic trainer should have the patient do active range of motion exercises in a pain-free range.

29–5 The patient appears to have iron-deficiency anemia. After verification by a physician, the patient should eat a diet rich in iron, avoid coffee and tea, eat foods high in vitamin C, and take a daily iron supplement.

29–6 This patient is experiencing insulin shock as a result of too much insulin and not enough blood sugar. Glucose should be administered to this patient as soon as possible in the form of sugar, candy, orange juice, or a glucose solution.

29–7 This situation must be handled with the strictest confidentiality. Because this condition could be gonorrhea, immediate medical referral must be made. The patient must avoid all sexual contact until this condition has been resolved.

29–8 These medical disorders make up the female athlete triad. Osteoporosis is the softening and increased porosity of bones with subsequent fracturing. Individuals who have anorexia nervosa or bulimia to establish a perceived body image are at risk. Individuals who train so hard that they stop menstruating also stop their estrogen production, which results in a loss of calcium in the bones.

# REVIEW QUESTIONS AND CLASS ACTIVITIES

1. Contrast the symptoms and signs of the following respiratory tract conditions: the common cold, influenza, and allergic rhinitis.
2. Discuss mononucleosis in detail, including prevention and etiology.
3. Discuss and contrast bronchial obstructive diseases, such as bronchitis and asthma. How do you care for a patient having an acute asthmatic attack?
4. Describe the most common gastrointestinal complaints. How are the conditions that produce them acquired and managed?
5. What is diabetes mellitus? What value might exercise have for the person with diabetes mellitus? How are diabetic coma and insulin shock managed?
6. What are some major indications that a patient has a contagious disease?
7. What is epilepsy? How should a general tonic/clonic or seizure be managed?
8. Define hypertension. What dangers does it present to the athlete?
9. Describe the anemias that most often affect the patient. How should each be managed?
10. What are the classic warning signs for cancer, according to the American Cancer Society?
11. Discuss the etiology, symptoms and signs, and management of the most common sexually transmitted diseases. How can they be prevented?
12. Discuss menstrual irregularities that occur in highly active individuals. Why do they occur? How should they be managed? How do they relate to reproduction?
13. What are the implications of pregnancy for extensive physical activity?

# REFERENCES

1. Acharya K: Attitudes and belief of sports medicine providers to sickle cell trait screening of student athletes, *Clin Sports Med* 21(6):480–85, 2011.
2. Artal R: Guidelines of the American College of Obstetricians and Gynecologists for exercise during pregnancy and the postpartum period, *Brit J Sports Med* 37(1):6, 2003.
3. Asplund C: 2010. Treatment of hypertension in athletes: An evidence-based review, *The Physician Sportsmed* 38(1):37–44.
4. Auwaerter PG: Infectious mononucleosis: Return to play, *Clin Sports Med* 23(3):485, 2004.
5. Bass S: Menstrual dysfunction and bone health in female athletes, *J Sports Med* 1(5):48, 2001.
6. Beck B: Osteoporosis: Understanding key risk factors and therapeutic options, *Physician Sportsmed* 28(2):69, 2000.
7. Birrer R: Exercise and diabetes mellitus, *Physician Sportsmed* 31(5):29, 2003.
8. Bonura F: Prevention, screening, and management of osteoporosis: An overview of the current strategies, *Postgraduate Medicine* 121(4):5–17, 2009.
9. Bushby K: Diagnosis and management of Duchene muscular dystrophy, Parts 1 and 2, *The Lancet* 9(1):77–93, 177–89.
10. Bushman B: Anaerobic power performance and the menstrual cycle: Eumenorrheic and oral contraceptive users, *J Sports Med Phys Fitness* 46(1):132, 2006.
11. Centers for Disease Control; Sexually transmitted diseases treatment guidelines, 2010, *Morbidity and Mortality Weekly Report*, 59(RR12):1–110, 2010.
12. Conti-Fine B: Myasthenia gravis: Past, present, and future, *Journal of Clinical Investigation* 116(11):2843–54, 2006.
13. De Souza M, et al.: Female athlete triad coalition consensus statement on treatment and return to play of the female athlete triad, *British Journal of Sports Medicine* 48, 289–309, 2014.
14. Dishuck J: Educating the asthmatic athlete, *Athletic Therapy Today* 6(5):26, 2001.
15. Dishuck J: Management and treatment of allergic rhinitis and sinusitis, *Athletic Therapy Today* 6(5):6, 2001.
16. Dugan D: Femoral-neck stress fracture in an amenorrheic runner, *Athletic Therapy Today* 6(4):40, 2001.
17. Eichner R: Iron deficiency anemia, *Current Sports Medicine Reports* 9(3):122–23, 2010.
18. Eichner R: Sickle cell trait in sports, *Current Sports Medicine Reports* 9(6):347–51, 2010.
19. Ewald A: Meningitis in the athlete, *Current Sports Medicine Reports* 7(1):22–27, 2008.
20. Feingold D: Female athlete triad and stress fractures, *Orthopedic Clinics North America*, 37(4):575–83, 2006.
21. Fiala K: A survey of team physicians on the participation status of hemophilic athletes in National Collegiate Athletic Association Division I athletics, *J Athl Train* 38(3):245–51, 2003.
22. Fiala K: Traumatic hemarthrosis of the knee secondary to hemophilia A in a collegiate soccer player: A case report, *J Athl Train* 37(3):315, 2002.
23. Fiala K: Medical care for athletes with hemophilia, *Athletic Therapy Today* 9(2):16, 2004.
24. Fields K: Wheezing and respiratory tract infection in athletes, *Current Sports Medicine Reports* 1(2):85–89, 2012.
25. Gamboa S: What's the best way to manage athletes with amenorrhea? *Journal of Family Practice* 57(11):749–50, 2008.
26. Hamann B: *Disease: Identification, prevention, and control*, New York, 2006, McGraw-Hill.
27. Hardiman O: Clinical diagnosis and management of amyotrophic lateral sclerosis, *Nature Reviews Neurology*, 7:639–49, 2011.
28. Harris M: Infectious disease in athletes, *Current Sports Medicine Reports* 10(2):84–89, 2011.
29. Hendrick D: The prevelance and current opinion of treatment of allergic rhinitis in elite athletes, *Current Opinion in Allergy and Clinical Immunology*, 11(2):103–08, 2011.
30. Hermansen C: Identifying exercise induced bronchospasm, *Physician Sportsmed* 33(12):25, 2005.
31. Hinton P: Iron deficiency in physically active adults, *ACSM's Health and Fitness Journal* 10(5):12, 2006.
32. Horodyski M: Returning to athletics after mononucleosis, *Athletic Therapy Today* 6(4):47, 2001.
33. Howe W: The athlete with chronic illness. In Birrer R, ed: *Sports medicine for the primary care physician*, ed 2, Boca Raton, FL, 1994, CRC Press.
34. Jimenez C: National Athletic Trainers' Association position statement: Management of the athlete with type 1 diabetes mellitus, *J Athl Train* 42(4):536, 2007.
35. Kawaguchi J: Redefining the female athlete triad, *Athletic Therapy Today* 13(1):11, 2008.
36. Knowles B: Athletes with seizure disorders, *Current Sports Medicine Reports* 11(1):16–20, 2012.
37. Kovan J: Exercise-induced asthma, *Athletic Therapy Today* 6(5):22, 2001.
38. Landry G: Common infectious diseases. In Landry G, ed: *Essentials of primary care sports medicine*, Champaign, IL, 2003, Human Kinetics.
39. Leaver-Dunn D: Assessment of respiratory conditions I athletes, *Athletic Therapy Today* 5(6):14, 2000.
40. Lively M: Sports participation and pregnancy, *Athletic Therapy Today* 7(1):11, 2002.
41. Loucks A: Introduction to menstrual disturbances in athletes, *Med Sci Sports Exerc* 35(9):1551, 2003.
42. Lovering R: The muscular dystrophies: From genes to therapies, *Phys Ther* 85(12):1372, 2005.
43. Luke A: Prevention of infectious diseases in athletes, *Clinics in Sports Medicine* 26(3):321–44, 2007.
44. MacKnight J: The daily management of athletes with diabetes, *Clinics in Sports Medicine* 28(3):479–95, 2009.
45. Martin S: Exercise and respiratory tract viral infections, *Exercise and Sport Science Reviews* 37(4):157–64, 2009.

46. Mata H: Influenza in athletes, *Athletic Therapy and Training* 16(2):24–26, 2011.

47. Mellion M: Medical problems in athletes. In Birrer R, ed: *Sports medicine for the primary care physician*, Boca Raton, FL, 2004, CRC Press.

48. Merrick M: Do nasal dilator strips help athletes? *Athletic Therapy Today* 6(2):42, 2001.

49. Merrick M: Managing type-1 diabetes in athletes, *Athletic Therapy Today* 6(5):40, 2001.

50. Miller M: National Athletic Trainers' Association position statement: Management of asthma in athletes, *J Athl Train* 40(3):224, 2005.

51. Millward D: The diagnosis of asthma and exercise-induced bronchospasm in Division 1 athletes, *Clin J Sports Med* 19(6):482–86, 2009.

52. Nixon P: Cystic fibrosis. In Moore G, ed: *ACSM's exercise management for persons with chronic diseases and disabilities,* Champaign, IL, 2016, Human Kinetics.

53. Olivera L: Hypertension update and cardiovascular risk reduction in physically active individuals and athletes, *Physician Sportsmed* 38(1):11–20, 2010.

54. Olson D: Exercise in pregnancy, *Current Sports Medicine Reports* 8(3):147–53, 2009.

55. Oosthuyse T: The effect of the menstrual cycle on exercise metabolism: Implications for exercise performance in eumenorrhoeic women, *Sports Medicine* 40(3):207–27, 2010.

56. Parks E: Seizure disorders in athletes, *Athletic Therapy Today* 11(4):36, 2006.

57. Parsons J: Exercise-induced asthma, *Current Opinion in Pulmonary Medicine* 15(1):25–28, 2009.

58. Pavarnik J: Impact of physical activity during pregnancy and postpartum on chronic disease risk, *Med Sci Sports Exerc* 38(5):989, 2006.

59. Porter R: *The Merck manual of diagnosis and therapy,* Hoboken, NJ, 2016, John Wiley and Sons.

60. Putukian M: Mononeucleosis and athletic participation: An evidence-based subject review, *Clin J Sports Med* 18(4):309–15, 2008.

61. Rand S: Complex regional pain syndrome in the adolescent athlete, *Current Sports Medicine Reports* 8(6):285–87, 2009.

62. Saladin K: *Anatomy and physiology: The unity of form and function,* New York, 2015, McGraw-Hill.

63. Sanborn C: Disordered eating and the female athlete triad, *Clin Sports Med* 19(2):199, 2000.

64. Scott S: Exercise in the postpartum period, *ACSM's Health and Fitness Journal* 10(4):40, 2006.

65. *Stedman's concise medical dictionary for the health professions,* Baltimore, MD, 2016, Lippincott, Williams and Wilkins.

66. Stuifbergen A: Exercise, functional limitations, and quality of life: A longitudinal study of persons with multiple sclerosis, *Arch Phys Med Rehabil* 87(7):935, 2006.

67. Swann E: Emergency management of allergic reactions, *Athletic Therapy Today* 6(5):11, 2001.

68. Velasquez B: When is a skin rash more than just a rash? Sexually transmitted diseases: A dermatological perspective, *Athletic Therapy Today* 7(3):16, 2002.

69. Venes D: *Taber's cyclopedic medical dictionary,* Philadelphia, PA, 2016, F.A. Davis.

70. Vinci D: Athletes and type 1 diabetes mellitus, *Athletic Therapy Today* 7(6):48, 2002.

71. Wahlers B: Management of exercise-induced bronchospasm in athletes, *American Journal of Medicine and Sports* 6(4):167, 2004.

72. Weaver J: Exercise induced asthma, *Athletic Therapy Today* 5(3):38, 2000.

73. Weidner T: Preventing the common cold and associated secondary problems in athletes, *Athletic Therapy Today* 6(4):44, 2001.

74. Wheatley C: Exercise is medicine in cystic fibrosis, *Exercise and Sport Science Reviews* 39(3):155–60, 2011.

## ANNOTATED BIBLIOGRAPHY

Colbert S, ed: *The diabetic athlete,* Champaign, IL, 2001, Human Kinetics.

*Describes the effects different sports and activities have on blood sugar and the body. Provides tables and advice on how to manage glucose levels depending on the sport and type of insulin being used.*

Cuppett M, Walsh K: *General medical conditions in the athlete,* New York, 2014, Mosby.

*A complete guide to physical examination and general medical conditions in athletes.*

Dirckx, JH, ed: *Stedman's concise medical dictionary for the health professions,* Baltimore, MD, 2011, Lippincott, Williams and Wilkins.

*Contains the medical terminology used in more than 30 of today's fastest growing health profession areas.*

Hamann B: *Diseases, identification, prevention, and control,* New York 2006, McGraw-Hill.

*An excellent reference guide for the health professional on the most common human diseases.*

O'Conner D, Fincher L: *Clinical pathology for athletic trainers: Recognizing systemic disease,* Thorofare, NJ, 2015, Slack.

*Written specifically for athletic trainers, this text emphasizes practical knowledge, development of clinical skills, including evaluation and treatment, and development of clinical decision-making abilities.*

Porter R, Jones T: *The Merck manual of medical information: Home edition,* Hoboken, NJ, 2016, John Wiley & Sons.

*One of the classic medicine references available to health care professionals, this text covers most medical conditions.*

Venes S, Venes D: *Tabor's cyclopedic medical dictionary,* Philadelphia, PA, 2016, F.A. Davis.

*A wealth of valuable information on various health conditions.*

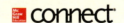

# Addresses of Professional Sports Medicine Organizations

American Academy of Family Physicians, 11400 Tomahawk Creek Parkway Leawood, KS 66211-2680. www.aafp.org

American Academy of Ophthalmology 655 Beach St., Box 7424, San Francisco, CA 94120-7424. (415) 561-8500.

American Academy of Orthopaedic Surgeons (AAOS), 9400 West Higgins Rd., Rosemont, IL 60018. www.aaos.org

American Academy of Pediatrics, Council on Sports Medicine and Fitness, 141 NW Point Blvd., Elk Grove Village, IL 60007-1098. www.aap.org

American Academy of Physical Medicine and Rehabilitation (AAPMR), 9700 W. Bryn Mawr Ave., Suite 200, Rosemont, IL 60018. (847) 737-6000. www.aapmr.org

American Academy of Podiatric Sports Medicine (AAPSM), 3121 NE 26th St., Ocala, FL 34470. www.aapsm.org

American Chiropractic Association Sports Council, (ACASC) 1720 S. Belluaire St., Suite 406, Denver, CO 80222. www.acasc.org

American College of Sports Medicine, 401 W. Michigan St., Indianapolis, IN 46202-3233. www.acsm.org

American Massage Therapy Association, 820 Davis St., Evanston, IL 60201. www.amtamassage.org

American Medical Athletic Association (AMAA), 4405 East West Highway, Suite 405, Bethesda, MD 20814. www.amaasportsmed.org

American Medical Society for Sports Medicine (AMSSM), 4000 W. 114th St., Suite 100, Leawood, KS 66211. (913) 327-1415. www.amssm.org

American Medical Tennis Association, 2414 43rd Ave. East, B-1, Seattle, WA 98112. www.mdtennis.org

American Optometric Association (AOA) Sports Vision Section (SVS), 243 N. Lindbergh Blvd., St. Louis, MO 63141-7881. www.aoa.org/optometrists/membership/aoa-sections/sports-vision-section

American Orthopaedic Society for Sports Medicine, 9400 W. Higgins Rd., Suite 300, Rosemont, IL 60018. www.sportsmed.org

American Osteopathic Academy of Sports Medicine, 2424 American Ln., Madison, WI 53704. (608) 2424 American Lane Madison, WI 53704. www.aoasm.org

Association, 1111 N. Fairfax St., Alexandria, VA 22314. www.apta.org

American Running Association, 4405 East West Hwy., Suite 405, Bethesda, MD 20814. www.americanrunning.org

American Society of Biomechanics (ASB), c/o Stacie Ringleb, Ph.D., Sec./Mem. Chair, Old Dominion University, Norfolk, VA 23529. (757) 683-5934. www.asbweb.org

American Sports Medicine Association, 660 W. Duarte Rd, Suite 1, Arcadia, CA 91007. (818) 445-1978.

Association of Volleyball Physicians, 1229 N. North Branch, Suite 122, Chicago, IL 60622. (708) 210-3112.

Canadian Academy of Sport and Exercise Medicine, 55 Metcalfe St., Suite 300, Ottawa, ON K1P 6L5. (613) 748-5851. http://casem-acmse.org

Canadian Athletic Therapists Association, Suite 300, 400 5th Ave. S.W., Calgary, AB, T2P 0L6. (888) 509-2282. www.athletictherapy.org

Canadian Sport Massage Therapists Association (CSMTA), Suite 208, 1518 Pandora Ave., Victoria, BC, V8R 1A8. (250) 590-9861. www.csmta.ca

College Athletic Trainers' Society, c/o Robert Murphy, PO Box 250325, Atlanta, GA 30325. www.collegeathletictrainer.org

Royal College of Chiropractic Sports Sciences (Canada), c/o Canadian Chiropractic Association, 1396 Eglinton Ave. W., Toronto, ON M6C 2E4. (416) 781-5656. http://rccssc.ca

Cooper Institute for Aerobics Research, 12330 Preston Rd., Dallas, TX 75230. (972) 341-3200. www.cooperinst.org

Gatorade Sport Science Institute, 617 W. Main St., Barrington, IL 60010. www.gssiweb.com

International Academy of Sports Vision (IASV), 200 S. Progress Ave., Harrisburg, PA 17109. (717) 652-8080. http://intlsportsvisionacademy.weebly.com

International Powerlifting Federation Medical Committee, Box 4160, Opelika, AL 36803. (334) 749-6222.

The International Society for Sport Psychiatry, 316 N. Milwaukee St., Suite 318, Milwaukee, WI 53202. (414) 271-2900. www.sportspsychiatry.org

Joint Commission on Sports Medicine and Science, 1620 Valwood Pkwy, Suite 115, Carrollton, TX 75006. (214) 637-6282. www.jcsmsonline.org

National Academy of Sports Medicine (NASM), 1750 E. Northrop Blvd., Suite 200, Chandler, AZ 85286-1744. (800) 460-6276. www.nasm.org

National Collegiate Athletic Association, Competitive Safeguards and Medical Aspects of Sports Committee, 700 W. Washington St., P.O. Box 6222, Indianapolis, IN 46206-6222. www.ncaa.org

National Athletic Trainers' Association, 1620 Valwood Pkwy, Suite 115, Carrollton, TX 75006. (214) 637-6282. www.nata.org

The National Council for Sports Medicine Education (NCSME), P.O. Box 3, Saratoga Springs, NY 12866. (518) 786-1529.

The National Federation of State High School Athletic Associations, PO Box 690, Indianapolis, IN 46206. (317) 972-6900. http://nfhs.org

National Strength and Conditioning Association, 1885 Bob Johnson Dr., Colorado Springs, CO 80906. (800) 815-6826. www.nsca.com

North American Society for Pediatric Exercise Medicine (NASPEM), Box 5076, 1607 N. Market St., Champaign, IL 61825-5076. (217) 351-5076. www.naspem.org

North American Society for the Psychology of Sport and Physical Activity (NASPSPA), c/o Quincy J. Almeida, qalmeida@wlu.ca.naspspa.com

Sports Medicine Council of British Columbia (SMCBC), 2350-3713 Kensington Ave., Burnaby, BC, V5B 0A7. (604) 294-3050.

U.S. Olympic Committee Sports Medicine Division, 1 Olympic Plaza, Colorado Springs, CO 80909-5760. (800) 933-4473 ext 2. www.teamusa.org/about-the-usoc/athlete-development/sports-medicine

Wilderness Medical Society, 2150 S 1300 E, Suite 500, Salt Lake City, Utah 84106. (801) 990-2988. www.wms.org

# NATA Position, Official, Consensus, and Support Statements

## POSITION STATEMENTS

www.nata.org/news-publications/pressroom/statements/position

- Exertional Heat Illnesses (Sept. 2015)
- Management of Sport Concussion (Mar. 2014)
- Preparticipation Physical Examinations and Disqualifying Conditions (Feb. 2014)
- Conservative Management and Prevention of Ankle Sprains in Athletes (Aug. 2013)
- Lightning Safety for Athletics and Recreation (Mar. 2013)
- Evaluation of Dietary Supplements for Performance Nutrition (Feb. 2013)
- Anabolic-Androgenic Steroids (Sept. 2012)
- Preventing Sudden Death in Sports (2012)
- Safe Weight Loss and Maintenance Practices in Sport and Exercise (2011)
- Prevention of Pediatric Overuse Injuries (2011)
- Skin Diseases (2011)
- Acute Management of the Cervical Spine Injured Athlete (2009)
- Environmental Cold Injuries (2008)
- Preventing, Detecting, and Managing Disordered Eating in Athletes (2008)
- Management of the Athlete with Type 1 Diabetes Mellitus (2007)
- Management of Asthma in Athletes (Sept. 2005)
- Head Down Contact and Spearing in Tackle Football (2004)
- Management of Sport-Related Concussion (2004)
- Emergency Planning in Athletics (2002)
- Exertional Heat Illnesses (2002)
- Fluid Replacement for Athletes (2000)

## OFFICIAL STATEMENTS

www.nata.org/news-publications/pressroom/statements/official

- Support of New NCAA Autonomous 5 (aka Power 5) Conferences' Independent Medical Care Rules (Feb. 2016)
- College Supervision of Student Aides (Jan. 2016)
- Meaningful Use Statement (Aug. 2014)
- Proper Supervision of Secondary School Student Aides (Jun. 2014)
- Prehospital Care of the Athlete with Cervical Spine Injury (May 2014)
- Friday Night Tykes (Jan. 2014)
- Calling Crown of the Helmet Violations (Aug. 2013)
- "Time Outs" Before Athletic Events Recommended for Health Care Providers (Aug. 2012)
- Providing Quality Health Care and Safeguards to Athletes of All Ages and Levels of Participation (Dec. 2011)

- Commotio Cordis (2007)
- Communicable and Infectious Diseases in Secondary School Sports (2007)
- Steroids and Performance Enhancing Substances (2005)
- Community-Acquired MRSA Infections (2005)
- Youth Football and Heat Related Illness (2005)
- Use of Qualified Athletic Trainers in Secondary Schools (2004)
- Full-Time On-Site Athletic Trainer Coverage for Secondary School Athletic Programs (2004)
- Automated External Defibrillators (2003)

## CONSENSUS STATEMENTS

www.nata.org/news-publications/pressroom/statements/consensus

- Inter-Association Recommendations for Developing a Plan to Recognize and Refer Student Athletes with Psychological Concerns at the Secondary School Level: A Consensus Statement (Mar. 2015)
- Appropriate Care of the Spine Injured Athlete (2015)
- Inter-Association Recommendations in Developing a Plan for Recognition and Referral of Student Athletes with Psychological Concerns at the Collegiate Level (Oct. 2013)
- Inter-Association Consensus Statement on Best Practices for Sports Medicine Management for Secondary Schools and Colleges (Jan. 2014)
- Inter-Association Task Force for Preventing Sudden Death in Secondary School Athletics (Jul. 2013)
- Inter-Association Task Force for Preventing Sudden Death in Collegiate Conditioning Sessions: Best Practices Recommendations (Aug. 2012)
- Managing Prescriptions and Non-Prescription Medication in the Athletic Training Facility (2009)
- Preseason Heat Acclimatization Guideline for Secondary School Athletics (2009)
- Inter-Association Recommendations on Emergency Preparedness and Management of Sudden Cardiac Arrest in High School and College Athletic Programs (Mar. 2007)
- Sickle Cell Trait and the Athlete (2007)
- Appropriate Medical Care for Secondary School-Age Athletes (2003)
- Inter-Association Task Force on Exertional Heat Illnesses (Jun. 2003)

## SUPPORT STATEMENTS

www.nata.org/news-publications/pressroom/statements/support

- American Medical Society for Sports Medicine Letter of Support for Athletic Trainers in Secondary Schools (2016)
- American Academy of Family Physicians' Support of Athletic Trainers for High School Athletes (2007)
- Recommendations and Guidelines for Appropriate Medical Coverage of Intercollegiate Athletics (2007)
- The Coalition to Preserve Patient Access to Physical Medicine and Rehabilitation Services (2005)
- Appropriate Medical Care for Secondary School-Age Athletes (manuscript) (2004)
- NCAA Support of Recommendations and Guidelines for Appropriate Medical Coverage of Intercollegiate Athletics (2003)
- American Medical Association's Support of Athletic Trainers in Secondary Schools (1998)

# Sports Medicine–Related Journals

Acta Orthopaedica Scandinavica
Adapted Physical Activity Quarterly
Advances in Orthopaedic Surgery
American Journal of Medicine and Sport
American Journal of Orthodontics and Dentofacial
   Orthopedics
American Journal of Sports Medicine
Archives of Orthopaedic and Trauma Surgery
Archives of Physical Medicine and Rehabilitation
Arthroscopy
Arthroskopie
Athletic Therapy and Training
Bone
British Journal of Sport Medicine
Canadian Journal of Applied Physiology
Clinical Exercise Physiology
Clinical Journal of Sports Medicine
Clinical Orthopaedics and Related Research
Clinics in Sports Medicine
Complications in Orthopedics
Current Opinion in Orthopedics
Current Orthopaedics
Current Sports Medicine Reports
European Journal of Orthopaedic Surgery and
   Traumatology
European Spine Journal
Exercise Immunology Review
Foot and Ankle International
Foot and Ankle Clinics
Hand Clinics
Hand Surgery
International Journal of Sport Nutrition
International Journal of Sports Medicine
International Orthopaedics
Internet Journal of Orthopedic Surgery and Related
   Subjects
Journal of Aging and Physical Activity
Journal of the American Academy of Orthopaedic
   Surgeons
Journal of Applied Biomechanics
Journal of Arthroplasty
Journal of Athletic Training

Journal of Back and Musculoskeletal Rehabilitation
Journal of Bone and Joint Surgery
Journal of Hand Surgery (American)
Journal of Hand Surgery (British and European volume)
Journal of Musculoskeletal Research
Journal of Orthopaedic Science
Journal of Orthopaedic Trauma
Journal of Orthopedic and Sports Physical Therapy
Journal of Pediatric Orthopaedics
Journal of Science and Medicine in Sport
Journal of Spinal Disorders
Journal of Sport Rehabilitation
Journal of Sports Chiropractic and Rehabilitation
Journal of Sports Medicine
Journal of Sports Medicine and Physical Fitness
Journal of Strength and Conditioning Research
Medicine and Science in Sport and Exercise
Medscape Orthopedics and Sports Medicine
Neuro-Orthopedics
Operative Techniques in Orthopaedics
Operative Techniques in Sports Medicine
Orthopaedic Physical Therapy Clinics
Orthopedic Clinics of North America
Orthopedics
Orthopedics Today
Orthopedic Surgery
Pediatric Exercise Science
Physical Medicine and Rehabilitation Clinics of
   North America
Physical Therapy Journal
Physical Therapy in Sport
Physician and Sportsmedicine
Scandinavian Journal of Medicine and Science in Sports
Seminars in Musculoskeletal Radiology
Skeletal Radiology
Spine
Sports Medicine
Sports Medicine and Arthroscopy Review
Strength and Conditioning
Techniques in Orthopaedics
The Knee
Training and Conditioning

# Sample Résumé

Joseph Q. Doe, ATC, LAT
jqdoe@email.unc.edu
100 Lexington CT
Chapel Hill, NC 27514
(919) 555-1234

**EDUCATION**

UNIVERSITY OF NORTH CAROLINA AT CHAPEL HILL
Graduation: Masters of Arts, May 2016
Major: Exercise and Sports Science
Specialization: Athletic Training (NATA Accredited Program)

UNIVERSITY OF NORTH CAROLINA AT CHAPEL HILL
Graduation: Bachelor of Arts, May 21, 2014, with Highest Honors
Major: Exercise and Sports Science    GPA: 3.456, Major: 3.644
Specialization: Athletic Training (CAATE Accredited Program)

**ATHLETIC TRAINING EXPERIENCE**

Graduate Assistant Athletic Trainer
   University of North Carolina Chapel Hill, NC, August 2014–Present
      Responsible for evaluation, treatment, and rehabilitation of injuries
      Coverage of practices and meets, record keeping, and updating coaches and medical
         staff for football, men's lacrosse, and fencing
      Advanced Clinical Instructor for undergraduate student athletic trainers
      Supervising undergraduate athletic trainers
      Head Trainer for the University of North Carolina's Junior Varsity Football Team
Athletic Training Student
   University of North Carolina Chapel Hill, NC, August 2010–2014
      Responsible for evaluation, treatment, and rehabilitation of injuries
      Coverage of practices and meets, record keeping, and updating coaches and medical
         staff for wrestling, women's lacrosse, and women's volleyball
University of North Carolina Summer Camp Athletic Training
      Served as Camp Coordinator for wrestling camp; in charge of ordering
         medical supplies and overseeing the athletic training staff
      Served as an athletic trainer at various camps, including men's and women's lacrosse,
         cheerleading, and soccer

**TEACHING EXPERIENCE**

Instructor
- Golf
- Bowling
- Racquetball
- Self-defense

Teaching Assistant
- Emergency Care class
- Gross Anatomy labs
- Guest lecture in Personal Health class

**CERTIFICATIONS AND MEMBERSHIPS**

- Certified Athletic Trainer
- Licensed Athletic Trainer (LAT)
- Responding to Emergency Instructor
- First Aid and Community CPR Instructor
- Automated External Defibrillator Instructor
- Epi-Pen Certified
- NATA member
- UNC Student Athletic Trainer member

**VOLUNTEER EXPERIENCES**

Coaching
- Chapel Hill YMCA, Basketball Coach, 2010–2012
- Carrboro Park and Rec., Baseball Coach, 2011–2013
- Rainbow Soccer, Soccer Coach, 2012–2014

**REFERENCES**

Available on Request

# NATA Code of Ethics

## PREAMBLE

The National Athletic Trainers' Association Code of Ethics states the principles of ethical behavior that should be followed in the practice of athletic training. It is intended to establish and maintain high standards and professionalism for the athletic training profession. The principles do not cover every situation encountered by the practicing athletic trainer, but are representative of the spirit with which athletic trainers should make decisions. The principles are written generally; the circumstances of a situation will determine the interpretation and application of a given principle and of the Code as a whole. When a conflict exists between the Code and the law, the law prevails.

## PRINCIPLE 1

Members shall respect the rights, welfare and dignity of all.

1.1 Members shall not discriminate against any legally protected class.
1.2 Members shall be committed to providing competent care.
1.3 Members shall preserve the confidentiality of privileged information and shall not release such information to a third party not involved in the patient's care without a release unless required by law.

## PRINCIPLE 2

Members shall comply with the laws and regulations governing the practice of athletic training.

2.1 Members shall comply with applicable local, state, and federal laws and institutional guidelines.
2.2 Members shall be familiar with and abide by all National Athletic Trainers' Association standards, rules and regulations.
2.3 Members shall report illegal or unethical practices related to athletic training to the appropriate person or authority.
2.4 Members shall avoid substance abuse and, when necessary, seek rehabilitation for chemical dependency.

## PRINCIPLE 3

Members shall maintain and promote high standards in their provision of services.

3.1 Members shall not misrepresent, either directly or indirectly, their skills, training, professional credentials, identity or services.

3.2 Members shall provide only those services for which they are qualified through education or experience and which are allowed by their practice acts and other pertinent regulation.
3.3 Members shall provide services, make referrals, and seek compensation only for those services that are necessary.
3.4 Members shall recognize the need for continuing education and participate in educational activities that enhance their skills and knowledge.
3.5 Members shall educate those whom they supervise in the practice of athletic training about the Code of Ethics and stress the importance of adherence.
3.6 Members who are researchers or educators should maintain and promote ethical conduct in research and educational activities.

## PRINCIPLE 4

Members shall not engage in conduct that could be construed as a conflict of interest or that reflects negatively on the profession.

4.1 Members should conduct themselves personally and professionally in a manner that does not compromise their professional responsibilities or the practice of athletic training.
4.2 National Athletic Trainers' Association current or past volunteer leaders shall not use the NATA logo in the endorsement of products or services or exploit their affiliation with the NATA in a manner that reflects badly upon the profession.
4.3 Members shall not place financial gain above the patient's welfare and shall not participate in any arrangement that exploits the patient.
4.4 Members shall not, through direct or indirect means, use information obtained in the course of the practice of athletic training to try to influence the score or outcome of an athletic event, or attempt to induce financial gain through gambling.
4.5 Members shall not provide or publish information, photographs, or any other communications related to athletic training that negatively reflects the profession.

# Manual Muscle Tests

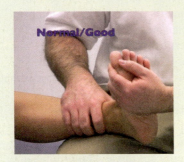

F–1    Ankle Dorsiflexion and Inversion

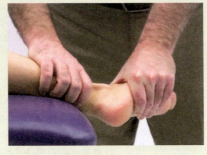

F–2    Ankle Eversion

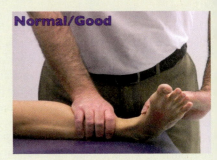

F–3    Ankle Inversion

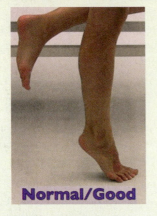

F–4    Ankle Plantarflexion

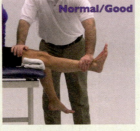

F–5    Knee Extension

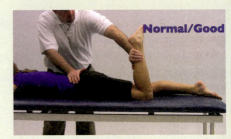

F–6    Knee Flexion

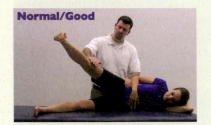

F–7    Hip Abduction with Hip Flexed

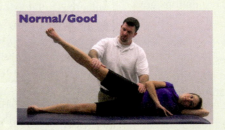

F–8    Hip Abduction

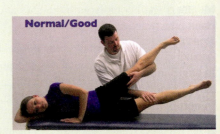

F–9    Hip Adduction

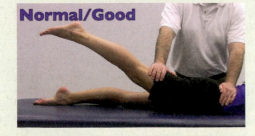

F–10    Hip Extension

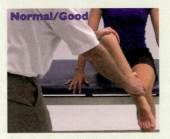

F–11    Hip Flexion, Abduction, Lateral Rotation

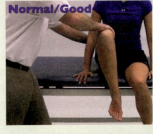

F–12    Hip Flexion

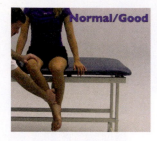

F–13    Hip Lateral Rotation

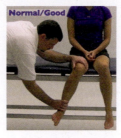

F–14    Hip Medial Rotation

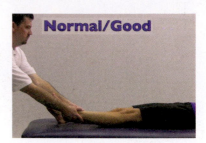

F–15    Pelvic Elevation

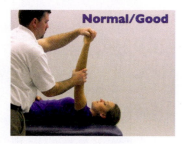

F–16    Scapular Abduction and Upward Rotation

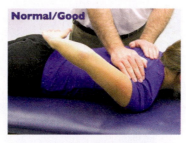

F–17    Scapular Adduction and Downward Rotation

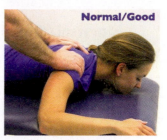

F–18    Scapular Adduction

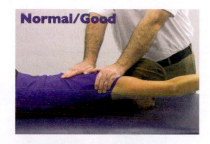

F–19    Scapular Depression and Adduction

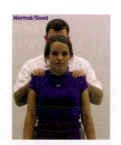

F–20    Scapular Elevation

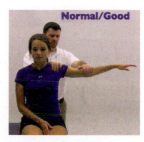

F–21    Shoulder Abduction to 90 Degrees

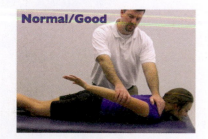

F–22    Shoulder Extension

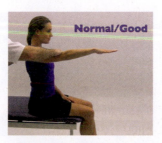

F–23    Shoulder Flexion

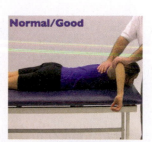

F–24    Shoulder Horizontal Abduction

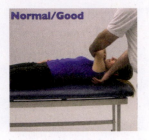

F–25    Shoulder Horizontal Adduction

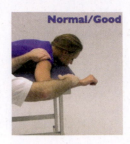

F–26    Shoulder Lateral Rotation

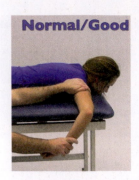

F–27    Shoulder Medial Rotation

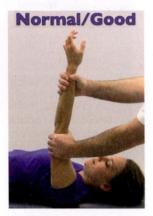

F–28    Elbow Extension

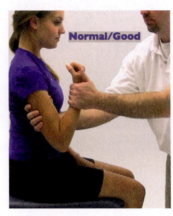

F–29    Elbow Flexion

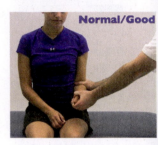

F–30    Forearm Pronation

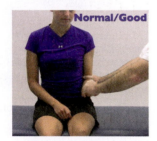

F–31    Forearm Supination

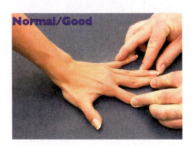

F–32    Finger Abduction

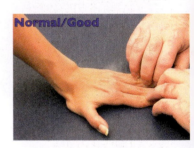

F–33    Finger Adduction

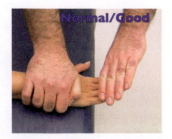

F–34    Hand Metacarpophylangeal
        Joint Extension

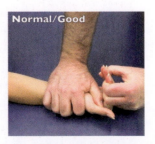

F–35    Hand Metacarpophylangeal
        Joint Flexion

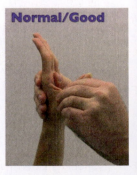

F–36    Thumb Abduction

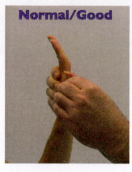

**Normal/Good**

F–37    Thumb Adduction

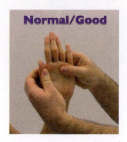

**Normal/Good**

F–38    Thumb Extension

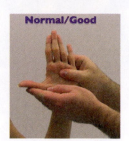

**Normal/Good**

F–39    Thumb Flexion

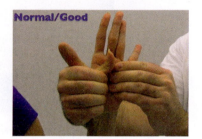

**Normal/Good**

F–40    Thumb Opposition

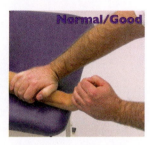

**Normal/Good**

F–41    Wrist Extension

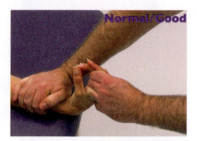

**Normal/Good**

F–42    Wrist Flexion

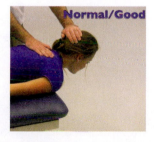

**Normal/Good**

F–43    Neck Extension

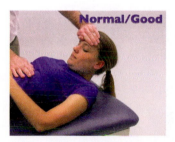

**Normal/Good**

F–44    Neck Flexion

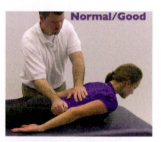

**Normal/Good**

F–45    Trunk Extension

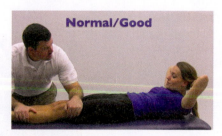

**Normal/Good**

F–46    Trunk Flexion

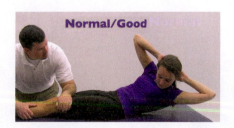

**Normal/Good**

F–47    Trunk Rotation

# Goniometric Measurements of Range of Motion

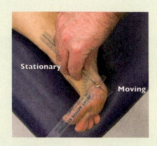

G–1    Toe MP Joint Extension

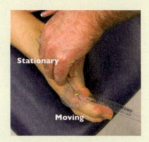

G–2    Toe MP Joint Flexion

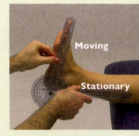

G–3    Ankle Dorsiflexion

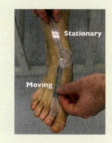

G–4    Ankle Eversion

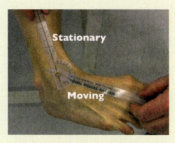

G–5    Ankle Inversion

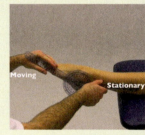

G–6    Ankle Plantarflexion

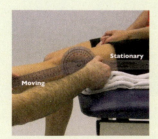

G–7    Knee Extension

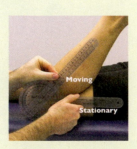

G–8    Knee Flexion

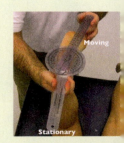

G–9    Tibial Rotation

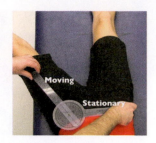

G–10    Hip Abduction

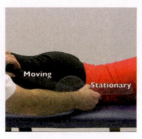

G–11    Hip Extension

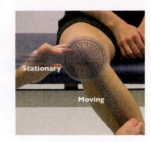

G–12    Hip External Rotation

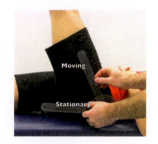

G–13    Hip Flexion

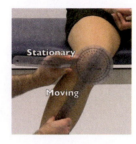

G–14    Hip Internal Rotation

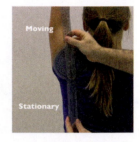

G–15    Shoulder Abduction

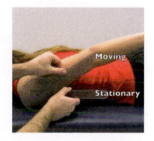

G–16    Shoulder Extension

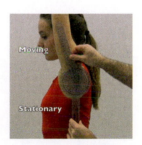

G–17    Shoulder Flexion

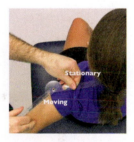

G–18    Shoulder Horizontal Abduction

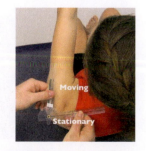

G–19    Shoulder Horizontal Adduction

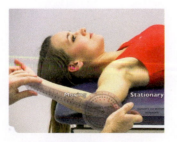

G–20    Shoulder Lateral Rotation

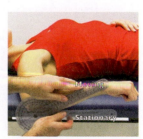

G–21    Shoulder Medial Rotation

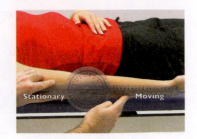

G–22    Elbow Extension

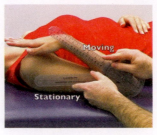

G–23    Elbow Flexion

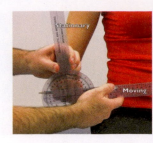

G–24    Forearm Pronation

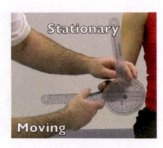

G–25    Forearm Supination

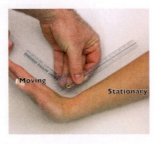

G–26    Wrist Extension

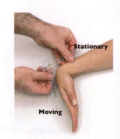

G–27    Wrist Flexion

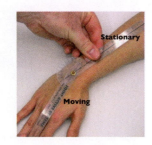

G–28    Wrist Radial Deviation

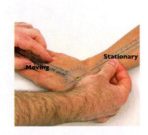

G–29    Wrist Ulnar Deviation

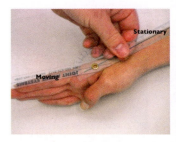

G–30    Finger MP Joint Extension

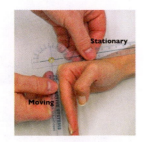

G–31    Finger MP Joint Flexion

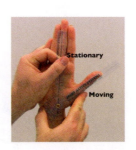

G–32    Thumb Abduction

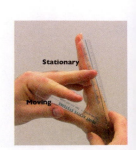

G–33    Thumb Flexion

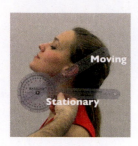

G–34   Neck Extension

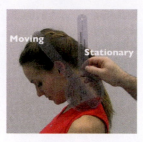

G–35   Neck Flexion

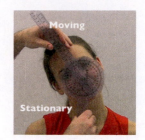

G–36   Neck Lateral Sidebending

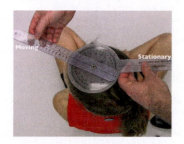

G–37   Neck Rotation

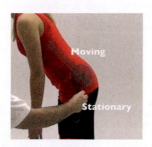

G–38   Trunk Isolated
        Lumbar Flexion

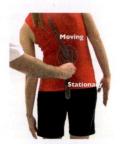

G–39   Trunk Lateral
        Sidebending

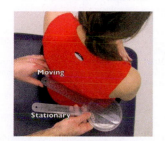

G–40   Trunk Rotation

# Glossary

## A

**abduction**   Movement of a body part away from the midline of the body.

**accident**   An act that occurs by chance or without intention.

**acclimatization**   A process by which an individual adapts to a gradual change in environmental conditions.

**accommodating resistance**   Change in resistance at different points in the range.

**active range of motion (AROM)**   Joint motion that occurs because of muscle contraction.

**acute injury**   An injury with sudden onset and short duration.

**adduction**   Movement of a body part toward the midline of the body.

**adipose cell**   Stores triglyceride.

**afferent nerves**   Nerves that transport messages toward the brain.

**Affordable Care Act**   Mandates the availability of affordable health care insurance for every American.

**agonist muscles**   Muscles directly engaged in contraction as related to muscles that relax at the same time.

**ambient**   Environmental (e.g., temperature or air that invests one's immediate environment).

**ambulation**   Move or walk from place to place.

**ameoboid action**   Cellular action like that of an amoeba, using protoplasmic pseudopod.

**amenorrhea**   Absence or suppression of menstruation.

**amino acids**   Basic units that make up proteins.

**ampere**   Volume or amount of electrical energy.

**analgesia**   Pain inhibition.

**analgesic**   Agent that relieves pain without causing a complete loss of sensation.

**anaphylaxis**   Increased susceptibility or sensitivity to a foreign protein or toxin as a result of previous exposure to it.

**androgen**   Any substance that aids the development and controls the appearance of male characteristics.

**anemia**   Lack of iron.

**anesthesia**   Partial or complete loss of sensation.

**ankle mortise**   Talocrural joint formed by the tibia, fibula, and talus.

**anomaly**   Deviation from the normal.

**anorexia**   Lack or loss of appetite; aversion to food.

**anorexia nervosa**   Eating disorder characterized by a distorted body image.

**anoxia**   Lack of oxygen.

**antagonist muscles**   Muscles that counteract the action of the agonist muscles.

**anterior**   Before or in front of.

**anteroposterior**   Refers to the position of front to back.

**anteversion**   Tipping forward of a part as a whole, without bending.

**antipyretic**   Agent that relieves or reduces fever.

**anxiety**   A feeling of uncertainty or apprehension.

**apnea**   Temporary cessation of breathing.

**apophysis**   Bony outgrowth to which muscles attach.

**apophysitis**   Inflammation of an apophysis.

**arrhythmical movement**   Irregular movement.

**arthrogram**   Radiopaque material injected into a joint to facilitate the taking of an X-ray.

**arthrokinematics**   Physiological and accessory movements of the joint.

**arthroscopic examination**   Viewing the inside of a joint through an arthroscope, which uses a small camera lens.

**assumption of risk**   An individual, through express or implied agreement, assumes that some risk or danger will be involved in a particular undertaking; a person takes his or her own chances.

**asymmetry (body)**   Lack of symmetry of sides of the body.

**ATC**   Certified Athletic Trainer.

**athletic training clinic**   Health care facility.

**atrophy**   Wasting away of tissue or of an organ; decrease in the size of a body part or muscle.

**attenuation**   A decrease in intensity as sound or any form of energy enters deeper tissues.

**aura**   Pre-epileptic phenomenon, involving visual sensation of fire or glow, along with other possible sensory hallucinations and dreamlike states.

**autogenic inhibition**   The relaxation of the antagonist muscle during contractions.

**automatism**   Automatic behavior before consciousness or full awareness has been achieved after a brain concussion.

**avascular**   Devoid of blood circulation.

**avascular necrosis**   Death of tissue caused by the lack of blood supply.

**avulsion**   Forcible tearing away of a part or a structure.

**axilla**   Armpit.

## B

***Bacillus***   Genus of bacteria which can cause major systemic damage.

**bacteremia**   Bacterial infection in the blood.

**bacteria**   Morphologically, the simplest group of nongreen vegetable organisms, various species of which are involved in fermentation and putrefaction, the production of disease, and the fixing of atmospheric nitrogen; a schizomycete.

**bacteriostatic**   Halting the growth of bacteria.

**ballistic stretching**   Older stretching technique that uses repetitive bouncing motions.

**beam nonuniformity ratio (BNR)**   Amount of variability in intensity of an ultrasound beam.

**bending**   Force on a horizontal beam or bone that places stresses within the structure, causing it to bend or strain.

**benign**   Of no danger to health.

**beta-endorphin**   Chemical substance produced in the brain.

**bioavailability**   How completely a particular drug is absorbed by the system.

**bioequivalent drugs**   Drugs having a similar biological effect.

**biomechanics**   Branch of study that applies the laws of mechanics to living organisms and biological tissues.

**biotransformation**   Transforming a drug so that it can be metabolized.

**bipedal**   Having two feet or moving on two feet.

**BMR**   Basal metabolic rate.

**body composition**   Percent body fat plus lean body weight.

**bradykinin**   Peptide chemical that causes pain in an injured area.

**bradypnea**   Slow breathing.

**buccal**   Pertaining to the cheek or mouth.

**bulimia**   Binge-purge eating disorder.

**buoyancy**   The tendency of a body to float or rise when placed in water.

**bursae**   Pieces of synovial membrane that contain a small amount of fluid.

**bursitis**   Inflammation of bursae at sites of bony prominences between muscle and tendon such as those of the shoulder and knee.

## C

**calcific tendinitis**   Deposition of calcium in a chronically inflamed tendon, especially the tendons of the shoulder.

**calisthenic**   Exercise involving free movement without the aid of equipment.

**calorie (large)**   Amount of heat required to raise 1 kg of water 1°C; used to express the fuel or energy value of food or the heat output of the organism; the amount of heat required to heat 1 lb of water to 4°F.

**cardiorespiratory endurance**   Ability to perform activities for extended periods of time.

**catastrophic injury**   Relates to a permanent injury of the spinal cord that leaves the athlete quadriplegic or paraplegic.

**catecholamine**   Active amines, epinephrine and norepinephrine, that affect the nervous and cardiovascular systems.

**cellulitis**   An inflammation of cells and connective tissue that extends deep into the tissues.

**cerebrovascular accident**   Stroke.

**chafing**   Superficial inflammation that develops when skin is subjected to friction.

**chemical mediator**   A chemical that causes or produces a specific physiological response.

**chemotaxis**   Response to influence of chemical stimulation.

**chiropractor**   One who practices a method for restoring normal condition by adjusting the segments of the spinal column.

***Chlamydia trachomatis***   A microorganism that can cause a wide variety of diseases in humans, one of which is venereal and causes nonspecific urethritis.

**chondromalacia**   Abnormal softening of cartilage.

**chronic injury**   Injury with long onset and long duration.

**cicatrix**   Scar or mark formed by fibrous connective tissue; left by a wound or sore.

**circadian dysrhythmia (jet lag)**   Disruption of the biological and biophysical time clock.

**circadian rhythm**   Biological time clock by which the body functions.

**circuit training**   Exercise stations that consist of various combinations of weight training, flexibility, calisthenics, and aerobic exercises.

**circumduct**   Act of moving a limb, such as the arm or hip, in a circular manner.

**clonic**   Involuntary muscle contraction characterized by alternate contraction and relaxation in rapid succession.

**clonic muscle contraction**   Alternating involuntary muscle contraction and relaxation in quick succession.

**closed fracture**   A fracture that does not penetrate superficial tissue.

**coenzymes**   Enzyme activators.

**collagen**   Main organic constituent of connective tissue.

**collision sport**   Sport in which athletes use their bodies to deter or punish opponents.

**colloid**   Liquid or gelatinous substance that retains particles of another substance in a state of suspension.

**commission (legal liability)**   Person commits an act that is not legally his or hers to perform.

**commotio cordis**   Cardiac arrest that occurs due to blue impact to the chest.

**communicable disease**   Disease that may be transmitted directly or indirectly from one individual to another.

**compression**   Force that crushes tissue.

**concentric (positive) contraction**   The muscle shortens while contracting against resistance.

**conduction**   Heating through direct contact with a hot medium.

**conjunctiva**   Mucous membrane that lines the eyes.

**contact sport**   Sport in which athletes do make physical contact but not with the intent to produce bodily injury.

**contrast bath procedure**   Technique that uses immersion in ice slush, followed by immersion in tepid water.

**contrecoup injury**   After head is struck, brain continues to move within the skull, resulting in injury to the side opposite the force.

**contusion**   Compression of soft tissue that results in bleeding into surrounding tissues.

**convection**   Heating indirectly through another medium, such as air or liquid.

**conversion**   Heating through other forms of energy (e.g., electricity).

**convulsions**   Paroxysms of involuntary muscular contractions and relaxations.

**core**   Muscles of the lumbar spine, abdomen, hips, and pelvis.

**core temperature**   Internal, or deep, body temperature monitored by cells in the hypothalamus, as opposed to shell, or peripheral, temperature, which is registered by that layer of insulation provided by the skin, subcutaneous tissues, and superficial portions of the muscle masses.

**corticosteroid**   Steroid produced by the adrenal cortex.

**coryza**   Profuse nasal discharge.

**counterirritant**   Agent that produces mild inflammation and acts, in turn, as an analgesic when applied locally to the skin (e.g., liniment).

**coup injury**   Injury that occurs on the same side of the brain as the impact.

**coupling medium**   Used to facilitate the transmission of ultrasound into the tissues.

**creep**   Deformation of tissues that occurs with application of a constant load over time.

**crepitus**   Crackling sound heard during the movement of ends of a broken bone.

**cryokinetics**   Cold application combined with exercise.

**cryotherapy**   Cold therapy.

**cubital fossa**   Triangular area on the anterior aspect of the forearm directly opposite the elbow joint (the bend of the elbow).

**cyanosis**   Slightly bluish, grayish, slate-like, or dark purple discoloration of the skin caused by a reduced amount of blood hemoglobin.

## D

**DAPRE**   Daily adjustable progressive resistance exercise.

**debride**   Removal of dirt and dead tissue from a wound.

**deconditioning**   State in which the athlete's body loses its competitive fitness.

**deformation**   Change in shape of a tissue.

**degeneration**   Deterioration of tissue.

**dermatome**   Area of skin innervated by a single spinal or cranial nerve.

**diagnosis**   Identification of a specific condition.

**diapedesis**   Passage of blood cells, via ameoboid action, through the intact capillary wall.

**diarthrodial joint**   Ball-and-socket joint.

**diastasis**   Separation of articulating bones.

**diastolic blood pressure**   The residual pressure when the heart is between beats.

**DIP**   Distal interphalangeal joint.

**diplopia**   Seeing double.

**dislocation**   A bone is forced out of alignment and stays out until surgically or manually replaced or reduced.

**distal**   Farthest from a center, from the midline, or from the trunk.

**DNA**   Deoxyribonucleic acid.

**doping**   The administration of a drug that is designed to improve the competitor's performance.

**dorsiflexion**   Bending toward the dorsum or rear; opposite of plantar flexion.

**dorsum**   The back of a body part.

**dressing**   Covering, protective or supportive, that is applied to an injury or a wound.

**drug**   A chemical agent used in the prevention, treatment, or diagnosis of disease.

**drug vehicle**   The substance in which a drug is transported.

**duty of care**   Part of an official job description.

**dynamic stretching**   Controlled stretches recommended prior to beginning an activity.

**dyspnea**   Difficult breathing.

**dysrhythmia**   Irregular heartbeats.

## E

**eccentric (negative) contraction**   The muscle lengthens while contracting against resistance.

**ecchymosis**   Black-and-blue skin discoloration caused by hemorrhage.

**ectopic**   Located in a place different from normal.

**edema**   Swelling as a result of the collection of fluid in connective tissue.

**effective radiating area**   Portion of the transducer that produces sound energy.

**efficacy**   A drug's capability of producing a specific therapeutic effect.

**effleurage**   Stroking.

**elasticity**   Property that allows a tissue to return to normal following deformation.

**electrolyte**   Solution that is a conductor of electricity.

**embolus**   A mass of undissolved matter.

**emetic**   Agent that induces vomiting.

**endurance**   Body's ability to engage in prolonged physical activity.

**enthesitis**   Group of conditions characterized by inflammation, fibrosis, and calcification around tendons, ligaments, and muscle insertions.

**enzyme**   An organic catalyst that can cause chemical changes in other substances without being changed itself.

**epidemiological approach**   Study of sports injuries that involves the relationship of as many factors as possible.

**epidemiology**   Study of factors affecting the health and illness of individuals and populations.

**epilepsy**   Recurrent paroxysmal disorder characterized by sudden attacks of altered consciousness, motor activity, sensory phenomena, or inappropriate behavior.

**epiphysis**   Cartilaginous growth region of a bone.

**epistaxis**   Nosebleed.

**ethics**   Principles of morality.

**etiology**   Science dealing with causes of disease.

**eversion of the foot**   To turn the foot outward.

**evidence-based practice**   Making clinical care decisions based on supporting evidence available in the literature.

**excoriation**   Removal of a piece or strip of skin.

**exotosis**   Benign bony outgrowth, usually capped by cartilage, that protrudes from the surface of a bone.

**external rotation gain (ERG)**   Significantly increased glenohumeral external rotation.

**extracellular matrix**   Collagen, elastin, ground substance, proteoglycans, and glycosaminoglycans.

**extraoral mouth guard**   Protective device that fits outside the mouth.

**extravasation**   Escape of a fluid from its vessels into the surrounding tissues.

**exudate**   Accumulation of fluid in an area.

## F

**facilitation**   To assist the progress of.

**fascia**   Fibrous membrane that covers, supports, and separates muscles.

**fasciitis**   Inflammation of fascia.

**fibrinogen**   Blood plasma protein that is converted into a fibrin clot.

**fibroblast**   Any cell component from which fibers are developed.

**fibrocartilage**   Type of cartilage (e.g., intervertebral disks) in which the matrix contains thick bundles of collaginous fibers.

**fibroplasia**   Period of scar formation.

**fibrosis**   Development of excessive fibrous connective tissue; fibroid degeneration.

**first intention**   Normal healing of a wound where new cells are formed to take the place of damaged cells, leaving little or no scar.

**flash-to-bang**   Number of seconds from lightning flash until the sound of thunder, divided by five.

**foot pronation**   Combined foot movements of plantar flexion, adduction, and eversion.

**foot supination**   Combined foot movements of dorsiflexion and inversion.

**force couple**   Depressor action by the subscapularis, infraspinatus, and teres minor muscles to stabilize the head of the humerus and to counteract the upward force exerted by the deltoid muscle during abduction of the arm.

**frequency**   Measured in hertz (Hz), cycles per second (cps), or pulses per second (pps).

**friction**   Heat producing.

**FSH**   Follicle-stimulating hormone.

## G

**GAS theory**   General adaptation syndrome.

**genitourinary**   Pertaining to the reproductive and urinary organs.

**genu recurvatum**   Hyperextension at the knee joint.

**genu valgum**   Knock-knee.

**genu varum**   Bowleg.

**GH**   Growth hormone.

**glenohumeral internal rotation deficit (GIRD)**   Significantly decreased glenohumeral internal rotation.

**glycemic index (GI)**   A scale that indicates how much different types of carbohydrate affect blood glucose levels.

**glycogen supercompensation**   High-carbohydrate diet.

**glycosaminoglycans**   Carbohydrate that partially composes proteoglycans.

**glycosuria**   Abnormally high proportion of sugar in the urine.

**Good Samaritan law**   Provides limited protection against legal liability to any individual who voluntarily chooses to provide first aid.

**granulation tissue**   Fibroblasts, collagen, and capillaries.

## H

**half-life**   Rate at which a drug disappears from the body through metabolism, excretion, or both.

**health insurance**   A contract between the insurance company and policyholder.

**hemarthrosis**   Blood in a joint cavity.

**hematolytic**   Pertaining to the degeneration and disintegration of the blood.

**hematoma**   Blood tumor.

**hematuria**   Blood in the urine.

**hemoglobin**   Coloring substance of the red blood cells.

**hemoglobinuria**   Hemoglobin in the urine.

**hemolysis**   Destruction of red blood cells.

**hemophilia**   Hereditary blood disease in which coagulation is greatly prolonged.

**hemopoietic**   Forming blood cells.

**hemorrhage**  Discharge of blood.

**hemothorax**  Bloody fluid in the pleural cavity.

**hertz (Hz)**  Number of sound waves per second.

**high intensity interval training (HIIT)**  Alternating periods of work with active recovery.

**hirsutism**  Excessive hair growth or the presence of hair in unusual places.

**homeostasis**  Maintenance of a steady-state in the body's internal environment.

**HOPS**  Evaluation scheme that includes history, observation, palpation, and special tests.

**hunting response**  Causes a slight temperature increase during cooling.

**hyperemia**  Unusual amount of blood in a body part.

**hyperextension**  Extreme stretching of a body part.

**hyperflexibility**  Flexibility beyond a joint's normal range.

**hyperhidrosis**  Excessive sweating; excessive foot perspiration.

**hyperkeratosis**  Excessive growth of the horny tissue layer.

**hypermobility**  Extreme mobility of a joint.

**hyperpnea**  Hyperventilation; increased minute volume of breathing; exaggerated deep breathing.

**hypertension**  High blood pressure; abnormally high tension.

**hyperthermia**  Elevated body temperature.

**hypertonic**  Having a higher osmotic pressure than a compared solution.

**hypertrophy**  Enlargement of a body part or muscle caused by an increase in the size of its cells.

**hyperventilation**  Labored breathing.

**hypoallergenic**  Low allergy producing.

**Hyponatremia**  Low blood sodium caused by consuming too much fluid, usually water.

**hypothermia**  Abnormally low body temperature.

**hypoxia**  Lack of an adequate amount of oxygen.

**I**

**idiopathic**  Cause of a condition is unknown.

**iliotibial band friction syndrome**  Runner's knee.

**immune system**  The body's defense system against invading microorganisms.

**injury**  An act that damages or hurts.

**innervation**  Nerve stimulation of a muscle.

**interosseous membrane**  Connective tissue membrane between bones.

**intertrigo**  Chafing of the skin.

**inunctions**  Oily or medicated substances (e.g., liniments) that are rubbed into the skin to produce a local or systemic effect.

**inversion of the foot**  To turn the foot inward; inner border of the foot lifts.

**ions**  Electrically charged atoms.

**ipsilateral**  Situated on the same side.

**ischemia**  Lack of blood supply to a body part.

**isokinetic exercise**  Resistance is given at a fixed velocity of movement with accommodating resistance.

**isokinetic muscle resistance**  Accommodating and variable resistance.

**isometric exercise**  Contracts the muscle statically without changing its length.

**isotonic exercise**  Shortens and lengthens the muscle through a complete range of motion.

**J**

**joint capsule**  Saclike structure that encloses the ends of bones in a diarthrodial joint.

**joint play**  Movement that is not voluntary, but accessory.

**K**

**keratolytic**  Loosening of the horny skin layer.

**keratosis**  Excessive growth of the horny tissue layer.

**kilocalorie**  Amount of heat required to raise 1 kg of water 1°C.

**kinesthesia; kinesthesis**  Sensation or feeling of movement; the awareness one has of the spatial relationships of one's body and its parts.

**kyphosis**  Exaggeration of the normal curve of the thoracic spine.

**L**

**labile**  Unsteady; not fixed and easily changed.

**lactase deficiency**  Difficulty digesting dairy products.

**laser**  Light amplification by stimulated emission of radiation.

**leukocytes**  Consist of two types–granulocytes (e.g., basophils and neutrophils) and agranulocytes (e.g., monocytes and lymphocytes).

**LH**  Luteinizing hormone.

**liability**  The state of being legally responsible for the harm one causes another person.

**load**  Outside force or forces acting on tissue.

**lordosis**  Abnormal lumbar vertebral convexity.

**luxation**  Complete joint dislocation.

**lymphocytes**  Cells that are the primary means of providing the body with immune capabilities.

**lysis**  To break down.

**M**

**macerated skin**  Skin that has been softened by exposure to wetting.

**macrophage**  A phagocytic cell of the immune system.

**macrotear**  Soft-tissue damage generally caused by acute trauma.

**malaise**  Discomfort and uneasiness caused by an illness.

**malfeasance (or act of commission)**  When an individual commits an act that is not legally his or hers to perform.

**malignant**  Dangerous to health; cells invade and destroy nearby tissue and potentially spread to other parts of the body.

**managed care**  Costs of health care are monitored closely by insurance carriers.

**margination**  Accumulation of leukocytes on blood vessel walls at the site of injury during early stages of inflammation.

**mast cells**  Connective tissue cells that contain heparin and histamine.

**MCP**  Metacarpophalangeal joint.

**mechanical failure**  Elastic limits of tissue are exceeded, causing tissue to break.

**mechanism**  Mechanical description of the cause.

**menarche**  Onset of menstrual function.

**metabolism**  Changing a drug into a water-soluble compound that can be excreted.

**metatarsalgia**  Pain in the ball of the foot.

**microtear**  Minor soft-tissue damage associated with overuse.

**microtrauma**  Microscopic lesion or injury.

**misfeasance**  When an individual improperly does something that he or she has the legal right to do.

**mm Hg**  Millimeters of mercury.

**muscle contracture**  Permanent contraction of a muscle as a result of spasm or paralysis.

**muscle cramps**  Involuntary muscle contractions.

**muscle guarding**  Muscle contraction in response to pain.

**muscle soreness**  Pain caused by overexertion in exercise.

**muscle strain**  A stretch, tear, or rip in the muscle or its tendon.

**muscular endurance**  The ability to perform repetitive muscular contractions against some resistance.

**muscular strength**  The maximal force that can be applied by a muscle during a single maximum contraction.

**myocarditis**  Inflammation of the heart muscle.

**myoglobin**  Respiratory protein in muscle tissue that is an oxygen carrier.

**myositis**  Inflammation of muscle.

**myositis ossificans**  Myositis marked by ossification of muscles.

**myotomes**  Muscle or groups of muscles innervated by motor fibers from a specific motor nerve.

**N**

**necrosin**  Chemical substance that stems from inflamed tissue, causing changes in normal tissue.

**negative resistance**  Slow, eccentric muscle contraction against a resistance.

**negligence**  The failure to use ordinary or reasonable care.

**nerve entrapment**  Nerve compressed between bone or soft tissue.

**neuritis**  Inflammation of a nerve.

**neuroma**  A bulging that emanates from a nerve.

**neuropraxia**  Disruption of normal nerve function without degeneration thus interrupting conduction of an impulse down the nerve fiber.

**neutrophils**  A type of leukocyte.

**nociceptor**  Receptor of pain.

**noncontact sport**  Sport in which athletes are not involved in any physical contact.

**nonfeasance (or an act of omission)**  When an individual fails to perform a legal duty.

**NSAIDs**  Nonsteroidal antiinflammatory drugs.

**nystagmus**  Constant, involuntary back and forth, up and down, or rotary movement of the eyeball.

**O**

**obesity**  Excessive amount of body fat.

**obstructed**  Blocked airway caused by either partial or complete obstruction.

**ohm**  Resistance.

**omission (legal)**  Person fails to perform a legal duty.

**open fracture**  Overlying skin is lacerated by protruding bone fragments.

**orthopedic surgeon**  One who corrects deformities of the musculoskeletal system.

**orthosis**  Used in sports as an appliance or apparatus to support, align, prevent, or correct deformities or to improve function of a movable body part.

**orthotics**  Field of knowledge relating to orthoses and their use.

**OSHA**  Occupational Safety and Health Administration.

**osteoarthritis**  Chronic disease involving joints in which there is destruction of articular or hyaline cartilage and bony overgrowth.

**osteoblasts**  Bone-producing cells.

**osteochondral**  Refers to relationship of bone and cartilage.

**osteochondritis**  Inflammation of bone and cartilage.

**osteochondritis dissecans**  Fragment of cartilage and underlying bone are detached from the articular surface.

**osteochondrosis**  Disease state of a bone and its articular cartilage.

**osteoblasts**  Bone-remodeling cells.

**osteoclasts**  Cells that resorb bone.

**osteoporosis**  A decrease in bone density.

**P**

**palpation**  Feeling an injury with the fingers.

**paraplegia**  Paralysis of lower portion of the body and of both legs.

**paresis**  Slight or incomplete paralysis.

**paresthesia**  Abnormal or morbid sensation, such as itching or prickling.

**passive range of motion**  Movement that is performed completely by the examiner.

**pathogenic**  Disease producing.

**patella alta**  Patella more superior.

**patella baja**  Patella more inferior.

**pathology**  Science of the structural and functional manifestations of disease.

**pathomechanics**  Mechanical forces that are applied to a living organism and adversely change the body's structure and function.

**patient**  Ill or injured athlete.

**pediatrician**  Specialist in the treatment of children's diseases.

**permeable**  Permitting the passage of a substance through a vessel wall.

**pes anserinus tendinitis**  Cyclist's knee.

**petrissage**  Kneading.

**phagocytes**  Neutrophils, macrophages, and leukocytes that ingest microorganisms, other cells, and foreign particles.

**phagocytosis**  Destruction of injurious cells or particles by phagocytes (white blood cells).

**phalanges**   Bones of the fingers and toes.

**phalanx**   Any one of the bones of the fingers and toes.

**pharmacokinetics**   The method by which drugs are absorbed, distributed, metabolized, and eliminated.

**pharmacology**   The study of drugs and their origin, nature, properties, and effects on living organisms.

**phonophoresis**   Introduction of ions of soluble salt into the body through ultrasound.

**photophobia**   Unusual intolerance to light.

**piezoelectric effect**   Electrical current produced by applying pressure to certain crystals.

**PIP**   Proximal interphalangeal joint.

**plastic**   Deformation of tissues that exists after the load is removed.

**platelet-rich plasma (PRP)**   Using blood plasma that has been enriched with platelets to stimulate healing of bone and soft tissue.

**plyometric exercise**   Type of exercise that maximizes the myotatic, or stretch, reflex.

**pneumothorax**   Collapse of a lung as a result of air in the pleural cavity.

**podiatrist**   Practitioner who specializes in the study and care of the foot.

**point tenderness**   Pain produced when an injury site is palpated.

**posterior**   Toward the rear, or back.

**potency**   The dose of a drug that is required to produce a desired therapeutic effect.

**power**   The ability to generate force rapidly.

**primary assessment**   Initial first-aid evaluation.

**primary survey**   An evaluation used to determine the existence of life-threatening, emergent conditions or illnesses.

**prognosis**   Prediction as to the probable result of a disease or an injury.

**prolotherapy**   Injecting an irritant solution into a tendon or ligament to facilitate healing.

**pronators**   Those who run on the inside of the foot.

**prophylaxis**   Guarding against injury or disease.

**proprioception**   The ability to determine the position of a joint in space.

**proprioceptive neuromuscular facilitation (PNF)**   Stretching techniques that involve combinations of alternating contractions and stretches.

**proprioceptor**   One of several receptors, each of which responds to stimuli elicited from within the body itself (e.g., the muscle spindles that invoke the myotatic, or stretch, reflex).

**prostaglandin**   Acidic lipid widely distributed in the body; in musculoskeletal conditions, it is concerned with vasodilation, a histamine-like effect; it is inhibited by aspirin.

**prosthesis**   Replacement of an absent body part with an artificial part; the artificial part.

**proteoglycans**   Molecule made of protein and carbohydrate.

**prothrombin**   Interacts with calcium to produce thrombin.

**proximal**   Nearest the point of reference.

**psychogenic**   Of psychic origin; that which originates in the mind.

**purulent**   Consisting of or containing pus.

**Q**

**quadriplegia**   Paralysis affecting all four limbs.

**R**

**radiation**   Transfer of heat through space from one object to another.

**Raynaud's phenomenon**   Condition in which cold exposure causes vasospasm of digital arteries.

**rebound tenderness**   Pain that is felt after the athletic trainer's hand is removed from an area.

**referred pain**   Pain that is felt somewhere other than its origin.

**regeneration**   Repair, regrowth, or restoration of a part, such as tissue.

**residual**   That which remains; often used to describe a permanent condition resulting from injury or disease (e.g., a limp or paralysis).

**resorption**   Act of removal by absorption.

**retroversion**   Tilting or turning backward of a part.

**retrovirus**   A virus that enters a host cell and changes its RNA to a proviral DNA replica.

**revascularize**   Restore blood circulation to an injured area.

**RICE**   Rest, ice, compression, and elevation.

**ringworm (tinea)**   Common name given to many superficial fungal infections of the skin.

**RNA**   Ribonucleic acid.

**rotation**   Turning around an axis in an angular motion.

**rubefacients**   Agents that redden the skin by increasing local circulation through the dilation of blood vessels.

**S**

**SAID principle**   Specific adaptation to imposed demands.

**scoliosis**   Lateral rotary curve of the spine.

**sebaceous cyst**   A cyst filled with sebum; usually found in the scalp.

**secondary assessment**   Follow-up; a more detailed examination.

**secondary survey**   An evaluation of existing signs and symptoms performed after the presence of life-threatening conditions has been ruled out.

**second intention**   Healing where granulation tissue replaces damaged cells, creating increased scar tissue, and delays the healing process.

**seizure**   Sudden attack.

**septic shock**   Shock caused by bacteria, especially gram-negative bacteria commonly seen in systemic infections.

**sequela**   Pathological condition that occurs as a consequence of another condition or event.

**serotonin**   Hormone and neurotransmitter.

**shearing**   Force that moves across the parallel organization of the tissue.

**sign**   Objective indicator of a disease.

**sovereign immunity**   States that neither the government or any individual who is employed by the government can be held liable for negligence.

**SPF**   Sun protection factor.

**spica**   A figure-eight bandage with one of the two loops larger than the other.

**stance phase**   Portion of the gait cycle from initial contact to toe-off.

**Staphylococcus**   Genus of gram-positive bacteria normally present on the skin and in the upper respiratory tract and prevalent in localized infections.

**stasis**   Blockage or stoppage of circulation.

**static stretching**   Passively stretching an antagonist muscle by placing it in a maximal stretch and holding it there.

**steady-state**   When the amount of the drug taken is equal to the amount that is excreted.

**stiffness**   Ability of a tissue to resist a load.

**strain**   Extent of deformation of tissue under loading.

**stretching**   Force that pulls beyond the yield point, leading to rupturing of soft tissue or fracturing of a bone.

**Streptococcus**   Genus of gram-positive bacteria found in the throat, respiratory tract, and intestinal tract.

**stress**   The internal reaction or resistance to an external load; also, the positive and negative forces that can disrupt the body's equilibrium.

**stressor**   Anything that affects the body's physiological or psychological condition, upsetting the homeostatic balance.

**subluxation**   Partial or incomplete dislocation of an articulation.

**supinators**   Those who run on the outside of the foot.

**swing phase**   Portion of gait cycle that is a period of non-weight bearing.

**symptom**   Subjective change that indicates injury or disease.

**syndesmotic joint**   An articulation in which the bones are united by a ligament.

**syndrome**   Group of typical symptoms or conditions that characterize a deficiency or disease.

**synergy**   To work in cooperation with.

**synovial joints**   Articulations of two bones surrounded by a joint capsule lined with synovial membrane.

**synovitis**   Inflammation of the synovium.

**synthesis**   To build up.

**systolic blood pressure**   The pressure caused by the heart's pumping.

**T**

**tachypnea**   Rapid breathing.

**tapotement**   Percussion.

**tendinitis/tendinosis**   Inflammation of a tendon.

**tendon**   Tough band of connective tissue that attaches muscle to bone.

**tenosynovitis**   Inflammation of a tendon synovial sheath.

**tension**   Force that pulls or stretches tissue.

**tetanus (lockjaw)**   An acute, often fatal condition characterized by tonic muscular spasm, hyperreflexia, and lockjaw.

**tetanus toxoid**   Tetanus toxin modified to produce active immunity against *Clostridium tetani*.

**tetany**   Maximum muscle contraction.

**thermotherapy**   Heat therapy.

**thrombi**   Plural of *thrombus*; blood clots that block small blood vessels or a cavity of the heart.

**tinea (ringworm)**   Superficial fungal infections of the skin.

**tonic**   Type of muscle contraction characterized by constant contraction that lasts for a period of time.

**tonic muscle spasm**   Rigid muscle contraction that lasts over a period of time.

**torsion**   Act or state of being twisted.

**torts**   Legal wrongs committed against a person.

**training effect**   Stroke volume increases while heart rate is reduced at a given exercise load.

**transitory paralysis**   Temporary paralysis.

**translation**   Refers to anterior gliding of tibial plateau.

**trauma**   A physical injury or wound sustained in sport and produced by an external or internal force.

**traumatic**   Pertaining to an injury or a wound.

**trigger points**   Small, hyperirritable areas within a muscle.

**V**

**valgus**   Position of a body part that is bent outward.

**varus**   Position of a body part that is bent inward.

**vasoconstriction**   Decrease in the diameter of a blood vessel.

**vasodilation**   Increase in the diameter of a blood vessel.

**vasospasm**   Blood vessel spasm.

**vehicle**   The substance in which a drug is transported.

**verruca**   Wart caused by a virus.

**vibration**   Rapid shaking.

**viscoelastic**   Any material whose mechanical properties vary depending on rate of load.

**viscosity**   Resistance to flow.

**volar**   Referring to the palm or the sole.

**voltage**   Force.

**volume of distribution**   The volume of plasma in which a drug is dissolved.

**W**

**Watt**   Power.

**wrap**   Strip of cloth or other material used to cover a wound or hold a dressing in place.

**Y**

**yield point**   Elastic limit of tissue.

# Index

Note: Page numbers followed by *f* or *t* indicate figures or tables, respectively.

# *Suggested Supplies*

*Tape*
White adhesive, 1½-inch
White adhesive, 1-inch
Liteguard, 2-inch
Proformula, 1½-inch
Elastic, 3-inch
Elastic, 2-inch
Elastic, 1-inch
Pre wrap
Deriform knitted tape
Medi-rip, 2-inch
Patellofemoral tape
Clothwrap, 2-inch

*Bandages*
Coverlet, 1½ × 2
Coverlet, 2 × 3
Coverlet knuckle
Coverlet strips
Telfa, 2 × 3
Telfa, 3 × 4
Band-Aid Clear Patches
Gauze, 4 × 4 (sterile)
Gauze, 3 × 3 (sterile)
Gauze, 2 × 2
Gauze cling, 4-inch (sterile)
Steri Strips, ⅛-inch
Steri Strips, ¼-inch
Steri Strips, ½-inch
Adaptic Dressing

*Wraps*
Ace wraps, 3-inch
Ace wraps, 4-inch single
Ace wraps, 4-inch double
Ace wraps, 6-inch single
Ace wraps, 6-inch double

*Foam and Felt*
1-inch felt

½-inch felt
¼-inch felt
¼-inch adhesive felt
⅛-inch adhesive felt
⅛-inch adhesive foam
⅛-inch firm foam (gray)
⅛-inch firm foam (black)
¼-inch firm foam (black)
Moleskin
½-inch blue memory foam
¼-inch adhesive foam
½-inch vinyl foam
¼-inch vinyl foam
¼-inch vinyl adhesive foam

*Braces and Splints*
Finger splints
Toe splints
Foam padded finger, ¾-inch
Wooden splints
Air splint, leg
Air splint, foot
Velcro, 1-inch (both sides)
Knee immobilizers
Foot boot (medium, large)
Aircast, left
Aircast, right
Hexalite, 4-inch
Cervical collar (small, medium,
  large)
Toe caps
Heel cups (medium, large)
Patella strap, large
Fibrifoam Patt strap
Fibrifoam wrist/hand strap
Wrist immobilizer (left, right, universal)
Ankle braces (xx-small, x-small, small,
  medium, large, x-large)

Triangular bandage
Slings
Nose guard
Elbow sleeves
Neoprene shorts
Thigh sleeves pro (small, medium,
  large, x-large, xx-large)
Back support (x-small, small, medium,
  x-large)
Moldable back supports
Knee sleeves (x-small, small, medium,
  large, x-large)
Knee brace post-op
Splint cement
Silicone rubber adhesive
Silicone, 1 lb
Cramerol
Readi-Cast
Cotton roll, 4-inch
Stockinet, 3-inch
Elastomer Kits

*Paper Products*
Towels (cases)
Cups (cases)
Scrub pants
Exam shorts
Pillowcases
Tampons

*Modalities*
Ultrasound gel, 5 lb
Flex All, 1 gal
Cramergesic, 5-lb tub
Skin lube, 5-lb tub
Skin lube, 25-lb tub
Gray T-band
Black T-band
Heat packs (medium, large)

Heat packs, neck
Standard terry cover
Neck terry cover
Fluorimethane
Cold spray
Ice bags
Ice bags, Cramer
Kwik-heat pack
Cramer Atomic Rub Down
Flexi-wrap (small, large)
Flexi-wrap handles
Lotion, 1 gal

*First Aid*
Cotton rolls (nose plugs)
Tongue depressors
Pocket masks
Cotton tip applicators
Cotton tip applicators (sterile)
Sani Cloths
Latex gloves (medium, large)
Cotton balls
Skin-preps
Save-A-Tooth
Penlights
Biohazard bags
Safety goggles

*Taping Accessories*
Heel and lace pads
Tape adherent spray
Tape remover

*Sharps*
Stainless steel prep blades
Scalpel blades, #10, #11 (sterile)
Scissors bandage
Scissors, small

Tweezers
Tweezers (sterile)
Suture sets
Nail clippers (large, small)
Tape cutters
Stethoscopes
Shark refill blades

*Inhalants*
Afrin

*Antiseptics*
Triadine
Peroxide
Rubbing alcohol
Betasept, small bottles
Betasept, 1-gal jug
Antimicrobial skin cleaner
Super Quin 9
Zorbicide Spray

*Skin Treatments*
Polysporin
Bacitracin
1% tolnaftate powder
Lamisil
1% hydrocortisone
Second skin
Collodion
2% miconazole
10% hydrocortisone
Baby powder
Tincture of benzoin

*Eye Treatment*
Dacriose Irrigation
Saline
Eye wash

ReNu contact cleaning agent
Penlights

*Teeth Treatment*
Blue mouth guards, 25/box
Clear mouth guards, 25/box

*Oral Medications*
Acetaminophen bottle
Acetaminophen, 2 pk
Cepastat
Chlorpheniramine, 4 mg
Diphenhydramine, 25 mg
Ibuprofen bottle
Ibuprofen, 2 pk
Imodium AD
Pepto-Bismol tabs
Q-fed pkg
Sudodrin, 2 pk
Titralac
Robitussin DM

*Crutches*
Large
Medium
Small
Large aluminum

*Water*
Bottle carriers
Water bottles
Coolers (3-, 7-, 10-gal)
Chest

*Other*
Stools
Spray bottles
Bucket
Cloth towels

## Field Kit Supplies

Adhesive bandages:
  regular (medium, large, X-large)
  knuckle
  patch
  sterile strips
Tape cutters
Scissors
Eye cover
Save-A-Tooth
Pseudoephrine (bottle and dose)
Acetominophen (bottle and dose)
Pepto-Bismol tablets
Imodium AD caplets
Ibuprofen tablets
Diphenhydramine
Dramamine
Hydrocortizone cream
A and D ointment
Petroleum jelly
Scalpels
Razor blades
Dacriose sterile eye irrigating solution
Latex gloves
Oral screw
QDA spray
Skin lube
Gauze pads: $2 \times 2$, $3 \times 3$, or $4 \times 4$
Heel cup
Sling
Hex-a-lite
Betasept
Titralac antacid
Hydrogen peroxide
Finger splints
Cotton-tipped applicators
Tongue depressors
Flex All
Lotion
EpiPen
Contact lens solution
CPR mask
Antiseptic hand cleaner
Sunscreen
Tape supplies: zonas, stretch, heel and
  lace pads, prewrap, 3-inch,
  2-inch, 1-inch brown, 1-inch white,
  blood tape
Ace wraps: 2-inch, 3-inch, 4-inch,
  6-inch, double 4-inch, double
  6-inch
Alcohol
Cramergesic
Flex-wrap
Adhesive foam

Adhesive felt
Moleskin
Penlight
Stethoscope
Ear thermometer
Pens
Self-stick notes
Polysporin ointment
Tongue forceps
Tweezers
Eye patch
Dental sponges
Ventolin inhaler
Contact lens cases
Contact lens wetting solution
Scalpel blades

## Bruise Bag

Adhesive foam: 1 sheet, 18 inch ×
  11 inch
Adhesive felt: 1 sheet, 18 inch ×
  11 inch
Knee sleeves: large, x-large, xx-large
  (2 each)
Elbow sleeves: large, x-large,
  xx-large (2 each)
Knee brace: 2 lateral hinge
Mouth guards: 25 moldable
Ice bags: 10
Air casts: right large, right x-large, left
  large, left x-large (1 each)
Ace wraps: 2-inch, 4-inch, 6-inch,
  double 4-inch, double 6-inch
  (1 each)
Back wraps: large, x-large (1 each)
Lace-up ankle braces: right large, right
  x-large, left large, left x-large (1 each)
Turf toe steel plates: right and left sizes:
  14 and 10 (2 each)
Foam padding: 24 inch × 24 inch
  roll
Philadelphia Collar
Neck roll
AC pads: 1 right, 1 left, 2 Lax pads
Soft neck collar: 1
Tape cutter: 2
Thigh sleeves: large, x-large, xx-large
  (2 each)
Spenco arch supports: size 5, size 3
  (2 each)
Spenco insoles: size 14, 11 (2 each)
Wrist splints: right and left, large,
  x-large (2 each)
Thigh pads: 2
Knee pads: 2

## Sideline Emergency Supplies for the Physician

Automatic electric defibrillator (AED)
Battery charger
Bag mask rescusitator with oxygen
  tube
Pocket mask
Alcohol prep pads
Adhesive tape
IV starter kit
IV bag solution
Solution set (IV line)
Latex gloves
18-gauge IV catheter
14-gauge IV catheter
20cc syringe
Epinephrine

## Items for the Field

6 10-gallon coolers for water and
  electrolyte drink
4 pitchers
Ice bags and ice chest with ice for ice
  bags
Field kit
Bruise bag
Spine board
Crutches
Flatbed cart
Personal kits (fanny packs)
Emergency kit with oxygen
Physio-Dyne
Vacuum splints
Water bottles
Towels
Water hose
Extension cords

## Seasonal Supplies

Ice towels
7-gallon coolers
Port-a-cools with needed supplies
Ice cans
Electrolyte drink
2 10-gallon coolers for electrolyte
  drink
Cups
7-gallon cooler with ice towels
2 extra pitchers
Bee and wasp spray
Extra trash bags

# Metric-English Conversions

## Length

| ENGLISH (USA) | = METRIC |
|---|---|
| inch | = 2.54 cm, 25.4 mm |
| foot | = 0.30 m, 30.48 cm |
| yard | = 0.91 m, 91.4 cm |
| mile (statute) (5,280 ft) | = 1.61 km, 1,609 cm |
| mile (nautical) (6,077 ft, 1.15 statute mi) | = 1.85 km, 1,850 m |

| METRIC | = ENGLISH (USA) |
|---|---|
| millimeter | = 0.039 in |
| centimeter | = 0.39 in |
| meter | = 3.28 ft, 39.37 in |
| kilometer | = 0.62 mi, 1,091 yd, 3,273 ft |

## Weight

| ENGLISH (USA) | = METRIC |
|---|---|
| grain | = 64.80 mg |
| ounce | = 28.35 g |
| pound | = 453.60 g, 0.45 kg |
| ton (short—2,000 lb) | = 0.91 metric ton (907 kg) |

| METRIC | = ENGLISH (USA) |
|---|---|
| milligram | = 0.002 grain (0.000035 oz) |
| gram | = 0.04 oz |
| kilogram | = 35.27 oz, 2.20 lb |
| metric ton (1,000 kg) | = 1.10 tons |

## Volume

| ENGLISH (USA) | = METRIC |
|---|---|
| cubic inch | = 16.39 cc |
| cubic foot | = 0.03 m$^3$ |
| cubic yard | = 0.765 m$^3$ |
| ounce | = 0.03 liter (3 ml)* |
| pint | = 0.47 liter |
| quart | = 0.95 liter |
| gallon | = 3.79 liters |

| METRIC | = ENGLISH (USA) |
|---|---|
| milliliter | = 0.03 oz |
| liter | = 2.12 pt |
| liter | = 1.06 qt |
| liter | = 0.27 gal |

1 liter ÷ 1000 = milliliter or cubic centimeter ($10^{-3}$ liter)
1 liter ÷ 1,000,000 = microliter ($10^{-6}$ liter)
*1 ml = 1 cc

# Fahrenheit-Celsius Conversion

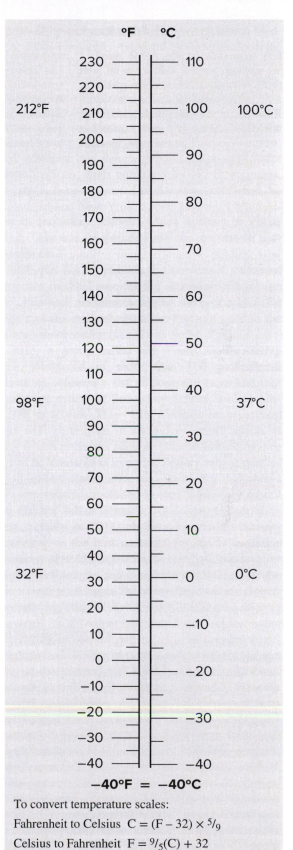

**−40°F = −40°C**

To convert temperature scales:

Fahrenheit to Celsius  $C = (F - 32) \times \frac{5}{9}$

Celsius to Fahrenheit  $F = \frac{9}{5}(C) + 32$